Diagnostic and Interventional Radiology in Surgical Practice

Edited by

Peter Armstrong MB BS FRCR
Professor of Radiology
St Bartholomew's Hospital
London, UK

Martin L. Wastie MB BChir FRCP FRCR
Consultant Radiologist
University Hospital
Nottingham, UK

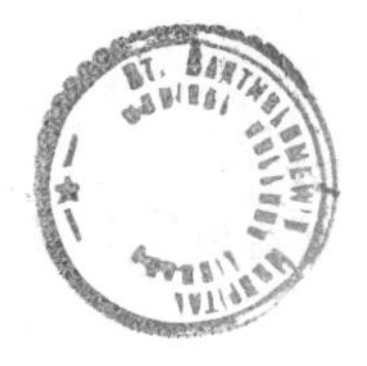

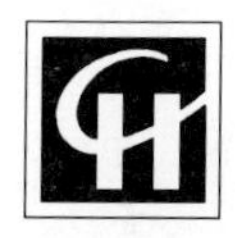

CHAPMAN & HALL MEDICAL
London · Weinheim · New York · Tokyo · Melbourne · Madras

Published by Chapman & Hall, 2–6 Boundary Row, London SE1 8HN, UK

Chapman & Hall, 2–6 Boundary Row, London SE1 8HN, UK

Blackie Academic & Professional, Wester Cleddens Road, Bishopbriggs, Glasgow G64 2NZ, UK

Chapman & Hall GmbH, Pappelallee 3, 69469 Weinheim, Germany

Chapman & Hall USA, 115 Fifth Avenue, New York, NY 10003, USA

Chapman & Hall Japan, ITP-Japan, Kyowa Building, 3F, 2–2–1 Hirakawacho, Chiyoda-ku, Tokyo 102, Japan

Chapman & Hall Australia, 102 Dodds Street, South Melbourne, Victoria 3205, Australia

Chapman & Hall India, R. Seshadri, 32 Second Main Road, CIT East, Madras 600 035, India

First edition 1997

Typeset in 10 on $11\frac{1}{2}$ pt Palatino by Genesis Typesetting, Rochester, Kent
Printed in Great Britain at the University Press, Cambridge

ISBN 0 412 61960 1 (HB) 0 412 61970 9 (PB)

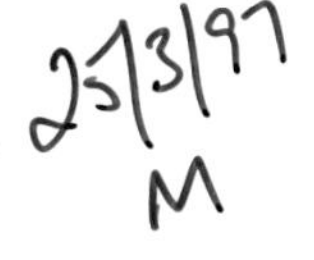

A catalogue record for this book is available from the British Library

Library of Congress Catalog Card Number: 96-86529

♾ Printed on acid-free text paper, manufactured in accordance with ANSI/NISO Z39, 48–1992 (Permanence of Paper).

Contents

Colour plates appear opposite pages 354 and 562.

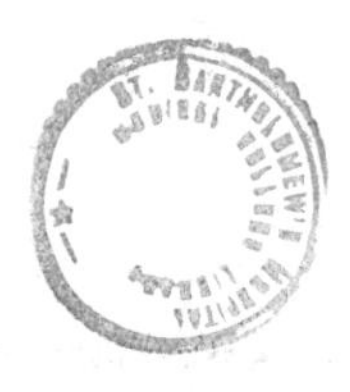

Foreword

All of us in practice have our favourite, wise, up-to-date radiologist to whom we go for advice and succinct judgement. Reading this textbook is just such an experience. Practising surgeons, surgical residents and fellows, and also other residents, medical students and physicians will find clear descriptions of the indications and limitations of diagnostic and interventional radiological procedures written by experienced radiologists. Each chapter conforms to a clear format, presenting normal radiological anatomy first, and then pathological radiological changes. The quality of the reproductions is excellent – reinforcing the narrative discussion in the text.

Clinical radiological judgement is the hallmark of this new textbook. One will not find endless encyclopaedic lists of diagnostic possibilities but rather succinct lists – often displayed within the text in an easily readable form – followed by a discussion of the most likely diagnoses and radiological signs to look for. Within the discussion of each organ system or anatomical area, there is an integrated discussion of the relative value of the use of conventional radiology, ultrasound, angiography, computed tomography, magnetic resonance imaging and radionuclear studies.

Those of us practising in the environment of increasing managed care will find the authors' attempts to suggest the most appropriate imaging modalities and to avoid the "wasteful use of radiology" particularly instructive and useful.

At the end of the textbook, there is a thorough, cross-referenced index, which will make the book useful to the very busy surgeon who wishes to use it as a resource for help with a specific clinical problem.

In summary, this new textbook supplies the reader with basic radiological wisdom and judgement, while at the same time, explaining and encompassing the very latest developments in radiological diagnostic studies and interventional procedures.

Thomas M. Daniel
Professor of Thoracic Surgery
University of Virginia School of Medicine
Charlottesville, Va, USA

Preface

The past two decades have seen the introduction of new imaging modalities which are now widely accepted and have indeed often replaced older methods of investigation. Moreover, the scope of interventional radiology has increased so that radiologists often perform therapeutic procedures that were formerly the province of the surgeon.

This book has been written by contributors expert in their own field, who work in close conjunction with their respective surgeons. The aim is to provide surgeons, particularly those in training, with an account of conditions that they are likely to encounter in every day practice. We also believe that the book will be of value to radiologists-in-training. A description is given of those imaging appearances which emphasize the most appropriate imaging modality. It is apparent that the newer imaging modalities of ultrasound, computed tomography and magnetic resonance are playing an increasingly important role in the investigation of the surgical patient.

It is not possible in a book of this size to give details of the pathological aspects of the various conditions nor is it appropriate for radiologists to discuss surgical treatment. Our aim has been to assist the surgeon in interpreting the images, to suggest the most appropriate imaging modalities and to explain the techniques and indications of modern interventional radiology.

Acknowledgements

Many individuals are involved in the production of a medical text book. Our heartfelt thanks go to the many contributors who, in spite of being hassled and cajoled, managed to keep to a strict timetable. Their various Audiovisual Departments have produced pictures of uniformly high quality. Our many thanks go to the secretaries who typed the manuscripts. In particular, Linda McGurk of Nottingham and Julie Jessop at Barts, the best personal secretaries anyone could ever hope to have, who typed the correspondence concerning the book and assisted with the preparation of the manuscripts. The chapter authors all wish to thank their respective secretaries. Secretarial assistance was also provided by Tiina Wastie, Natasha Armstrong and Veronica Nettleship; Rachel Vincent gave much help with word processing. Our good colleague Dr Tim Jaspan of Nottingham gave generously of his time and provided much specialist help.

Finally our thanks go to Anne Waddingham and the staff of Chapman & Hall for their assistance during all stages in the production of the book.

Contributors

Andreas N. Adam, MB BS FRCP FRCR,
United Medical and Dental Schools of Guy's & St Thomas's Hospitals,
London, UK

Peter Armstrong, MB BS FRCR,
Academic Department of Radiology,
St Bartholomew's Hospital,
London, UK

Sarah Burnett, MB BS MRCP FRCR MBA,
St Mary's Hospital,
London, UK

Iain R. Colquhoun, MB BS FRCS FRCR,
Charing Cross Hospital,
London, UK

Andrew J. Evans, MB ChB MRCP FRCR,
City Hospital,
Nottingham, UK

Richard Farrow, BSc MB BS MRCP FRCR,
Treliske Hospital,
Truro, UK

Stuart Field, MA MB BChir DMRD FRCR,
Kent & Canterbury Hospital,
Canterbury, UK

Roger H. S. Gregson, BSc MB BS FRCR,
University Hospital,
Nottingham, UK

Donald M. Hadley, PhD MB ChB FRCR DMRD,
Institute of Neurological Sciences,
Glasgow, UK

Jane M. Hawnaur, MB ChB MRCP DMRD FRCR,
University of Manchester,
Manchester, UK

Jeremiah C. Healy, MB BChir MRCP FRCR,
Chelsea and Westminster Hospital,
London, UK

Tim Jaspan, BSc MB ChB MRCP FRCR,
University Hospital,
Nottingham, UK

James McIvor, FDSRCS FRCR,
Charing Cross Hospital and
Eastman Dental Institute,
London, UK

Ivan Moseley, MD PhD FRCP FRCR,
Moorfields Eye Hospital,
London, UK

Rodney H. Reznek, FRCP FRCR,
St Bartholomew's Hospital,
London, UK

Asif Saifuddin, BSc MB ChB MRCP FRCR,
Royal National Orthopaedic Hospital,
Stanmore, UK

Giles W. Stevenson, FRCP FRCR FRCP (C),
Department of Radiology,
McMaster University Medical Center,
Hamilton, Ontario, Canada

Martin L. Wastie, MB BChir FRCP FRCR,
University Hospital,
Nottingham, UK

Anthony F. Watkinson, BSc MSc MB BS FRCS FRCR,
Royal Free Hospital,
London, UK

Judith A.W. Webb, BSc MD FRCP FRCR,
St Bartholomew's Hospital,
London, UK

Simon C. Whitaker, MB BChir MRCP FRCR,
University Hospital,
Nottingham, UK

Brian K. Wignall, MB ChB MRCP FRCR,
Charing Cross Hospital,
London, UK

A. Robin M. Wilson, MB ChB FRCR FRCP(E),
City Hospital,
Nottingham, UK

CHAPTER 1

Imaging techniques

Peter Armstrong,
Jane M. Hawnaur,
Rodney H. Reznek,
and Martin L. Wastie

USE OF THE IMAGING DEPARTMENT

X-ray and imaging departments need to be efficiently utilized in order to minimize radiation hazard and be cost-effective. Good communication between clinician and radiologist is vital: the radiology staff need to know and understand the clinical problem in order to carry out appropriate tests and to interpret the results in a meaningful way; the clinicians need to understand the strengths and limitations of the investigations they request.

Sensible selection of investigations is most important. Laying down precise guidelines for requesting the various imaging examinations is difficult because patients are managed differently in different centres and the information required varies significantly. The Royal College of Radiologists has published a very useful booklet *Making the Best Use of a Department of Clinical Radiology: Guidelines for Doctors*, (3rd edn, 1995, Royal College of Radiologists, London, UK). It gives the following advice:

> A useful investigation is one in which the result – positive or negative – will alter management or add confidence to the clinician's diagnosis. A significant number of radiological investigations do not fulfil these aims. Unnecessary investigations increase waiting times, waste limited resources, lower standards and may add unnecessarily to patient irradiation.

The chief causes of the wasteful use of radiology are:

1 Investigation when results are unlikely to affect patient management: because the anticipated 'positive' finding is usually irrelevant, e.g. degenerative spinal disease (as 'normal' as grey hairs from early middle age) or because a positive finding is so unlikely. DO I NEED IT?

2 Investigation too often: i.e. before the disease could have progressed or resolved or before the results influence treatment. DO I NEED IT NOW?

3 Repeating investigations which have already been done: e.g. at another hospital, in an Outpatient Department, or in Accident & Emergency. HAS IT BEEN DONE ALREADY?

4 Failing to provide appropriate clinical information and questions that the radiological investigation should answer. Deficiencies here may lead to the wrong radiographs being obtained (e.g. the omission of an essential view). HAVE I EXPLAINED THE PROBLEM?

5 Doing the wrong investigation. Imaging techniques are developing rapidly. It is often helpful to discuss an investigation with a radiologist before it is requested. IS THIS THE BEST INVESTIGATION?

Diagnostic and Interventional Radiology in Surgical Practice. Edited by P. Armstrong and M. L. Wastie. Published in 1997 by Chapman & Hall, London. ISBN 0 412 61960 1 (HB), 0 412 61970 9 (PB)

X-RAY PRODUCTION

The production of X-rays is the same for both conventional radiography and computed tomography (CT). X-rays are produced when a stream of electrons from a heated tungsten filament, the cathode, hits a target anode, usually made of tungsten. The electrons are accelerated by applying a high voltage in the range of 70–140 kV between the anode and cathode both of which are enclosed in a vacuum tube. Metal shielding around the X-ray tube absorbs unwanted X-rays and allows a beam of X-rays to emerge. (Fig. 1.1) Less than 1% of the energy of the electrons is converted into X-rays; the rest is converted into heat and the dissipation of heat is an important factor in the design of X-ray tubes, especially those used for CT.

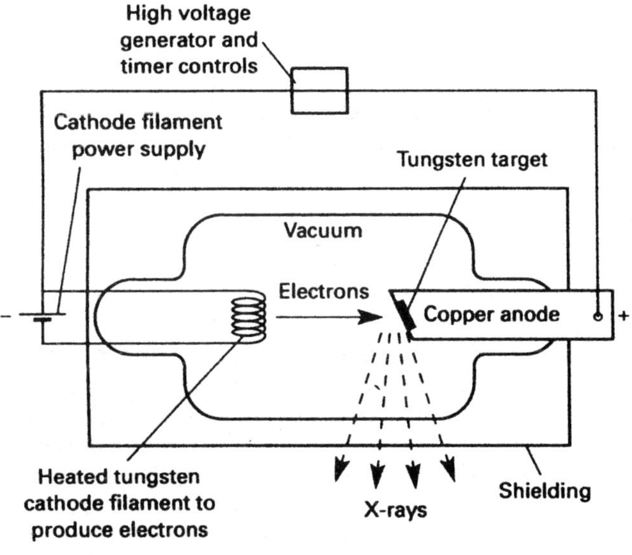

Fig. 1.1 X-ray tube.

CONVENTIONAL RADIOGRAPHY

PHOTOGRAPHIC EFFECT

The formation of images in a conventional radiograph is dependent on the differential absorption of X-rays by calcified structures, soft tissues, fat and gas. The resulting unabsorbed X-rays passing through the body cause blackening of a photographic film that is then processed. The film, which is sensitive to both light and radiation, is enclosed in a light-proof cassette and the film is sandwiched between two intensifying screens. These screens convert the radiation to light that is detected by the film. It is mainly the light emitted from these intensifying screens that cause blackening of the developed film. The use of intensifying screens allows lower exposures and, therefore, a reduction in radiation dose to the patient.

GRIDS

Grids are employed to improve the image quality by removing scattered radiation which would otherwise cause blurring of the film. A grid consists of thin strips of lead separated by transparent material.

PROJECTION

By convention the projection assigned to a radiograph is determined by the direction of the X-ray beam through the body. Hence in a postero-anterior (PA) film, which is the normal projection for a chest X-ray, the patient has the sternum against the X-ray cassette and the X-ray beam traverses from the back to the front of the chest, whereas for an antero-posterior (AP) film the beam passes from front to back and the patient's back is against the film.

HORIZONTAL BEAM

For the detection of air–fluid levels or free abdominal gas, the film must be taken with a horizontal beam. The analogy can be made with a glass of water: the only way to see the fluid level is to look from the side in a horizontal direction. Another use of a horizontal beam is in a lateral decubitus film for which the patient lies on either the right or left side. The result is an AP projection, but with a horizontal beam.

PORTABLE FILMS

Films taken on the ward with the use of portable X-ray equipment should be avoided if possible. The films tend to be of inferior quality as positioning of the patient is difficult and longer exposures are needed resulting in blurring from respiratory movement. Also, the radiation dose to patients and staff is higher than with films taken in the radiology department.

FLUOROSCOPY

X-rays striking a fluorescent screen cause it to emit a minute amount of light. By means of an image intensifier the image can be made sufficiently bright to be viewed on a television monitor and, if necessary, a permanent record may be made of the image. Fluoroscopy has had a profound impact on imaging as it allows interventional procedures such as biopsy, catheterization and orthopaedic manoeuvres to be performed under direct vision. All examinations of the gastrointestinal tract are performed with fluoroscopy as peristalsis can be observed and the patient positioned for the optimum images to be recorded.

SUBTRACTION

This technique of removing unwanted images from a film is normally used in angiography to eliminate the bone and soft tissue images, so leaving the contrast-filled vessels clearly visible. Nowadays this is performed electronically and is widely used in the form of digital subtraction angiography (DSA).

RADIATION HAZARDS

Because of the energy they possess, X-rays cause ionization and so alter molecules in tissue leading to adverse biological effects. Most ionizing radiation comes from the sun and from the earth's core; medical radiation accounts for about 12% of the total radiation received by humans. Other artificial sources, such as nuclear fallout, account for only 1% of the total amount.

Some organs are more sensitive to radiation than others. The gonads are highly sensitive and are irradiated in X-rays of the lumbar spine and pelvis; they receive a particularly high dose from a barium enema and pelvic CT.

The major adverse effects of radiation are the induction of cancer and genetic effects. There is no dose threshold below which no harmful effect will occur; thus all ionizing radiation is potentially harmful.

Irradiating the fetus *in utero* is especially hazardous as rapidly dividing cells are particularly radiosensitive. The main risk is the induction of childhood cancer and leukaemia. The natural risk in childhood is 1:650 but a high radiation examination such as barium enema or pelvic CT during pregnancy doubles this risk. The natural frequency of genetic disease manifesting at birth is between 1–3%. A high radiation examination in pregnancy increases this risk by only 0.1%.

DOSE MEASUREMENT

The maximum radiation dose limit for the general public and occupationally exposed workers has been determined by the International Commission on Radiological Protection (ICRP). Hospital personnel can wear small dosemeters to measure the radiation they receive. This may be a film badge, which will show blackening when exposed to radiation, or a thermoluminescence dosemeter (TLD), which stores the energy from the radiation. TLD monitors may be sufficiently small to enable the dose to the fingers to be measured.

DOSE LIMITATION

Because all ionizing radiation is harmful and there is no safe lower threshold of radiation, everyone must strive to keep the radiation dose to the patient as low as reasonably achievable. Much of this is the province of the radiology department with the use of a meticulous radiographic technique and up-to-date equipment. However, the referring clinician can contribute by:

- avoiding unnecessary examinations or examination not of direct relevance, e.g. there is no indication for a routine preoperative chest X-ray;
- ensuring the examination has not already been performed and waiting an appropriate time before requesting a repeat examination, e.g. a week should elapse before requesting a follow-up film in an uncomplicated pneumonia;
- using an alternative technique such as ultrasound or MRI which does not involve ionizing radiation;
- avoiding whenever possible the use of X-rays during pregnancy.

It has been calculated in the UK that if these radiation reducing methods were implemented, including the elimination of unnecessary examinations, it would be possible to reduce the number of radiation-induced cancer fatalities by over 100 cases a year.

PICTURE ARCHIVING AND COMMUNICATION SYSTEMS (PACS)

Over the past two decades, digital recording has developed dramatically. CT, ultrasound, MRI, nuclear medicine, fluoroscopy and angiography are all now recorded in a digital format. Even conventional radiographs, which currently use analog film/screen combinations, can be based on digital information. For digital radiography, the radiograph is produced on a special phosphor screen and read by a laser which then writes the image onto film or the image can be displayed on a TV monitor. A TV image can be altered by adjusting the window level or width as described (see p.10) in the section on CT.

One of the advantages of digital data is that it can be processed by a computer and allows electronic transmission between sites, buildings and even countries, and most importantly, allows computer storage. Another advantage of digital data is that computers can be used to manipulate the images, an ability most dramatically illustrated by 3-dimensional or multiplanar reconstructions.

A fully digital department would obviate the need for X-ray films with a potential saving in film costs. Also, images with their report could be viewed in the wards and clinics on television monitors. Outlying hospitals could send images into a central radiology department. Lost films would become a thing of the past. The inability to lose images, the simultaneous display of different studies and the ability to enhance these images are all great advantages of a digital system, but further technical developments will be needed before filmless radiology departments become widespread and cost-effective.

INTRAVENOUS CONTRAST AGENTS FOR UROGRAPHY, ANGIOGRAPHY AND CT

The intravenous and angiographic contrast agents rely on iodine in solution to absorb X-rays. The same agents are used for urography, angiography and contrast enhancement at computed tomography. Usually they are given in large doses, often with rapid rates of injection. Since their only purpose is to produce opacification, ideally they should be pharmacologically inert. This has not yet been totally achieved, though the introduction of low-osmolality agents, such as the non-ionic media, has been a great advance in reducing adverse effects. The advantage of the newer agents is that they have a lower osmolality than the ionic contrast media previously in general use and are therefore safer. The disadvantage of the newer agents is that they are considerably more expensive than their predecessors. The following discussion applies particularly to the older ionic agents: the same complications occur with the newer low-osmolality agents, but with lesser frequency.

Patients may experience a feeling of warmth spreading over the body as the contrast medium is injected; a few find this feeling objectionable. Sometimes, particularly with slow injections of the more concentrated solutions, pain occurs in the upper arm and shoulder due to stasis in the veins. When this occurs it is helpful to raise the patient's arm at the end of the injection.

Nausea, vomiting or light-headedness are experienced by a few patients and some will develop an urticarial rash. All these phenomena usually subside spontaneously. Contrast inadvertently injected outside the vein can be very painful and should be carefully guarded against.

Bronchospasm, laryngeal oedema or hypotension occasionally develop and may be so severe as to be life-threatening. It is, therefore, essential to be prepared for these dangerous reactions and to have available the equipment and drugs to cope with them. Approximately one in 160 000 patients dies as a consequence of ionic contrast agents, a risk which, although small, should not be ignored.

Patients with known allergic manifestations, particularly asthma, are more likely to have an adverse reaction. Similarly, patients who have had a previous reaction to contrast agents have a higher than average risk of problems during the examination. Such patients are usually premedicated with steroids, preferably for at least 18 hours prior to the examination. Antihistamine drugs may also be given shortly before the contrast injection.

High-risk groups are given low-osmolality agents to help minimize complications from contrast injections. Patients with a higher than average risk of complications from intravenous contrast injections include:

- **infants**, who are at risk from a rapid rise in plasma osmolality because of the high osmolality of the injected contrast agent; even with low-osmolality agents the injection rate in infants should, when possible, be slow;
- **elderly patients**, who often tolerate the injected contrast medium poorly;
- **those with known heart disease**; arrhythmias are a risk in these patients;
- **those with renal failure, myeloma or severe diabetes**; even the non-ionic agents have a temporary adverse effect on renal function. (Patients are more likely to show a deterioration of renal function due to the contrast medium if they are deprived of fluids prior to the examination.)

RADIONUCLIDE IMAGING

Radionuclide imaging depends on the fact that radionuclides can be tagged to certain substances which concentrate selectively in different parts of the body. These substances are known as radiopharmaceuticals and are most often administered by intravenous injection (Fig. 1.2). For most diagnostic tests in nuclear medicine, radionuclides emitting gamma radiation are used. The gamma radiation can be detected and an image produced by means of a gamma camera. When a photon of gamma radiation strikes an activated sodium iodide crystal, the crystal scintillates emitting a small flash of light. A gamma camera consists of a large activated sodium iodide crystal with a large number of photomultiplier tubes facing the crystal. Each photomultiplier tube generates a signal proportional to the amount of light it receives. The location of the scintillations can be determined and so an image can be produced which, if desired, may be recorded on X-ray film. Each detected photon is recorded as a count. Between 300 000 and 500 000 counts are needed to produce a satisfactory image, necessitating about 3–5 minutes to obtain the image.

EMISSION TOMOGRAPHY

In this technique the gamma camera moves around the patient. A computer can analyse the information and produce sectional images which, as in MRI, may be reconstructed in any plane. However, the spatial resolution of emission tomography is inferior to both CT and MRI. Since only one usable photon is emitted

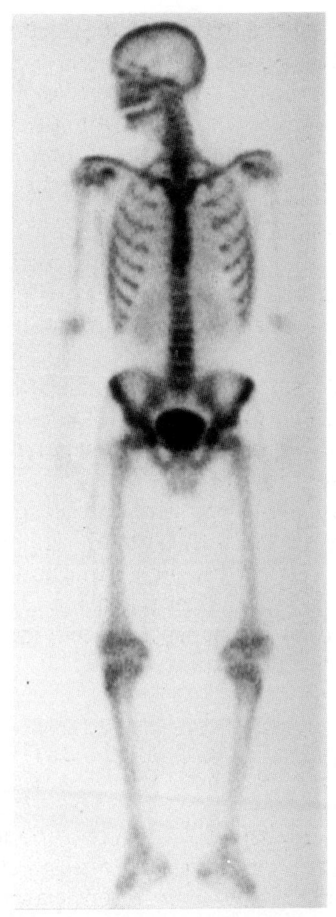

Fig. 1.2 Radionuclide bone scan. The patient has received an intravenous injection of a ^{99m}Tc-labelled complex organic phosphate. This agent is taken up by the bones in proportion to bone turnover and blood flow so that an image of the skeleton can be produced.

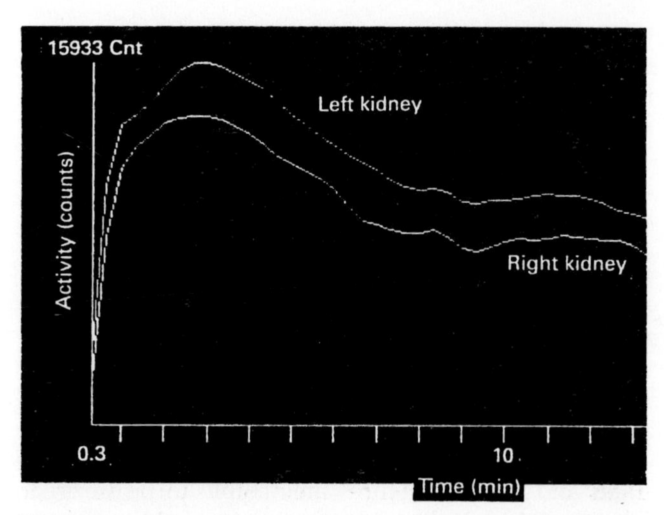

Fig. 1.3 Renogram. When rapid serial images are taken after an intravenous injection of ^{99m}Tc-DTPA, which is excreted by the kidneys, an activity – time curve is produced giving information on renal function.

for each disintegration the technique is also known as single photon emission computed tomography (SPECT). Conventional radionuclides such as technetium-99m or thallium-201 are used.

DYNAMIC IMAGING

Another advantage of radionuclide imaging is that not only are anatomical images produced, dynamic scans may also be performed so that function may be measured. With the use of a computer, rapid serial images may be taken and an activity/time curve produced. This technique is employed in renography to measure renal function. (Fig. 1.3).

RADIOPHARMACEUTICALS

Radiopharmaceuticals must be regarded from both their biological and radiation standpoint. The radiopharmaceutical must localize safely in a certain organ or compartment within the body and stay there long enough to be imaged. Technetium-99m is the most commonly used radionuclide. It has a convenient half-life of 6 hours which is short enough to limit the radiation dose to the patient but sufficiently long to enable the imaging study to be completed. Technetium-99m emits only gamma radiation and this radiation is of a suitable energy for detection by the gamma camera. Moreover it is easily prepared at any time from a molybdenum-99 generator. Because of its chemical nature it can be incorporated into various radiopharmaceuticals in order to localize in different parts of the body.

Other radionuclides in common use include iodine-123, thallium-201, gallium-67, indium-111 and the gases krypton-81m and xenon-133.

Cell labelling, usually with technetium-99m, has become an important technique. Labelled leucocyte scanning is employed for the detection of inflammation and abscesses. Labelling of the red blood cells enables gastrointestinal blood loss to be detected and, because it provides blood pool imaging, it permits cardiac imaging to be performed.

SAFETY OF RADIONUCLIDE IMAGING

Although radionuclide imaging employs ionizing radiation, the patient dose in most examinations is quite low.

ULTRASOUND

Ultrasound has become a readily available and much used examination in a wide variety of situations. Ultrasound imaging is based on the fact that if high frequency sound is directed into the body from a transducer placed on the skin, some of the sound is reflected by tissue interfaces in the body to produce echoes which are picked up by the same transducer and converted into an image. All ultrasound examinations are now performed with real time imaging, a system which produces images fast enough to allow motion to be followed. In any position of the transducer, the image obtained is that of a slice; thus to obtain information about the whole of an organ or region, the transducer must be moved and angled to produce a number of slices. Hence there are no fixed projections and the image acquisition and subsequent interpretation depends greatly on the skill of the operator.

Since air and bone absorb the ultrasound beam, gas-filled and bony structures are unable to be imaged. Ultrasound is unable to cross a tissue–gas or tissue–bone boundary; therefore deeper structures may be obscured. Bowel gas frequently limits visualization of abdominal structures and ultrasound plays little part in the diagnosis of lung or bone pathology.

Ultrasound is produced by a transducer constructed of a piezoelectric crystal which changes thickness when a voltage is applied across it. When electrically pulsed, the crystal resonates, producing high frequency sound depending on the thickness of the crystal. Not only is the transducer the transmitter, it also acts as the receiver producing a small electric signal when an ultrasound wave strikes it. Very short pulses of sound lasting about a millionth of a second are transmitted by the transducer about a thousand times a second.

For diagnostic use the frequency of the ultrasound ranges from 3.5 MHz to 10 MHz. The skin is smeared with a jelly-like substance in order to effect acoustic coupling between the skin and the transducer. The ultrasound beam travels through tissue at a near constant velocity of 1540 m/s. The time delay between the initiation of a pulse and the return of an echo is proportional to the distance the beam has travelled. This distance can be calculated from the velocity of sound in tissues. Distance is essential information needed to place the echoes in the correct position. It also allows accurate measurement to be made from ultrasound images.

Reflection of sound is greatest when there is a large difference between the acoustic impedance of two structures which explains why cysts and cystic structures such as the gallbladder and the fetus in its sac of amniotic fluid are so well demonstrated with ultrasound. Strong echoes are produced from the cyst walls but no echoes arise from the fluid within the cyst. As more sound traverses the cyst, more echoes are received from the area behind the cyst, a feature known as **acoustic enhancement** (Fig. 1.4). Conversely with a calcified structure, such as a stone, there is a reduction in the sound passing through, causing a band of reduced echoes beyond the stone, known as **acoustic shadowing** (Fig. 1.5).

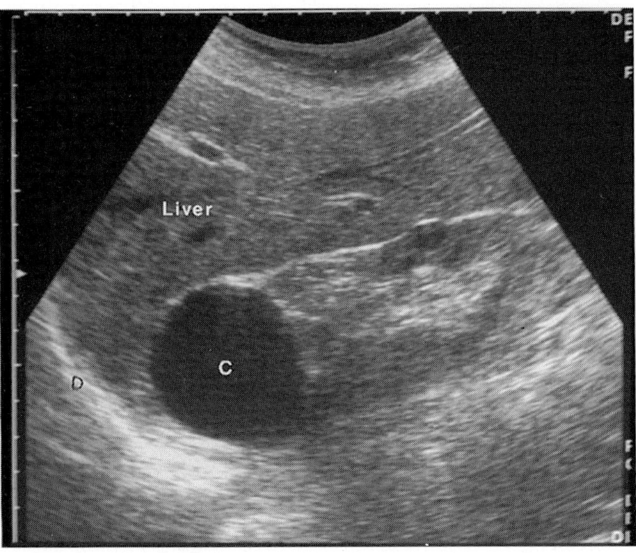

Fig. 1.4 Acoustic enhancement. The area behind the cyst (C) in the upper pole of the right kidney shows brighter echoes as more sound traverses the cyst. No echoes are seen from the cyst itself. D = diaphragm.

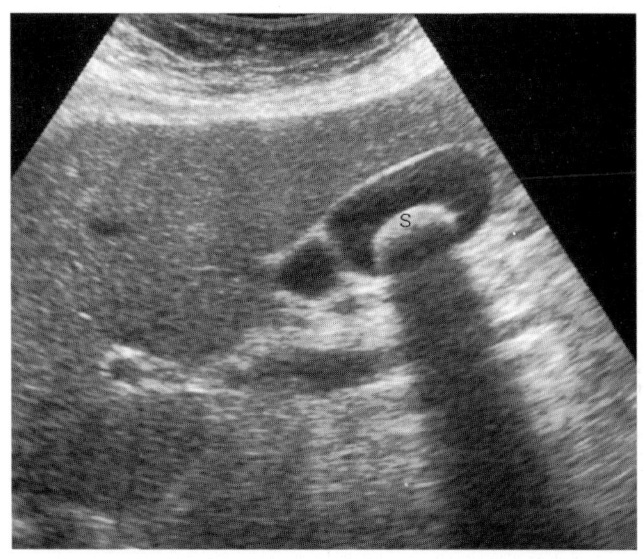

Fig. 1.5 Acoustic shadowing. The area behind the stone (S) in the gall bladder shows reduced echoes as sound does not pass through the stone.

As sound waves pass through the body the amount of reflection is determined by the difference in the acoustic impedance of the tissues. A liver metastasis may have a different acoustic impedance from the surrounding normal liver, so the sound is reflected differently to enable the metastasis to be visualized.

DOPPLER EFFECT

The Doppler effect is the shift in frequency of a wave when the source moves relative to the receiver. The rise in pitch of a train whistle as a train approaches is a familiar example. The assessment of blood flow is based on the Doppler effect as sound is reflected from the blood cells flowing in the vessels. When blood flows towards the transducer, the received signal is of higher frequency than the transmitted frequency (Fig. 1.6) whilst the opposite occurs if blood is flowing away from the transducer. This frequency shift can be measured and blood flow velocity calculated from the formula:

$$\text{frequency shift} = \frac{2 \times \text{Fi} \times v \times \cos\theta}{\text{C}}$$

where C equals the speed of sound in tissues and Fi, the incident frequency of the beam. As these are constant and if the Doppler angle Θ is kept constant, the frequency shift depends on the blood flow velocity v.

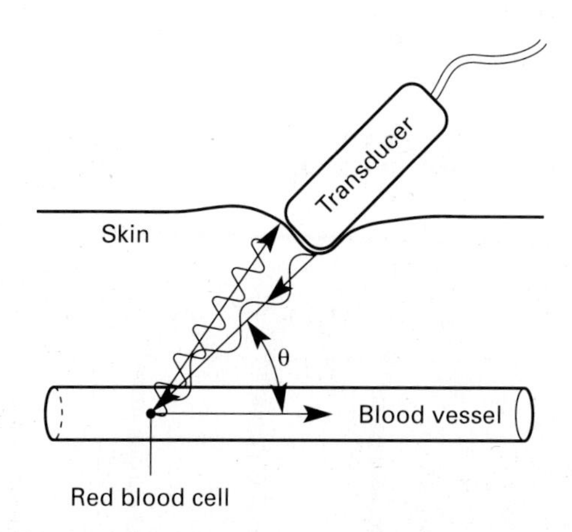

Fig. 1.6 Principle of Doppler ultrasound. With blood flowing towards the transducer the frequency of the received sound is increased. The difference in frequency between the transmitted and received sound is known as the Doppler shift. θ = angle between the vessel and the transmitted sound wave: an angle known as the Doppler angle.

The Doppler signals fall in the audible range so, when amplified, they give a characteristic sound for arterial and venous flow that may be altered if flow is disturbed. In addition the flow velocity wave form may be recorded by plotting the Doppler signal against time. These waveforms from specific arteries and veins have a characteristic shape; this may change if, for example, there is a stenosis causing a flow abnormality. Further information about these waveforms can be obtained by spectral analysis which evaluates the spectrum of frequencies making up the waveform.

Pulsed Doppler is now employed. It uses repetitive bursts of sound which enable a Doppler trace to be available simultaneously with an ultrasound image and the position of the Doppler gate from which the signal arises can be chosen at will. This combined system of Doppler and an ultrasound image is known as **duplex scanning**. A further development is **colour Doppler** which shows flow patterns over the whole ultrasound image. Direction of blood flow towards or away from the transducer can readily be determined and can be assigned a colour, usually red or blue (Plate 1 opposite p. 354).

A recently introduced technique is **power Doppler** which is based on the Doppler signal strength and is not frequency dependent. This technique gives no information on direction or velocity of flow but it is able to demonstrate low flow and has the potential to show tissue perfusion to advantage (Plates 2a and b opposite page 354).

ULTRASOUND CONTRAST AGENTS

The action of ultrasound contrast agents depends on microscopic air bubbles that scatter the ultrasound energy so causing echo enhancement. These contrast agents are injected intravenously and are used in cardiac and Doppler studies. Their use in clinical practice is yet to be determined.

INTERVENTIONAL PROCEDURES

Percutaneous biopsies can conveniently be performed under ultrasound control because the course of the needle can be viewed as it passes to the target. Similarly, abscess aspiration and placement of drainage tubes can readily be performed using ultrasound. Intraoperative ultrasound can be valuable in certain situations such as in localizing an endocrine tumour of the pancreas during surgery.

SAFETY OF ULTRASOUND

Although high power ultrasound can inflict damage to tissues, no harmful effects have been recorded at the intensities used for diagnostic purposes. Follow-up has failed to detect any abnormality resulting from ultrasound scans performed during pregnancy, despite the many millions of such scans that have been performed.

COMPUTED TOMOGRAPHY

Computed tomography (CT) overcomes some of the limitations of plain radiography by removing the problem of superimposition of structures and by enabling very small density difference between tissues to be shown.

The problem of superimposition of structures is achieved by collimation of the X-rays into a thin beam that only passes through the 'slice' of tissue being imaged. Having passed through the patient, the X-ray beam strikes very sensitive detectors which can distinguish and quantify subtle differences in tissue density.

Compared to conventional plain radiography, the range of densities recorded is increased from approximately 20 to 2000 or more. CT scanning is a digital imaging system based on three essential components:

- data acquisition
- data processing
- image display, manipulation, storage and recording.

DATA ACQUISITION

There are two methods of data acquisition, 'slice-by-slice' and 'volume-acquisition'. The X-ray detectors measure the radiation transmitted through the patient from all the different locations of the X-ray tube, in both the slice-by-slice and volume-acquisition techniques.

Relative transmission values (or penetration measurements) can then be calculated. The **relative transmission** depends almost entirely on the attenuation of the X-rays by the body, which in turn depends on the number of atoms in the path of the beam, and their atomic number.

In the conventional slice-by-slice method, data are collected by the X-ray tube rotating around the patient, thus giving information from a single slice. The tube comes to a stop and the patient is then moved into position so that the next slice can be scanned (Fig. 1.7). This process continues until all slices have been scanned.

In the newer method of volume acquisition, a special X-ray beam geometry, referred to as **spiral or helical CT**, is used to scan a volume of tissue rather than one slice at a time (Fig. 1.8).

The patient is transported continuously through the scanner. As the X-ray tube rotates continuously around the patient, the X-ray beam traces a spiral or helical path with respect to the moving patient while data are acquired continuously through each 360° rotation. This images a volume of tissue (rather than a slice) so the technique is also referred to as **volume scanning**.

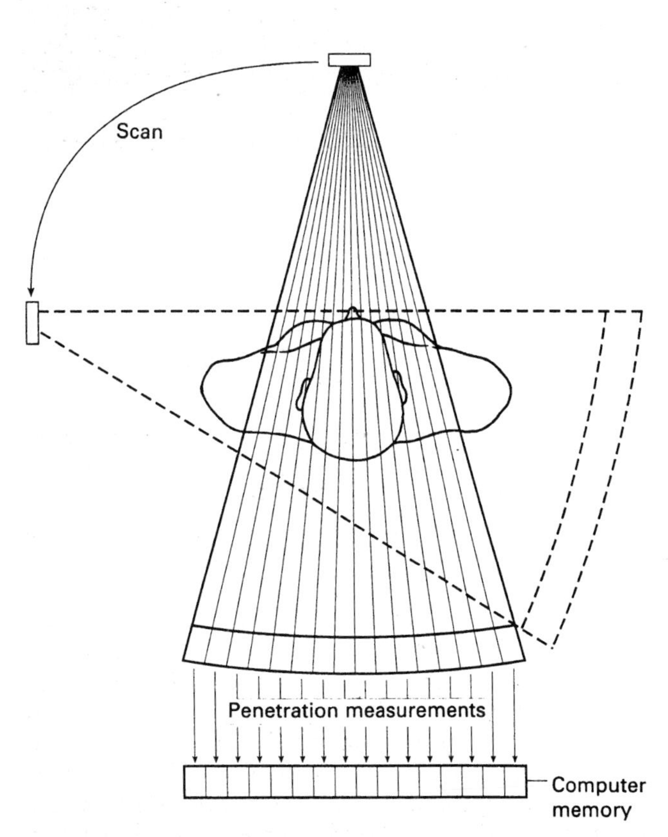

Fig. 1.7 Scanning the patient. This involves rotating the X-ray tube and detectors around the patient to collect transmission or penetration measurements; these are stored in the computer memory.

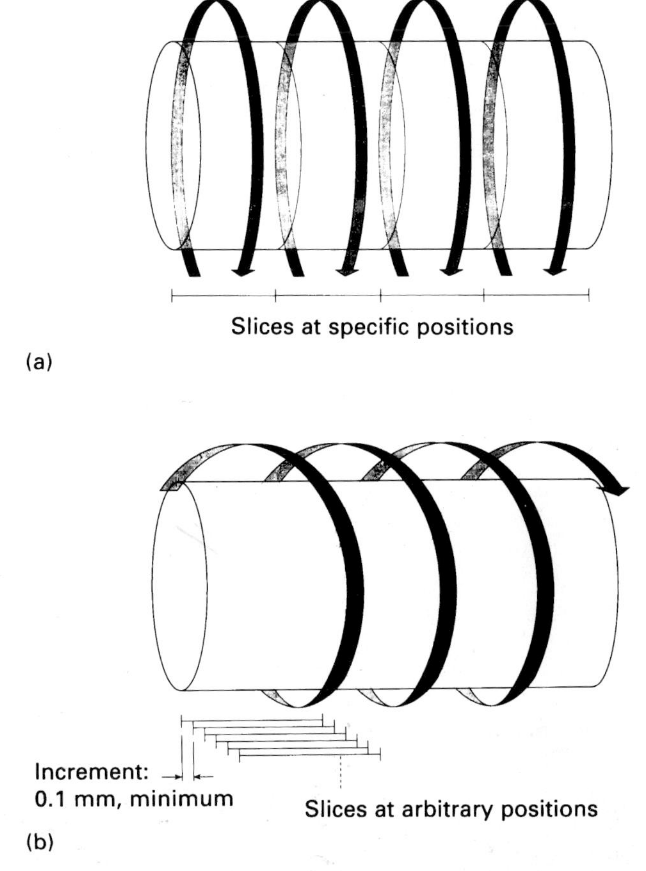

Fig. 1.8 Two methods of data collection in CT (a) through conventional scanning and (b) through spiral scanning.

A major requirement of spiral scanning is an increase in the capacity of the X-ray tube which has to deliver X-rays continuously during the time it takes to scan the volume of tissue. Usually patients are moved by 10 mm/s so that a typical 24-s scan covers 240 mm (24 cm). The maximum scanning time is usually in the order of 32 s. Slice thickness may range between 1 mm and 1 cm (Fig. 1.8).

THE ADVANTAGES OF SPIRAL (HELICAL) CT

Several advantages are associated with the use of spiral (helical) CT.

- The examination time is reduced by elimination of an interscan delay so that whole organs can be scanned on a single breath-hold.
- The potential for a gap between slices is removed because a volume of tissue is scanned rather than scans being obtained slice by slice.
- The effect of different depths of respiration is removed as there is no shifting of anatomical structures between the slices and lesions can be localized accurately.
- Slices can be reconstructed at any arbitrary position within the volume after the data have been acquired.
- There is greater accuracy in multiplanar and 3D reconstruction; this has proved particularly valuable in studying the facial bones (Fig. 1.9), complex joints such as the elbow, and in demonstrating the vascular system (Fig. 1.10).

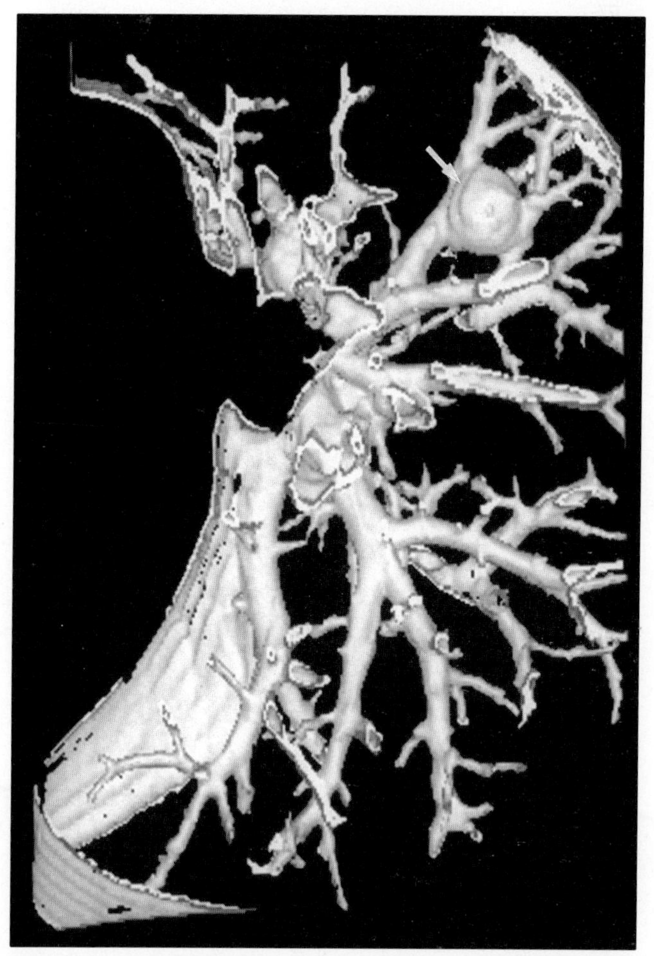

Fig. 1.10 3D reconstruction of the pulmonary vasculature. The relationship of a small nodule to the adjacent vessels is clearly seen (arrow).

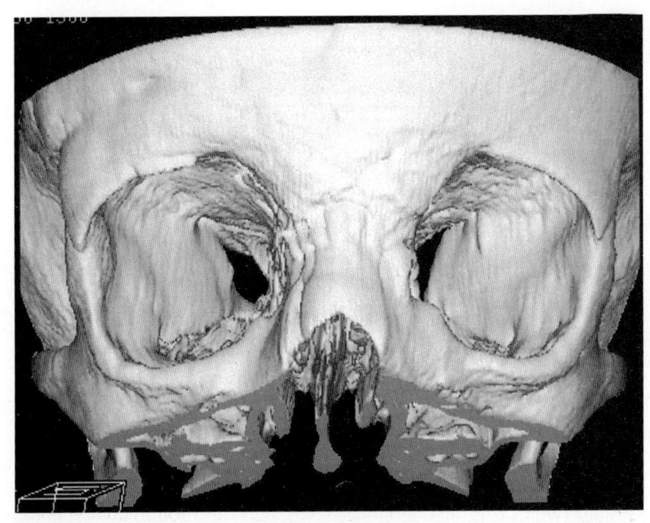

Fig. 1.9 3D reconstruction of the facial bones.

DATA PROCESSING AND CT NUMBERS

The X-ray transmission values collected during scanning are stored as raw data in the computer and then converted into numbers – CT (Hounsfield) numbers or attenuation values – by a mathematical process referred to as a reconstruction technique or algorithm. The computer prints images based on these CT numbers. Thus X-rays passing through bone/calcification (+1000) undergo the most attenuation and those passing through air (–1000) are least attenuated (Fig. 1.11). The final image is converted to a grey-scale image by relating the attenuation value of the tissues to that of water, the CT number of which is designated zero. The relationship of CT numbers to brightness level is shown in Fig. 1.12, in which the upper (+1000) and lower (–1000) limits of the scale represent white and black respectively.

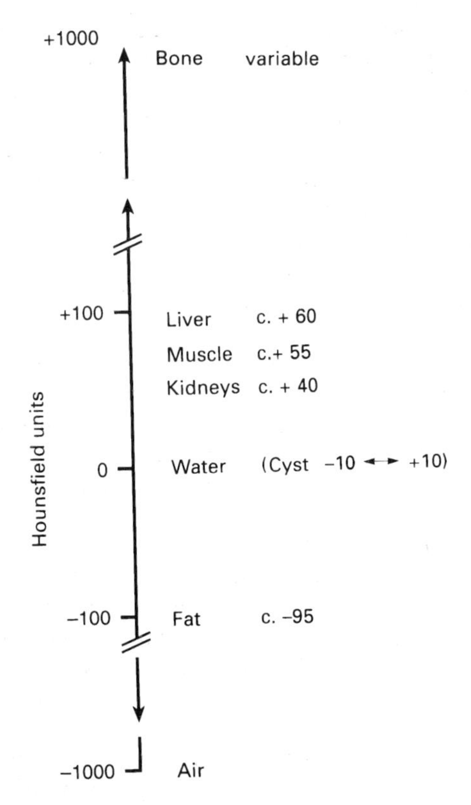

Fig. 1.11 Chart depicting the Hounsfield scale, showing the values for some normal structures.

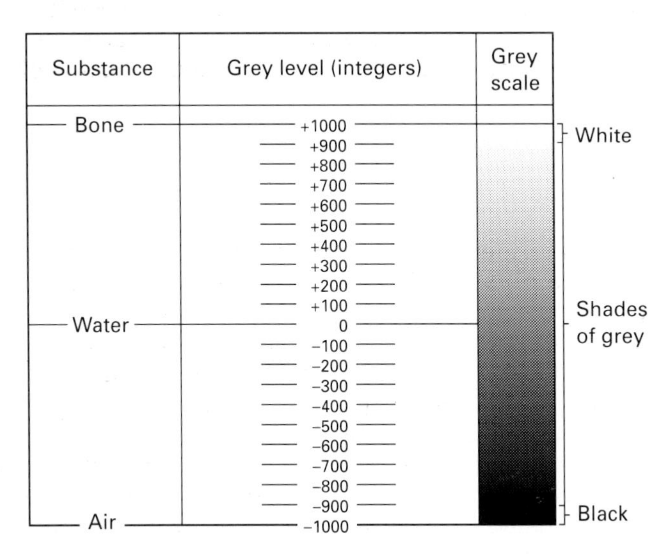

Fig. 1.12 Relationship between CT numbers and the brightness level (grey scale).

IMAGE DISPLAY

The image so obtained consists of a matrix of picture elements (**pixels**), each representing the degree of attenuation of X-rays at a particular point in the body. Since each image represents a certain thickness of tissue, the attenuation value recorded at a point represents the mean value obtained from a tiny volume of tissue (the **voxel**). This image is displayed on a television monitor. An important parameter of the grey-scale display monitor is resolution, which is related to the size of the pixel matrix (**matrix size**).

Windowing

Since only a limited number of grey-scale steps can be appreciated by the human eye, only a limited range of values can be distinguished simultaneously. For this reason, the viewing console is provided with controls which enable the observer to select a range of values for display and recording appropriate to the tissue being examined. The centre of the range is known as the window level, and the range of density, the window width. The smaller the range of density values represented by each grey-scale step, the greater the contrast. For this reason, a narrow width is used when structures such as the liver or brain are being examined where small differences in density can be important.

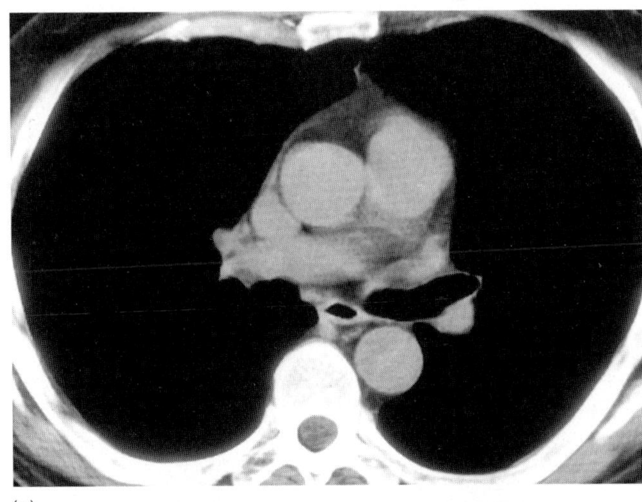

(a)

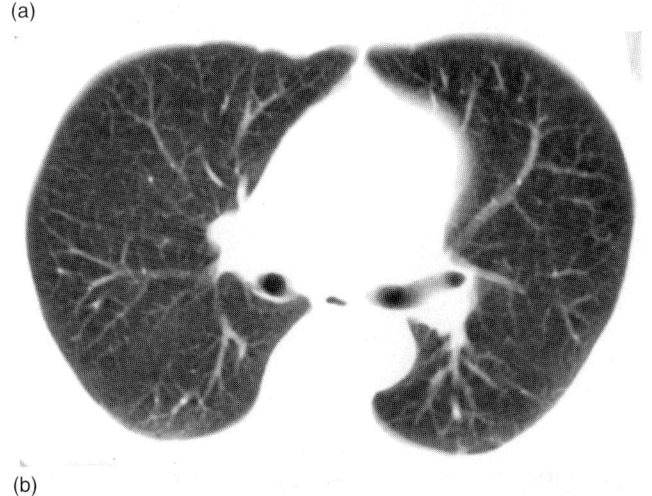

(b)

Fig. 1.13 An example of varying the window width and level by manipulating the data of one thoracic image. (a) At conventional soft tissue settings (width 400 HU, level 40 HU) the normal mediastinal soft tissue striations are shown but the lung detail is not seen. (b) At lung settings (width 1000 HU, level −700 HU), bone and soft tissue detail are now all lost as they all appear white. Lung detail is well seen.

Relatively wider widths are commonly used in body scanning when the shape and contours of structures are the main criteria for diagnosis (Fig. 1.13).

ARTEFACTS

Partial volume effect

When CT numbers are computed, the calculations are based on the measurement of attenuation for an entire voxel of tissue. If the voxel contains only one tissue type then the calculations give the true attenuation of the tissue. On the other hand, if the voxel contains more than one tissue type, then the CT number for that voxel is based on an average of those tissues. This is known as **partial volume averaging** and may lead to inaccuracies when tissues are being characterized and their size estimated (Fig. 1.14). This potential artefact can be minimized by scanning thinner slices so that the likelihood of different tissues being present in a given voxel is reduced.

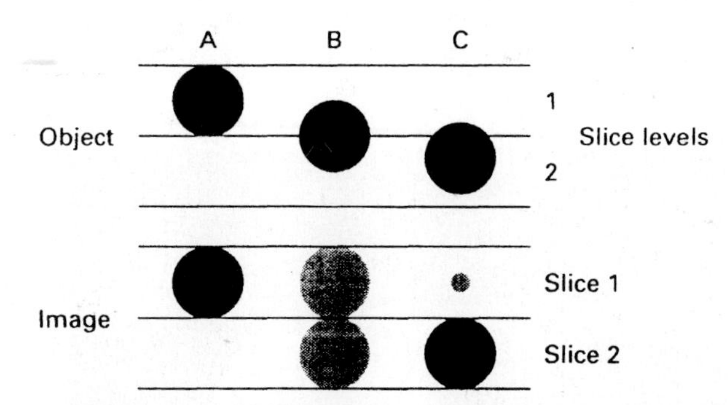

Fig. 1.14 Partial volume effect. Object A occupies the full height of the slice and so its diameter and density are accurately represented on the images. Object B lies half in slice 1 and half in slice 2 so the images will indicate its correct size but the density on each image slice will be half its true value. Object C lies partly in slice 1 but mainly in slice 2 and so the upper slice of the image will underestimate both its diameter and density.

Streak artefacts

Movement, either voluntary or involuntary, such as peristalsis or cardiac motion, during scanning can result in the appearance of streak artefacts on the image which are tangential to the high density difference edges of the moving part. Very high density materials, including metals, barium, surgical clips and electrodes, can also give rise to streak artefacts on the image.

THE USE OF CONTRAST MEDIUM

Oral contrast medium

The use of dilute oral contrast material to opacify the gastrointestinal tract is essential when scanning the abdomen, so that homogeneous fluid-filled bowel loops are not confused with masses or abscesses. Proper opacification of the gastrointestinal tract is especially valuable in patients who are extremely thin and lack the usual amount of intra-abdominal fat necessary to outline structures. Gastrografin (an iodine-containing compound) diluted to 2% solution or dilute barium sulphate are the most commonly used contrast agents for abdominal and pelvic scans. If the examination is being performed primarily to study the stomach, the patient is given 300–500 ml contrast medium immediately before the study. If the examination extends to the remainder of the abdomen, then the small bowel is opacified by the patient being given contrast medium to drink 45 minutes to 1 hour before the examination. Rectal contrast medium may also be administered before pelvic examination.

Intravenous contrast agents

Intravenous contrast medium is most frequently used to increase the density difference between the normally enhancing parenchyma of an organ (such as the liver, pancreas or kidney) and a focal abnormality (such as a tumour or an abscess) which takes up the contrast medium to a lesser extent. This improves the sensitivity with which focal abnormalities are detected. Contrast is also useful for distinguishing between vessels and a mass, and for identifying the extent of vascular displacement or invasion. Intravenous contrast material may be used to opacify blood vessels to determine the relative vascularity of a mass. The contrast media are the same as those used for angiography and urography.

RADIATION DOSE FROM CT

When a CT examination is requested, consideration must be given to the radiation dose to the patient, particularly in view of the potential for high patient doses. Examinations on children require an even higher level of justification since children are at greater risk from radiation than adults. When clinically appropriate, the alternative use of safer non-ionizing techniques (such as ultrasound and MRI) or of low dose X-ray techniques must always be considered. Currently, in the United Kingdom, by far the highest collective patient dose arises from the use of CT. The effective dose of a chest or abdomen CT (which includes a weighting for the relative risks of fatal malignancy) is equivalent to 200 chest X-rays, approximately the same as the dose for a barium enema.

MAGNETIC RESONANCE IMAGING

Magnetic resonance imaging (MRI) depends on the magnetic properties of the nuclei of certain elements. The basic physical principles centre on the concept that the nuclei of hydrogen behave like small, spinning bar magnets and align with the magnetic field when placed in a strong magnetic field. Hydrogen nuclei (**protons**) are present in large numbers in water molecules and lipids. If a radiofrequency pulse at an appropriate frequency (**resonant frequency**) is beamed into the patient, a proportion of the protons change their alignment, flipping through a preset angle, and rotate in phase with one another. Following this radiofrequency pulse, the protons return to their original positions. As the protons realign (relax) they induce a radio signal which, though very weak, can be detected by coils placed around the patient. The site of origin of this radio signal can be determined and an image representing the distribution of the hydrogen protons can be built up. The strength of the signal depends not only on proton density but also on two relaxation times, T1 and T2: T1 depends on the time the protons take to return to the axis of the magnetic field and T2 depends on the time the protons take to dephase. A T1-weighted image is one in which the contrast between tissues is due mainly to their T1 relaxation properties, while in a T2-weighted image the contrast is due to the T2-relaxation properties (Fig. 1.15). Some sequences produce mixed (often called 'balanced') images which approximate to proton density. Most pathological processes show increased T1 and T2 relaxation times which appear lower in signal (blacker) on a T1-weighted scan and higher in signal (whiter) on a T2-weighted scan than the surrounding normal soft tissues. The T1 and T2 weighting of an image can be selected by appropriately altering the timing and sequence of radiofrequency pulses.

MRI pulse sequences are a very important but complicated subject. The complexity is compounded by a series of acronyms and technical names, several of which appear from time to time in the chapters in this book. The term STIR (short-term inversion recovery) refers to a sequence that makes fat appear dark so that many pathological processes stand out as bright white regions. An alternative method of reducing the signal from fat is a special fat-suppression pulse. The types of sequences, such as spin-echo and gradient-echo, are of great importance to the radiographer and radiologist because they influence image contrast and affect speed of acquisition, but are of less importance to the practising clinician.

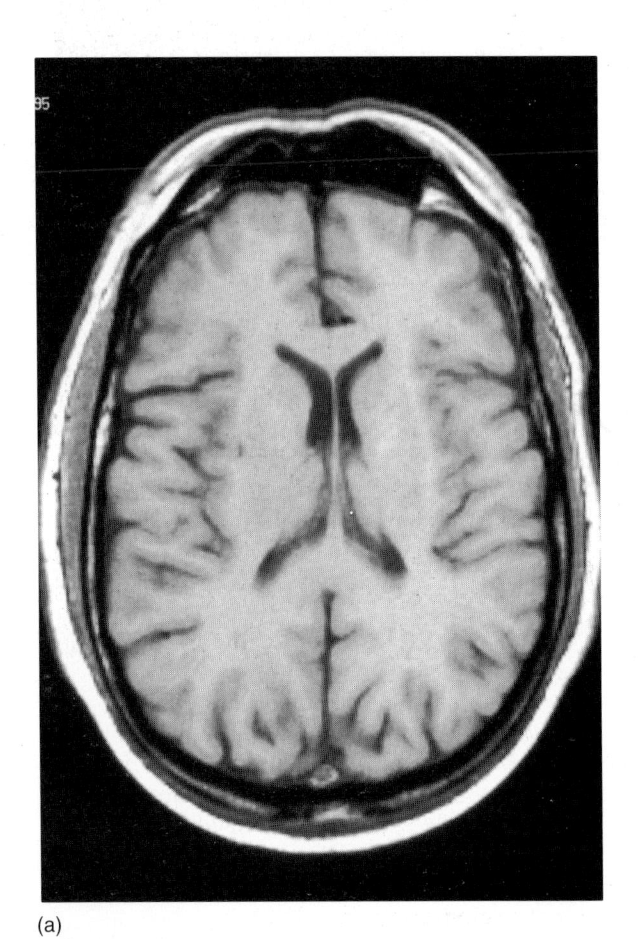

(a)

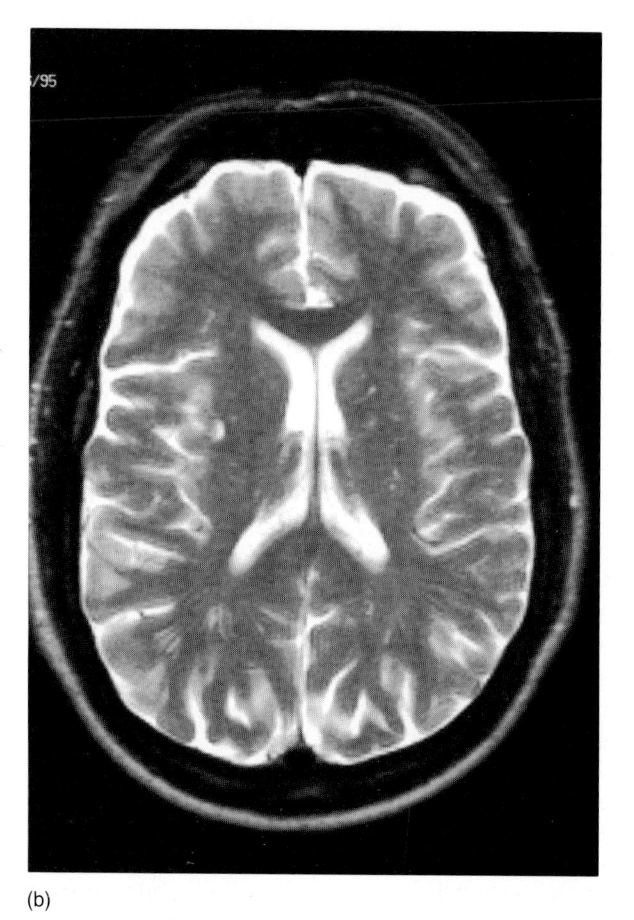

(b)

Fig. 1.15 MRI of brain. Axial sections through the lateral ventricles of a normal brain. (a) T1-weighted image. (b) T2-weighted image. The CSF is low signal on the T1-weighted image but high signal on the T2-weighted image. Note the different signal intensity of the grey and white matter on the two images.

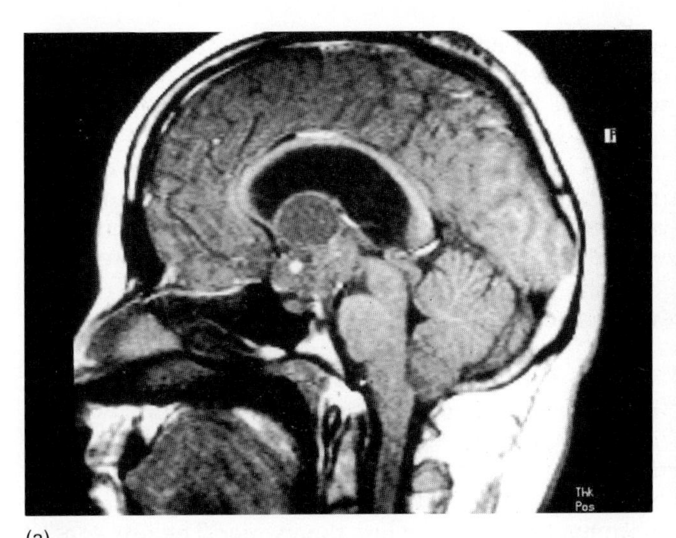

(a)

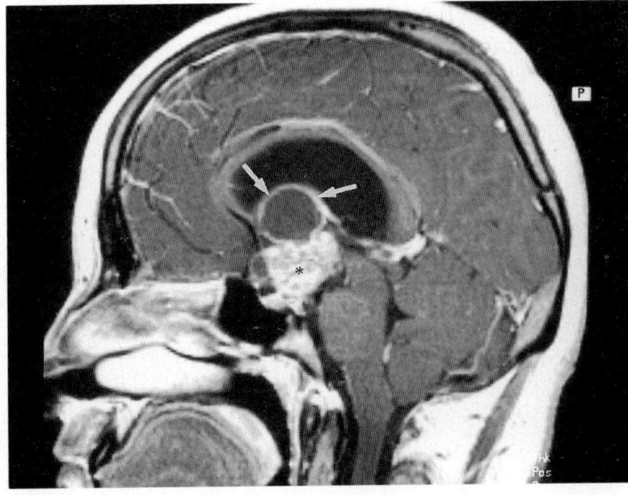

(b)

Fig. 1.16 MRI contrast enhancement of craniopharyngioma. Sagittal T1 weighted scans (a) precontrast and (b) postcontrast with gadolinium. There is contrast enhancement of the tumour (*). The rim of the cystic component of tumour also enhances (arrows).

An MRI scanner consists of a large, strong magnet. Inside the magnet are the radiofrequency transmitter and receiver coils, as well as gradient coils to allow spatial localization of the MRI signal. Ancillary equipment converts the radio signal into a digital form which is then processed by a computer to form a final image. One advantage of MRI over CT is that the information can be directly reconstructed in any plane. Currently MRI is, in most instances, a slow process (often several minutes) requiring a long scan time compared to CT, with the disadvantage that it is necessary to keep the patient still during the scanning procedure. Unavoidable movements due to breathing, cardiac pulsation and peristalsis often degrade the image. Techniques for limiting the effect of such motion with significantly shorter scan times and various electronic gating devices are being actively developed. **Cardiac gating** is already widely available.

In the same way that contrast media have been of great value in CT, magnetic contrast media are providing useful diagnostic information with MRI. These agents depend on magnetic and paramagnetic properties to produce contrast. The most widely used agent is gadolinium DTPA which dramatically decreases the T1 relaxation time (Fig. 1.16).

MRI is now widely used to scan the brain and spinal cord, where it has significant advantages over CT and few disadvantages. It is also an established technique for imaging the spine, bones, joints and pelvis.

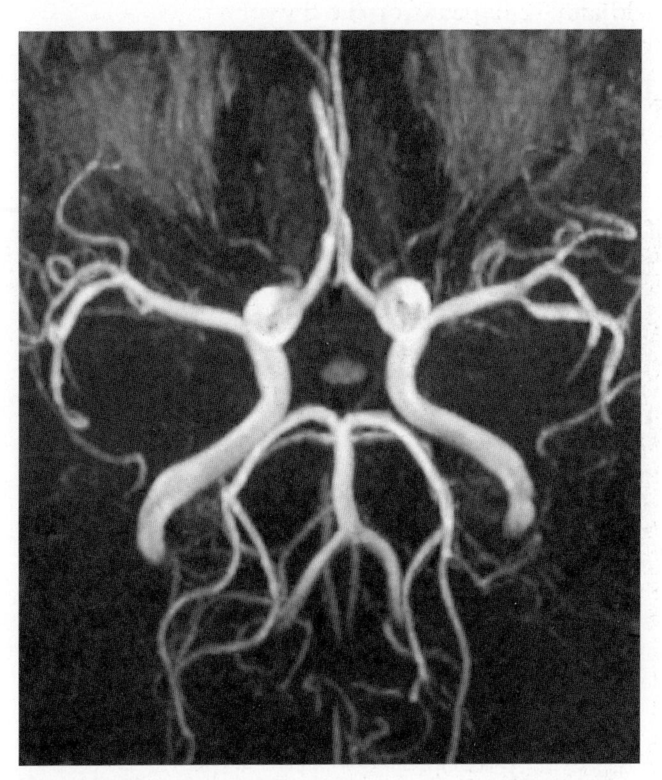

Fig. 1.17 MR angiogram of the cerebral arteries. This flow sequence produces images of the arteries forming the circle of Willis at the base of the brain without the need for contrast media.

The physical basis of vascular MRI is complicated and beyond the scope of this book. With some sequences, fast-flowing blood produces no signal, whereas with others it produces a bright signal. This 'motion effect' can be exploited to image the vascular system; for example, large arteriovenous malformations can be readily demonstrated without contrast media, hilar vessels can be distinguished from masses, and even stenoses of blood vessels can be demonstrated. Recently, special flow sequences have been developed which give images of vessels, resembling a conventional angiogram without the need for contrast media. This technique is known as **magnetic resonance angiography** and it may eventually replace conventional angiography (Fig. 1.17).

MRI of the heart uses electronic gating to obtain images during a specific proportion of the cardiac cycle. With this technique it is possible to limit the degradation of the image by cardiac motion and, therefore, demonstrate the cardiac chambers, valves and myocardium. Recently developed rapid scanning techniques allow the beating heart to be directly visualized as a cine image.

SAFETY OF MRI

One of the advantages of MRI is that it involves no ionizing radiation; also no adverse biological effects from diagnostic MRI have been demonstrated. It is, however, contraindicated in patients with metallic intraocular foreign bodies, certain types of aneurysm clips and cardiac pacemakers, because of the strong magnetic fields involved.

GENERAL PRINCIPLES OF ULTRASOUND, CT AND MR IMAGE INTERPRETATION

Familiarity with the appearance of component tissues in pathological processes on the various cross-sectional imaging modalities is vital to provide a useful differential diagnosis. In many situations, however, different diseases have similar appearances radiologically and a specific histological diagnosis cannot be given.

The ultrasound appearance is dictated by the pattern of transmission and reflection of a beam of high-frequency sound waves, determined by tissue interfaces and the acoustic impedance of tissues in the path of the beam. Structures containing watery fluid, such as the bladder or simple cysts, transmit ultrasound extremely well, appearing echo-free and allowing a high proportion of the beam to reach deeper structures, resulting in posterior acoustic enhancement. Tissues such as fat and bone, calcification and gas reflect a high proportion of the ultrasound beam, appearing echogenic, with reduced ultrasound transmission to deeper structures, i.e. acoustic shadowing. Complex cystic masses, solid organs and soft tissue masses produce a variable echo pattern.

On CT, the appearance of tissues depends on their electron density and atomic number: the higher the value of these parameters, the more X-rays are absorbed by the tissue and the whiter the tissue appears on the grey-scale image. The CT density, measured in Hounsfield units (HU), ranges from –1000 for air to +1000 for compact bone. Water has a value of 0 HU, but most fluids *in vivo* contain electrolytes and protein increasing the range up to about 20 HU. Most soft tissues are denser than water, in the range 20–50 HU, overlapping in density with proteinaceous or haemorrhagic fluid. Fat is an exception, having a density less than water. The presence of blood, calcium or administered contrast medium increases the density of tissues. Cortical bone has an extremely high density, measuring several hundred HUs.

On MRI, signal intensity of tissue can be made to reflect many variables, but for the purpose of clinical diagnosis, image interpretation is based on changes in proton density, T1 and T2 relaxation times. Many pathological processes are associated with an increased number of mobile protons which provides more signal, and prolongation of relaxation times which reduces signal intensity on T1-weighted sequences and increases signal on T2-weighted sequences. Muscle, including that in the walls of viscera such as the bladder and rectum, has a low signal on T2-weighted sequences, but increases in signal if inflamed or involved by tumour. Fat is characterized by a short T1 relaxation time, causing high signal intensity on T1-weighted sequences, a pattern also seen in certain components of haemorrhage. Signal voids occur in gas, bone and calcification (where hydrogen protons are absent or unable to generate signal), in flowing blood on certain sequences and when there is local distortion of the magnetic field caused by metal or haemosiderin.

CHAPTER 2

Plain abdomen

Stuart Field

In patients presenting with acute abdominal pain, plain films remain one of the most valuable initial investigations. The main purpose of the plain radiograph is to try and establish a diagnosis so that the clinician can decide whether or not a patient with acute abdominal pain needs an operation and, if an operation is needed, whether it needs to be performed immediately or whether time can be spent resuscitating or performing other investigations to confirm the diagnosis.

NORMAL APPEARANCES

The formation of a radiographic image depends on the structure and size of the organs within the abdomen. Gas which absorbs least X-rays appears black or dark grey, fat is usually seen as dark grey lines, the soft tissues appear very light grey with large soft tissue masses appearing almost white and finally calcification, which absorbs most X-rays, appears white (Fig. 2.1).

Relatively large amounts of gas are normally present in the stomach and colon, but only a small amount of gas is usually seen in the small bowel. The duodenum often contains air and a fluid level is frequently seen in it on horizontal X-ray films. The presence of bowel gas is important in assessing the diameter and position of the bowel and judging the amount of fluid within it.

When the stomach is empty it is usual to be able to identify the gastric rugae on a radiograph taken with the patient supine and to see a relatively long air–fluid

Diagnostic and Interventional Radiology in Surgical Practice. Edited by P. Armstrong and M. L. Wastie. Published in 1997 by Chapman & Hall, London, ISBN 0 412 61960 1 (HB), 0 412 61970 9 (PB)

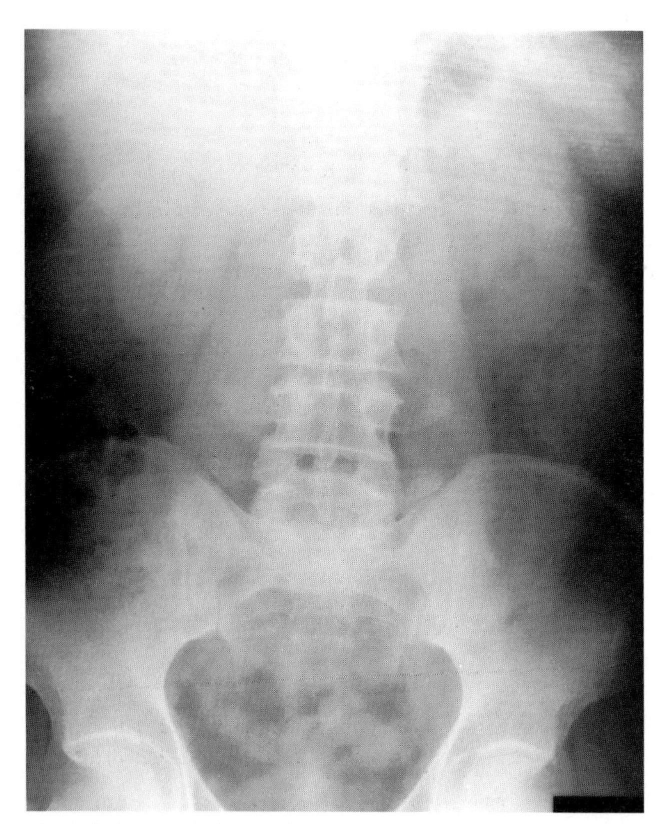

Fig. 2.1 Normal abdomen. A relatively gasless bowel and good fat lines outlining the psoas muscles, kidneys, liver, spleen and bladder can be seen.

level in the fundus of the stomach when the patient is erect. Because the antrum and body are normally contracted, small amounts of fluid and air result in a relatively long fluid level in the fundus on the erect film. There is rarely sufficient gas present in the small bowel to outline more than a short length and although the mucosal pattern may be seen, the thin bands of the valvulae conniventes, which extend across the full width of the jejunum, are seldom identified in a normal patient. However, air and fluid are normal contents of the small bowel and short fluid levels are not abnormal. The significance of air fluid levels is often overstated. Fluid levels may occur in the colon in normal people. Three to five fluid levels less than 2.5 cm in length may be seen, particularly in the right lower quadrant without any evidence of intestinal obstruction or paralytic ileus. However, more than two fluid levels in dilated small bowel (calibre > 2.5 cm) is abnormal and usually indicates paralytic ileus or intestinal obstruction but may also be seen in normal radiographs. Most of the gas seen within bowel has been swallowed and it normally reaches the colon within 30 minutes. However, when severe pain is present anywhere in the body or when respiration is laboured, such as in pneumonia or asthma, more air is swallowed producing a dramatic plain abdominal radiograph showing gas-filled, slightly dilated loops of bowel throughout the abdomen. The term 'meteorism' is sometimes given to this appearance (Fig. 2.2). It is sometimes difficult to differentiate air swallowing, produced for example by renal colic, from intestinal obstruction. The clinical history and examination frequently enable the radiological findings to be correctly interpreted.

The amount of gas present in a normal colon is extremely variable from almost none to what may appear to be pathological gaseous distension. Sufficient gas is usually present for colonic haustra, which form thick incomplete bands extending across most of the large bowel, to be readily identified. Numerous colonic fluid levels, some several centimetres in length, may be a common finding and up to 20% of normal people may have a fluid level in the caecum.

Large bowel calibre is very variable with considerable overlap between the normal and abnormal: a reliable measurement for the upper limit of normal diameter of the large bowel cannot be given. However, a transverse colonic diameter of 5.5 cm has been suggested as the upper limit of normal in patients with colitis and, if the diameter of the transverse colon is greater, then megacolon should be suggested. The caecum is readily distensible, particularly in large bowel obstruction, and it has been suggested that a

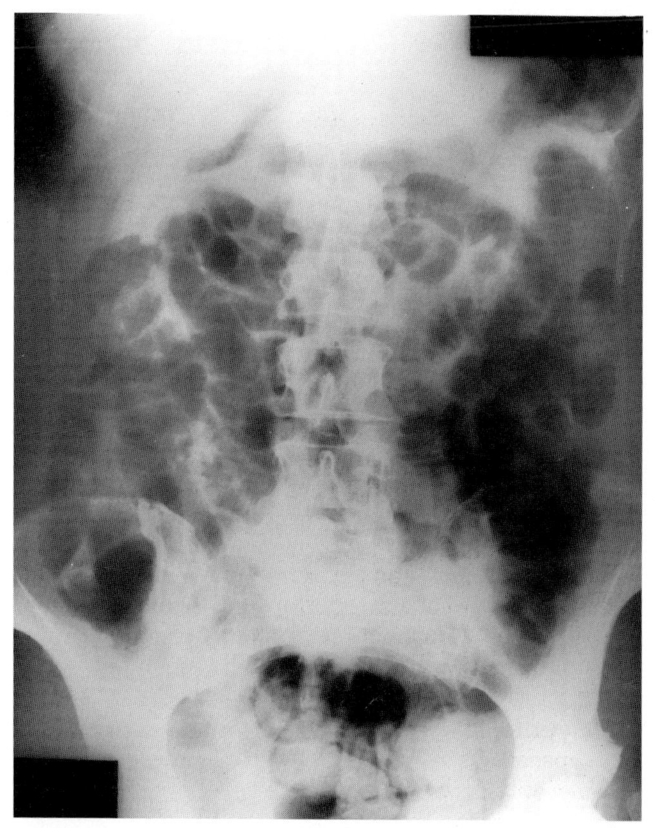

Fig. 2.2 Normal abdomen. The entire alimentary tract is gas-filled due to air swallowing. The stomach, duodenal cap, varying lengths of small bowel and entire left half of colon are filled with gas but not unduly distended.

diameter of 9–10 cm is a critical level beyond which there is a great risk of perforation.

The outlines of the kidneys, psoas muscles, bladder and the posterior borders of the liver and spleen can often be identified by the fat which surrounds them (Fig. 2.1). These fat lines can be displaced by enlargement of these organs or effaced by inflammation or fluid. It is, however, important to realize that in a number of normal people these fat lines may be blurred or even absent. The outline of the spleen cannot be identified in around 40% of normal individuals and the right psoas is blurred in nearly 20%. In children, due to the small amount of body fat, loss of the psoas outlines may occur in up to 50% of normal individuals and the properitoneal fat lines may not be visible in almost 20% of normal children. These factors must be considered carefully before undue emphasis is placed on fat line changes.

ABDOMINAL CALCIFICATION

Although the history and clinical examination may contribute important clues, the finding of calcification on a plain abdominal radiograph is often unexpected and it may not be possible to elucidate the exact cause.

The commonest types of abdominal calcification are non-visceral and often unrelated to the presenting clinical problem:

- **Common**
  - atherosclerosis
  - mesenteric lymph nodes
  - phleboliths
  - aneurysm
  - rib cartilage (normal)
  - injections in the buttocks
- **Uncommon**
  - infestations
    - Armillifer armillatus
    - cysticercosis
    - guinea worm
    - hydatid
  - tumours
    - lipoma
    - haemangioma
    - neuroblastoma
    - osteo/chondrosarcoma
    - retroperitoneal sarcoma
    - peritoneal metastases
    - phaeochromocytoma
  - tuberculosis
    - peritonitis
    - psoas abscess
  - meconium peritonitis
  - pseudomyxoma peritonei
  - dermoid cyst
  - mesenteric cyst
  - pancreatitis with saponification
  - lithopaedion
  - appendices epiploicae
  - ligaments
  - foreign bodies
  - post-traumatic buttock cysts.

Abdominal calcification associated with an acute abdomen is relatively uncommon. The associations are summarized below:

- **Gallstones**
  - cholecystitis
  - pancreatitis
  - biliary colic (stone may be close to spine)
  - empyema of gallbladder
  - gallstone ileus (stone in abnormal location)
- **Calcified gallbladder wall**
  - cholecystitis
- **Limey bile**
  - cholecystitis
- **Appendix calculus**
  - appendicitis
- **Calculus**
  - Meckel's diverticulum
  - jejunal diverticulum
  - colonic diverticulum

  } Showing acute inflammation or perforation
- **Pancreatic calculi**
  - pancreatitis – chronic and acute (rare)
- **Ureteric calculus**
  - renal colic
- **Calcified aneurysms** (aortic, splenic, hepatic)
  - rupture
- **Teeth/bone in ovarian dermoid**
  - torsion.

THE ACUTE ABDOMEN

Patients with acute abdominal pain form one of the largest groups presenting as an emergency to the general surgeon. Plain radiographs have become established as an essential investigation in these patients. Interpretation of the radiographs may present a formidable challenge. While in many cases a specific diagnosis can be made, plain radiographs are often non-specific or occasionally even misleading, and further investigations with contrast agents, ultrasound, radionuclides or computed tomography may be necessary. When the radiological diagnosis is specific or supports the clinical diagnosis, surgery is often indicated. If immediate surgery is indicated on clinical grounds, negative or equivocal radiological findings should be ignored.

RADIOGRAPHIC TECHNIQUE

A supine abdomen and erect chest can be regarded as the basic standard radiographs. The bladder should be emptied before the supine radiograph is taken and the film should include the area from the diaphragm to the hernial orifices.

A horizontal ray abdominal radiograph, either erect or left lateral decubitus (right side raised), is frequently taken to add information and to demonstrate fluid levels. The clinical condition of the patient will determine whether erect radiographs are taken with the patient standing or sitting. In a patient who is too ill even to sit, it may only be possible to obtain a lateral decubitus or supine radiograph with a horizontal ray. Ideally the patient should always remain in position for 10 minutes prior to the horizontal ray radiograph to allow time for any free gas to rise to the highest point.

A chest radiograph is essential because the following chest diseases may mimic an acute abdomen:

- pleurisy
- pneumonia
- pulmonary infarction
- myocardial infarction
- leaking or dissecting thoracic aneurysm
- congestive cardiac failure
- pericarditis
- pneumothorax.

Furthermore the erect chest radiograph is superior to the erect abdominal view for the demonstration of free intra-abdominal gas under the diaphragm and, therefore, it is essential that the chest film includes the diaphragmatic area. Up to one third of patients presenting with acute abdominal pain may have an abnormal chest X-ray: either pleural effusions or evidence of pneumonia and occasionally the chest condition may actually simulate an acute abdomen. It is also helpful to have a chest radiograph as a baseline because chest complications and subphrenic abscess are frequent postoperative complications in patients presenting with acute abdominal pain and who proceed to emergency surgery.

Further abdominal views may be needed to obtain additional information when the standard radiographs have been viewed or a specific diagnosis is suspected. A left lateral decubitus radiograph (one taken with the patient lying on their left side and with the use of a horizontal ray) may be taken to confirm equivocal free gas suspected on an erect chest radiograph. A left lateral decubitus film may also demonstrate a dilated gas-filled duodenum in acute pancreatitis. However, the supine abdominal radiograph is the most useful single view and, in many conditions, it is the only plain film of the abdomen that is required. Although in some centres as many as six different plain film views have been suggested, this is time-consuming and expensive if done on every patient with abdominal pain! There is a body of opinion which believes that an erect chest and supine abdomen should be taken and viewed, and additional films taken only if the clinical story warrants it or abnormalities are identified which require further elucidation. A management change as a result of information gleaned from radiographs of the chest and abdomen can be expected in 10–15% of patients presenting with an acute abdomen.

DILATATION OF BOWEL

Dilatation of bowel occurs in mechanical intestinal obstruction, pseudo-obstruction, paralytic ileus and air-swallowing. However, in some individuals, particularly those who are institutionalized or intellectually impaired, the diameter of the colon may be enormous without any evidence of obstruction. Differentiation of the causes of dilated bowel will depend on the clinical history and examination together with the determination of the size and distribution of the various loops of bowel.

GASTRIC DILATATION

An enlarged stomach can be caused by any of the following conditions.

- **Mechanical gastric outlet obstruction**
  - duodenal or pyloric canal ulceration
  - carcinoma of pyloric antrum
  - extrinsic compression, e.g. annular pancreas
- **Paralytic ileus**
  - postoperative
  - trauma
  - peritonitis
  - pancreatitis
  - cholecystitis
  - diabetes
  - hepatic coma
  - drugs
- **Gastric volvulus**
- **Intubation**
- **Air swallowing**.

Mechanical gastric outlet obstruction caused by peptic ulceration or a carcinoma of the pyloric antrum usually leads to a huge fluid-filled stomach or a stomach which contains inspissated food (Fig. 2.3). The dilated stomach may occupy most of the upper abdomen and may be identified as a soft tissue mass containing bubbles of air with little or no bowel gas in the remainder of the bowel. Usually, however a little gas is present in the stomach which allows the organ to be identified, particularly if a long fluid level is visible in the fundus on the erect chest radiograph. Paralytic ileus (often referred to as acute gastric dilation) may predominantly affect the stomach, particularly in old people (Fig. 2.4). Acute gastric dilatation is associated with considerable fluid and electrolyte disturbance and carries a high mortality.

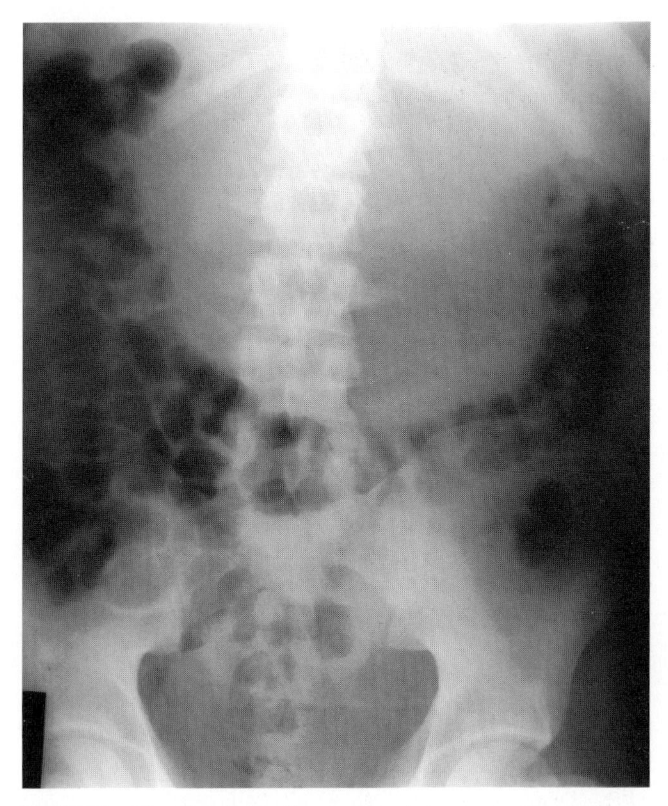

Fig. 2.3 Gastric outlet obstruction, supine abdomen position. The gas- and fluid-filled stomach gives rise to an upper abdominal soft tissue mass which is indenting the gas-filled transverse colon. The patient had chronic duodenal ulceration.

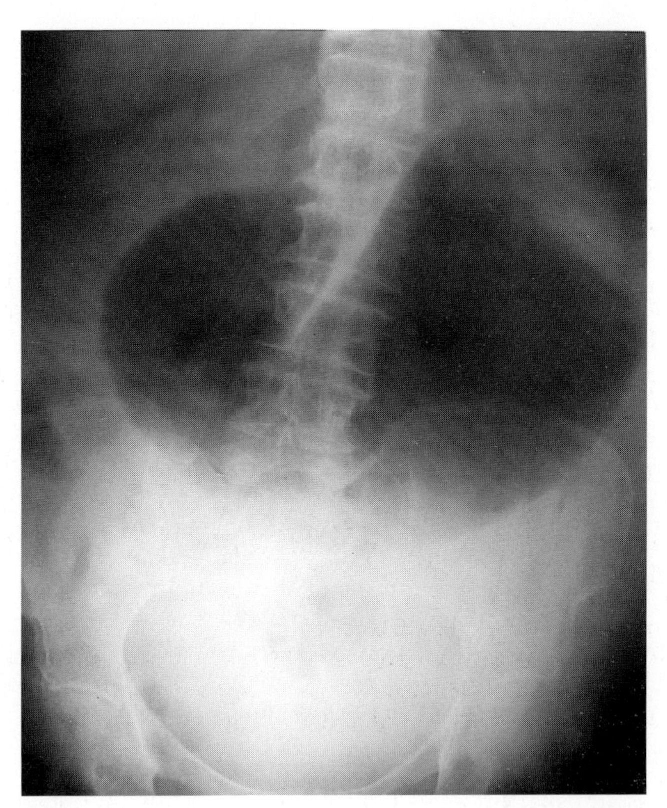

Fig. 2.4 Acute gastric dilatation. Air swallowing has produced a hugely distended gas-filled stomach in a patient with acute cholecystitis. (Source: S. Field, in D. J. Nolan, *A Radiological atlas of gastro-intestinal disease*; published by John Wiley, Chichester, 1983.)

A **gastric volvulus** is relatively rare and may result from the stomach twisting around the longitudinal, transverse or mesenteric axis. The dilated stomach due to a gastric volvulus is frequently spherical and may contain a long fluid level. The stomach is displaced upwards and is often associated with elevation of the left hemidiaphragm. The small bowel is usually collapsed and it is unusual to see any gas shadows beyond the stomach. If oral contrast medium is given there may be complete obstruction at the lower end of the oesophagus or if contrast does enter the stomach it may not pass beyond the obstructed pylorus.

Gastric dilation sometimes occurs simply due to air swallowing. After the patient has been resuscitated and intubated, large amounts of gas frequently enter the stomach, often leading to massive dilation. On the supine radiograph a gas-filled stomach can usually be identified with the wall of the greater curvature appearing convex caudally and the pyloric antrum pointing cranially.

It is important to differentiate a distended stomach from a caecal volvulus which may also be positioned beneath an elevated left hemidiaphragm.

SMALL AND LARGE BOWEL DILATATION

When a radiograph shows dilated bowel it is important to try and determine whether the small or large bowel or both are dilated. Useful differentiating features depend on the size, distribution and markings of the loops, features summarized in Table 2.1. The presence of solid faeces is the only reliable differentiating sign, the others being sometimes

Table 2.1 The distinction between small bowel and large bowel dilation

	Small bowel	*Large bowel*
Haustra	Absent	Present
Valvulae conniventes	Present in jejunum	Absent
Number of loops	Many	Few
Distribution of loops	Central	Peripheral
Radius of curvature of loop	Small	Large
Diameter of loop	30–50 mm	50 mm +
Solid faeces	Absent	May be present

misleading. Dilated lower ileum may be difficult to distinguish from the sigmoid colon because both may be smooth in outline and occupy a similar position low in the central abdomen. Although haustra usually form thick incomplete bands across the colonic gas shadow they sometimes form complete transverse bands. However, these can usually be differentiated from valvulae conniventes because haustra are thicker and further apart than the small bowel folds. Haustra may be absent from the descending and sigmoid colon but can usually still be identified in other parts of the colon even when it is massively distended.

The small bowel folds or valvulae conniventes form thin complete bands across the bowel gas shadow, prominent in the jejunum but becoming less marked as the ileum is reached. The valvulae conniventes are much closer together than colonic haustra and become thinner when stretched but still remain relatively close together even when the small bowel calibre increases. However, if the small bowel blood supply is compromised and the bowel becomes oedematous or gangrenous, the valvulae conniventes may become thickened and then be difficult to differentiate from colonic haustra.

Although the bowel calibre is extremely variable, it is unusual in small bowel obstruction for the small bowel diameter to exceed much more than 5 cm. In large bowel obstruction it is unusual for the large bowel calibre to be less than 5 cm, indeed, it usually greatly exceeds this value.

SMALL BOWEL OBSTRUCTION

Mechanical obstruction of the small bowel normally causes small bowel dilation with an accumulation of both gas and fluid and a reduction of the calibre of the large bowel (Fig. 2.5).

The amount of gas present in the large bowel depends on the duration and the completeness of the small bowel obstruction. Valvulae conniventes are more prominent in the jejunum and the knowledge of this together with an assessment of the number and position of the dilated loops allow an estimate to be made as to the site of the obstruction. Plain film changes may appear after 3–5 hours with complete small bowel obstruction, and changes are usually very marked after 12 hours. However, with incomplete obstruction the plain radiographic changes may take hours or days to appear and even then may be undramatic. Barium studies or ultrasound may be required to establish the diagnosis. The dilated, gas-filled loops of small bowel are readily identified on the supine radiograph with multiple fluid levels present

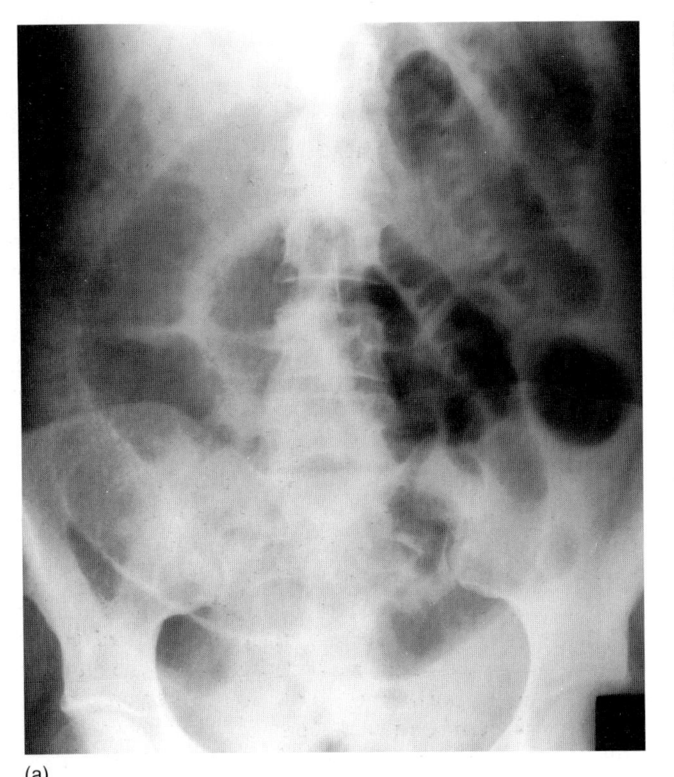

(a)

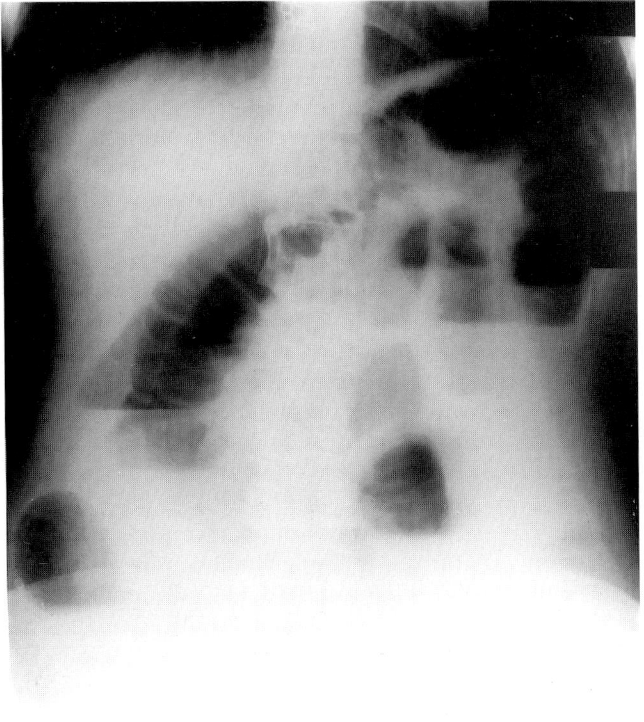

(b)

Fig. 2.5 Small bowel obstruction seen on (a) supine abdomen and (b) erect abdomen. The gas-filled loops of small bowel clearly identified by the valvulae conniventes can be seen filling the central part of the abdomen. There is no gas in the colon. Multiple fluid levels are present on the erect film.

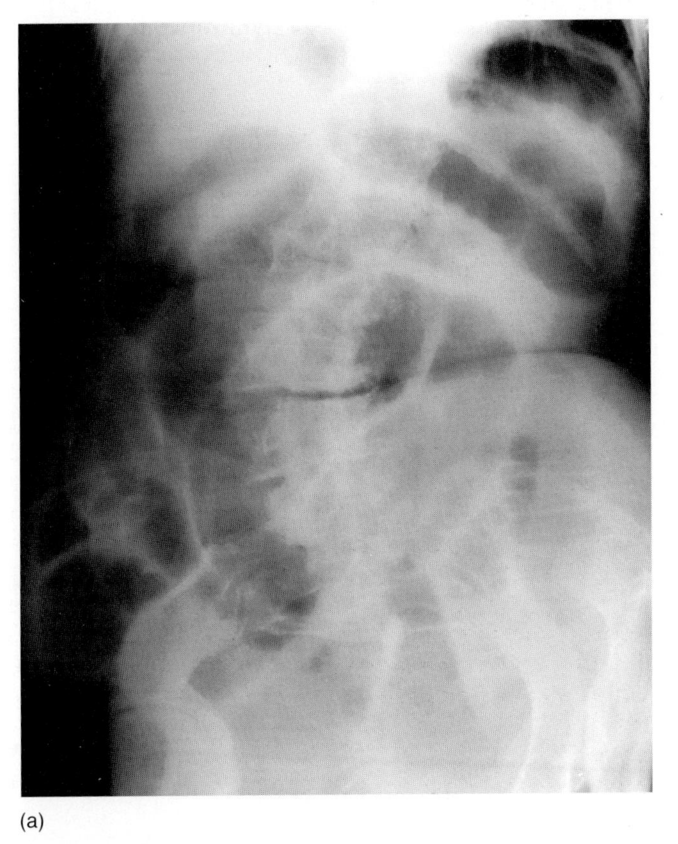

(a)

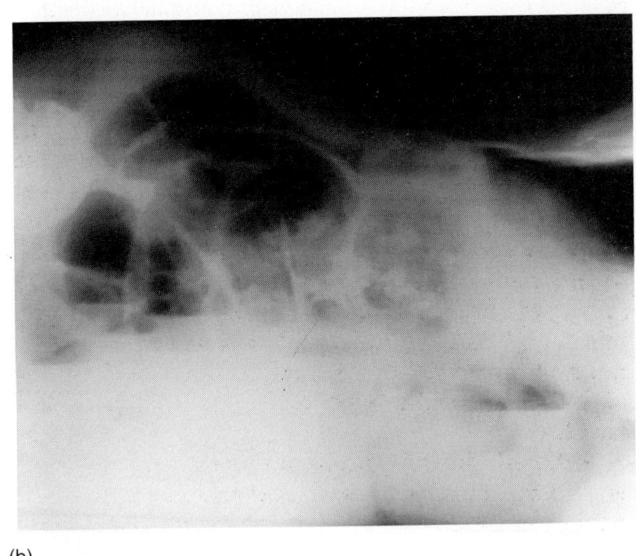

(b)

Fig. 2.6 Small bowel obstruction seen on (a) supine abdomen and (b) left lateral decubitus abdomen. In patients who are unfit to sit or stand for an erect film the left lateral decubitus is a valuable alternative horizontal ray film to an erect abdomen.

on the erect or lateral decubitus radiographs. In most cases there is little difficulty in diagnosing small bowel obstruction (Fig. 2.6); there are, however, many causes of small bowel fluid levels:

- normal (always < 25 mm in length)
- small bowel obstruction
- large bowel obstruction
- paralytic ileus
- gastroenteritis
- hypokalaemia
- uraemia
- jejunal diverticulosis
- mesenteric thrombosis
- saline cathartics
- peritoneal metastases (usually < 25 mm in length)
- cleansing enemas.

In some cases of small bowel obstruction relatively little air is swallowed and the small bowel is predominantly filled with fluid. Dilated fluid-filled loops of small bowel may then be identified as sausage-shaped, oval, or round soft-tissue densities that change position in different views. The **string of beads sign**, which is due to bubbles of gas trapped between valvulae conniventes, occurs when very dilated small bowel is almost completely filled with fluid, and this appearance is virtually diagnostic of small bowel obstruction (Fig. 2.7). Normal or equivocal initial radiographs that may result in delayed diagnosis are found in a proportion of patients with small bowel obstruction, particularly those with high obstruction (Fig. 2.8). There may be no gas fluid visible in the small bowel of patients with high jejunal obstruction who have substantial vomiting. As a result the small bowel diameter cannot be assessed and the diagnosis from the plain film is difficult or impossible to make. If there are suggestive clinical findings, repeat plain films after a few hours, ultrasound or barium studies should be performed (Fig. 2.9).

In the developed world about 80% of individuals with mechanical small bowel obstruction will have adhesions due to previous surgery. The obstruction will be caused by a strangulated hernia in less than 10% of cases. However, in developing parts of the world nearly three-quarters of cases of small bowel obstruction are caused by a strangulated hernia (Fig. 2.10). It is important to look for a hernia on the radiograph which may be identified as a small gas-filled viscus below the level of the inguinal ligament. However, visualization of a hernia does not always mean it is the cause of the small bowel obstruction. If, however, a dilated small bowel loop can be identified,

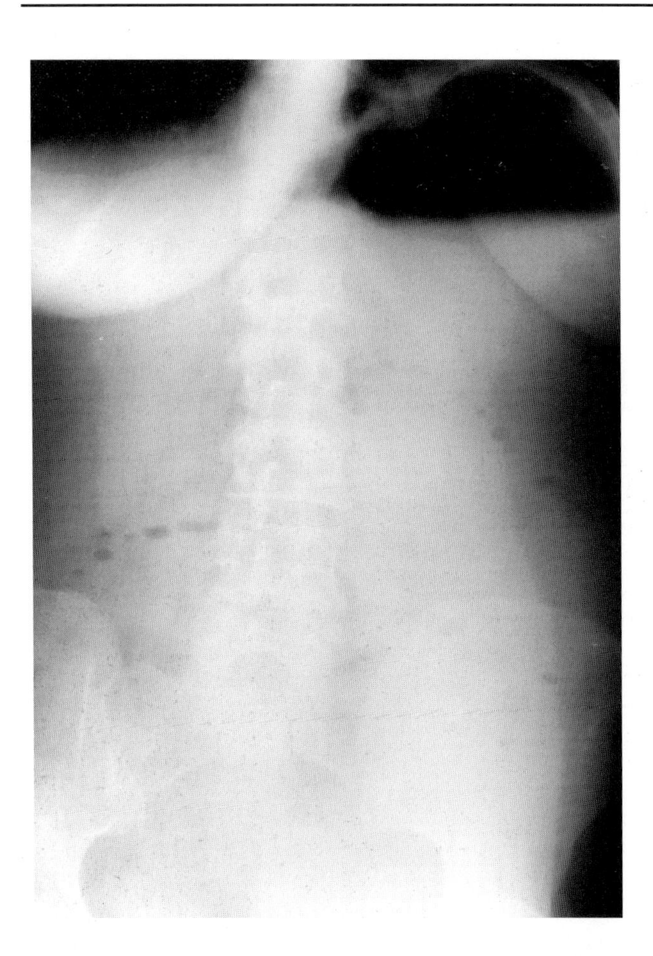

Fig. 2.7 'String of beads' sign. This is a valuable sign indicating a predominantly fluid-filled small bowel obstruction. Tiny bubbles of gas trapped between the valvulae conniventes are identified on this erect film. (Source: S. Field, in D. J. Nolan, *A Radiological atlas of gastrointestinal disease*; published by John Wiley, Chichester, 1983.)

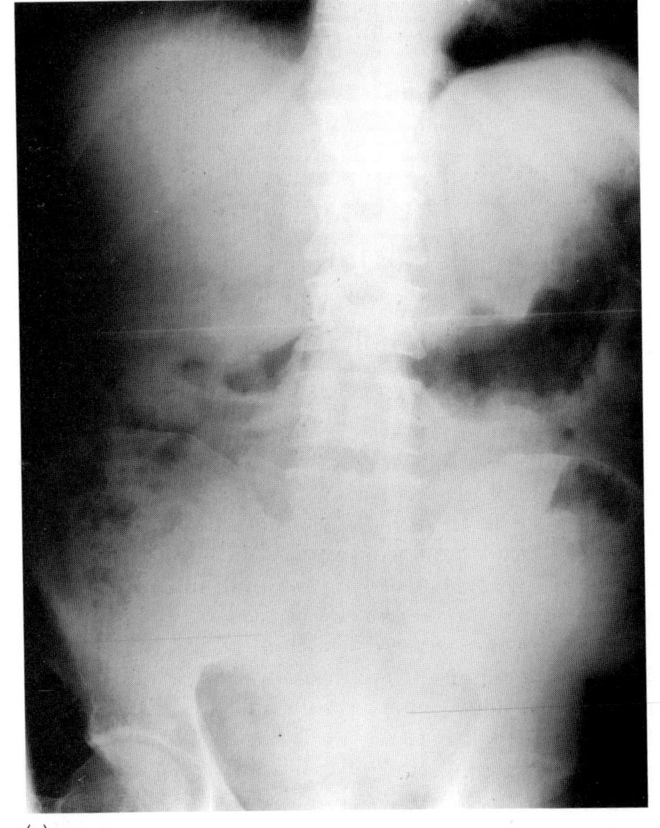

(a)

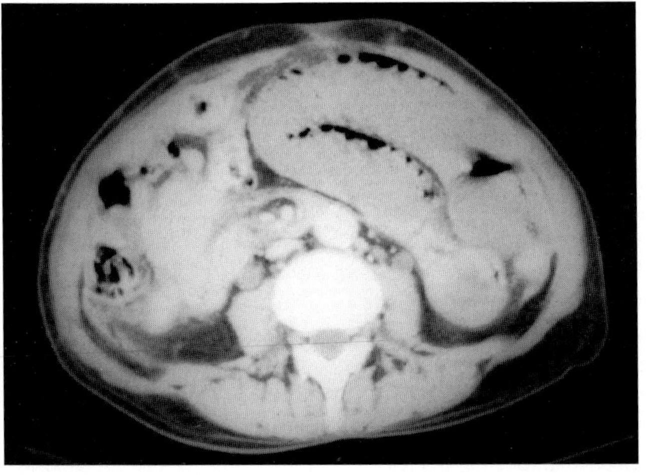

(b)

Fig. 2.8 Small bowel obstruction seen on (a) supine abdomen and (b) CT scan. The abdominal radiograph is within normal limits. The CT scan, however, clearly demonstrates a grossly dilated loop of small bowel with bowel with bubbles of gas trapped beneath the valvulae conniventes, the CT equivalent of the 'string of beads' sign.

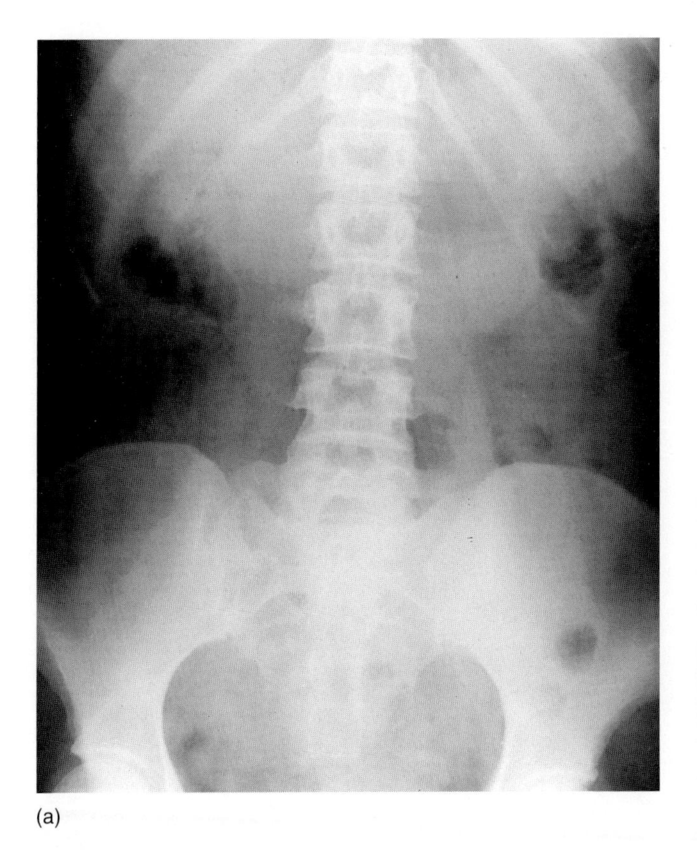

(a)

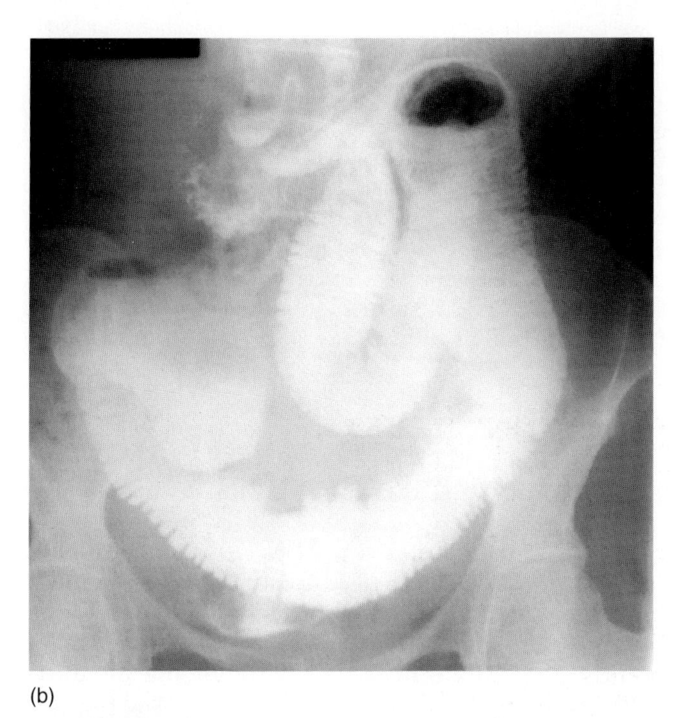

(b)

Fig. 2.9 Small bowel obstruction seen on (a) supine abdomen and (b) barium small bowel examination. The abdominal radiograph demonstrates borderline dilation of one or two loops of bowel in the left upper quadrant. The barium study clearly demonstrates markedly dilated small bowel which is obstructed proximally due to small bowel lymphoma. (Source: S. Field, in D. Sutton (ed), *Textbook of radiology and imaging*, published by Churchill Livingstone, Edinburgh, 1992.)

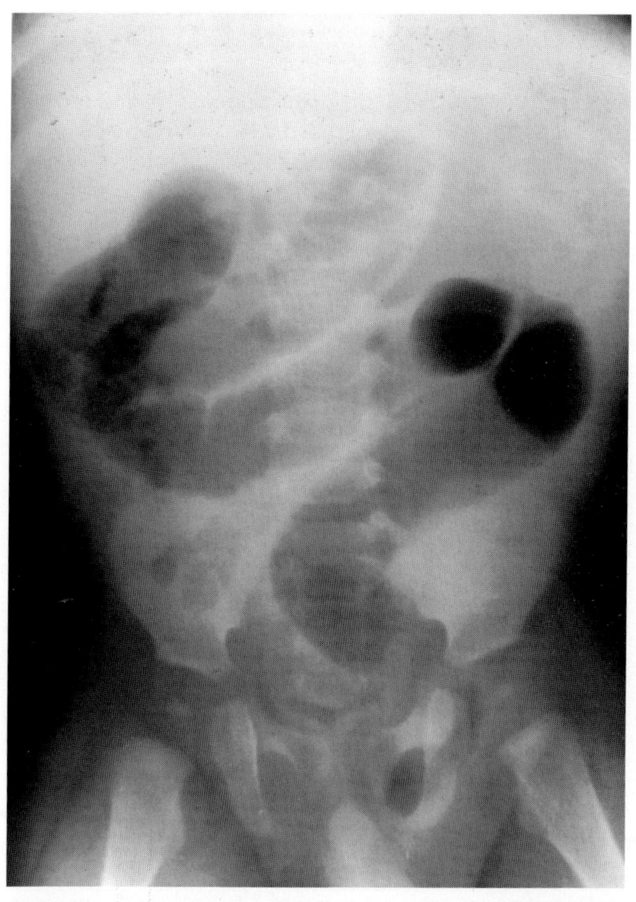

Fig. 2.10 Strangulated left femoral hernia seen on supine abdomen. Markedly dilated loops of small bowel can clearly be identified passing into the left femoral region in child aged 4 months with persistent vomiting.

which points directly to the inguinal region and which also contains an abnormally located gas shadow, a confident diagnosis of obstruction due to the hernia can be made.

Although hernias other than inguinal or femoral hernias may cause intestinal obstruction, it is extremely uncommon for these hernias to be identified on plain abdominal radiographs. Rarely a hernia through the foramen of Winslow, an umbilical or incisional hernia can be identified on the abdominal radiograph.

Causes of small bowel obstruction which may be identified on a plain abdominal radiograph include:

- hernia
- volvulus
- gallstone ileus
- intussusception
- constipation
- tumour
- mesenteric infarction
- foreign body
- malrotation.

STRANGULATING OBSTRUCTION

Strangulating obstruction occurs when a loop of obstructed small bowel becomes incarcerated by a band or by the neck of a hernial sac in such a way as to compromise the blood supply by compression of the mesenteric vessels (Fig. 2.11). The closed loop thus formed may fill with fluid, be palpable and be visible on a radiograph as a soft tissue mass or 'pseudo-tumour'. The strangulated loop may contain gas and the arms of the loop, separated only by thickened intestinal walls, may resemble a large coffee bean. If gangrene occurs, mucosal nodularity, small bubbles and linear gas shadows may be seen in the wall of the bowel (Fig. 2.12). However, the appearances in strangulating obstruction, with all its lethal potential, may be indistinguishable from simple small bowel obstruction. A raised white cell count is a pointer that strangulation may have occurred.

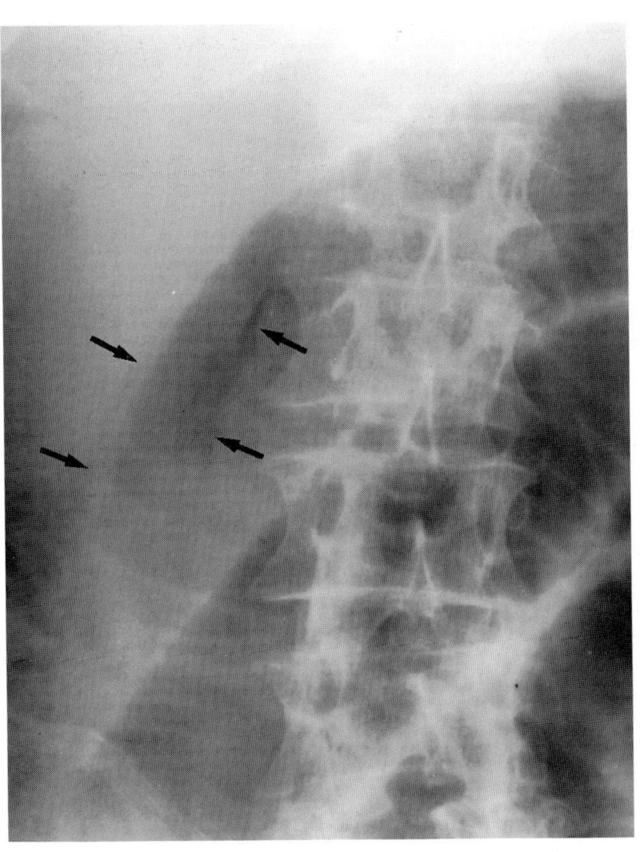

Fig. 2.12 Gangrene of small bowel in obstruction secondary to adhesions. Linear gas can be identified within the wall of the small bowel (arrows). (Source: S. Field, in *Clinics in Gastroenterology* 1984; **13**: 1.)

VOLVULUS OF THE SMALL INTESTINE

Volvulus of the small bowel may occur as an isolated abnormality or in combination with obstruction due to adhesive bands. It may be associated with anomalies of the mesentery and there is often associated malrotation of the bowel. In children incomplete rotation, malrotation or non-rotation of the gut may be associated with a massive small bowel volvulus that may occur in the neonatal period or sometimes months or even years after birth. Impairment of the blood supply frequently occurs in small bowel volvulus so that intramural gas or nodular thickening of the bowel wall may be seen. It is not usually possible to differentiate between strangulating obstruction, small bowel volvulus or simple small bowel obstruction from plain radiographs alone.

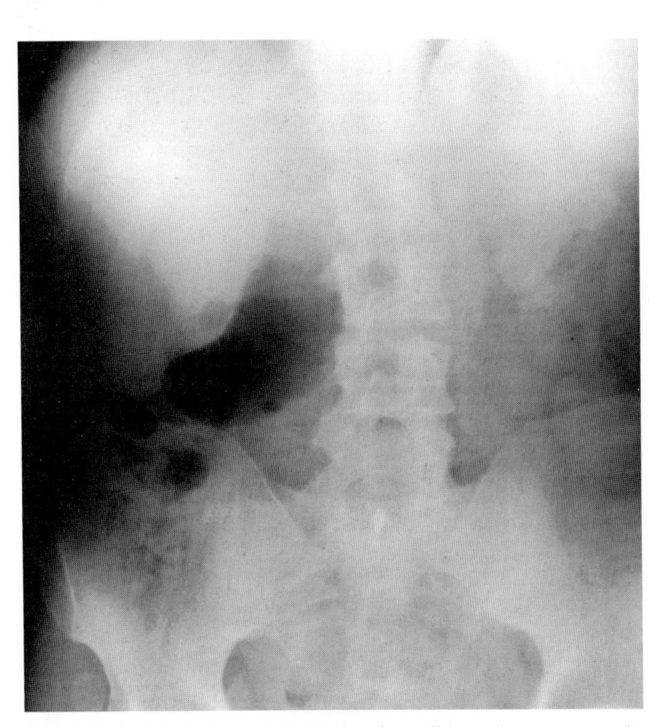

Fig. 2.11 Isolated strangulated loop of small bowel seen on supine abdomen. An isolated loop of small bowel can be identified in the right upper quadrant. Closed loop obstruction was secondary to band adhesions.

GALLSTONE ILEUS

Gallstone ileus is the term given to mechanical intestinal obstruction caused when one or more gallstones impact in the intestine. This usually occurs in the distal ileum at its narrowest point just proximal to the ileocaecal valve but may also rarely occur in the duodenum or colon. Following an attack of cholecystitis, a gallstone may pass through the inflamed gallbladder wall and into the duodenum. The patient, who is most commonly a middle-aged or elderly woman, will frequently have had recurrent episodes of right hypochondrial pain characteristic of cholecystitis. However, the most recent attack will usually have been more severe and associated with prolonged vomiting. Gallstone ileus accounts for around 2% of

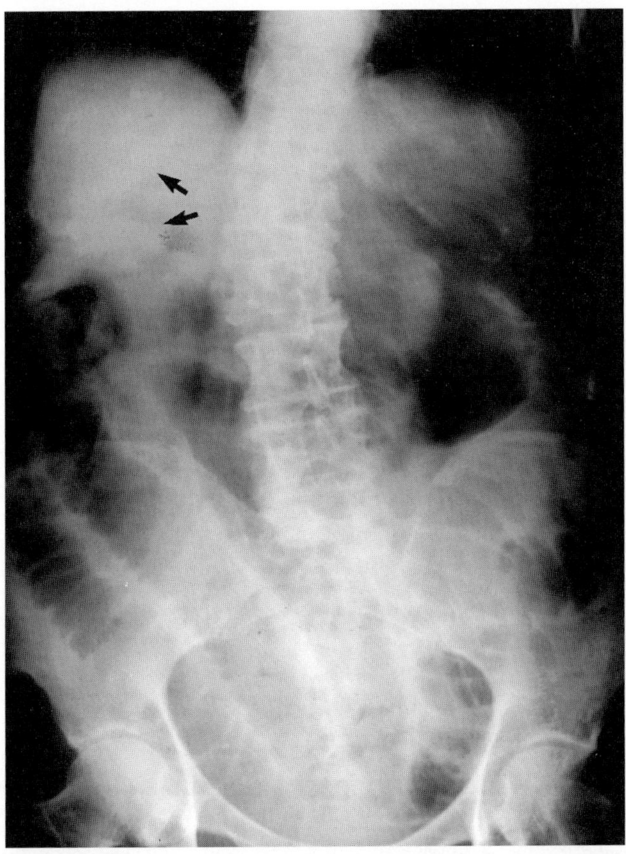

Fig. 2.13 Gallstone ileus seen on supine abdomen. Small bowel obstruction is present. Gas can be identified within the bile ducts in the right upper quadrant (arrows). (Source: S. Field, in D. J. Nolan, *A radiological atlas of gastrointestinal disease*; published by John Wiley, Chichester, 1983.)

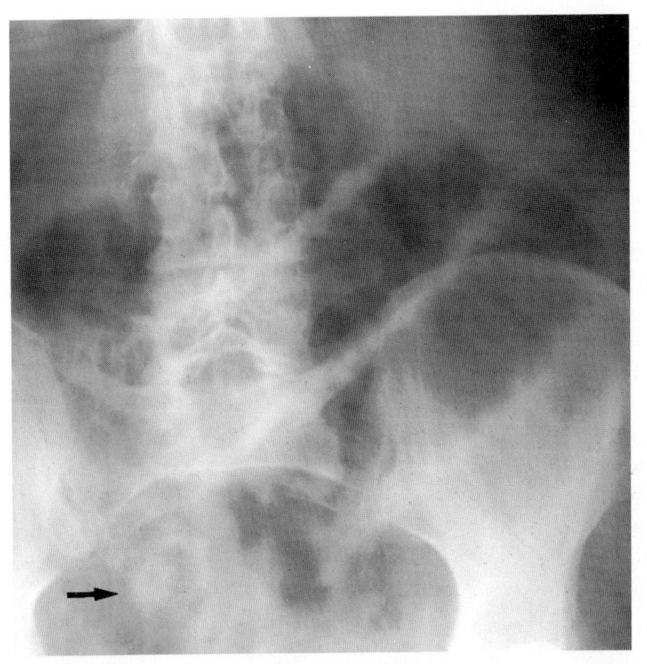

Fig. 2.14 Gallstone ileus seen on supine abdomen. Oedematous dilated loops of small bowel can be identified in the lower abdomen. The calcified ring shadow of the obstructing gallstone can be identified, with difficulty, overlying the sacrum (arrow).

patients presenting with small bowel obstruction. The diagnosis is frequently delayed or missed even though the characteristic radiological features of gallstone ileus are present in nearly 40% of cases. Over half of the patients will have evidence of intestinal obstruction and about one third will have gas present in the biliary tree (Fig. 2.13). The radiological features of gallstone ileus include:

- incomplete or complete small bowel obstruction;
- gas within the gallbladder and/or bile ducts;
- abnormal location of a gallstone;
- change in position of a gallstone;
- relatively large fluid-to-gas ratio in distended bowel.

Gas in the biliary tree can be recognized by its branching pattern with the gas being more prominent centrally. Gas in the biliary tree has to be differentiated from gas in the portal vein which tends to be more peripherally located in small veins around the edge of the liver. The gallstone that is causing obstruction usually lies in the loops of ileum overlying the caecum and, therefore, is often difficult to identify (Fig. 2.14). However, the gallstone can be seen in around one third of patients either on plain radiographs or on subsequent barium examinations. Although the obstructing gallstone is usually larger than 2.5 cm in size it may be difficult to identify on plain films because it is frequently composed almost entirely of cholesterol and may possess only a thin rim of calcification. The changing position of a previously observed gallstone is a rare sign. Gas in the biliary tree may also be seen in a number of other conditions:

- fistula between gallbladder and bowel from passage of a gallstone;
- following biliary surgery or endoscopic sphincterotomy;
- following percutaneous or endoscopic cholangiography;
- malignant fistula;
- perforated peptic ulcer (into bile duct);
- emphysematous cholangitis (gallbladder usually enlarged);
- physiological – due to lax sphincter.

Small bowel obstruction may develop following biliary surgery and the radiological appearances may mimic gallstone ileus.

INTUSSUSCEPTION

Two groups of patients develop small bowel intussusception. It is most frequently seen in children under the age of 2 years when the most usual form of

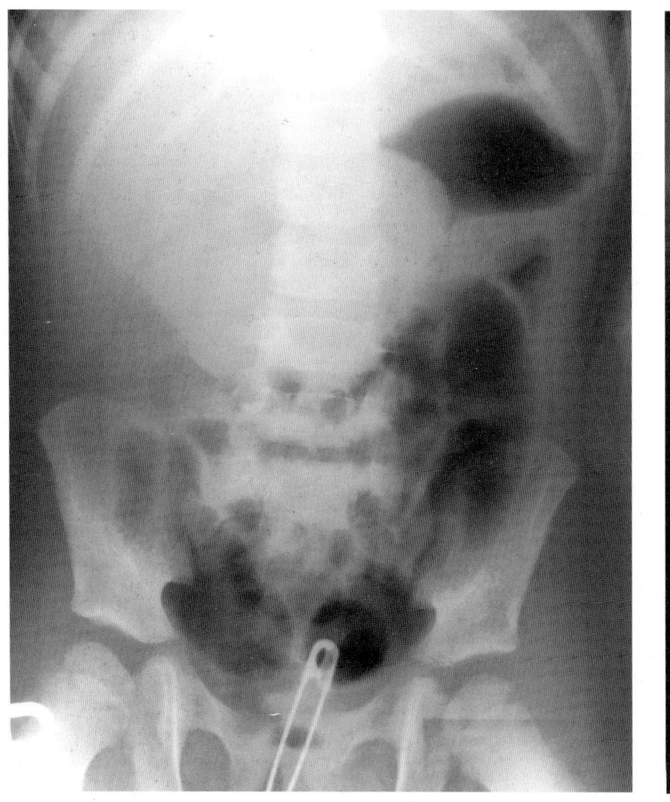

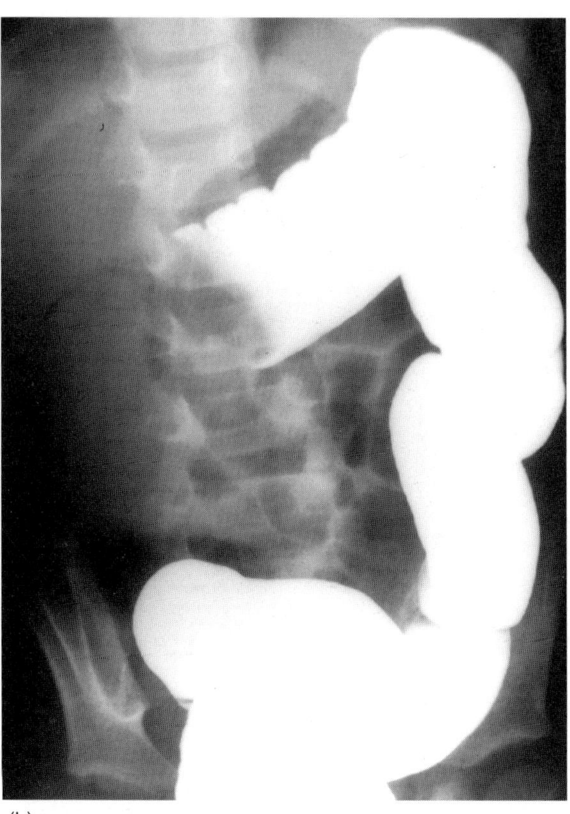

(a) (b)

Fig. 2.15 Ileocolic intussusception seen on (a) supine abdomen and (b) barium enema. A soft-tissue mass can be clearly identified within the transverse colon on the plain abdominal radiograph with a crescent of gas outlining the head of the intussusception in a child aged 2 years. These findings are confirmed on the barium study.

intussusception is the ileum invaginating into the colon. Inflammation of the lymphoid tissues in the ileum causes enlarged lymphatic patches to project into the lumen of the bowel and peristaltic movement then pushes one part of the lumen into another (Fig. 2.15). In adults intussusception is almost invariably associated with a tumour arising either in the small bowel or colon.

Intussusception is usually recognized clinically by pain, vomiting, blood in the stool and a palpable abdominal mass although the diagnosis is sometimes difficult to make.

Plain film radiographs in infants often show evidence of small bowel obstruction. The intussusception itself may be identified as a soft-tissue mass, frequently situated in the right hypochondrium. This mass may sometimes be surrounded by a crescent of gas giving rise to the 'crescent' sign whereas the 'target' sign consists of two concentric circles of fat density. Although visualization of a mass is the most common sign of intussusception, the crescent and target signs are more specific. The target sign is seen almost twice as frequently as the crescent sign. Depending on local practice, ultrasound or a barium or gas enema are frequently performed to confirm the diagnosis of intussusception. The gas or barium enema may be used in an attempt to reduce the intussusception.

Intussusception in adults develops either as a result of surgery, e.g. following gastroenterostomy, or more commonly secondary to a tumour in the bowel. Plain film diagnosis depends on identifying the soft-tissue mass which may be either spherical or oval, the cresent-shaped gas shadow at the apex of the mass or gas within the intussuscepting bowel resembling a 'coiled spring'.

SMALL BOWEL PSEUDO-OBSTRUCTION

Although pseudo-obstruction most commonly affects both the large and small bowel, it may occur in small bowel alone and simulate small bowel obstruction (Fig. 2.16).

MESENTERIC THROMBOSIS – SMALL BOWEL INFARCTION

Infarction of the small bowel is a most serious abdominal condition caused by thrombosis or embolism of the superior mesenteric artery. The clinical

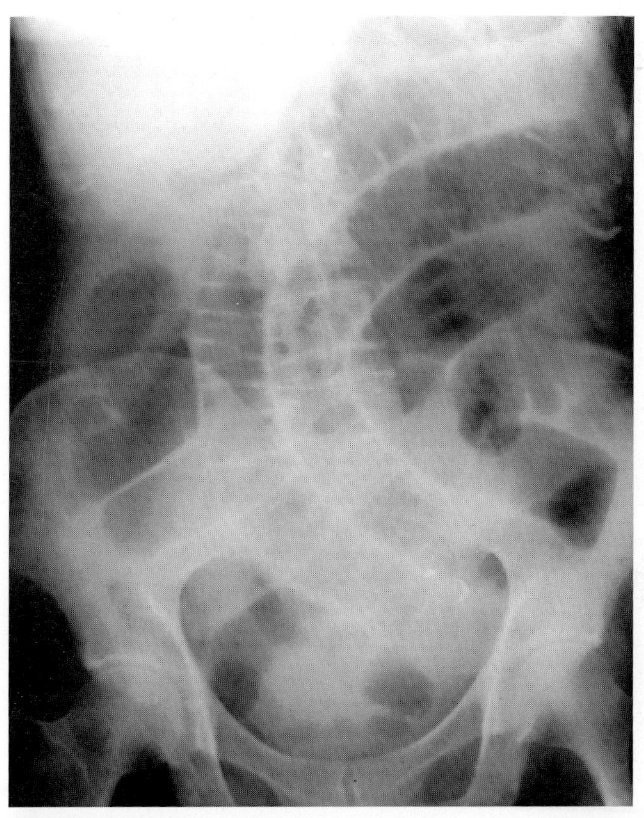

Fig. 2.16 Small bowel pseudo-obstruction seen on supine abdomen. Numerous loops of small bowel and gas-filled, but not unduly dilated, ascending colon can be identified in a patient aged 82. History of abdominal pain and vomiting for 3 weeks accompanied by marked abdominal tenderness. No obstructing lesion was found at laparotomy.

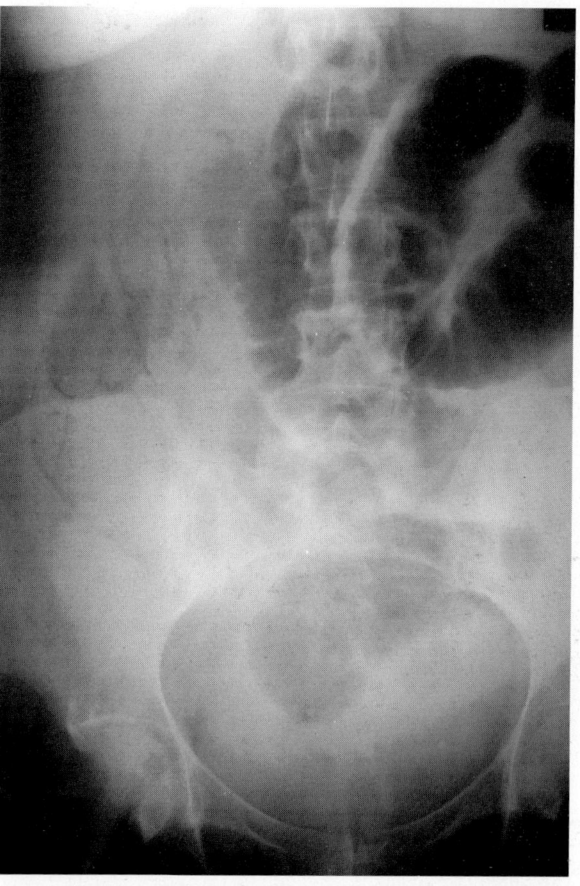

Fig. 2.17 Mesenteric embolus with small bowel infarction seen on supine abdomen. Multiple small bubbles of gas and linear intramural gas lie within infarcted small bowel in the right side of the abdomen. This caused functional obstruction; gas-filled loops of distended proximal small bowel can also be seen. The patient was aged 79 yrs and reported sudden onset of right hypochondrial pain. (Source: S. Field, in Patrick C. Freeney and Giles W. Stevenson (eds), *Margulis and Burhenne's Alimentary tract radiology*, published by Mosby, St Louis, 1994.)

diagnosis is often uncertain until laparotomy but the sudden onset of severe abdominal pain, sometimes associated with bloody diarrhoea, in an elderly person who may have other stigma of atherosclerosis, is very suggestive of small bowel infarction (Fig. 2.17). Gas-filled, slightly dilated loops of small bowel with multiple fluid levels, or fluid-filled loops of small bowel, are the most common plain film findings. However, the walls of the small bowel loops may become thickened and nodular, secondary to submucosal haemorrhage and oedema. Bubbles of gas and linear gas streaks may be identified within the bowel wall if gangrene develops and free gas may be present if perforation has occurred. Frequently there is also a generalized peritonitis, which may also cause colonic distension. In advanced cases intraluminal gas in the mesenteric or portal veins may be identified, which indicates a very grave prognosis.

MECHANICAL LARGE BOWEL OBSTRUCTION

Although adhesive bands are the commonest cause of small bowel obstruction, only very rarely do they cause obstruction in the colon. Common causes of colonic obstruction include tumour, particularly carcinoma of the sigmoid colon, abscesses secondary to perforated diverticular disease, large bowel volvulus and, more rarely, extrinsic compression from a pelvic tumour (Fig. 2.18). In the developed world over 80% of mechanical large bowel obstruction is caused by a carcinoma and most of these are situated in the sigmoid colon. Diverticulitis, commonly associated with a small pericolic abscess, is the next most common cause. In the developed world volvulus accounts for only around 10% of cases of colonic

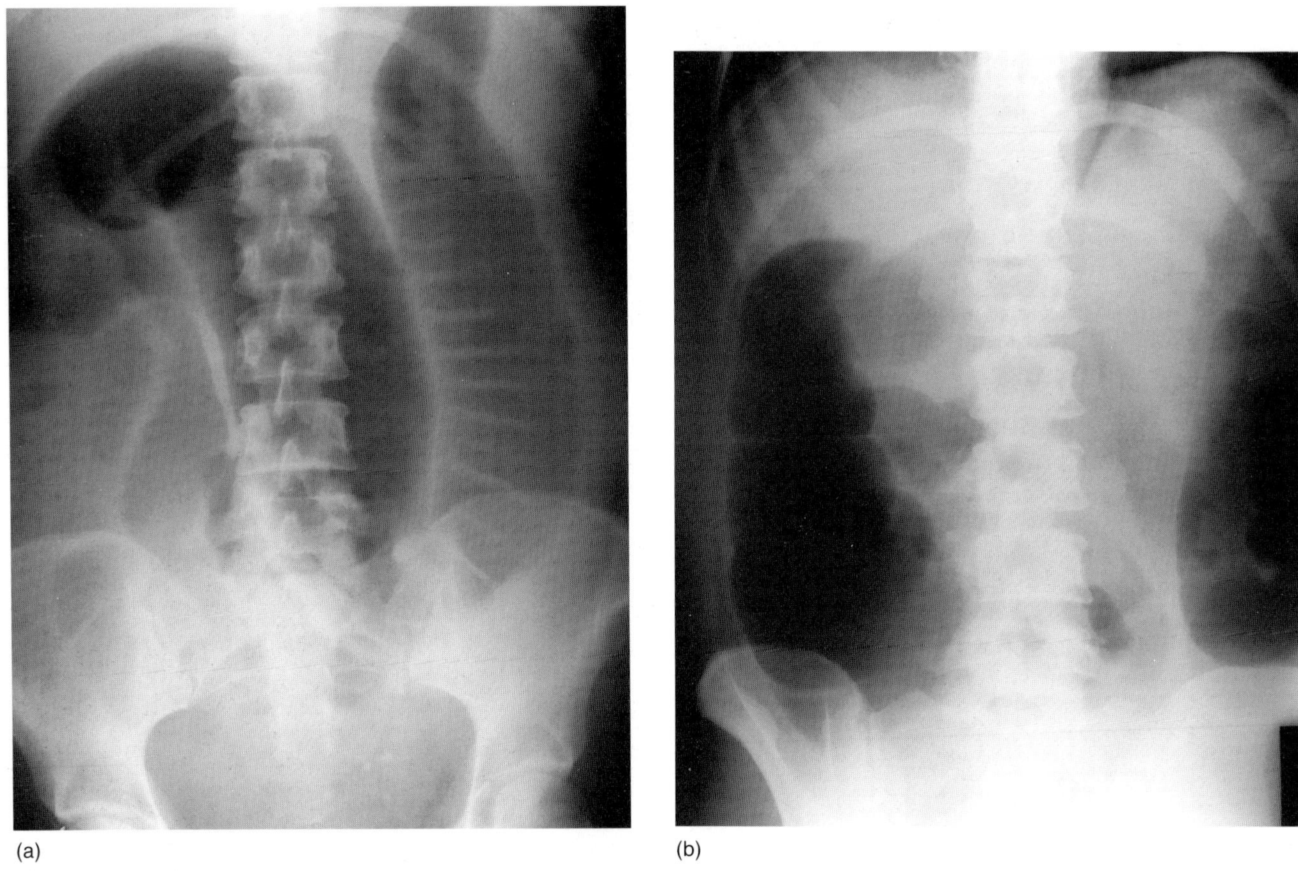

Fig. 2.18 Large bowel obstruction seen on (a) supine abdomen and (b) prone abdomen. In the supine position gas rises to the most superior part of the bowel which is the transverse colon, fluid fills the ascending and descending colon. In the prone radiograph fluid fills the transverse colon. This cannot be visualized but gas has filled the ascending and descending colon. It is important to recognize how different positions affect the distribution of gas.

obstruction, but in Iran and Africa volvulus may comprise more than 80% of cases of large bowel obstruction.

Obstruction to the left side of the colon is more common than to the right. The plain film findings depend on the site of obstruction and whether or not the ileocaecal valve is competent. If the ileocaecal valve remains competent, marked distension of the caecum will occur. The competent ileocaecal valve may also result in small bowel distension. Consequently in large bowel obstruction both small and large bowel dilation may be seen. However, if the ileocaecal valve is incompetent, the caecum and ascending colon do not become distended but there is marked small bowel distension. When the ileocaecal valve is competent massive caecal distension may occur and the caecum is then 'at risk' of perforation secondary to ischaemia (Fig. 2.19). It has been suggested that a caecal diameter of >10cm renders the caecum increasingly liable to perforation.

The obstructed colon almost invariably contains large amounts of gas and can usually be identified by the presence of haustra and by its position in the periphery of the abdomen. When both small and large bowel dilation are present the radiographic appearances may be indistinguishable from paralytic ileus. The variation in colonic diameter in normal individuals is very considerable and some people with large bowel obstruction may have colonic diameters that are less than those observed in some normal individuals.

There are numerous causes of colonic distension without obstruction and all causes of paralytic ileus may also lead to massive colonic distension. In many centres a single contrast barium enema is performed as an emergency investigation to differentiate between mechanical obstruction and pseudo-obstruction or colonic ileus. A barium study increases both the sensitivity and specificity of the plain film findings in large bowel obstruction. Although obstructed large bowel usually contains varying amounts of gas, a fluid-filled caecum can simulate small bowel obstruction (Fig. 2.20) and a completely fluid-filled large bowel can simulate ascites (Fig. 2.21).

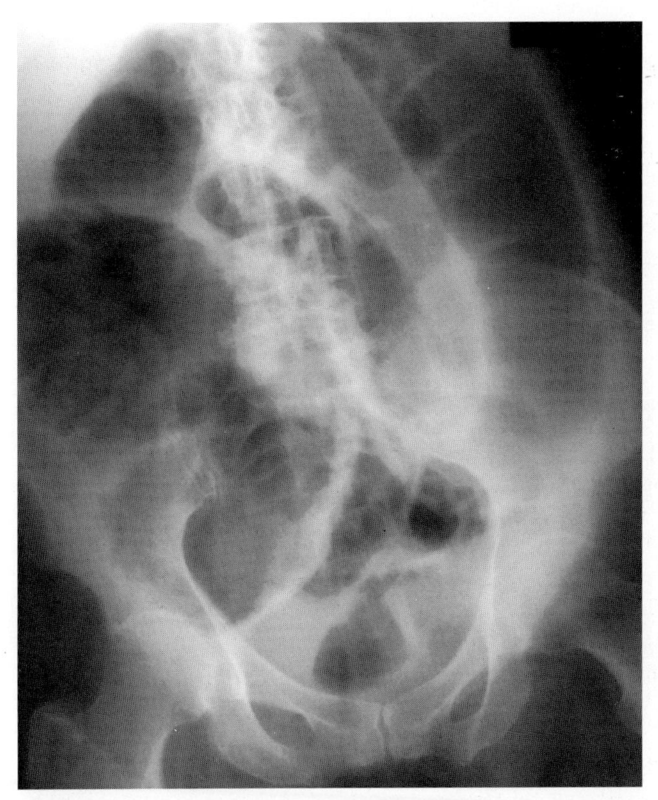

Fig. 2.19 Large bowel obstruction causing impending perforation of the caecum. The ileocaecal valve is competent and the caecum and small bowel are distended. There is gaseous distension of both small and large bowel. The transverse caecal diameter measures 11 cm and the wall of the caecum is oedematous and thickened auguring impending perforation. An ischaemic caecum was confirmed at surgery for carcinoma of the sigmoid colon. (Source: S. Field, in *Clinics in Gastroenterology* 1984; **13**: 1.)

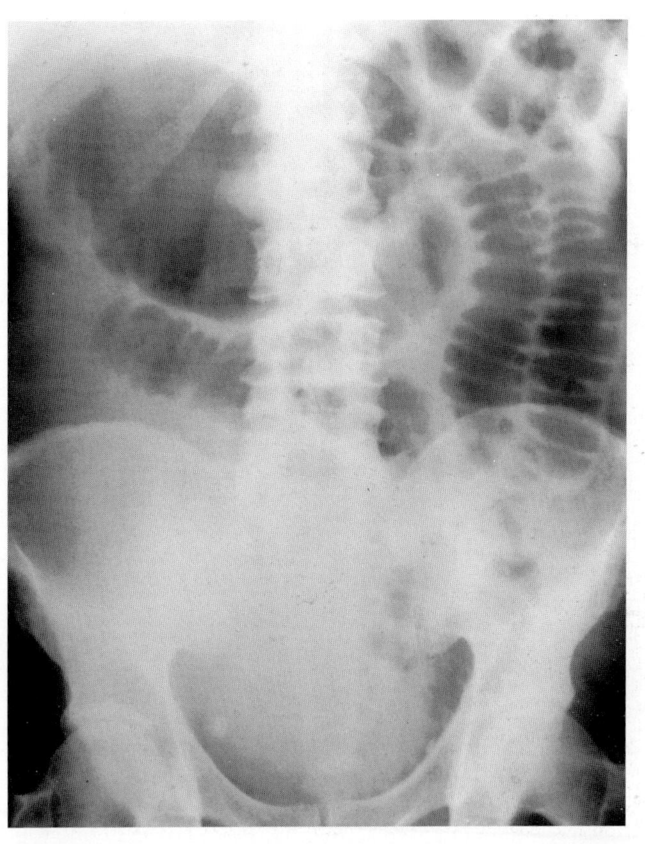

Fig. 2.20 Large bowel obstruction with a large fluid-filled caecum. A carcinoma of transverse colon was found at laparotomy. The hepatic flexure is gas-filled but the caecum, although markedly distended, is filled with fluid. There is obvious gas-filled small bowel distension. This radiograph could be misinterpreted as small bowel obstruction.

LARGE BOWEL VOLVULUS

Volvulus of the large bowel is relatively common in developing countries but is less frequent in the developed world where it comprises about 10% of all cases of large bowel obstruction. Volvulus of the colon can only occur where there is a long freely mobile mesentery. The sigmoid colon and caecum are, therefore, the most commonly affected sites and torsion of other parts such as the flexures or transverse colon is rare. A compound volvulus involving the intertwining of two loops of bowel such as an ileosigmoid knot is very rare in developed countries but is not uncommon in Africa, Iran and parts of Russia.

CAECAL VOLVULUS

Caecal or right colonic volvulus can only occur when there is a degree of malrotation and the caecum and ascending colon are on a mesentery. Compared with sigmoid volvulus it occurs in a relatively young age group, 30–60 years being most common. In around half the cases, the caecum twists and inverts so that the pole of the caecum and the appendix occupy the left upper quadrant (Fig. 2.22). In the other half of cases, the twist occurs in an axial manner without inversion and the caecum still occupies the right half of the abdomen, usually the right lower quadrant. Even though there is considerable distension of the rotated caecum in a caecal volvulus, one or two haustral markings can usually be identified. The distended caecum can usually be identified as a very large gas- and fluid-filled viscus that may be situated almost anywhere in the abdomen. Identification of the attached gas-filled appendix confirms the diagnosis. Marked gaseous or fluid distension of small bowel is often present and may sometimes obstruct the caecum itself. The left side of the colon is usually collapsed.

SIGMOID VOLVULUS

Sigmoid volvulus is the classic large-bowel volvulus normally occurring in old age. The usual mechanism is twisting of the sigmoid loop around the mesenteric

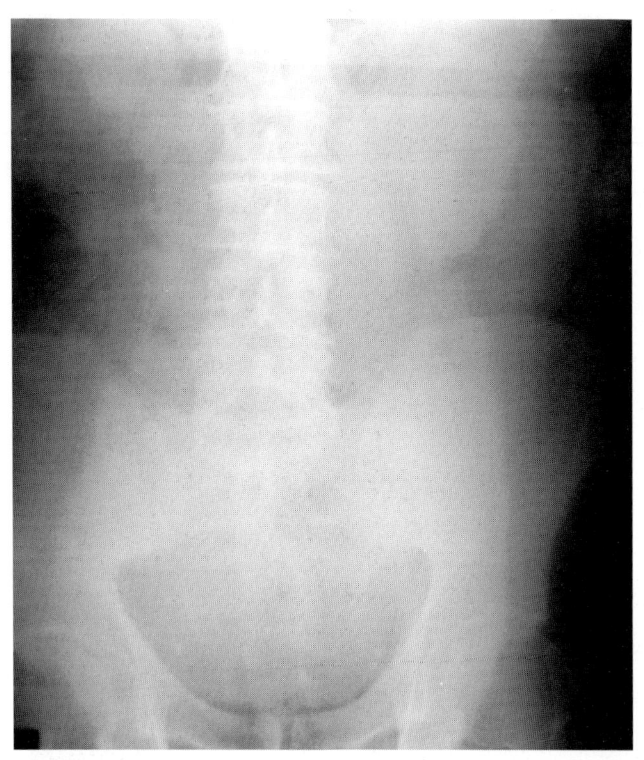

Fig. 2.21 Fluid-filled large bowel obstruction seen on supine abdomen. The walls of the distended fluid-filled descending colon are outlined by fat in this patient with carcinoma of the sigmoid. (From Field S in: Patrick C Freeney and Giles W Stevenson (eds.) *Margulis and Burhenne's Alimentary tract radiology* published by Mosby, St. Louis, 1994.)

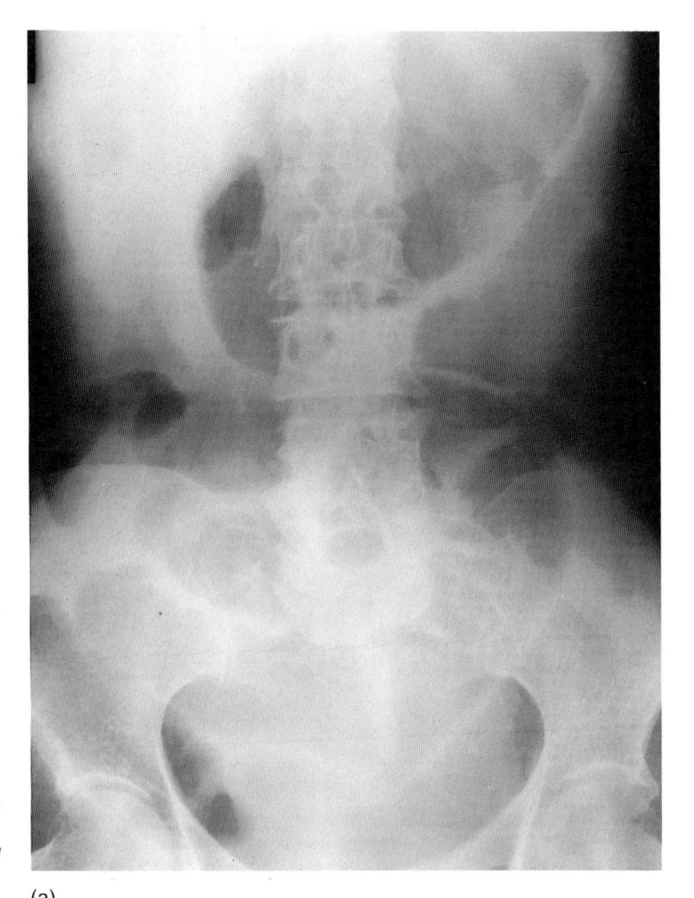

(a)

(b)

Fig. 2.22 Caecal volvulus seen on (a) supine abdomen and (b) erect abdomen. A dilated gas-filled caecum can be identified in the left upper quadrant; there is also evidence of small bowel obstruction. (From S Field in: *Clinics in Gastroenterology* 1984; 13: 1.)

axis; only rarely does one limb twist in axial torsion. Sigmoid volvulus is usually chronic with intermittent acute attacks although a true acute torsion may occur. Although plain film diagnosis may be easy, up to one third of cases are difficult to diagnose radiologically and further investigations may be needed. Signs of a sigmoid volvulus include:

- ahaustral margin
- left flank overlap sign
- liver overlap sign
- apex under left hemidiaphragm
- apex above 10th thoracic vertebra
- inferior convergence on left
- pelvis overlap sign.

When a sigmoid volvulus occurs the inverted 'U' shaped loop is usually massively distended and commonly devoid of haustra – an important diagnostic feature (Fig. 2.23). The margin of this ahaustral loop can often be identified overlapping:

- the haustrated dilated descending colon – **the left flank overlap sign**
- the lower border of the liver shadow – **the liver overlap sign**
- the left iliac bone – **the pelvis overlap sign**.

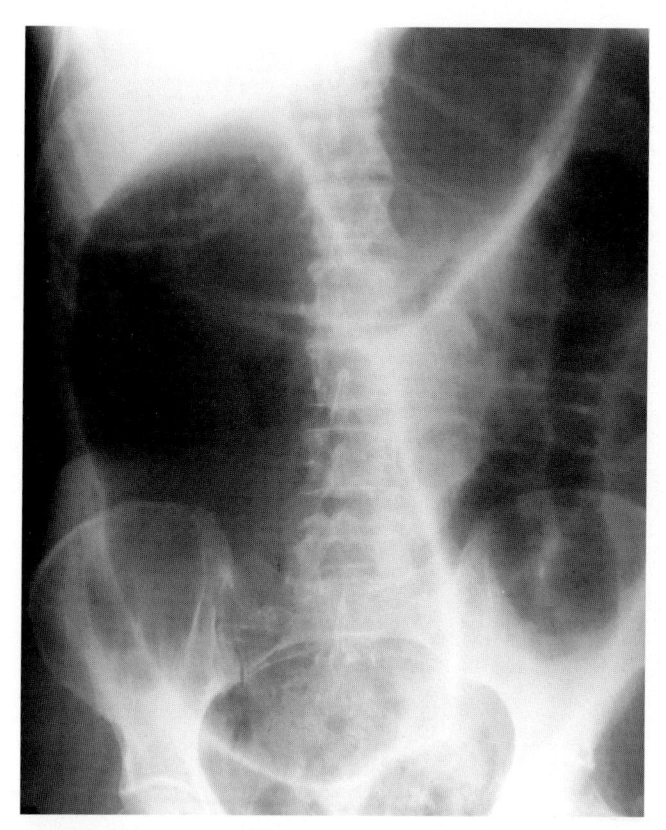

Fig. 2.23 Sigmoid volvulus seen on supine abdomen. A huge mainly ahaustral loop of sigmoid can be identified rising out of the pelvis. The ahaustral margin can be seen overlapping the liver (liver overlap sign) and overlapping the haustrated descending colon (left flank overlap sign).

The superior aspect of the sigmoid volvulus usually lies very high in the abdomen, above the level of D10 with its apex lying on the left side beneath the left hemidiaphragm. Sometimes the gas in the sigmoid loop may simulate free intraperitoneal gas.

Inferiorly, where the two limbs of the volved loop converge, three white lines meet representing the two outer walls and the contiguous inner walls of the twisted loop. This point is called the inferior convergence – it is usually on the left side of the pelvis at the level of the upper sacral segments. It is usual for a large amount of air to be present in the volvulus. A recent evaluation of the radiological signs suggested that apex of the loop under the left hemidiaphragm, inferior convergence on the left and the left flank overlap signs were highly specific as well as being very sensitive.

The initial management of a sigmoid volvulus frequently involves the insertion of a rectal tube (Fig. 2.24). If this fails and there is still doubt about the diagnosis on plain radiographs, a barium enema should be performed. Features seen at the point of torsion include smooth curved tapering like a hooked beak (the *'bird of prey sign'*) and the mucosal folds often showing a 'screw' pattern at the point of torsion (Fig. 2.25).

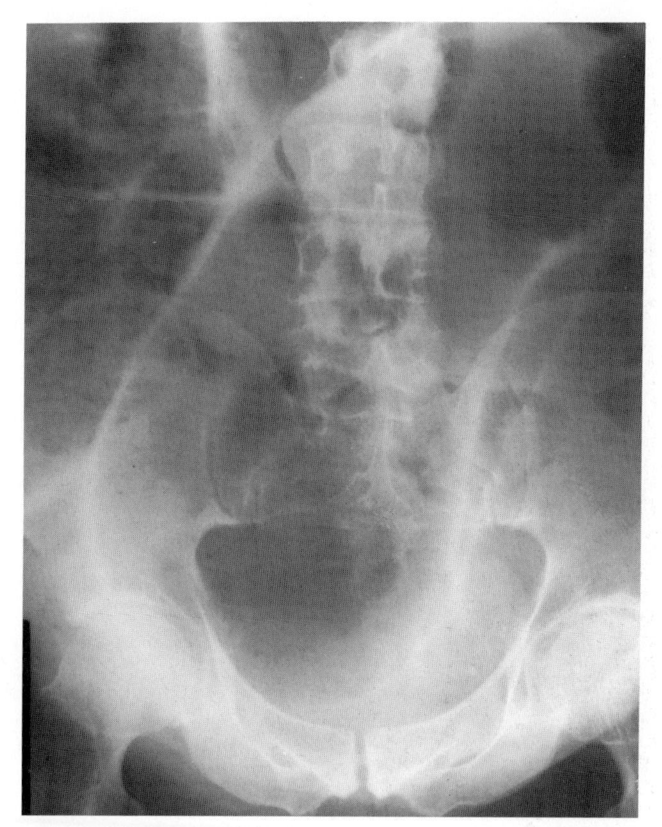

(a)

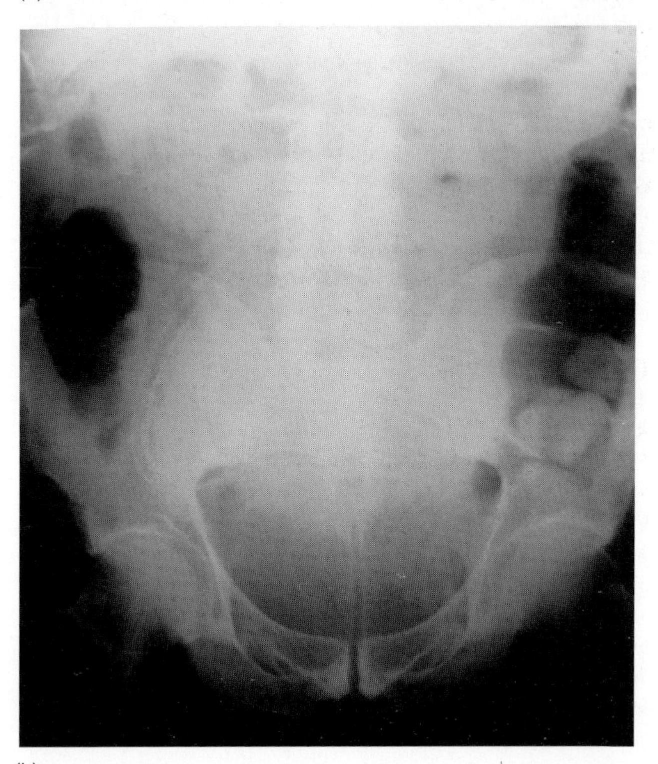

(b)

Fig. 2.24 Sigmoid volvulus seen on (a) supine abdomen and (b) following passage of a flatus tube. The massively distended ahaustral sigmoid loop can clearly be identified on the plain film. Following the passage of a rectal tube there has been dramatic deflation of the volvulus with gas remaining in a relatively undistended descending colon.

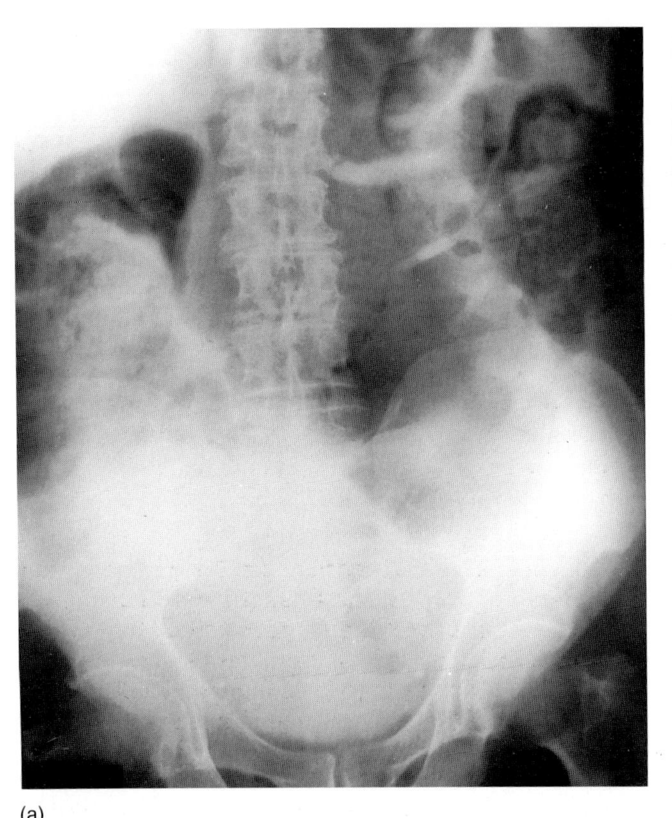

(a)

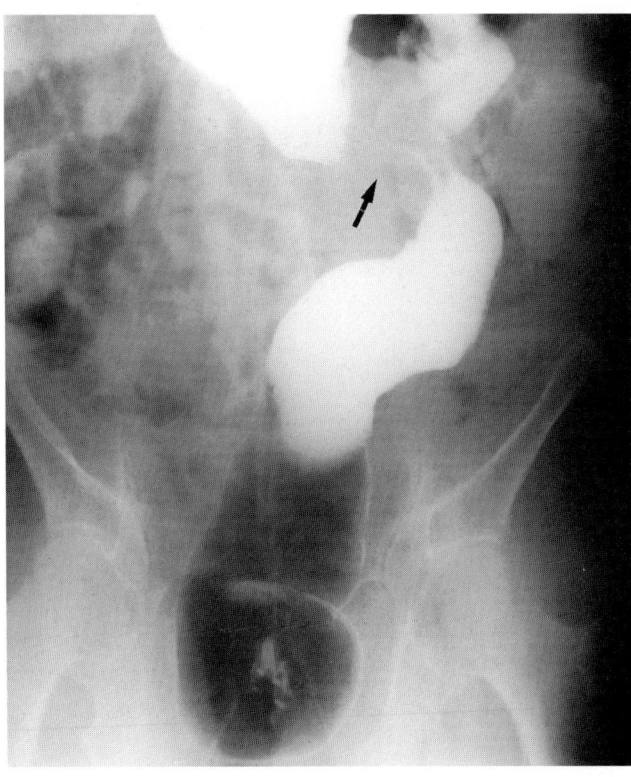

(b)

Fig. 2.25 Sigmoid volvulus seen on (a) supine abdomen and (b) emergency barium enema. There is marked distension of large bowel which contains faeces and air. The diagnosis cannot be made from the plain films alone. The barium enema demonstrates tapering of the sigmoid at the point of twist where the 'cork-screw' appearance of the mucosal folds is also seen (arrow). (Source: S. Field in Patrick C. Freeney and Giles W. Stevenson (eds), *Margulis and Burhenne's Alimentary tract radiology*, published by Mosby, St Louis, 1994.)

VOLVULUS OF TRANSVERSE COLON AND COLONIC FLEXURES

These types of volvulae are rare but careful evaluation of the plain film findings can often suggest the diagnosis.

COMPOUND VOLVULUS – ILEOSIGMOID KNOT

A compound volvulus – specifically an ileosigmoid knot – is well recognized in developing countries but is rare elsewhere. An abnormally mobile loop of small bowel passes around the base of the pelvic colon below the attachment of the pelvic mesocolon and forms a knot. The clinical onset is abrupt with a fulminating course and intense pain in the abdomen and back. The key radiological features are a dilated loop of pelvic colon and evidence of small bowel obstruction with retained faeces in an undistended proximal colon.

ISCHAEMIC COLITIS

Ischaemic colitis is characterized clinically by the sudden onset of abdominal pain followed by bloody diarrhoea. The splenic flexure and proximal descending colon are most frequently involved although other areas may be affected (Fig. 2.26). The wall and mucosa of the colon are thickened due to haemorrhage and oedema; this can sometimes be detected on plain radiographs but in most cases a barium enema is necessary. The term **thumb printing**, showing cresentic margins, has been used to describe the appearance of the submucosal haemorrhage. The part of colon, normally on the left side, involved by the ischaemia acts as an area of functional obstruction, so that the right side of the colon is frequently distended although the bowel wall and mucosa usually appear normal.

PARALYTIC ILEUS

Paralytic ileus occurs when intestinal peristalsis ceases and there is an accumulation of fluid and gas in the bowel. It is very common, occurring most frequently in the postoperative period and in peritonitis (Fig. 2.27). However, numerous conditions, many of which are not intra-abdominal, can cause bowel paralysis:

- peritonitis
- postoperative

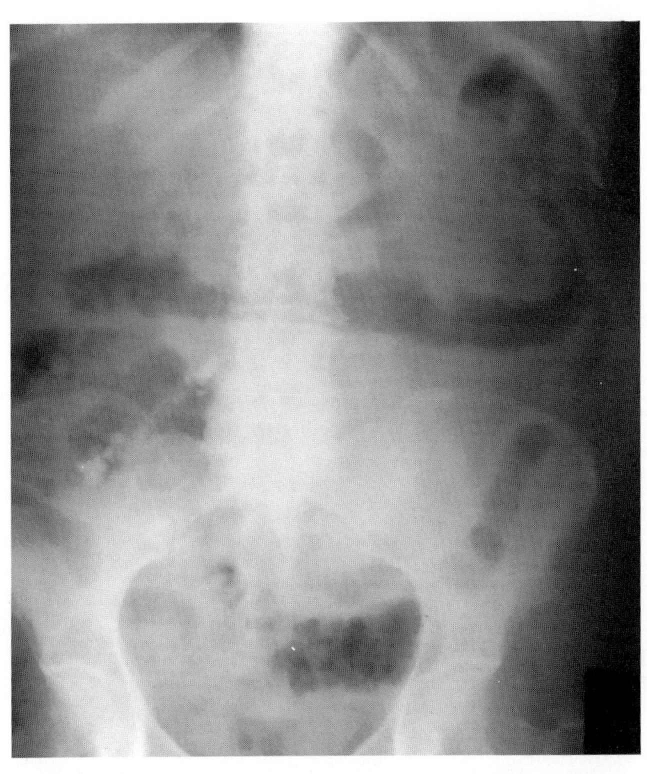

Fig. 2.26 Ischaemic colitis seen on supine abdomen. There is extensive mucosal abnormality with irregular outline and wall thickening ('thumb printing') involving the entire transverse colon and proximal descending colon. (Source: S. Field in Patrick C. Freeney and Giles W. Stevenson (eds), *Margulis and Burhenne's Alimentary tract radiology*, published by Mosby, St Louis, 1994.)

- trauma
- inflammation
  - appendicitis
  - pancreatitis
  - cholecystitis
  - salpingitis
- congestive heart failure
- pneumonia
- renal colic
- renal failure
- leaking abdominal aortic aneurysm
- low serum potassium
- drugs, e.g. morphine
- spinal lesions
- infection
- vascular occlusion.

The degree of distension of bowel may vary considerably from a short length of dilated small bowel to distension of the entire intestinal tract. When there is distension of both small and large bowel the appearances cannot usually be distinguished on plain radiographs from low large bowel obstruction. When there is local inflammation such as pancreatitis, cholecystitis or appendicitis, the ileus may affect only one or two adjacent loops of small bowel – **sentinel loops** – but the appearances are non-specific and in some cases may have features indistinguishable from small bowel obstruction.

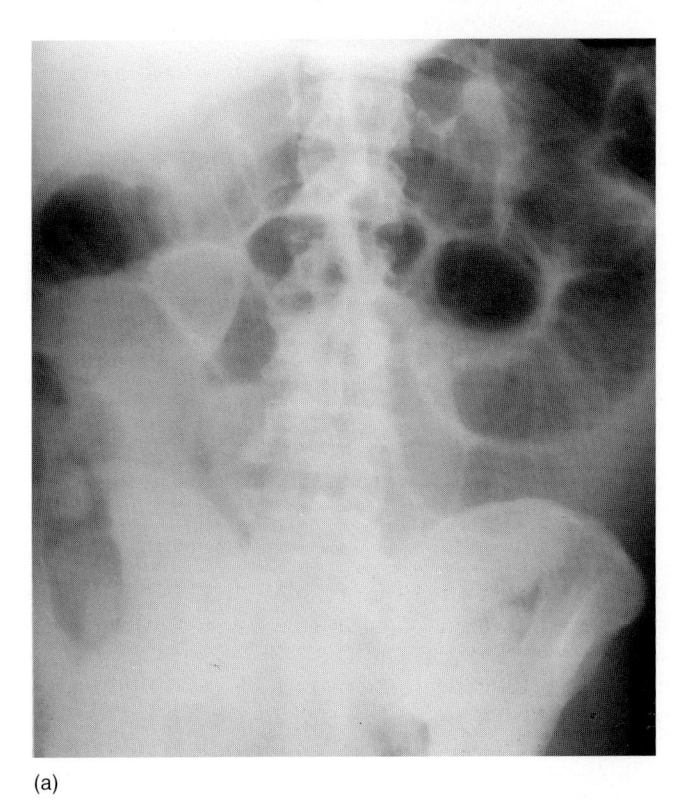

(a)

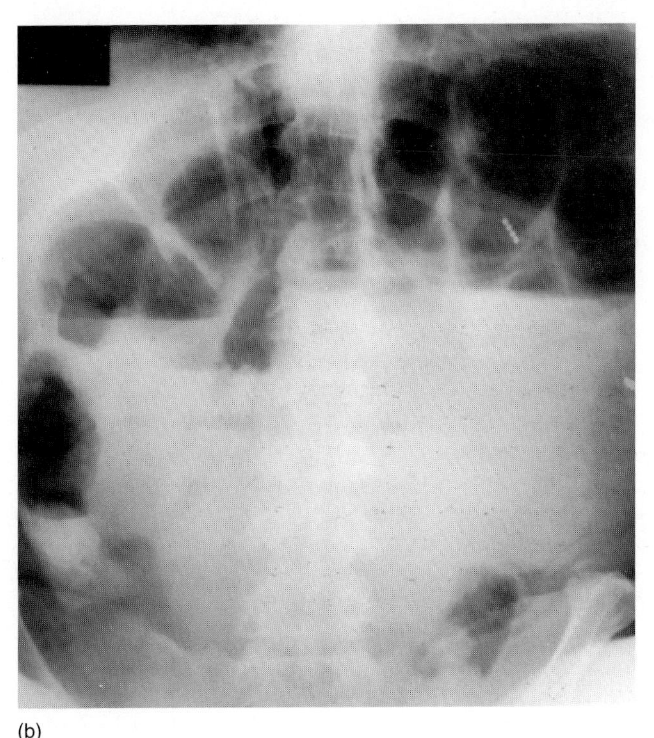

(b)

Fig. 2.27 Paralytic ileus seen on (a) supine abdomen and (b) erect abdomen. Multiple loops of distended small and large bowel are present in this patient aged 57, who had profuse vomiting three days after open cholecystectomy.

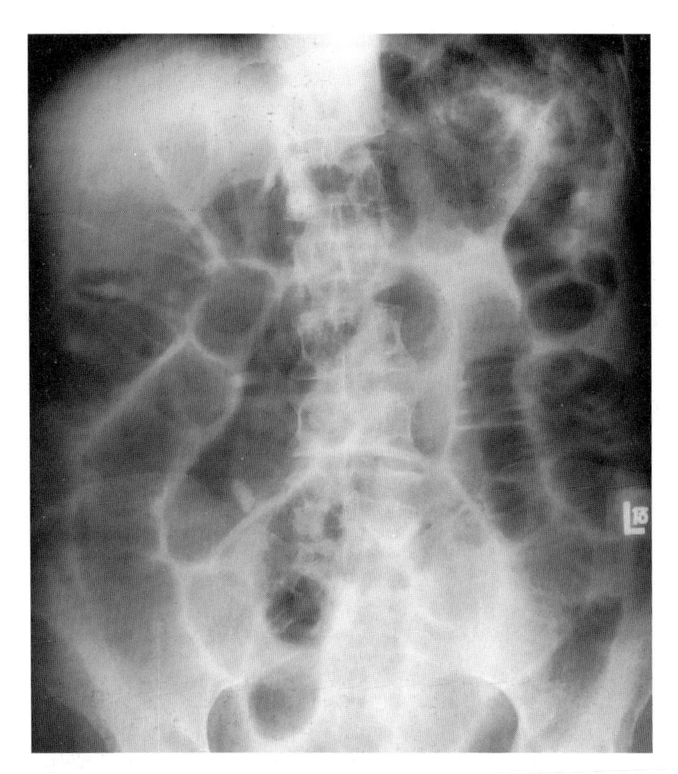

Fig. 2.28 Pseudo-obstruction seen on supine abdomen. This 58-year-old patient developed abdominal distension and obstructive bowel sounds seven days after a pin and plate operation for a fracture through the femoral neck. The distension settled following the insertion of a rectal tube and conservative treatment.

LARGE BOWEL PSEUDO-OBSTRUCTION

Pseudo-obstruction is a condition which clinically and radiologically mimics true intestinal obstruction. It is more commonly seen in elderly patients. It may be acute and self-limiting, for example when associated with pneumonia or myocardial infarction, or may be chronic in patients with myxoedema or abnormalities of the musculature of the bowel. Plain radiographic appearances can be dramatic showing very dilated colon and sometimes distended small bowel as well (Fig. 2.28). A contrast enema is usually required to exclude mechanical obstruction so preventing an unnecessary laparotomy. Sometimes, however, the caecum may exceed the critical diameter of 10 cm when perforation is imminent and a caecostomy or right-sided colostomy may be required to prevent perforation.

PNEUMOPERITONEUM

The presence of free intra-abdominal gas almost always indicates that perforation of a viscus has occurred (Fig. 2.29). The commonest cause is the **perforation of a peptic ulcer.** Other less common causes are perforation of a diverticulum and malignant tumour (Fig. 2.30).

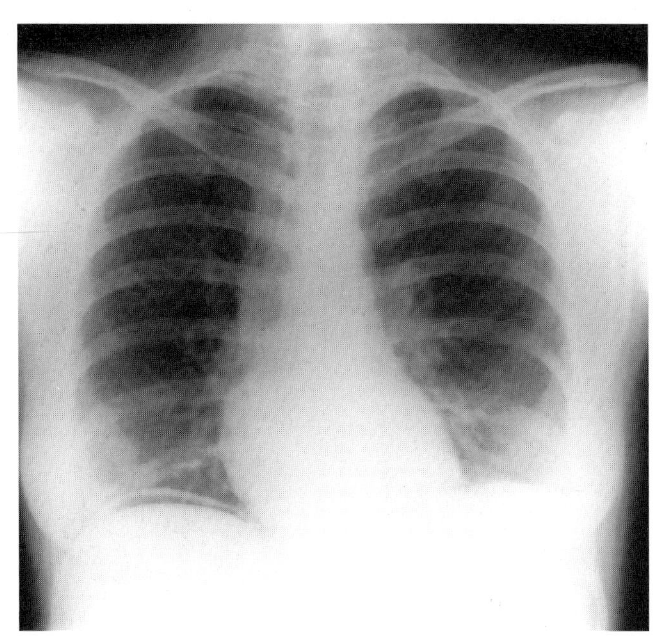

Fig. 2.29 Pneumoperitoneum seen on erect chest. A small amount of free intra-abdominal gas is clearly visible under the right hemidiaphragm.

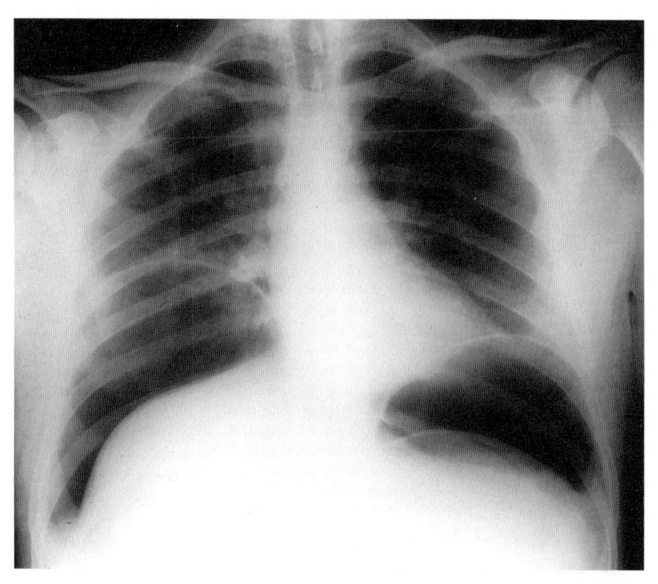

Fig. 2.30 Large pneumperitoneum seen on erect chest. On the right side the raised hemidiaphragm with free gas beneath it simulates a thickened lesser fissure. A large pneumoperitoneum can sometimes be more difficult to diagnose than a small one.

Around 70–80% of perforated ulcers will demonstrate free intra-abdominal gas but free gas is almost never seen in perforated appendicitis. By experimenting on himself, Rosco Miller demonstrated that as little as 1 ml of free gas can be detected on an erect chest or left lateral decubitus abdominal film. Studies on patients with free intra-abdominal gas following surgery have demonstrated that a patient should remain in position for 5–10 minutes prior to the horizontal ray radiograph

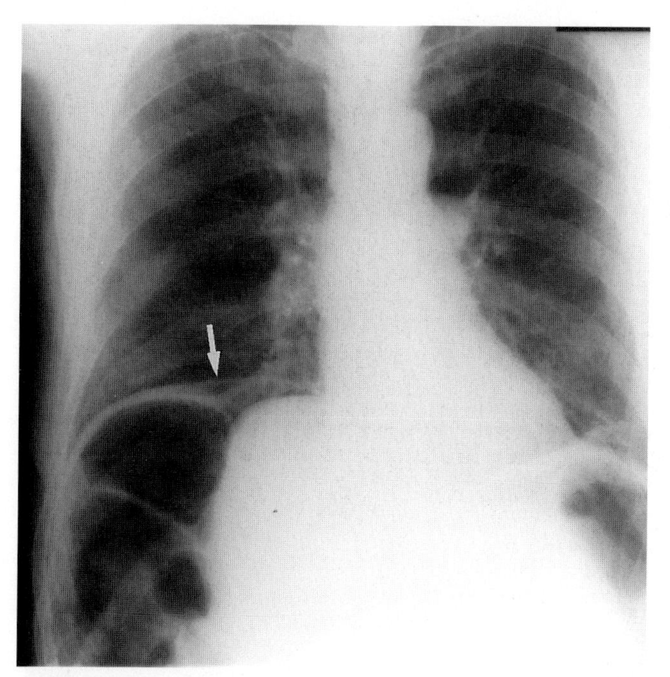

Fig. 2.31 Pneumoperitoneum and Chilaiditi's syndrome. A small triangle of gas (arrow) can be identified beneath the right hemidiaphragm adjacent to the hepatic flexure of the colon.

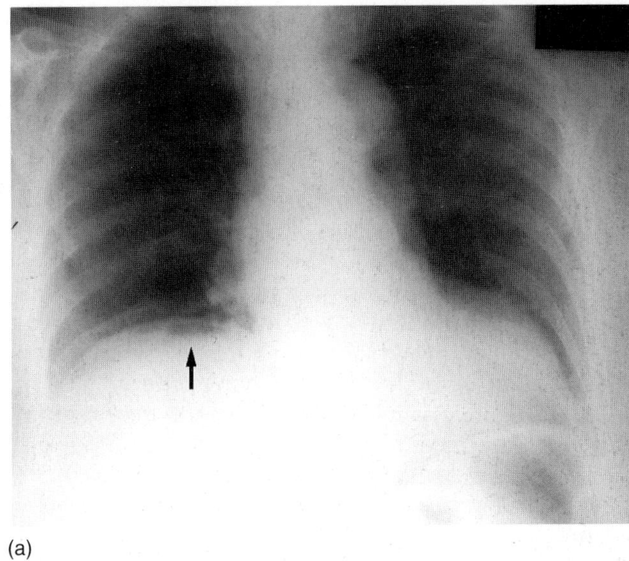

(a)

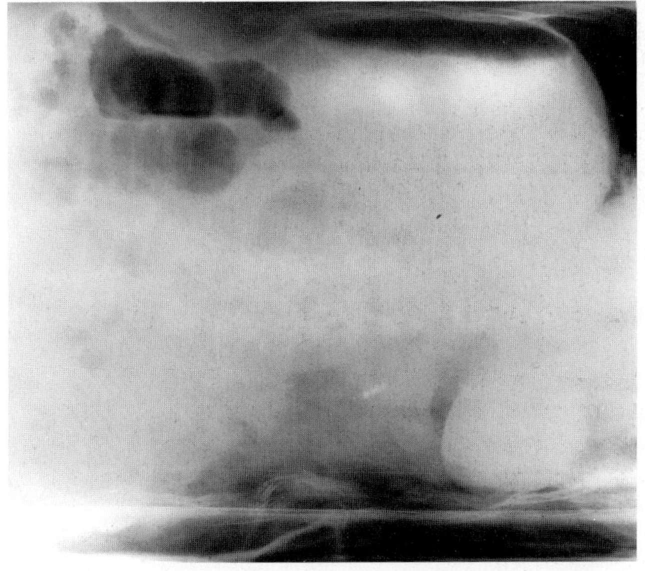

(b)

Fig. 2.32 Pneumoperitoneum seen on (a) erect chest and (b) left lateral decubitus abdomen. A small amount of gas (difficult to ascertain whether it is intraluminal or free) lies beneath the right hemidiaphragm on the erect chest radiograph (arrow). The left lateral decubitus radiograph taken after the patient had been lying on their left side for ten minutes clearly demonstrates the pneumoperitoneum. (Source: S. Field, in D. J. Nolan *A Radiological atlas of gastrointestinal disease*; published by John Wiley, Chichester, 1983.)

being taken, to ensure that any free gas present has time to rise and accumulate in the highest point (Fig. 2.31).

If a perforated viscus is suspected, then a horizontal ray radiograph – either an erect chest or left lateral decubitus abdomen – is mandatory. On the erect chest radiograph, gas is relatively easy to detect under the right hemidiaphragm, but, on the left side, free gas can be difficult to differentiate from stomach and colonic gas. In the left lateral decubitus position, free gas is readily demonstrated lying between the liver and the lateral abdominal wall (Fig. 2.32).

Horizontal ray radiographs may be difficult to obtain in some patients, particularly those who are unconscious, who have suffered trauma or are critically ill. It is, therefore, important to be able to recognize the signs of a pneumoperitoneum on supine radiographs particularly as perforation of a viscus may be clinically silent and be overshadowed by other serious medical or surgical conditions. A supine abdominal film, often taken using portable equipment, may be the only radiograph that can be obtained in these situations.

In nearly 60% of patients with a pneumoperitoneum, gas may be detectable on the supine radiograph:

- right upper quadrant gas
  - perihepatic
  - subhepatic
  - Morrison's pouch
  - visible fissure for the ligamentum teres
- Rigler's (double wall) sign
- ligament visualization
  - falciform (ligamentum teres)
  - umbilical (inverted 'V' sign)
- triangular air sign
- cupola sign
- football or air-dome sign
- scrotal air (in children).

Almost half the patients with free gas will have an oval or linear collection of gas visible in the right upper quadrant adjacent to the liver lying mainly in the subhepatic space and hepatorenal fossa (Morrison's pouch) (Fig. 2.33). The liver shadow appears darker when it is surrounded by free gas. A less common sign of free gas on a supine radiograph is the visualization of the outer wall of a loop of bowel (Rigler's sign) (Fig. 2.34). However, this sign may be misleading if several loops of bowel lie close together or if fat lies outside the bowel wall. The visualization of the falciform (Fig. 2.35) or umbilical ligaments may be demonstrated by the free gas lying on each side of these ligaments. Air in the fissure for the ligamentum teres may produce a band of air in the right upper quadrant. Free gas between loops of bowel may take on a triangular configuration and large amounts may accumulate under the diaphragm (cupola sign) or anterior abdominal wall simulating an American football.

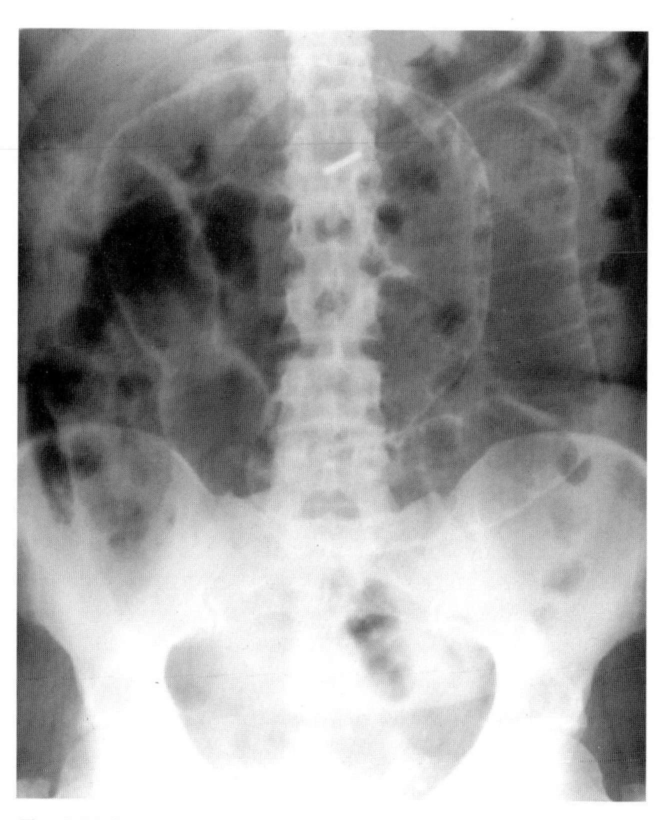

Fig. 2.34 Pneumoperitoneum ('Rigler's sign') seen on supine abdomen. Both sides of the bowel wall can clearly be identified in the distended small bowel loops. There is also free gas in the right upper quadrant. (Source: S. Field in Patrick C. Freeney and Giles W. Stevenson (eds), *Margulis and Burhenne's Alimentary tract radiology*, published by Mosby, St Louis, 1994.)

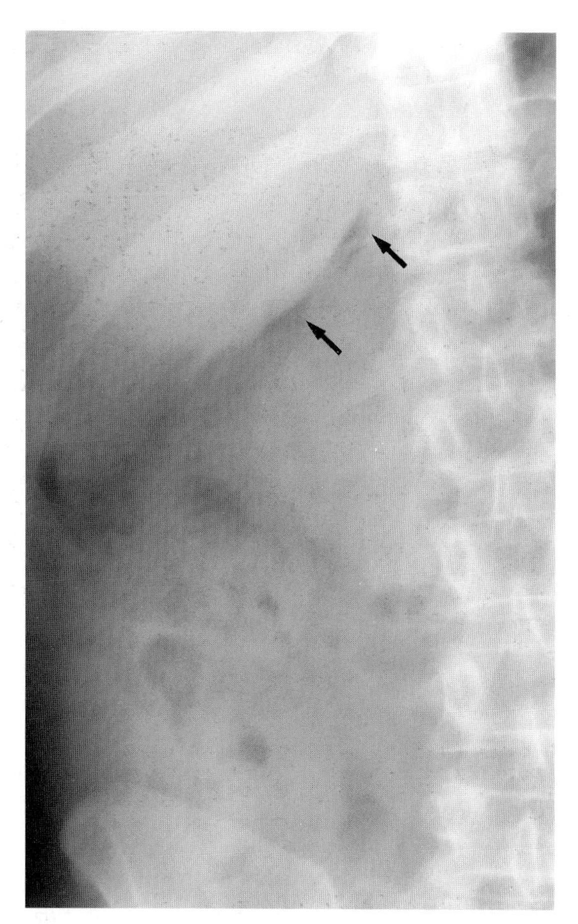

Fig. 2.33 Pneumoperitoneum seen on supine abdomen. Streaks and bands of linear gas can be identified in the right subhepatic region (arrows), in this patient with perforated duodenal ulcer. (Source: S. Field in D. J. Nolan, *A Radiological atlas of gastrointestinal disease*; published by John Wiley, Chichester, 1983.).

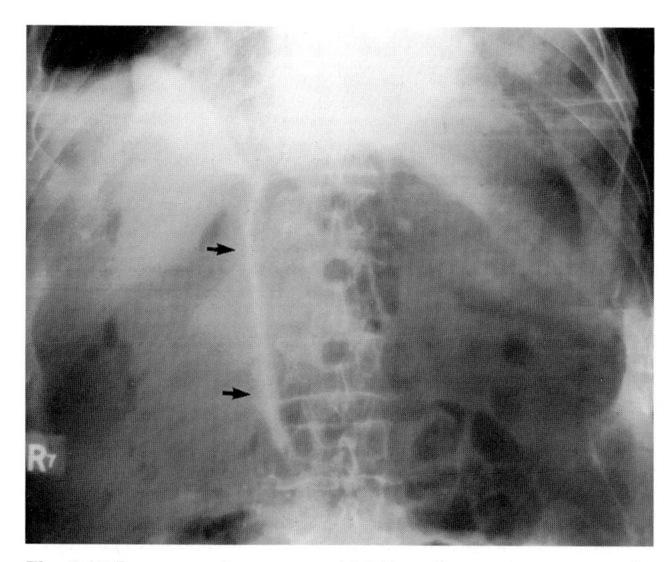

Fig. 2.35 Pneumoperitoneum, and falciform ligament seen on supine abdomen. The falciform ligament is clearly identified by the large amount of free gas which lies of either side of it (arrows). Small extra luminal bubbles of gas lie in multiple intraperitoneal abscesses in this case of perforated gastric ulcer.

PNEUMOPERITONEUM WITHOUT PERITONITIS

Rarely patients who present with vague clinical symptoms have unequivocal evidence of a pneumoperitoneum on chest or abdominal radiographs:

- silent perforation of a viscus which has sealed itself in:
  - the elderly
  - patients on steroids
  - unconscious patients
  - patients being ventilated
  - presence of other serious medical conditions
- postoperative
- peritoneal dialysis
- perforated jejunal diverticulosis
- perforated cyst in pneumatosis intestinalis
- tracking down from a pneumomediastinum
- stercoral ulceration
- leakage through a distended stomach (e.g. endoscopy)
- vaginal – tubal entry of air.

However, clinical examination may demonstrate that there is no evidence of peritonitis or indication for immediate surgery. Most of these patients will have perforated a viscus which has released gas and then sealed itself. Other causes of a pneumoperitoneum under these circumstances include pneumatosis intestinalis, recent abdominal surgery and other iatrogenic causes such as fallopian tube insufflation or peritoneal dialysis. Embolization of an intra-abdominal viscus has also been implicated and some physical activities in women such as water skiing are also well documented causes.

There are a number of rare but important conditions which on first appearances may look remarkably similar to a pneumoperitoneum and these must be considered in every doubtful case:

- intestine between liver and diaphragm (Chilaiditi's syndrome)
- subphrenic abscess
- curvilinear supradiaphragmatic pulmonary collapse
- subdiaphragmatic fat
- diaphragmatic irregularity
- cysts in pneumatosis intestinalis.

An error of interpretation may lead to an unnecessary laparotomy in search of a perforated viscus. The commonest of these is interposition of bowel between the liver and the diaphragm on the right side, **Chilaiditi's syndrome** (Fig. 2.36). Although this occurs in a small number of people with chronic lung disease or with postnecrotic cirrhosis of the liver and ascites, it is most commonly an incidental finding. **Subdiaphragmatic fat** can usually be distinguished from air by the slightly more lateral situation of the curvilinear radiolucent lines. Small amounts of gas giving this appearance are normally found under the highest point of the diaphragm. A thin band of curvilinear **pulmonary atelectasis**, situated just above and parallel to the diaphragm with a band of normally aerated lung

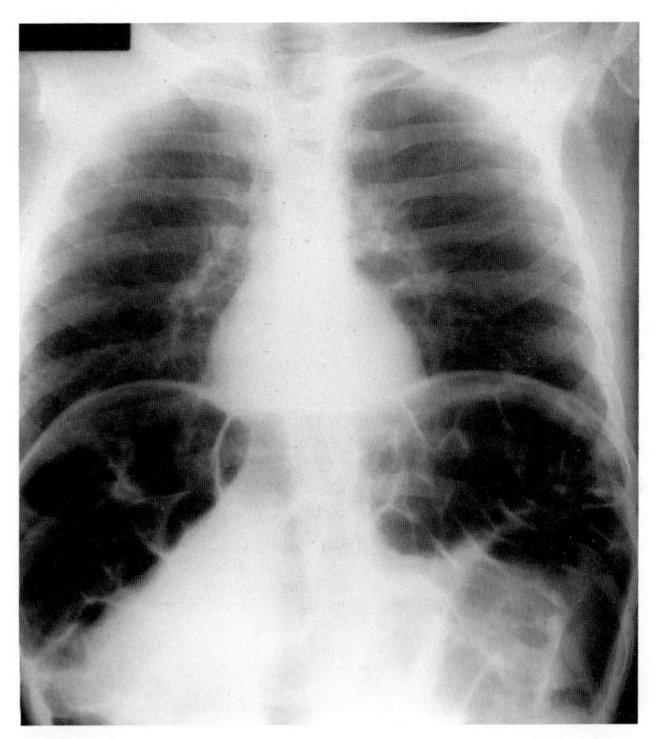

Fig. 2.36 Pseudopneumoperitoneum, (Chilaiditi's syndrome). Gas-filled loops of predominantly large bowel beneath both hemidiaphragms simulate a pneumoperitoneum.

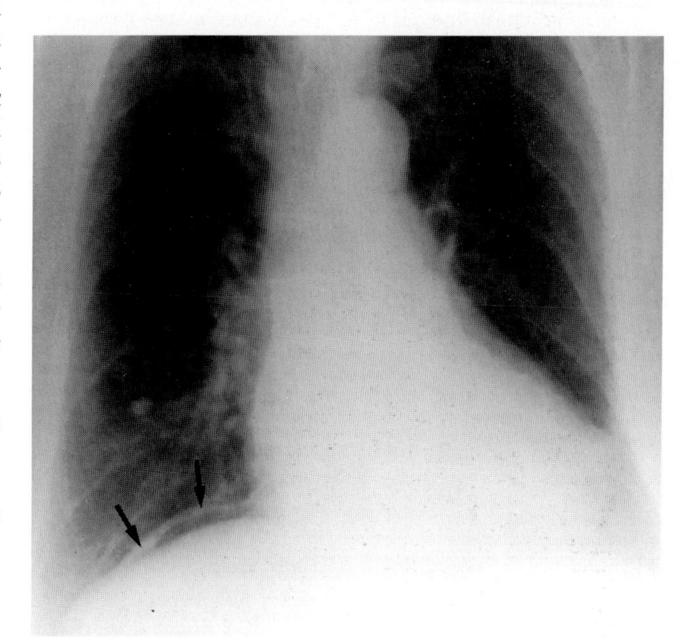

Fig. 2.37 Pseudopneumoperitoneum and curvilinear pulmonary collapse seen on erect chest. A band of curvilinear pulmonary collapse (arrows), with aerated lung beneath it, exactly simulates a small pneumoperitoneum.

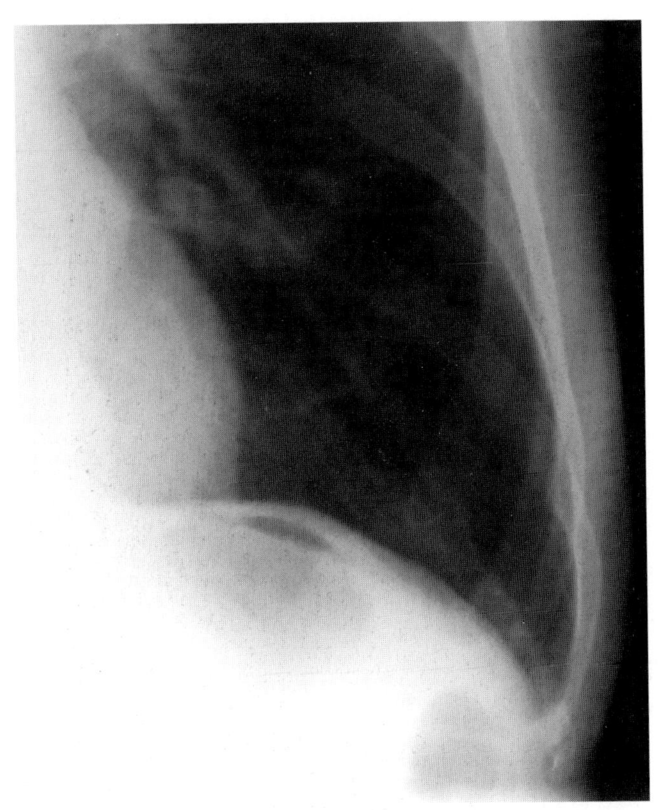

Fig. 2.38 Pseudopneumoperitoneum and double diaphragmatic hump seen on erect chest. The gastric fundal air shadow seen through an uneven diaphragm simulates a pneumoperitoneum. (Source: S. Field, in Patrick C. Freeney and Giles W. Stevenson (eds), *Margulis and Burhenne's Alimentary tract radiology*, published by Mosby, St Louis, 1994.)

between the atelectasis and the diaphragm can simulate a pneumoperitoneum almost exactly (Fig. 2.37). Gas within a **subphrenic abscess** can also simulate a pneumoperitoneum. When the left hemidiaphragm is slightly irregular, the stomach fundal gas shadow may be seen between two humps and the crescent of gas thus formed simulate a pneumoperitoneum (Fig. 2.38). Gas cysts in pneumatosis intestinalis lying between the diaphragm shadow and the intestinal wall may also form a trap for the unwary.

THE POSTOPERATIVE ABDOMEN

The same general principles for diagnosis apply for the postoperative as to the preoperative abdominal radiograph. However, because of recent surgical intervention the radiological signs may be modified and more difficult to interpret. **Postoperative paralytic ileus** is common and may simulate and coexist with obstruction. Sometimes obstruction due to adhesions may occur within a few days of a laparotomy.

Around 60% of all postlaparotomy patients will have evidence of a **pneumoperitoneum** and this will take 1–24 days to be reabsorbed. However, normally, postoperative gas is absorbed within three days. The patient's body habitus is the most important factor influencing the occurrence and duration of postoperative pneumoperitoneum. Gas is absorbed more rapidly in obese patients who normally have no residual gas after the fourth postoperative day. Providing an identical radiographic technique is used and adequate time is spent in the position for the horizontal ray radiograph (usually 10 minutes), any increase in the amount of gas occurring postoperatively indicates either an anastomotic leak or the perforation of a viscus. Very rarely, gas may track into the peritoneal cavity along an abdominal drain.

RETROPERITONEAL PERFORATION

Retroperitoneal perforation of a viscus occurs most commonly secondary to duodenal ulceration or diverticular disease. In the latter condition gas may track down into the leg.

INTRAPERITONEAL FLUID

Usually fluid within the peritoneal cavity collects in the most dependent part, namely the pelvis. As more fluid accumulates it passes up the paracolic gutter on each side and on the right reaches the subhepatic and subphrenic spaces.

The first radiological sign of fluid is a soft tissue density lying within the pelvis or 'dog ears' – soft tissue masses visualized lateral to the rectal gas shadow. More fluid causes the ascending and descending colon to be displaced medially and separate from the flank fat stripe (Fig. 2.39). As fluid enters the subhepatic space it causes loss of visualization of the hepatic angle and, finally, when large amounts of fluid are present, separation of small bowel loops, which move centrally, and thinning of the flank stripes may occur. Large amounts of intra-abdominal fluid causes a generalized haze over the abdomen resulting in poor visualization of normal structures such as the psoas and renal outlines.

INFLAMMATORY CONDITIONS

ACUTE APPENDICITIS

Acute appendicitis is the commonest acute surgical condition in the developed world and has an overall mortality of around 1%. When the clinical history and findings are typical, abdominal radiographs are not indicated. However, in a number of patients, particularly the young and old, clinical features may be obscure and the diagnosis difficult or sometimes impossible without further investigations, including a laparotomy. In complicated appendicitis radiographs may play a significant role in suggesting the diagnosis.

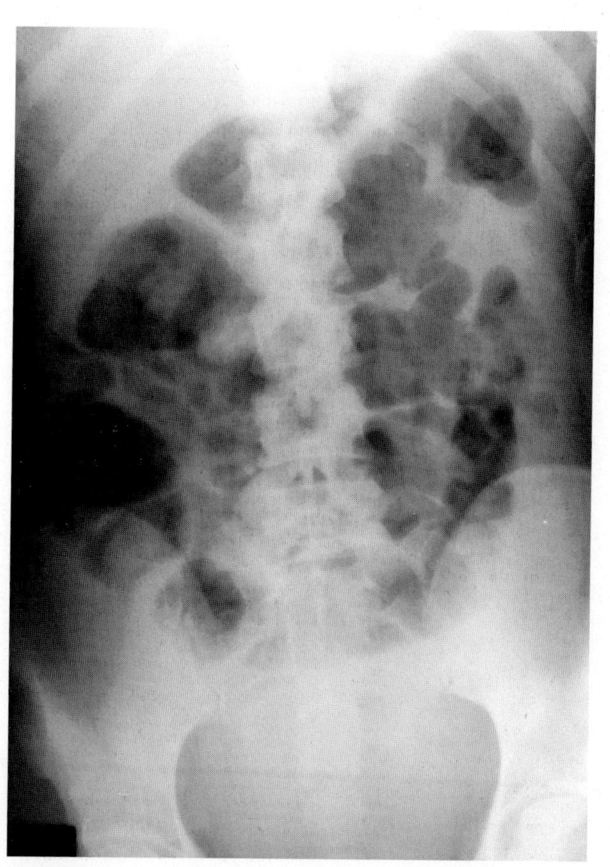

Fig. 2.39 Ascites seen on supine abdomen. Fluid density within the pelvis obliterates the fat line of the superior part of the bladder. Fluid within the flanks displaces the ascending and descending colon medially. The diagnosis was spontaneous intraperitoneal haemorrhage after childbirth. (Source: S. Field in Patrick C. Freeney and Giles W. Stevenson (eds), *Margulis and Burhenne's Alimentary tract Radiology*, published by Mosby, St Louis, 1994.)

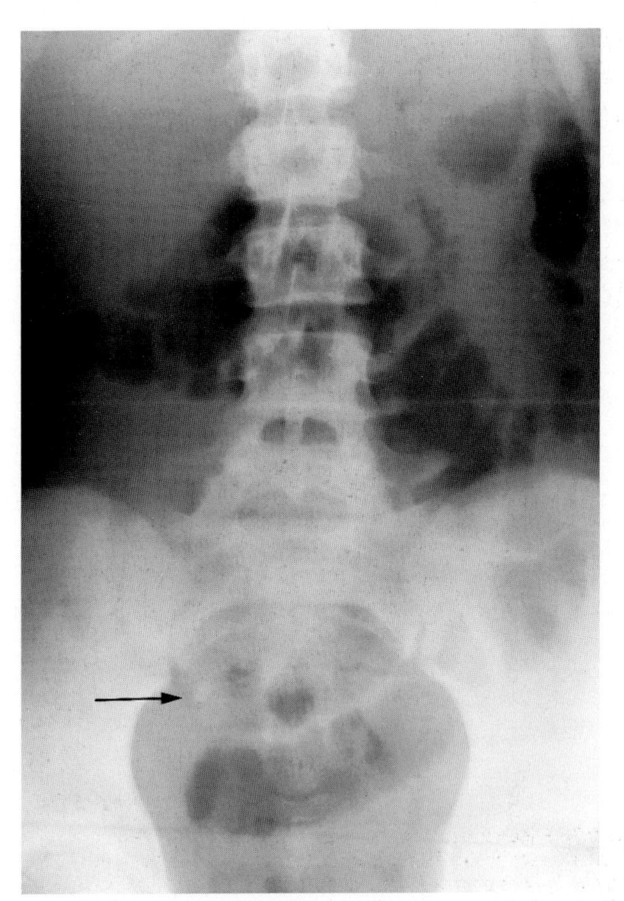

Fig. 2.40 Acute appendicitis seen on supine abdomen. An appendix calculus can be identified in the right side of the pelvis overlying the caecum (arrow). There is also small bowel distension.

There are no specific plain radiographic signs of acute appendicitis but features which frequently may be found include:

- appendix calculus 5–60 mm (appendolith);
- sentinel loop (dilated atonic ileum containing fluid level);
- widening of properitoneal fat line;
- blurring of properitoneal fat line;
- right lower quadrant haze due to fluid and oedema;
- scoliosis concave to the right;
- mass indenting the caecum.

Unfortunately many of these features are relatively non-specific. The radiographic signs result from localized inflammatory change leading to an associated paralytic ileus. The signs may change if the appendicitis leads to perforation and abscess formation. The abscess may result in the indentation of the caecum on its medial border and, when the inflammation permeates into the adjacent fat, may lead to loss of the lower part of the properitoneal fat line and the right psoas muscle shadow. Small bowel obstruction may occur as several loops of bowel become matted together or stuck to the inflamed appendix. An appendix calculus which can often be identified as an oval calcific ring shadow often with multiple rings, is associated with appendicitis, particularly in children (Fig. 2.40). Although air may be seen within the appendix in acute appendicitis this may also be seen in normal subjects, large bowel obstruction and paralytic ileus, particularly when the appendix is high and retrocaecal in position.

The use of other imaging techniques for the diagnosis of appendicitis is discussed on pages 93–94.

ACUTE CHOLECYSTITIS

Plain radiographic signs of acute cholecystitis include:

- gallstones, visualized in only 20%;
- right hypochondrial mass due to enlarged gallbladder;
- duodenal ileus;
- ileus of hepatic flexure of colon;
- gas within the biliary system.

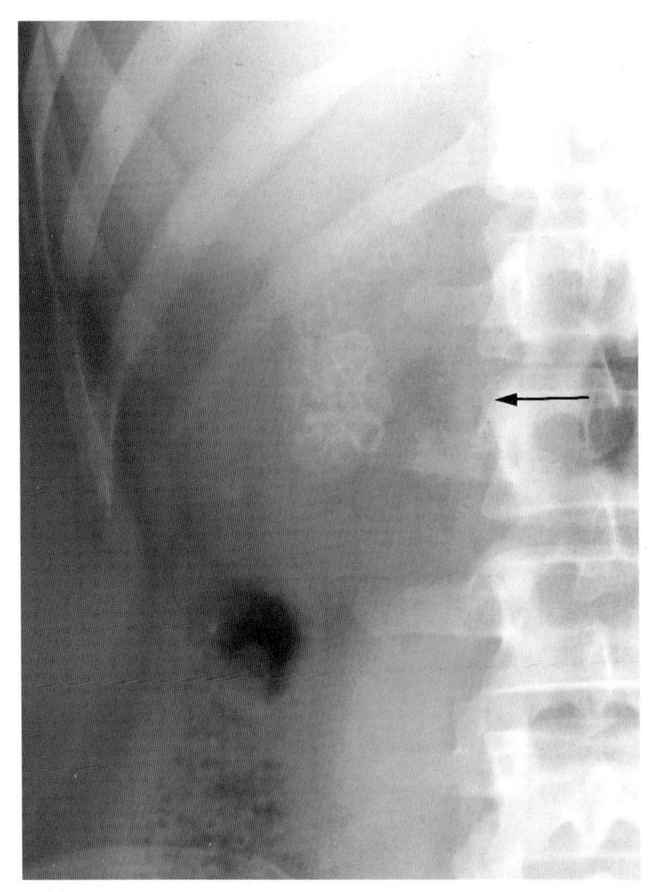

Fig. 2.41 Acute cholecystitis seen on supine abdomen. The gallbladder is full of faceted calcified stones. In addition, several calculi to the right of L2 lie within the common bile duct (arrows).

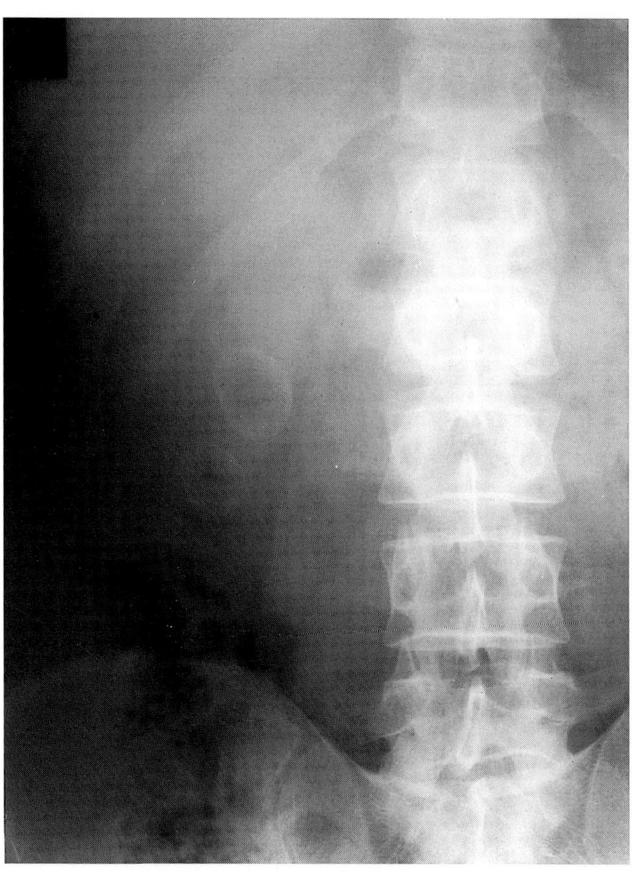

Fig. 2.42 Empyema of the gallbladder seen on supine abdomen. Several calcified gallstones can be identified, some containing gas ('Mercedes' sign). One calculus lies over the neck of the right twelfth rib and lies in Hartmann's pouch. Two others lie some distance away in the fundus of the gallbladder. An estimate of the gallbladder size can be made from the separation of the gallstones.

About 90% of cases of acute cholecystitis are associated with gallstones (Fig. 2.41). Acute cholecystitis is usually caused by a stone obstructing the cystic duct (Fig. 2.42). However, only around 20% of gallstones contain sufficient calcium to be visible on plain radiographs and only rarely does the wall of the gallbladder itself calcify. The majority of patients with gallstones, however, never develop acute cholecystitis. It is uncommon to identify a normal sized gallbladder on plain films because it is not surrounded by fat and has the same radiographic density as the adjacent structures. However, if the gallbladder enlarges due to obstruction of the cystic duct, it may then be visualized by the displacement of adjacent gas-filled structures (Fig. 2.43). In acute cholecystitis the duodenum and hepatic flexure of the colon may show a localized paralytic ileus secondary to inflammation. However, in most patients with acute cholecystitis the plain films may be completely normal or only demonstrate minimal dilation of small or large bowel.

Scintigraphy using ^{99m}Tc-labelled derivatives of iminodiacetic acid (IDA) is a simple and reasonably accurate method of diagnosing acute cholecystitis. However, enthusiasm for the technique is variable and usually ultrasound is performed (see p.139).

Tenderness of the gallbladder as it lies immediately beneath the ultrasound transducer is also a very reliable sign that the gallbladder is acutely inflamed – the 'ultrasound Murphy's sign'.

ACUTE PANCREATITIS

The pathological changes occurring in acute pancreatitis include oedema, haemorrhage, infarction of the pancreas, fat necrosis and sometimes acute suppuration. The inflammatory process may extend into the gastrocolic ligament or the paraduodenal area, or follow the root of the mesentery or extend into the anterior pararenal space. The clinical diagnosis of acute pancreatitis can be difficult and often rests on

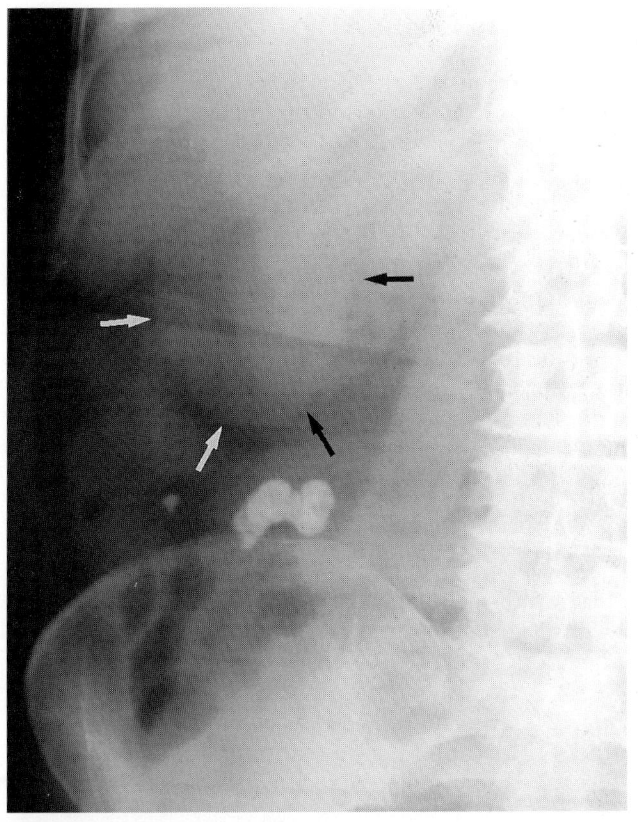

Fig. 2.43 Empyema of the gallbladder seen on supine abdomen. The greater omentum containing large amounts of fat was found to surround the inflamed gallbladder. This has rendered the distended gallbladder visible on the plain film (arrows).

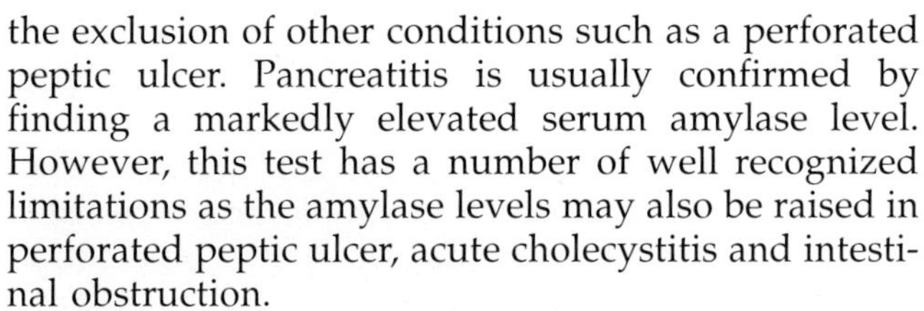

the exclusion of other conditions such as a perforated peptic ulcer. Pancreatitis is usually confirmed by finding a markedly elevated serum amylase level. However, this test has a number of well recognized limitations as the amylase levels may also be raised in perforated peptic ulcer, acute cholecystitis and intestinal obstruction.

A plain abdominal radiograph is frequently taken in patients suspected of having acute pancreatitis. Although a large number of radiological signs have been described many of these are of little or no value in the diagnosis of acute pancreatitis.

- **Most common and sometimes useful**
  - gas-filled duodenal cap and loop
  - single dilated small bowel loop (sentinel loop)
  - small bowel ileus
  - dilated colon, particularly transverse and ascending
  - dilated terminal ileum
  - loss of the left psoas outline
- **Rare but diagnostic**
  - gas within the pancreas
  - faint mottling due to fat necrosis.

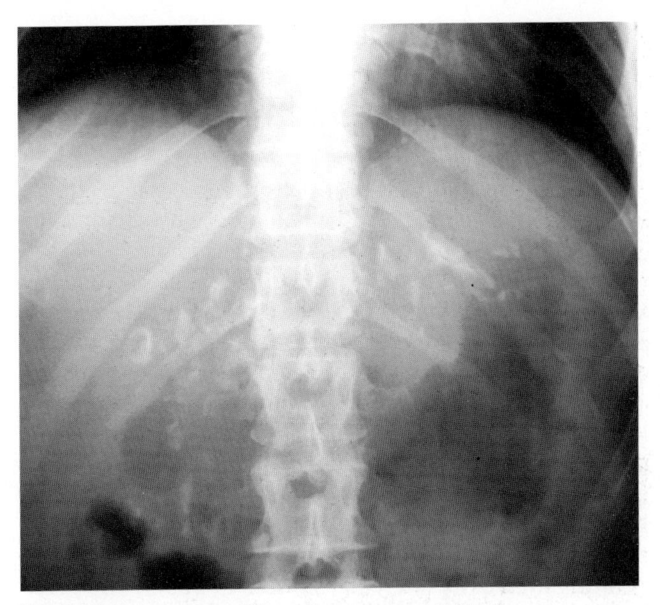

Fig. 2.44 Acute pancreatitis and pancreatic calcification.

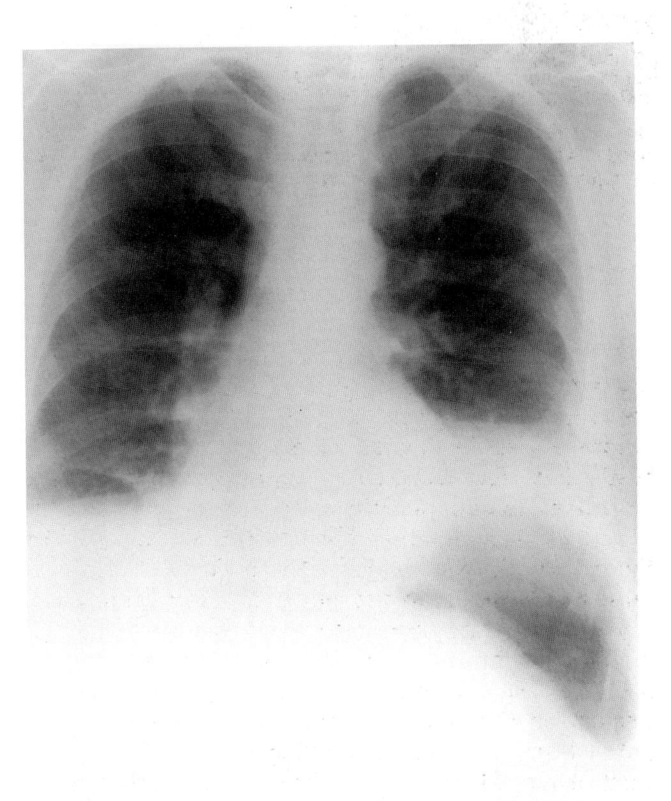

Fig. 2.45 Subphrenic abscess seen on erect chest. The left hemidiaphragm is raised and there is a left-sided pleural effusion associated with some collapse and consolidation in the left lower lobe. The gas-filled abscess is clearly visible beneath the left hemidiaphragm. The radiograph was taken ten days following a Hartmann's procedure for diverticular disease.

Gas in the duodenum is best demonstrated in the left lateral decubitus position. A dilated transverse colon and isolated dilated loops of proximal small bowel (sentinel loops) are frequent findings but they are non-specific. A gasless abdomen may be caused by persistent vomiting. Occasionally pancreatic calcification is identified in those patients who also have chronic pancreatitis (Fig. 2.44).

Demonstration of gas within the pancreas, usually seen as multiple small bubbles giving a mottled appearance, is diagnostic of a pancreatic abscess heralding a grave prognosis. In acute pancreatitis ultrasound may demonstrate an oedematous pancreas but gas-filled loops of small bowel resulting from the paralytic ileus may make ultrasound difficult or impossible. In these circumstances CT may demonstrate the pancreas but both CT and ultrasound may be normal in the early stages of acute pancreatitis. Complications of acute pancreatitis such as a pancreatic abscess or pancreatic pseudocyst may produce plain film findings such as a soft tissue mass but such complications are usually diagnosed by ultrasound or CT scanning (see p.153).

Pleural effusions, mainly left-sided, may occur in acute pancreatitis. The presence of a left-sided effusion in a patient with proven acute pancreatitis indicates a more severe disease process with a worse prognosis.

INTRA-ABDOMINAL ABSCESSES

Abscesses act as mass lesions displacing adjacent structures, for example elevation of a hemidiaphragm by a subphrenic abscess or displacement of the colon by a paracolic abscess. Abscesses are of soft-tissue density but frequently they contain gas. This gas may form single or multiple small bubble-like radiolucencies, produce radiolucent bands following fascial planes or outline an anatomical space. Sometimes there is a single or loculated large gas/fluid collection in the abscess giving an air–fluid level on an erect film. The inflammatory process and oedema usually cause ill-defined tissue margins and loss of fat lines outlining the adjacent anatomical structures. Plain film diagnosis of abscesses depends on a number of factors but a detailed knowledge is essential of the peritoneal reflections and spaces together with the normal anatomical landmarks. Meticulous attention to detail in viewing the radiograph is also needed as recognition of small bubbles of gas outside the bowel lumen, often unchanged in position on sequential films, strongly suggests an abscess. Although a high proportion of abscesses, particularly if large, may be identified on plain films, ultrasound, CT or radionuclide scanning with labelled leucocytes are more sensitive techniques (see p.107).

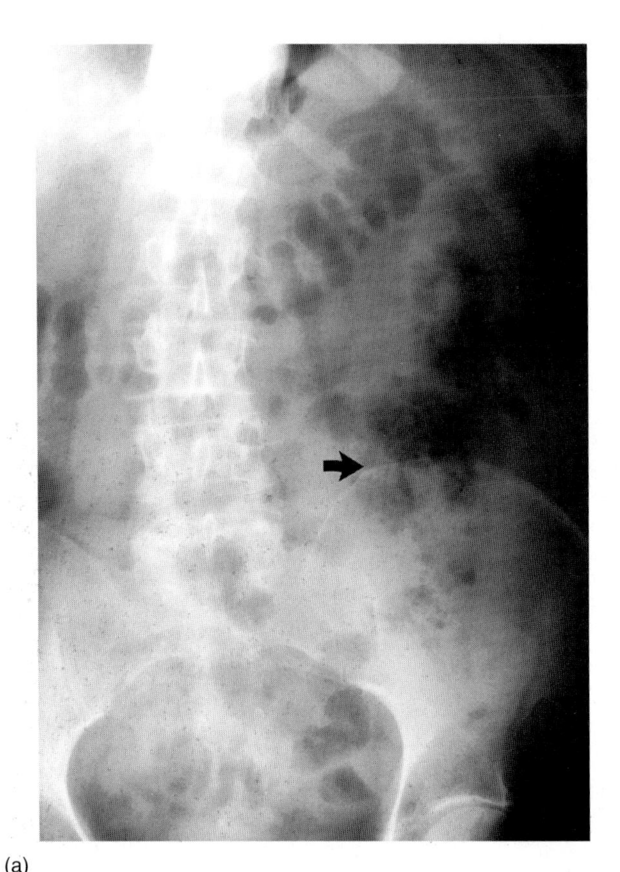

(a)

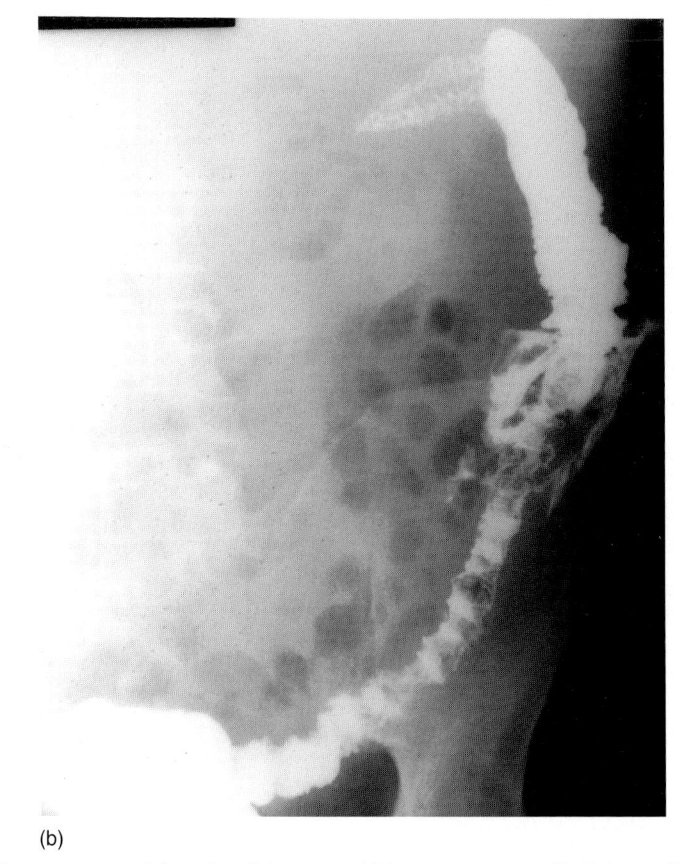

(b)

Fig. 2.46 Left paracolic abscess secondary to perforated diverticular disease seen on (a) supine abdomen and (b) contrast enema. Multiple small gas bubbles can be identified in the abscess on the plain film (arrow). The contrast enema clearly demonstrates leak outside the bowel lumen.

SUBPHRENIC ABSCESS

A subphrenic abscess is nearly always a consequence of surgery (Fig. 2.45). Subphrenic abscesses can be expected to show a raised hemidiaphragm on the affected side in 80% of cases; about 70% will show evidence of basal pulmonary consolidation or collapse and 60% will have an associated pleural effusion. In postlaparotomy patients, a subphrenic abscess is the commonest cause of unilateral pleural effusion. Abscesses may be identified as a soft tissue mass which may contain irregular pockets of gas and a gas-fluid level on the erect film.

PARACOLIC ABSCESS

Usually a paracolic abscess lies close to the causative lesion. Right paracolic and left paracolic abscesses most commonly follow appendicitis and diverticulitis (Figs 2.46, 2.47). Sometimes, however, infection may spread away from its origin and produce an abscess elsewhere either within the pelvis or in the subphrenic space. Soft-tissue masses, often containing bubbles of gas and causing colonic displacement, are the most common plain film findings.

PELVIC ABSCESS

The pelvis is the most dependent part of the abdomen and is the commonest site of abscesses in postlaparotomy patients. A pelvic abscess may occur following localized pelvic inflammatory disease or following appendicitis or diverticulitis. A soft-tissue mass sometimes containing gas may be identified superior to the bladder outline and the fat interface between the mass and the bladder is usually absent.

GAS WITHIN THE BOWEL WALL

CYSTIC PNEUMATOSIS (PNEUMATOSIS INTESTINALIS)

In this uncommon condition cyst-like collections of gas are seen both subserosally and submucosally in the intestine, with the colon being most commonly affected (**pneumatosis coli**) (Fig. 2.48). Pneumatosis intestinalis is a relatively benign condition usually occurring in the middle-aged and elderly and associated most commonly with chronic obstructive airways disease. The gas-filled cysts in the bowel vary in size from 1 cm to 3 cm and symptoms include vague abdominal pain,

(a)

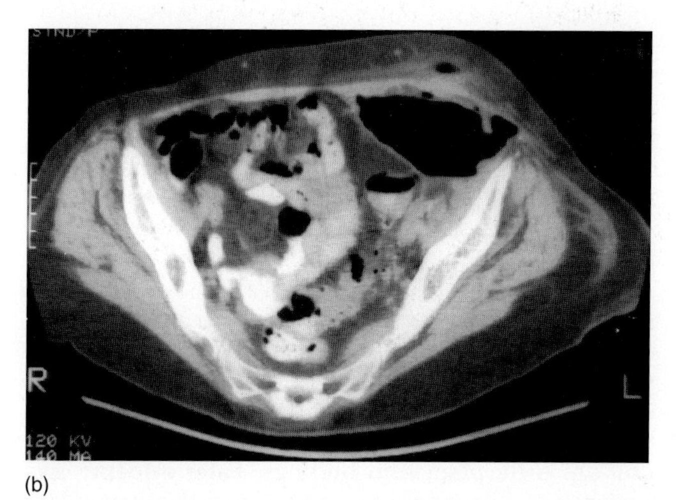

(b)

Fig. 2.47 Left paracolic abscess following perforated diverticular disease seen on (a) abdomen and (b) CT scan. On the plain film the abscess is identified as a large gas-filled viscus overlying the left iliac bone. On the CT scan its close association with the sigmoid colon is demonstrated. In addition the muscles of the abdominal wall have become involved and are being destroyed by the infective process.

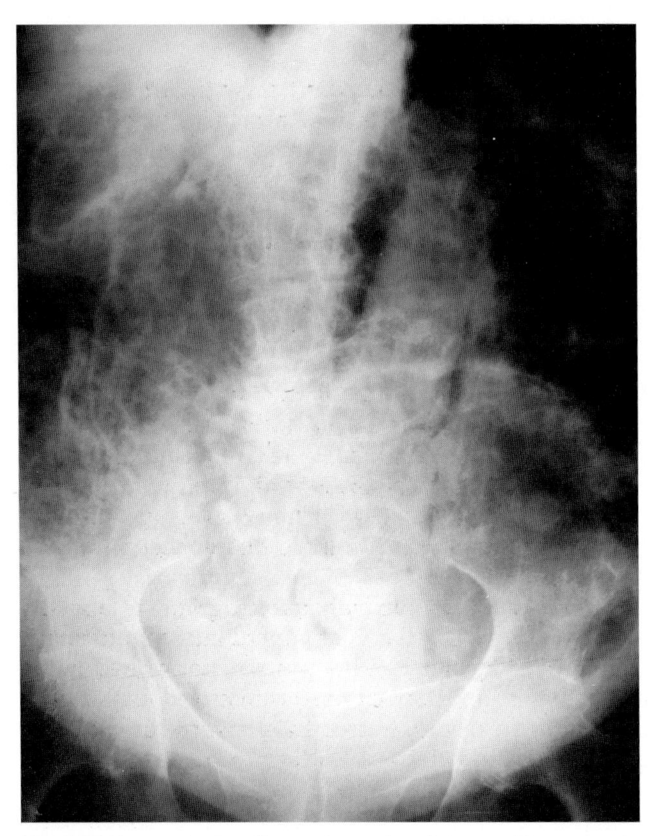

Fig. 2.48 Pneumatosis coli seen on supine abdomen. Numerous ring shadows of varying size can be identified arising from most of the large bowel in this patient aged 87 with abdominal pain and diarrhoea.

diarrhoea, constipation and mucus discharge. The plain film findings are characteristic: the gas-containing cysts give rise to an appearance quite different from normal gas shadows. Occasionally these cysts rupture producing a chronic pneumoperitoneum without evidence of peritonitis.

INTERSTITIAL EMPHYSEMA

In this rare condition linear bubbles of gas can be identified in the bowel wall and there is often associated oedema of the bowel. It occurs in ischaemia, severe infections or inflammatory bowel disease and in these situations it is associated with bowel necrosis and perforation.

Neonates, especially if premature, can develop severe inflammation of the gut – necrotizing enterocolitis. The diagnosis is based on clinical and radiological signs. The infants typically develop abdominal distension, vomiting and bloody diarrhoea. Generalized bowel dilation, wall thickening and bowel loop separation are early plain film findings. Later a foamy gas pattern and a linear or crescentic appearance caused by gas may be seen in the bowel wall when mucosal necrosis and autolysis have developed.

INFECTIONS WITH GAS-FORMING ORGANISMS

Many bacteria are capable of producing gas but those most commonly responsible in humans are *Escherichia coli, Clostridium welchii* and *Klebsiella aerogenes*. Such infections usually give rise to severe constitutional disturbance and toxaemia with a high mortality rate; they produce a localized abnormal collection of gas in the abdomen or pelvis. However, over half of all gas-forming infections occur in diabetics when the infecting organism is usually *E. coli*; in this group the constitutional disturbance is usually less than in non-diabetics.

EMPHYSEMATOUS GASTRITIS

Emphysematous gastritis is a severe infection resulting in a contracted stomach with frothy or mottled radiolucencies visible within the stomach wall in the left upper abdomen.

EMPHYSEMATOUS CHOLECYSTITIS

Emphysematous cholecystitis is caused by a gas-forming infection of the gallbladder which results in gas in the lumen and/or wall of the gallbladder (Fig. 2.49). It tends to occur in older patients, half of whom are diabetic, and with clinical findings suggestive of acute cholecystitis. It occurs with equal frequency in males and females and, unlike ordinary cholecystitis, gallstones may be absent.

EMPHYSEMATOUS CYSTITIS

Emphysematous cystitis causes gas cysts and linear gas streaks within the wall of the urinary bladder and is sometimes associated with gas within the lumen of the bladder (Fig. 2.50). The condition is most common in diabetics. Emphysematous cystitis must be distinguished from gas confined to the lumen of the bladder caused by a **vesicocolic fistula** which is not associated with gas within the wall of the bladder.

EMPHYSEMATOUS PYELONEPHRITIS

Emphysematous pyelonephritis is recognized by the demonstration of bubbles of gas within the kidney or linear streaks of gas beneath the renal capsule. The condition occurs in uncontrolled diabetics or in patients with obstructive uropathy.

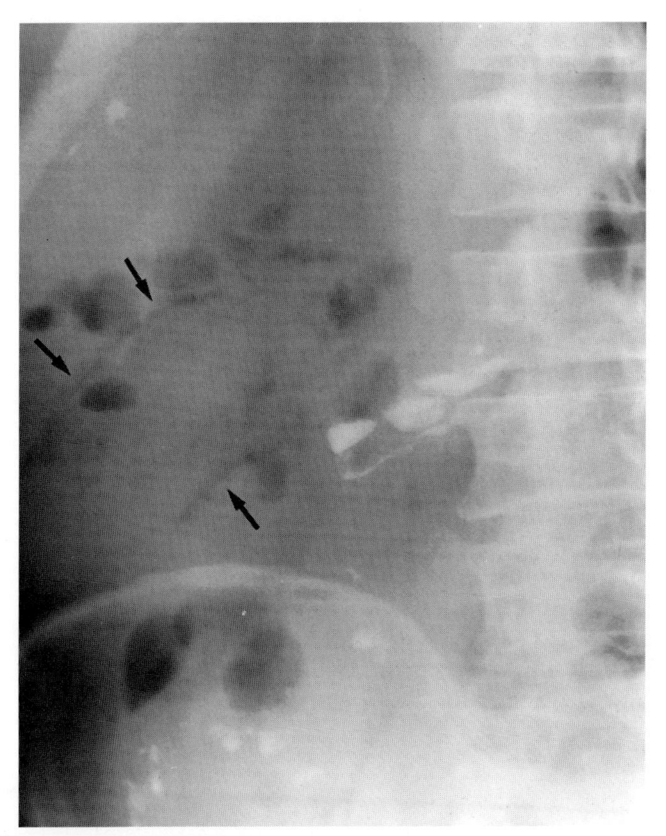

Fig. 2.49 Emphysematous cholecystitis seen on prone abdomen following oral cholecystographic contrast media. Linear gas shadows can be identified within the wall of the gallbladder (arrow) in this diabetic patient aged 62. (Source: S. Field in R. G. Grainger and D. J. Allison (eds), *Diagnostic radiology*; Published by Churchill Livingstone, Edinburgh, 1991.)

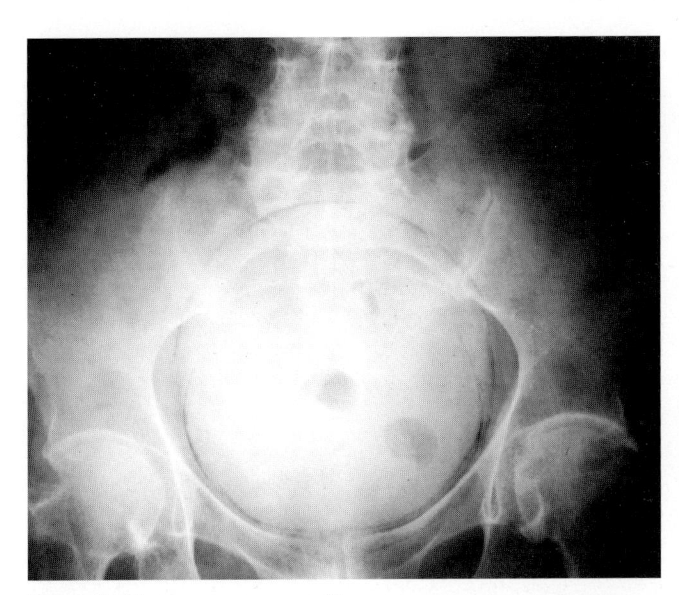

Fig. 2.50 Emphysematous cystitis seen on supine abdomen in a 78-year-old diabetic with *E. coli* urinary tract infection. The bladder is distended and linear streaks of gas can be clearly identified within its wall. (Courtesy Dr A. R. Carter.)

RENAL COLIC

A proportion of patients admitted with acute abdominal pain have acute ureteric obstruction. Although the calculus maybe situated in any part of the ureter it is frequently found at its lower end. Although nearly 90% of all ureteric calculi causing obstruction are radiopaque, they are often extremely small and difficult to identify on plain radiographs alone or, if identified, impossible to establish as being located within the ureter. **Phleboliths** within the pelvis are a source of potential confusion but their radiolucent centre and smooth spherical outline help to distinguish them from ureteric stones which are frequently oval, slightly irregular in outline and without a radiolucent centre. The pain of renal colic often leads to air swallowing and an associated paralytic ileus which results in dramatic gas-filled loops of small and large bowel that may also contain fluid levels.

An emergency intravenous urogram is usually required to make a diagnosis and identify the point of obstruction; in many centres this is performed as an emergency soon after hospital admission. Occasionally ureteric colic is complicated by the spontaneous rupture of the renal pelvis, leading to a retroperitoneal accumulation of urine known as a **urinoma**. This can be identified on plain radiographs as a soft-tissue mass

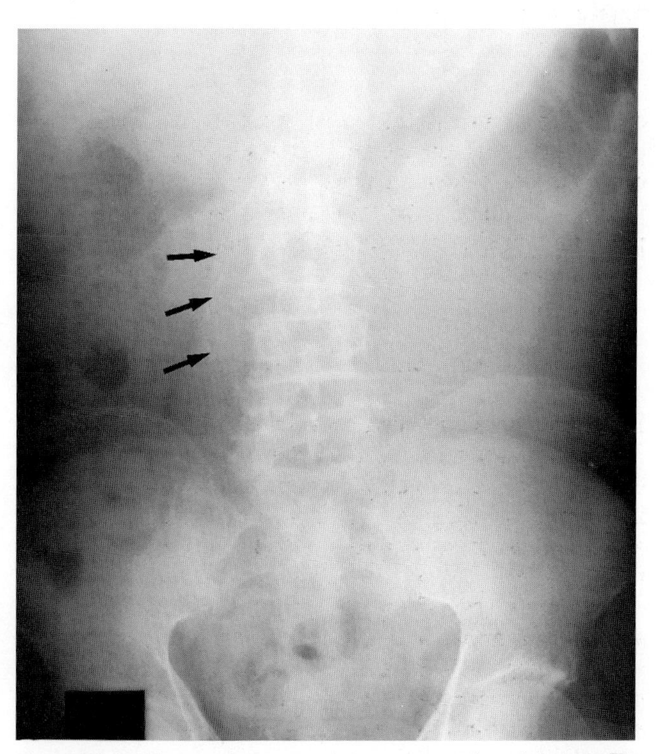

Fig. 2.51 Leaking aortic aneurysm seen on supine abdomen. The calcified wall of the aneurysm can be identified on the right (arrows) but the psoas margin can be seen. The is a soft-tissue mass on the left with obliteration of renal and psoas outlines and bulging in the flank. There was a left-sided leak with 5 litres of blood in the left retroperitoneal region.

with loss of the renal and psoas outline and is often associated with a marked paralytic ileus. Diagnosis is usually only confirmed following emergency urography or CT.

LEAKING ABDOMINAL AORTIC ANEURYSM

Signs include:

- soft tissue retroperitoneal mass;
- curvilinear calcification in the wall;
- loss of psoas outline;
- loss of renal outline;
- displacement of kidney.

A leaking abdominal aortic aneurysm usually presents as a an acute abdomen and may sometimes simulate renal colic. The clinical diagnosis may be obvious and if the patient is in a state of shock resuscitation followed by urgent surgery is indicated and further investigations are not usually required. If confirmation of a leaking aneurysm is required then ultrasound or CT (see p.113) will establish the diagnosis of an aneurysm and may demonstrate a retroperitoneal haematoma. However, sometimes a leaking aneurysm is not suspected clinically and chest and abdominal radiographs taken to investigate the pain may show an aneurysm as a central soft-tissue mass obscuring the psoas or renal shadows, particularly on the left side. Curvilinear calcification is a useful observation as it will indicate the size of the aorta and the presence of an aneurysm. Aortic calcification may be seen on an AP radiograph but is best detected on a lateral view. A soft-tissue mass identified outside the calcified aneurysm indicates haematoma caused by the leaking aneurysm. Loss of psoas or renal outlines or displacement of a kidney are strong presumptive evidence of a leak from the aneurysm (Fig. 2.51). An aneurysm is sometimes detected following emergency urography for suspected ureteric colic. The enlarging aneurysm causes displacement and compression of the ureter with resulting back pressure changes in the kidney. There is often an associated secondary paralytic ileus associated with the leaking aneurysm and the dilated bowel may completely obscure the aneurysm itself.

CHAPTER 3

Gastrointestinal tract

Richard Farrow
and Giles W. Stevenson

INTRODUCTION: TECHNIQUES AVAILABLE

PLAIN RADIOGRAPHS

Plain abdominal radiographs retain an important role in the evaluation of suspected obstruction, perforation, infection, inflammatory bowel disease and calcifications, but often the information available from the radiograph is not specific enough to permit a full diagnosis. A wide array of techniques is available either to supplement the plain film, or in many cases to serve as the initial imaging study. One of the challenges facing radiologists and surgeons is to identify those patients in whom newer techniques should replace plain abdominal radiographs as the initial imaging examination.

CONTRAST FLUOROSCOPY

The first contrast examination of the upper gastrointestinal (GI) tract using metallic salts introduced into the stomach of guinea-pigs was published in 1896, only months after the initial description of the X-ray by Roentgen. Initially clinical studies of the upper and lower GI tract used a single contrast technique with dense heavy metal salts. Attempts to obtain a more detailed mucosal view by means of a double contrast technique (radiopaque barium and radiolucent gas) date back to 1906 when a combination of bismuth and effervescent agents were used to visualize the stomach. Publications from Sweden and Japan led to the gradual acceptance of the double contrast technique in most departments around the world for both upper and lower GI studies. Initially air was used as the negative contrast agent for the colon, but more recently CO_2 has been utilized in an attempt to reduce postprocedural pain. For double contrast studies the ideal barium is non-flocculating, non-toxic, cheap, has a high radiographic density, gives good mucosal coating and is palatable and easy to administer. For single contrast the radiographic density must be much lower and a premium is placed on non-sedimentation of the barium suspension which is achieved by the use of more uniform and smaller barium particles.

Barium is an excellent contrast agent for the GI tract provided that is where it stays. Barium aspirated into the lungs is usually harmless and can be expectorated either spontaneously or with help from a physiotherapist. If there is a suspicion that contrast will not remain within the lumen of the GI tract, either because of the presence of a fistula, sinus, perforation or anastomotic leak, a water-soluble contrast agent should be used, since intraperitoneal barium causes a peritoneal reaction and adhesions, even if sterile. The

Diagnostic and Interventional Radiology in Surgical Practice. Edited by P. Armstrong and M. L. Wastie. Published in 1997 by Chapman & Hall, London. ISBN 0 412 61960 1 (HB), 0 412 61970 9 (PB)

first water-soluble contrast agents were both ionic and of high osmolality but more recently low osmolar ionic and non-ionic agents have become available. The high osmolar agents retain a place where leaks are suspected but there is no risk of aspiration into the lungs. These high osmolality agents are pneumotoxic, and in situations where aspiration is a possibility a low osmolar agent should be used.

In infants the low osmolar agents should be used in all situations to reduce fluid shifts from the intravascular to extravascular spaces that occur due to the osmotic effect of the high osmolar agents. The exception to this rule is when contrast is being introduced as a therapeutic measure in cases of neonatal meconium ileus. In this situation, the fluid shift caused by the high osmolality of the contrast agent within the bowel is an asset. The shift of fluid into the bowel lumen helps to soften the meconium and makes it easier to pass, but scrupulous attention to fluid balance is then required.

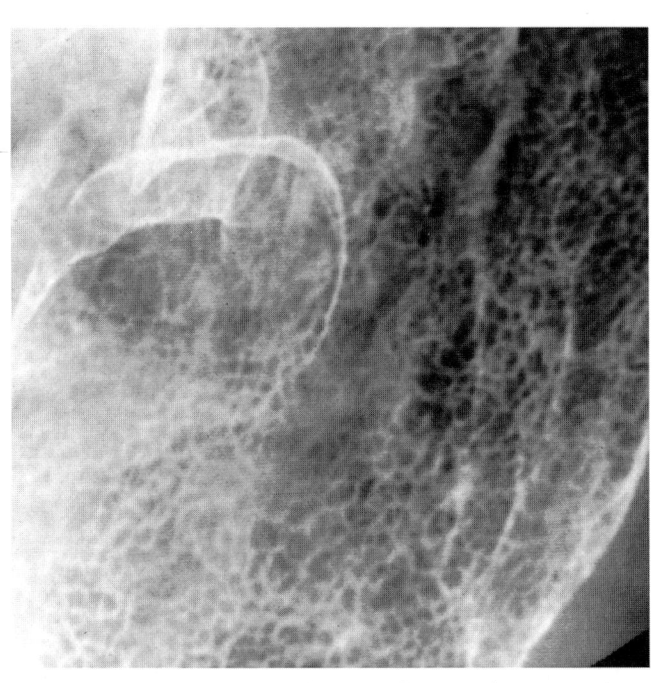

Fig. 3.2 Normal upper GI study demonstrating normal areae gastricae. Areae gastricae are not always visible on a barium study. Areae over 4 mm in size are statistically associated with duodenal ulcer disease and probably with *H. pylori* infection.

IMAGING EQUIPMENT

There have been many changes in equipment since the early days of GI radiology when the available X-ray tubes produced only a low and inconsistent output. Today high definition digital techniques are used which allow the fluoroscopic image to be stored and printed, with good spatial resolution, without the

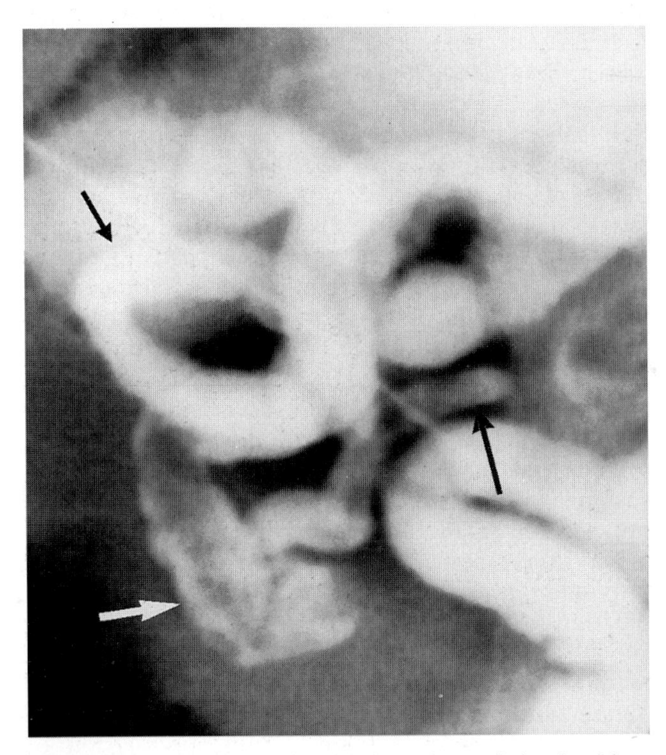

Fig. 3.1 Fluoro-record image (to minimize patient radiation dose) from a water-soluble enema study demonstrating a microcolon (small black arrow) and caecum (white arrow), and an abrupt termination to the ileum (long black arrow) due to ileal atresia.

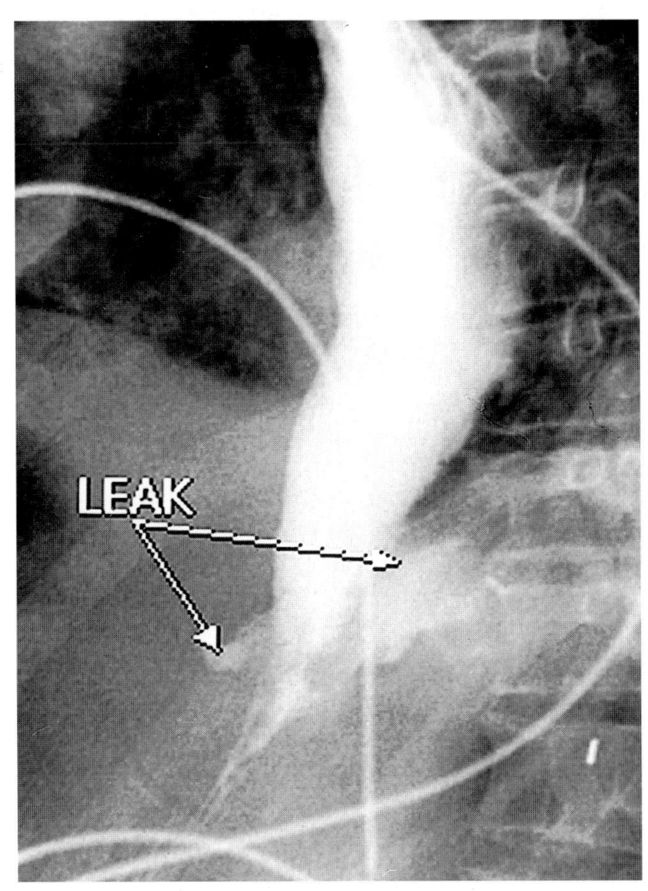

Fig. 3.3 Postoperative anastomotic leak demonstrated using non-ionic contrast swallow. Image annotation at the digital work station has been used to indicate the abnormality.

need for the additional radiation required for a conventional radiographic exposure (Fig. 3.1). When high detail resolution is required, a radiographic exposure can be made in the usual way (Fig. 3.2), and this image can then be further manipulated digitally. Most paediatric and interventional work can be done with the stored fluoroscopic images, with reductions in radiation dose of up to one half. The next ten years will see a revolution in digital imaging as TV monitors become more common in hospitals and outside clinics. Original images and images annotated by the radiologist (Fig. 3.3) will become available in operating theatres, outpatient clinics and on wards, with hard-copy films limited to a few relevant images of the major pathology, perhaps printed on high quality paper rather than the film which is used today.

COMPUTED TOMOGRAPHY

By 1975 whole body CT scanners capable of abdominal scanning were available. Further advances reduced scan times, enabling a single CT axial image to be acquired during the space of one breath-hold. More recently spiral scanners have become available which have produced a dramatic reduction in scan times such that the whole of the upper abdomen can now be imaged in one breath-hold. These new scanners also allow for 3D reconstruction of the structures imaged. This raises many exciting possibilities including image processing to obtain a display of the inside of the colon which could be traversed on the computer monitor, much as if an on-screen endoscopy was being performed. This technique has the potential to replace both barium studies and endoscopy for detection of colonic neoplasia, and may have a great future as a screening technique.

When assessing the alimentary tract with CT the bowel must be distended and opacified, usually with dilute water-soluble contrast or 1% barium, given in divided doses. The first dose is designed to opacify the large and lower small bowel, and a second dose of contrast is given just before the scan to opacify the stomach and upper small bowel. If this oral contrast is not given, loops of bowel may be misdiagnosed as abscess, lymphadenopathy or tumour. Regular barium is not used to opacify the bowel as the high density causes image artefact, and results in degradation of the image. Barium remaining within the bowel from a previous contrast study causes similar problems. CT is useful in the diagnosis and staging of alimentary tract tumours and in the assessment of inflammatory bowel disease and complications of Gl disease or surgery, such as fluid collections and abscesses. In general, CT is at its best in patients with sufficient body fat to delineate all the abdominal organs, both solid and hollow (Fig. 3.4), in contradistinction to ultrasound where excess fat may make examination difficult.

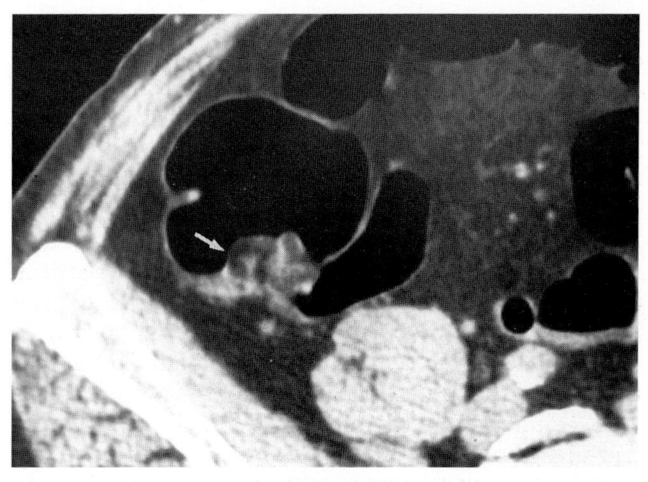

Fig. 3.4 CT scan of the caecum. The caecum has been distended with air, in order to evaluate the ileocaecal valve. Barium enema (after a failed colonoscopy) had shown a large valve with a differential diagnosis of cancer or fatty infiltration. The CT scan shows a prominent valve due to fatty infiltration (arrow) and no evidence of tumour.

ULTRASOUND

The Japanese, in 1949, were the first to report a medical use for ultrasound, describing falx localization to detect shift of intracranial midline structures. General acceptance of ultrasound awaited the introduction of high-resolution, hand-held, grey-scale scanners which provide a real-time image of the structure under evaluation. Ultrasound is readily available with machines that are both relatively inexpensive and mobile, and uses no ionizing radiation. These advantages mean that

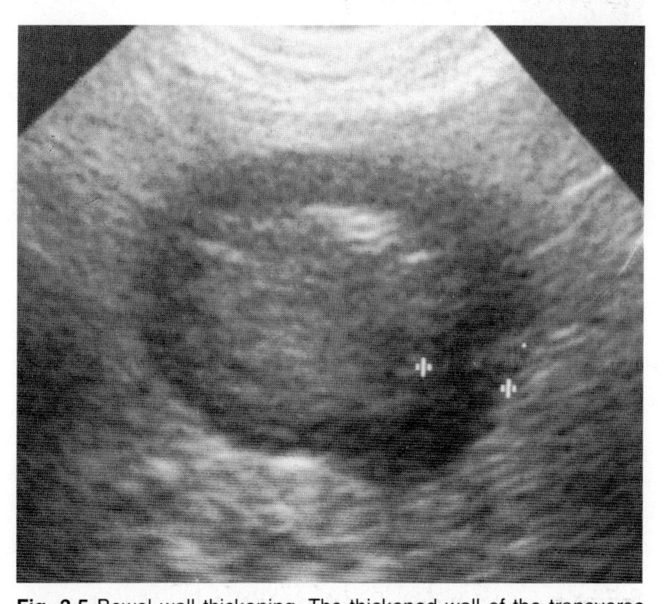

Fig. 3.5 Bowel wall thickening. The thickened wall of the transverse colon is demonstrated on ultrasound (the bowel wall thickness is measured using the calipers). This thickening was due to extensive pseudomembranous colitis but thickening can also be seen with Crohn's disease, ulcerative colitis, ischaemia, Campylobacter infection and diverticulitis.

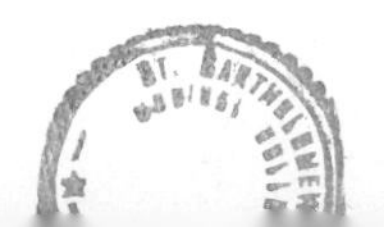

ultrasound should generally be considered for the initial cross-sectional examination in most patients with suspected abdominal pathlogy. The use of graded compression with real-time scanning allows evaluation of both bowel wall movement and wall thickness (Fig. 3.5). This, combined with the sensitivity of ultrasound to assess fluid collections and free fluid within the abdomen, has led to its use in a wide range of diseases affecting the bowel and mesentery. Endoluminal ultrasound probes provide information about the extent and location of disease within the layers of the bowel wall. Intraoperative probes are becoming available for both open and laparoscopic surgery, and therapeutic focused ultrasound for tumour ablation is moving from the laboratory to the operating theatre, and will in due course move to the radiology department's interventional suite.

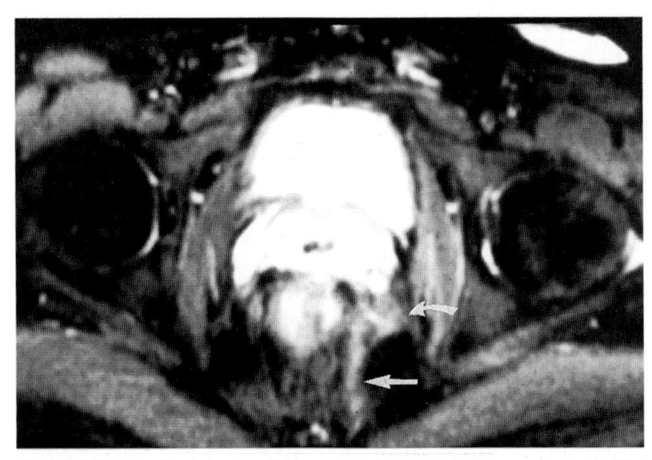

Fig. 3.6 Perianal abscess. This abscess is seen as an area of high signal (curved arrow) in this pelvic MR scan which uses a fat suppression sequence. Connecting with this abscess is a fistula, seen as a high signal track (straight arrow) which communicates with the skin by the ischiorectal fossa. (Courtesy of S. Somers.)

RADIONUCLIDE IMAGING

Radionuclide imaging provides images which are of lower spatial resolution than those provided by other imaging techniques but does provide information on function which may be impossible to achieve by other means. Most studies are now performed using technetium-99m as the radionuclide; ^{99m}Tc is incorporated into a variety of compounds to provide information on motility and the presence or extent of disease. The labelling of tumour-specific antigens is still being developed but raises the possibility of diagnostic scans for a specific primary tumour and also for assessment of involved but normal-size lymph nodes.

MAGNETIC RESONANCE IMAGING

MRI has traditionally had a very limited place in the assessment of the GI tract. This is largely due to the long scan times required and the intrinsic motility of the bowel which leads to poor resolution. In addition there is little difference in signal between the bowel wall and bowel contents on scans taken without contrast. Both these difficulties are gradually being resolved. The images while still improving do remain poor and inferior to other methods at the present time but MRI is of proven value in pelvic inflammatory disease and the relationship of fistulae to the sphincter complex (Fig. 3.6).

ENDOSCOPY

Endoscopy provides an alternative technique to contrast studies in the assessment of the GI tract. It provides indirect but highly detailed visual assessment of intestinal mucosa and also permits therapeutic interventional procedures and biopsies. Both endoscopy and barium studies can detect lesions missed by the other technique. Sensitivity for detecting tumours, polyps and ulcers is operator-dependent for both methods but is generally slightly better for endoscopy. Endoscopy does allow a better assessment of erythematous and angiodysplastic lesions. However, endoscopy has a higher morbidity and mortality than the corresponding barium study, and the need for sedation and postprocedural care are further relative disadvantages. There is less patient movement required for endoscopy and this can be an important consideration in patients with reduced mobility from whatever cause; older patients, for example, tend to prefer endoscopy. Selection between endoscopy or a barium study will thus depend on mobility of the patient, the local availability and quality of the two procedures and on the exact question that needs to be answered in any particular patient.

UPPER GI TRACT (OESOPHAGUS, STOMACH AND DUODENUM)

EXAMINATIONS AVAILABLE

Three different fluoroscopic examinations may be performed to evaluate the upper GI tract, each with some variations depending on the nature of the clinical problem. This section is organized to illustrate the role of each of the examinations: the swallowing assessment, the barium swallow and the barium meal.

Swallowing assessment

This study is used to assess patients who have difficulty with swallowing, and those who choke on or aspirate food.

The normal process of swallowing is complex and incorporates oral, pharyngeal and oesophageal phases which link together in a coordinated fashion to propel the food bolus from the mouth to the stomach. This process requires the coordination of many muscles, six cranial nerves (V, VII, IX, X, XI, XII) and the first, second and third cervical nerves. Afferent information is processed within the medulla, with the motor response coordinated through the motor ganglia of the appropriate cranial nerves. Thus neuronal or muscular dysfunction at many levels can result in eating difficulties.

Pharyngeal dysfunction may present with drooling, choking, a nasal voice, cough, recurrent chest infections and hoarseness as well as dysphagia, and it may be difficult to decide the most appropriate specialty for patient management. This has led to the introduction of a multidisciplinary team approach in the evaluation and treatment of these patients, with input from various specialties including speech therapy, radiology, gastroenterology, thoracic surgery and ENT. The presence of a speech therapist during the radiological assessment provides vital information on the exact clinical problems so that the examination can be tailored to answer the relevant questions. The radiologist and speech therapist should work as a team, issuing a joint report on the findings and the therapeutic implications. The speech therapist can get immediate feedback on the success of any therapeutic manoeuvres instigated. Video (which has largely replaced cineradiology) is an important component of pharyngeal fluoroscopy and allows the image to be frozen for more detailed assessment, as well as slow-motion viewing. Pharyngeal rings and webs may only be visible for a few frames on a long study and can be missed without slow-motion review. The swallowing assessment is performed mainly in the lateral and AP projections. Barium sulphate is the usual contrast agent and is made up to a variety of viscosities to simulate different foodstuffs. In addition barium can be incorporated into, for example, biscuit and pasta to allow a full assessment of swallowing of both liquids and solids.

Swallowing can be divided into five separate but interconnecting stages. The first is oral control of the bolus and control at the junction of mouth and pharynx, followed in sequence by closure of the palatopharyngeal isthmus, compression of the bolus by the tongue base and the constrictor muscles, closure of the larynx and finally opening of the pharyngo-oesophageal segment. Deficiency at any of these sites initially leads to compensation either by a modification of the type of food eaten or by changes in body habitus (head flexion to compensate for failure of pharyngo-oesophageal opening) or by changes in the action of the involved muscles (tongue and larynx displaced posteriorly to compensate for failure of the constrictor muscles to compress the bolus). Decompensation occurs when compensatory mechanisms no longer suffice. At this point there may be retention of the bolus. The bolus may be retained in the valleculae or piriform sinuses due to a suboptimal tongue push, weakness of the stripping wave or a relative obstruction such as a pharyngeal web or prominent cricopharyngeus. Alternatively, instead of retention, leakage may occur in one or more of the following ways:

- Weakness, atrophy or resection of the tongue, paralysis of the soft palate or missing teeth can lead to leakage of food from the mouth.
- Nasal regurgitation can occur due to weakness of the soft palate or superior constrictor.
- Penetration, which is the presence of contrast in the laryngeal vestibule or ventricle, or aspiration, defined as contrast in the trachea, may both occur due to poor epiglottic tilt, poor elevation of the larynx or poor laryngeal closure.

In infants with suspected pharyngeal dysfunction, tracheo-oesophageal fistula without atresia (the H-type fistula) must be considered and investigated first with low osmolar contrast agents (Fig. 3.7).

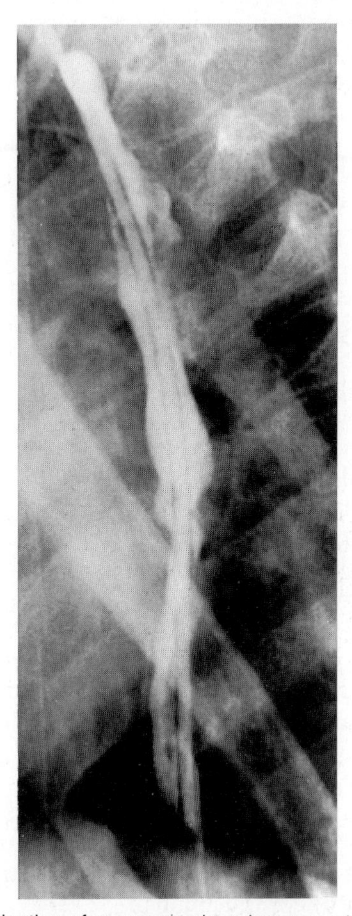

Fig. 3.7 Investigation of a suspected tracheo-oesophageal fistula. A nasogastric feeding tube is positioned in the distal oesophagus and the infant placed prone. Non-ionic contrast is injected as the tube is withdrawn and lateral fluoroscopy will show any tracheo-oesophageal fistula that is present. With this technique, any contrast seen in the bronchial tree must be due to an 'H' fistula, as pharyngeal aspiration has been excluded. No tracheo-oesophageal fistula was demonstrated in this particular study.

Barium swallow

When a barium swallow is requested the radiologist will usually perform a barium meal since diseases in stomach and duodenum may cause or exacerbate oesophageal symptoms. The exception is where the examination is being tailored to a specific question such as the presence or not of an oesophageal perforation. Both barium swallow and endoscopy may be falsely negative in patients with dysphagia. While barium swallow is probably the best initial examination, if this is negative the patient should proceed to endoscopy. Conversely if endoscopy is used as the initial investigation and is negative, barium swallow with a marshmallow to act as a solid bolus may prove helpful.

Oesophageal symptoms include heartburn, globus, dysphagia, odynophagia and chest pain. The study will be modified by the presence of these symptoms as the standard study will overlook many of the causes of these oesophageal symptoms. It is important therefore that the radiologist be aware of these symptoms so that appropriate modifications in technique can be made.

The routine study includes images of the whole length of the oesophagus in single contrast, in mucosal relief (barium-coated but collapsed and empty) and in double contrast. It is important to achieve good oesophageal distension when performing barium studies, as webs, rings and strictures may otherwise be missed. Conversely the length of strictures may be overestimated if the distal normal oesophageal segment is not adequately distended. In addition the oesophagus should routinely be assessed by observing swallowing in the prone or supine position.

In the presence of globus, films and video of the pharynx in the AP and lateral projections may reveal webs and epiglottic abnormalities. In dysphagia, if the routine films are normal, fluoroscopy while the patient swallows a 15 mm marshmallow, acting as a solid food bolus, followed by liquid barium, can highlight the site of stricture. In odynophagia (pain on swallowing), additional double contrast views are taken to detect oesophagitis. With heartburn, a more detailed assessment of motility and reflux is carried out. With chest pain, a detailed assessment of motility and reflux is made, and a provocative drug such as edrophonium chloride, may be used for diffuse spasm or nutcracker oesophagus.

If there is a concern about perforation, either due to trauma or secondary to endoscopy or surgery, a water-soluble contrast should be used initially followed by barium. This subject is discussed further in the section on postsurgical complications.

There are five types of contractile activity that can be observed in the oesophagus, two are peristaltic and three non-peristaltic.

- Primary peristalsis starts with a swallow and travels smoothly down the oesophagus taking about seven seconds, stripping all the contents into the stomach. Normal individuals may have a very small amount of contrast left behind around the level of the aortic arch on two or three out of five swallows (a phenomenon called **proximal escape**).
- Secondary peristalsis is the same type of contraction, but is initiated in mid-oesophagus by distension.
- Tertiary contractions are of low amplitude manometrically, and radiologically are non-lumen-obliterating and non-peristaltic contractions, most commonly seen in reflux disease.
- Lumen-obliterating, non-peristaltic contractions (higher amplitude) also occur in reflux disease, especially in old age, and are also seen in diffuse spasm, nutcracker oesophagus and in vigorous achalasia.
- Transient transverse ripples in the oesophagus are called the feline oesophagus, because the cat oesophagus constantly has such striations. These are seen mainly in people with reflux disease, moments after an episode of reflux, but may also occur in normal people.

Barium meal

With a double-contrast or multiphasic examination of the stomach, CO_2 forming granules are given as well as high-density barium and the patient is rolled to achieve good coating of the gastric mucosa by the barium. With the stomach distended with gas, supine, oblique and lateral views are taken to show all parts of the stomach in both barium-filled and double contrast modes. The radiologist also compresses the accessible parts of stomach and duodenum as this is a sensitive way of detecting small polypoid and marginated lesions. Once views of the stomach have been obtained, sufficient barium to coat the duodenum is run through the pyloric canal. A smooth muscle relaxant such as 20 mg of hyoscine-*N*-butyl bromide (Buscopan) or 0.1 mg of glucagon may be given by intravenous injection which has the effect of causing duodenal hypotonicity, relieving any spasm and allowing better distension. Magnified spot views of the duodenal cap are then obtained in various degrees of obliquity. At least one film is taken showing the whole of the duodenal loop and proximal jejunum to detect the occasional distal abnormality, such as unexpected coeliac disease or giardiasis. An adequate examination should include not less than five views of the stomach, two of the duodenal bulb and the whole of the duodenal loop.

OESOPHAGEAL DISORDERS

Gastro-oesophageal reflux

This is the most common motility disorder involving the oesophagus and can cause all of the symptoms described above. Endoscopy is the best method to assess mild oesophagitis, but barium studies provide a broader view of the disease, associated motility disturbances and complications. Either investigation is adequate but endoscopy will overlook the pharyngeal changes associated with globus symptoms, minor strictures and Schatzki rings, and does not provide such a good view of the motility dysfunction, though this is seldom important in deciding treatment.

When acid is instilled into the normal oesophagus, the resting tone of the cricopharyngeus rises. Patients with reflux disease show a variety of abnormalities of the cricopharyngeus such as incomplete relaxation, delayed relaxation, premature contraction after a bolus passes, and transient mini-Zenker's diverticula. The relation of these changes to globus symptoms is not yet clear, but they often coexist. The primary oesophageal peristaltic wave often becomes inefficient in reflux disease resulting in major proximal escape, and both tertiary contractions and lumen-obliterating non-peristaltic activity can be seen. In old age the latter is sometimes so marked as to cause a corkscrew appearance and may be called presbyoesophagus. This is probably one of the manifestations of reflux disease.

While most patients with severe gastro-oesophageal reflux do have a coexisting hiatus hernia, many patients are seen with hiatus hernia but no reflux and many with reflux but no hiatus hernia. The primary abnormality in gastro-oesophageal reflux is in the lower oesophageal sphincter which exhibits inappropriately frequent and prolonged transient relaxations, and in severe disease reduced resting tone. The para-oesophageal variety of hiatus hernia makes up only 1% of the hernias seen and is not associated with reflux. Radiologically, the presence of a sliding hiatus hernia is assessed by observing the position of the diaphragmatic hiatus which can be seen to compress the intrahiatal structures if the patient gives a sniff. This is compared to the position of the gastro-oesophageal junction.

Gastro-oesophageal reflux itself is also assessed with barium studies but the presence of reflux does not correlate well with the presence of reflux oesophagitis. Only 40% of patients with endoscopic evidence of oesophagitis have reflux demonstrated on barium studies. To check for reflux the patient is given barium to drink and the lower oesophagus is visualized with the patient lying supine. If no reflux is seen in this position the patient is rolled slightly on to the right side to bring the pool of barium in direct contact with the gastro-oesophageal junction and the patient given sips of water, the water siphon test. This test can demonstrate slight reflux even in normal patients but if marked reflux is seen the test is positive. The test also permits the assessment of clearance of refluxed liquid.

In patients with reflux oesophagitis, 50% have abnormal oesophageal motor function resulting in delayed clearing of the barium within the oesophagus and an increase in non-peristaltic contractions seen on the supine swallowing assessment. The best way to assess reflux in difficult cases, or for research purposes is 24-hour monitoring with a pH probe in the lower oesophagus. Reflux may also be assessed dynamically with a food bolus labelled with a radiopharmaceutical, usually technetium. This can provide semi-quantitative data on reflux as well as oesophageal motility and gastric emptying. With the use of labelled solid and liquid boluses, data on differential handling of these can be obtained.

When gastro-oesophageal reflux is complicated by moderate to severe reflux oesophagitis, morphological changes can be seen on the barium study in 80–90% of patients. Changes are usually not seen in patients with mild superficial oesophagitis. The changes of oesophagitis seen on barium swallow are those of irregularity in the outline of the oesophagus, thickened longitudinal folds with linear ulceration, transverse oesophageal folds, strictures and inflammatory polyps at the top of gastric rugal folds (Fig. 3.8). The inflammatory gastro-oesophageal polyps are an indication of chronic reflux disease and appear as a continuation of a single prominent mucosal fold that

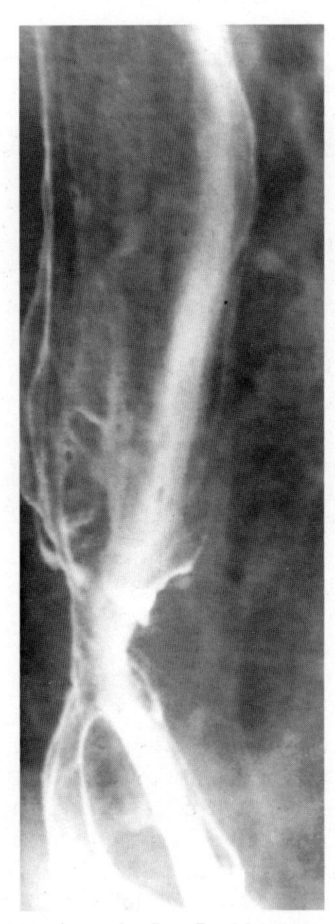

Fig. 3.8 Gastro-oesophageal reflux. Double contrast barium swallow showing a stricture and oesophagitis. Note the linear folds and scarring. This appearance can occasionally be caused by carcinoma. Endoscopic biopsy should be postponed until the oesophagitis has healed to facilitate endscopic and histological interpretation.

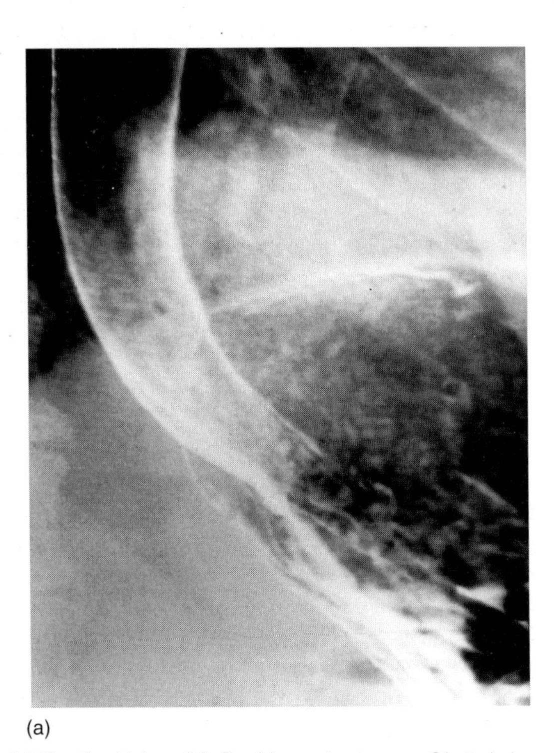

(a)

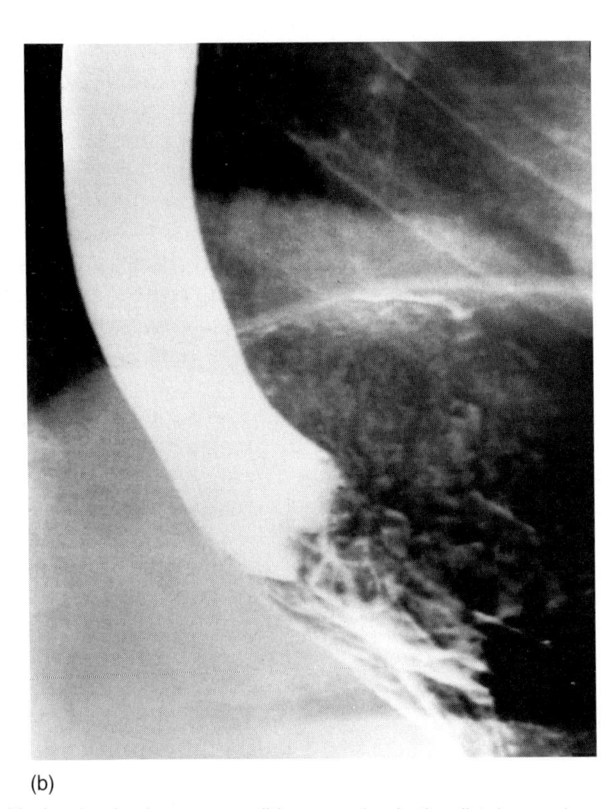

(b)

Fig. 3.9 Peptic stricture (a). Double contrast upper GI study in a patient with dysphagia shows a possible narrowing in the distal oesophagus (b). A marshmallow swallowed with a mouthful of barium lodges at the site of the stricture. The stricture supports a column of barium and reproduces the patient's symptoms, confirming the stricture which was shown to be a peptic stricture as a cause of the patient's dysphagia.

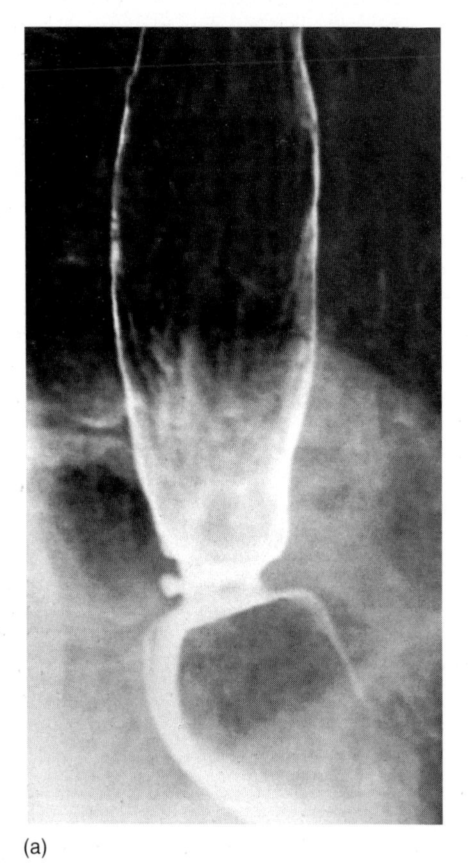

(a)

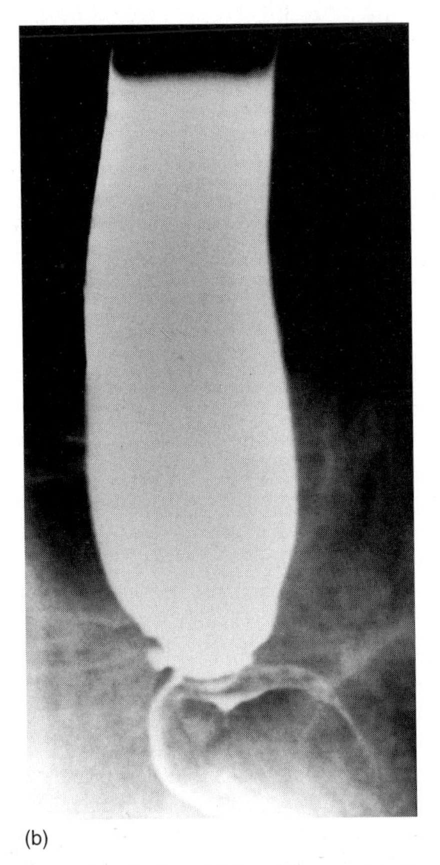

(b)

Fig. 3.10 Peptic stricture (a) in a patient with dysphagia (b). A small (7 mm) marshmallow was used to size the stricture. The marshmallow stuck at the stricture which supports a column of barium and reproduces the patient's symptoms.

originates in the gastric fundus and extends into the distal oesophagus. These folds are inflammatory and have no malignant potential, but cannot be distinguished radiologically from neoplasm, and therefore have to be biopsied.

Strictures are seen as a complication in 10–20% of patients with reflux oesophagitis, and may be circumferential and symmetrical (Fig. 3.9) or asymmetrical with sacculation and irregular borders (Fig. 3.10). When seen just above a hiatus hernia, a smoothly tapering stricture is virtually pathognomonic of a benign reflux-associated stricture. However, when all of these features are not present, endoscopic biopsy is advisable to rule out a malignant lesion. Chronic reflux may lead to a change in the distal oesophageal mucosa, from the usual squamous type to a columnar type known as Barrett's oesophagus. The columnar epithelium may be of the gastric type, or be specialized columnar or a junctional type: all three types can coexist at the same level. The presence of Barrett's oesophagus predisposes to the development of dysplasia and this can progress to frank adenocarcinoma (Fig 3.11). The risk of malignant transformation in a Barrett's oesophagus is one per 300 patient years. The presence of Barrett's oesophagus should be suspected when there is oesophagitis, an oesophageal stricture or a punched-out ulcer at a distance from the gastro-oesophageal junction especially if this is seen in the presence of a hiatus hernia and reflux. A distinctive reticular pattern is described on double contrast barium examination, but is not always seen. If a Barrett's oesophagus is suspected, endoscopy with brushings and biopsies of the oesophagus should be performed, both to establish the diagnosis and to allow an assessment of dysplasia.

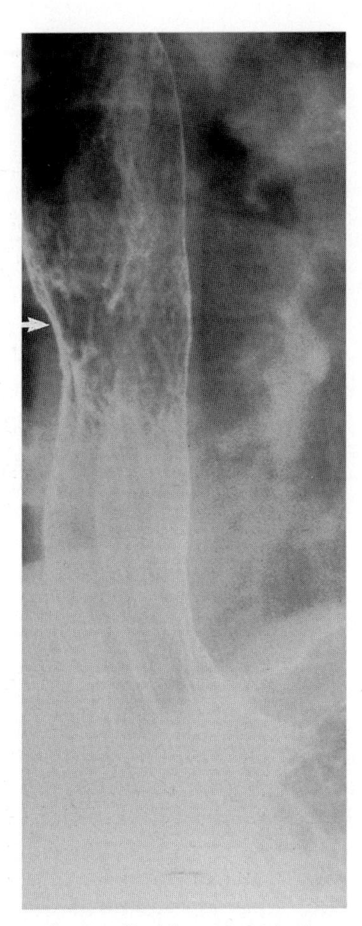

Fig. 3.11 Adenocarcinoma. Double contrast barium swallow showing narrowing and mucosal irregularity in the lower oesophagus some distance from the gastro-oesophageal junction in a patient with Barrett's oesophagus. The area of narrowing and mucosal abnormality (arrow) is due to adenocarcinoma.

Other oesophageal motility disorders

These may be of striated muscle or smooth muscle. Striated muscle is only present above the aortic arch where myasthenia and Eaton – Lambert syndrome are the main considerations, though these conditions are very rare.

There is a zone of transition where both types of muscle are present, and in the lower two thirds of the oesophagus, there is only smooth muscle. There may be too much motility as in **diffuse spasm** and **nutcracker oesophagus** in which chest pain and dysphagia coexist. Nutcracker oesophagus is hard to diagnose radiologically being characterized by fluoroscopically normal peristalsis with very high amplitude contractions (up to 1200 mm Hg) with delayed relaxation, and sometimes with associated non-peristaltic activity which can be seen spontaneously or provoked with edrophonium chloride. Diffuse spasm characteristically exhibits severe lumen-obliterating non-peristaltic activity, but it may be episodic and therefore overlooked. Manometry is a better way to diagnose these two disorders.

Diminished peristalsis may be seen in **achalasia**. In the early phase, vigorous achalasia may be seen. This condition is halfway between diffuse spasm and achalasia and shows vigorous lumen-obliterating contractions as well as a poorly or non-relaxing lower oesophageal sphincter. The characteristic finding in established achalasia is marked reduction or absence of the primary peristaltic wave from the aortic arch downwards, and failure of relaxation in the lower oesophageal sphincter. This soon leads to dilation of the oesophagus above the lower oesophageal sphincter, and the oesophagus may contain a considerable volume of food residue leading to a risk of aspiration and chronic recurrent chest infections. On barium studies there is slow emptying of the barium from the oesophagus into the stomach with the tight lower oesophageal sphincter producing a bird's beak appearance to the lower oesophagus (Fig. 3.12). Administration of gas granules will usually force open the sphincter and allow rapid emptying of the oesophagus in patients with primary achalasia. While these features are diagnostic of achalasia, they do not

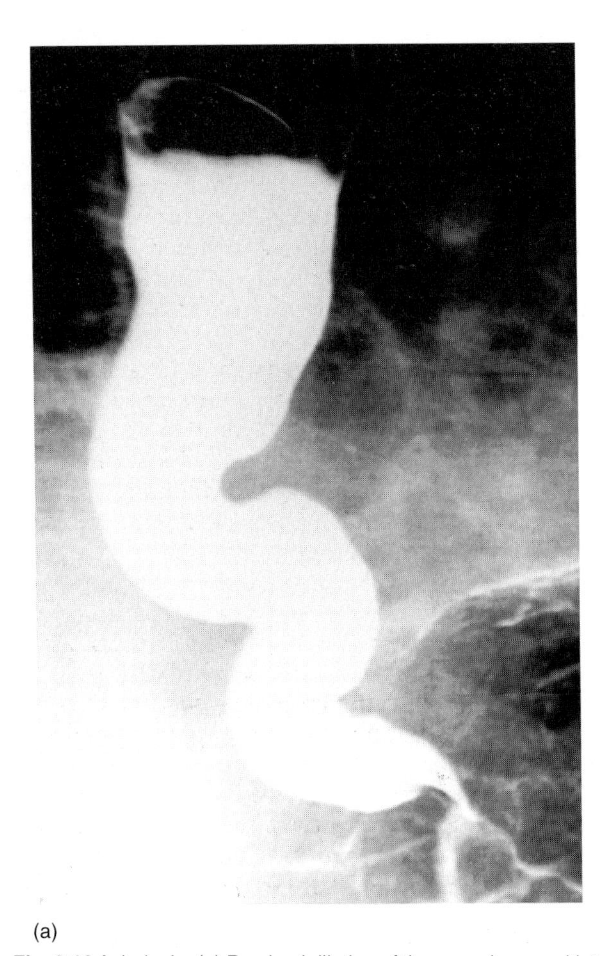

(a)

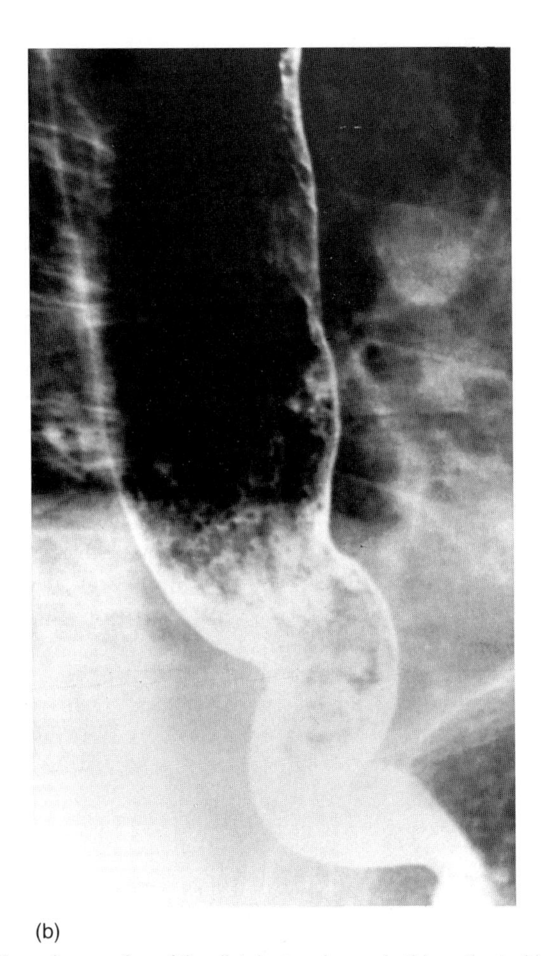

(b)

Fig. 3.12 Achalasia. (a) Proximal dilation of the oesophagus with tortuosity and narrowing of the distal oesophagus in this patient with dysphagia. The distal oesophagus is tapered and there is hold up of barium. (b) When gas granules are given, the distal oesophagus opens and allows the barium to pass into the stomach. There is no primary oesophageal peristalsis. A careful examination of the fundus is important to exclude secondary achalasia due to tumour.

distinguish between primary and secondary achalasia. Secondary achalasia is caused by gastric adenocarcinoma, or metastatic tumour, such as from breast carcinoma, infiltrating the submucosal oesophageal neural plexus and producing non-relaxation of the sphincter and diminished peristalsis. This may be suspected radiologically by the demonstration of a mass in the fundus, by the failure of the lower oesophageal sphincter to open with a gas-granule bolus by mouth, or by failure of the lower oesophageal sphincter to relax when the patient sniffs amyl nitrite. Endoscopy and biopsy are required to exclude or document such a secondary achalasia. Achalasia itself predisposes the oesophagus to malignant transformation with the risk of oesophageal squamous carcinoma being approximately 10 times greater than in a control population.

Oesophageal dysmotility may also occur in **scleroderma**, which involves the oesophagus in approximately 80% of cases. The smooth muscle of the oesophagus is replaced by collagen which results in reduced or absent lower oesophageal peristalsis and a low resting lower oesophageal sphincter tone. These abnormalities lead to marked gastro-oesophageal reflux, reflux oesophagitis and stricture formation. These radiological findings, in combination with the reduced primary peristalsis seen on fluoroscopy, suggest the diagnosis of scleroderma. Radiologists should ask about Raynaud's phenomenon in any patient with severely reduced primary peristalsis. It is important to differentiate between scleroderma and idiopathic reflux disease: patients with scleroderma respond badly to fundoplication because the feeble peristalsis cannot push food through the wrap.

The dermatological skin conditions of **epidermolysis bullosa dystrophica** and **pemphigoid** can also affect the oesophagus. Oesophageal involvement with epidermolysis bullosa dystrophica is a disease of childhood which should be investigated with double contrast barium studies because endoscopy carries an unacceptable risk of perforation. The study may show bullae involving the oesophageal mucosa which appear as discrete filling defects within the oesophagus. These may be extensive and produce areas of ulceration in the mucosa when they burst. Disordered motility also occurs and in severe cases strictures develop. Pemphigoid is a disease affecting older patients in whom bullae may also rarely be observed but the more usual finding is superficial ulceration. At a later stage strictures develop in the upper oesophagus.

Oesophageal webs and rings

Webs and rings may be found as incidental findings but may also produce dysphagia. The most common abnormal oesophageal ring in the lower oesophagus is at the gastro-oesophageal junction, and was described by Richard Schatzki (Fig. 3.13). The symptomatic **Schatzki ring** is associated with a hiatus hernia and responds well to balloon dilatation. The characteristic history is of intermittent dysphagia for meat in a patient with mild to moderate reflux symptoms. Luminal narrowing to below 12 mm causes dysphagia in almost all cases, while narrowing above 20 mm rarely causes symptoms. The rings are only visible on maximal distension which is why the mild ones are readily overlooked at endoscopy and on barium studies unless a marshmallow bolus is used. It is unknown why some patients with reflux disease develop extensive oesophagitis with stricture but no ring, and others develop a Schatzki ring with little or no oesophagitis.

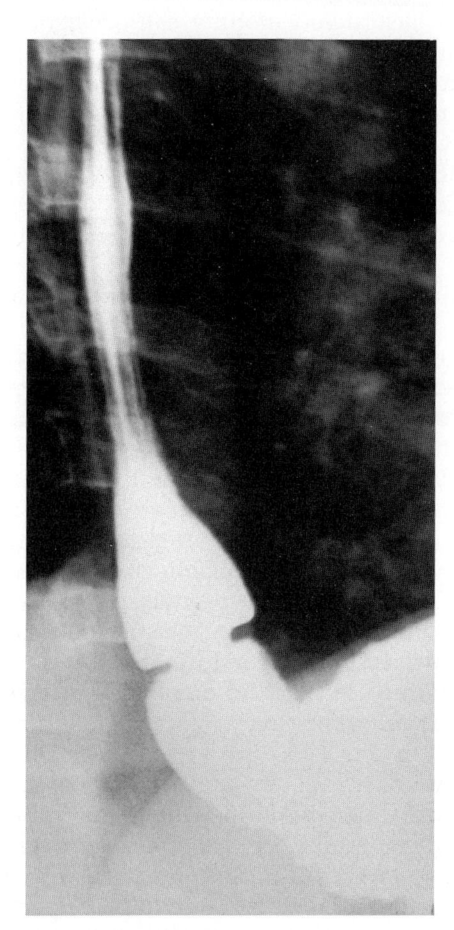

Fig. 3.13 Schatzki ring causing dysphagia, demonstrated on the single contrast phase of a barium swallow.

Oesophageal webs may be idiopathic, or part of the **Paterson–Kelly–Plummer–Vinson syndrome**. Webs are 1–2 mm thick structures, usually occurring in the cervical oesophagus in older patients. The idiopathic variety is very common, being seen in up to 8% of patients referred for barium examination of the oesophagus. In some patients the webs contain heterotopic gastric mucosa leading to the possibility of peptic ulcer disease. Isolated patches of gastric mucosa are often observed in the cervical oesophagus endoscopically but their significance is unknown. Other webs are seen in the lower oesophagus associated with gastro-oesophageal reflux. The association of cervical oesophageal webs, iron-deficiency anaemia and pharyngeal or oesophageal carcinoma in the Paterson–Kelly–Plummer–Vinson syndrome remains controversial.

Non-reflux oesophagitis

Oesophagitis is most frequently due to gastro-oesophageal reflux, but there are many other causes.

Infectious oesophagitis usually presents with odynophagia in contrast to the heartburn or dysphagia of reflux disease. Infectious oesophagitis may be caused by a wide range of pathogens, the most common being candida, herpes simplex and cytomegalovirus (CMV) but tuberculosis, diphtheria, cryptococcus and other organisms are occasionally responsible. Cases of infectious oesophagitis are most often seen in patients with reduced immunocompetence due to diabetes mellitus, chemotherapy, radiotherapy and treatment with steroids or antibiotics. Increasingly, infectious oesophagitis is encountered in patients immunosuppressed following transplantation or with depressed T-cell function due to HIV infection.

By far the most common cause for infectious oesophagitis is candidal infection, usually from *Candida albicans*. At endoscopy, adherent white plaques are seen on a background of erythematous, friable mucosa. Double-contrast barium studies have a sensitivity of 90% in the diagnosis of candidal oesophagitis. The appearance of multiple well-defined slightly raised nodules that run in a longitudinal fashion, interspersed between normal-looking mucosa, is a highly suggestive pattern. Other patterns include a cobblestone appearance due to coalescing plaques, and prominence of the longitudinal oesophageal folds or granular pattern due to oedema. In more severe cases pseudomembrane formation and deeper ulceration lead to a shaggy appearance of the oesophagus or even a double-barrelled oesophagus due to undermining of the mucosa (Fig. 3.14). Areas of narrowing are usually due to oedema but true strictures can occur and tend to be long and smoothly tapering.

Herpes oesophagitis causes small vesicles which later burst leaving a shallow ulcer. In a more advanced state pseudomembrane formation occurs giving a similar appearance to that seen with candida. In 50%

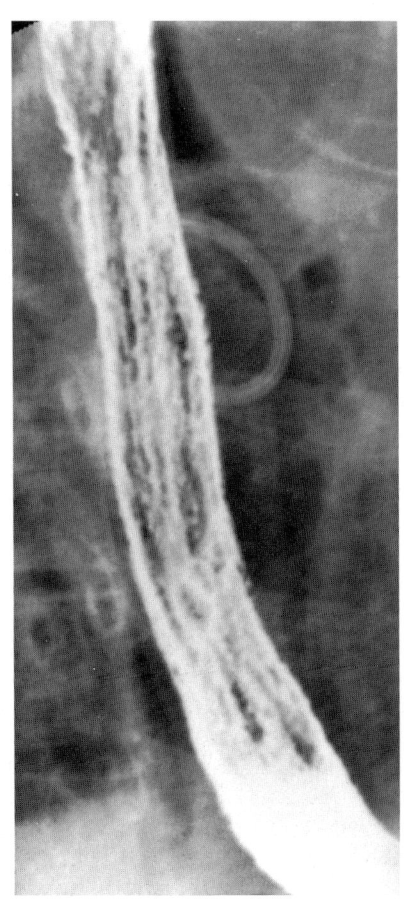

Fig. 3.14 Candida oesophagitis. Patient with lymphoma undergoing chemotherapy showing shaggy appearance of the oesophagus due to ulceration. (Courtesy of S.S. Amar.)

of patients with endoscopic herpes oesophagitis, double contrast barium studies show discrete ulcers, usually in the mid-oesophagus. These ulcers are often surrounded by a ring of surrounding oedema giving a halo appearance on the barium study.

CMV oesophagitis appears endoscopically as discrete ulceration with normal surrounding mucosa. On double contrast barium studies CMV may appear as large superficial ulcers measuring a few centimetres in diameter, a finding rarely seen with the other forms of infectious oesophagitis. Less common are superficial ulcers similar to those seen with herpes. Granular mucosa and thickened longitudinal folds from CMV infection occasionally mimic reflux oesophagitis.

Oesophagitis leading to stricture formation may also be caused by **ingestion of drugs** particularly doxycycline, tetracycline, potassium chloride and quinidine, especially when tablets remain in the oesophagus for longer than usual. This prolonged transit may be due either to reduced motility or because tablets are taken in the supine position or without a water chaser. The oesophagitis is usually mid-oesophageal as this is where tablets tend to stick because of the slight narrowing caused by external compression from the aorta and left main bronchus, and also because this is the site of least effective peristalsis, the point where striated and smooth muscle merge and where the manometric pressure during peristalsis is lowest. A large left atrium can cause a further area of oesophageal compression and predispose to tablet hold-up and subsequent oesophagitis. On double contrast barium studies there are ulcers usually in the mid-oesophagus. The ulcers are often shallow and may be single or multiple.

Radiotherapy to the thorax used in the treatment of malignancy affecting the lung, mediastinum or thoracic spine can also lead to oesophagitis. The oesophagitis presents with substernal burning pain, dysphagia or odynophagia, two to three weeks after the radiotherapy. The symptoms may last several weeks or subside over a 48-hour period. Most patients are treated empirically but if double-contrast barium studies are performed in the acute phase they will demonstrate superficial ulceration in the segment corresponding to the radiation field. With higher radiation doses the appearance may be more striking, with large ulcers and areas of mucosal sloughing and the possible development of fistula formation. The fistulae are usually to the left main bronchus and are caused by radiation necrosis due to end arteritis obliterans. Disordered motility can occur one to two months after the completion of therapy. Stricture formation within the irradiated segment may occur later, usually four to eight months after the radiotherapy.

Sclerotherapy is another cause of oesophageal injury, occasionally leading to an incompetent lower oesophageal sphincter, reflux, severe ulceration and stricture.

Corrosive chemicals, such as acids, alkalis and phenols, when ingested can cause injury to the oesophagus. The damage caused by alkalis tends to be more severe than that seen with acids. The oesophagitis progresses through an acute necrotic stage followed by ulceration and sloughing of necrotic mucosa which then heals with granulation tissue. Later there is fibrosis with resultant strictures which are smoothly tapering and occur in the region of the carina, although the whole oesophagus may be involved. Steroids, antibiotics and prophylactic dilatation are employed but despite these measures up to 40% of patients proceed to stricture formation. In the patients who do proceed to stricture there is an increased risk of oesophageal carcinoma.

Neoplasms

Dysphagia with or without weight loss may be the presenting symptom of oesophageal malignancy, which is squamous cell carcinoma in 90% of cases. Adenocarcinoma accounts for about 10%, particularly in the presence of Barrett's oesophagus, and carcinosarcoma about 1%. Oesophageal carcinomas occur in the distal oesophagus in 40%, in the mid-oesophagus in 40% and in the proximal oesophagus in 20%. Tumours can be detected on the mucosal relief phase of a barium study but the best method is with double contrast. On barium studies early oesophageal carcinomas may appear as an area of mucosal irregularity, a sessile polyp or a zone in the oesophagus which does not distend as well as the rest. Barium swallow is not a reliable method to detect early and asymptomatic carcinoma. Cytology appears to be the most sensitive technique for early lesions. Barium swallow, properly performed, remains a sensitive investigation for those carcinomas which are causing dysphagia. Large tumours may give the appearance of irregular sessile polyps often with ulceration, or as an apple-core stricture. Advanced tumours may appear as smoothly tapering strictures, irregular strictures or as coarse nodular lesions. A varicoid variety resembling oesophageal varices may also be seen.

Once the diagnosis is established a CT scan provides information with regard to staging (Fig. 3.15), but CT is not completely reliable for the detection of aortic invasion or for local lymph node involvement. Endoscopic ultrasound is under investigation as an alternative method, but its place is not yet established. Prognosis is good for patients with early stage disease but such patients are very rare. By the time dysphagia is present there is little hope of cure, with 5-year survival figures remaining stubbornly below the 5% level.

The oesophagus can be involved by **secondary malignant disease** either by direct invasion, invasion from adjacent lymph nodes or by blood-borne metastases. Bronchogenic carcinoma is the most common primary to affect the oesophagus. With direct invasion the appearances are similar to those seen in primary malignant disease. Nodal involvement causes focal narrowing usually of the anterior oesophageal wall in the mid-oesophagus.

Benign tumours of the oesophagus can cause dysphagia although most are detected as incidental findings on barium studies performed for other indications. The most common benign tumour is the **leiomyoma** accounting for about 50% of benign tumours. Leiomyomas predominantly occur in middle-aged men and histologically they resemble uterine fibroids in appearance. Leiomyomas develop in the smooth muscle of the muscularis externa usually in the distal two-thirds of the oesophagus. Leiomyomas in the oesophagus are usually between 1 and 6 cm in size although they can grow very large and weigh up to 5 kg. Despite this, they rarely ulcerate and so are seldom a cause of blood loss. The leiomyoma may be seen as a soft-tissue density mass projecting from the wall of the oesophagus and with double contrast barium studies these submucosal lesions appear as a filling defect.

Foreign bodies

Dysphagia, odynophagia or chest pain may be caused by intraluminal obstruction secondary to a swallowed foreign body. This is most often seen in infants, children or patients with psychiatric problems. Smooth foreign bodies such as coins, buttons and batteries may pass freely into the stomach but if they do lodge in the oesophagus they tend to do so in areas of normal narrowing, at the thoracic inlet, the aortic arch and the diaphragmatic hiatus. These swallowed foreign bodies may stick elsewhere in the oesophagus, particularly if there is an underlying and perhaps subclinical stricture. Sharp foreign bodies do not lodge in such a predictable fashion and may snag at any level. The most common swallowed foreign body causing dysphagia is a partially chewed meat bolus. Metallic foreign bodies are easily seen on a plain film but for other objects contrast studies may be needed. Again the use of a marshmallow swallow can be very

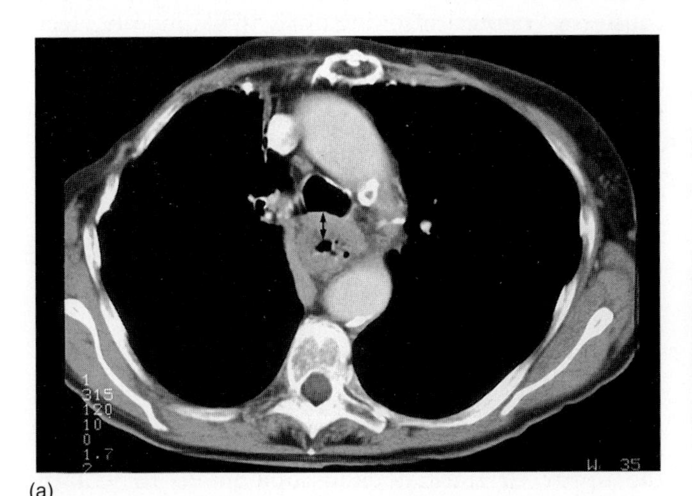

(a)

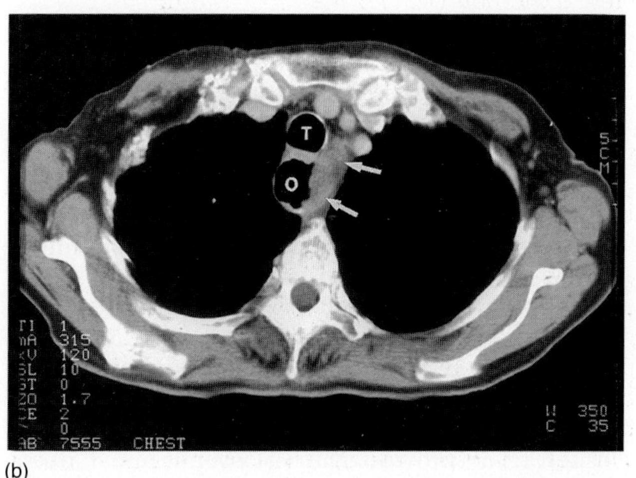

(b)

Fig. 3.15 Carcinoma of the oesophagus. (a) The tumour is causing marked thickening of the wall of the oesophagus (arrows); (b) a more cranial section shows tumour (arrows) extending alongside the trachea (T) and dilated oesophagus (O).

useful for showing small, otherwise hard-to-demonstrate foreign bodies. If there is any chance of a perforation caused by the swallowed foreign body water-soluble contrast should be used initially. Water-soluble contrast should also be used if there is any chance that endoscopy may be needed afterwards, since barium clogs the suction and biopsy channels of an endoscope. The use of atropine to relax the oesophageal musculature or of glucagon to relax the lower oesophageal sphincter may help to encourage the passage of a lodged foreign body, as will swallowed gas granules in selected patients.

Trauma

The oesophagus may be perforated spontaneously by vomiting, iatrogenically during endoscopy, and sometimes by closed or penetrating trauma. Vomiting causes gastric fundal mucosa to intussuscept into the lower oesophagus, which may cause a tear in the mucosa of either the oesophagus or the stomach. This is the **Mallory–Weiss tear**, which presents with haematemesis. These longitudinal tears are almost impossible to see on barium swallow and are best diagnosed by endoscopy. Vomiting against a closed throat or with a full stomach may cause a tear in the oesophagus that is full thickness (**Boerhaave's syndrome**). Typically this tear occurs in the left posterior wall of the lower 5 cm of the oesophagus, and leads to a leak that goes directly between the leaves of the inferior pulmonary ligament, where it may be contained for a while, appearing on the plain film as a triangular-shaped air collection behind the heart. Once the ligament gives way, gastric contents escape into the left pleural cavity as well as up into the mediastinum. Plain films may be sufficient for diagnosis, but if there is doubt, a water-soluble contrast swallow will reveal the leak.

GASTRIC AND DUODENAL DISEASE

Barium meal, endoscopy, ultrasound and CT can be used to examine the stomach and duodenum. Both barium and endoscopy miss about 5% of lesions over 1 cm in diameter, but endoscopy is far more accurate for small lesions. Erosive gastritis can be detected readily on good barium meals and severe gastritis and duodenitis can also be diagnosed with some reliability. Endoscopy also has the advantage of permitting biopsies but has a higher associated morbidity and mortality. The inability to visualize oesophageal motility limits the endoscopic assessment of reflux disease by comparison with a barium study. Thus young mobile adults will have most serious pathology adequately demonstrated on a good barium meal and barium study provides the best overall initial assessment of gastro-oesophageal reflux disease. On the other hand, patients with GI bleeding, or previous gastric surgery as well as those who are elderly or immobile are best assessed for gastroduodenal disease with endoscopy. Overall, endoscopy is more sensitive than barium for gastric and duodenal pathology, and is easier to perform well in the old and immobile, so that it is the initial examination of choice for suspected gastric and duodenal disease.

Disease of the stomach and duodenum may present with dyspepsia, abdominal pain, weight loss, anorexia, vomiting or symptoms of acute or chronic blood loss.

Dyspepsia which affects up to 40% of the population, may be defined as pain or discomfort in the upper abdomen or chest which is relieved or exacerbated by eating. Many would insist that it should be present for not less than three weeks before any investigation is performed. Dyspepsia has numerous causes including gastro-oesophageal reflux disease, oesophageal and gastric motility disorders, peptic ulcers, gastric carcinoma, pancreatitis and biliary pathology. Patients with these symptoms are often investigated with barium studies or endoscopy of the upper GI tract together with abdominal ultrasound. Performing all of these investigations on the 40% of the population with symptoms would be a huge financial drain and also result in a large number of deaths on the basis of current postendoscopy mortality data (one death in 10 000 procedures). The main concern with not investigating these patients is that a gastric carcinoma will be missed but a carcinoma is rare in patients under the age of 50 years and in those without weight loss or anaemia. A rational approach is to treat with a trial of H_2-receptor or proton pump blockers those patients suffering dyspepsia for three weeks in whom the suspicion of gastric carcinoma is low, i.e. those without weight or blood loss. Further investigation may be confined to patients with little or no response after 10 days and those whose symptoms have improved but not resolved at 10 weeks. The discovery of the key role of *Helicobacter pylori* as the cause of peptic ulcer disease will modify this approach. Serum or saliva testing will soon be available allowing the presence of *H. pylori* infection to be established at initial presentation.

Gastritis and duodenitis

Inflammation of the stomach and duodenum has numerous causes, but a major discovery of the last decade has been that a newly recognized organism, *H. pylori* infects the stomach of perhaps 40% of the population in developed countries and 85% of the population in less developed countries. Children living in poor or overcrowded conditions acquire the infection during the first few years of life. *H. pylori* is a gram negative, spiral bacillus isolated from biopsy of the upper GI tract at endoscopy in up to 95% of patients with chronic antral gastritis. *H. pylori* is also found in 80% of patients with gastric ulcers and in virtually 100% of patients with duodenal ulcers. *H. pylori* causes an acute antral superficial gastritis, increased gastrin output, hyperchlorhydria, and duodenal or gastric ulceration. It sometimes causes a hypertrophic gastritis, progressing to Ménétrier's disease; it may also cause a lymphoid response in antral mucosa progressing to lymphoid hyperplasia and mucosa-associated lymphoid tissue (MALT) lymphoma. In some patients the gastritis progresses to atrophy and intestinal metaplasia. The organism count then declines as it cannot live on intestinal cells, but the metaplasia may progress on to dysplasia and carcinoma. There is therefore considerable interest in treatment aimed at eradication of *H. pylori*, and effective identification and elimination of the organism may lower the need for barium meal or endoscopy for dyspepsia. However, eradication is not entirely without risk, and there have been deaths from pseudomembranous colitis in patients on drug therapy. The treatment is expensive and often with minor side effects but the cost of eradication is substantially less than that of repeated treatment for recurrent duodenal ulceration. Radiologically, *H. pylori* infection may be suspected when antral gastritis is diagnosed on the basis of thickened folds and/or erosions in the antrum in the absence of non-steroidal anti-inflammatory drugs (NSAIDs) or aspirin (Fig. 3.16). Findings of duodenitis such as thickened folds, poor coating and erosions in the absence of Crohn's disease and coeliac disease, are also suggestive of *H. pylori* infection, as is the recognition of heterotopic gastric mucosa in the duodenal bulb (Fig. 3.17).

There are other important causes of gastritis. Erosive gastritis and duodenitis occur in over 20% of

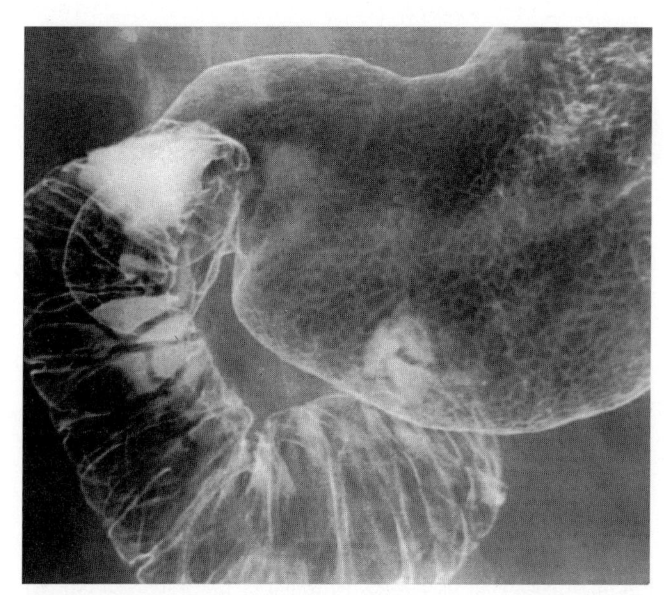

Fig. 3.16 Large areae gastricae. Enlarged areae gastricae in the antrum are associated with duodenal ulcer disease and this is now known to arise on the basis of *H. pylori* infection and increased gastrin production.

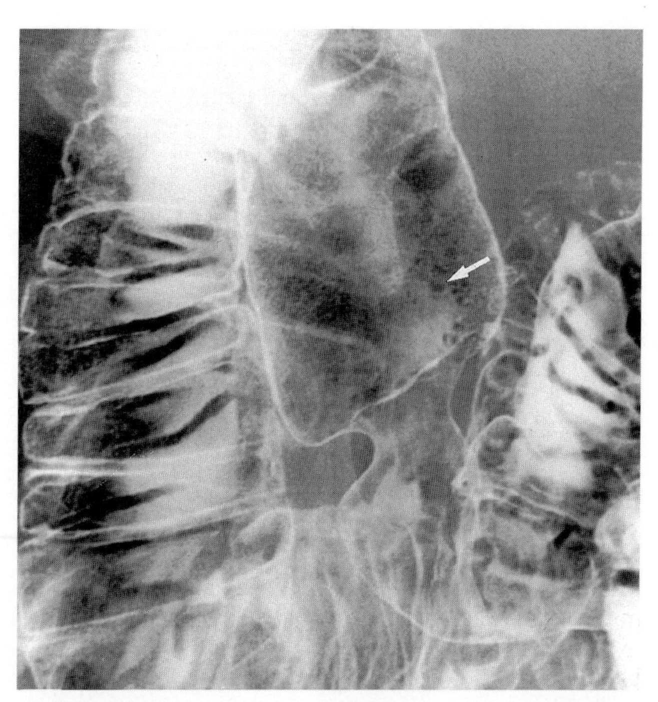

Fig. 3.17 Heterotopic gastric mucosa in the base of the duodenal cap seen as small polygonal filling defects (arrow). Originally described radiologically as a normal variant, they are now readily visible endoscopically. Such heterotopia is often associated with *H. pylori* infection, but the strength of this association is unknown.

patients with Crohn's disease, but disease in these sites is rarely the cause of initial presentation. Sarcoidosis and certain infectious agents, in particular tuberculosis and syphilis cause gastritis. Eosinophilic gastritis, usually in the antrum, is associated with a blood eosinophilia, but is seldom an isolated lesion and is usually seen in association with ulceration or strictures in the small bowel. Ulcerations and erosive gastritis may be idiopathic or due to a direct toxic action on the stomach by corrosives, certain medications and following radiotherapy.

Ménétrier's disease presents clinically with epigastric pain, weight loss and peripheral oedema secondary to protein loss from the stomach. On barium studies it is characterized by marked thickening of the gastric folds (Fig. 3.18) but involvement of the antrum does not preclude the diagnosis. The mucosal detail is often poor because of the copious amounts of mucus seen in this condition. It is associated with low or absent acid production in 75% of patients and represents a late stage of *H. pylori* infection.

Peptic ulcer disease

Duodenal ulcers are almost always benign but both benign and malignant gastric epithelium may ulcerate.

Both gastric and duodenal ulcers are typically seen as round collections of barium usually < 1 cm in diameter, and mucosal folds radiating outward indicate some degree of chronicity. During healing, ulcers

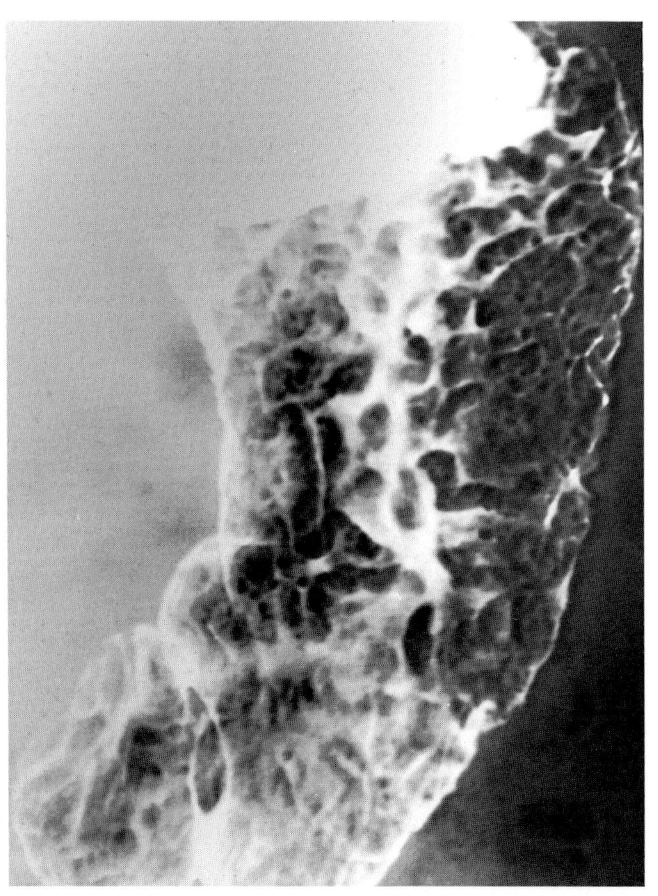

Fig. 3.18 Ménétrier's disease. Double contrast seen on barium meal as thick rugal folds. Thick folds may also be seen in Crohn's disease, lymphoma and Zollinger–Ellison syndrome. Patients with thick folds should have an upper GI endoscopy with biopsy to obtain the definitive diagnosis and to test for *H. pylori*.

Duodenal ulcers are seen in the cap in 95% of cases and most postbulbar ulcers are seen proximal to the ampulla of Vater (Fig. 3.19). The anterior wall of the duodenal bulb is the site of 50% of duodenal ulcers and is the area most difficult to examine radiologically. Duodenal ulcers distal to the papilla are infrequently seen and suggest the diagnosis of Zollinger – Ellison syndrome. Multiple ulcers are also suggestive of the Zollinger – Ellison syndrome but are seen in up to 15% of patients with peptic ulcer disease. Duodenal ulcers heal quickly with appropriate treatment but may lead to bulbar deformity or an ulcer scar with radiating folds originating at the site of the original ulcer crater. The ulcer scar may have a small central depression, which when seen with surrounding radiating folds can be mistaken for an active ulcer. When bulbar deformity is produced through scarring, the unaffected parts of the duodenal cap balloon outward as pseudodiverticula. When these pseudodiverticula are multiple the classic 'cloverleaf' appearance of the duodenal cap is produced. Scarring from ulcers in the pyloric canal, distal antrum and postbulbar region can lead to outflow obstruction. Endoscopy is the preferred examination in dyspeptic patients with previous duodenal ulcer disease.

When trying to assess whether gastric ulcers are benign or malignant, it is important to obtain images of the ulcer in profile and *en face*. The profile views are often improved by imaging the patient erect and the *en face* views by the use of compression. Benign ulcers penetrate through the gastric mucosa and cause more extensive destruction in the submucosa leading to an undermining of the overlying mucosa. In malignant sometimes become serpiginous or linear. In the past **gastric ulcers** were often larger on initial presentation but now with earlier treatment large ulcers are rare in countries where there is ready access to medical care. When giant gastric ulcers, defined as larger than 3 cm, are seen, they are associated with a higher complication rate from perforation and bleeding but not with a higher malignancy rate. Most gastric ulcers occur on the lesser curve or the posterior wall of the antrum or body and the distribution tends to be more distal in young patients, since gastric ulcers occur in transitional epithelium. The level of the junctional epithelium migrates up the stomach with increasing age, so that the elderly often have their gastric ulcers high on the lesser curve near the cardia. Benign ulcers in the fundus or in the proximal part of the greater curve are very rare and any ulcer in this position should be biopsied in case of malignancy. Most ulcers are single but multiple ulcers are seen in 20% of cases and each of the ulcers must be assessed individually to determine the aetiology, as benign and malignant ulcers can coexist.

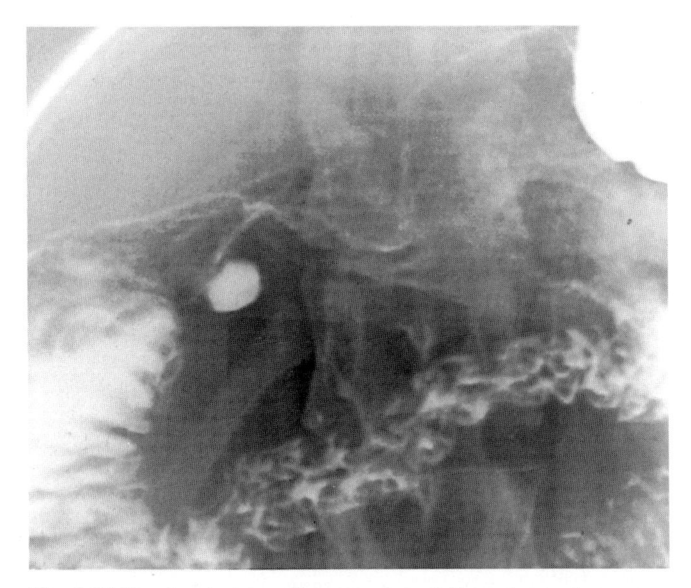

Fig. 3.19 Duodenal ulcer with narrowing of the pylorus shown on water-soluble contrast study to rule our perforation. Endoscopy is not required for ulcers that are clearly in the duodenal cap (bulb), but is prudent for pyloric channel ulcers which may represent ulceration in a distal gastric carcinoma.

ulceration, the ulcer occurs within an area of malignant epithelium. Ulcers which penetrate beyond the wall of the stomach are likely to be benign but this can be seen with early gastric carcinoma. The radiating folds with benign ulceration tend to be regular and are seen up to the edge of the ulcer crater, while in malignant disease the radiating folds end before reaching the ulcers and are irregular or amputated in appearance. Two careful studies have shown that a gastric ulcer which has the characteristic radiological features of a benign ulcer is histologically benign. Ulcers of indeterminate status on radiological criteria (about 25% of which prove to be malignant) and ulcers that are clearly radiologically malignant (about 95% confirmed as malignant) should be biopsied without delay. Since gastric ulcers should be followed to complete healing in order to reduce the likelihood of relapse, it makes sense to make endoscopy the follow-up procedure to assess for healing, and to biopsy for dysplasia and *H. pylori*. An ulcer that fails to heal on treatment must be biopsied.

Peptic ulcers can also lead to perforation which may be free or confined. Free perforation occurs when an ulcer erodes into the peritoneal cavity which typically occurs with ulcers on the anterior wall of the stomach or duodenum. Anterior gastric wall ulcers are rare and most free perforations are caused by duodenal ulcers. If there is free peritoneal air on plain films then no further imaging is usually required, but when there is a suspicion of perforation but no free air, water-soluble contrast studies may be indicated. When there has been a perforation but there is no free air, the perforation is not shown on a contrast examination in 50% of cases because of spontaneous sealing. Of those in whom perforation is shown, 50% show a free leak into the peritoneal cavity and the other 50% a contained leak within a walled-off cavity. Posterior wall ulcers occasionally perforate through to the lesser sac or into the anterior pararenal space. Water-soluble contrast studies can show these leaks but the extent of any abscess formation is better assessed by abdominal CT or ultrasound examination. Confined perforation of posterior wall ulcers involves the pancreas in up to 75% of cases but may also penetrate surrounding organs to produce an abscess in the liver, spleen or transverse mesocolon. These confined leaks show as abnormal gas collections on plain films or cavities on water-soluble contrast examination in 50% of cases. CT can demonstrate the presence of the abscess cavity even after the leak has sealed off and should be considered whenever there is a deep posterior wall ulcer. Fistulae may develop secondary to peptic ulcer disease and include gastroduodenal (seen as a double-channel pyloric canal on barium studies), gastrocolic, gastropericardial, duodenocolic, choledochoduodenal and duodenorenal fistulae. Barium studies can usually determine the site, size and communication of the fistulous track.

Zollinger – Ellison syndrome should be suspected when postbulbar ulcers and ulcers in the fourth part of the duodenum or jejunum are demonstrated either on barium meal or endoscopy especially if accompanied by large quantities of resting fluid in the stomach and duodenum. The syndrome is caused by hypersecretion of gastrin either from an autonomous tumour or, rarely, from primary G-cell hyperplasia which results in the production of large quantities of gastric acid. The tumour is usually malignant and is situated in the pancreas in 75% of cases, in the duodenum in 15% and in other sites in 10%. Some 25% of gastrinomas are associated with multiple endocrine neoplasia (MEN type 1) and are seen in combination with tumours of the parathyroids, pituitary and adrenal. The large quantities of gastric acid leads to peptic ulcers in 90% of patients and the volume of gastric secretions produces diarrhoea in 50%. The ulcers are often multiple and resistant to treatment with H_2-receptor blockers although the proton pump inhibitor omeprazole can lead to healing. When the Zollinger – Ellison syndrome is strongly suspected on biochemical and clinical grounds, the patient should be assessed for metastatic disease using ultrasound, CT or MRI. When there is no widespread metastatic disease and surgical cure is being considered radiology may help with tumour localization. In addition to the cross-sectional imaging, additional information may be obtained preoperatively by endoscopic ultrasound and selective angiography. This may be supplemented by arterial stimulation with secretin and venous sampling for gastrin. During surgery intraoperative ultrasound is an excellent localization technique and should increasingly be used in these complex cases.

Benign tumours

Gastric polyps are hyperplastic in 75–90% of cases. **Hyperplastic polyps** have no malignant potential and if positively identified require no further follow-up. They appear radiologically as smooth sessile lesions, usually measuring <1 cm in size, and occur mainly in the gastric fundus or body. When in the dependent part of the barium pool they appear as filling defects but when seen on the non-dependent surface they are outlined by a ring or crescent of barium at the junction between the polyp and the normal mucosa. Hyperplastic polyps can grow larger, and then may be pedunculated or lobulated, in which case the diagnosis of a hyperplastic polyp cannot be made with certainty and endoscopic excision biopsy is required. There is evidence in some cases that hyperplastic polyps regress following eradication of *H. pylori*.

Adenomatous polyps do have malignant potential, with carcinomatous foci being found in 50% of those >2 cm in size. They occur most commonly in the antrum appearing as filling defects in the dependent barium pool and may be sessile or pedunculated. Adenomatous polyps tend to be more lobulated than

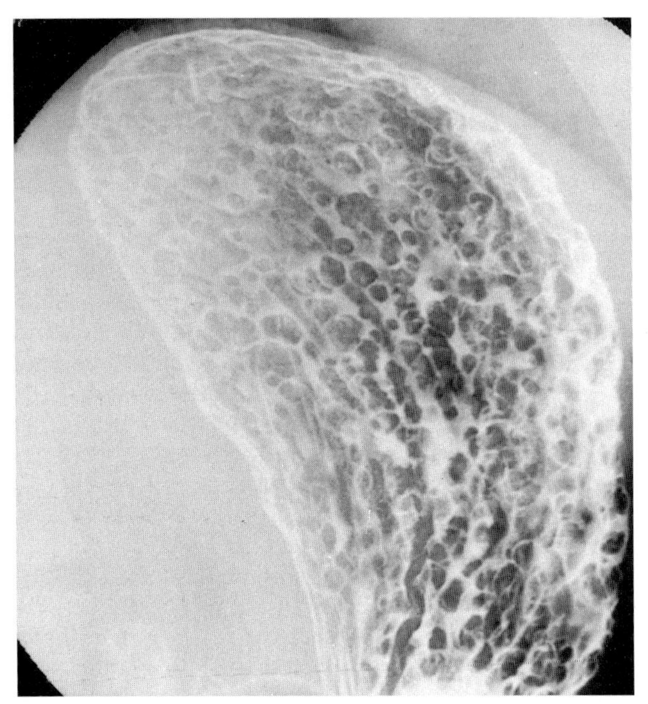

Fig. 3.20 Hyperplastic gastric polyps in a patient with familial polyposis coli. The polyps spare the antrum and are benign.

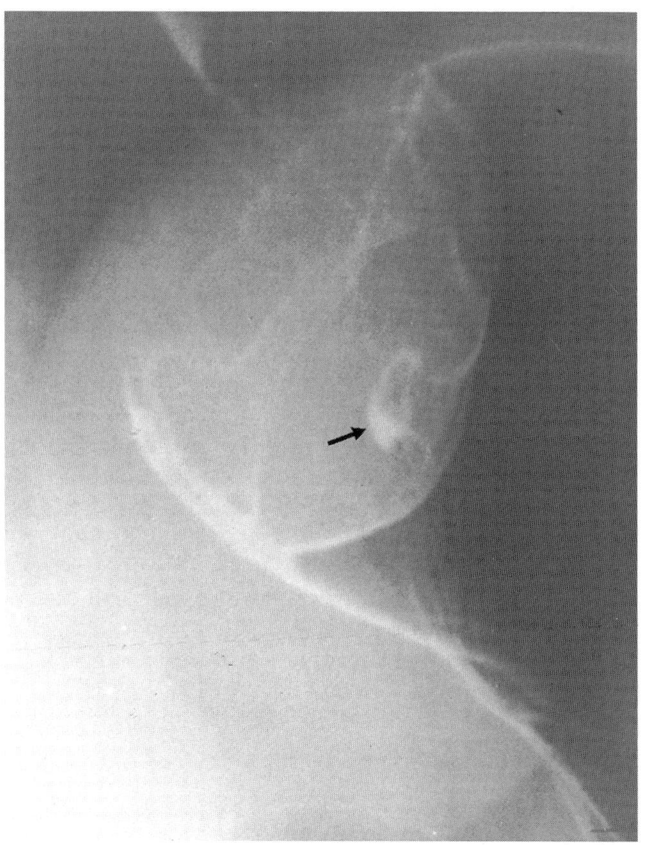

Fig. 3.21 Leiomyoma. The barium study shows a large smooth mass at the cardia with a central depression containing a pool of barium (arrow). The patient presented with a haematemesis due to bleeding from the ulcer.

hyperplastic polyps and are usually larger measuring > 1 cm. In view of the malignant potential adenomatous polpys should undergo endoscopic excision biopsy. Adenomatous polyps are also found in the stomach and duodenum in both familial polyposis coli and Gardner's syndrome, but most gastric polyps in these conditions are hyperplastic and occur in the gastric fundus (Fig. 3.20).

In Peutz – Jeghers' syndrome, the gastric polyps are **hamartomas** with almost no malignant potential and appear as sessile or pedunculated polyps measuring up to 3 cm in size. Hamartomatous polyps are also seen in juvenile polyposis. Cronkhite – Canada and Cowden's syndrome also have gastric hamartomatous polyps and these have a small malignant potential. Cronkhite – Canada syndrome in contrast to the others is characterized by a carpet of small, subcentimetre, gastric polyps.

Leiomyomas account for about 40% of benign gastric tumours and may cause problems due to haemorrhage, a palpable mass, nausea or, in the case of pedunculated tumours, gastric outflow obstruction due to prolapse into the antrum or duodenum. Leiomyomas may rarely be recognized on plain films as a soft-tissue mass but are more commonly picked up on barium studies of the stomach or by endoscopy. Small leiomyomas are covered with normal gastric mucosa, indent the normal gastric outline and have well-defined margins when seen *en face*. With larger tumours there is often ulceration, seen radiographically as a barium-filled crater on the surface of the tumour mound (Fig. 3.21).

Ectopic pancreatic rests can mimic leiomyomas. They are usually single, measure up to 3 cm in size and are located on the greater curve of the gastric antrum or between the duodenal cap and the ampulla of Vater (Fig. 3.22). Like leiomyomas, they may have a central puddle of barium. This is due to a rudimentary ductal system producing a dimple on the surface of the rest. If the duct system is more advanced it may appear as multiple small pouches filled with barium and this appearance is pathognomonic of ectopic pancreatic rests.

Malignant tumours

Gastric carcinoma has been in decline over the last fifty years but in those who have the disease the outlook remains poor with a 20% 5-year survival rate. Gastric carcinoma is predominantly a disease of middle-to-old age but the proportion of young patients affected is increasing. The fundus, body and antrum are affected equally with about 10% of tumours being diffusely infiltrating. Over 90% of cases are due to adenocarcinoma and most are detected in an advanced stage, i.e. they have invaded the muscularis propria. There are two types of the disease: a diffuse (signet cell) type which affects younger people

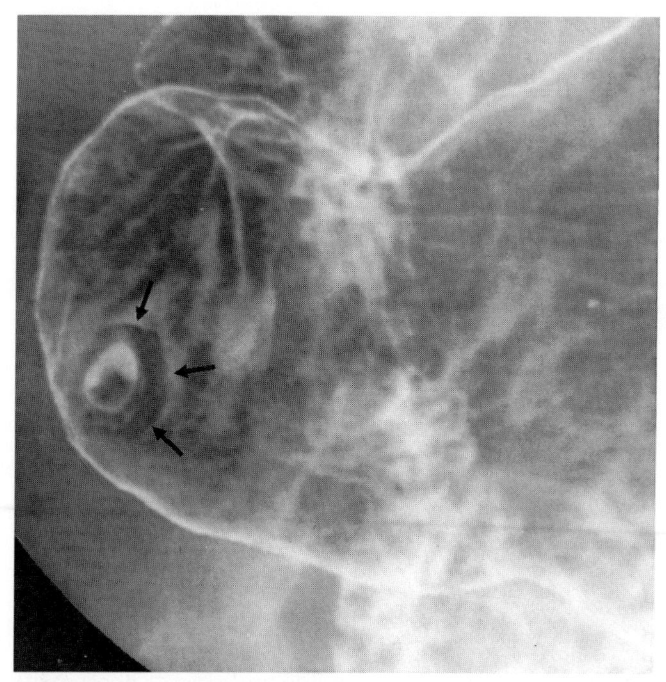

Fig. 3.22 Ectopic pancreas. This raised lesion (arrows) in the antrum with central depression could be an ulcer, an ulcerated carcinoma or, most likely at this site, ectopic pancreas, which was the final diagnosis. Endoscopy is required to confirm the diagnosis.

and has an incidence that has not changed over the years, and an intestinal type that is associated with intestinal metaplasia and is due largely to *H. pylori* infection and its sequelae. Pernicious anaemia and the associated autoimmune gastritis is also associated with gastric carcinoma but *H. pylori* is no more common in these patients than in the general population. Gastric carcinoma remains common in several countries and the precise role of genetic and environmental factors, including *H. pylori*, remains unclear, although the World Health Organisation has now accepted *H. pylori* as a primary carcinogen for gastric cancer. Partial gastrectomy, particularly the Bilroth II variety, is associated with later development of gastric carcinoma in the gastric remnant.

The Japanese Endoscopy Society has classified early gastric carcinoma (Table 3.1). Type I lesions are seen on barium studies as polypoid masses projecting into the lumen of the stomach. These may be of considerable size and still be early carcinoma histologically, because many of these lesions represent malignant change in a adenomatous polyp. Type II lesions may appear as areas of mucosal irregularity, nodularity or loss of the normal mucosal pattern, and may be slightly elevated or depressed. Type III lesions are areas of ulceration with barium pooling, but, in contrast to the features seen with benign ulcers, the Type III early gastric cancers tend to have shallow ulcers with radiating folds which stop abruptly at some distance from the ulcer. The radiating folds may be fused or clubbed.

Table 3.1 Early Gastric Cancer (Japanese Classification)

Type	*Description*	*Appearance*
I	Polypoid (>0.5 cm in height)	
IIa	Superficial, elevated (<0.5 cm in height)	
IIb	Superficial, flat or minimal elevation	
IIc	Superficial, depressed	
III	Excavated	

Early lesions, particularly in the region of the cardia, are not easily demonstrated and subtle changes in the gastric fold pattern should be sought. Lesions under 1 cm are usually missed, and even 1–2 cm Type II lesions are very hard to detect unless ulcerated. Endoscopy is a little more sensitive than barium for detection of small early gastric

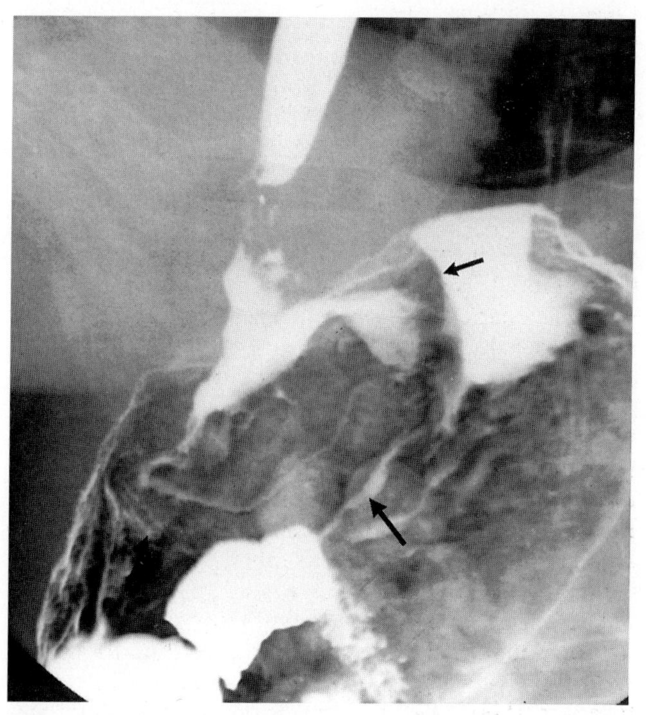

Fig. 3.23 Carcinoma of the cardia (arrows) invading the oesophagus. The prevalence of carcinoma at this site is increasing, possibly due to short segment Barrett's disease.

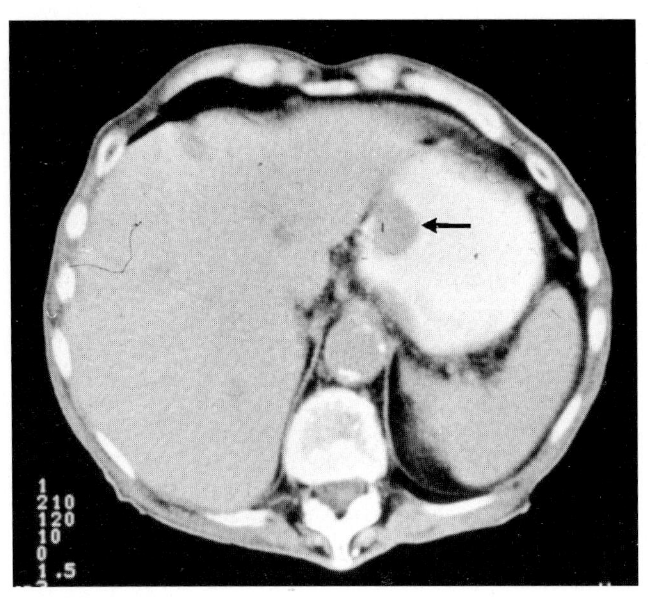

Fig. 3.24 Malignant gastric polyp shown on CT examination in an elderly patient with anaemia as a filling defect in the contrast-filled stomach (arrow). (Courtesy of E. Jurriaans.)

carcinomas, but the flat non-ulcerated lesions are still very easily overlooked.

Advanced carcinomas are more obvious on double-contrast studies, and Borrmann has described four types:

Type 1: A non-ulcerating polypoid mass which projects into the lumen of the stomach. These lesions may become very large (Fig. 3.23) but are usually well-differentiated (Fig. 3.24). When the mass lies in the barium pool in the dependent portion of the stomach, it appears as an irregularly polypoid, nodular filling defect and, when on the non-dependent surface, it is outlined by a ring of barium.

Type 2: A fungating tumour which is closely related to a Type 3 lesion.

Type 3: An ulcerating gastric carcinoma which may show tumour nodules in the surrounding mucosa. The folds radiating out from the ulcer are fused, clubbed and amputated, stopping at a distance from the actual ulcer crater.

Type 4: A scirrhous carcinoma which infiltrates the stomach producing a shrunken or non-distensible stomach known as linitis plastica or water-bottle stomach. There is often antral sparing with the tumour seen as an area of non-distensibility in the body and/or fundus (Fig. 3.25). Adequate gaseous distension is needed if this is to be recognized. Scirrhous tumours may also produce slight mucosal irregularity or nodularity.

CT and endoscopic ultrasound are used to stage gastric carcinomas, with assessment of direct and lymphatic spread. CT findings of enlarged local nodes or local invasion are unreliable and do not necessarily

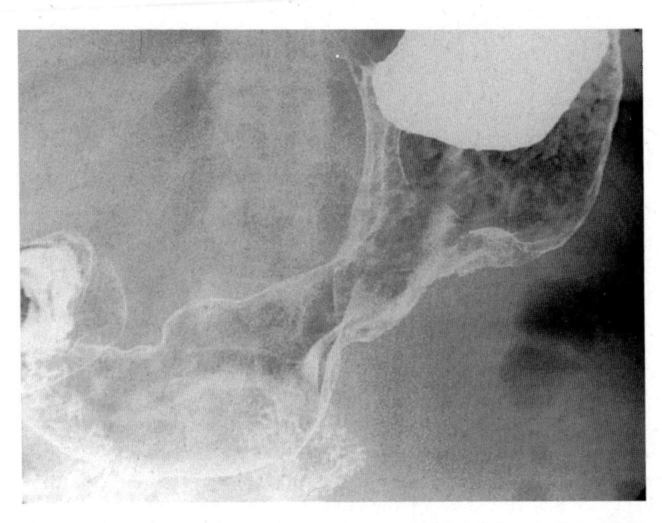

Fig. 3.25 Advanced gastric carcinoma. Lack of local distensibility draws attention to a tumour of the greater curve of the stomach. There is also compression of the lesser curve. CT scan showed that this was due to simple liver cysts and not to metastases.

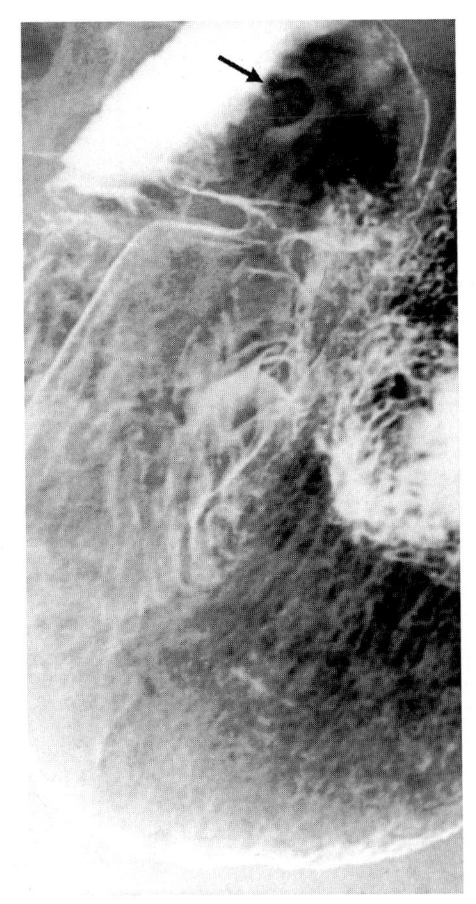

Fig. 3.26 Normal variants are common and can be confusing. This 'polyp' (arrow) at the apex of the duodenal bulb is normal and is produced by bulking of mucosa at the acute angle between the distended first and second parts of the duodenum. (Courtesy S. Laplante.)

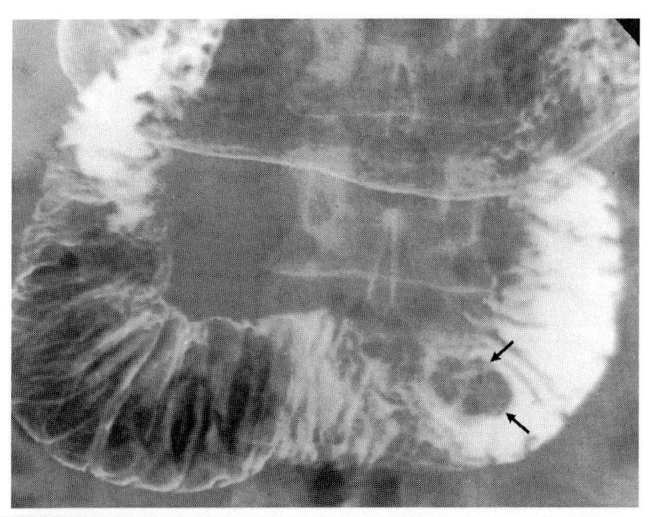

Fig. 3.27 Adenomatous polyp in the third part of the duodenum (arrows). Barium study performed with Buscopan as hypotonic agent.

indicate advanced disease. CT is more accurate at showing distant metastatic disease, but minor findings should not be accepted without biopsy confirmation. With these provisos, CT scanning may be useful in surgical planning for these patients, especially in directing the approach to a palliative rather than curative resection.

Other duodenal lesions

The duodenum may be affected by disease of neighbouring organs such as the pancreas, and there are also uncommon duodenal primary tumours, such as leiomyoma, leiomyosarcoma, neurofibroma and carcinoma. These neoplasms may present with bleeding or obstruction and are readily shown on barium studies, but they must be distinguished from pseudopolyps which are due to redundant mucosa when there is acute angulation of the intestine, most commonly at the junction of the first and second parts of the duodenum (Fig. 3.26). Lesions that appear primarily duodenal require endoscopy and biopsy (Fig. 3.27) while extrinsic compression or invasion is best assessed by CT examination (Fig. 3.28).

An unusual cause of vomiting occurs in obstruction of the third part of the duodenum by the root of the superior mesenteric artery. This occurs in patients who have lost a great deal of weight, and once it has developed, the obstruction leads to further weight loss. Enteral or parenteral nutrition and regaining weight will cure the condition in those who do not have a serious underlying disease. Barium study shows a dilated second and third part of duodenum with vigorously peristals is and sudden cut-off in front of the aorta (Fig. 3.29). Turning the patient prone results in flow of barium past the obstruction, indicating that it is not a stricture.

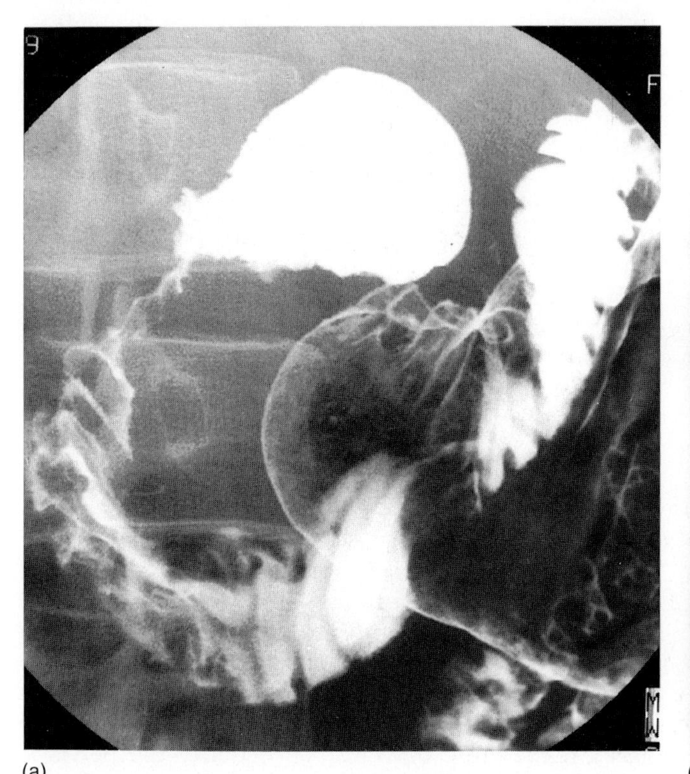

(a)

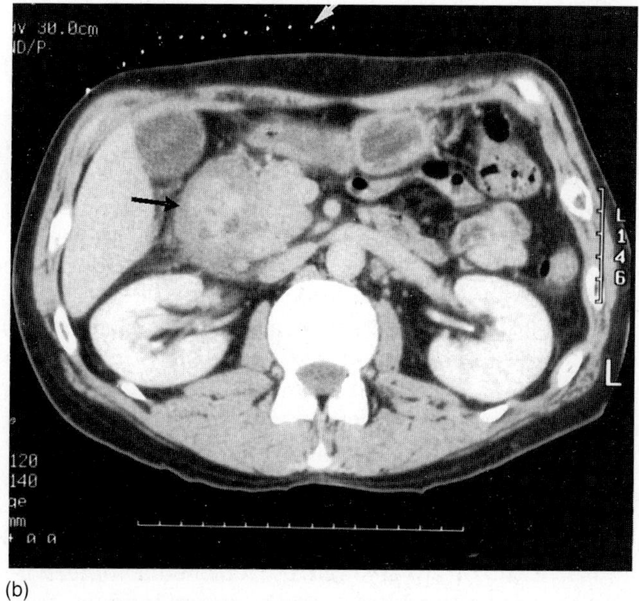

(b)

Fig. 3.28 Chronic pancreatitis. (a) Barium meal and (b) CT scan in 49-year-old patient with vomiting and elevation of serum alkaline phosphatase. The compression of the duodenum could be due to pancreatitis or carcinoma. CT scan was chosen to confirm the pancreatic origin of the mass (black arrow), and to guide percutaneous biopsy. Note the anterior abdominal wall skin markers as an aid to biopsy (white arrow). Biopsy was negative for cancer and the clinical course remained consistent with chronic pancreatitis.

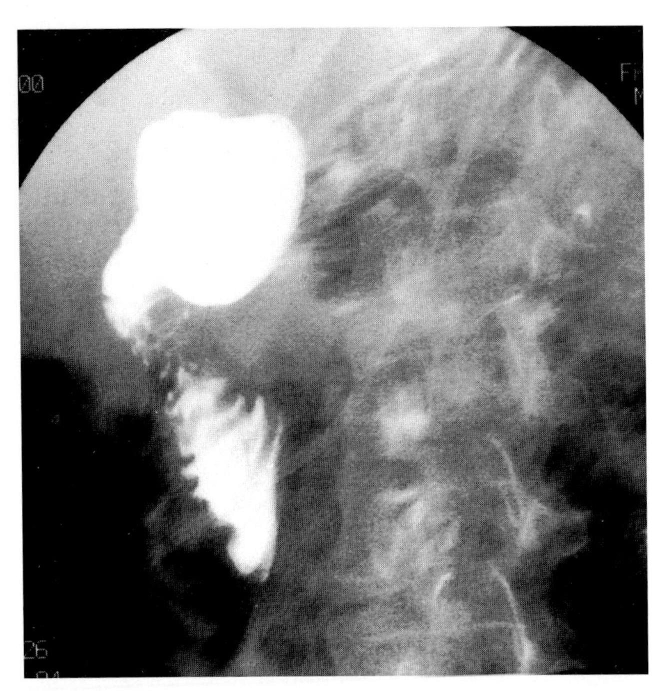

Fig. 3.29 Superior mesenteric artery syndrome. Abrupt termination to the barium column in the third part of the duodenum is seen in a patient with marked weight loss secondary to an eating disorder. There was active peristalsis in the more proximal duodenum. Following the passing of a jejunal tube for feeding and weight gain the obstruction in the third part of the duodenum resolved.

LOWER GI TRACT

SMALL BOWEL

Examination

Only the first and last 15 cm of the small bowel are within reach of the endoscopist. Investigation relies heavily on barium-based studies either single or double contrast, though ultrasound and CT are proving to have an increasingly valuable role. Examination of the stomach and duodenum requires a relatively small volume of high-density barium and the injection of an agent to reduce motility (such as Buscopan), while investigation of the small bowel requires a large volume of low-density barium and often the oral administration of metoclopramide to shorten transit time. The examination of the stomach and duodenum therefore has requirements which are in direct contrast to those needed for adequate examination of the small bowel.

Clinical findings should be used to decide whether to request a barium meal or a small bowel study. Examination of the small bowel may be by means of a small bowel meal or by a small bowel enema, otherwise known as enteroclysis. Both examinations have strengths and weaknesses. The small bowel meal is quicker, easier to perform, is less uncomfortable for the patient and has minimal complications. Enteroclysis allows better evaluation of the exact site of pathology and gives more bowel distension, facilitating assessment of adhesions.

For a **small bowel meal** the patient drinks a mixture of low-density barium and metoclopramide syrup, and plain films of the abdomen are obtained at intervals until the barium has reached the colon. Once contrast has reached the colon, spot views of the terminal ileum are taken. The rest of the small bowel is also carefully examined fluoroscopically with compression applied to separate loops of bowel and to assess for tethering. Following this an attempt may be made to view the distal ileum in double contrast by inserting a small tube into the rectum and insufflating carbon dioxide until it refluxes around the colon into the ileum (Fig. 3.30).

Optimal distension of the small bowel requires a high barium flow rate which can be achieved by **enteroclysis**. Rapid delivery of fluid to the stomach or duodenum increases the risk of gastro-oesophageal reflux and pulmonary aspiration. These risks are minimized by infusing barium directly into the jejunum. The patient's nose and throat are anaesthetized and intravenous sedation and metoclopramide administered. The tube is placed into the patient's nostril and advanced to the jejunum, with the help of a stiffening wire and changes in patient position. Once in the jejunum a balloon at the end of the catheter may be inflated to further reduce reflux. Enteroclysis can be performed as a single contrast study using dilute barium (Fig. 3.31) or as a double contrast study using higher density barium and a methylcellulose chaser. The column of barium is visualized using fluoroscopy as it advances through the small bowel and images are recorded for later study. The procedure is unpleasant for the patient but serious complications such as perforation are extremely rare.

The small bowel can be imaged with **transabdominal ultrasound**. The bowel can be assessed for peristalsis and wall thickening which is greatly helped by the use of a graded compression technique. Focal or generalized bowel wall thickening may be detected particularly if the appropriate clinical history and physical signs are given to guide the conduct of the examination.

CT examination is used in the assessment of the small and large bowel. A double dose of oral contrast is needed to opacify both distal and proximal intestine in order to distinguish intestinal loops from pathology. The first dose is given approximately 60 minutes before the CT examination and the second dose 10 minutes before. Rectal and vaginal contrast should be given if the large bowel or particularly the pelvis is being examined. Intravenous contrast is important if an abscess is suspected or if demonstration of mesenteric vessels is required to distinguish them from lymph nodes or metastases.

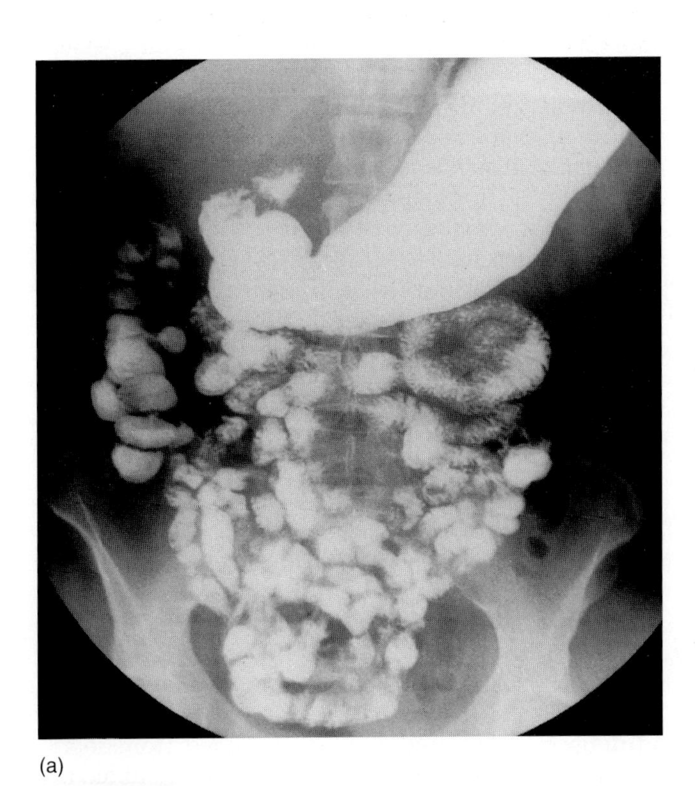

(a)

Fig. 3.30 Normal small bowel meal. (a) Digital image of the whole abdomen with the patient prone. Spot views of the terminal ileum are obtained in single (b) and double contrast (c). The mucosa in the terminal ileum is shown in exquisite detail.

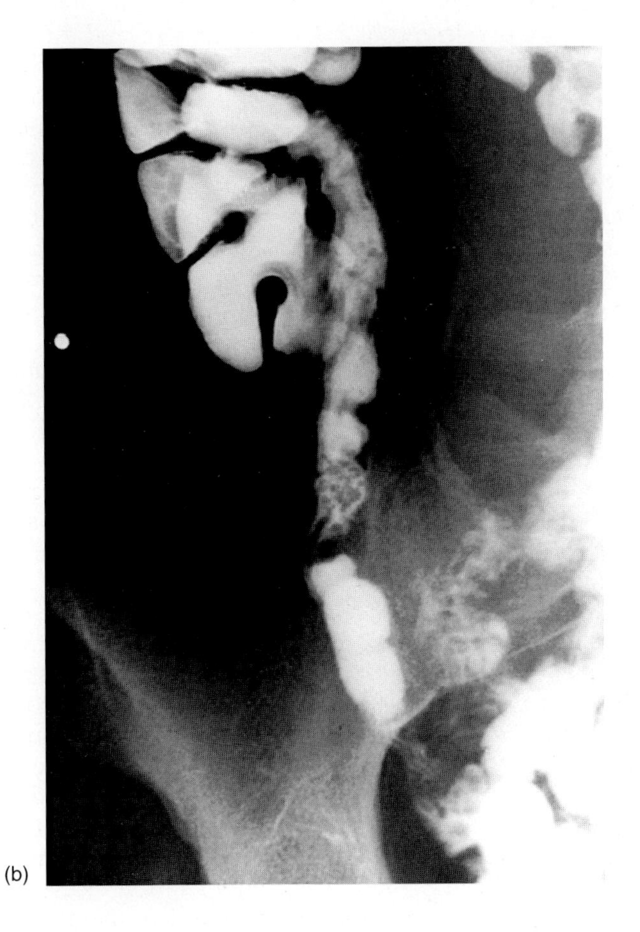

(b)

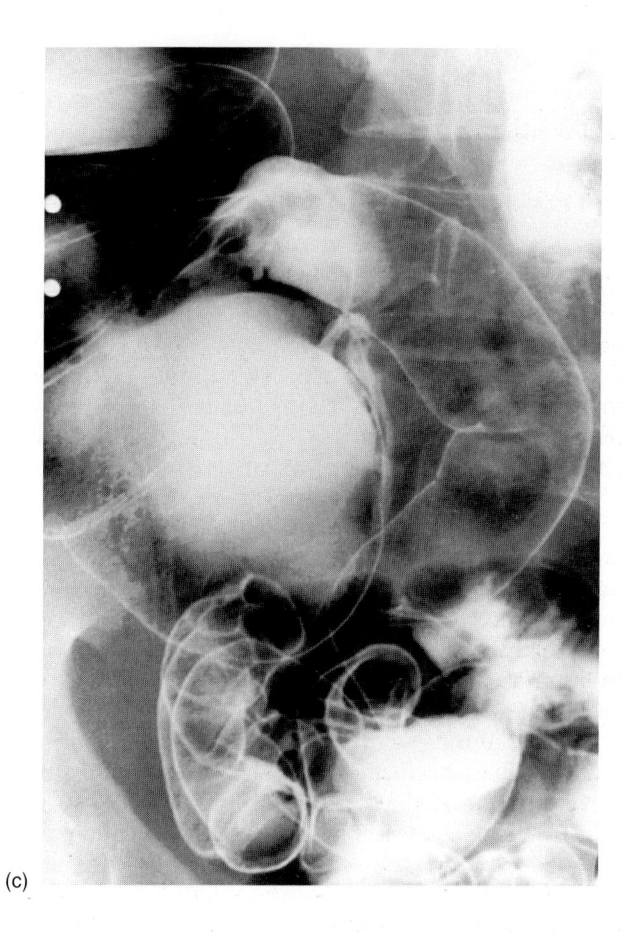

(c)

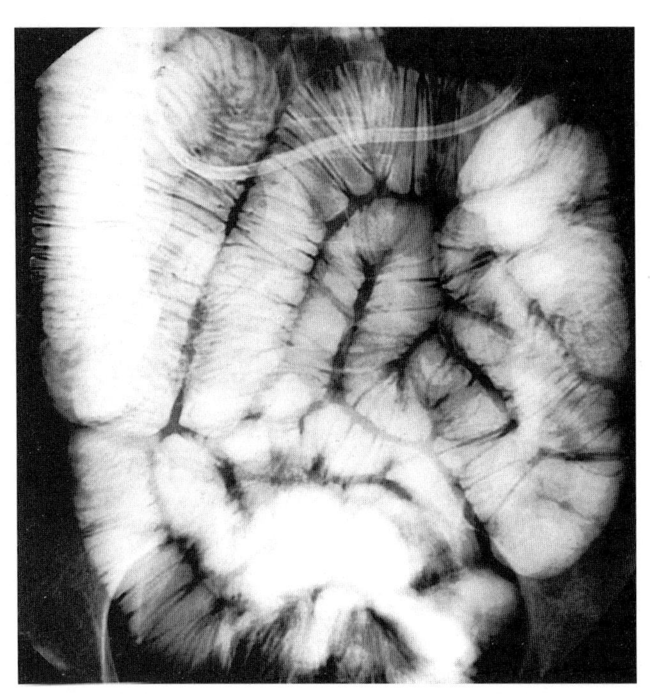

Fig. 3.31 Normal small bowel enema (enteroclysis) demonstrating normal valvulae conniventes and good distension of the small bowel. The use of a low-density barium and a high kilovoltage ensures that overlapping loops of bowel are not obscured.

One of the most common indications for investigation of the small bowel is the diagnosis or follow up of inflammatory bowel disease, in particular Crohn's disease (see p. 80).

Diseases of the small bowel

Malabsorption The diagnosis of malabsorption is made clinically and is often confirmed by biopsy of the distal duodenal or jejunal mucosa at upper GI endoscopy or by using a peroral biopsy technique under X-ray control, such as the Crosby capsule. Malabsorption may be due to a primary disorder of the bowel such as coeliac disease or may be secondary to infection or altered immunity. Barium studies remain helpful in equivocal cases to assess the extent of disease and to investigate for complications of the underlying disease. Tropical sprue shows similar appearances on barium studies to those seen with coeliac disease although the aetiology is very different.

Coeliac disease is particularly prevalent in northern Europe and is due to a sensitivity to alpha-gliadin. The complications of malabsorption include osteomalacia and there may be radiological evidence of this on the abdominal radiograph. The barium study is abnormal in 90% of patients and shows dilation of the jejunum, especially the more distal part. The valvulae conniventes are most often normal but, due to the dilation of the bowel, the margins may lose their rounded appearance and appear rather square (Fig. 3.32). Rarely, in advanced coeliac disease the valvulae may be completely absent. This is known as the 'moulage sign'. More commonly the number of valvulae increases in the ileum and decreases in the jejunum to the extent that there is a reversal of the normal pattern of distribution. The hypersecretion of fluid seen in coeliac disease may give the barium a rather granular appearance but the classic radiological sign of flocculation is rarely seen with the new barium preparations. Complications of coeliac disease may also be shown, including entero-enteric intussusception, lymphoma and carcinoma, which may affect the small bowel or the oesophagus.

Intestinal infections such as **giardiasis** can also cause malabsorption. Giardiasis is usually an acute illness but may become chronic with inflammation of the proximal small bowel. If it is suspected, diagnosis is by endoscopy and jejunal fluid aspiration. On barium studies there is thickening of the valvulae conniventes, spasm of the bowel and oversecretion of fluid, giving the barium a rather granular appearance. This abnormal appearance is confined to the jejunum and definitive diagnosis may be obtained from stool culture or distal duodenal/jejunal biopsies obtained at endoscopy.

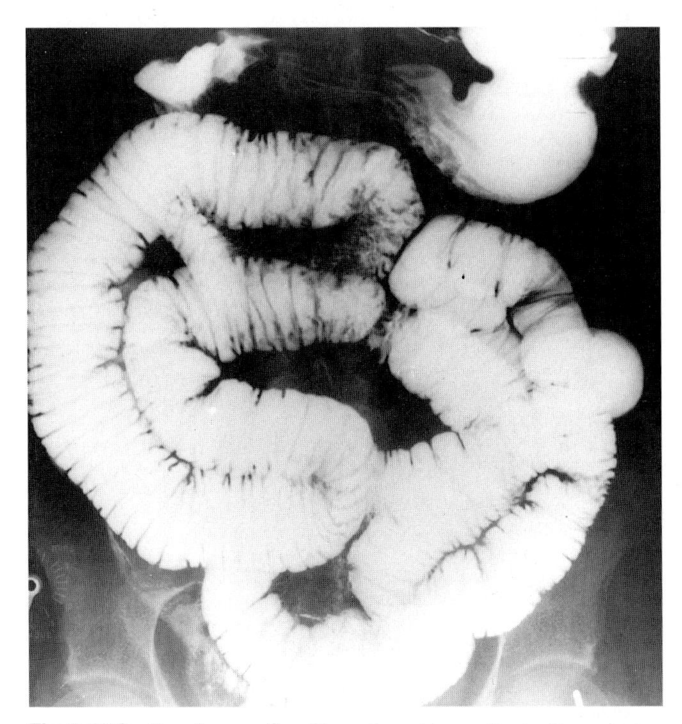

Fig. 3.32 Coeliac disease. Small bowel meal in a patient with anaemia. There is small bowel dilation and ileojejunal fold reversal. The left upper quadrant loops have fewer valvulae (like ileum), while those in the right lower quadrant have closely packed valvulae (like jejunum). Dilation is the most common finding and often the only abnormality, but fold reversal is not uncommon and is diagnostic.

Tumours These are much less common than those of the large bowel and are of different cell types.

Intestinal lymphoma constitutes about one-third of all small bowel malignant tumours and is most commonly of the non-Hodgkin variety. Lymphoma is also seen with an increased frequency in patients with AIDS and possibly in patients with Crohn's disease. Small bowel lymphoma has a variety of appearances on barium studies:

- Thickening of the bowel wall is the most common appearance due to lymphomatous infiltration. When this is diffuse, the abnormal bowel merges into normal bowel with no clear margin of transition. In the abnormal segment the mucosal folds may be absent or thickened. Bowel wall involvement and extramural disease are recognized by the separation of adjacent bowel loops, as only the lumen is filled with barium. Often there are slight strictures within the involved segment of bowel. Alternatively the involvement can be more localized and circumferential with well-defined margins.
- Mucosal abnormalities are produced by lymphomatous infiltration of the bowel and appear as loss of the valvulae and nodularity. The involved segment may be of normal diameter, narrowed or dilated. A lymphomatous mass may ulcerate, the ulceration appearing on barium study as a pool of contrast. The ulceration may be so extensive as to leave only a thin rim of viable lymphomatous cells at the base of the ulcer and in this case the barium study often shows a focally dilated segment of bowel. If the lymphoma is predominantly intraluminal it appears as a polypoid filling defect and can lead to obstruction. Less commonly, lymphoma causes multiple nodules which may carpet the bowel. These nodules may ulcerate and show a central depression filled with barium.
- Extramural spread may lead to fistulous connections between the affected bowel and adjacent normal loops of bowel. If the lymphoma is predominantly extramural and affecting the mesenteric nodes, the bowel outlined by barium may have a scalloped margin due to the external indentation. Although barium studies, particularly enteroclysis, show small bowel lymphoma to good effect, the extent of the disease, bowel wall thickening and involvement of regional lymph nodes are best seen with abdominal CT (Fig. 3.33). These advantages make CT an excellent technique for following the progress of the disease and its response to treatment. Follow-up scans should be performed to a set protocol so that direct comparisons can be made with previous studies.

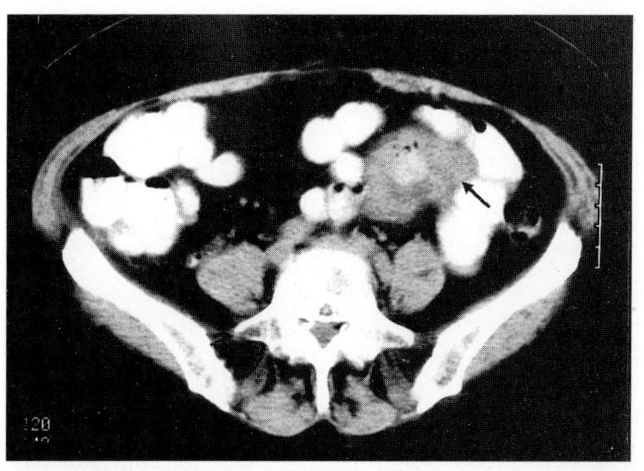

Fig. 3.33 Lymphoma showing bowel wall thickening. On this CT scan there is marked bowel wall thickening (arrow) in one of the ileal loops with contrast confined to the lumen. The stomach and a few other bowel loops also showed wall thickening due to lymphomatous involvement.

Adenocarcinoma may arise in the small bowel, the frequency decreasing with distance from the ligament of Treitz, with most tumours seen in the duodenum and jejunum. As in the colon, small bowel adenocarcinomas arise from malignant transformation within an adenoma. In families with Lynch II hereditary non-polyposis colon cancer the incidence of small bowel adenocarcinoma is 50 times greater than in the general population. On barium studies an adenocarcinoma commonly appears as a well-defined region of luminal narrowing with loss of the normal mucosal pattern and overhanging edges. The narrowing causes progressive obstruction with dilation of the bowel proximal to the carcinoma. The bowel wall thickening and involvement of regional lymph nodes may be seen to good effect with abdominal CT.

Carcinoid tumour most often originates in the bowel with 40% occurring in the appendix and about 30% in the small bowel. The histology of these tumours does not correlate well with the behaviour of the tumour. Tumours < 1 cm in diameter are unlikely to have distant metastases. On barium studies the tumours are often small and appear as nodules often in the distal ileum. The tumour can induce a fibrotic reaction in the adjacent mesentery resulting in kinking or acute angulation of bowel loops with straight segments of intervening bowel similar to that seen with postoperative adhesions. The bowel lumen may be narrowed either as a result of the desmoplastic reaction or due to compression from a mesenteric tumour mass. CT is proving useful in the assessment of carcinoid tumours and the liver can also be imaged for the presence of metastases (Fig. 3.34).

Metastases can spread from distant tumours to involve the small bowel via the blood, through the peritoneal cavity, by direct invasion from adjacent tumours or via lymphatics. Although malignant melanoma is a rare tumour it frequently spreads to involve the bowel. The metastases appear as multiple polypoid luminal filling defects, but there is often a sizeable extraluminal component as well. In the

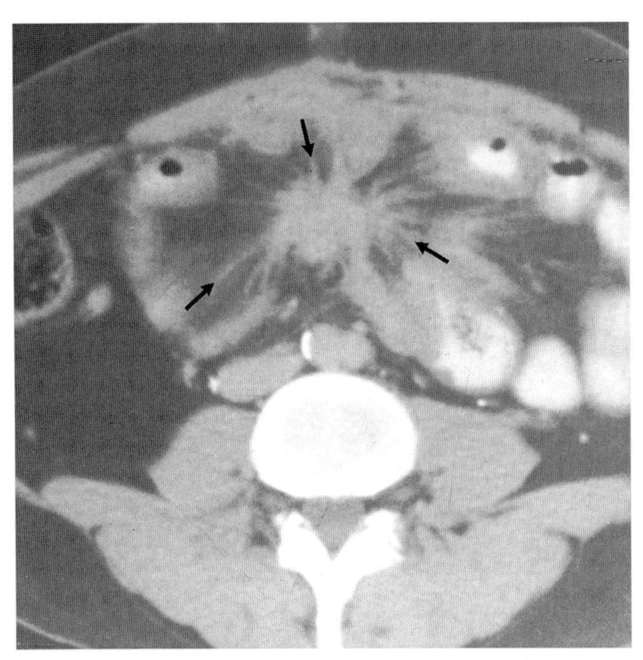

Fig. 3.34 Carcinoid. CT scan in a patient with diarrhoea showing a soft tissue mass and multiple radiating soft tissue strands (arrows) extending into the mesentery. This spoke wheel pattern indicates a desmoplastic reaction and is most commonly seen in carcinoid.

stomach and duodenum these intraluminal polyps show central depressions which fill with a pool of barium but this feature is rarely seen in the jejunum and ileum. These polypoid masses can act as a lead point for an intussusception (Fig. 3.35). Tumour nodules can also occur in the mesentery which cause external compression on the bowel. Metastatic melanoma can also appear as a large mass, in which ulceration can occupy almost the entire volume of the tumour resulting in a dilated segment of bowel which is prone to haemorrhage.

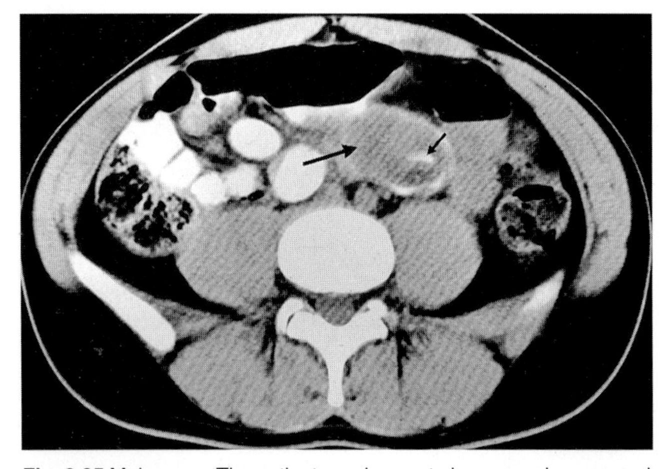

Fig. 3.35 Melanoma. The patient was known to have a melanoma and presented with an acute abdomen. The CT scan shows a large filling defect (long arrow) in the contrast-filled bowel, due to an intussusception which contains oral contrast in its centre (small arrow). At surgery the patient had a melanoma metastasis as the lead point of the intussusception. (Courtesy E. Jurriaans.)

Benign tumours of the small bowel are often asymptomatic but may cause bleeding or act as a lead point for an intussusception. **Leiomyomas** arising in the submucosa appear on barium studies as smooth filling defects with stretched but otherwise normal mucosal covering. If they arise in the subserosa then there may be no intraluminal component but adjacent loops of bowel will be displaced. On CT the leiomyoma is seen as a mass in which there may be central necrosis. **Adenomas** account for about 25% of benign tumours and can arise throughout the small bowel but are most often seen in the duodenum and proximal jejunum. **Lipomas** constitute the only other common small bowel benign tumour and they usually arise in the ileum. Lipomas appear as rounded filling defects on barium studies and it may be possible to change their shape by manual compression on the abdomen. The appearance on CT is a mass related to the small bowel, which has the attenuation value of fat.

LARGE BOWEL

Examination

Detailed imaging of the large bowel is by means of colonoscopy, contrast enema, CT, ultrasound and MRI. Endoscopy allows biopsy material to be obtained but is a more lengthy procedure with an associated higher morbidity and mortality. For routine colonoscopy and barium enema the patient must have bowel preparation so that the colonic mucosa can be well visualized. The bowel preparation is achieved by means of oral laxatives taken the day before the procedure. The routine radiographic study is the double contrast barium enema using high density barium. An antispasmodic agent such as Buscopan may be used if there is colonic spasm. Carbon dioxide or air is insufflated through the rectal tube once enough barium has been introduced and the patient is turned repeatedly to achieve double contrast views of the entire colon. Traditionally air has been used as the negative contrast agent but there may be considerable postprocedural pain which is largely abolished by the use of carbon dioxide. The double contrast barium enema examination provides excellent mucosal detail of the colonic mucosa but does require considerable agility on the part of the patient. Simplified techniques have been described to facilitate double contrast examinations in frail patients but alternative techniques, particularly abdominal CT (Fig. 3.36), can often provide the necessary information with less patient discomfort.

The strengths of endoscopy and the double contrast barium enema can be combined by a biphasic examination using flexible sigmoidoscopy and a modified double contrast barium enema. Flexible sigmoidoscopy can image the sigmoid and descending colon, sometimes to the splenic flexure. This is less painful

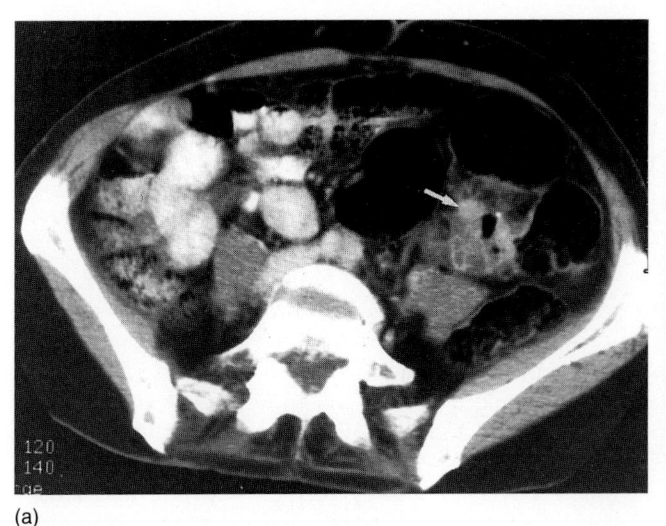

(a)

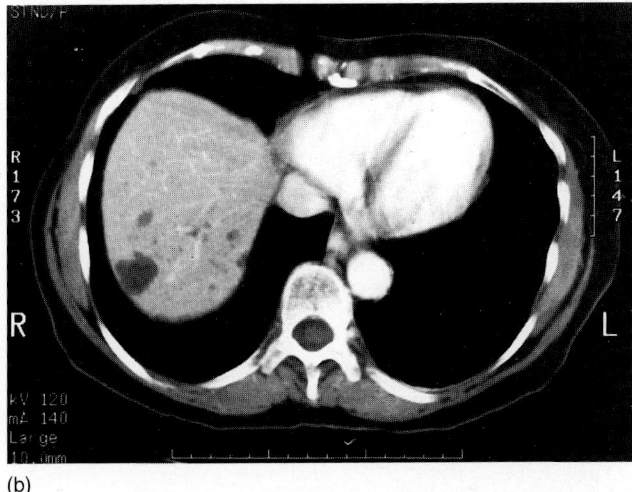

(b)

Fig. 3.36 Carcinoma of the colon. (a) CT scan shows an area of thickened wall in the sigmoid (arrow) with marked narrowing of the lumen. (b) CT scan of liver shows low attenuation lesions representing metastases from the colonic primary. Thus with a single examination, the patient's primary tumour and the metastases were diagnosed.

for the patient than formal colonoscopy and can be performed without the need for intravenous analgesia and sedation. It also permits mucosal biopsy and the detection of subtle vascular changes associated with colitis in the distal colon. Immediately following the flexible sigmoidoscopy, a modified double contrast barium enema is performed. This allows assessment of the colon not visualized by endoscopy, around to the caecum. As the sigmoid has already been visualized, this area can be omitted from the barium study and the radiologist can concentrate on the remainder of the colon.

Patients with perianal disease, particularly Crohn's, may have exquisite local tenderness, such that barium enema, colonoscopy or even simple digital rectal examination may be impossible due to pain. A caudal block administered by an anaesthetist takes only five minutes to perform and will provide at least half an hour of complete perianal anaesthesia, allowing comfortable radiological and endoscopic examinations that would othewise require a general anaesthetic.

Faeces, air bubbles, mucus or foreign bodies can cause confusing filling defects on double contrast barium enema which may resemble a polyp. These can generally be moved along the bowel by flowing barium or gas over them and can thus be differentiated from a true polyp. Diverticula can also have appearances similar to a polyp but can usually be filled with barium or be seen on an oblique view projecting outside the bowel rather than into the lumen.

In a case of suspected large bowel obstruction the diagnosis can be confirmed using a single contrast technique which requires no bowel preparation and much less patient movement than the double contrast technique. Dilute barium is run in until it reaches the obstruction or is seen refluxing into the terminal ileum. If a perforation is suspected water-soluble contrast should be substituted for the barium. If pseudo-obstruction (Ogilvie's syndrome) is suspected, the diagnosis is best made using a water-soluble single contrast enema. Pseudo-obstruction can be treated by decompression which can be either colonoscopic or fluoroscopic using specially designed coaxial catheters.

Diseases of the large bowel

Adenoma and adenocarcinoma Most adenocarcinomas arise in pre-existing adenomas. The presence of a familial polyposis syndrome greatly increases the risk that one of the polyps present will progress to an adenocarcinoma but these cases account for only 1% of all colonic carcinomas. Hereditary non-polyposis colon cancer is responsible for about 5% of colorectal cancer, and hereditary factors play a part in a further 15% of cases with family clusters of colonic adenocarcinoma. A further risk factor is total ulcerative colitis. After the first 10 years of colitis, the risk increases with about 10% of patients developing carcinoma in 25 years.

Both adenomas and carcinomas are most commonly found in the rectosigmoid area, although with increasing age there is a shift of this distribution, with more lesions being seen in the ascending colon. Adenomatous polyps are often multiple and if one is found there is an approximately 50% chance that a further synchronous polyp will be present (Fig. 3.37). If more than a dozen polyps are found it is likely that the patient has a polyposis syndrome. Carcinomatous foci may be present in adenomatous polyps that are macroscopically indistinguishable from benign adenomas. The size of the lesion is the single most important predictor

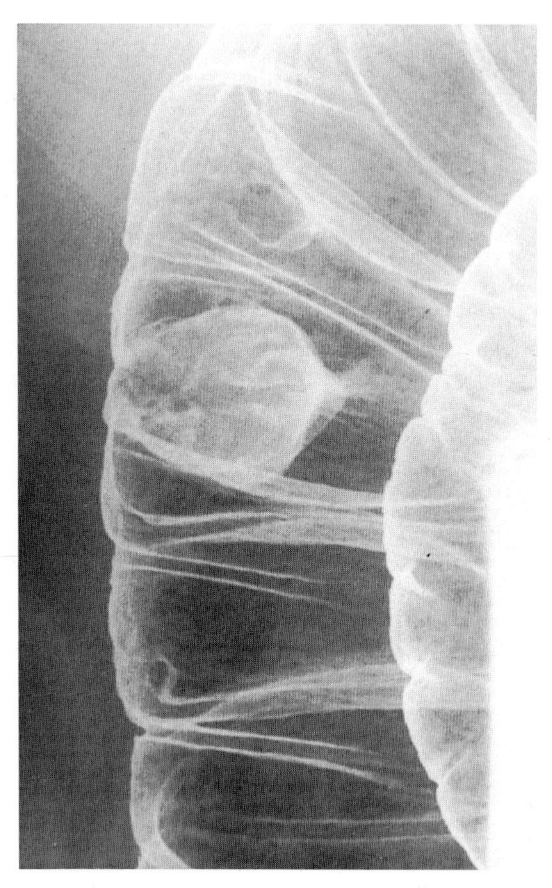

Fig. 3.37 Adenoma. Three adenomas in the right colon of a 48-year-old man, who also had a 5 mm rectosigmoid polyp. When a colonic adenoma is discovered there is a 34–53% chance of further adenomas being present. Thus the finding of one polyp should stimulate the search for more.

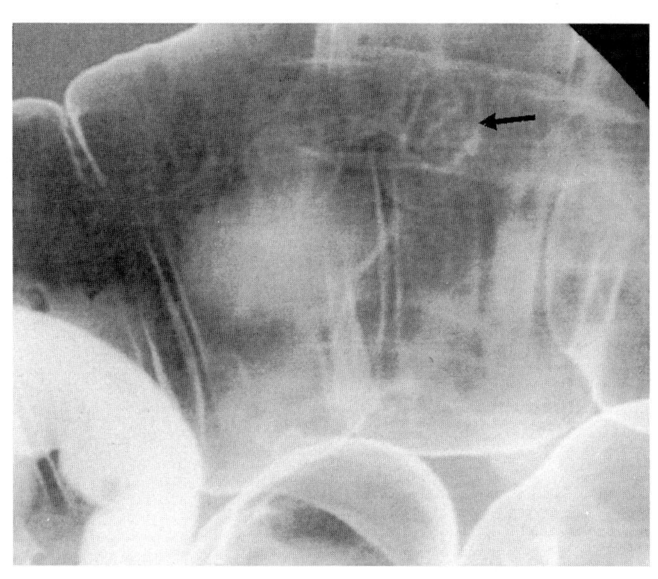

Fig. 3.38 Adenoma. Subtle flat adenoma in the transverse colon (arrow). When this quality of display can be provided, barium enema will miss fewer lesions than colonoscopy in the right colon, but endoscopy has better sensitivity in the sigmoid colon. (Courtesy A. O'Donovan.)

of malignancy, but, for a given size. Carcinoma is virtually unknown in polyps < 5 mm, is present in 1% of polyps measuring between 5 and 10 mm and in 50% of those > 2 cm. Polyps > 5 mm seen on barium studies should be removed especially if the polyp is lobulated or has an irregular outline. Patients with adenomas < 5 mm in diameter are statistically at no increased risk for later development of carcinoma. Detection of lesions of this size is therefore not of clinical importance. Only about 40% of these small polyps are detected on double contrast barium enema examinations while colonoscopy detects about 60%. Polyps > 1 cm have a 90% detection rate by colonoscopy and 75–85% rate by double contrast barium enema.

Cancer detection rates can be as high as 98% by both techniques but this is rarely achieved in practice. Most cancers missed on double contrast barium enema are visible on the films. Double reading of films provides the best chance of avoiding diagnostic error and surgeons should be in the habit of looking at the double contrast barium enema films rather than relying completely on the radiological report.

Polyps appear on double contrast barium studies as sessile plaques, sessile hemispheres, pedunculated spheres or as carpet lesions (Fig. 3.38). Carpet lesions which are often tubulovillous adenomas are flat, may be quite large and produce a change in the normal mucosal pattern of the bowel. The plaque-like lesions appear as slight elevations of the bowel wall when seen tangentially. The sessile hemispheres are seen as larger protrusions into the bowel lumen. This can be confused with a diverticulum although the diverticulum points away from the bowel lumen whereas the polyp points into the bowel lumen. Seen *en face* the sessile hemispheric polyp appears as a ring of barium (Fig. 3.39). Pedunculated polyps when seen in profile appear as a polypoid mass attached to a stalk of variable length. When seen *en face* the appearance of a pedunculated polyp with a short stalk is that of a 'Mexican hat' or 'target'.

Some adenocarcinomas have a large intraluminal component while others infiltrate deeply with a smaller intraluminal mass. In both cases narrowing

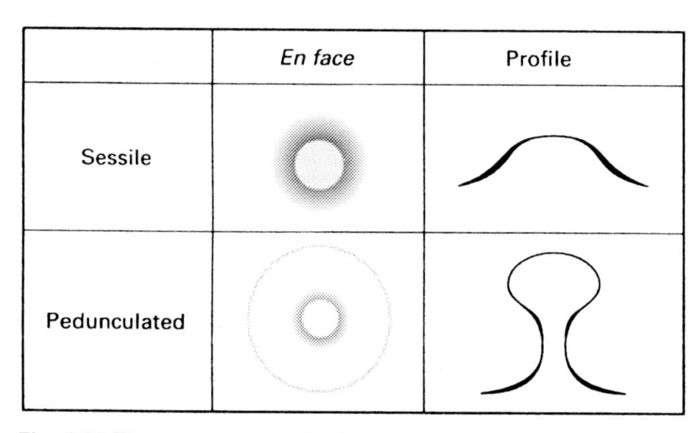

Fig. 3.39 The appearances of polyps.

occurs and there is replacement of normal colonic mucosa by tumour which often ulcerates. As the tumour advances around the circumference of the bowel, it resembles a saddle but with further growth the advancing edges meet, causing a circumferential stricture of the classic applecore type (Fig. 3.40). Polypoidal tumours can be very difficult to recognize if they are oblique to the X-ray beam, i.e. neither seen *en face* or in profile. In this situation the only clue to their presence may be a fine line of barium paralleling the bowel wall. The appearance in patients with ulcerative colitis is often atypical with carcinomas appearing as smooth, apparently benign-looking strictures. These strictures should be biopsied in all cases.

Staging of colorectal cancer requires the determination of the depth of invasion of the tumour, presence of lymph node metastases and the presence of other remote metastases, particularly to the liver. With rectal cancer, local invasion is best assessed by endorectal ultrasound; with more proximal tumours, assessment is best by CT. However, the sensitivity of CT is only 50–60% for local extension. For distant spread, either CT or MRI can be used but immunoscintigraphy is more sensitive than either of these for nodal and peritoneal metastases. When metastatic liver disease is assessed, ultrasound is often used as an initial investigation but CT and MRI are more sensitive. Intraoperative ultrasound may show lesions that have been overlooked by the preoperative evaluation.

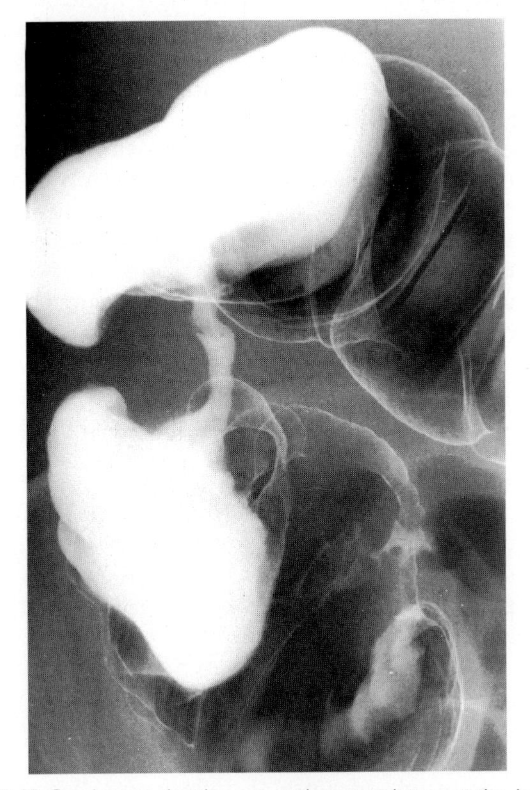

Fig. 3.40 Carcinoma showing an applecore stricture at the hepatic flexure.

Villous adenomas appear as areas of mucosal irregularity or a frond-like mass, with the individual fronds of the tumour covered in barium. True villous lesions tend to occur in the rectum and caecum and can cause diarrhoea with electrolyte loss due to the large surface area of these tumours. Villous adenomas often secrete mucus which may be inadequately cleared by bowel preparation. The mucus coats poorly with barium and these tumours may, therefore, easily be overlooked if the possible significance of an area of poor coating and mucus is not recognized at fluoroscopy.

A villous adenoma is 10 times more likely to harbour carcinoma than is a tubular adenoma.

There are number of hereditary and non-hereditary polyposis syndromes. The best known is **adenomatous polyposis coli** in which there is hereditary transmission, multiple polyps and the development of colonic carcinoma in untreated individuals. The mode of transmission is autosomal dominant with high penetration but about one-third of cases occur as a result of new mutations. The polyps vary in size from under 1 mm to 1 cm or more and are more numerous in the descending colon and rectosigmoid than in the more proximal colon. The whole colon can be affected such that no normal mucosa can be identified and the bowel is carpeted by multiple polyps. The colonic polyps develop before the age of 20 in most patients but polyps can appear for the first time in older individuals. The polyps develop into colonic carcinomas after about 15 years. Double contrast barium studies are useful for diagnosis, to assess the extent of the disease and the presence of carcinoma. As all of these patients eventually develop colonic carcinoma, a prophylactic colectomy should be performed, which can usually be deferred without penalty until the patient has reached the late teens. Patients with adenomatous polyposis coli may also develop hyperplastic and adenomatous polyps in the stomach, duodenum and small bowel. These patients have a higher incidence of duodenal carcinoma than non-polyposis-affected individuals.

Metastatic disease can involve the large bowel either by direct extension, peritoneal implantation or the haematogenous route. Direct invasion from contiguous tumours occurs most frequently from an ovarian primary in females and from a prostatic carcinoma in males. In females a primary tumour of the left ovary can extend to involve the inferior margin of the sigmoid colon. On barium examination this appears as sharp angulation of the sigmoid loops with spiculation and tethering of the mucosa. With involvement from a prostatic primary, the rectum is the involved segment of bowel. Initially a prostatic primary will extend superiorly to involve the seminal vesicles and at this point may appear as an extrinsic mass indenting the outline of the rectosigmoid but causing no mucosal derangement. With further posterior extension the anterior rectal mucosa is involved and will appear on barium studies as spiculation and tethering of the mucosal folds. With more advanced disease the tumour can completely encircle the rectum, mimicking both the symptoms and the radiological appearance of a primary rectal carcinoma. On barium examination this is seen as a circumferential rectal narrowing with enlargement of the presacral space but there is, in addition, spiculation of the mucosa which differentiates the condition from a primary rectal tumour. CT and MR scans of the pelvis can be very helpful to differentiate between primary bowel tumours and secondary involvement. Tumours can also involve the bowel via extension along a peritoneal fold. In this way pancreatic carcinoma can spread to the inferior surface of the transverse colon along the transverse mesocolon whereas gastric carcinoma spreads along the gastrocolic ligament to involve the superior surface of the transverse colon. In both cases the affected border of the transverse colon shows evidence of fixation, irregularity and spiculation while the uninvolved border may appear sacculated.

Blood-borne metastases may also involve the bowel. Secondaries from a breast primary are the most common but are usually small and asymptomatic, appearing on barium studies as an area of nodularity. Less often breast secondaries cause strictures of the bowel with irregular mucosa on barium examination. Melanoma can also involve the large bowel and usually appears as a mass protruding into the bowel lumen covered with normal colonic mucosa that is frequently ulcerated. A similar appearance can, however, be seen with lymphoma, Kaposi's sarcoma and carcinoid tumour. Intraperitoneal seedlings, most commonly from ovarian carcinoma, may also be detected on double contrast barium studies (Fig. 3.41). They may appear as an external mass on the large bowel but with more extensive disease there is angulation of bowel loops, tethering and spiculation of the mucosa and scalloping of ileal loops. CT is useful in confirming omental involvement and may also demonstrate the primary tumour and the extent of other secondary disease.

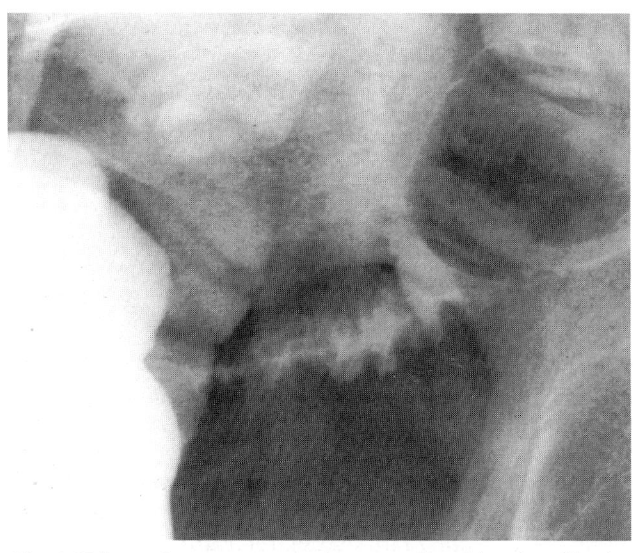

Fig. 3.41 Serosal metastases causing narrowing of the sigmoid colon due to invasion by drop metastases from the stomach. The serrated edges are characteristic. The appearances should not be mistaken for diverticulitis. Note the absence of diverticula.

Endometriosis A change in bowel habit, a reduction in stool calibre and abdominal pain may also be the presenting symptoms in endometriosis. This is a disorder affecting women between the ages of 20 to 45 years who most frequently present with dyspareunia, dysmenorrhoea and infertility. It is due to heterotopic endometrium in extrauterine locations. This endometrium remains under hormonal control and secretes and proliferates with the menstrual cycle, producing cysts filled with new and old blood, so-called 'chocolate cysts'. Involvement of the bowel affects the rectosigmoid in 95% of cases but may be seen in any part of the large or small bowel or even rarely the stomach. On double contrast barium enema examination, the endometrial implants appear as submucosal or serosal deposits with intact overlying mucosa. It is often difficult to distinguish confidently between endometriosis and metastatic disease to the bowel but sometimes MRI can help in this respect. Metastatic disease is generally low signal (dark) on T1 sequences and high signal (bright) on T2 sequences. Endometriomas are often multilocular containing both solid and cystic areas. The signal on MRI varies characteristically depending on the age of the blood.

Diverticular disease This is the most common disease affecting the colon in the western world, primarily as a result of the low fibre content of diets in these countries. It affects about 5% of the population under the age of 40 but this figure has increased to over 50% by the age of 80. The sigmoid colon is mainly affected with the curious exception of Japan where the right colon is affected more frequently than the left. Complications occur in approximately 5% of all patients with diverticula and require surgical or radiological intervention in 0.5%. The outpouchings from the bowel contain mucosa and submucosa and occur at the site where the nutrient arteries pass through the submucosa. On double contrast barium studies viewed in profile the diverticula appear as protrusions from the bowel filled with a variable amount of barium. *En face* they appear as a ring shadow or as a hat, the dome of which points away from the bowel lumen. Diverticula may be mistaken for polyps especially if they invert into the bowel lumen. Changes in the calibre of the bowel are often seen in the presence of diverticular disease and may appear before true diverticula develop. Calibre changes are usually due to thickening of the circular muscle layer with shortening of the taenia. On barium enema radiographs, deep haustral clefts are seen arising from both sides of the bowel which interdigitate with each other to produce a concertina appearance to the bowel.

Diverticulitis occurs in 20% of patients with diagnosed diverticular disease (Fig. 3.42). Inflammation and mucosal erosion at the apex of a diverticulum may progress to erosion of the muscle wall of the diverticulum causing perforation and abscess formation either in the wall of the bowel or more commonly in the pericolic fat. This can subsequently lead to frank perforation, haemorrhage, fistula formation or a pericolic abscess. The radiological signs of diverticulitis depend on the demonstration of deformed diverticular sacs, extravasation of contrast or of the presence of an abscess, and CT is the examination of choice in a sick patient with diverticulitis. Deformity of the sac is an early sign of diverticulitis but may also be due to the presence of previous disease causing fibrosis around the sac, so that although sometimes useful it is by no means a specific sign. The demonstration of extravasation of contrast material is a more useful sign and easier to recognize. The leak of contrast may be into an abscess cavity or may connect with another pelvic organ such as the bladder. The contrast may also appear as a track running parallel to the long axis of the colon. In this situation the contrast is situated in a subserosal abscess and often connects up with several diverticular sacs, giving a double lumen appearance to the bowel. The diagnosis of a pericolic abscess is often difficult with barium investigation, though the abscess may sometimes be identified as an indentation in the outline of the colon. These abscesses are more reliably demonstrated using CT, which may also show inflammatory change in the surrounding pericolic fat. CT may also show thickening of the bowel wall or small fluid collections in the paracolic spaces. Ultrasound is less useful for full assessment of acute complicated diverticulitis, as pathological details are frequently obscured by gas. CT and ultrasound can also be used to guide interventional procedures. Diverticulitis also causes strictures and obstruction. These strictures may resemble a carcinoma radiologically but the margin between narrowed and normal calibre bowel is more tapering in nature than that seen with malignant strictures. Also with a diverticular stricture the mucosa is intact and the diameter of the narrowed lumen is more variable. A diverticular sac in the middle of a narrowed segment is strong evidence against a carcinoma as the cause of the narrowing. Carcinomatous strictures tend to be < 7 cm long. In the final analysis double contrast barium enema is not a reliable method to exclude carcinoma in the presence of suspected acute diverticulitis and any suspicious stricture should be biopsied for histological confirmation. Diverticulitis and cancer can coexist.

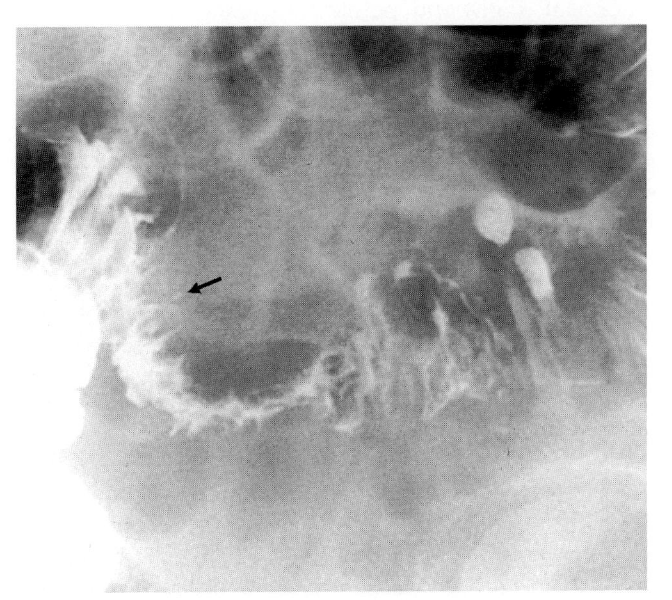

Fig. 3.42 Barium enema shows narrowing of the sigmoid, compression of the adjacent diverticula (arrow) and an absence of mucosal destruction. These features are suggestive of acute diverticulitis. CT scan provides a much better overall picture of the colon and adjacent organs in the assessment of acute diverticulitis.

A further complication of diverticulitis is bleeding which can be very brisk. Angiography has shown that in many cases the actual source of the bleeding is an angiomatous malformation rather than the diverticulitis itself. Angiography allows the site of the bleeding to be identified permitting either embolization of the bleeding source or a localized surgical resection. A giant sigmoid diverticulum, which is in fact a large cyst, can also arise as a complication of diverticulitis, and clinically these present with abdominal pain and a mass. On plain films a pelvic mass is seen which may have an air – fluid level. On barium studies contrast enters the cyst in almost 70% of cases and the cysts are associated with radiologically demonstrable diverticula in 80% of patients.

RECTUM

Examination

The rectum may be affected by the same inflammatory, infective and malignant processes as the rest of the large bowel and the appearance of these disorders is covered elsewhere. However, the presence of the anal sphincters makes the demonstration of bowel fistulae particularly important in this area. Fistulae can be investigated by injecting water-soluble contrast into the sinus tract or into the rectum. Often a more detailed assessment of a fistula, including the relationship to the internal and external sphincters, is required but this is difficult to provide with traditional contrast studies as the position of the sphincters is not visualized. Anorectal ultrasound can be very useful for demonstrating fistulous tracts and their relationship to the bowel wall and the surrounding sphincters. MRI is also useful, particularly as most of these patients have a very tender perineum and the introduction of an anorectal ultrasound probe can cause considerable discomfort. The fistulous tract has a high signal on T2-weighted and fat-suppression scans, and the entry points on to the two epithelial-lined surfaces may be clearly demonstrated. MRI can provide images in any plane which is a great advantage over CT.

Rectal disorders

Constipation and incontinence Constipation is a term that may be used loosely by patients to refer to symptoms that may result from either delayed transit or difficulty with evacuation. Tumours and metabolic disorders should be considered, but the majority of patients have transit disorders or pelvic floor dysfunction. Most patients respond to simple management. For those who do not respond, it is useful to assess colonic transit in order to detect major transit problems. Patients who are shown to have major transit delay may not need detailed assessment of pelvic floor function. A convenient transit study is a shape study in which the patient swallows each day for 5 days a capsule containing 24 radiopaque rings. A single abdominal radiograph on day 6 allows determination of bowel transit time (Fig. 3.43). With the patient on a usual diet, a transit time of up to three days is acceptable, corresponding to 72 shapes on the radiograph.

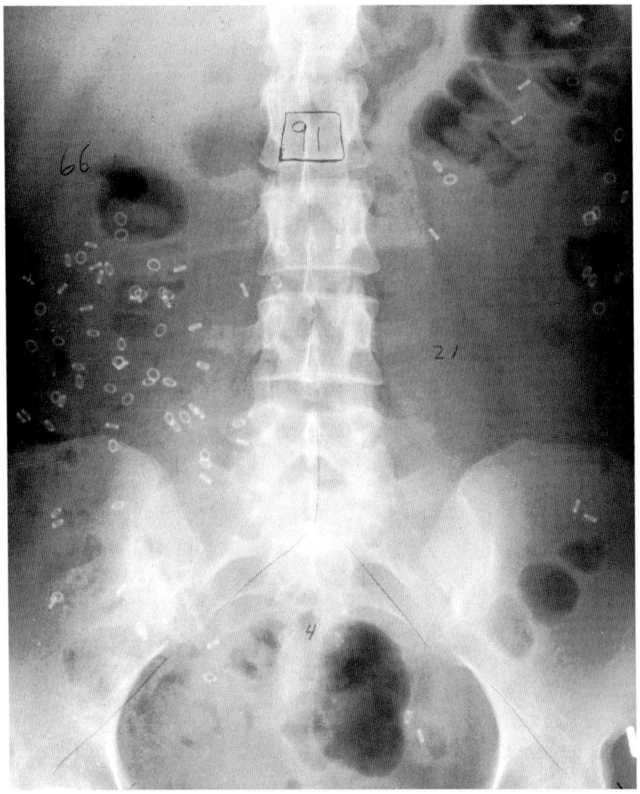

Pelvic floor dysfunction leading to problems with defecation is predominantly seen in female patients who comprise about 80% of the referred population. Patients may present with incontinence which can take the form of a constant leak of faeces or an ability to hold only a small volume of stool before defecation occurs with little or no warning. Alternatively patients can present with constipation which can take the form of excessive straining to initiate or complete defecation, difficulty in starting defecation or inability to completely empty the rectum. Imaging evaluation of these patients depends largely on defecating proctography but this is complemented by endorectal ultrasound and MRI which provide exquisite anatomical detail of the sphincter musculature.

To perform defecating proctography the small bowel should first be opacified with oral water-soluble contrast. Thick barium paste is instilled into the rectum and, in female patients, the vagina is also opacified using a contrast – gel mixture. Fluoroscopic imaging is carried out with the patient sitting on a radiolucent commode. The patient is asked to contract the pelvic floor musculature, which decreases the anorectal angle and increases the anal canal length. When the patient strains (without defecating), the anorectal angle increases, the anal canal lengthens and the anorectal junction descends. Measurements of anorectal angle and pelvic floor excursion have not been found to be associated consistently with any

Fig. 3.43 Colon transit study in 27-year-old woman with 'constipation'. The finding on day 6, that 91 of 120 shapes remain within the patient, indicates a transit time of almost 4 days. Moreover, as the majority of the shapes are in the right colon there is probably segmental dysmotility.

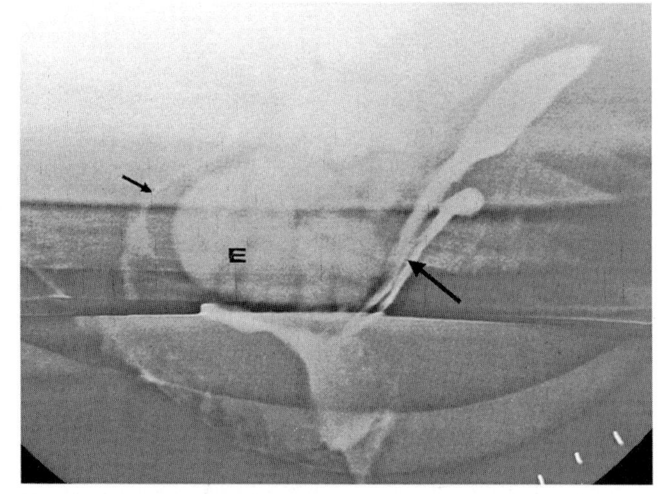

Fig. 3.44 Enterocoele. Defecogram in a patient with constipation demonstrates a large enterocoele (E) with contrast-filled loops of small bowel separating the vagina (small arrow) from the rectum. There is also a rectal intussusception with a linear filling defect (long arrow) in the column of rectal contrast caused by the intussuscepting rectal wall.

disease entities in recent reports. Imaging is performed during defecation. Patients who need to adopt various positional changes or use digital techniques to defecate are filmed while performing these procedures.

Rectocoeles are relatively common in the normal population, but are large in some patients with weakened pelvic floors and then are often associated with other abnormalities. They usually appear on defecating proctography as anterior outpouchings of the rectal mucosa. These may be associated with rectal intussusception which usually starts 5–10 cm above the anal canal. The intussusception is usually anterior and can descend to obstruct the anal canal causing symptoms of obstruction or of the solitary rectal ulcer syndrome.

Patients may also show evidence of an **enterocoele**, which appears as a separation between the vagina and the anterior wall of the rectum during straining and defecation. This gap may fill with opacified loops of small bowel descending into the pouch of Douglas (Fig. 3.44).

In patients with constipation but with normal colonic transit, abnormalities of the puborectalis muscle are not uncommon. On straining and defecation there may be either no change or a decrease in the anorectal angle instead of the normal increase. Alternatively, the puborectalis muscle may relax normally but there is no relaxation of the external anal sphincters. This is often associated with painful anal conditions such as anal fissure or painful haemorrhoids but can also be secondary to central neuronal abnormalities often caused by compressive lesions within the spinal canal or demyelination.

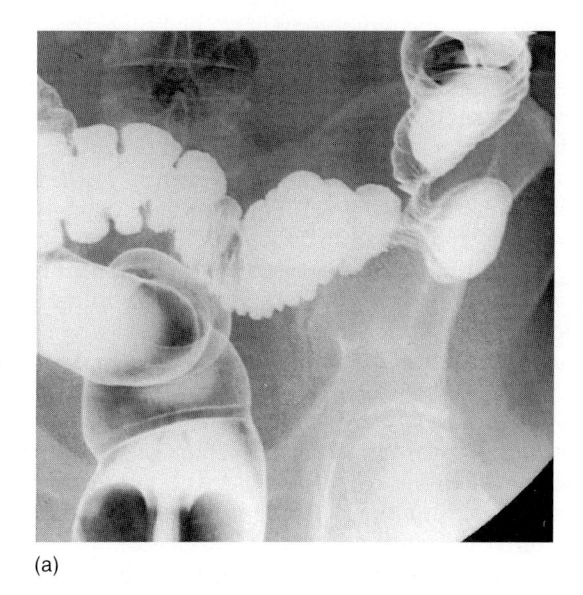
(a)

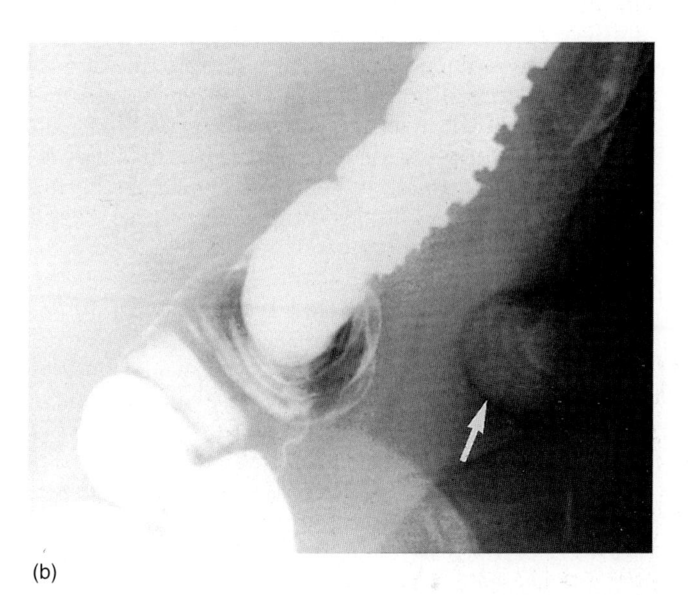
(b)

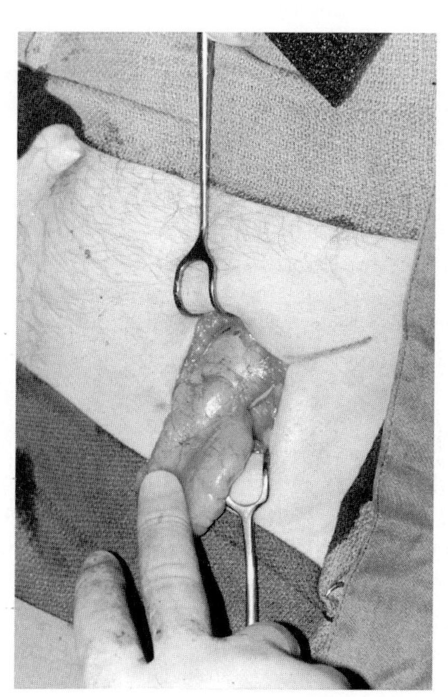
(c)

Fig. 3.45 Spigelian hernia. (a) The hernia is seen as a focal outpouching in the sigmoid colon. (b) The hernia was reducible with digital pressure by the patient's thumb (arrow). (c) The hernia was identified at surgery and repaired. (Courtesy Dr J. Gately.)

Defecating proctography may also be useful in patients with incontinence due to rectal prolapse; the incontinence in this condition may be partly due to dilation of the external sphincter by the prolapsing mucosa. When this is present on the barium study the patient may benefit from rectopexy or posterior anal repair. When the incontinence is due to sphincter trauma, the defecating proctogram is less useful as it merely documents a lax and leaking anal canal without indicating the cause. In such patients anorectal ultrasound is the examination of choice as it can demonstrate the location of the damage and thus determine whether the sphincters are completely disrupted or whether there is focal damage which is more likely to be amenable to surgical repair.

Hernia

Hernias rarely need radiological investigation but occasionally patients present with symptoms suggestive of an inguinal hernia but in whom no hernial sac can be felt clinically. Herniograms in these patients can detect small symptomatic hernias or prevent unnecessary exploratory surgery when no evidence of a hernia is shown. Herniography may also be helpful in the assessment of recurrent hernias following surgical repair. The examination is contraindicated when an incarcerated hernia is suspected, because the examination will fail to show a hernial sac.

To perform herniography, the peritoneal cavity is opacified with water-soluble contrast. Five folds can be identified, the median umbilical fold, two medial umbilical folds and two lateral umbilical folds. These divide the inguinal area into six fossae, three on each side of the midline comprising a supravesical fossa, and a medial and lateral inguinal fossa. Direct inguinal hernias originate from the supravesical fossa or from the medial inguinal fossa, while indirect inguinal hernias are seen as outpouchings from the lateral inguinal fossa. Femoral hernias have narrower necks than inguinal hernias and appear as pear-shaped protrusions. Generalized weakness of the groin can also be identified at herniography and is a condition that affects young athletes as well as older men. Rare hernias may require tailored examinations (Fig. 3.45).

INFLAMMATORY BOWEL DISEASE

CROHN'S DISEASE

Crohn's disease was originally known as terminal ileitis but it is now recognized that any part of the bowel from the mouth to the anus can be involved and there may be widespread manifestations in non-intestinal body systems. The disease is uncommon on a worldwide basis with a prevalence of between 10 to 70 per 100 000, but the incidence has been increasing by up to 400% in the last 40 years. The highest incidence is in Western Europe, the United States and Israel and it is very rare in Africa. The sex distribution is equal but Crohn's disease is more common in Caucasians and Jews. Patients typically present between the ages of 15 to 25 years or between 50 to 80 years. Crohn's disease can present with a variety of symptoms, the most common of which are abdominal pain, bleeding and diarrhoea. Abdominal pain is a symptom in 75% of patients on initial presentation. This can be a lower abdominal colicky pain or a more severe pain in the right iliac fossa, mimicking appendicitis. Rectal bleeding is seen in about 50% of patients when the disease is active but profuse bleeding or blood mixed with mucus is more suggestive of ulcerative colitis. Physical examination may reveal an abdominal mass and/or tenderness, and sigmoidoscopy often shows areas of inflammatory change interspersed with normal mucosa. As well as involvement of the bowel there are many extraintestinal diseases associated with Crohn's disease, some of which can precede the bowel-related symptoms, such as low back pain from an associated sacroiliitis. Skin complaints such as pyoderma gangrenosum, erythema nodosum, dermatitis herpetiformis or vitiligo are also seen. The cardiovascular system can also be affected with thrombophlebitis or cardiac failure resulting from myocarditis or a cardiomyopathy. Finger clubbing occurs in up to 40% of patients particularly with proximal small bowel involvement, and can be associated with hypertrophic osteopathy with periosteal reaction seen on plain radiographs of the wrist.

Crohn's disease can affect the whole of the GI tract. Small bowel involvement, in particular the terminal ileum, is the commonest site of involvement but pure colonic involvement is also seen. Disease of both colon and terminal ileum is common but the stomach, duodenum and oesophagus can also be affected. Involvement of the bowel is characteristically patchy in nature with segments of normal bowel being interspersed between diseased segments ('skip lesions'). Even in areas of disease, bowel involvement is usually asymmetrical with disease on the mesenteric border predominating, leaving the antimesenteric border relatively spared. As the small bowel is the commonest involved site, small bowel investigations are frequently requested. These can visualize the small bowel in single contrast and the terminal ileum in double contrast by means of a pneumocolon technique.

Radiological changes of Crohn's disease

Mucosal granularity and enlargement of the lymphoid follicles These are early changes which appear as nodular sessile protrusions into the bowel lumen. Lymphoid follicles are, however, seen as a normal finding in young patients and in this population great care must be taken to avoid overdiagnosing disease.

Ulceration Larger lymphoid nodules may develop mucosal ulceration producing aphthoid ulcers. These appear as small barium-filled craters measuring 1–2 mm in diameter surrounded by a lucent halo produced by the lymphoid nodule. The appearance is that of ring and dot lesions, where the ring represents a meniscus of barium around a follicle and the dot represents the ulcer crater (Fig. 3.46). These lesions are known as aphthous ulcers and are difficult to see on single contrast views of the small bowel even with a meticulous compression technique. They may be more clearly seen when a pneumocolon technique demonstrates the terminal ileum in double contrast. Aphthous ulcers may also be seen in the colon on double contrast barium enemas, and in the stomach or duodenum on barium meal examination. These aphthous ulcers may occur singularly or in groups, and tend to occur at the edge of more severe established disease. The surrounding mucosa in the colon is usually normal in contrast to ulcerative colitis.

The ulcers may remain unchanged for long periods but can also be seen to enlarge or to regress completely. Alternatively the ulcers may coalesce to give a wide area of lattice-type ulceration, in which the ulcers are surrounded by inflamed oedematous bowel. It is the combination of the ulceration and the raised surrounding mucosa which gives a cobblestone appearance to the bowel. The areas surrounding the ulcers appear as raised irregular areas and, as the ulceration extends, the islands of inflamed but non-ulcerated mucosa give a false appearance of polyps. The inflammation in Crohn's disease spreads to involve the full thickness of the bowel wall, although this is usually asymmetrical and can affect only part of the circumference of the bowel. When the active episode of Crohn's disease remits, the ulcerated mucosa begins to heal and inflamed hyperplastic mucosa may remain as postinflammatory pseudopolyps. These may be small and round or oval in shape but long filiform polyps may also occur. Fronds of proliferating mucosa can be seen which may be mistaken for a villous adenoma.

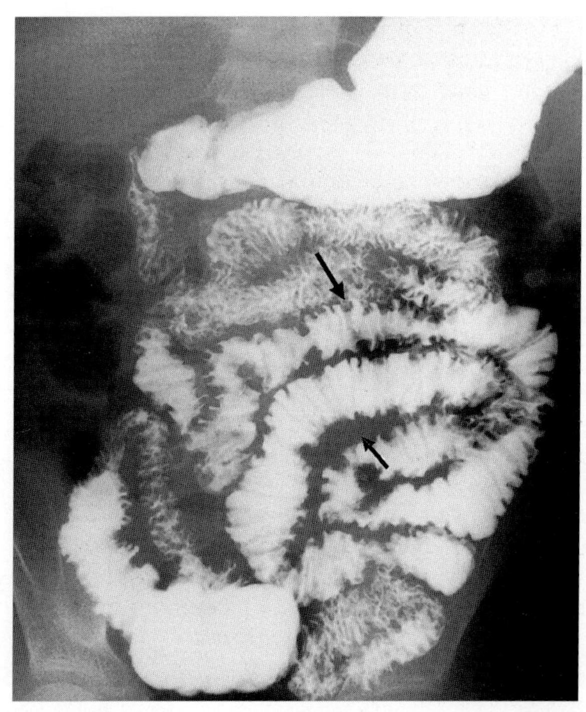

Fig. 3.47 Crohn's disease. Small bowel meal in a patient with jejunal Crohn's disease, demonstrating some thickened valvulae conniventes (long arrow) and patchy wall thickening (small arrow). The distal bowel appears normal.

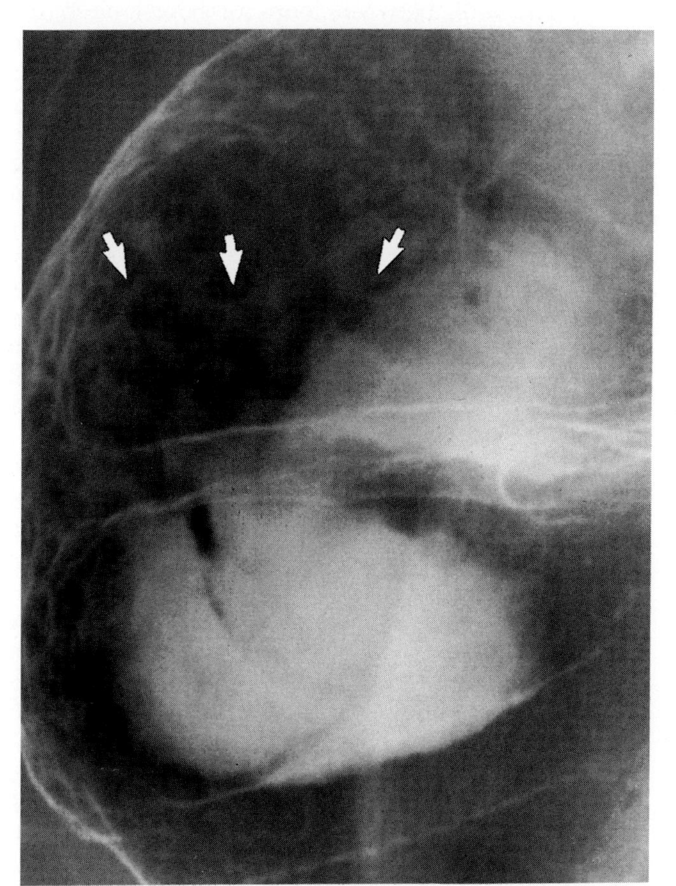

Fig. 3.46 Apthous ulceration. Double contrast barium examination of the rectum in a patient with Crohn's disease, showing ring and dot lesions; the dots (arrows) represent tiny ulcers.

Bowel wall thickening During an acute flare-up of the disease, the oedema and inflammation leads to bowel wall thickening which on barium studies is seen as separation of adjacent loops of bowel (Fig. 3.47). The barium-filled lumen of normal loops of bowel are closely applied or can be made to approximate with abdominal compression, whereas the barium in an inflamed section of diseased bowel may be separated from adjacent loops by a distance of several centimetres.

These areas of bowel wall thickening are more directly shown by CT (Fig. 3.48) or by ultrasound; the

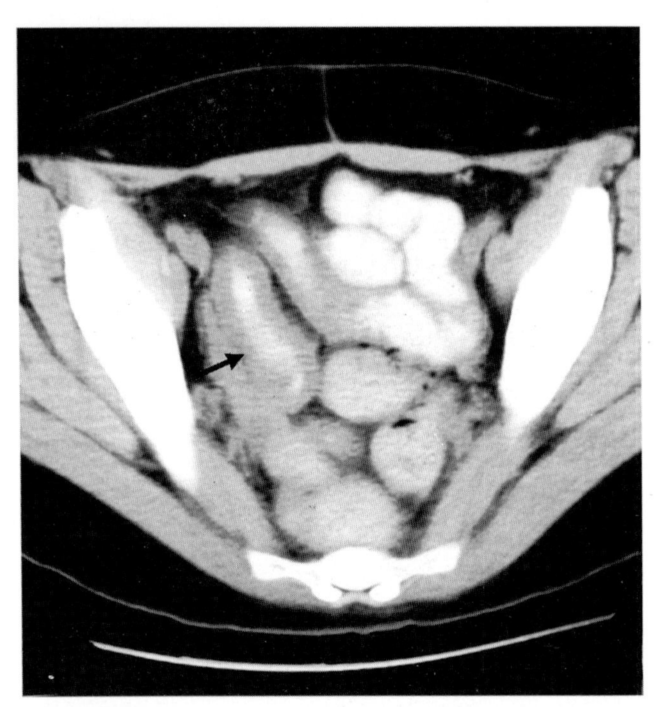

Fig. 3.48 Crohn's disease showing thickened bowel wall in loops of distal ileum (arrow). This patient has active disease but there is no dilation of the proximal bowel loops to suggest obstruction.

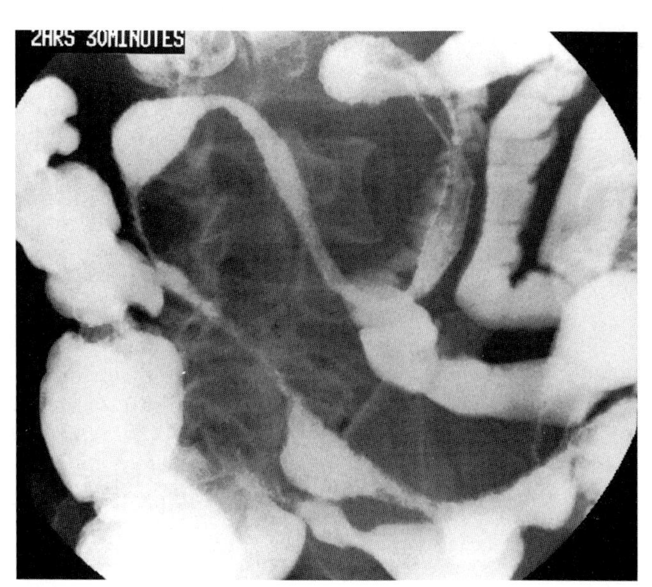

Fig. 3.49 Crohn's disease. Small bowel meal showing multiple strictures of varying lengths in the small bowel.

latter shows a target lesion when the bowel is imaged in transverse plane. Separation of bowel loops can also be due to fibrofatty infiltration into the mesentery, which becomes thickened from oedema and fibrous tissue; it is seen on CT as streaky high attenuation areas in the normally low attenuation mesentery. CT with oral contrast is an excellent initial radiological examination in a patient with an acute flare-up of Crohn's disease showing the mucosal thickening as well as abscess formation.

Strictures Strictures are seen in approximately 20% of cases of Crohn's disease due to oedema and inflammatory tissue or to fibrosis. The narrowing can be very marked and result in the 'string sign', the narrowed segment containing only a string-like thread of barium. A stricture can be associated with a fistula which tends to originate at the proximal end of the narrowed segment. Fibrotic strictures can be very tight and are irreversible and often require surgical resection. These strictures can be long or short and there are frequently segments of normal-calibre bowel interspersed between the strictures (Fig. 3.49). The ends of these strictures can be very abrupt and can mimic malignant strictures in the colon. In these cases biopsy is usually required for diagnosis.

Abscess The detection of an abscess is very important as clinical diagnosis is often difficult especially as many of these patients are on steroids. On CT with intravenous contrast enhancement abscesses characteristically show a non-enhancing centre composed of necrotic tissue with an enhancing wall, while phlegmonous masses enhance more uniformly. While abscesses can occur spontaneously they are often related to surgery and occur in about 20% of Crohn's disease patients at some point. They can occur in the abdominal wall, between loops of bowel or in the retroperitoneum. CT is also helpful in planning the most appropriate skin access site for percutaneous drainage.

Fistula A wide range of imaging tests may be required to assess the full extent of fistulae depending on their site. For ileo-ileal fistula, small bowel barium investigation often shows the site and course, but detailed compression views of suspicious areas may be needed. Ileocolic fistulae can be shown in an antegrade fashion using a small bowel barium technique, or retrogradely by means of a barium enema. Enterocutaneous fistulae can be demonstrated by a sinogram. It is important to take the time to manoeuvre the sinogram catheter as deeply as possible into the sinus tract in order to demonstrate a fistula and to show all significant connections. Vaginal fistulae may be demonstrated by barium enema techniques but occasionally require a vaginogram. Perianal and perineal fistulae are difficult to demonstrate using conventional contrast studies. CT is a very useful technique to investigate this area and can demonstrate about 90% of lesions. CT provides information not only on the site of fistulous tracks but also on the presence of any associated abscesses. Endorectal ultrasound can be useful in identifying the presence of a perianal track and its relationship to the sphincters. An alternative examination is MRI which can show the fistulous track as a high signal on the T2-weighted and fat-suppression sequences and can sometimes provide additional information in the region of the ischiorectal fossa.

Remote complications of Crohn's disease

A non-erosive **arthropathy** can occur in peripheral joints as part of the extraintestinal manifestations of Crohn's disease. About one-fifth of patients are affected at some time and this type of arthritis usually occurs at or soon after the onset of intestinal symptoms. Patients can also develop a symmetrical bilateral sacroiliitis similar to that seen in ankylosing spondylitis and 75% of patients are HLA B27 positive. Radiographically the sacroiliac joint space appears irregular with erosions particularly affecting the iliac side of the joint; sclerosis is also seen at the joint margins. With time there may be complete fusion of the joint. Late changes are easily seen on a plain radiograph of the pelvis and can usually be seen on an abdominal film taken because of bowel symptoms. Early changes are harder to visualize but a limited number of narrow section CT scans through the sacroiliac joints can detect these subtle changes (Fig. 3.50). The radiation dose from a conventional three-view radiographic examination of the sacroiliac joints is approximately three times that of the thin-section CT mini-series.

Extraintestinal manifestations of Crohn's disease may be secondary to **malabsorption** caused by the diseased bowel and include weight loss, anaemia of chronic disease and a fatty liver appearing hyperechoic on ultrasound and with a low attenuation on CT.

Gallstones occur in up to 50% of patients especially following terminal ileal resection and are best imaged with upper abdominal ultrasound. **Pericholangitis** is also seen but usually follows a benign course. **Sclerosing cholangitis** is uncommon. **Amyloidosis** affecting the liver and kidneys is also seen resulting in enlargement of these organs.

Urinary calculi occur in 5–10% of patients. These are most often urate stones because of fluid loss particularly in patients with an ileostomy which may lead to an increased risk of dehydration and acidosis. Oxalate stones also occur; oxalate is usually bound to calcium in the small bowel. In malabsorption fatty acids bind the calcium and soluble sodium oxalate enters the colon where it is passively absorbed.

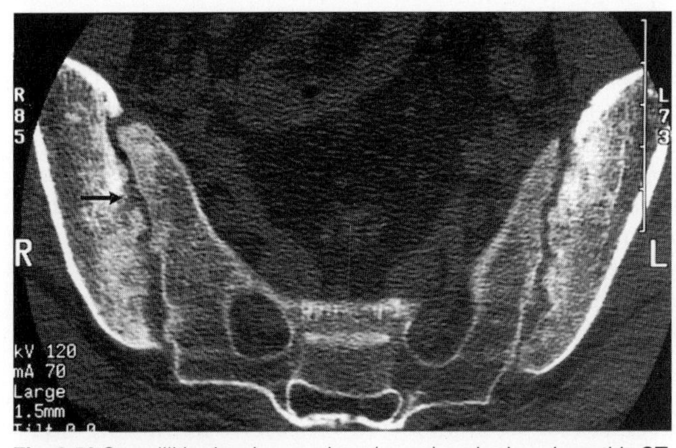

Fig. 3.50 Sacroiliitis showing erosions (arrow) and sclerosis on this CT scan of a patient with inflammatory bowel disease. A sacroiliitis CT protocol provides excellent definition of the sacroiliac joints at a lower radiation dose than from a conventional sacroiliitis plain film series. (Courtesy L. Friedman.)

Patients with Crohn's disease have an increased incidence of small and large bowel **carcinoma** though less than that of chronic total ulcerative colitis. The tumours frequently develop in surgically bypassed loops of large or small bowel and tend to occur at an earlier age than carcinomas which are not Crohn's related. The carcinomas are usually of colloid or mucinous type. There are problems with the diagnosis of carcinoma in Crohn's disease, as strictures are in most cases the result of the Crohn's disease rather than a complicating tumour. The incidence of **lymphoma** and **leukaemia** in patients with Crohn's disease is also increased.

ULCERATIVE COLITIS

Ulcerative colitis is most common in westernized countries where there is an incidence of 1 in 1000. Presentation below the age of 5 years or above the age of 75 is rare and most cases present between the ages of 15 and 25 years. Up to 25% of patients have a close relative who is also affected by the disease. Patients typically present with bloody diarrhoea with or without mucus, and may also complain of weight loss, abdominal pain and extraintestinal problems with joint pain, skin and eye complaints.

An assessment of the extent of the disease is important in regard to complications but it is known that double contrast barium enema underestimates the extent of disease compared to both colonoscopy and histology. Barium enema examination is unable to detect the loss of vessel pattern that is the earliest endoscopic pattern of ulcerative colitis. Colonoscopy also underestimates the extent of disease compared with histology. In the 1960s Goligher showed that disease extending to the hepatic flexure on barium studies should be assumed to be an extensive colitis causing histological change throughout the colon.

It is important to distinguish between Crohn's disease and ulcerative colitis and this distinction may be made in most cases by a careful consideration of all of the clinical, radiological and histological data, but approximately 10% of cases show intermediate features preventing a clear separation. In acute disease the macroscopic pathological features as displayed in radiographs may be more helpful in differentiation than the histology, which can be difficult to analyse in the face of an acute colitis, the histology becoming more reliable in the quiescent phase. The bowel in ulcerative colitis is affected in a uniform fashion both circumferentially and continuously, in contrast to the discontinuous disease involvement characteristic of Crohn's colitis. The diseased segment in ulcerative colitis usually extends from the rectum proximally, but in patients on treatment the rectum may be normal endoscopically and radiologically in the presence of active proximal disease. A small group of patients appear to progress over the space of a few years from classic ulcerative colitis to classic Crohn's disease, both radiologically and histologically.

Main features of ulcerative colitis

Granularity and ulceration On double contrast barium enema the early changes of ulcerative colitis are those of mucosal granularity (Fig. 3.51). The normal smooth pencil-thin line of barium coating is replaced with multiple rings of barium, representing focal mucosal elevation, and dots of barium due to superficial ulceration. This combination of small rings and dots gives the appearance of mucosal granularity when seen *en face* and of a slightly fuzzy appearance to the barium coating when seen tangentially. In the majority of patients the colon is the only part of the bowel to be affected, with disease extending proximally for a variable distance from the rectum.

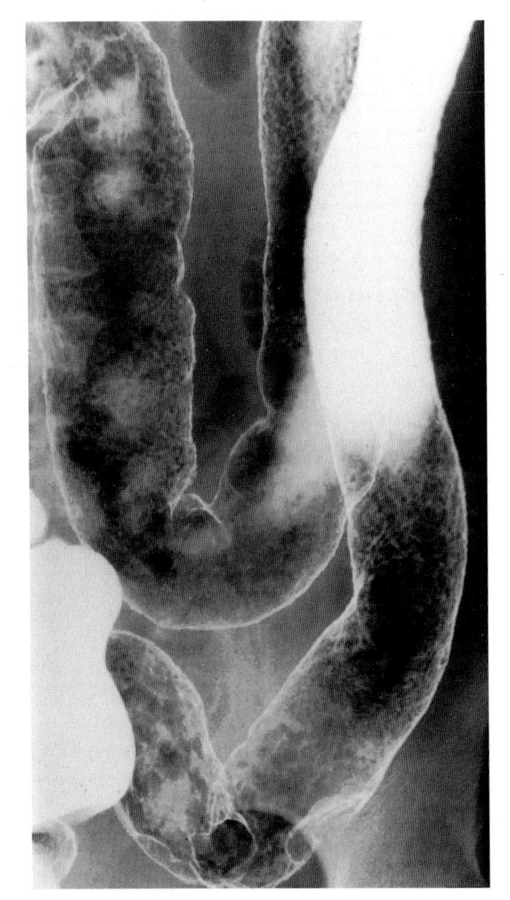

Fig. 3.51 Ulcerative colitis showing a granular mucosa in the transverse and descending colon.

During a more severe acute attack of ulcerative colitis extensive superficial ulcerations occur with more marked focal oedema giving a stippled and nodular appearance to the mucosa on barium studies; linear ulcers may also be seen. In contrast to Crohn's disease these changes are circumferential and affect the bowel in continuity without skip lesions. The ulcers tend to be shallower than those seen with Crohn's disease.

Terminal ileal changes In total ulcerative colitis the terminal ileum may show abnormalities in up to 40% which include a granular mucosa, giving a diagnosis of backwash ileitis, but the most common change is of a patent ileocaecal valve and a dilated terminal ileum. The more proximal small bowel is not affected. Ulceration does not, however, occur in the terminal ileum in ulcerative colitis, and ulceration extending into the small bowel therefore prompts the search for an alternative diagnosis such as Crohn's disease or a secondary diagnosis of superadded infection such as tuberculosis, yersinia or campylobacter.

Polyps Various types of polyps are seen in ulcerative colitis. Inflammatory polyps and pseudopolyps occur during an acute attack of ulcerative colitis, and postinflammatory polyps in the quiescent phase. Inflammatory polyps appear as filling defects on a granular mucosa and are typically multiple. Pseudopolyps are seen during severe acute attacks of ulcerative colitis. The polyps are in fact islands of oedematous mucosa surrounded by areas in which the colon has been denuded of mucosa by extensive confluent ulceration. Once an acute severe attack has subsided, postinflammatory polyps can develop and are seen in approximately 10% of patients with ulcerative colitis. These postinflammatory polyps may be sessile or may project into the bowel lumen as finger-like processes known as filiform polyps. Clues to the postinflammatory nature of these polyps are usually provided by other changes in the mucosa but occasionally these polyps are seen on a background of normal mucosa.

Shortening and narrowing of the colon with loss of haustra This develops in total chronic ulcerative colitis, an appearance sometimes called the 'lead pipe' colon.

Presacral thickening This occurs when there is an increase in the gap between the anterior margin of the sacrum and the posterior wall of the rectum on lateral radiographs of the pelvis. This gap is known as the **presacral space** and in normal patients is usually less than 1 cm in size.

Strictures Strictures are common in chronic ulcerative colitis, usually benign in aetiology and may be reversible or permanent. Reversible strictures are due to muscle hypertrophy but appear similar to permanent strictures on barium studies with smoothly tapering ends and smooth mucosa. Differential diagnosis should be made between benign and malignant strictures and, particularly when multiple strictures are present, from cathartic colon.

Megacolon Ulcerative colitis is an important but not the sole cause of toxic megacolon which can also be seen in Crohn's disease, ischaemic colitis, Behçet's disease and infective causes including amoebiasis and pseudomembranous colitis. Toxic megacolon is an important condition to recognize because of the high associated mortality. The diagnosis rests on a combination of clinical and radiological findings. Clinically the patient presents with abdominal pain, fever, raised white cell count and acute phase proteins. On plain abdominal films the striking abnormality is colonic dilation beyond the 6 cm upper limit of normal. It is important to perform a plain film before embarking on barium studies as barium enema can precipitate colonic perforation. The dilation of the colon is secondary to transmural inflammation with neuromuscular degeneration. Perforation, which usually occurs in the sigmoid colon is not uncommon in toxic megacolon and is associated with a very high mortality.

Colonic tumours These can complicate ulcerative colitis and, as in Crohn's disease, tend to be of the colloid or mucinous type. The risk of tumour development increases with an early onset of disease and can be recognized in patients with extensive or pancolitis who have had ulcerative colitis for 10 years. On double contrast barium studies dysplastic changes appear as irregularity and nodularity of the mucosa and nodular filling defects (Fig. 3.52). Dysplastic areas may herald and/or progress to carcinoma. These dysplastic changes are, however, difficult to demonstrate unless the bowel preparation is optimal, and may be difficult to differentiate from active disease. It is not possible to exclude a carcinoma in a stricture which appears radiologically benign. For several years routine colonoscopic surveillance of patients with ulcerative colitis at high risk for colon cancer has been recommended but the usefulness of this has recently been questioned, and there is still no clear evidence that surveillance improves survival. However, colonoscopic biopsy of suspicious lesions seen on barium studies is very useful, particularly for those patients with radiologically visible areas of dysplasia.

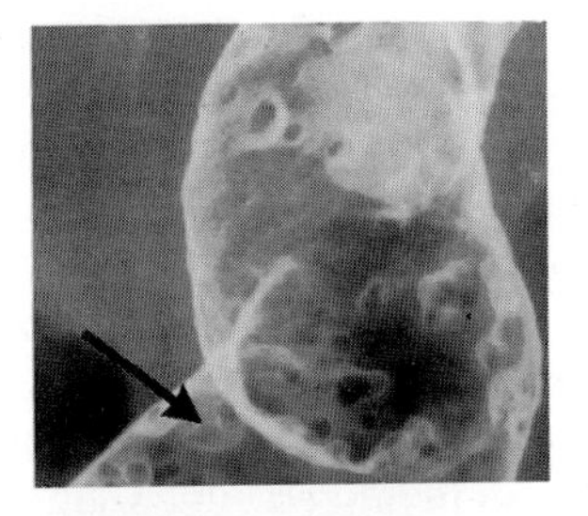

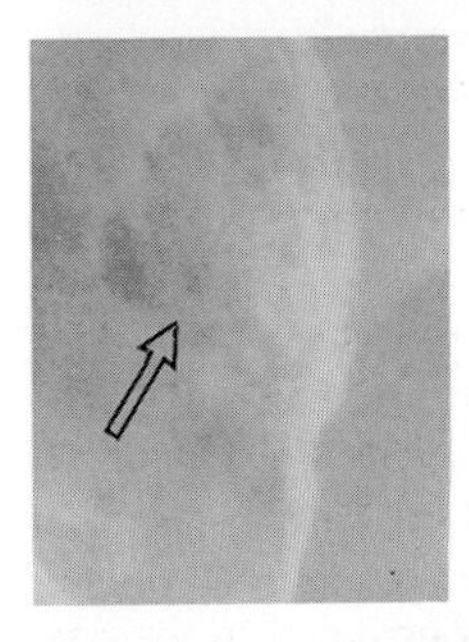

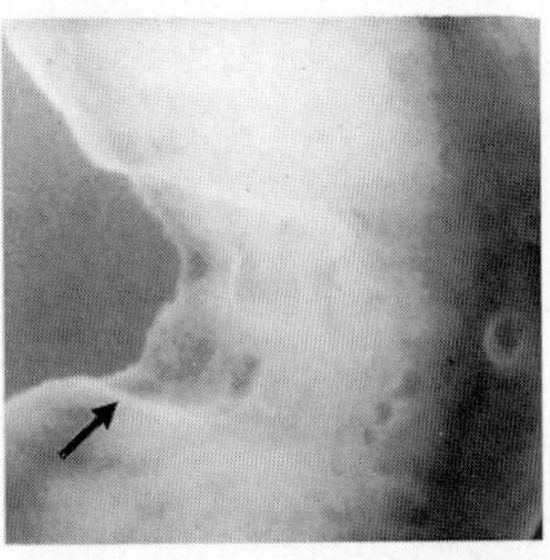

Fig. 3.52 Double contrast barium enema in a patient with a past history of ulcerative colitis showing multiple filiform polyps (long black arrow), a dysplasia-associated lesion (open arrow) and a carcinoma (small black arrow). The presence of a dysplasia-associated lesions means that there is a strong likelihood of a co-existing carcinoma.

Remote manifestations of ulcerative colitis

Ulcerative colitis is also associated with extraintestinal disease:

- anaemia, common from blood loss, malnutrition and the effects of drug therapy;
- deep venous thrombosis or pulmonary emboli;
- iritis and uveitis, often in combination with skin and joint symptoms;
- pyoderma gangrenosum or erythema nodosum, often coinciding with an acute attack of colonic disease;
- symmetrical sacroiliitis and spinal changes identical to ankylosing spondylitis sometimes antedating the onset of colonic symptoms;
- arthritis, occuring with a peripheral joint involvement, which typically migrates from one joint to another;
- liver abnormalities, occuring in about 5% of patients with ulcerative colitis and including fatty change secondary to malnutrition. Pericholangitis, sclerosing cholangitis and cholangiocarcinoma also occur, sclerosing cholangitis predisposing to cholangiocarcinoma.

ISCHAEMIC BOWEL DISEASE

Ischaemia of the bowel may be due to arterial or venous causes and can be generalized or localized to a short segment of bowel.

Acute occlusive ischaemia This is usually caused by embolic occlusion in the territory of the superior mesenteric artery and is particularly common in the elderly population. The extent of the ischaemia may include the whole of the small bowel as well as the right side of the colon. Patients usually present with ill-defined abdominal pain. Rectal bleeding, acidosis, pyrexia and a raised white cell count may also occur but are similarly non-specific. The high mortality of up to 90% from this type of ischaemia is largely due to the frequent delay in diagnosis. Plain-film findings in acute mesenteric ischaemia tend to occur late. They include a generalized ileus and bowel wall thickening. More specific signs such as air in the wall of the bowel and air in the portal vein are only seen in later stages when there is bowel necrosis. Air in the portal vein visible on plain film carries a very poor prognosis.

CT scanning is diagnostic in about a third of cases and can demonstrate relatively early on the non-specific signs of dilated bowel loops, thickened bowel wall and ascites. When a loop of affected bowel is imaged in cross-section, a double halo appearance can be seen due to low-attenuation bowel content and wall oedema separated by a ring of hyperaemic enhancing bowel wall. Intramural gas and portal vein gas can also be identified at an earlier stage than is possible with plain films. Air may be seen in the mesenteric vessels and is a highly specific sign of acute mesenteric ischaemia.

Ultrasound can also provide clues to the diagnosis by demonstrating thickened bowel wall and ascites. Barium examinations have little place when acute ischemia is suspected because the findings are non-specific and more importantly residual barium within the bowel lumen interferes with the other imaging modalities.

CT is often useful as a screening procedure in a patient with an acute abdomen in whom bowel ischaemia is just one of several possibilities. However, the sensitivity of CT and ultrasound is low, and when the clinical likelihood of acute intestinal ischaemia is high, angiography should be performed urgently. Angiographic assessment includes aortography and selective superior mesenteric arterial injection. At angiography the occlusion may be complete or partial. When complete the vessel is seen to come to an abrupt end (Fig. 3.53) and, when partial, an intraluminal filling defect is seen. Emboli tend to lodge distal to the first three centimetres of the superior mesenteric artery, whereas thrombi tend to occur within the first two centimetres of the origin of the superior mesenteric artery. The occlusion from both emboli and thrombi leads to a reflex vasoconstriction of the distal mesenteric vessels which can mimic non-occlusive mesenteric ischaemia. This distal vasoconstriction is probably responsible for the progression of bowel ischaemia and bowel infarction that may develop despite a technically successful surgical embolectomy. Therefore, surgery should be supplemented with transcatheter papaverine infusion to treat the mesenteric vasoconstriction. The papaverine infusion should start at the time of the angiography and continue during and after surgery.

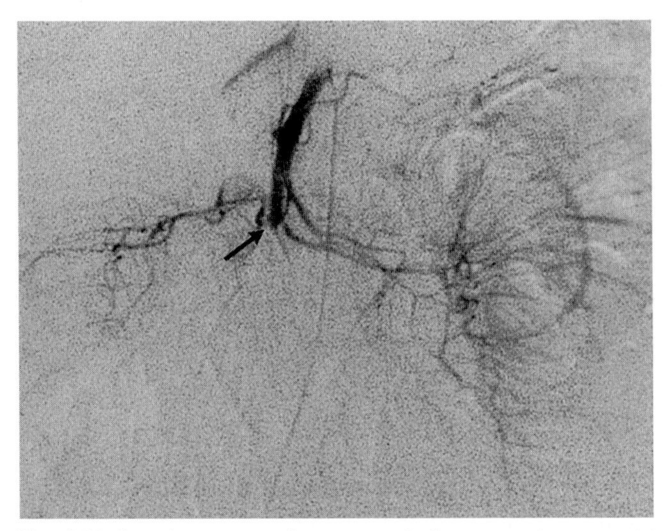

Fig. 3.53 Superior mesenteric artery embolism secondary to atrial fibrillation. The selective mesenteric arteriogram shows an abrupt cut off (arrow) to the contrast a few centimetres from the origin of the vessel. (Courtesy of J. Mernagh.)

Acute non-occlusive mesenteric ischaemia This is the most common type of mesenteric ischaemia and caries a high morbidity particularly if diagnosis is delayed. In this condition there is no evidence of vessel occlusion but ischaemia occurs due to marked mesenteric vasoconstriction. The differentiation of occlusive from non-occlusive mesenteric ischaemia is important as surgical treatment is usually required for the former but not for the latter, unless bowel infarction has occurred. Non-occlusive mesenteric ischaemia is usually secondary to a low cardiac output from a variety of causes. The reduced cardiac output leads to a reflex vasoconstriction of the mesenteric vessels causing bowel hypoxia. As this progresses, further bowel necrosis may occur leading to septicaemia and a further reduction in cardiac output. This condition can also develop in patients on vasopressive drugs due to the vasoconstriction they cause.

Patients in whom non-occlusive mesenteric ischaemia is the likely diagnosis should have an initial chest and abdominal plain film to exclude other pathology, followed by early angiographic assessment consisting of an aortogram, followed by selective superior mesenteric arterial injection. These images should be carefully studied to exclude a proximal obstructing thrombus or embolus, as distal vasoconstriction is commonly seen secondary to occlusive mesenteric ischaemia.

The angiographic diagnosis of non-occlusive mesenteric ischaemia is made when there is diffuse mesenteric vasoconstriction in the absence of proximal occlusive disease. Systemic hypotension or vasopressive agents will also cause this appearance and therefore correction of hypotension is vital before the angiogram is performed. The diagnosis should also be made with much caution if the patient is on vasopressive medication. The vasocontriction in non-occlusive mesenteric ischaemia appears as vessel narrowing. Once the diagnosis has been established, treatment is by transcatheter infusion of a vasodilator and correction of the underlying abnormality leading to the low-flow state. Papaverine is the most commonly used vasodilator and is infused directly into the superior mesenteric artery. The infusion can be continued for up to 5 days but 24 hours is usually enough to reverse the vasoconstriction provided that supportive measures are implemented to correct the underlying abnormality. Digoxin and vasopressive agents should be avoided if at all possible in these patients. Despite optimal treatment some patients do progress to bowel necrosis and urgent surgery will be required.

Chronic mesenteric ischaemia This is due to arterial narrowing and is also hard to diagnose; however, the urgency of diagnosis is not so great. The typical presenting complaint is upper abdominal pain starting approximately 15 minutes following food and lasting for about 2 hours. Weight loss is a frequent consequence as patients reduce the frequency of food intake. The cause of the ischaemia is usually atherosclerotic stenosis of the mesenteric vessels causing ischaemia at times of maximal flow following meals. The rich collateral blood supply to the bowel and the slow progressive nature of the vessel narrowing usually protects against ischaemia until at least two of the mesenteric vessels are affected by at least a two-thirds reduction in blood flow. Unfortunately many asymptomatic patients both young and old have flow reductions on ultrasound which limits the usefulness of this technique as a screening tool. Angiography is usually required when the diagnosis is suspected clinically in order to demonstrate the exact extent of the flow reduction. Traditionally treatment has been surgical, but it carries a significant morbidity and mortality and angioplasty is increasingly being used. Usually only one vessel needs to be dilated to produce a clinical improvement.

Mesenteric vein ischaemia This is a rare cause of mesenteric ischaemia which was probably confused with non-occlusive mesenteric ischaemia in the past. Patients present with gradually increasing abdominal pain which may be associated with other pathology such as trauma, portal hypertension or hypercoagulable states. Selective superior mesenteric arterial injection may show a diffuse vasoconstriction with marked opacification of the small intramural vessels. Non-visualization of the venous phase of the study is also suggestive of the diagnosis but intravenous filling defects are more specific (Fig. 3.54).

Ischaemic colitis This is an important cause of colitis in the elderly population. The cause is unclear in most cases but is thought to be due to a combination of a low-flow state and small vessel disease. Most patients are over the age of 60 and present with abdominal pain or rectal bleeding. The region of the splenic flexure is most commonly involved as it is a watershed zone between the superior mesenteric artery and inferior mesenteric artery territories. The left colon and sigmoid are not uncommonly involved and no part of the colon is immune.

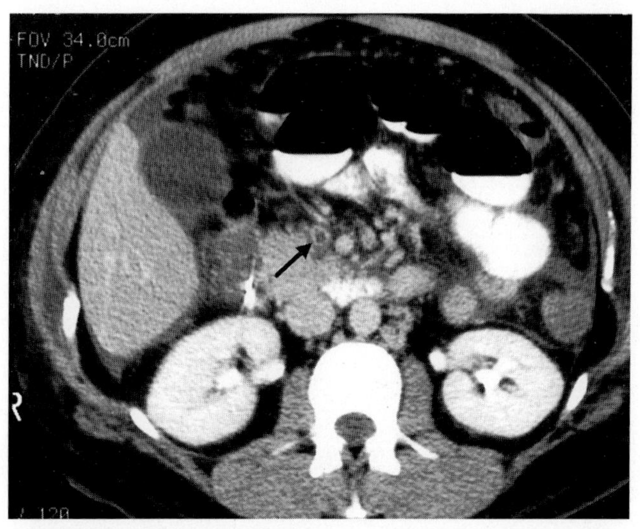

Fig. 3.54 Superior mesenteric vein thrombosis demonstrated during an i.v. contrast-enhanced CT. The thrombus is seen as a filling defect (arrow) in the superior mesenteric vein. (Courtesy G. Gill.)

Ischaemic colitis mostly affects the mucosa but can be transmural increasing the risk of gangrene and perforation. The ischaemic episode may be self-limiting resulting in complete healing which occurs in about a third of cases. An intermediate group of patients develop strictures or chronic colitis. Plain films may show no abnormalities or a non-specific ileus. More specific signs such as submucosal haemorrhage and oedema, visible as thumbprinting, are sometimes seen (Fig. 3.55). The diagnosis can be established in most cases with a double contrast barium enema. If there is a clinical suspicion of perforation or gangrenous bowel, barium is contra-indicated. When barium enema is performed early in the course of the disease, the most common finding is thumbprinting, seen as smooth polypoid filling defects which protrude into the bowel lumen. Another sign is thickened parallel folds running in a transverse fashion in the affected segment due to oedema and accentuated by the spasm which frequently coexists. At a later stage there may be sloughing of the necrotic mucosa and a barium examination at this stage will show evidence of ulceration. The ulcers tend to run in a longitudinal fashion and can mimic the ulcers of inflammatory bowel disease but ischaemic ulcers change over a few weeks as the disease progresses. These ulcers may heal completely or persist as chronic

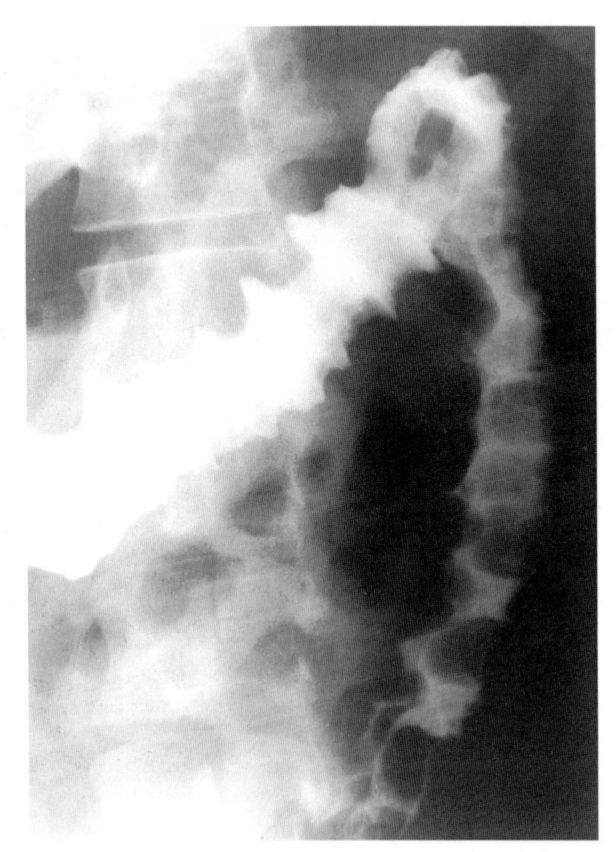

Fig. 3.55 Thumbprinting at the splenic flexure. Single contrast barium examination in a patient with rectal bleeding. The appearance may be due to haemorrhage or oedema secondary to ischaemic colitis, intramucosal haemorrhage (as in Henoch – Schönlein syndrome) and less likely pseudomembranous colitis, ulcerative colitis, Crohn's disease and amoebic colitis.

ulcerative ischaemic colitis with persistent symptoms. Alternatively the ulceration can heal leaving a stricture. Strictures can be seen as early as 3 weeks after the acute ischaemic episode; they are usually smooth in outline on barium studies with tapering ends but there may be associated lobulated outpouchings. The strictures may be seen without a clear history of precipitating ischaemia but rarely give rise to obstructive symptoms.

INFECTIVE BOWEL DISEASE

Tuberculous infection of the GI tract is a rare occurrence in western countries, but may be expected to rise with the increase in tuberculous disease at other sites which is now being reported, especially in the USA. Pulmonary disease accompanies GI involvement in about 20% of cases and the terminal ileum remains the area most commonly affected. At all sites tuberculosis is often accompanied by weight loss, loss of appetite and malaise. Malignant disease is usually the initial clinical diagnosis.

Oesophageal disease tends to affect the upper third and results in shallow ulcers and mucosal thickening causing disruption of the normal primary and secondary peristaltic waves. In the stomach the antrum is most frequently involved and ulceration and fibrosis predominate. In both oesophagus and stomach, fibrosis and luminal narrowing occur and may mimic carcinoma. Occasionally a large mass, a **tuberculoma,** appears as a filling defect on barium studies. Caseating lymph nodes around the stomach can be identified on both CT and ultrasound and may help in the diagnosis. In the duodenum and small bowel ulceration, wall thickening and fistulae can develop but a common final stage is fibrosis with narrowing. These features are best demonstrated with enteroclysis but even then are hard to separate from the findings in Crohn's disease.

The terminal ileum and caecum are by far the most common sites for intestinal tuberculous disease and require examination with both double contrast barium enema and small bowel meal with pneumocolon technique for complete evaluation. In the early stages the terminal ileum may show spasm but later deep ulcers, which are partially or completely circumferential, develop as well as fibrosis leading to a narrowed ulcerated terminal ileum with a widely patent, gaping ileocaecal valve. The combination of strictures in the caecum and terminal ileum can lead to partial or complete obstruction with dilation of the proximal loops of bowel, usually in association with caecal distortion and shortening of the right side of the colon. Enteroliths may develop proximal to these strictures and are seen on plain films of the abdomen as small or lamellated areas of calcification within the bowel.

Peritonitis can also develop which is initially associated with ascites (Fig. 3.56) with bowel wall and mesenteric thickening, best shown on ultrasound or CT. Later there is lymphadenopathy particularly in the

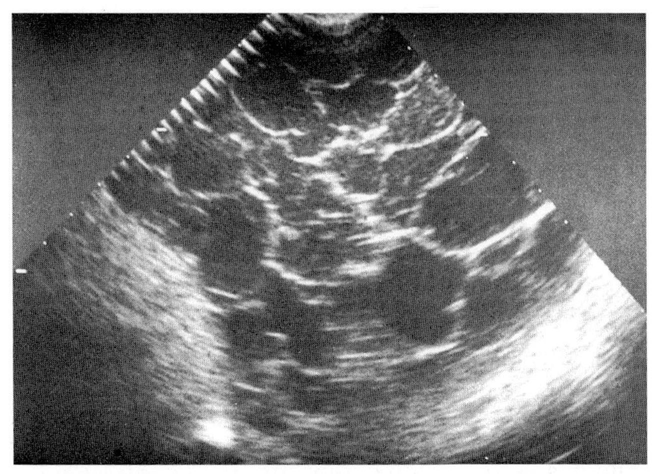

Fig. 3.56 Tuberculous peritonitis. Ultrasound of the abdomen showing multiple fibrous peritoneal strands giving a lattice-like appearance. (Courtesy V. Patel.)

right iliac fossa. The nodes tend to mat together and central caseation develops, which causes adhesions and often a degree of bowel obstruction.

POSTRADIOTHERAPY CHANGES

Radiotherapy can be complicated by both acute and chronic injury to any part of the GI tract. Complications are more likely with higher doses covering large areas at short intervals. Previous surgery increases the chance of complications as the bowel is less mobile because of adhesions resulting in the same part of bowel being exposed to each radiation fraction. Chemotherapy also increases the chance of injury, as do conditions which compromise the blood supply to the bowel such as diabetes or cardiac failure.

The acute radiation changes are rarely investigated radiologically and resolve by 6 weeks. Chronic damage can occur due to small vessel injury and patients may present months to years later. Acute damage to the **oesophagus** usually presents with odynophagia, although it is rarely investigated. Barium studies show mucosal fold thickening and abnormal motility. Chronic radiation damage to the oesophagus can present with dysphagia due to stricture which must be differentiated from tumour recurrence. Radiotherapy strictures are smooth in appearance on double contrast barium studies with gently tapering margins while tumour recurrence is typically irregular in outline. Endoscopy and multiple biopsies are often needed to make the distinction. Ulceration may occur in the oesophageal wall and these ulcers can progress to fistula formation. Fistulae most often communicate with the bronchus but can also involve other mediastinal structures.

Radiation damage to the **stomach** leads to a higher incidence of peptic ulcer disease. Narrowing and fibrosis of the antrum can lead to outflow obstruction, and endoscopy and biopsy are usually necessary to differentiate the effects of radiation from tumour, lymphoma, tuberculosis and Crohn's disease.

Acute radiation damage to the **small bowel** usually leads to malabsorption and diarrhoea. In the long term, patients can present with abdominal pain, diarrhoea, which is often bloody, and obstruction. The terminal ileum and pelvic loops are most frequently involved and on small bowel meal examination or enteroclysis the loops of bowel are relatively fixed with sharp angulation instead of the usual smooth turns. Smooth tapering strictures can also be seen with dilation of loops of proximal bowel. Fistulae can develop either between adjacent loops of bowel or to the skin or pelvic organs, and abscesses are not uncommon. Thickened bowel wall, fistulous tracks and abscesses can be demonstrated on CT.

Acute **colonic involvement** is common and presents with diarrhoea. Chronic involvement can also present with diarrhoea and abdominal pain. A double contrast barium study may show narrowing with smoothly tapering margins (Fig. 3.57). The underlying mucosa may be normal or show thick folds and thumbprinting secondary to oedema and haemorrhage from ischaemia. Fistulae can develop either to the skin, the bladder or the vagina.

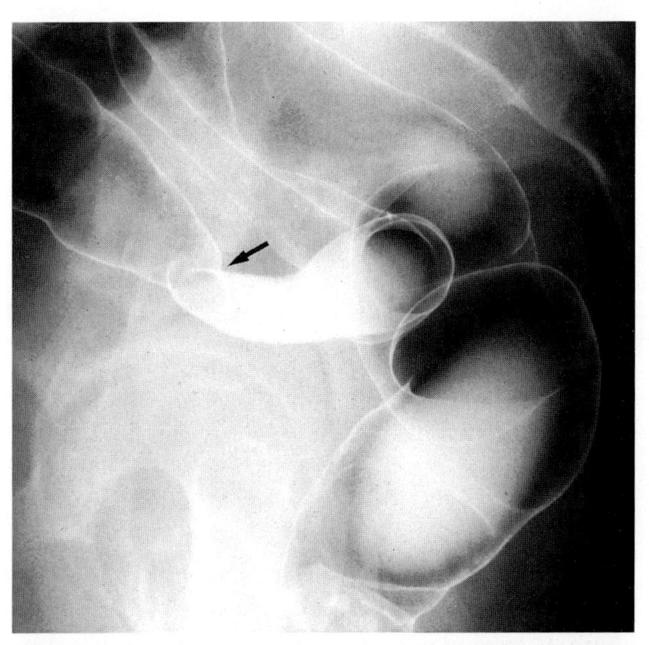

Fig. 3.57 Radiation stricture. Smoothly narrowed sigmoid loop (arrow) without shouldering or evidence of mucosal disease. This is characteristic of chronic radiation ischaemia; in this case it is associated with treatment for carcinoma of the cervix. The small bowel is often also involved and the ischaemia may cause ulceration and long-standing minor blood loss.

Rectal perforation from a balloon enema tip is more likely in a patient with fragile narrowed bowel secondary to radiotherapy. It is therefore very important that the clinician inform the radiologist about previous radiotherapy if a patient is referred for barium enema, so that an appropriate enema catheter can be selected. The same considerations make endoscopy hazardous.

CATHARTIC COLON

In patients with chronic laxative abuse a cathartic colon can develop which, in its later stages, mimics the features seen in ulcerative colitis. The first changes in laxative abuse are colonic dilation and lengthening, but after many years haustra are lost and the colon shortens and narrows. The colon shows shallow ulcers seen as small pools of contrast on barium studies. In contrast to ulcerative colitis the caecum and right side of the colon are predominantly affected with cathartic colon. Multiple narrowed segments are seen in motility dysfunction but they are permanent with cathartic colon. Multiple narrowed fibrotic strictures may also be present. The differentiation from ulcerative colitis can usually be made on barium studies combined with appropriate clinical information, and may be supported by melanosis seen on endoscopy.

GI BLEEDING

Acute gastrointestinal bleeding may require immediate resuscitative measures before any diagnostic tests can be brought to bear. Bleeding, however, may be chronic, necessitating infrequent but repeated blood transfusion and/or oral iron. Chronic blood loss is often more difficult to diagnose due to the slow nature of the haemorrhage. The investigative strategy is usually similar in both cases, and begins with endoscopy but, when this is not diagnostic, close liaison with the radiology department is essential in order to optimize the sequence of investigations needed. Acute GI bleeding carries a mortality rate of 8–10%. This figure has changed little over the past fifty years despite the advances in diagnostic and therapeutic techniques, partly because many people with gastrointestinal bleeding have severe associated medical conditions, and perhaps also because of the increasing age of the population.

ACUTE

Acute upper GI bleeding

The type and severity of the bleed dictate the choice and timing of the first investigation. If there is haematemesis of either bright blood or 'coffee grounds' and/or melaena, it is likely that the bleeding source is from the upper GI tract, proximal to the jejunum. Conversely, if there is rectal bleeding, which is not black and tarry (melaena), then the bleeding is likely to be coming from the lower GI tract or from a huge upper GI bleed when associated haematemesis may be expected, but is not always present. GI bleeds which appear to be small should not be dismissed as these may represent the warning before a catastrophic bleed occurs. It is often difficult to judge the size of a GI bleed especially in young patients who have a remarkable ability to compensate haemodynamically for a large blood loss, most of which can lie hidden within the bowel for some time.

The causes of upper GI haemorrhage are wide ranging, but include Mallory–Weiss tears, hiatal hernias, oesophagitis, varices, gastric ulcers, carcinoma, gastritis, the Dieulafoy lesion, duodenal ulcers, duodenal diverticula and aortoduodenal fistula. Haematological disorders with clotting abnormalities and collagen disorders, such as Ehlers–Danlos syndrome, can cause bleeding from the upper or lower GI tract.

If a perforation of the oesophagus, stomach or duodenum is clinically suspected but not confirmed on plain films of chest and abdomen then a water-soluble contrast study of the upper GI tract should be performed. This may confirm either a free or confined perforation and obviate the need for further investigation. If there is no suspicion of perforation either clinically or on initial radiographs, an upper GI endoscopy should be performed. The timing of endoscopy remains controversial, and depends on both the severity and likely cause of the bleeding. Some authorities advocate placement of a nasogastric tube to assess continuing bleeding while others undertake clinical assessment. In patients with cirrhosis early endoscopy is helpful, once the patient is stabilized, both because patients with variceal bleeding require specific endoscopic treatment and because a peptic ulcer is often the cause of bleeding in cirrhotic patients with varices. In any patient with continued active bleeding, assessed clinically or by nasogastric tube aspiration of fresh blood, urgent endoscopy should be performed. The majority of patients do not require immediate endoscopy, although endoscopy should be performed within 24 hours. These difficult endoscopies deserve the attention of the full endoscopy team including dedicated endoscopy nurses and the most experienced endoscopists.

Endoscopy correctly identifies the source of bleeding in 80–90% and is also very useful in predicting rebleed rates, particularly in patients who are bleeding from a peptic ulcer. The visualization of a blood vessel at the bottom of the ulcer crater predicts a high risk of early rebleeding. Endoscopic Doppler detection of an artery under the ulcer is an even stronger predictor of rebleeding, but has not come into general use. Early endoscopy is particularly important in patients who have a prosthetic graft and should be followed by contrast-enhanced CT scanning to evaluate integrity of the graft and to ensure that there is no aortoenteric fistula.

If upper GI endoscopy fails to demonstrate a cause for the bleeding the next investigation depends on the local availability of different imaging modalities and whether radiological intervention is being considered. The current options are angiography or nuclear medicine scanning with either ^{99m}technetium-labelled colloid or technetium-labelled erythrocytes. If the patient is actively bleeding and endoscopy has failed to show a bleeding point, angiography is the investigation of choice. Angiography is performed using a standard femoral artery approach with selective catherization of the coeliac and superior mesenteric arteries. Angiography will detect an actively bleeding site in about 90% of cases in whom the blood loss is greater than 0.5 ml/min and may also demonstrate the angiographic features of the responsible tumour even if it is not actively bleeding (Fig. 3.58).

If endoscopy has demonstrated the site of bleeding, but the bleeding is persisting despite optimal medical and endoscopic treatment, surgery or therapeutic

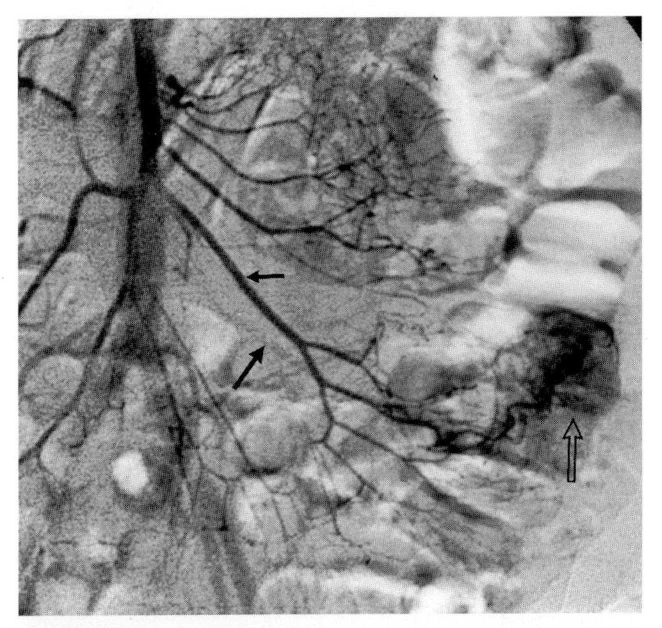

Fig. 3.58 Massive GI bleeding due to a leiomyoma of the mid-small bowel. The angiogram shows a large feeding artery (small arrow), an abnormal tumour blush (open arrow) and an early filling vein (long arrow).

angiography are required. Interventional radiological procedures to avert bleeding include a variety of transcatheter embolization procedures and vasopressin administration.

Radionuclide imaging has an established place in the diagnosis of acute upper GI bleeding as a sensitive and non-invasive technique: ^{99m}Tc-labelled colloid scans can detect the source of bleeding with rates down to 0.1 ml/min but this potential is seldom realized and, in practice, such slow bleeding rates are seldom detected. Colloid scans should be used when endoscopy does not show the bleeding site and when the rate of bleeding is not so brisk that it requires immediate transcatheter therapy. Radionuclide scans are often unable to distinguish between small and large bowel bleeding so that angiography is usually required to localize further the site of haemorrhage. The colloid scan is performed by giving the patient a single intravenous injection of technetium-labelled colloid and images of the abdomen are acquired over 15 minutes. Active bleeding is shown as a gradual increase in activity within the abdomen as the background activity falls.

Acute lower GI bleeding

Bleeding from the GI tract distal to the ligament of Treitz may be caused by a wide variety of conditions including inflammatory, ischaemic or infective bowel disease, Meckel's diverticulum with ectopic gastric mucosa, angiodysplasia, small bowel and colonic tumours, diverticulitis and haemorrhoids. These patients usually present with rectal bleeding. When the blood is bright red the source of the bleeding is usually in the left side of the colon and more proximal bleeding is often plum-coloured. However, rapid blood loss from anywhere within the GI tract can produce bright red rectal bleeding. While seldom diagnostic, an initial chest X-ray and supine abdominal film are prudent initial investigations in these patients, especially in those who are old, on steroids or have abdominal pain. In most cases of lower GI haemorrhage there is no indication as to the specific diagnosis. In contrast to upper GI haemorrhage, endoscopy is not indicated as the first investigation in these cases. This is because endoscopy in an unprepared colon is difficult and often unsatisfactory, as blood tracks in both directions and the view is poor. Colonoscopy is also unable to evaluate the great majority of the small bowel and may, therefore, not reach the site of the blood loss. Colonoscopy can be useful if the patient is prepared with a lavage solution with 1–2 l of solution given orally or via a nasogastric or preferably nasojejunal tube. In acute lower GI bleeding selective superior and inferior mesenteric angiography or radionuclide scans using ^{99m}Tc-labelled colloid are the best initial imaging modalities.

CHRONIC

Chronic upper GI bleeding

If bleeding is chronic and/or intermittent the investigative strategy needs to be changed. Endoscopy remains an excellent first-line investigation and, if negative in a stable patient with no signs of continuing bleeding, should be complemented by double contrast barium studies of the upper GI tract. If these investigations fail to identify the source of the bleeding, radionuclide scans again have a role. A technetium-labelled red cell scan is the more useful radiopharmaceutical as it is possible to monitor the patient for bleeding over a 24-hour period by a single intravenous injection. The erythrocytes can be labelled *in vitro* or *in vivo* and following injection, images of the abdomen are acquired every 10 minutes for the first hour and then every 2 hours for up to 24 hours. The rate of bleeding needs to be greater than 0.2 ml/min and at least 10 ml needs to have bled into the bowel during the course of the study. There is more background vascular activity with the red cell scan than with the colloid scan as the technetium is bound to the circulating erythrocytes and is not cleared by the liver as occurs with colloid. Consequently vascular structures as well as the richly vascularized liver and spleen can obscure the bleeding site or be misinterpreted as bleeding bowel. Bleeding is shown as a region of increased activity in the abdomen, which may move on consecutive images due to peristalsis. Once a bleeding site has been identified angiography is usually required to localize more precisely the source of bleeding and provide further information as to the underlying cause.

Chronic lower GI bleeding

If the blood loss is chronic or intermittent and thought to arise from the colon, patients should have a colonoscopy or double contrast barium study. Indeed, in patients who have a particularly elusive bleeding site, both investigations are required as well as upper GI endoscopy. Colonoscopy can be used as a therapeutic as well as a diagnostic technique as polyps can be removed and isolated arteriovenous malformations can be treated with diathermy or laser. If the bleeding site remains obscure then the patient will require a radiological small bowel study. This may be with a dedicated small bowel meal with pneumocolon technique, reserving enteroclysis for those patients with a negative small bowel meal. Some authorities recommend omitting the small bowel meal and proceeding directly to enteroclysis, claiming this is more sensitive for the detection of small tumours, but this approach does subject all such patients to the more invasive procedure.

Nuclear medicine studies can also be used at this stage using either a red cell-labelled scan to detect the site of intermittent blood loss or a pertechnetate scan to look for ectopic gastric mucosa within a Meckel's diverticulum. Ectopic gastric mucosa can lead to peptic ulceration and blood loss particularly in younger patients (Fig. 3.59). If the site of haemorrhage still remains obscure a contrast enhanced abdominal CT scan should be performed to look for bowel-related masses and involvement of the mesentery. Finally angiography may be performed. The inferior mesenteric artery should be examined first before the bladder fills with contrast, followed by the superior mesenteric and coeliac arteries. Superselective catheterization may be required to show a small lesion. If angiography also fails to show a bleeding site, consideration should be given to provocative testing, which needs careful discussion with all involved parties (surgeon, patient and radiologist) as it is not without risk, but it can provide the answer when all else has failed. Provocative testing involves pretreating the patient with heparin and then performing the angiogram. Enteroscopy is a relatively new and very invasive procedure in which a narrow non-steerable endoscope is passed through the nose and manoeuvred into the small bowel. In one study enteroscopy revealed the source of bleeding in one third of patients in whom all other tests had been negative. Its place in clinical practice is not yet clear and probably awaits further technical improvements.

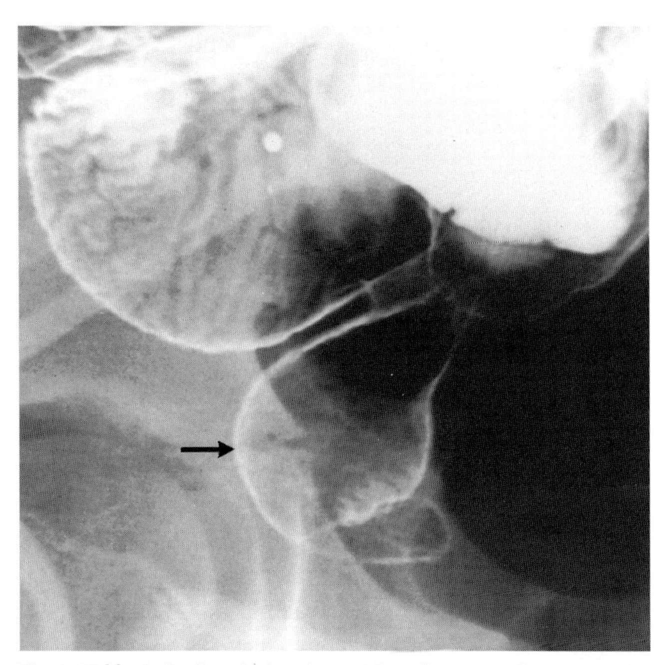

Fig. 3.59 Meckel's diverticulum (arrow) found on peroral pneumocolon at the end of a small bowel meal examination. These small sacs are seldom obvious on routine films.

THE ACUTE ABDOMEN

Patients presenting with an 'acute abdomen' present a formidable diagnostic challenge. A detailed history and examination, combined with blood tests and plain radiographs of the chest and abdomen may lead to a specific diagnosis. More often a list of possible diagnoses is formulated. Often the most pressing decision is whether the patient needs immediate operation based on the patient's condition and the likely diagnosis. Additional imaging can help to narrow the differential diagnosis and aid in this decision process in a select group of patients. While conventional contrast studies still have a place, the most useful additional investigations in these patients are abdominal and pelvic ultrasound and CT. Disease affecting any of the abdominal systems may cause or contribute to an acute abdomen and these include pancreatic, renal, gynaecological, hepatic, splenic and alimentary tract disease. Non-abdominal causes also need to be considered, in particular cardiac and pulmonary disease, and specifically lower lobe infection. Diseases causing a generalized disturbance, such as the vasculitides, can affect multiple end organs and present with an acute abdomen; more obscure pathology such as familial Mediterranean fever can also present in this way.

PERFORATION

Patients with a suspected perforation, which is not confirmed on plain radiographs, may benefit from water-soluble contrast studies which can show a small free leak or the cavity of a contained perforation. CT scanning is also useful to confirm small amounts of extraluminal gas, particularly in the retroperitoneum where the ability to show the location of this gas can help in determining the site of the perforation. The perforation is likely to be from the sigmoid if free gas is seen low in the abdomen and from the duodenum if seen only in the upper abdomen.

TRAUMA

CT with intravenous contrast enhancement is particularly useful in patients with solid organ trauma but can also be helpful in the identification of bowel trauma. Bowel trauma produces focal bowel wall thickening or soft-tissue density collections around the site of traumatized bowel due to local haematoma. Air in the peritoneal cavity or in the retroperitoneum is detected with a greater sensitivity than on plain radiographs. Air is, however, not always seen in the presence of a small perforation and oral water-soluble contrast is, therefore, advisable. This may confirm a leak by appearing in an extraluminal location and can also localize the site of the perforation. A haemoperitoneum appears as high attenuation fluid collection within the peritoneum which differentiates it from serous fluid which has a low attenuation. Haemoperitoneum is usually the result of solid organ damage but can also be seen with damage to the hollow viscera.

OBSTRUCTION

In cases of obstruction the clinical findings and plain films usually provide the diagnosis but CT can sometimes be useful by showing a transition zone between proximal dilated loops of bowel and collapsed bowel distally. Thus the site of the obstruction is usually demonstrated, and the cause for the obstruction may often be shown by the demonstration of a bowel-related mass or a more specific finding such as intussusception.

If findings suggest a distal colonic obstruction, an enema should be performed to differentiate mechanical obstruction from pseudo-obstruction (Ogilvie's syndrome). A single contrast enema suffices and in pseudo-obstruction barium flows freely past the site of apparent obstruction. With a colonic obstruction a single contrast study is usually quite adequate to detect an obstructing lesion. In the middle-to-old-age adult population obstruction is usually due to diverticular disease and/or carcinoma, but the differentiation between them is not always possible on the barium study.

DIVERTICULAR DISEASE

Diverticular disease can present in a variety of ways, including an acute abdomen. A barium enema examination will confirm the presence of diverticular disease and in patients without clinical evidence of complications, may be all that is required. Barium studies are not very accurate in the evaluation of collections around the colon and, in patients in whom an abscess is suspected on clinical findings, a CT scan is the preferred examination (Fig. 3.60); this will confirm the presence of colonic diverticula but will also demonstrate the size, shape and position of any pericolonic collection. Patients with single or few distinct abscess collections may benefit from initial percutaneous abscess drainage under ultrasound or CT control.

APPENDICITIS

Imaging may also help in the diagnosis and treatment of appendicitis and suspected appendicitis. Traditionally it has been prudent to operate to remove an appendix suspected of being the cause of an acute abdomen. There is, however, often uncertainty about the cause of right lower quadrant pain especially in young female patients in whom a gynaecological origin for the pain must also to be considered. Transabdominal or transvaginal ultrasound is the preferred examination when the differential includes a gynaecological cause for the pain as the visualization of the uterus, ovaries and adnexae is superior to that from CT. The appendix itself is examined using the technique of graded ultrasound compression. Bowel loops in the right lower quadrant are imaged and compressed using the ultrasound transducer as a pressure device. Normal bowel will compress but an inflamed appendix will show minimal compression

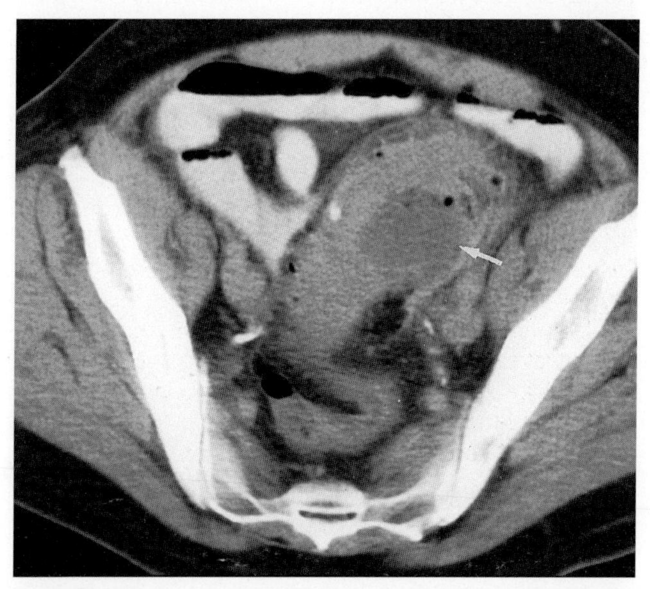

Fig. 3.60 Abscess as a complication of diverticular disease. The abscess is seen as a low attenuation mass lesion (arrow) on this pelvic CT scan. Air within sigmoid diverticula is also seen. The abscess was drained percutaneously under CT guidance. (Courtesy A. O'Donovan.)

and be greater than 7 mm in diameter while being compressed (Fig. 3.61). The wall will be hypoechoic and the lumen hyperechoic so giving a target appearance on transverse section; when seen in longitudinal section the thickened bowel appears as a tube-like structure of varying length. An appendicolith may also be seen as a highly reflecting focus within the appendix which casts an acoustic band seen as a dark shadow lying behind the bright appendicolith reflection. If no abnormality is detected in the right iliac fossa the rest of the abdomen should be examined for other causes of abdominal pain. This includes the pelvis, the upper abdomen and an assessment of free fluid. Ultrasound is about 90% accurate in the diagnosis of acute appendicitis but problems arise with retrocaecal appendix and in patients with large amounts of subcutaneous fat which causes considerable image degradation. In these cases and when there is a clinical suspicion of an appendix abscess a CT scan is the preferred examination.

INTUSSUSCEPTION

Intussusception usually presents in babies between the ages of three months and two years with abdominal pain, vomiting and blood and mucus in the stools. The commonest type of intussusception is the ileocolic when small bowel invaginates into the colon. The diagnosis may be made on plain films. Ultrasound shows a mass with a hyperechoic centre surrounded by concentric hyper- and hypoechoic rings. The diagnosis is confirmed with a single contrast enema using carbon dioxide or air as the contrast agent. For this, gas is insufflated under fluoroscopic control and if an intussusception is present an attempt at pneumatic reduction can be made (Fig. 3.62). Reduction should only be attempted if there are no signs of peritonitis.

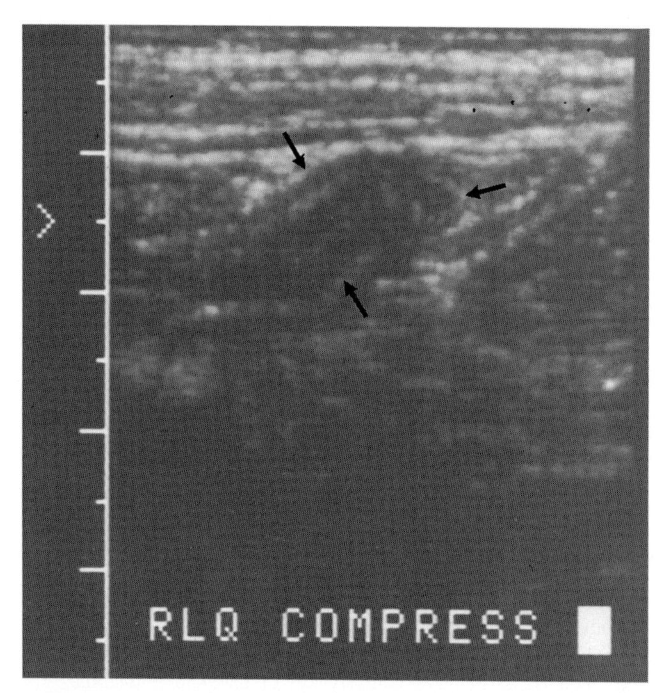

Fig. 3.61 Appendicitis. Ultrasound carried out on a child with abdominal pain reveals a blind-ending oedematous loop of bowel (arrows), almost a centimetre in diameter, that was not compressible – the diagnostic ultrasound features of appendicitis.

THE POSTSURGICAL PATIENT

Patients are often referred for radiological assessment of the GI tract following surgery, either as a precautionary measure or to determine the cause of a postoperative complication. The radiological technique employed will depend on the type of surgery performed and the question which is to be addressed. It is extremely helpful if the surgeon provides the radiologist with a detailed diagram of the surgery undertaken so that the postsurgical anatomy is known. If the radiologist has this knowledge the examination can be devoted to answering the clinical question rather than working out the anatomy. The contrast agents used in the immediate postoperative period are generally water-soluble. Patients in whom perforation has not been shown on water-soluble contrast studies may then require a barium study to provide better anatomical detail.

THE OESOPHAGUS

Tumour surgery

Various palliative surgical procedures are employed for oesophageal carcinoma all of which may require postoperative imaging. One week after oesophagogastrectomy a routine non-ionic contrast study is usually performed. The oesophagogastrectomy may be combined with an antireflux procedure and complications from both parts of the operation may therefore be present simultaneously. Ideally the patient drinks the contrast in various positions, as an anastomotic leak may only be demonstrated when the site of the leak is on the dependent part of the oesophagus, although such an examination is not always possible due to patient discomfort or immobility. As well as contrast leaks, aspiration into the trachea may be demonstrated. There may also be obstruction, either at the anastomosis due to oedema or haemorrhage, or at the distal part of the intrathoracic stomach. Such distal obstructions may be due to oedema, around the site of the antireflux procedure, or gastric volvulus. Many of these patients present with dysphagia after an interval and this may be due to tumour recurrence or a benign stricture, either at the anastomosis or in the low neo-oesophagus secondary to reflux oesophagitis. While

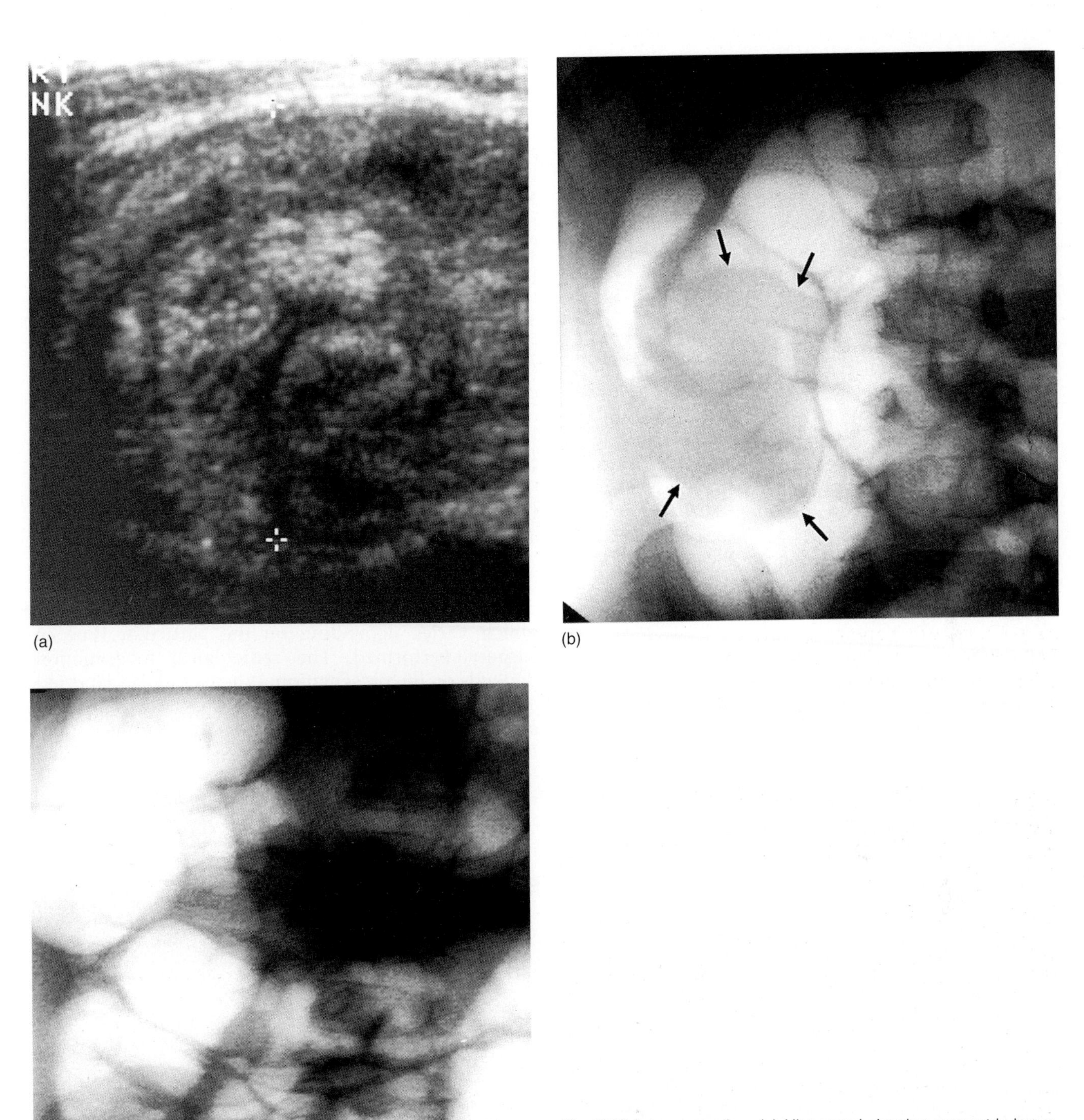

(c)

Fig. 3.62 Intussusception. (a) Ultrasound showing concentric hyperechoic and hypoechoic rings in an infant with abdominal pain. A diagnosis of intussusception was made and a carbon dioxide enema (b) shows the colon filled with gas, with a large filling defect (arrows) in the ascending colon representing the partially reduced intussusception. (c) Keeping the pressure of CO_2 between 80 and 120 mm Hg, the intussusception was completely reduced and gas was seen to enter the small bowel (arrow). The two fluoroscopy images were obtained using a fluororecord technique keeping radiation dose to the absolute minimum. The images were manipulated so that gas appears white.

most of these patients will require endoscopy to provide a histological diagnosis, a preliminary barium study will identify the site of the problem, and lead to a safer and more focused endoscopic examination.

Colonic interposition may also be used as an alternative to oesophagogastrectomy. Complications from colonic interposition are higher than with oesophagogastrectomy, with anastomotic leaks occurring in up to 40% of patients. Mediastinal complications such as haematoma or abscess are also seen and best imaged by CT scans. At a later stage a stricture may develop, particularly at the proximal anastomosis, leading to delay in emptying and dilatation of the interposed colon.

Gastro-oesophageal reflux

The oesophagus may also be operated on in an attempt to reduce gastro-oesophageal reflux. In the postoperative period, dysphagia may occur due to oedema or haemorrhage at the gastro-oesophageal junction which appears on contrast studies as a fundal mass with a tapering lower oesophagus supporting a column of contrast. These appearances usually resolve as the oedema subsides over a few weeks but a persistent narrowing may be demonstrated due to an overtight fundal wrap.

Achalasia

Patients with achalasia who have had a cardiomyotomy or pneumatic dilation also require postoperative assessment. Following a cardiomyotomy, perforation is the most frequent immediate postoperative complication. In about 50% of cases the oesophagus is seen to have an eccentric outpouching at the site of the myotomy and it is important that this is not mistaken for a leak. Delayed complications are those of gastro-oesophageal reflux and complications related to reflux. Patients who have had pneumatic balloon dilation have a perforation risk of up to 4%. A limited water-soluble contrast swallow and a chest X-ray are usually performed as some of these perforations can be clinically silent. If no leak is seen on this initial study, a barium contrast study should be performed to assess the anatomy of the area more thoroughly and to detect subtle leaks. There is considerable oedema immediately following balloon dilation and small leaks can therefore be missed. A contrast study should be repeated if the patient's condition deteriorates in the postoperative period. If a contrast swallow is negative in a patient in whom there is a high index of suspicion of an oesophageal leak, an urgent CT should be organized.

THE STOMACH AND DUODENUM

Common to almost all surgery to the stomach and duodenum is the risk of postoperative **perforation** which varies depending on the particular type of surgery performed. The radiological investigation depends on the presentation. When a leak is suspected a single contrast water-soluble study is helpful, with careful attention being taken to ensure that the patient is examined in several positions. Fever, leucocytosis

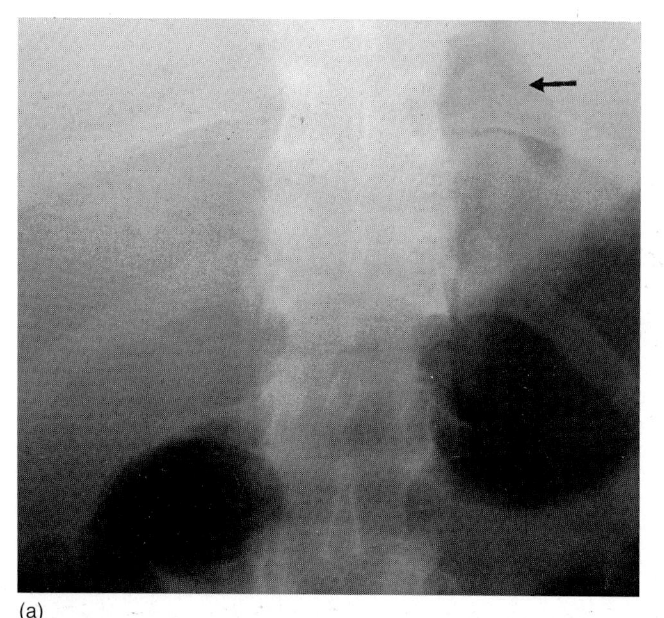

(a)

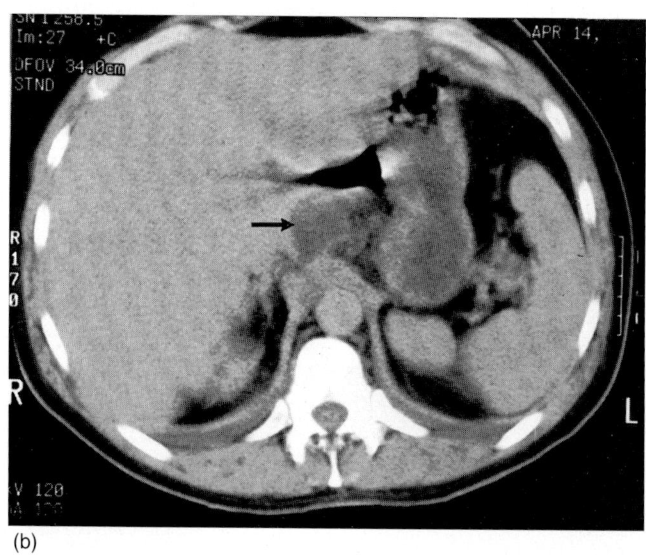

(b)

Fig. 3.63 Postoperative abscess. (a) An abdominal film 5 days after laparoscopic fundoplication shows a gas collection in the mediastinum (arrow). (b) CT scan revealed that the abscess (arrow) involved the upper abdomen and further cuts showed that it extended into the mediastinum. The abscess was drained percutaneously with an approach through the left lobe of the liver and the catheter tip was later manoeuvred up into the mediastinum.

and/or pain occurring a few days following surgery suggest an **abscess**. Ultrasound is an excellent tool to investigate this potential complication although the presence of a postoperative ileus may result in too much bowel gas for proper evaluation. In this setting a CT scan of the upper abdomen is indicated with intravenous contrast to determine the size and site of the collection (Fig. 3.63). Most abscesses are suitable for percutaneous drainage and again ultrasound or CT may be used to guide the drainage procedure. In patients with an abscess after surgery a contrast study is also indicated to detect a continuing leak.

In patients who have had operations for peptic ulceration, recurrent **ulcers** can occur. These are best investigated by endoscopy, as is local recurrence in patients who have had surgery for carcinoma. Due to the distorted anatomy, adequate endoscopic evaluation is not always possible and in this situation a barium study may provide valuable information. Double contrast barium examination of the postoperative stomach is more difficult than in a native stomach due to problems of flooding of the distal bowel. Postoperative problems are similar for patients who have had surgery for peptic ulcer disease or gastric carcinoma, and the complications also overlap; the following discussion therefore applies to both groups.

Barium studies are useful to assess anastomotic strictures which can lead to outlet obstruction. Gastric emptying can be quantified using a radiolabelled solid and/or liquid feed by recording the gastric activity over time. The radionuclide study is usually reserved for patients who have symptoms of **gastric outflow obstruction**, but no structural abnormality on barium studies or at endoscopy. Gastric stasis is not uncommon after gastric surgery and may lead to problems with bloating, vomiting and weight loss, in a similar fashion to that seen with mechanical obstruction. Gastric outlet obstruction can also occur due to intussusception of gastric remnant mucosa, or the entire gastric wall thickness may prolapse through the anastomosis. Outflow obstruction in the immediate postoperative period may be due to stomal oedema which may persist for two to three weeks. At endoscopy the stoma appears oedematous and closed, but once the endoscope has been passed through it, gastric drainage often improves. Pancreatitis is another cause of postoperative outflow obstruction, and clinical features guide the diagnosis.

Patients can also develop **retrograde intussusception** of the small bowel into the gastric remnant, which typically involves the efferent loop. This can be seen in the immediate postoperative period but tends to occur as a delayed complication after many years. If seen in the immediate postoperative period the presentation is usually dramatic with upper abdominal pain, an upper quadrant mass, vomiting and haematemesis. Plain radiographs are often unrewarding but barium studies show a mass lesion within the gastric remnant consisting of jejunal loops which have oedematous compressed folds giving a coiled spring appearance. In the delayed form symptoms are less severe, the intussusception is often intermittent and barium studies give the greatest yield if performed during an acute attack.

Gastric surgery may also be complicated by the **dumping syndrome** but this is generally a clinical diagnosis and imaging has little to offer. Radionuclide studies however can quantitate the speed of gastric emptying.

Malabsorption can also occur as a postoperative complication in patients who have had gastric surgery. Malabsorption can occur due to bacterial overgrowth secondary to stasis in an afferent loop which can be diagnosed by carbon-14 breath tests. Alternatively the malabsorption can be due to coeliac disease which can be precipitated by gastric surgery. The diagnosis of malabsorption may be made by the appearance of the small bowel loops during barium studies but the diagnosis is confirmed with endoscopic biopsy of the distal duodenum or jejunum. Malabsorption may also occur due to an inadvertent gastroileal anastomosis at surgery when a gastrojejunal anastomosis was intended. This is uncommon and tends to occur when the surgery has been particularly difficult.

Patients may also develop **obstruction of the afferent loop** leading to vague pains relieved by vomiting. This is difficult to investigate with routine barium studies because in 20% of normal postoperative patients the afferent loop is not opacified. Ultrasound can be useful in demonstrating a dilated loop of bowel in the upper abdomen. A CT scan with oral contrast is an alternative technique demonstrating

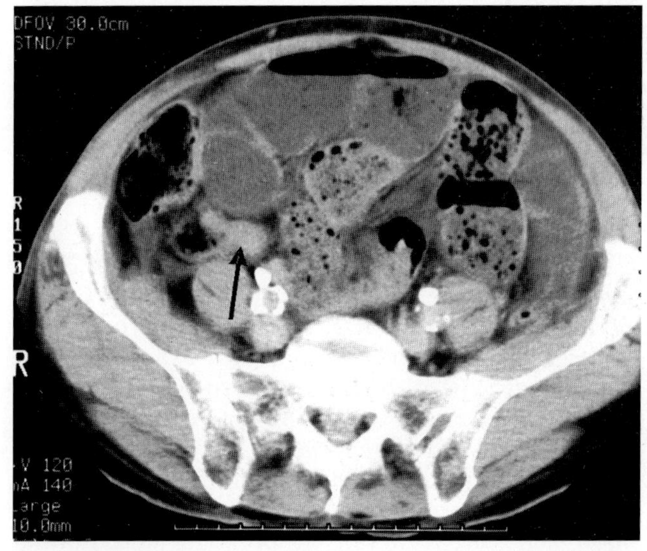

Fig. 3.64 Small bowel obstruction due to adhesions. The CT scan shows multiple loops of dilated small bowel but a collapsed terminal ileum (arrow) and caecum. No bowel-related masses were seen at the transition point.

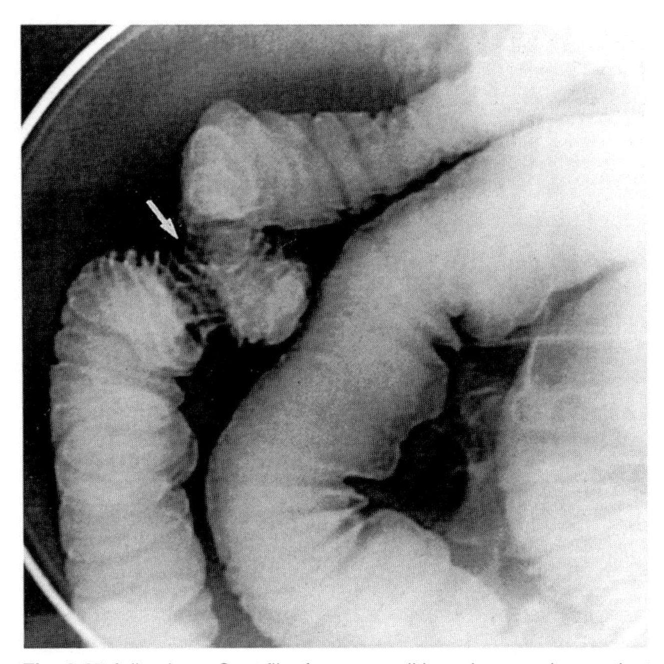

Fig. 3.65 Adhesions. Spot film from a small bowel enema in a patient with repeated adhesions with postprandial pain and distension. The kink (arrow) in the distal ileum was constant and due to an adhesion. Surgical lysis of this adhesion stopped the attacks.

a U-shaped dilated loop of bowel containing no contrast; this may be associated with dilated bile ducts.

Gastric surgery is also performed as a weight control procedure in patients with morbid obesity using either a stapling procedure to reduce the volume of the stomach, or a bypass operation. **Gastritis** or **ulceration** at the suture or staple line may occur. The gastritis and proximal ulceration is best assessed endoscopically but ulceration within the narrowed gastric channel may be difficult to evaluate and in this situation double contrast barium techniques may show the ulcer crater. Outlet obstruction is not a rare complication in the immediate postoperative period due to oedema and generally settles without investigation or specific treatment. In the immediate postoperative period the anastomosis may leak causing an abscess.

In the later postoperative period following any gastric surgery **small bowel adhesions** can cause obstruction. There is a paucity of good data on the merits of CT, small bowel meal and enteroclysis in these patients but practice is moving toward CT in the acute situation (Fig. 3.64) and enteroclysis in chronic recurrent obstruction (Fig. 3.65). Enteroclysis may not be possible with some types of gastric surgery because of difficulty in cannulating the jejunum. CT with oral water-soluble contrast demonstrates a transition zone between dilated proximal and normal distal bowel with acute angulation of bowel loops at the site of the adhesion. Barium meal examination or enteroclysis can show a sharp angulation of bowel loops, and often reproduces the patient's symptoms when a large volume of barium reaches the diseased segment.

THE SMALL BOWEL

Surgery on the small bowel can be complicated by **postoperative leak** which should be investigated by water-soluble contrast delivered as close to the leak as possible. The initial administration of contrast should be through a nasogastric, nasojejunal tube or by ileostomy depending on whether the leak is thought clinically to be from proximal or distal small bowel. When clinical suspicion persists after a negative or suboptimal fluoroscopic examination, abdominal CT following oral water-soluble contrast will often show both the leak and any associated abscess.

In patients with **enterocutaneous fistula** a sinogram can be performed using a small-bore feeding tube passed from the skin opening deeply into the track using water-soluble contrast to demonstrate any connection with the bowel.

Feeding jejunostomy tubes can be placed for long- or short-term feeding. The position of the feeding tube can be checked before starting feeding by injecting water-soluble contrast to confirm that the tube is within the bowel lumen and that the contrast flows freely into distal loops. If there is tube displacement, either initially or due to later tube migration, the contrast will be seen to enter a cavity or outline a track. The tip of the tube may be seen to lie outside of the bowel loops. If the tube has migrated it is often possible to reposition it using catheters and guidewires under radiological control and thus avoid a repeat operation. Small bowel obstruction distal to the feeding tube can also be investigated by injecting barium down the tube.

Ileostomies may not function well in the immediate postoperative period or develop problems later. Most abnormalities occur close to the ostomy and include adhesions or stenosis causing obstruction. Herniation around the stoma can also occur, as can disease recurrence in the remaining small bowel. These problems are best investigated by retrograde barium studies. Ileal stenosis close to the ostomy site can cause obstruction and appear as a narrowed segment of bowel with proximal dilation. This can occur very close to the ostomy site so it is important not to pass catheters too far into the bowel or these lesions will be missed. Recurrent disease usually gives similar findings to those seen with the primary disease. Insufflation of CO_2 or air to obtain a double contrast study of the distal bowel can be very helpful in recurrent mucosal disease, especially with Crohn's disease. Alternatively an endoscope can be passed retrogradely through the ostomy, which has the advantage of allowing biopsies of suspicious areas. Adhesions can also cause obstruction and may appear as sharply angulated loops of bowel associated with dilation proximal to the adhesion. If para-ileostomy herniation is suspected CT is probably the best imaging modality and only limited thin sections are required through the site of the ostomy. Para-ileostomy herniation is seen as a loop of bowel lying beside the stoma and protruding out of the abdominal cavity into the subcutaneous tissues.

Patients with small bowel surgery may also develop a **blind loop or pouch syndrome** and present with malabsorption, diarrhoea and abdominal pain. The malabsorption, which is due to bacterial overgrowth in the blind loop or pouch, can be investigated by carbon-14 breath tests. The anatomy of these loops can be demonstrated with a barium meal, although enteroclysis often provides more detailed information.

Patients with a small bowel bypass operation frequently develop complications which are difficult to investigate due to non-opacification of the bypassed loop. Conventional antegrade barium studies can show abnormalities such as stricture and adhesions and thus help in the distinction between structural abnormalities and bypass enteritis. Abnormalities in the diseased segment such as intussusception are best evaluated by ultrasound or CT.

Patients may also develop small bowel problems following the formation of a **ileo-anal pouch**. The pouch is initially protected with a proximal ileostomy, and before this is reversed, the pouch is usually checked using water-soluble contrast for anastomotic leaks. These pouchograms are performed with soft catheters and can demonstrate leaks, displacement of the bowel by a collection and abnormal gas collections within an abscess. An abscess can be further studied with contrast-enhanced CT scan. At a later date patients can develop pouchitis with diarrhoea and pain. Pouchitis appears on barium studies as mucosal fold thickening within the pouch, associated with spasm. The inflammation in the pouch can also be detected by endoscopy with biopsy or most easily with a technetium-labelled leucocyte scan. The clinical symptoms, however, are sufficiently clear that in many cases antibiotic treatment will be given on clinical diagnosis and no imaging is needed.

THE LARGE BOWEL

Following colorectal surgery, postoperative leaks and fistulae are investigated in similar ways to those used for the small bowel. Recurrent disease and postoperative strictures may be evaluated by double contrast barium studies or endoscopy. Complete obstruction is best studied with a low density single contrast technique as patients are often sick and this technique requires little patient movement. Studies through colostomies are performed in much the same way as for ileostomies. If the defunctioning limb of the colostomy is cannulated and contrast injected the colon typically appears to have a small lumen and may show features of diversion colitis with nodular mucosa giving the appearance of focal nodular hyperplasia. These patients are generally asymptomatic and the findings are of no clinical significance.

CHAPTER 4

Peritoneum and retroperitoneum

Jeremiah C. Healy
and Rodney H. Reznek

NORMAL ANATOMY
PATHOLOGY

Before the introduction of cross-sectional imaging, the peritoneum, mesentery and retroperitoneal structures could only be imaged with difficulty, often requiring invasive techniques. Ultrasound, and more particularly computed tomography (CT) and magnetic resonance imaging (MRI), have allowed the accurate demonstration of the anatomy of these regions and detailed detection of pathology; even minor changes can be reliably shown.

NORMAL ANATOMY

PERITONEUM

The peritoneum is the largest and most complex serous membrane in the body. In the male it forms a closed sac, whereas in the female it is penetrated by the lateral ends of the fallopian tubes. The peritoneal cavity is the potential space between the visceral and parietal layers of peritoneum consisting of a main region, termed the greater sac, and a diverticulum, the omental bursa or lesser sac, situated behind the stomach.

The radiological anatomy of the peritoneum is illustrated using axial CT with the peritoneal space demonstrated using positive contrast medium (Fig. 4.1).

Diagnostic and Interventional Radiology in Surgical Practice. Edited by P. Armstrong and M. L. Wastie. Published in 1997 by Chapman & Hall, London. ISBN 0 412 61960 1 (HB), 0 412 61970 9(PB)

Peritoneal spaces

The peritoneal cavity is divided into two main compartments by the transverse colon and its mesentery which connects the colon to the posterior abdominal wall (Fig. 4.2); the

- **supramesocolic compartment**
- **inframesocolic compartment**.

Supramesocolic compartment The supramesocolic compartment can be divided into right and left peritoneal spaces, which in turn are arbitarily divided into a number of subspaces, which are normally in communication, but often become separated by adhesions:

The right supramesocolic space has three subspaces:

- **The right subphrenic space** extends over the diaphragmatic surface of the right lobe of the liver to the right coronary ligament postero-inferiorly and the falciform ligament (Fig. 4.1a) medially, which separates it from the left subphrenic space.
- **The right subhepatic space** (Fig. 4.1b) can be further divided into anterior and posterior compartments. The anterior subhepatic space (Fig. 4.1b) is limited inferiorly by the transverse colon and its mesentery. The posterior subhepatic space (Fig. 4.1b), also known as the **hepatorenal fossa** or **Morrison's pouch**, extends posteriorly to the parietal peritoneum overlying the right kidney. Superiorly the subhepatic space is bounded by the

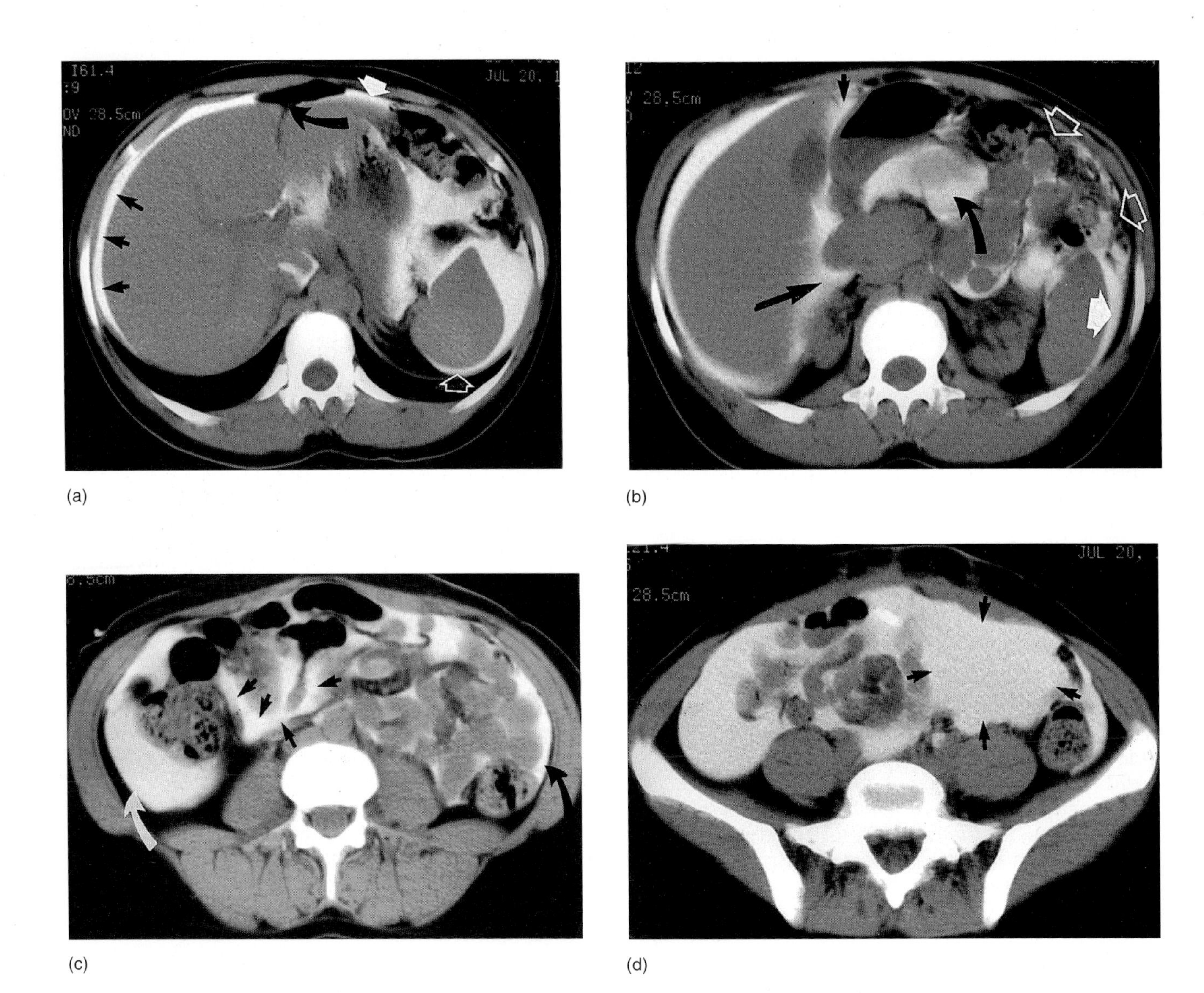

(a) (b)

(c) (d)

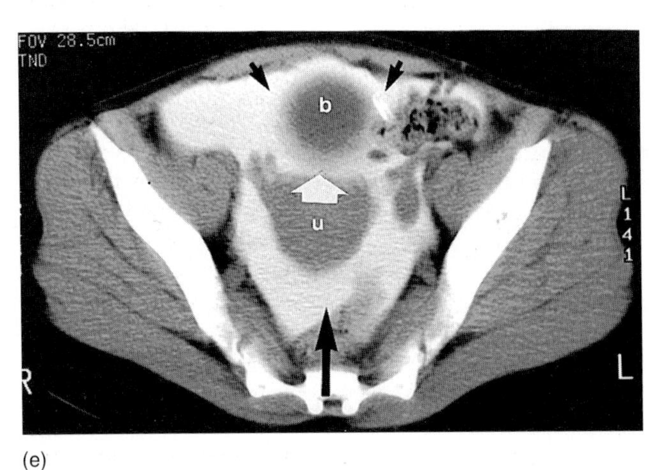

(e)

Fig. 4.1 Normal anatomy shown on CT after intraperitoneal injection of contrast medium. (a) CT with intraperitoneal contrast, at the level of the porta hepatis, demonstrating the right subphrenic space (small black arrows), the left anterior subphrenic space (white arrow), the left posterior subphrenic space (open white arrow) and the falciform ligament (curved black arrow). (b) CT with intraperitoneal contrast, at the level of the renal hilum, demonstrating the lesser sac (curved black arrow), anterior right subhepatic space (small black arrow), Morrison's pouch (large black arrow) and the left posterior subphrenic space (white arrow). Fat lies within the greater omentum (open white arrows). (c) CT with intraperitoneal contrast, just above the aortic bifurcation, demonstrating the right paracolic gutter (curved white arrow), left paracolic gutter (curved black arrow) and right infracolic space (small black arrows). (d) CT with intraperitoneal contrast, at the level of the iliac crests, demonstrating the left infracolic space (small black arrows). (e) CT with intraperitoneal contrast, at the level of the uterus (u) and bladder (b), demonstrating the paravesical (small black arrows), uterovesical (white arrow) and rectovesical (large black arrow) spaces.

inferior surface of the right lobe of the liver. The right subphrenic space and right subhepatic space communicate freely with the right paracolic gutter (Fig. 4.2).

- **The lesser sac** extends behind the stomach, anterior to the pancreas, communicating with the rest of the peritoneal cavity through a narrow inlet, the **epiploic foramen** (foramen of Winslow). A prominent oblique fold of peritoneum is raised on the posterior wall of the lesser sac by the left gastric artery, dividing it into two major recesses. The smaller superior recesss completely encloses the caudate lobe of the liver. It extends superiorly deep into the fissure for the ligamentum venosum and lies adjacent to the right diaphragmatic crus. The larger inferior recess (Fig. 4.1b) lies between the stomach and the visceral surface of the spleen. It is bounded inferiorly by the transverse colon and its mesentery, but can extend for a variable distance between the leaves of the greater omentum.

The left supramesocolic space has four arbitary communicating subspaces:

- **The left anterior perihepatic space** (Fig. 4.1b) is bounded medially by the falciform ligament, posteriorly by the liver surface, and anteriorly by the diaphragm.
- **The left posterior perihepatic space**, also called the gastrohepatic recess, follows the inferior surface of the lateral segment of the left hepatic lobe.
- **The left anterior subphrenic space** (Fig. 4.1a) lies between the anterior wall of the stomach and the left hemidiaphragm, communicating inferiorly with the left anterior perihepatic space.
- **The posterior subphrenic (perisplenic) space** (Fig. 4.1a) covers the superior and inferolateral surfaces of the spleen.

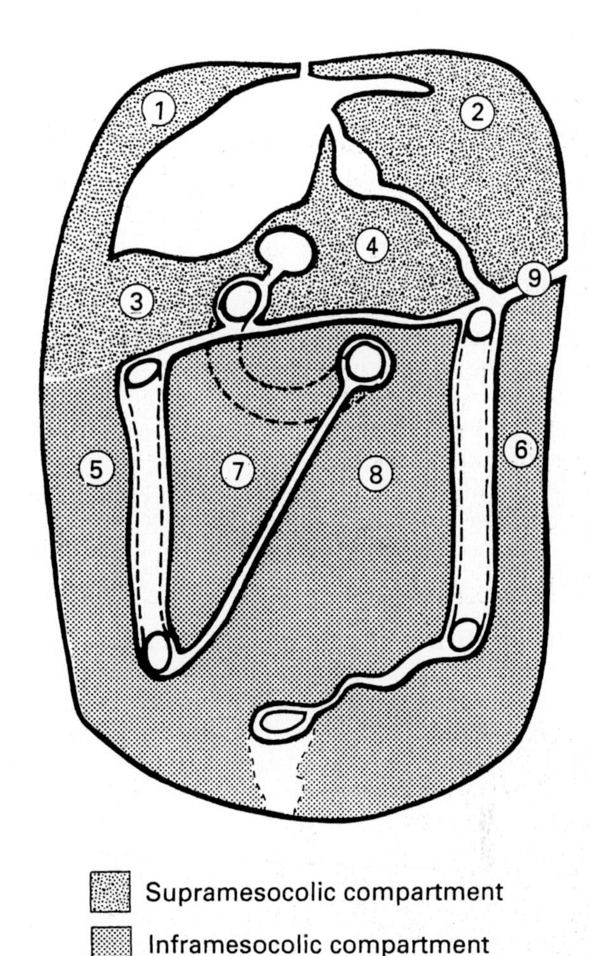

Fig. 4.2 Diagram to show the posterior peritoneal spaces and the peritoneal attachments to the posterior abdominal wall. (1) Right subphrenic space; (2) left subphrenic space; (3) right subhepatic space; (4) lesser sac; (5) right paracolic gutter; (6) left paracolic gutter; (7) right infracolic space; (8) left infracolic space; (9) the phrenicocolic ligament.

The **phrenicocolic ligament** (Fig. 4.2), extending from the splenic flexure of the colon to the diaphragm, partially separates the perisplenic space from the rest of the peritoneal cavity. It forms a partial barrier to the spread of fluid from the left paracolic gutter into the left subphrenic space, explaining why left subphrenic collections are less common than right-sided collections.

Inframesocolic compartment The inframesocolic compartment (Fig. 4.2) is divided into two unequal spaces by the root of the small bowel mesentery, as it runs from the duodenojejunal flexure in the left upper quadrant to the ileocaecal valve in the right lower quadrant:

- The smaller **right infracolic space** (Fig. 4.1c) is bounded inferiorly by the small bowel mesentery, extending from the duodenojejunal flexure to the ileocaecal valve.
- The larger **left infracolic space** (Fig. 4.1d) is in free communication with the pelvis except where it is bounded by the sigmoid mesocolon.

The **paracolic gutters** are the peritoneal recesses on the posterior abdominal wall lateral to the ascending and descending colon. The right paracolic gutter (Fig. 4.1c) is larger than its counterpart on the left (Fig. 4.1c) and is continuous superiorly with the right subhepatic and subphrenic spaces. Both paracolic gutters are in continuity with the pelvic peritoneal space.

Inferiorly the peritoneum is reflected over the fundus of the bladder, the anterior and posterior surface of the uterus in females, and on to the superior part of the rectum. The urinary bladder subdivides the pelvis into right and left paravesical spaces (Fig. 4.1e). In men there is only one potential space for fluid collection posterior to the bladder, the rectovesical pouch. In women there are two potential spaces posterior to the bladder, the uterovesical pouch (Fig. 4.1e), and posterior to the uterus, the rectouterine pouch (pouch of Douglas) (Fig. 4.1e).

Peritoneal reflections

In early fetal life as the abdominal cavity divides into the retroperitoneum and peritoneum, the parietal peritoneum is reflected over the peritoneal organs to form a series of supporting ligaments, mesenteries and omenta. Consequently a natural connecting pathway for the extension of intra-abdominal disease is formed between the retroperitoneum and structures enveloped by peritoneum, which has been termed the **subperitoneal space**.

The small bowel mesentery, sigmoid mesocolon, and greater omentum are frequently involved in disease processes, and can sometimes be identified in normals.

- **The small bowel mesentery** (Fig. 4.3) is a broad fan-shaped fold of peritoneum connecting the loops of jejunum and ileum to the posterior abdominal wall, extending obliquely from the duodenojejunal flexure to the ileocaecal valve.
- **The sigmoid mesocolon** is a fold of peritoneum which attaches the sigmoid colon to the posterior pelvic wall.
- **The greater omentum** (Fig. 4.1b) is the largest peritoneal fold in the abdomen. It descends from the stomach and proximal duodenum, passing inferiorly, anterior to the small bowel, before turning superiorly again to insert into the anterosuperior aspect of the transverse colon.

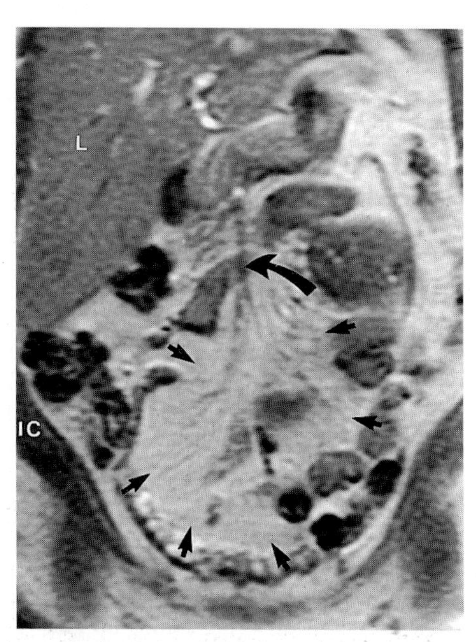

Fig. 4.3 T1-weighted coronal MRI demonstrating the liver (L), the normal small bowel mesentery (small black arrows), the right iliac crest (IC) and the superior mesenteric artery to the small bowel (curved black arow).

RETROPERITONEUM

The retroperitoneal space is bounded anteriorly by the parietal peritoneum, posteriorly by the transversalis fascia and laterally by the lateral conal fascia. It is largest posteriorly but continues anteriorly as the properitoneal fat compartment. It extends from the diaphragm to the pelvic brim. The retroperitoneum contains the true retroperitoneal organs (the adrenal glands, kidneys, ureters and pancreas), and those structures that are closely applied to the posterior abdominal wall and only covered in part by parietal peritoneum (the aorta, the inferior vena cava, portions of the duodenum and colon, lymph nodes and nerves).

The retroperitoneal space can be divided into five separate components:

- a poorly defined space surrounding the aorta, inferior vena cava, their branches and tributaries;
- the psoas spaces;
- the kidneys and perirenal spaces;
- the posterior pararenal spaces;
- the complex anterior pararenal space produced by fusion of the dorsal mesenteries of the stomach, duodenum, and colon with the posterior body wall.

Plain radiography only identifies advanced pathology in the retroperitoneal space indirectly by its effect on adjacent structures, e.g. loss of the psoas shadows, erosion of the adjacent lumbar vertebrae and deviation of the calcified wall of the aorta.

Cross-sectional imaging, in the form of ultrasound, CT and MRI, allows exquisite, non-invasive imaging of the normal and pathological retroperitoneal anatomy.

The great vessels

The aorta, inferior vena cava, their branches and their tributaries course within a loosely defined space just anterior to the vertebral bodies. This space is in continuity with the posterior mediastinum and thus pathological processes can spread between these regions. The **abdominal aorta** begins at the hiatus of the diaphragm and extends inferiorly to its bifurcation into the common iliac arteries at the fourth lumbar vertebra. The calibre of the aorta decreases as it progresses caudally to its bifurcation. At the level of the diaphragmatic crura the aorta measures up to 2.5 cm in diameter on imaging, tapering to 1 cm at the bifurcation. Ultrasound demonstrates the aorta well in thin patients, but bowel gas may obscure some portions especially in the lower abdomen. The major branches including the coeliac trunk, the superior mesenteric, the renal, and the very proximal inferior mesenteric arteries can sometimes be identified on ultrasound, but are more consistently demonstrated on contrast enhanced CT.

The **inferior vena cava** (IVC) is formed by the two common iliac veins at the level of the fifth vertebral body. It ascends to the right of the aorta to the level of the diaphragm, initially adjacent to the lumbar vertebrae, but as it moves in a cephalad direction it becomes more ventral in position. Its calibre varies greatly depending on the phase of respiration. The IVC is well seen on both ultrasound and CT. Ultrasound is particularly well-suited to demonstrating the intrahepatic portion of the IVC but the infrahepatic portion of the IVC is obscured by bowel gas in as many as 30% of cases. However, the accuracy of ultrasound exceeds that of CT in demonstrating the intrahepatic and supradiaphragmatic portions of the IVC. Demonstrating patency of the IVC on CT requires intravenous contrast medium. MRI identifies the aorta and IVC as flow voids on spin-echo techniques (Fig. 4.4), whereas with other motion-sensitive sequences these vessels can be shown as high signal structures.

Variants of IVC anatomy are relatively common, because of its complex embryological development from several primitive segments. Awareness of these variations is important to avoid misdiagnosising pathology in the retroperitoneum. A left-sided IVC occurs in 0.2% of the general population and may be confused with lymph node enlargement. The usual form consists of a left cava draining into a large left renal vein that crosses in front of the aorta to a normal caval segment above the renal vein.

Para-aortic and paracaval lymphatics and lymph nodes accompany these vessels in their entire course. In normal patients these nodes are usually less than 1 cm in short axis dimension on CT; however in the retrocrural location 6 mm is taken to be the upper limit for normal nodes.

The psoas major and minor muscles

The relationship of these muscles to nerves, lumbar arteries and the sympathetic trunks, are best demonstrated on CT and MRI (Fig. 4.5) rather than on ultrasound.

Retroperitoneal spaces

On CT and MRI, the normal retroperitoneal spaces are well demonstrated. The posterior renal fascia is seen in continuity with the lateral conal fascia, which extends anteriorly just lateral to the ascending or descending colon. The thinner less well-defined anterior renal fascia intersects with the posterior renal fascia at an acute angle. Lateral to the lateral conal fascia, posterior to the renal fascia, but within the transversalis fascia, lies the **posterior pararenal space**, continuous with the properitoneal fat stripe. It contains no organs but is closely related to the posterior surfaces of the ascending and descending colon. Consequently inflammatory conditions from the large bowel can extend into this area.

The dorsal mesenteries of the stomach (pancreatic tail and splenorenal ligament), duodenum (mesoduodenum and head of the pancreas), and ascending and descending colon fuse to form the **anterior pararenal space**. This space contains duodenum, ascending colon, descending colon and pancreas. CT and MRI can elegantly demonstrate pathologic processes affecting any of these organs and the retroperitoneal space.

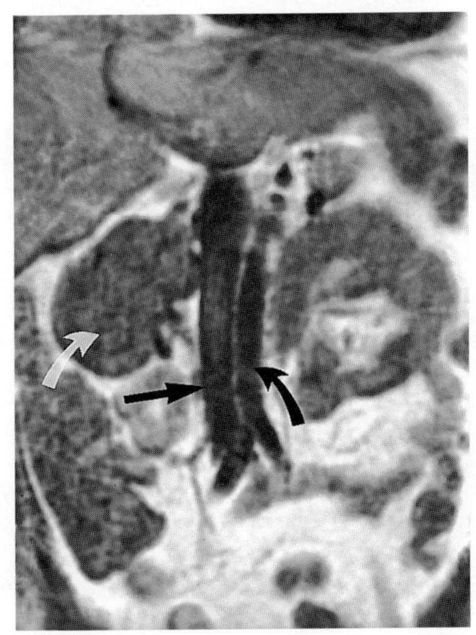

Fig. 4.4 Coronal T1-weighted MRI scan showing a signal void of flowing blood in a patent aorta (curved black arrow) and IVC (straight black arrow). Note the large right-sided renal tumour (curved white arrow).

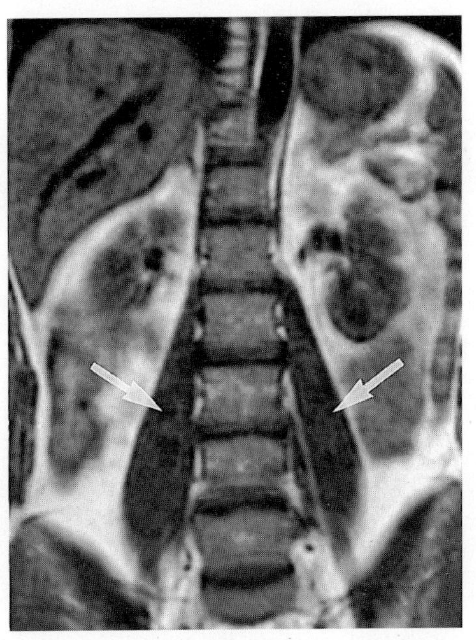

Fig. 4.5 Coronal T1-weighted MRI scan showing the upper parts of normal psoas muscles (arrowed).

PATHOLOGY

THE PERITONEUM

Ascites

Ascites results from increased fluid production in, or reduced fluid removal from, the peritoneal cavity. The fluid may be a transudate, for example, secondary to hypoproteinaemia, congestive heart failure and cirrhosis. Alternatively it may be an exudate, for example, secondary to carcinomatosis, peritonitis and pancreatitis. Peritoneal fluid collects initially within the pelvis. As more fluid collects flow occurs in a cephalad direction in either paracolic gutter to reach the subphrenic and subhepatic spaces. Ascites is more common in the right subphrenic and subhepatic spaces as flow to the left subphrenic space from the left paracolic gutter is impeded by the phrenicocolic ligament.

Plain film radiography is an insensitive technique for the detection of ascites. The topic is discussed on page 38.

Ultrasound is an extremely sensitive technique for detecting free fluid in the peritoneal cavity, detecting as little as 10 ml of free fluid in the pouch of Douglas. Uncomplicated ascites is typically echo-free and mobile within the peritoneal cavity. The gas-containing bowel loops float anteriorly within this fluid, which consequently may obscure the para-aortic and retroperitoneal structures. If the ascites is due to infection or malignant neoplasm, the fluid may become loculated by adhesions from bowel and peritoneal ligaments tethered to the abdominal wall. The mesentery may be thickened and bowel peristalsis may be diminished or abolished. Infective or malignant ascites may contain echoes due to pus, other cellular material or septa.

CT can also demonstrate very small amounts of ascites and allows visualization of fluid within the leaves of the mesentery and lesser sac, a relatively blind spot for ultrasound. The distribution of ascites varies according to aetiology: transudate ascites usually has a smaller lesser than greater sac component, carcinomatosis has similar sized collections in both sacs, and pancreatitis gives large lesser sac collections which may extend into the greater omentum or even into the mediastinum.

On MRI, most fluid has a low signal on T1-weighted images and a very high signal on T2-weighted images. Infective and malignant fluid often has a higher protein content than transudate ascites and therefore may have recognizably higher signal on T1-weighted images. However, the MRI appearances are not specific and needle aspiration, which can be guided by ultrasound, is needed to confirm the nature of the ascites.

Peritonitis

Peritoneal inflammation may be secondary to bacterial or granulomatous infection, or to a variety of chemical substances, as in biliary peritonitis. The response of the peritoneum is consistent, producing oedema and inflammation, followed by a fibroblastic exudate forming adhesions between peritoneal surfaces in an attempt to contain the infection.

In the presence of peritonitis ultrasound may identify free fluid in the peritoneal cavity and the mesenteric fat may appear very echogenic but visualization may be obscured by free gas and distended loops of bowel.

On CT there may be thickening of the mesentery, increased density in the mesenteric fat, and ascites.

Tuberculous peritonitis This is rarely encountered in the developed world, but there is an increased

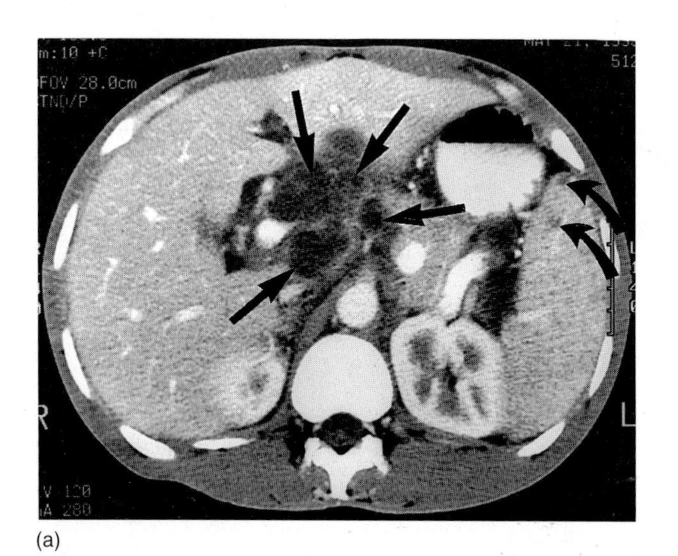

(a)

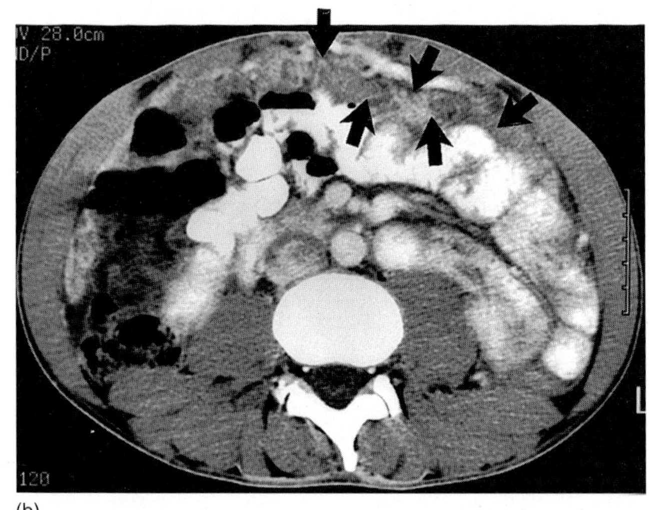

(b)

Fig. 4.6 Intra-abdominal tuberculosis. (a) CT with intravenous contrast showing ring enhancing low density lymph nodes at the porta hepatis (straight arrows). Note also focal abnormalities in the spleen (curved arrows). (b) CT showing nodular soft-tissue thickening in the greater omentum (arrowed).

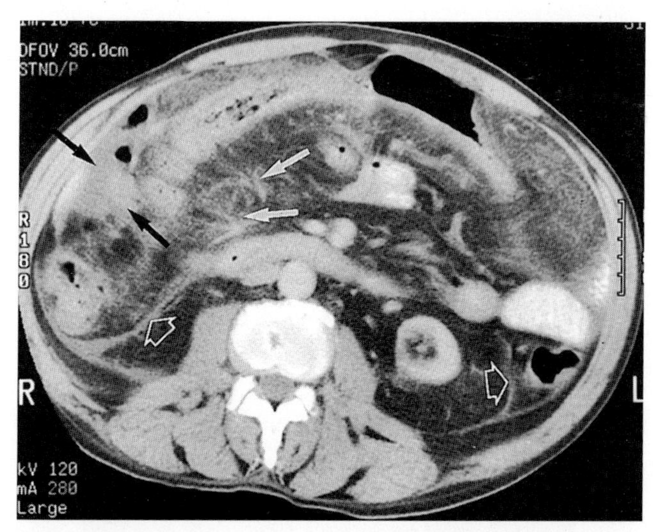

Fig. 4.7 CT showing high density ascites (black arrows) and soft-tissue thickening in the mesenteric fat (white arrows) in this patient with tuberculosis. Also notice the inflammatory thickening of the perirenal fascia bilaterally (open white arrows).

incidence in patients with AIDS and in immigrant populations. On CT, the following signs are highly suggestive of tuberculous peritonitis:

- enlarged lymph nodes with central low density due to caseous necrosis (Fig. 4.6a), seen in up to 40% of patients in the mesenteric and peripancreatic areas;
- nodular thickening of the peritoneal surfaces (Fig. 4.6b), and
- associated ascites, which is characteristically of relatively high density due to its high protein content (Fig. 4.7).

Associated features of intra-abdominal tuberculosis may also be present, such as thickening of the bowel wall, particularly the terminal ileum, focal abnormalities in the liver or spleen due to granulomata (Fig. 4.6a), and occasionally adrenal pathology. The chest radiograph is abnormal in only 50% of patients with tuberculous peritonitis.

Meconium peritonitis This sterile chemical peritonitis occurs *in utero* following perforation of the bowel as a consequence of small or large bowel obstruction. The perforation seals *in utero* due to the resultant inflammatory response. Obstetric ultrasound may show polyhydramnios, fetal ascites or dilated bowel. The plain film on delivery shows marked intra-abdominal calcifications scattered throughout the peritoneal cavity with distended bowel indicating obstruction. If the obstruction involves the lower small bowel, a barium enema examination may reveal a microcolon as the colon is underused.

Intraperitoneal abscess

Intraperitoneal abscess remains a major cause of morbidity and mortality following surgery despite modern surgical techniques and antimicrobial therapy. The symptoms and signs are usually non-specific and thus early diagnosis and effective management are essential.

Prompt diagnosis depends on understanding the dynamic anatomy of the peritoneal spaces and the peritoneal reflections (pages 101–105). The most common sites for abscess formation include the pelvis, the right subphrenic and the right subhepatic spaces.

Plain film diagnosis is discussed on page 42. If a fistula or sinus has formed to the skin surface, opacification with an iodinated contrast agent will visualize the abscess cavity.

The accuracy of ultrasound for the detection of intraperitoneal abscess is not as high as CT, since successful ultrasound examination depends on the patient's body habitus and abscesses are often obscured or confused with bowel loops. However, ultrasound is a rapid, inexpensive and readily available first-line technique. It is best suited for diagnosing abscesses in the right and left upper quadrants, especially subphrenic collections (Fig. 4.8), because the ability to image in the longitudinal plane allows easy distinction between fluid above and below the diaphragm. It is also very good for detecting pelvic collections using the distended bladder as an acoustic window. The ability to perform portable ultrasound examinations on the ward or on ITU in critically ill patients is a major benefit.

On ultrasound the abscess cavity may appear echo-free, mimicking a cyst, or it may contain low level echoes or solid elements. The margin of the collection is usually thick and irregular depending on its age. As ultrasound is completely reflected at soft tissue – air interfaces, the abscess may be obscured if it contains bubbles of gas. Similarly, abscess collections within the mesentery are poorly visualized as they are obscured by the surrounding loops of bowel containing gas.

CT, which is much less operator-dependent than ultrasound, is the most sensitive technique for the

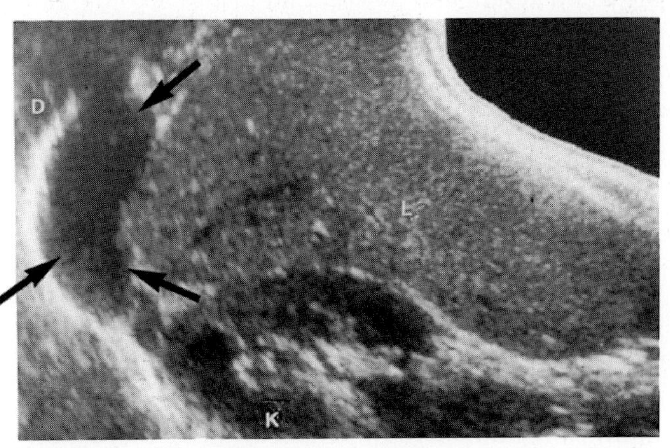

Fig. 4.8 Longitudinal ultrasound in the right upper quadrant, showing the liver (L), the kidney (K) and the diaphragm (D). There is a hypoechoic right subphrenic collection (arrowed) above the liver and right kidney, consistent with an abscess.

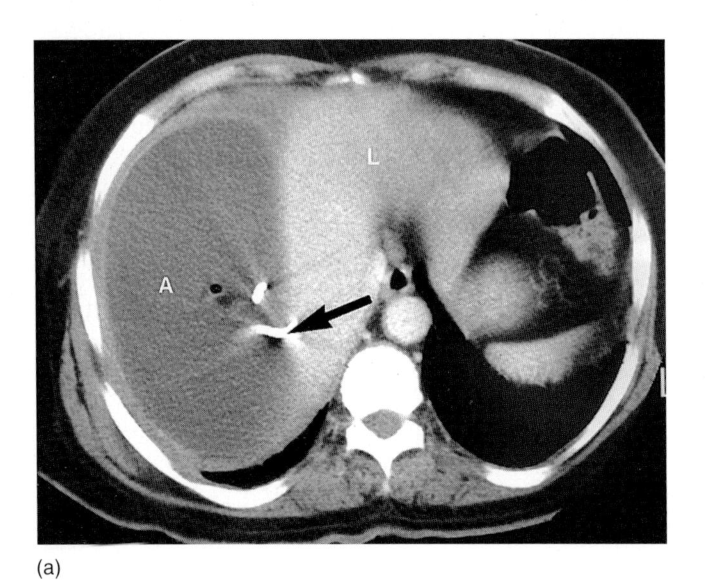

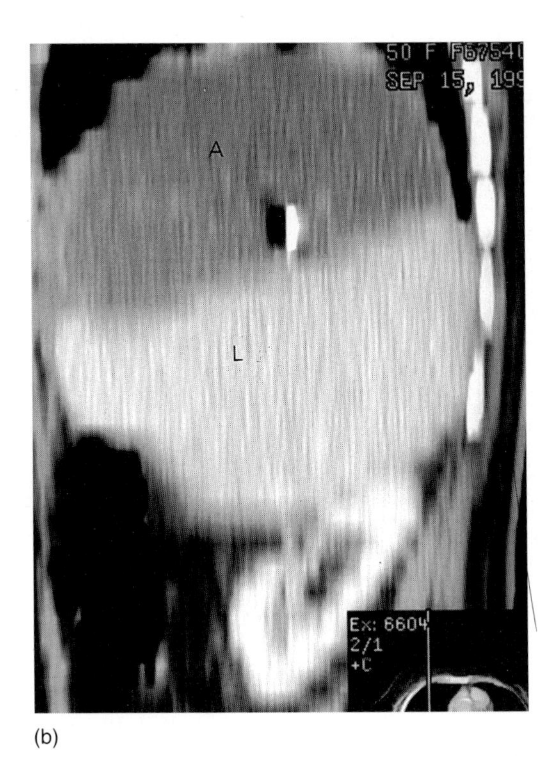

(a) (b)

Fig. 4.9 Subphrenic abscess on spiral CT. (a) Axial CT showing the liver (L) and a large encapsulated fluid collection containing a pocket of air, consistent with a right subphrenic abscess (A). The abscess contains a drain (arrowed). (b) Sagittal reformation from axial spiral CT showing the liver (L) and a right subphrenic abscess (A).

detection of intraperitoneal abscess. The entire abdomen and pelvis can be surveyed. The CT appearances depend to some extent on the age of the abscess. In the earliest stages the abscess may appear as a mass, representing the swollen tissues or viscera colonized by neutrophils and bacteria. As the process advances, its centre undergoes liquefactive necrosis, producing a region of fluid attenuation, the margin of which enhances following intravenous contrast enhancement. About 30% of abscesses contain air which appears as dark bubbles on CT or produces an air–fluid level. Displacement of adjacent stuctures and thickening or obliteration of adjacent fat planes accompanies abscess formation. Most abscesses are round or oval in shape on CT but those adjacent to solid organs may be lenticular or cresenteric in configuration. The CT appearances may suggest the cause of the abscess; for example, a right lower quadrant mass containing a calcific density is likely to represent an appendix abscess with an associated appendicolith.

The accuracy of CT for detecting abscesses in the subphrenic spaces and pelvis is similar to ultrasound. Subphrenic abscesses have the same features on CT as abscesses elsewhere. However, it can occasionally be extremely difficult to determine whether fluid lies above or below the diaphragm. Spiral CT, which allows longitudinal reconstruction, allows this distinction to be made with greater ease (Figs 4.9a, b). CT is much better than ultrasound for detecting collections centrally within the abdomen and those closely related to bowel. Additionally, unlike ultrasound, CT is not dependent on body habitus and the position of drains and dressings.

Both ultrasound and CT have significant roles to play in needle aspiration and percutaneous drainage of abscesses, thus reducing the morbidity of reoperation. Radionuclide imaging using gallium-67 or leucocytes labelled with indium-111 is quite sensitive for detecting intraperitoneal abscess formation; however, the specificity of this technique is much poorer than CT or ultrasound. Even when radionuclide imaging is positive, ultrasound or CT is required to localize collections anatomically.

MRI does not offer any benefit over ultrasound and CT for the diagnosis of intraperitoneal abscess. At present, MRI of the abdomen is degraded by respiratory and peristaltic bowel movement and fluid in the bowel can be difficult to differentiate from extraluminal collections. Also MRI contrast opacification of the bowel is not as effective as in CT.

Other intraperitoneal fluid collections

Intraperitoneal haemorrhage Haemorrhage secondary to anticoagulation, a bleeding diathesis or visceral trauma can be specifically identified on CT due to the high attenuation value of fresh blood. Within several days, however, clot lysis occurs and the attenuation of the haemorrhage decreases, approaching the density of water by 2–4 weeks.

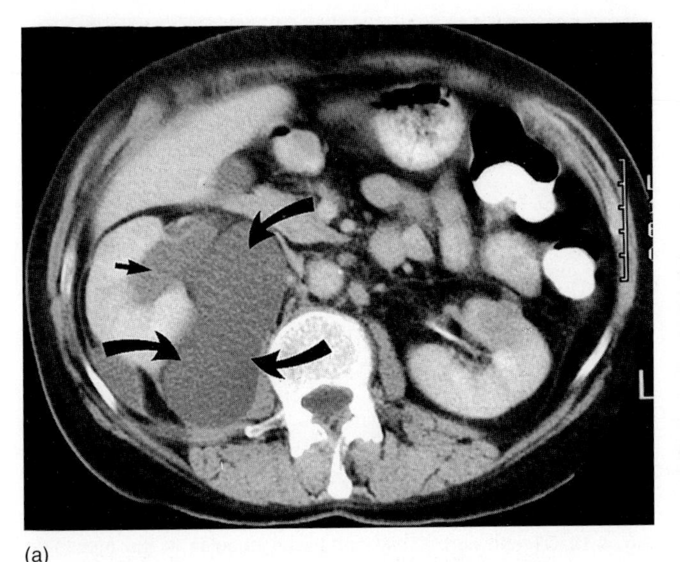

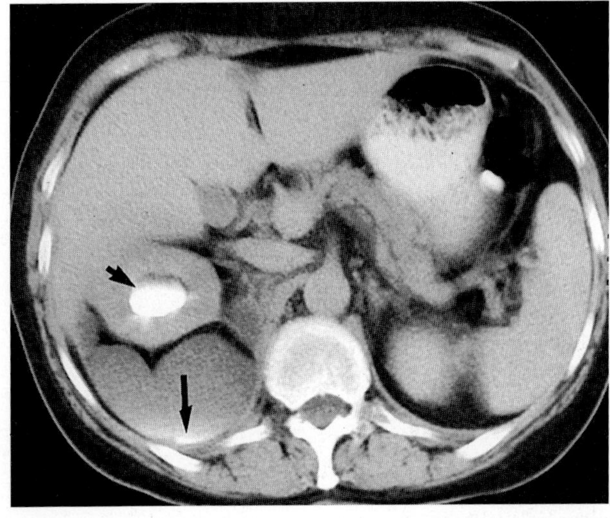

(a) (b)

Fig. 4.10 Perirenal urinoma. (a) Axial CT showing a markedly dilated right renal pelvis prior to excretion of contrast (small arrow). Fluid has accumulated in the perirenal space medially and laterally as a large right-sided perirenal urinoma (curved arrows). (b) More superior axial CT scans following intravenous contrast show contrast in the upper pole collecting system (small arrow), and in the perirenal urinoma posteriorly (large arrow).

The haemorrhagic fluid may appear inhomogeneously dense on CT due to irregular clot formation and resorption, or because of intermittent bleeding. In the case of haemoperitoneum due to trauma, contrast-enhanced CT helps to identify the injured viscera.

Perirenal urinomas These usually occur in the retroperitoneum, but can occur intra-abdominally if the tissue planes are disrupted by trauma or surgery (Fig. 4–10a). Delayed contrast-enhanced CT may show filling of the urinoma with iodinated contrast (Fig. 4.10b).

Chylous ascites This can occur as a consequence of disruption to the lymphatic vessels by tumour or surgery. Occasionally on CT the Hounsfield numbers of chylous ascites may be negative due to its high fat content, thus allowing a specific diagnosis to be suggested by imaging.

Intraperitoneal bilomas These occur following trauma, surgery and spontaneous rupture of the biliary tree. Bile elicits a low-grade inflammatory reaction that walls off the collection within the mesentery and omentum. On CT most bilomas have low attenuation except when complicated by infection or haemorrhage. They are usually located in the right upper quadrant, but can be found in the left upper quadrant in 30% of cases.

Neoplasms

Metastases The most common malignant process involving the peritoneum is metastatic disease. Peritoneal metastases usually originate from intra-abdominal primary neoplasms, including the stomach, colon, ovary and pancreas. Prior to the advent of CT, peritoneal metastases were not radiographically detectable until late in the disease, when they displaced adjacent organs, caused intestinal obstruction, or produced radiological signs due to massive ascites on plain films. Conventional barium studies only provide indirect signs of peritoneal and mesenteric disease due to displacement of bowel, mucosal tethering, or invasion into the bowel itself. Abnormal findings on CT often eliminate the need for a barium study, or at least suggest the region to examine in detail.

In patients with large amounts of ascites, ultrasound is capable of demonstrating superficial peritoneal and omental tumour nodules as small as 2–3 cm, but ultrasound will not detect small peritoneal deposits if there is only minimal ascites. Also ultrasound will not identify centrally located tumour deposits as these are obscured by bowel gas and by the increased acoustic impedance of mesenteric fat.

Although MRI may offer superior soft-tissue contrast to CT, the spatial resolution of the technique, at present, is diminished by movement artefact caused by bowel peristalsis and respiration. Therefore CT is the imaging procedure of choice for evaluating patients known to have, or suspected of having peritoneal or mesenteric neoplasms.

Metastatic neoplasms disseminate throughout the peritoneum in four ways:

- direct spread along the peritoneal ligaments, mesenteries and omenta;
- intraperitoneal seeding through the ascitic fluid;
- lymphatic extension;
- embolic haematogenous spread.

However, it must be stressed that none of these appearances is specific for the malignancies mentioned and can be mimicked by other metastatic tumours, primary peritoneal tumours such as mesothelioma, and inflammatory conditions, such as pancreatitis and tuberculous peritonitis. Also many of the distinct patterns of metastatic disease described often coexist.

Peritoneal spread of neoplasms Intraperitoneal seeding of neoplasms depends on the normal flow of fluid within the peritoneal cavity. This flow is facilitated by gravity, and in the upper abdomen by changes in intra-abdominal pressure caused by respiration. The pouch of Douglas, the lower small bowel mesentery near the ileocaecal junction, and the right paracolic gutter are the most common sites for pooling of ascites and subsequent fixation and growth of peritoneal metastases.

On barium examination, peritoneal metastases may produce angulation and kinking of bowel loops and spiculation and tethering of their mucosal folds.

On CT early peritoneal involvement produces increased density within the fat adjacent to the primary neoplasm. Subsequently, a mass contiguous with the primary neoplasm may be seen extending along the expected course of the peritoneal reflection. As these peritoneal reflections are in continuity with the posterior abdominal wall, spread may also occur to the retroperitoneum. Neoplastic infiltration of the greater omentum can produce soft-tissue nodular thickening within the omental fat (Fig. 4.11). Early in the disease, this will appear as an ill-defined loss of the normal clarity of the fat. With more advanced disease a large mass may separate the colon from the anterior abdominal wall in a phenomenon known as 'omental caking' (Fig. 4.12). Widespread peritoneal metastases and omental caking, which occasionally calcify, are most frequently associated with metastatic ovarian cancer.

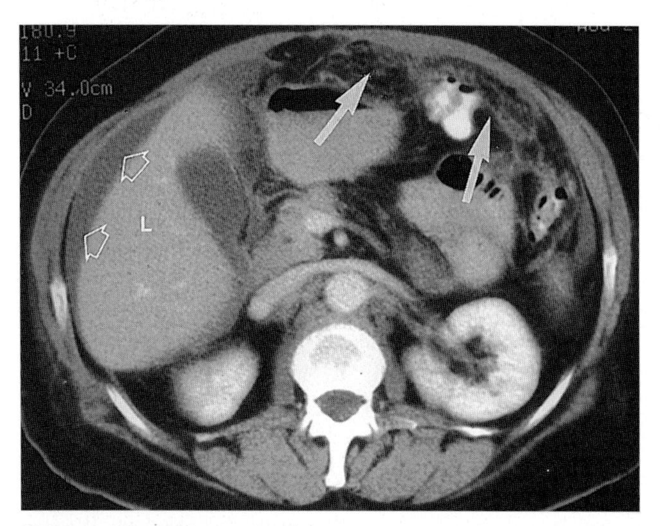

Fig. 4.11 CT showing ascites (open arrows) lateral to the liver (L) and soft-tissue stranding in the omental fat (solid arrows) in this patient with disseminated ovarian cancer.

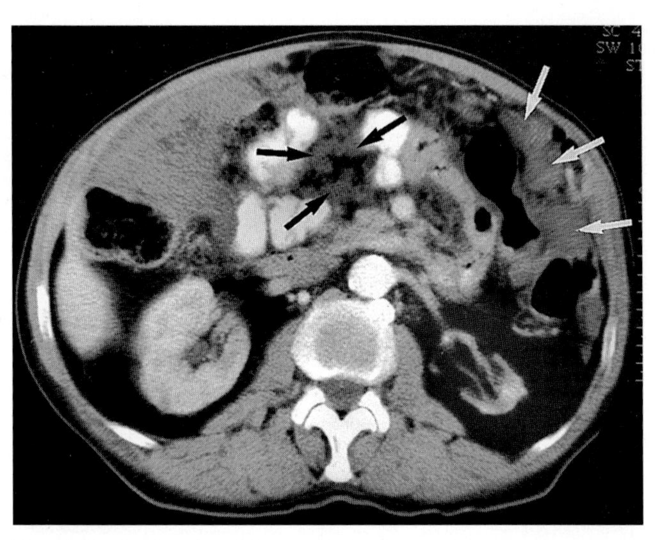

Fig. 4.12 CT showing diffuse soft-tissue nodules in the mesentery (black arrows) and omental caking (white arrows) in this patient with peritoneal metastases from colonic cancer.

Specific neoplasms often spread by anatomically predictable routes and give characteristic CT appearances:

- Malignant neoplams of the stomach, colon, pancreas and ovary can spread directly along the visceral peritoneal reflections to affect other peritoneal structures.
- Neoplasms of the colon, stomach and pancreas use the transverse mesocolon and greater omentum as conduits for spread.
- Gastric malignancies can spread to the spleen via the gastrosplenic ligament.
- Neoplasms of the pancreatic tail spread via the phrenicocolic ligament to the splenic flexure of the colon.
- Biliary and hepatic malignancies usually spread via the lesser omentum and hepatoduodenal ligaments.
- Ovarian cancer spreads along all of its adjacent mesothelial surfaces to produce marked peritoneal thickening, nodularity and rounded masses (Fig. 4.13). It also frequently produces cake-like masses and cystic mesenteric masses.
- Carcinoid and lymphoma produce marked soft-tissue thickening in the small bowel mesentery, with shortening of the mesentery, perivascular soft-tissue encasement and tethering of the bowel.
- Pancreatic, breast and colonic metastases commonly produce stellate masses, with radiating mesenteric extensions along the vessels.

Lymphatic dissemination Lymphatic spread is the primary route of metastasis for lymphoma. Approximately 50% of patients with non-Hodgkin's

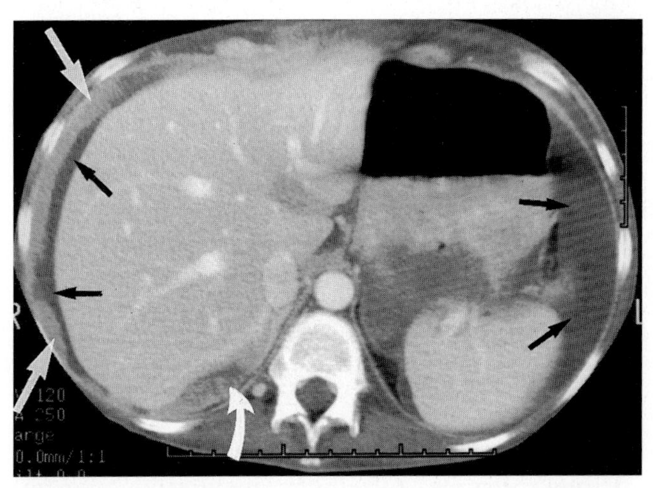

Fig. 4.13 CT showing diffuse peritoneal deposits (white arrows) and ascites (black arrows) from ovarian cancer. The irregular liver surface is also due to peritoneal disease (curved white arrow).

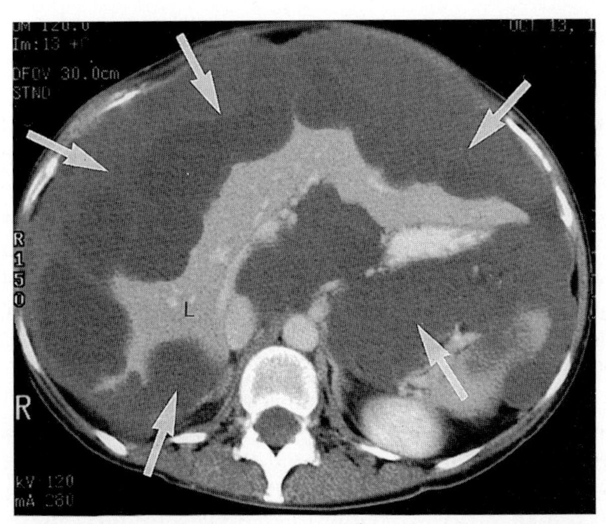

Fig. 4.14 Contrast-enhanced CT showing low density masses (arrowed) causing characteristic scalloping of the liver (L) margin in this patient with pseudomyxoma peritonei.

lymphoma have enlarged mesenteric lymph nodes at presentation. These nodes may be confluent producing large mass lesions in the mesentery. Characteristically, these nodal masses surround and encase vessels, particularly the superior mesenteric vessels. It is important to note, however, that enlargement of mesenteric lymph nodes can be due to inflammatory causes such as Crohn's disease, Whipple's disease and tuberculosis. In these conditions individual lymph nodes generally remain more discrete and rarely become a conglomerate mass.

Embolic metastases Metastases may spread via the mesenteric arteries to the antimesenteric border of the bowel, where malignant cells can implant and subsequently grow into submucosal nodules. On barium studies these deposits appear as 'bull's eye' or 'target' lesions with central ulceration as the deposit outgrows its blood supply. This type of deposit is characteristic of malignant melanoma metastases. Embolic metastasis to the stomach may produce a 'linitis plastica' appearance on barium meal examination, with marked narrowing of the lumen and scirrhous thickening of the bowel wall. This type of appearance is seen particularly with embolic breast metastases. On CT these metastases produce thickening of the adjacent mesenteric leaves or focal bowel wall thickening with associated ulceration.

Pseudomyxoma peritonei In pseudomyxoma peritonei the peritoneal surfaces become diffusely involved with large amounts of mucinous material as a consequence of rupture of a mucinous cystadenocarcinoma or cystadenoma usually of the ovary or appendix. It occurs more frequently in females than in males. On CT there may be low attenuation masses surrounded by discrete walls, which may contain calcification. The low attenuation masses may contain septa and often fill the peritoneal spaces, causing scalloping of the liver margins. (Fig. 4.14). The inability of the bowel to float anteriorly in this gelatinous material, along with the other CT features, are characteristic of the condition.

Primary neoplasms Primary neoplasms of the peritoneum are rare and are usually of mesenchymal origin.

Mesothelioma (Fig. 4.15) arises in the serosal lining of the pleura, peritoneum and pericardium associated with asbestos exposure. Peritoneal involvement may occur alone or in combination with pleural involvement. On CT there is marked thickening of the peritoneum, mesentery and omentum, which may show an irregular or nodular appearance. Peritoneal calcification (which may be seen on plain films) and

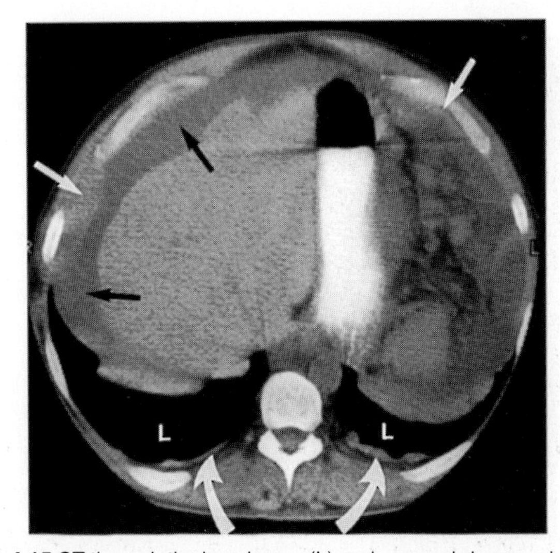

Fig. 4.15 CT through the lung bases (L) and upper abdomen, showing peritoneal deposits (white arrows) and ascites (black arrows) in this patient with peritoneal mesothelioma; note also the bilateral pleural plaques (curved white arrows).

associated ascites are seen on CT. The amount of ascites may be disproportionately small in relation to the peritoneal disease when compared to other peritoneal neoplasms. The mesenteric involvement may produce a stellate appearance due to thickening of perivascular bundles. These appearances, however, are not specific for mesothelioma and may be indistinguishable from metastases, lymphoma or tuberculous peritonitis. The diagnosis is strongly suggested if there is concomitant thickening and calcification of the pleura in a patient with a history of asbestos exposure (Fig. 4.15).

Lipomatous tumours occasionally involve the peritoneal cavity and have typical CT and MRI appearances. Benign lipomas are well-defined and composed entirely of fat except for very thin septa. Liposarcomas (Figs 4.16, 4.17) are distinguished from lipomas by the presence of soft-tissue elements within the fatty material and their locally invasive nature.

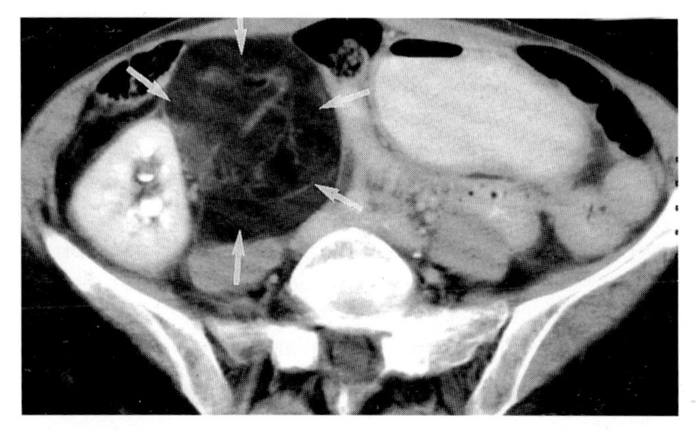

Fig. 4.16 Liposarcoma. CT showing a well-defined retroperitoneal liposarcoma (arrowed) intimately related to the right perirenal space, containing soft-tissue stranding.

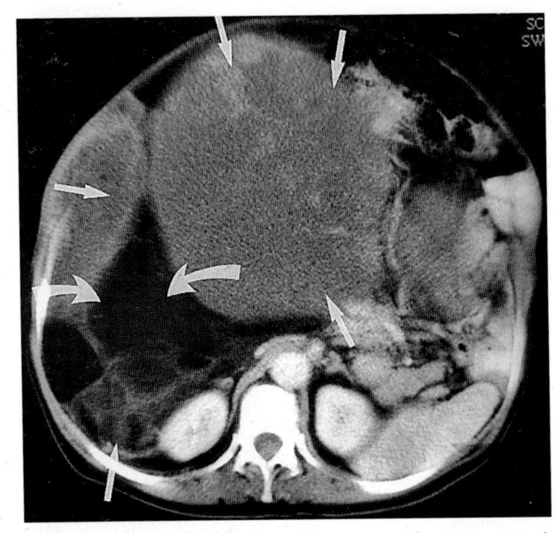

Fig. 4.17 Liposarcoma. CT showing a massive mesenteric liposarcoma; note that some parts have the attenuation of normal fat (curved white arrows), but other regions have soft-tissue density and fluid density (straight arrows).

THE MESENTERY

CT, with appropriate bowel contrast opacification, is the best modality for identification of mesenteric abnormalities because of the presence of a relatively large amount of fat in the normal mesentery. Pathological conditions infiltrating the mesentery increase the attenuation of the fat, obscure the mesenteric vessels and distort the associated bowel loops.

Currently MRI is less valuable for detecting and characterizing mesenteric pathology because respiratory and peristaltic bowel movements degrade the images.

Inflammation

Crohn's disease CT allows identification of extramural abnormalities in the mesentery due to Crohn's. The associated fibrofatty proliferation increases the density of the mesenteric fat, as does diffuse inflammation within the mesentery. Mesenteric abscesses are well shown on CT as fluid-filled masses, but may be obscured on ultrasound by surrounding bowel gas. CT, with adequate bowel contrast, can also demonstrate fistulae from the bowel to abscess collections. Demonstrating these changes in the mesentery on CT, may help in distinguishing between causes of inflammatory bowel disease, as mesenteric complications do not occur in ulcerative colitis.

Tuberculous peritonitis This commonly affects the mesentery. The CT findings include thickening and nodularity within the mesentery (Fig. 4.7) and marked mesenteric lymphadenopathy. The nodes may have central low attenuation because of caseous necrosis (Fig. 4.6a).

Diverticulitis CT accurately defines the extracolonic disease within the sigmoid mesentery. Inflammation appears as increased attenuation and stranding in the fat. Complications such as pericolic and more distant abscess formation, ureteral obstruction and bladder involvement are also well demonstrated with CT.

Desmoid tumour

Mesenteric desmoid tumours (aggressive fibromatosis) are infiltrating fibroblastic proliferations which do not show the features of an inflammatory response or neoplasia. They occur in 9–18% of patients with familial adenomatous polyposis. In this condition, desmoid tumours arise either in musculoskeletal sites or in the mesentery. Unlike muscular desmoids which seldom cause symptoms, mesenteric desmoids are potentially life-threatening. On CT, the earliest changes are an ill-defined loss of clarity of the normal mesenteric fat, which with time acquires a 'whorled' appearance as linear soft tissue is interleaved with fat. This retractile mesenteritis results in tethering, angulation and then encasement of bowel. Finally, this

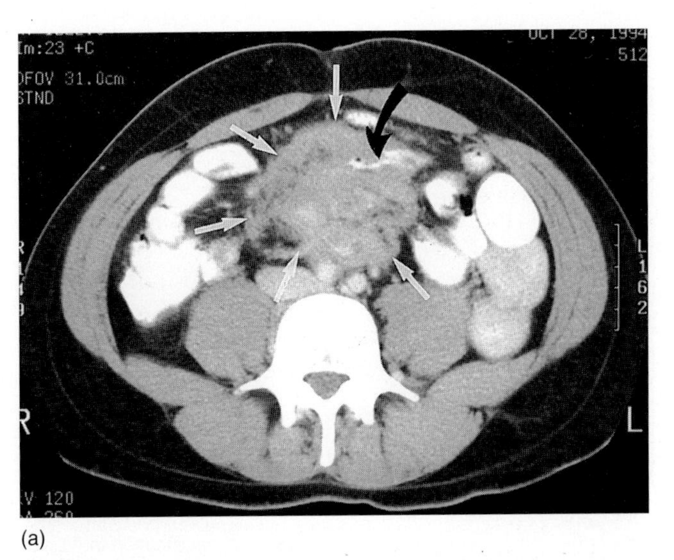

(a)

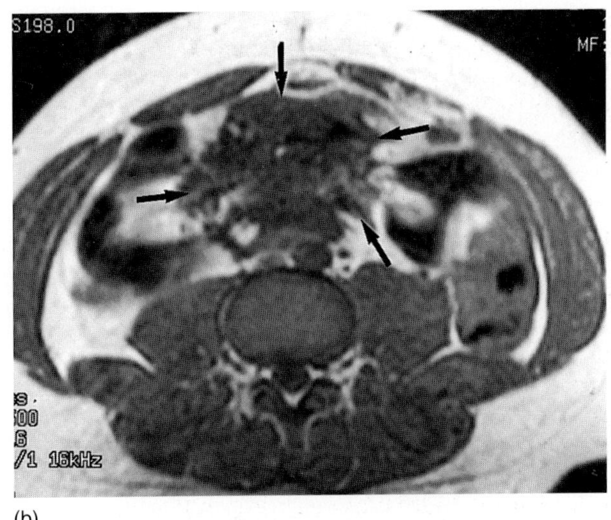

(b)

Fig. 4.18 Mesenteric desmoid tumours. (a) CT showing an ill-defined mesenteric desmoid tumour (white arrows) encasing a loop of small bowel centrally (curved black arrow). (b) Axial T1-weighted MRI, at the same level of the CT scan, showing an ill-defined mesenteric desmoid of low-signal intensity (arrowed).

desmoplastic response results in an irregular mass-like lesion often encasing loops of bowel (Fig. 4.18a), which is also well-demonstrated on barium follow through examination. Depending on the stage of development, these masses vary in size between 2 and 20 cm. Up to 50% of the masses will be 10 cm or larger at the time of presentation. The infiltrative nature of desmoids commonly results in obstruction of, or damage to, local bowel loops and vascular structures, as well as the urinary tract. On MRI, desmoid tumours generally have low signal on T1-and T2-weighted scans (Fig. 4.18b) due to their large fibrous component.

Mesenteric/omental cysts

Mesenteric and omental cysts can be lymphatic harmartomas, lined by mesothelial cells with serous or chylous fluid within them, or enterogenous cysts, derived from a sequestered intestinal diverticulum. The radiological appearance is the same irrespective of the aetiology. They appear as centrally placed soft-tissue masses displacing adjacent bowel around them on the plain abdominal film. On ultrasound they are well-defined, echo-free fluid collections in the central abdomen. On CT they are well-defined, single (occasionally multiple) fluid-filled structures found most commonly in the small bowel mesentery. Occasionally, if there is a significant amount of chylous fluid present, there may be a fat – water fluid level within them. On MRI mesenteric cysts show the typical signal characteristics of fluid, namely low signal intensity on T1-weighted images and very high signal intensity on T2-weighted images.

Mesenteric venous thrombosis

Superior mesenteric vein thrombosis, which is well seen on CT, is the cause of intestinal ischaemia in 5–15% of cases. The typical appearances of chronic superior mesenteric vein thrombosis are enlargement of the vein, with a central low density surrounded by a higher density wall. The thrombus may be of high attenuation in the acute state. Mesenteric oedema may be visible. It may be severe enough to cause bowel infarction, in which case intramural, portal vein or mesenteric vein gas may be identified. CT is also of great value in establishing an underlying local cause of venous thrombosis, such as pancreatic cancer, pancreatitis or a bowel neoplasm.

Mesenteric lymphadenopathy

Lymphatic dissemination plays a minor role in the dissemination of intraperitoneal metastatic carcinoma, but is the primary mode of spread of lymphoma to mesenteric nodes. Approximately 50% of patients with non-Hodgkin's lymphoma have mesenteric node involvement at presentation, as opposed to 5% with Hodgkin's disease. On CT these nodes range from small discrete nodules in the mesenteric fat to large confluent masses surrounding the superior mesenteric vessels. Non-neoplastic causes of mesenteric lymphadenopathy include Crohn's disease, sarcoidosis, Whipple's disease, tuberculous peritonitis, giardiasis and AIDS.

RETROPERITONEUM

Aorta – atherosclerosis, aneurysm formation and dissection

Atherosclerosis and aortic aneurysms can be detected on plain radiographs in a large number of cases by identifying mural calcification. Ultrasound is the diagnostic procedure of choice in confirming the

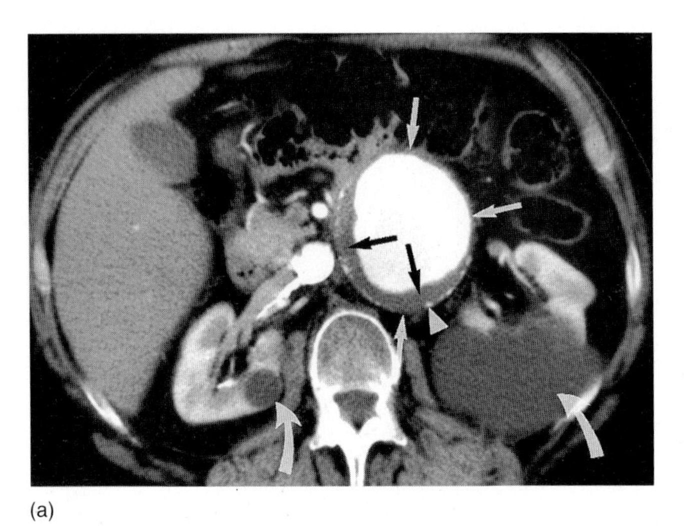

(a)

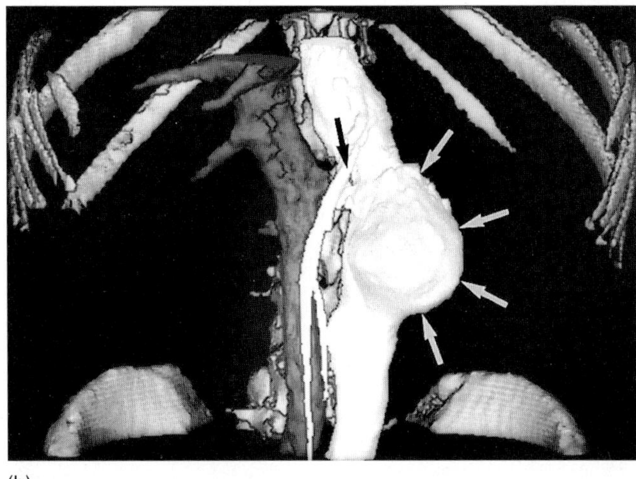

(b)

Fig. 4.19 Aortic aneurysm on spiral CT. (a) Contrast enhanced CT showing a large aortic aneurysm (white arrows) with calcification in its wall (arrowhead) and intraluminal thrombus (black arrows). Incidental note is also made of bilateral simple renal cysts (curved white arrows). (b) 3D CT reformation of the aortic aneurysm in the same patient (white arrows), arising below the superior mesenteric artery (black arrow).

diagnosis of a clinically suspected aortic aneurysm as it is relatively inexpensive and readily available. It allows differentiation of aneurysmal dilatation from a tortuous atheromatous aorta of normal diameter, a hyperdynamic aorta in a thin patient, and transmitted pulsation from a para-aortic mass. Unlike angiography, which measures the lumen of flowing blood only, ultrasound demonstrates both the size of the lumen and any associated thrombus. An aneurysm with a true diameter $\geq$ 5 cm has an increased risk of rupture. Progressive enlargement of an aneurysm, which is easily followed on ultrasound, at a rate >1 cm per annum is often regarded as an indication for surgery. Ultrasound sometimes allows visualization of the renal arteries, which is important because their relationship to the aneurysm affects the surgical treatment and the associated morbidity and mortality. The exact extent of an aortic aneurysm and its relation to any branches, however, is most accurately demonstrated using dynamic contrast-enhanced spiral CT (Figs 4.19a,b).

Acute rupture of the aorta is a surgical emergency with a high mortality and imaging studies are not usually appropriate as they serve only to delay surgery. Imaging is useful in subacute or chronic rupture. On ultrasound a pulsating haematoma or a periaortic collection extending into the flanks may be seen.

Aortic dissection gives a characteristic ultrasound appearance with a 'flapping' inner wall representing the intimal flap. However, CT is a more accurate technique as it is less operator-dependent than ultrasound and surveys the entire abdominal aorta, an important factor in the evaluation of aortic rupture or dissection. The accuracy of CT for detecting both abdominal aortic dissection and extension of thoracic dissection into the abdominal aorta is high, comparable to aortography. Initial non-contrast CT scans may be helpful to detect medial displacement of intimal calcification, but the definitive CT finding of aortic dissection is a contrast-filled double channel with an intervening intimal flap. If one channel is completely thrombosed, differentiating a dissection from a fusiform aneurysm with adherent clot may be difficult. Associated findings in dissection are intraluminal thrombosis, dilatation of the aorta with compression of the true lumen, irregular contour of the contrast-filled part of the aorta and differential flow to the kidneys. CT, preferably with a spiral scanning technique and dynamic contrast enhancement, can demonstrate false aneurysms, retroperitoneal haematomas and even contrast leaking

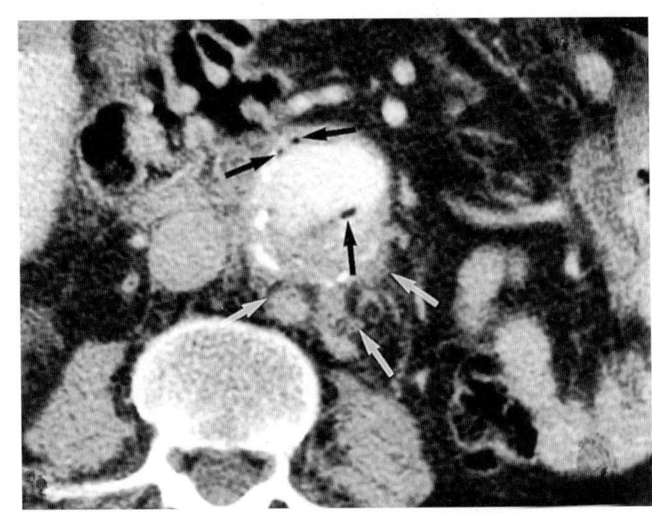

Fig. 4.20 CT showing an infected aortic graft, with bubbles of air in the anterior wall and in the posterior thrombus (black arrows). Note the periaortic ill-defined soft tissue consistent with inflammation (white arrows).

from a rupture. Ultrasound and CT can also effectively evaluate the postoperative complications of aortic grafts, which include occlusion, infection, false aneurysm formation, haemorrhage and aorto-enteric fistula. Infection is particularly well evaluated on CT as pockets of air can be identified in the aortic lumen (Fig. 4.20).

MRI is rapidly becoming an accurate investigation for examining abdominal aortic disease. It is at least as accurate as CT and aortography for the diagnosis of aortic dissection. Furthermore the diagnosis can be made reliably without the use of iodinated contrast material, an important advantage for a patient who risks complications from iodinated contrast injection. However, MRI generally remains a less clinically useful investigation than ultrasound or CT because it is still relatively expensive and time-consuming, and there are also considerable difficulties in monitoring critically ill patients.

Inferior vena cava thrombosis

Tumoral and non-tumoral thrombosis of the IVC can be identified using ultrasound from the level of the renal veins to the right atrium. Below this level the IVC is usually obscured by bowel gas. On ultrasound, thrombosis within the IVC is highly reflective and the IVC is distended. Fresh thrombus, however, may have lower echogenicity. Doppler ultrasound allows characterization of flow or lack of flow within the IVC. It also aids the identification of recanalization following anticoagulant treatment.

Contrast-enhanced CT demonstrates the entire abdominal IVC and its tributaries. On CT a fresh thrombus distends the IVC and has a density similar to circulating blood; an older thrombus is of lower density. When the occlusion is complete, the involved segment does not enhance on postcontrast images. Ultrasound is more accurate than CT in defining the superior limit of the intracaval thrombus. The IVC is invaded in approximately 10% of patients with renal cancer and the superior extent of tumour thrombus must be determined since it influences the surgical approach. The distinction between tumour thrombus and bland non-tumour thrombus is seldom possible. CT and ultrasound are both relatively inaccurate for predicting invasion of the wall of the IVC by tumoral thrombus.

Venous thrombosis produces intraluminal signal on spin-echo MRI sequences with focal dilation of the IVC similar to the findings on CT and ultrasound. MRI is as accurate as CT in displaying normal flow and thrombus within the IVC. Its major advantage is that it does not need intravenous contrast enhancement. It can therefore be used in patients with contraindications to iodinated contrast agent administration, or when CT and ultrasound are equivocal. CT, MRI and Doppler ultrasound can also be used to document the patency of portocaval or mesocaval shunts.

Lymphadenopathy

CT is the most widely used method of detecting retroperitoneal lymph node pathology and is the standard method for staging disease in patients with **lymphoma** and **testicular tumours**. In these diseases CT demonstrates all the enlarged nodes and also demonstrates any extranodal pathology. For tumours such as renal cell, cervical and prostatic carcinoma, CT can rapidly evaluate the primary site, any lymph node metastases and the liver in one examination. It is, therefore, the first choice investigation for oncologic staging and for follow-up after treatment or surgery.

As with ultrasound and MRI, CT relies on an increase in size to diagnose nodal pathology. Retroperitoneal nodes are considered enlarged on CT if they measure >10 mm in their shortest axis. In the retrocrural area, nodal enlargement is diagnosed when the shortest axis is >6 mm (Fig. 4.21). On CT, malignant nodal enlargement may follow one of the following patterns: discrete lymph node enlargement, conglomerate lymph node enlargement or large masses in which separate nodes are no longer visible. Massive enlargement of the retroaortic or retrocaval nodes may cause anterior displacement of the aorta and vena cava.

The accuracy of CT for detecting intra-abdominal and pelvic lymphadenopathy in malignant disease is reported to be as high as 90%. Difficulty in interpretation can result from non-opacified bowel or vessels, which can be resolved with meticulous attention to bowel opacification and vascular enhancement. False-positive results largely relate to lymph-node enlargement due to other causes, for example infection. False-negative results occur when infiltrated lymph nodes are not enlarged. CT is extremely useful in following response of nodal disease to treatment and in diagnosing remission, especially in lymphoma.

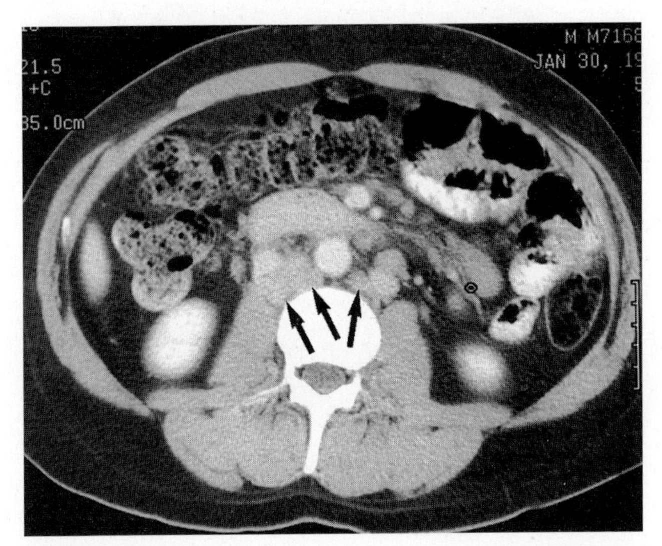

Fig. 4.21 Contrast-enhanced CT showing enlarged retroperitoneal lymph nodes (arrowed) in this patient with non-Hodgkins lymphoma.

However, patients with massive lymphadenopathy at presentation may not revert completely to normal, as bulky fibrosis may persist within the successfully treated lymph nodes following chemotherapy and radiotherapy, particularly in Hodgkin's disease and testicular tumours. Biopsy of such masses can be achieved using CT guidance.

On MRI, abnormal nodes are diagnosed on the basis of size rather than by any alteration in signal intensity. They are best seen on T1-weighted sequences as their signal intensity is usually higher than that in muscle but lower than in fat (Fig. 4.22). On T2-weighted sequences nodes may be difficult to distinguish from surrounding fat which can be of similar signal intensity. Generally, abnormal nodes show homogeneous signal intensity but they may appear inhomogeneous when calcified or necrotic.

MRI is as accurate as CT for evaluating the retroperitoneum for lymphadenopathy, but at present is not as good a survey technique for the rest of the abdomen. The images may be degraded by movement artefacts from respiration or peristalsis and inadequate bowel opacification may cause confusion in separating bowel from lymph-node masses. Also poorer spatial resolution may compromise visualization of minimally enlarged lymph nodes. Similarly, a cluster of normal-sized nodes that are readily defined by CT as discrete normal structures may be misdiagnosed as a solitary enlarged node on MRI. MRI thus offers no substantial benefit over CT for routine staging and follow-up. However, MRI is a useful problem-solving technique in certain situations. It can, for example, distinguish vascular structures as flow voids without the use of iodinated contrast agents, and thus may help to separate nodes from vessels in difficult areas, such as the internal iliac nodal area. Surgical clips do not degrade MRI images to the same extent as they degrade CT images and thus MRI may be useful in follow-up after surgery.

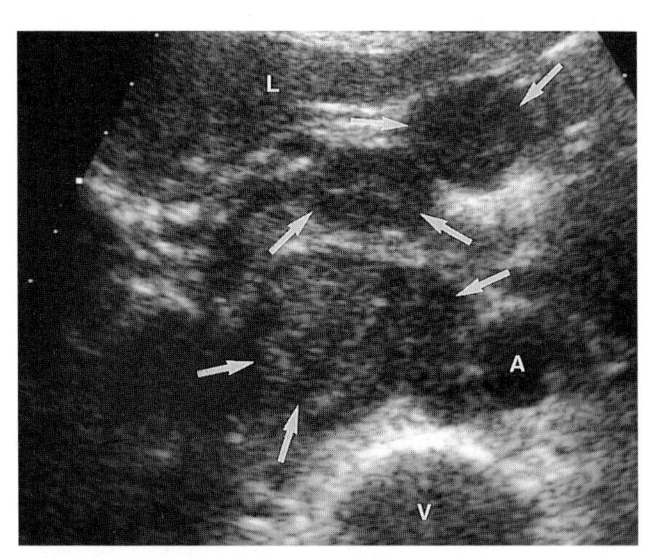

Fig. 4.23 Transverse abdominal ultrasound scan showing enlarged hypoechoic retroperitoneal lymph nodes in this patient with metastatic carcinoid (arrowed). These lie to the right of the aorta (A) and anterior to the vertebral body (V). Nodes are also seen lying posterior to the left lobe of the liver (L).

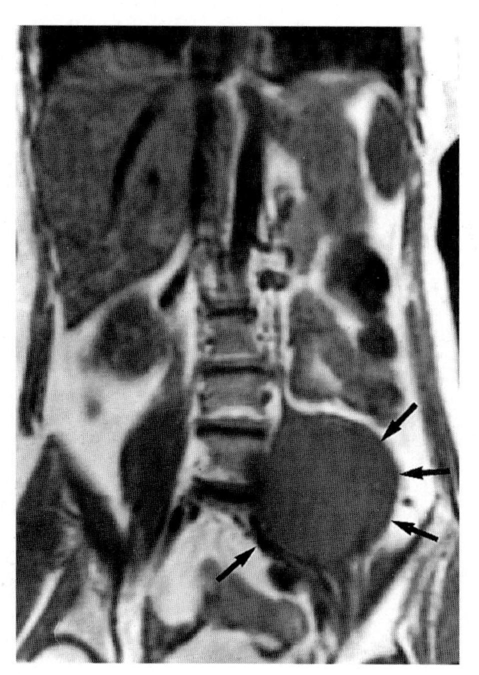

Fig. 4.22 Coronal T1-weighted MRI showing a large nodal metastasis to the left psoas (arrowed) from ovarian cancer.

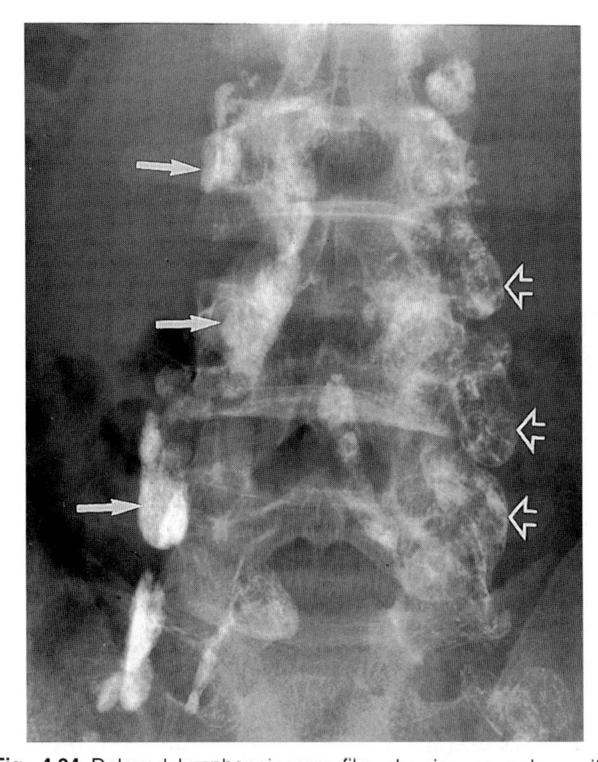

Fig. 4.24 Delayed lymphangiogram film showing normal opacified nodes on the right of the spine (closed arrows). On the left the nodes are abnormal as they are enlarged and show multiple filling defects (open arrows).

On ultrasound, enlarged nodes typically show uniformly low echogenicity, sometimes appearing almost echo-free (Fig. 4.23). Ultrasound can detect abnormal nodes as small as 1.5 cm and can be used to direct needle biopsy. However, with the inability to penetrate bowel gas, which may obscure the retroperitoneum in about a third of cases, ultrasound is not a useful survey technique.

Gallium scintigraphy has proved disappointing for identifying abdominal malignant lymph nodes, with a true positive rate of only 48%.

Bipedal lymphangiography was previously used universally to investigate possible lymph-node abnormalities (Fig. 4.24). The procedure is often time-consuming, sometimes difficult to perform, and uncomfortable for the patient. It does not demonstrate all nodal groups, and lymph nodes totally replaced by disease may not be opacified. However, bipedal lymphangiography is of some value in the investigation of patients whose cross-sectional imaging is equivocal, as lymphangiography can detect abnormality in normal-sized nodes that would otherwise be overlooked.

Tumours

Approximately 80% of retroperitoneal tumours are malignant. In adults, most are mesenchymal in origin, the commonest being liposarcoma, leiomyosarcoma (Fig. 4.25) and malignant fibrohistiocytoma (Fig. 4.26). They tend to be quite large at presentation, only producing symptoms when they compress adjacent structures. Plain films will identify these neoplasms at an advanced stage by detecting erosion of lumbar vertebrae or displacement of the renal shadows and psoas outlines. Diagnosis is readily achieved on CT even when these tumours are quite small.

CT illustrates the extent and effect on adjacent structures and may suggest the histological diagnosis.

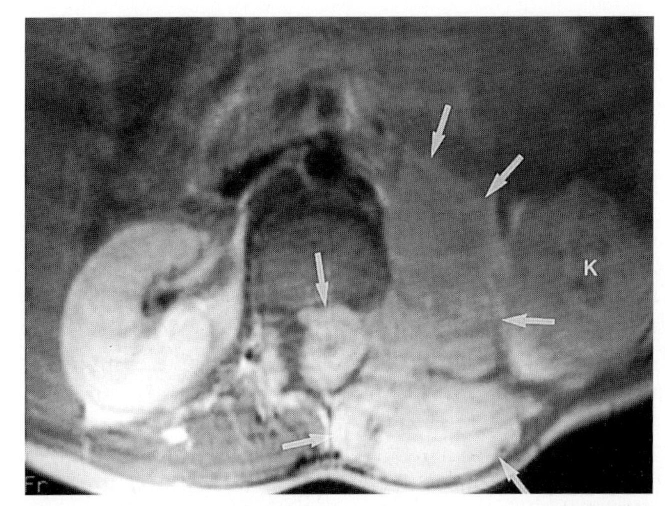

Fig. 4.26 Axial T1-weighted MRI following contrast enhancement showing a left-sided malignant fibrohistiocytoma (arrowed) occupying the left psoas and erector spinae muscles, invading the spinal canal and displacing the left kidney (K) laterally.

Retroperitoneal lipomas appear as sharply marginated, homogeneous masses with a CT attenuation value equivalent to normal fat. The other tumours are predominantly of soft tissue density though they may show calcification. Liposarcomas may, however, have areas of low attenuation consistent with normal fat, especially when well-differentiated (Fig. 4.17a). Leiomyosarcomas often have areas of necrosis and cystic degeneration which appear as areas of fluid density on CT. Other retroperitoneal neoplasms include neurogenic tumours such as neurofibromas (Fig. 4.27), extra-adrenal phaeochromocytomas and paragangliomas. Neurogenic tumours sometimes extend through a widened neural foramen into the extradural space, where they can produce nerve root or cord compression.

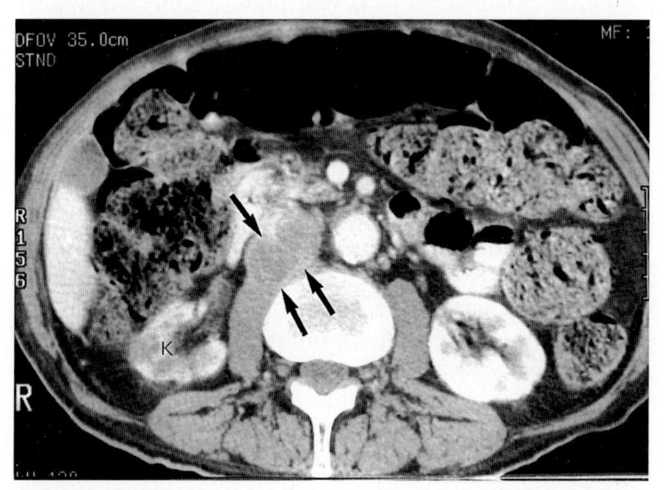

Fig. 4.25 Contrast-enhanced CT showing a retroperitoneal leiomyosarcoma arising from the IVC (arrowed). Incidental note is made of a scarred atrophic right kidney (K).

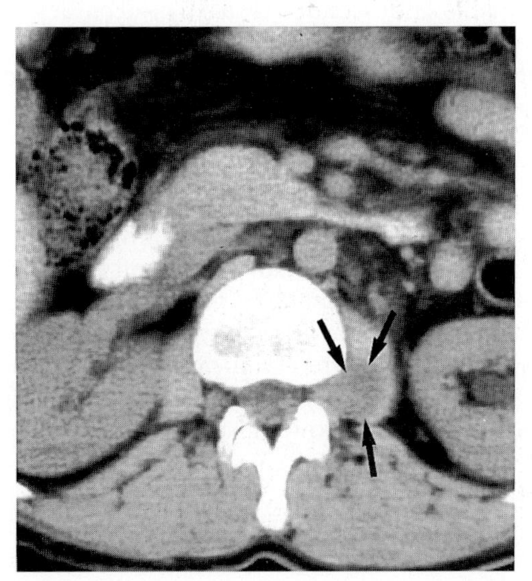

Fig. 4.27 Axial CT showing a low-density left retroperitoneal neurofibroma at the left L2 exit foramen (arrowed).

In children the commonest retroperitoneal tumours are rhabdomyosarcomas, neuroblastoma and teratomas. On CT most of these tumours show soft-tissue density; neuroblastomas classically also have diffuse stippled calcification within their substance. Teratomas may have areas of fatty density and calcifications within them. MRI in general offers little additional information but can be useful in selected cases. For example, it can diagnose lipomas and liposarcomas on the basis of their signal characteristics, as fatty tumours have very high signal on T1-weighted images. MRI may be more useful than CT in differentiating neoplastic tissue from normal psoas muscle; this can help to exclude psoas invasion. The psoas muscle is well demonstrated on MRI and has a lower signal intensity than retroperitoneal tumours on T2-weighted images. MRI may also be of value in identifying extension of retroperitoneal tumours into the spinal canal (Fig. 4.26), as the intrathecal space, spinal cord, and nerve roots are exquisitely demonstrated on MRI.

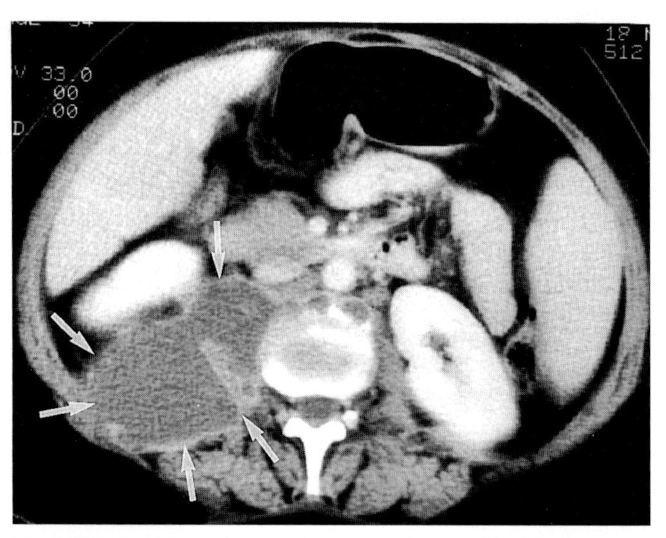

Fig. 4.28 Tuberculous abscess. Contrast-enhanced CT showing a rim-enhancing tuberculous abscess occupying the right psoas muscle (arrowed).

Undescended testis

The testes originate as paired retroperitoneal structures, arising from the gonadal ridge on the medial aspect of the mesonephros and descend into the scrotum during the eighth month of gestation. Normal testicular descent may be arrested at any point along a path extending from the renal hilum to the scrotum.

About 80% of maldescended testes are found distal to the inguinal ring and thus can be palpated. However, 20% are not palpable either because of congenital absence, as happens in 4%, or because they are located within the abdominal cavity.

The undescended testis is 12–40 times more likely to harbour foci of malignancy than a normal testis, therefore finding a testis within the abdominal cavity is important. Several series show that both CT and MRI are sensitive techniques for preoperative localization in non-palpable undescended testes. The accuracy of both techniques is greater for the identification of low-lying than it is for high intra-abdominal testes. Accurate localization requires careful attention to pelvic anatomy, as the undescended testis is typically smaller and more elliptical than the normally descended testis and is most frequently identified near the inguinal ring adjacent to the iliac vessels. On CT, atrophic and dysplastic testes appear as small foci of soft tissue similar in density to the adjacent abdominal wall musculature. MRI provides distinct advantages over CT in detection due to its multiplanar imaging capabilities. Undescended tests are usually of high signal on T2-weighted images, but may be of low signal if atrophic.

Fluid collections

Retroperitoneal abscesses The common sites for retroperitoneal abscesses are the psoas muscle and perirenal spaces. Many retroperitoneal abscesses are due to direct extension of infection from contiguous structures such as the spine, kidney, bowel and pancreas. Most are due to pyogenic bacterial pathogens, but occasionally they can be tuberculous in nature (Fig. 4.28).

CT best demonstrates the extent of the abscess and any associated abnormalities in contiguous structures. On CT the psoas muscle is enlarged, usually having lower density centrally, representing the abscess. Visualization of the abscess is made more conspicuous by intravenous contrast enhancement, which enhances the rim of the abscess (Fig. 4.28). Gas bubbles may be seen within the abscess if it is caused by a gas-forming organism or if it communicates with the bowel.

Ultrasound can demonstrate psoas abscesses in the upper retroperitoneal space as echo-free areas within the psoas muscle surrounded by an irregular thick wall. However, if gas is present, the abscess may be obscured as ultrasound is completely reflected at soft tissue – gas interfaces.

MRI shows psoas abscesses to have a very high signal on T2-weighted images but, in general, does not offer any substantial advantage over CT or ultrasound for detection or management. However, MRI may demonstrate spinal pathology more elegantly, using sagittal and coronal scanning planes.

Retroperitoneal haemorrhage Retroperitoneal haemorrhage is usually due to anticoagulant therapy, trauma or bleeding from an aortic aneurysm or retroperitoneal tumour. Spontaneous psoas haemorrhage may also occur in patients with a bleeding diathesis such as haemophilia. CT is the most accurate, non-invasive technique for detecting retroperitoneal haemorrhage. The exact location depends on the cause of the haemorrhage, for example a haematoma from a leaking aneurysm will surround the aorta before extending into the adjacent retroperitoneum. The

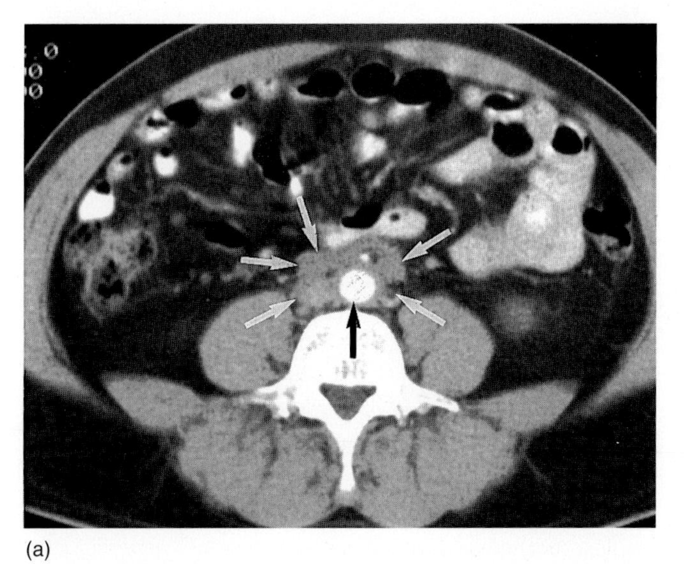
(a)

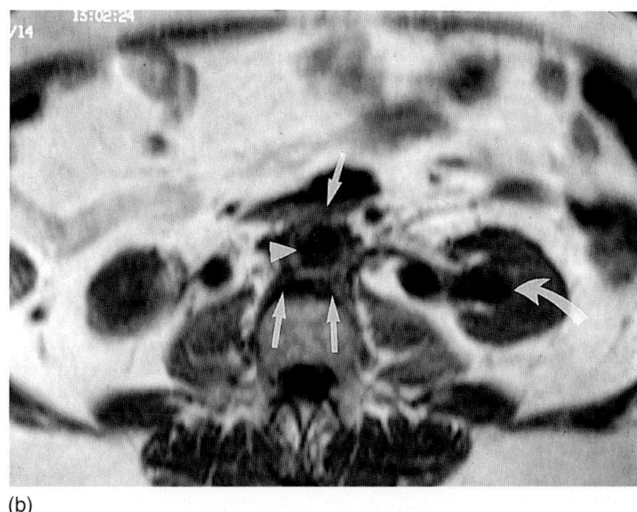
(b)

Fig. 4.29 Retroperitoneal fibrosis. (a) Axial contrast-enhanced CT showing the aorta (black arrow) surrounded by periaortic retroperitoneal fibrosis (white arrows). (b) Axial T1-weighted MRI showing a signal void in the aorta (arrowhead), and low-signal periaortic retroperitoneal fibrosis (straight arrows). There is dilation of the left renal pelvis (curved arrow).

attenuation value depends on the age of haemorrhage. **Acute haematomas** show higher attenuation than circulating blood, because clot formation and retraction causes a greater concentration of haemoglobin. A **chronic haematoma**, which may have associated calcification, appears as a low density mass as clot lysis takes place. The appearance of a subacute or chronic haematoma can thus be confused with a retroperitoneal tumour, abscess, lymphocoele or cyst.

Ultrasound shows acute haematomas as echo-free fluid collections. Chronic haematomas may appear as complex multiseptate structures or even solid masses. The appearance of haemorrhage on MRI is complex and depends on the field strength of the magnet and the age of the haemorrhage. It may have a characteristic appearance on MRI, but occassionally bleeding into a tumour or abscess may be indistinguishable from a simple bleed.

Retroperitoneal cysts Retroperitoneal cysts are rare and include lymphatic cysts, inclusion cysts, embryonic gastrointestinal cysts and genitourinary tract remnants. Their imaging features are similar, namely a well-defined, thin-walled, fluid-filled mass.

Fibrosis

Retroperitoneal fibrosis is characterized by fibrous tissue proliferation along the posterior aspect of the retroperitoneal cavity, generally confined to the central and paravertebral regions. The tissue is sharply delineated and tends to envelop rather than displace adjacent structures, such as the ureters and blood vessels. The histological features range from an active inflammatory process to a more acellular, hyalinized reaction. Most cases are idiopathic but retroperitoneal fibrosis can be secondary to certain drugs (such as methysergide), primary and secondary tumours, aneurysms and aneurysm surgery.

On intravenous urography there is medial deviation and obstruction of the ureters, typically at about L4/5 bilaterally.

On ultrasound an ill-defined echo-poor mass of fibrous tissue can sometimes be identified together with any associated hydronephrosis.

CT, however, offers the best delineation of the process, demonstrating a periaortic soft-tissue mass of similar attenuation to muscle (Fig. 4.29a), which may show enhancement following intravenous contrast. Retroperitoneal fibrosis tends to encase the aorta anteriorly and laterally, distinguishing it from retroperitoneal malignancy which may occur behind the aorta displacing it anteriorly. Retroperitoneal fibrosis most commonly encases the infrarenal aorta and common iliac arteries and is often predominantly left-sided. Hydronephrosis is well demonstrated on CT when the ureters are obstructed. Insidious disease progression is the general rule. Shrinkage of retroperitoneal fibrosis in response to treatment with steroids is sometimes demonstrated using CT, however residual periaortic tissue is common following treatment and CT has no value in determining disease activity in such circumstances. It may not always be possible to distinguish retroperitoneal fibrosis from other retroperitoneal masses and CT can be used to guide percutaneous biopsy, which should be generous in size to differentiate from malignancy.

MRI is as accurate as CT in demonstrating retroperitoneal fibrosis. The soft tissue is of low signal intensity on both T1- (Fig. 4.29b) and T2-weighted imaging. As with ultrasound and CT, hydronephrosis is readily demonstrated.

CHAPTER 5

Liver, biliary system, pancreas and spleen

Rodney H. Reznek

LIVER

Prior to the development of high quality ultrasound and computed tomography, imaging the liver, biliary system, pancreas and spleen depended on indirect visualization, primarily through nuclear medicine and angiography. Ultrasound, MRI and CT now allow direct demonstration of these organs. The choice of the most appropriate technique will always depend on a consideration of several factors including the clinical indication, the accuracy of any particular modality, cost and availability.

IMAGING TECHNIQUES

ULTRASOUND

Most focal intrahepatic masses are detected by echo patterns that differ from those of surrounding normal liver parenchyma. The smallest structure that can be

Diagnostic and Interventional Radiology in Surgical Practice. Edited by P. Armstrong and M. L. Wastie. Published 1997 by Chapman & Hall, London. ISBN 0 412 61960 1 (HB), 0 412 61970 9 (PB)

resolved depends on the contrast in reflectivity between the mass and the surrounding parenchyma. For example, metastases as small as 10 mm can be detected if a large difference in reflectivity exists between normal parenchyma and the focal lesion.

Diffuse hepatic abnormalities may also result in alteration of hepatic contour and echo pattern. These changes are usually appreciated by comparing the echo pattern of the liver and the adjacent right renal cortex. The size and patency of the portal and hepatic venous systems can also be assessed.

COMPUTED TOMOGRAPHY

Although CT is only slightly more accurate than ultrasound in showing focal hepatic lesions, it has several advantages. All the upper abdominal anatomy is displayed on the CT image, providing information about extrahepatic processes that can influence interpretation. Also, intravenous injection of water-soluble contrast medium increases the detection rate of small masses.

Liver lobes and segments are accurately delineated by CT provided the liver is imaged both before and after the intravenous injection of contrast medium. This also increases the contrast between most focal lesions and normal liver parenchyma and thus increases the sensitivity of the technique in detecting focal pathology. The best method of enhancing normal hepatic parenchyma is to use a rapid and sustained delivery of a large intravenous bolus of contrast medium followed by rapid scanning.

CT angiography can be used in patients being assessed for partial hepatectomy as it may demonstrate additional lesions undetected by standard scanning after an intravenous bolus. Contrast medium can be injected selectively into the hepatic artery or, as in CT arterioportography, into the superior mesenteric artery.

MAGNETIC RESONANCE IMAGING

MRI of the liver is used predominantly as a problem-solving technique rather than as a survey procedure. The normal appearance of the liver depends on the pulse sequence used. Several different pulse sequences have been advocated depending on the clinical problem. With spin-echo sequences the liver parenchyma has a low signal intensity and blood vessels appear dark.

SCINTIGRAPHY

Technetium-99m tin or sulphur colloid or albumin colloid is selectively trapped by the hepatic and splenic reticuloendothelial cells to give an image of the liver and spleen. Characteristic abnormalities are seen in patients with diffuse and focal liver disease. However, both ultrasound and CT have supplanted colloid scintigraphy due to their superior sensitivity in detecting small lesions within the liver parenchyma and because these modalities yield more information about extrahepatic structures. The widespread use of percutaneous liver biopsies has also resulted in far less frequent use of scintigraphy to diagnose diffuse liver disease.

ARTERIOGRAPHY

Arteriography is now largely performed as part of an interventional procedure and is only rarely performed for diagnostic purposes, usually as part of the pre-operative assessment of primary and secondary neoplasm.

NORMAL INTRAHEPATIC SEGMENTAL ANATOMY (Figs 5.1a–d)

The lobes, segments and subsegments of the liver are defined by the branching pattern of the structures entering and leaving its porta with the hepatic veins coursing in the interlobar and intersegmental planes, dividing the liver into two lobes, four segments and eight subsegments. These segments and subsegments (Figs 5.1a–d) can be identified readily on cross-sectional imaging techniques including sonography, CT and MRI. An appreciation of segmental anatomy is a prerequisite for accurate localization of lesions before surgical intervention. The easiest method of classifying segmental liver anatomy is based on the hepatic vascular and fissural landmarks. The anatomical landmarks are variable depending on the level of the scan.

At the most cephalad level (Figure 5.1a), hepatic veins are clearly identified converging towards the inferior vena cava and, at this level, the middle hepatic vein separates the right and left lobes; the right hepatic vein separates the anterior and posterior segments of the right lobe and the left hepatic vein separates the lateral and medial segments of the left lobe.

Slightly more inferiorly (Fig. 5.1b), the left portal vein separates the medial and lateral segments of the left lobe. A line along the right portal vein, extended laterally, separates the anterior and posterior segments of the right lobe. The medial and lateral segments of the left lobe are separated by the ligamentum teres. The caudate lobe is separated from the lateral segment of the left lobe by the ligamentum venosum (Fig. 5.1c).

At the level of the gallbladder fossa (Fig. 5.1d) an imaginary line constructed between the gallbladder fossa and the inferior vena cava, divides the liver into right and left lobes. The ligamentum teres fissure

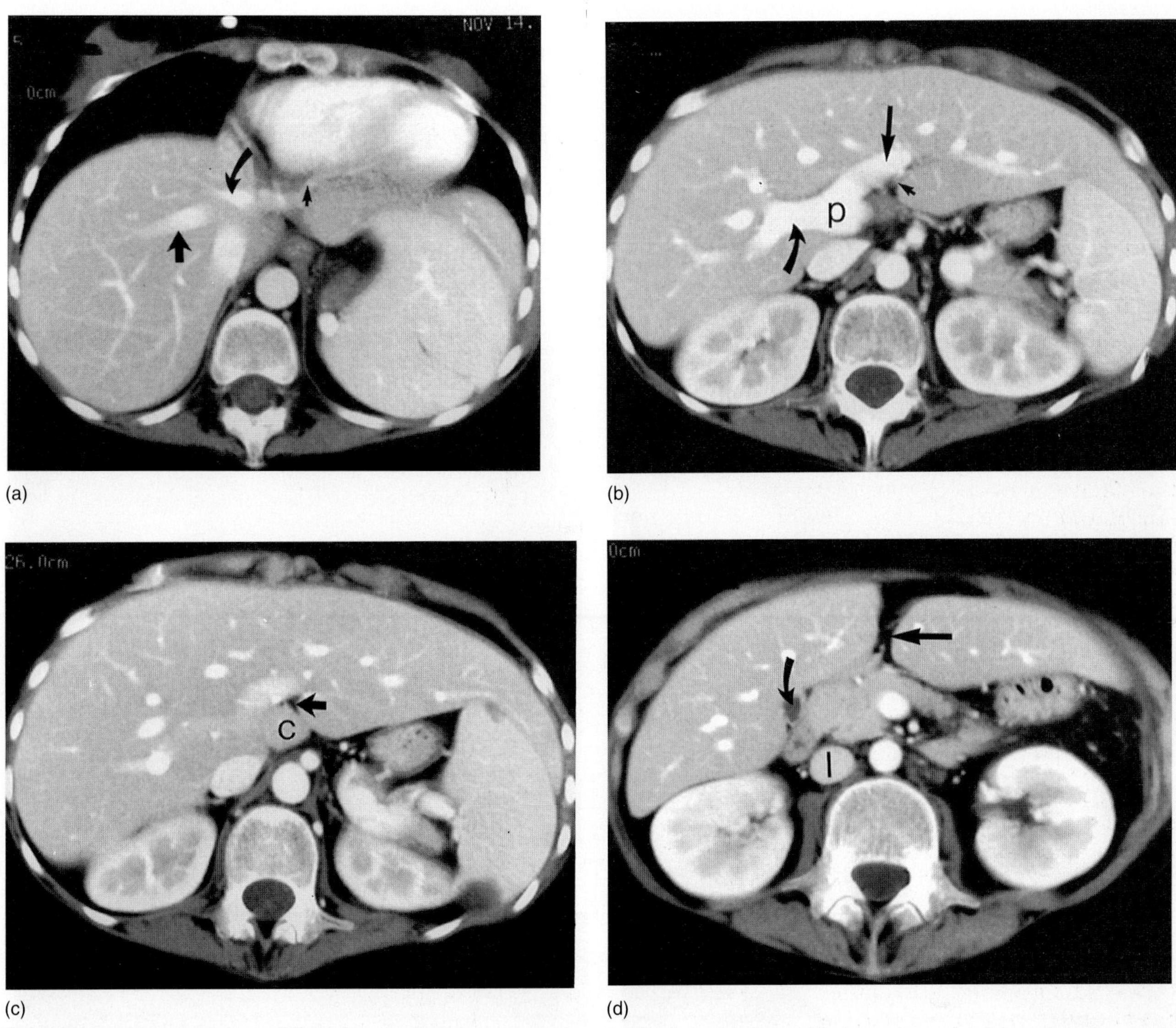

(a) (b) (c) (d)

Fig. 5.1 Normal liver anatomy on CT. (a) Scan through the superior aspect of the liver showing middle (curved arrow), left (arrowhead) and right (arrow) hepatic veins. (b) Scan through the level of the portal vein (P) showing the left portal (arrow) and right portal (curved arrow) veins. The inferior aspect of the ligamentum teres (arrowhead) separates the medial and lateral segments of the left lobe. (c) Scan through the caudate lobe of the liver (C) separated from the lateral segment of the left lobe of the liver by the ligamentum venosum (arrow). (d) Scan through the gallbladder fossa (curved arrow). A line joining the inferior vena cava (I) divides the liver into right and left lobes at this level. The ligamentum teres (arrow) divides the left lobe into medial and lateral segments at this level.

separates the medial and lateral segments of the left lobe.

Readily visible landmarks for all segments are not visualized on every section. However, when taken as a composite, highly accurate segmental landmarks can be established.

DIFFUSE HEPATOCELLULAR DISEASE

CIRRHOSIS AND FATTY CHANGE

Ultrasonography

Because of the opposing effects of fatty change and fibrosis, the liver is either enlarged or of normal size in the early stages of cirrhosis. A small, shrunken liver is seen only in advanced stages. Criteria for the sonographic diagnosis of cirrhosis include increased parenchymal echogenicity, decreased beam penetration through the liver and poor depiction of intrahepatic portal vein walls. Similar findings are encountered with fatty change and therefore, in the early stages, fatty change cannot be distinguished from cirrhosis. In more advanced cirrhosis, the left lobe is relatively preserved or enlarged, the caudate lobe hypertrophied, and both are relatively large compared to the right lobe. Advanced cirrhosis results in contour indentations, nodularity and occasionally regenerating nodules, usually 0.5–1.5 cm in diameter, which are isoechoic with the parenchyma.

Computed tomography

Fatty liver is the most common CT feature in early cirrhosis and results in lowering of the CT density of the liver parenchyma, usually to below 40 Hounsfield units (HU) (Fig. 5.2). Hepatomegaly is frequent but the liver contour is normal. In advanced cirrhosis, an overall decrease in liver volume is accompanied by atrophy of the right lobe and medial segment of the left lobe, and hypertrophy of the caudate lobe and lateral segment of the left lobe (Fig. 5.3). Caudate lobe enlargement is present early in cirrhosis and roughly parallels the degree of cirrhosis thereafter. Regenerating nodules cause nodularity of the liver contour (Fig. 5.4). Non-uniform attenuation, often striking, can result from chronic fatty infiltration or fibrosis.

MRI

Common findings in MRI, as with other cross-sectional imaging modalities, include contour nodularity, relative right lobe atrophy and hypertrophy of

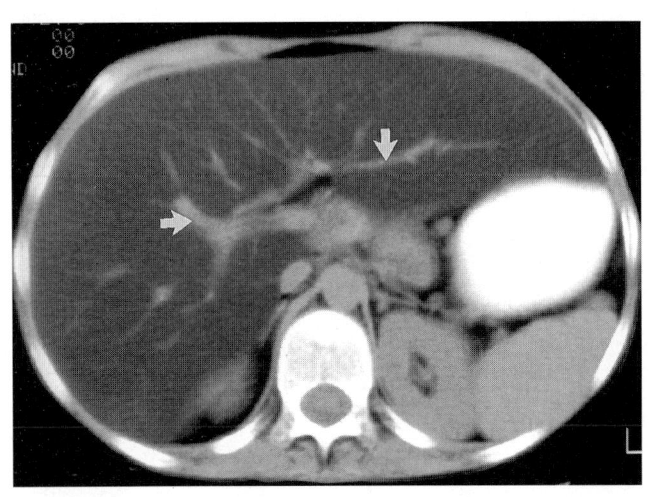

Fig. 5.2 Severe fatty change in a liver of normal size shown on CT. The presence of a marked amount of fat has lowered the density of the liver to such an extent that the blood vessels appear of higher density than the liver parenchyma (arrows).

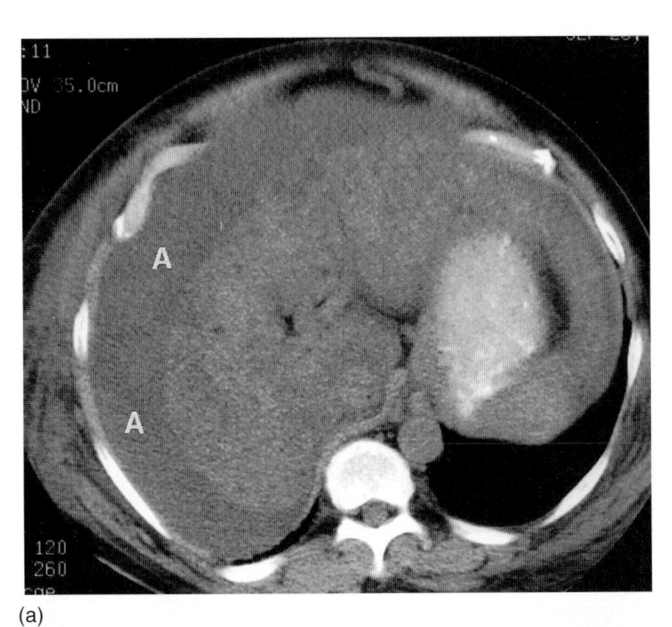

(a)

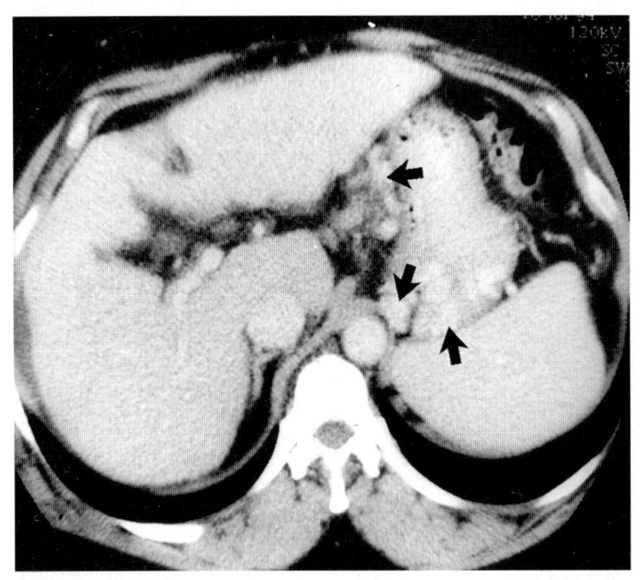

Fig. 5.3 Cirrhosis with portal hypertension shown on CT after intravenous injection of contrast medium. There is atrophy of the right lobe and medial segment of the left lobe with hypertrophy of the caudate and lateral segment of the left lobe. The liver surface is irregular and there is a small amount of ascites. Large collateral vessels are seen in the region of the splenic hilum, around the gastro-oesophageal junction and along the lesser curve of the stomach (arrows).

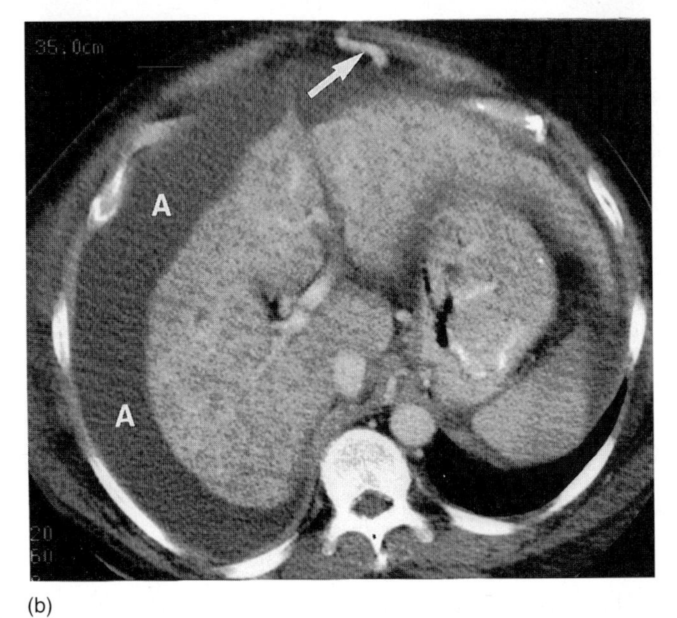

(b)

Fig. 5.4 Cirrhosis of the liver. (a) Scan without intravenous contrast medium showing a small shrunken liver containing multiple small nodules. A large amount of ascites (A) is seen. (b) Scan taken after intravenous injection of contrast medium, showing irregularity of the liver contour and inhomogeneous attenuation due to multiple regenerating nodules. A collateral vessel due to portal hypertension is seen anteriorly (arrow).

the left and caudate lobes. Vascular distortion is better demonstrated on MRI than ultrasound or CT. Available data on the signal characteristics are conflicting, and clear-cut, clinically useful, diffuse alterations in signal intensity induced by cirrhosis have yet to be elucidated.

PORTAL HYPERTENSION

In most cases, portal hypertension is secondary to liver disease and imaging of the liver is helpful in providing confirmatory evidence of diffuse pathology. Where the cause of portal hypertension is uncertain, imaging of the portal venous anatomy is crucial.

Portal or splenic vein enlargement, or both, is easily detected on CT or ultrasound. Portosystemic collaterals are often readily seen as tortuous, tubular or round masses of soft tissue attenuation on unenhanced scans; scans after injection of a bolus of contrast medium may be necessary to confirm their vascular nature (Fig. 5.3). Oesophageal varices can be suggested on CT by a thickened oesophageal wall with a lobulated outer contour and a scalloped lumen with intraluminal protrusions that exhibit marked contrast enhancement.

Assessment of portal vein size and patency can also be made sonographically. A portal vein exceeding 16 mm in diameter on deep inspiration in the supine position has been shown to be diagnostic of portal hypertension in a high percentage of cases. Lack of the normal distension of the portal, splenic or superior mesenteric veins on deep inspiration, and loss of the normal respiratory fluctuation in the Doppler signal are other signs indicating portal hypertension. Indirect signs such as splenomegaly, the opening of collaterals and ascites are also reliably demonstrated by ultrasound.

Portal or splenic vein thrombosis is seen on contrast-enhanced CT scans as a lucent blood clot surrounded by an enhanced vessel wall together with inhomogeneous enhancement of the periportal parenchyma (Fig. 5.5). When the vein is occluded and enlarged, it is likely that tumour thrombus is present – hepatocellular carcinoma, cholangiocarcinoma, pancreatic carcinoma and gastric carcinoma are the likely causes. Numerous collateral veins by-passing the occluded portal vein are recognized on CT by the appearance of serpentine, opacified collaterals in the hepatoduodenal ligament.

In most cases, ultrasound can demonstrate portal vein thrombosis in the main portal vein or its larger branches as echogenic material within the vascular lumen. In older thrombus, when the obstruction is complete, and the lumen entirely filled with echogenic material, it may be difficult to identify the vein at all.

Conventional spin-echo MRI is comparable to CT and arterial portography for demonstrating the presence or absence of portosystemic collaterals and portal vein thrombus. MR angiography can also provide images of the thrombosed portal vein. The exact signal characteristics of the thrombus will vary with age, pulse sequence and field strength.

Direct preoperative demonstration of the portal venous anatomy is now best achieved by **arterial portography** which has replaced the traditional

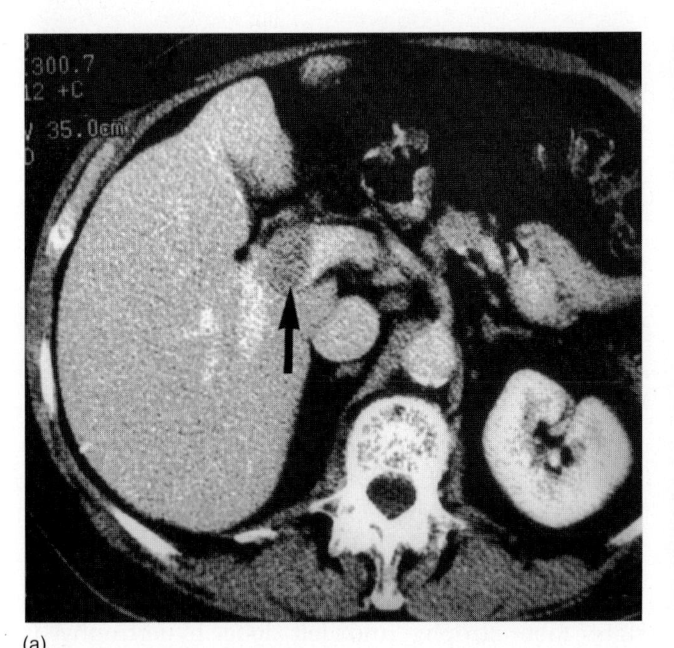

(a)

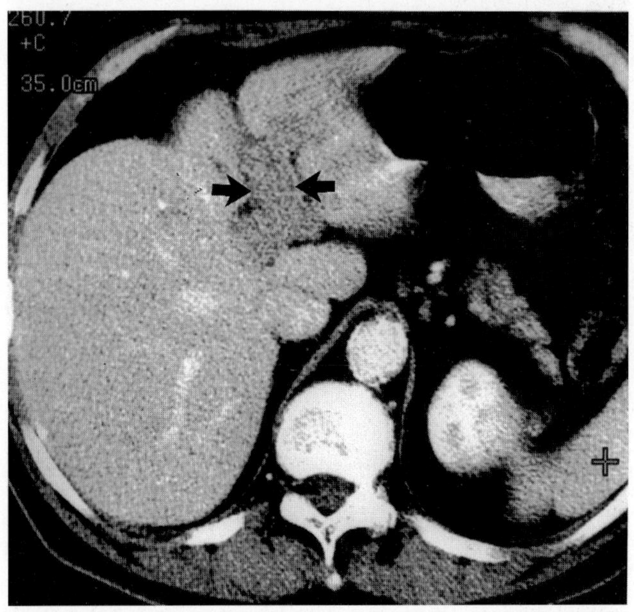

(b)

Fig. 5.5 CT and ultrasound in portal vein thrombosis. (a) CT scan taken after intravenous injection of contrast medium showingt a filling defect within the portal vein (arrow). (b) A scan at a level superior to (a) shows extension of the filling defect into the left portal vein (arrows) which is also expanded. (*continued overleaf*)

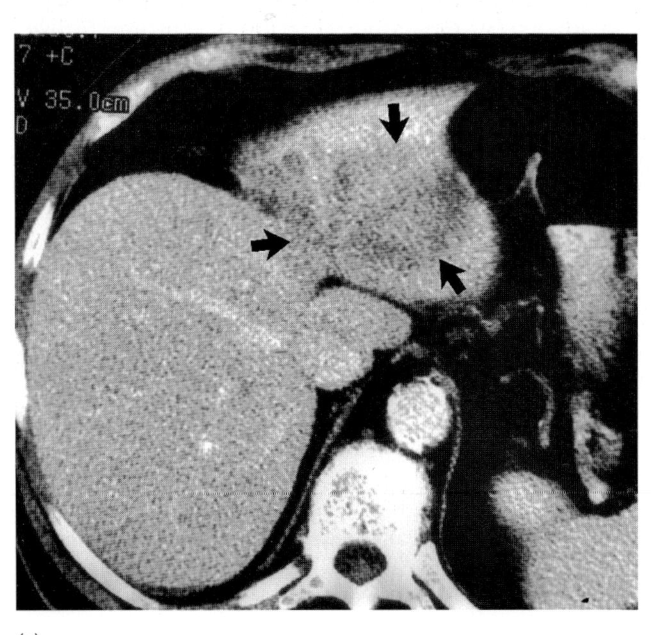

(c)

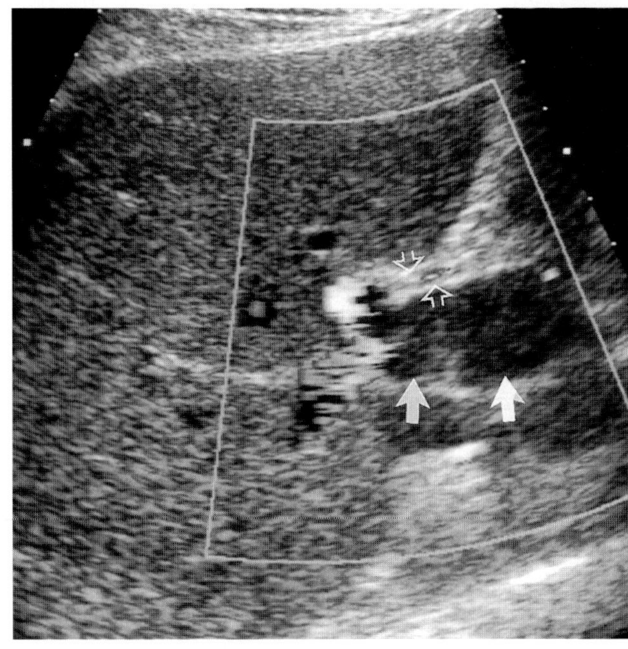

(d)

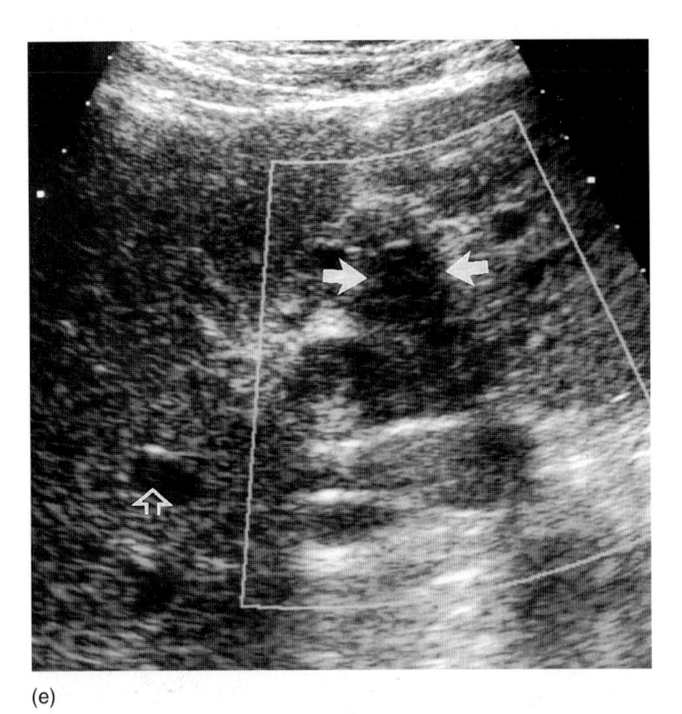

(e)

Fig. 5.5 (*continued*) (c) CT scan at a level superior to (b) showing a defect in the enhancement of the parenchyma in the left lobe (arrows) due to the presence of thrombus. (d) Longitudinal ultrasound scan in the same patient showing numerous echoes within the portal vein (arrows) consistent with thrombus. The normal common duct is seen lying anterior to the portal vein in this projection (open arrows). (e) Transverse ultrasound scan showing thrombus within the left portal vein (arrows). A patent vein is shown in the right lobe of the liver, free from any internal echoes (open arrow).

technique of splenoportography as it is safer and gives additional information about the vascular tree. Selective catheterization of the splenic, hepatic and superior mesenteric arteries gives a full demonstration of the arterial supply to the liver as well as showing the portal venous anatomy. The position and patency of the mesenteric, splenic and portal veins, IVC and renal veins can be assessed in order to help decide which form of shunt to use.

BUDD–CHIARI SYNDROME

Ultrasound, CT and MRI will amost invariably show ascites, hepatomegaly and mild splenomegaly in Budd–Chiari syndrome. Caudate hypertrophy with right lobe atrophy and left lobe hypertrophy is common. Thrombus within the hepatic veins in the acute phase, or non-visualization in the chronic phase, can be detected on ultrasound (with or without

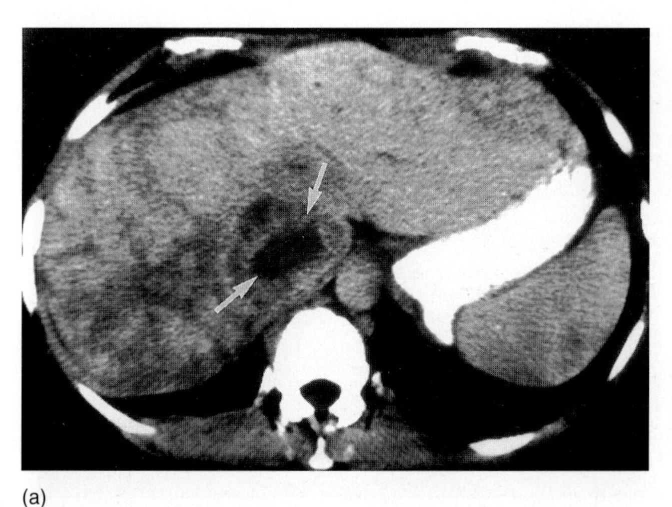

(a)

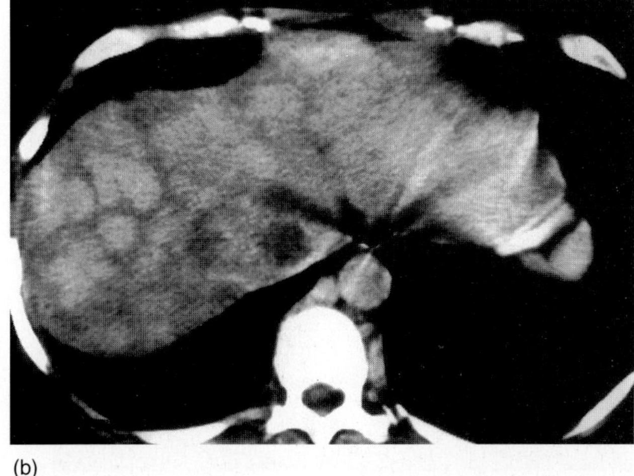

(b)

Fig. 5.6 Budd–Chiari syndrome on CT. (a) CT scan after intravenous contrast medium showing inhomogeneous enhancement of the liver parenchyma with focal areas of increased and decreased enhancement. Thrombosis can be seen within the inferior vena cava (arrows). (b) Scan taken slightly superior to (a) showing relative sparing of the left lobe and extension of the thrombus superiorly. The hepatic veins are not opacified.

Doppler), CT or MRI, as can intrahepatic and extrahepatic venous collaterals. In chronic cases of Budd–Chiari syndrome, the typical CT pattern is inhomogeneous enhancement due to a mixture of normal or hypertrophied hepatic parenchyma with regions of liver atrophy (Fig. 5.6).

Hepatic scintigraphy may demonstrate a characteristic pattern in Budd–Chiari syndrome: a central region of normal activity (appearing 'hot') in the caudate lobe, the rest of the liver showing greatly diminished activity. This characteristic pattern is seen only when the veins draining the caudate lobe (which enter separately into the vena cava) are spared.

FOCAL LIVER DISEASE

METASTATIC NEOPLASMS

Signs and symptoms of metastases occur in only 50% of patients with hepatic metastases. Biochemical hepatic function tests can be misleading: they may be normal in 25–50% of cases with metastases and elevated in numerous benign abnormalities. Carcinoembryonic antigen measurements and visual inspection of the liver at laparoscopy or surgery are also generally considered insufficiently sensitive or specific for detecting metastases.

Radionuclide liver/spleen scanning has significant false-negative and false-positive rates ranging from 15 to 25%. Lesions <2 cm are rarely detected and central lesions >2 cm can be missed frequently. Although tomography has brought about improvement, ultrasound, CT and MRI predominate in the evaluation for metastatic disease in most institutions.

Ultrasound

High-resolution, real-time ultrasound is a highly sensitive and specific modality for detecting small liver metastases. Drawbacks remain, such as the unfavourable body habitus of some patients and the poor visibility of small lesions near the dome of the

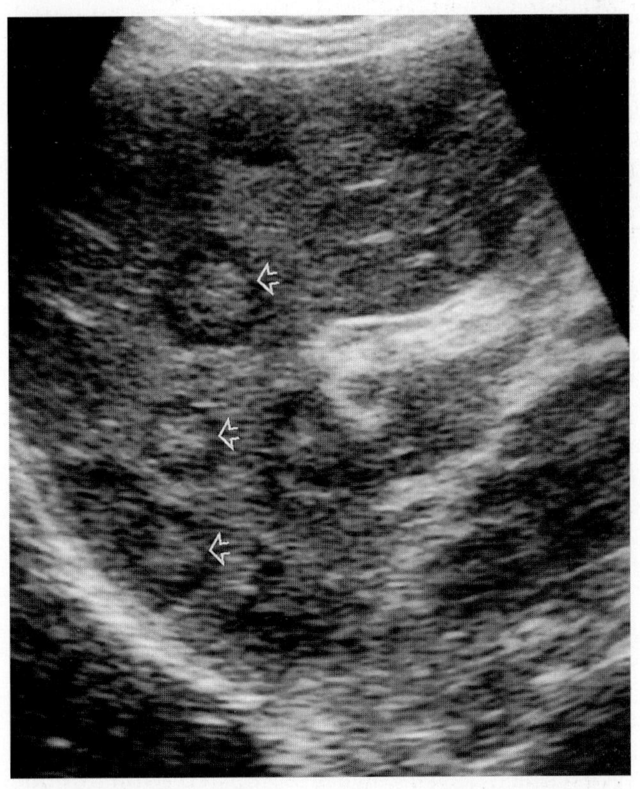

Fig. 5.7 Multiple liver metastases shown on a longitudinal ultrasound scan. Multiple hyperechoic lesions are seen in a patient with colonic carcinoma. A typical lucent 'halo' is seen around most of the lesions (open arrows).

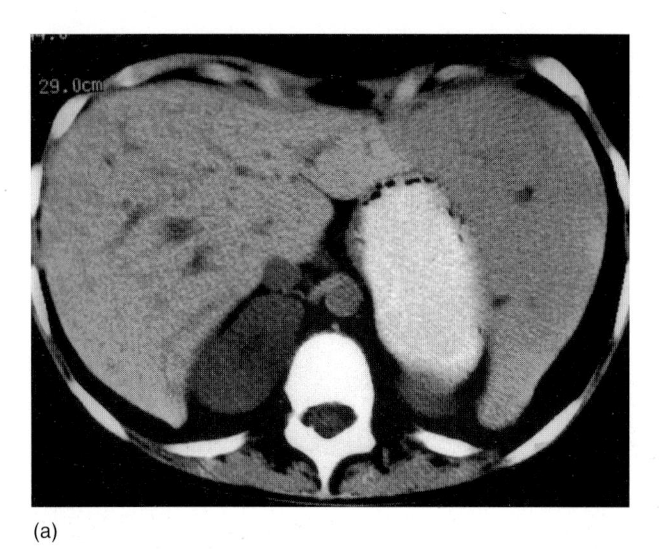

(a)

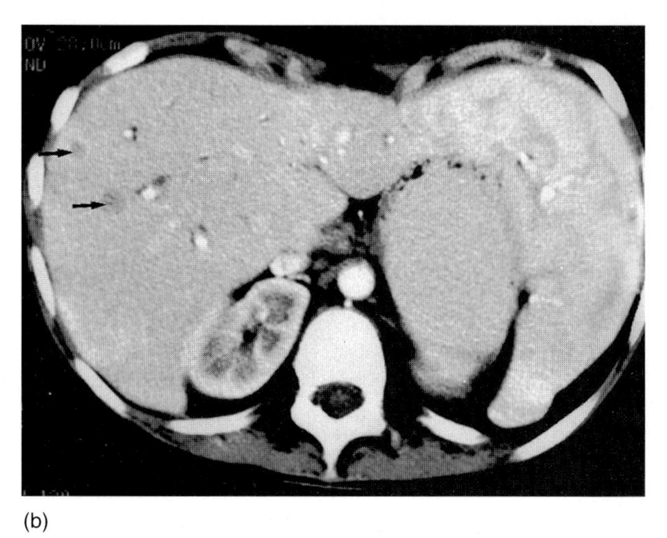

(b)

Fig. 5.8 Liver deposits best demonstrated on CT after intravenous injection of contrast medium. (a) A CT scan through the liver without contrast medium showing no obvious focal abnormality. (b) After intravenous injection of contrast medium, a scan at the same level as (a) shows two small focal abnormalities enhancing to a lesser extent than the adjacent normal liver parenchyma (arrows).

liver and the liver surface. Also, the segmental anatomy is more readily appreciated on CT or MRI for liver resection evaluation.

Metastases can be hyperechoic, hypoechoic or isoechoic compared to the surrounding parenchyma. A thin hypoechoic rim may be seen (the 'halo' sign) (Fig. 5.7). Multiple, large, poorly demarcated hyperechoic masses are usually metastases from colorectal carcinoma.

The development of high frequency transducers has led to the use of ultrasound for intraoperative use. Intraoperative sonography, performed immediately before metastectomy, has been shown to yield additional information compared with preoperative CT and ultrasound.

Computed tomography

CT is the preferred single imaging technique for screening the abdomen for metastatic disease. Incremental bolus dynamic CT (rapid liver scanning after intravenous injection of a bolus of contrast medium) is a very accurate means of detecting focal liver masses >1 cm in size but its sensitivity for lesions <1 cm is only about 50%.

Most hepatic metastases are hypovascular and therefore hypodense on contrast-enhanced scans (Fig. 5.8). Calcification can occur within liver deposits, particularly in patients with colon carcinoma (Fig. 5.9). Computed tomographic hepatic arteriography and CT arterial portography maximize differential contrast enhancement between liver parenchyma and metastases and thus improve the detection of liver metastases by as much as 50% when compared with routine contrast-enhanced CT. These are, however, invasive procedures requiring catheter placement in the hepatic, superior mesenteric or splenic artery, and are only justified in evaluating patients being considered for major hepatic surgery.

MRI

MRI is having an increasing impact on the evaluation of the liver in both the screening and staging of malignant disease, and may eventually become the definitive method for the evaluation of hepatic metastases. Comparisons of MRI with both ultrasound and CT are sparse but it is difficult to distinguish statistically significant differences between the accuracies of CT and MRI. Most metastases, being hypovascular, exhibit a low-to-intermediate signal intensity on T1-weighted images and an increased signal on T2-weighted images.

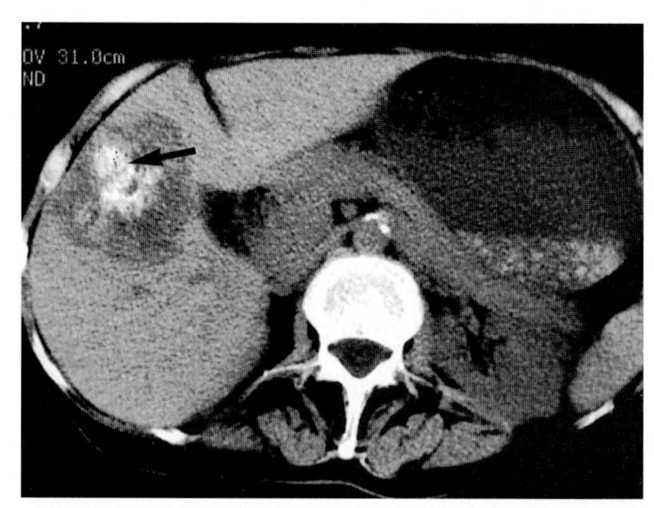

Fig. 5.9 A CT scan without intravenous injection of contrast medium showing the typical appearance of calcification within a focal liver deposit (arrow) in a patient with colonic carcinoma.

Arteriography

Since the introduction of ultrasound and CT, arteriography of the liver has a very limited role in diagnosis. However, therapeutic manoeuvres can be conducted through a catheter placed percutaneously in the hepatic artery. This method has been effectively used, for example, in metastatic carcinoid tumours.

PRIMARY LIVER TUMOUR (HEPATOCELLULAR CARCINOMA)

Plain films may show generalized hepatomegaly or a localized bulge in the contour of the diaphragm. Calcification may be seen on the plain film but is very unusual in untreated hepatocellular carcinoma.

The appearance of hepatocellular carcinoma on ultrasound, CT and MRI is variable but can be divided into three major categories that correlate well with pathological data. The most common appearances are discrete lesions (solitary or multiple), diffuse parenchymal infiltration and a combination of the discrete and diffuse hepatic patterns.

On **ultrasound**, discrete lesions are usually hypoechoic, only occasionally isoechoic, and detected by a thin, hypoechoic halo. The diffuse pattern results in disorganization of the normal echo pattern with multiple areas of increased and decreased echogenicity without distinct masses. Unfortunately, these ultrasound patterns can also be seen with other entities such as metastases, fatty liver, cirrhosis or lymphoma, making guided biopsy necessary for definitive diagnosis. Ultrasound demonstration of venous involvement favours hepatocellular carcinoma over metastases as it has a propensity to invade the portal and hepatic veins. Such features, including ascites and splenomegaly, are well demonstrated on ultrasound.

On **CT**, discrete solitary or multiple lesions are seen as well-defined low-density areas of decreased attenuation, usually 20–30 HU lower than adjacent normal liver (Fig. 5.10). Foci of calcification may be seen within the tumour. Most primary liver tumours enhance after intravenous injection of contrast medium owing to their hypervascularity, but they still show a lower CT number than the normal enhanced liver parenchyma (Fig. 5.11). As with ultrasound, the solitary or multiple discrete pattern of hepatocellular carcinoma cannot be distinguished from metastases. Diffuse parenchymal infiltration results in irregular, poorly defined areas of decreased density within the liver. After intravenous injection of contrast medium, they enhance inhomogeneously and to a lesser extent than the surrounding normal parenchyma (Fig. 5.12).

The sensitivity of ultrasound and CT for detecting hepatocellular carcinoma is similar and both exceed 80%. CT is, however, useful for early detection of extrahepatic metastases, most commonly to the lung. Metastases to the adrenal glands, peritoneal cavity, lymph nodes and skeleton are also readily detected by CT. Thus, when hepatocellular carcinoma is being staged, it is important to use the two techniques in conjunction. CT surpasses ultrasound in showing the distribution of the tumour within the liver as well as extrahepatic spread, while ultrasound is superior in the evaluation of the portal and hepatic veins.

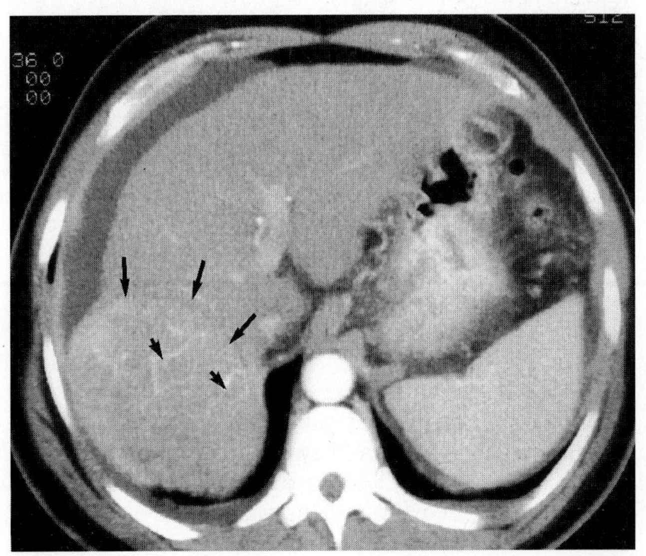

Fig. 5.10 CT scan showing a unifocal hepatocellular carcinoma (arrows) in a patient with cirrhosis. The tumour can be seen to enhance inhomogeneously after intravenous injection of contrast medium and to contain abnormal vessels (arrowheads).

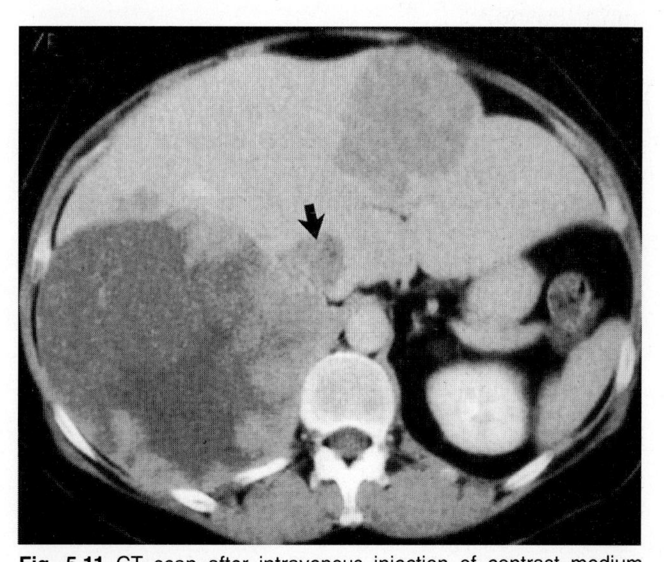

Fig. 5.11 CT scan after intravenous injection of contrast medium showing a multifocal hepatocellular carcinoma. The liver lesions are seen to enhance to a lesser extent than the adjacent normal liver parenchyma. There is also tumour extension into the inferior vena cava (arrow).

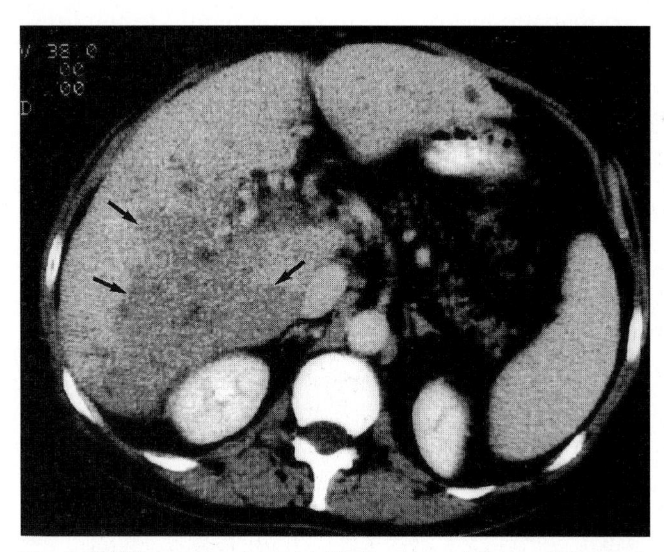

Fig. 5.12 Diffuse parenchymal infiltration due a hepatocellular carcinoma, shown as an irregular 'geographical' area of abnormal enhancement after intravenous injection of contrast medium (arrows).

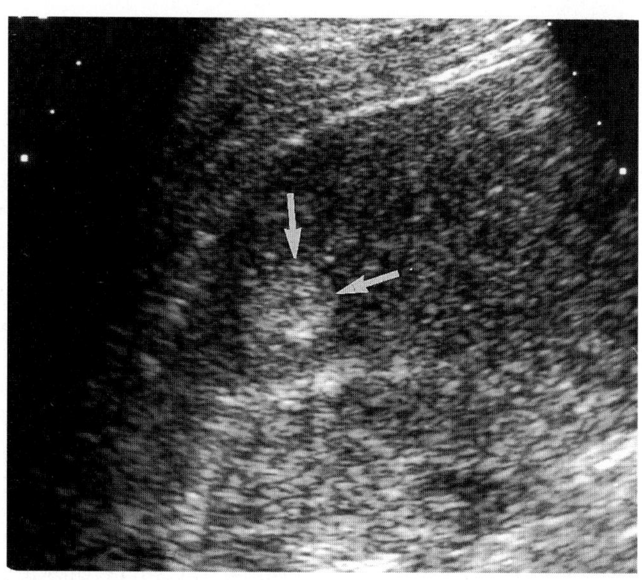

Fig. 5.13 Transverse ultrasound scan through the posterior segment of the right lobe of the liver showing a well-defined area of uniformly increased echogenicity (arrows).

The **MRI** appearance depends on the type of disease (solitary, multiple or diffuse), degree of fibrosis, the possibility of necrosis or haemorrhage and the sequences used. Typically, lesions are of decreased signal intensity on T1-weighted images and moderately increased on T2-weighted images. Data are not yet available on the accuracy of MRI for the detection or staging of hepatocellular carcinoma.

HAEMANGIOMAS

Haemangiomas are found in up to 3% of patients undergoing routine CT scanning of the liver and can often be confused with other focal liver pathology. The majority are small, capillary lesions and are seen on ultrasound as clearly defined, highly reflective lesions close to the periphery of the liver (Fig. 5.13). Cavernous haemangiomas are less common and have a varied appearance, being hyper- or hypoechoic. Duplex or colour Doppler sonography has not contributed significantly to establishing the diagnosis. Most haemangiomas do not change substantially over time although a few may become less echogenic. In about 55% of cases, haemangiomas will display specific morphological findings on CT allowing a diagnosis to be made with close to 90% probability, namely low-density compared to normal liver on the precontrast scan, peripheral contrast enhancement on the immediate postcontrast phase and progressive 'fill-in' on delayed scans up to 30 minutes following intravenous administration of contrast medium, until the haemangioma becomes the same density as the adjacent normal parenchyma (Fig. 5.14). This pattern can, however, also be seen in 5% of metastases and, if the patient is known to have a primary malignancy, follow-up is usually advised.

Scintigraphy with ^{99m}Tc-sulphur colloid depicts haemangiomas as non-specific focal regions of decreased activity. Technetium-99m-labelled red blood cell scanning is very specific. Typically, dynamic scanning seconds after injection of a bolus of labelled red blood cells, shows hypoperfusion with gradually increasing activity due to red blood cell accumulation on serial delayed imaging which peaks within 30 to 50 minutes after injection. This pattern of radioactivity is considered diagnostic of haemangioma.

MRI has also been used in diagnosing haemangiomas. The characteristic appearance is a sharply defined homogeneous hyperintense mass on T2-weighted images and a hypointense appearance on T1-weighting. Unfortunately, there is overlap of the signal characteristics with other conditions, notably necrotic tumours and hypervascular metastases. Gadolinium-enhanced MRI produces a pattern of enhancement similar to that seen with contrast-enhanced CT.

Thus, when typical imaging features are present in a patient with normal liver function tests and no known primary malignancy, the diagnosis of haemangioma is statistically very likely and can be made with a high degree of accuracy. Patients with known primary malignancies are slightly more problematic, especially when the typical CT appearance is not present. If needed, fine-needle aspiration can be performed.

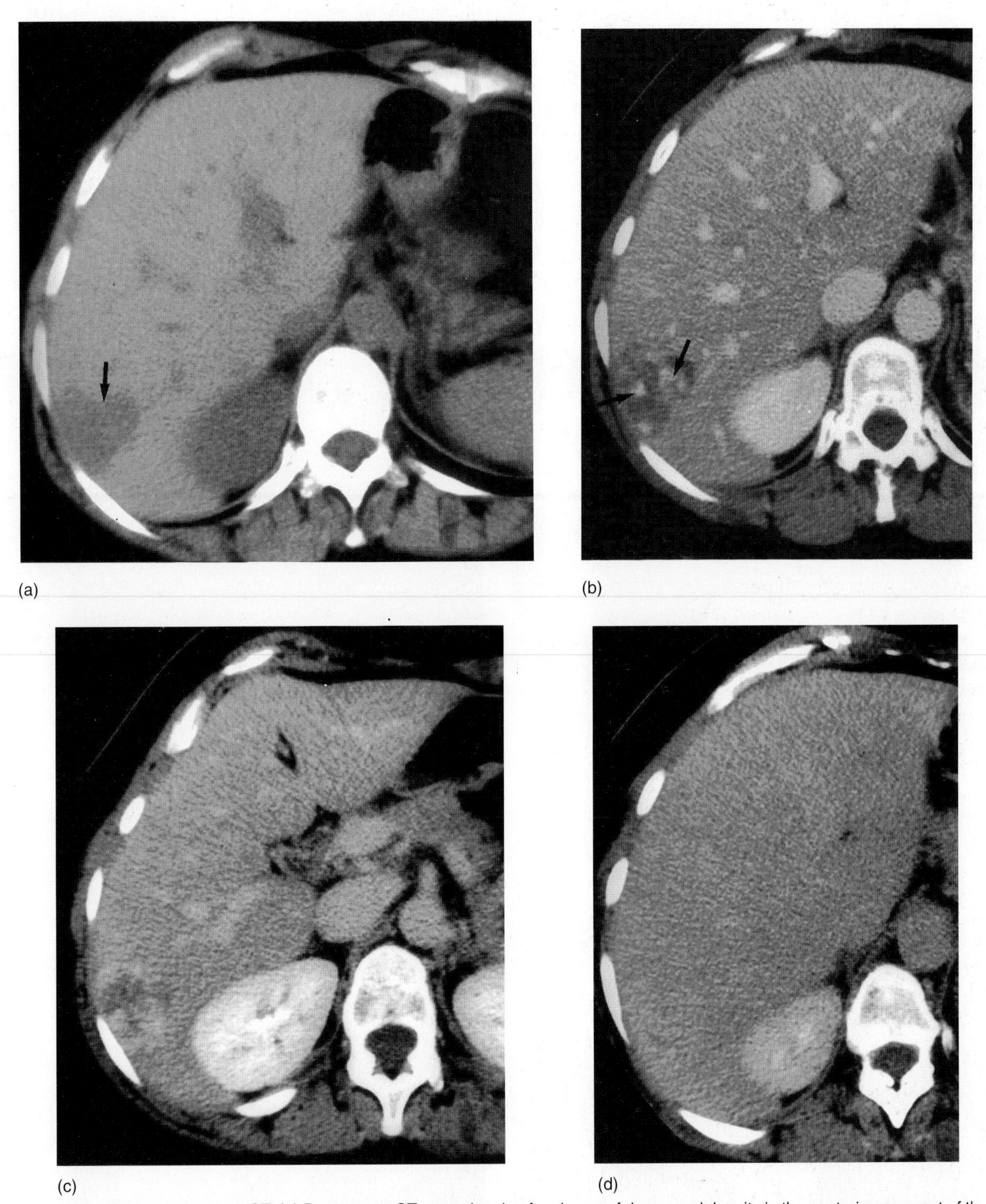

Fig. 5.14 Cavernous haemangioma on CT. (a) Precontrast CT scan showing focal area of decreased density in the posterior segment of the right lobe of the liver (arrow). (b) Scan at the same level as (a) taken during intravenous injection of contrast medium showing pools of contrast medium on the periphery of the lesion (arrows). (c) Scan at same level 3 minutes after intravenous injection of contrast medium showing progressive 'filling in' of the lesion with dense contrast medium. (d) CT scan at 30 minutes after intravenous injection of contrast medium showing that the lesion has become the same density as the adjacent liver parenchyma.

FOCAL NODULAR HYPERPLASIA AND ADENOMAS

Ultrasound, CT and MRI cannot reliably distinguish focal nodular hyperplasia or adenomas from other hepatic masses. The presence of a central fibrous scar, recognized as a central radiolucency on a non-contrast CT scan, an area of increased echogenicity on ultrasound, or a hyperintense area on T1-weighted MR images may strongly suggest the diagnosis (Fig. 5.15). However, a similar appearance may be seen in fibrolamellar hepatocellular carcinomas.

The capsule of an adenoma may contain an excess of lipid-laden hepatocytes permitting a low-density peripheral ring to be identified on CT. Areas of increased density on non-contrast scans representing haemorrhage are a common finding on CT in patients whose adenomas have bled (Fig. 5.16).

BENIGN CYSTS

Soliary or multiple congenital liver cysts are a frequent incidental finding. On ultrasound, they appear as rounded, smooth-walled, echo-free areas with distal enhancement owing to the low attenuation of ultrasound by the clear fluid within the cyst (Fig. 5.17). The presence of internal echoes should raise the suspicion that the lesion is not a simple cyst. On CT, cysts are seen

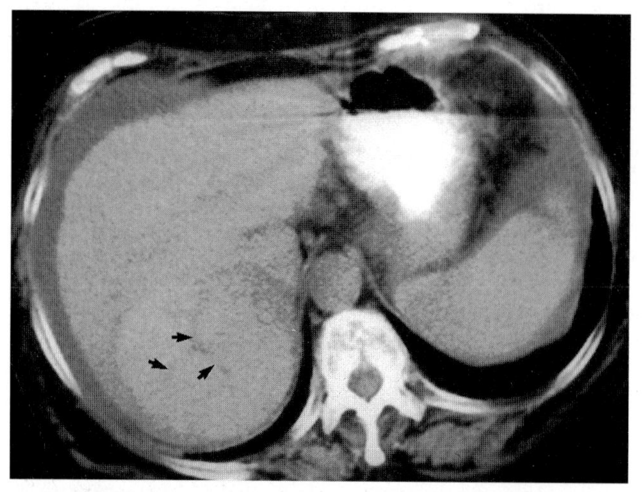

Fig. 5.15 Focal nodular hyperplasia. A CT scan without intravenous contrast medium showing a well-defined focal abnormality in the posterior segment of the right lobe. A central stellate radiolucency can be identified (arrowheads) corresponding to a central fibrous scar. Ascites and an irregular liver margin due to cirrhosis are noted.

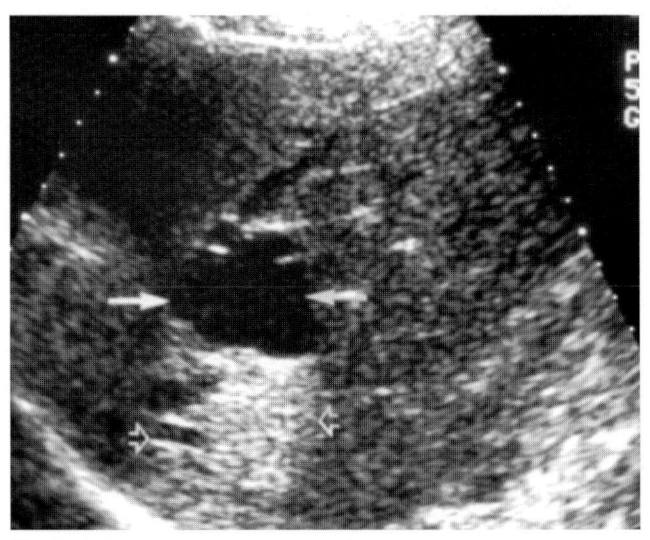

Fig. 5.17 Benign liver cyst on ultrasound. A longitudinal ultrasound scan of the liver showing an anechoic lesion (arrows) with a sharp posterior margin and distal enhancement (open arrows).

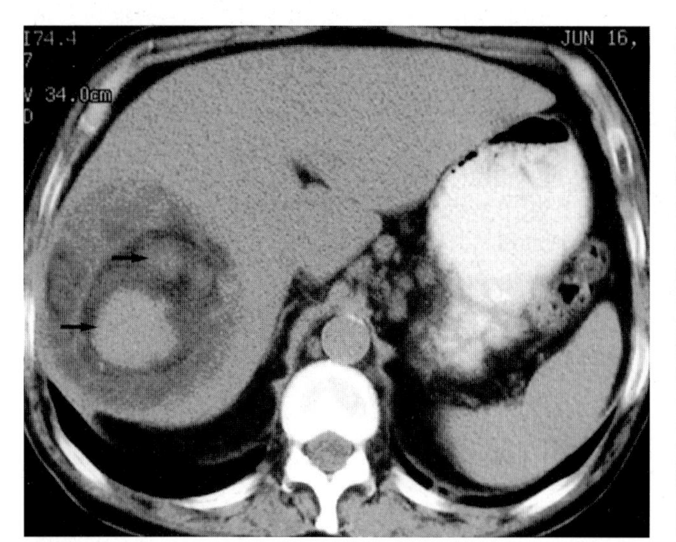

Fig. 5.16 Adenoma of the liver. A large inhomogeneous focal abnormality is seen in the posterior aspect of the right lobe of the liver on an unenhanced CT scan. Areas of high density (arrows) can be seen within it corresponding to a spontaneous bleed within the adenoma.

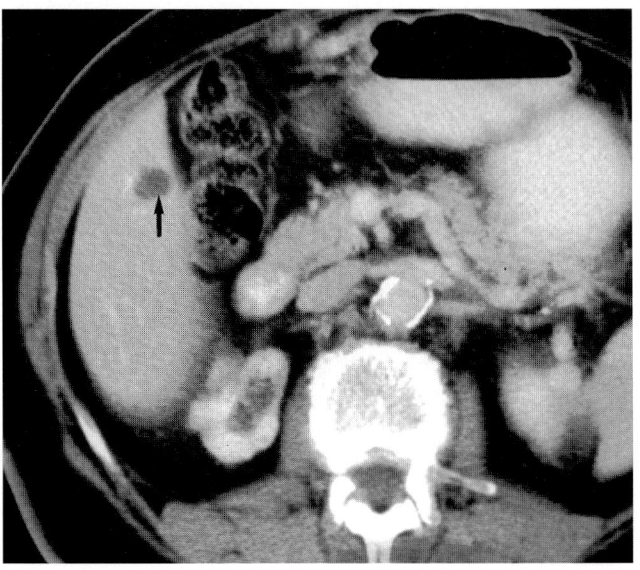

Fig. 5.18 Liver cyst on CT. CT scan after intravenous injection of contrast medium showing a well-defined, small, fluid-filled focal lesion that does not enhance (arrow).

as sharply defined homogeneous areas, the contents of which have a density nearer to that of water and do not enhance after intravenous injection of contrast medium (Fig. 5.18). The contents of the cyst influences the appearance on MRI but usually the signal is low on T1-weighted images and high on T2-weighted images. The differential diagnosis of benign congenital cysts includes hydatid disease, abscesses, degenerating tumours and 'cystic' metastases.

INFLAMMATORY LESIONS

Abscesses

CT is more sensitive than ultrasound for the detection of abscesses, most of which are solitary and occur in the posterior part of the right lobe of the liver. Their imaging appearance depends on the stage of development. At an early stage an abscess appears as a focal area of altered echogenicity on ultrasound, which then

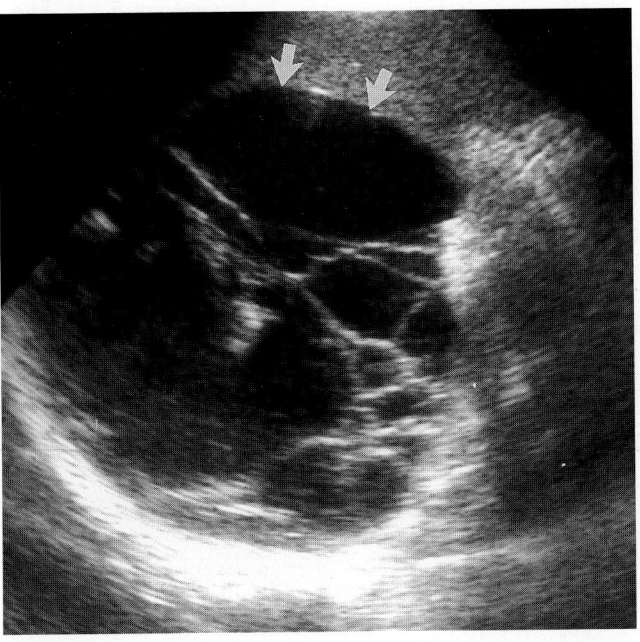

Fig. 5.19 Liver abscess on ultrasound. This longitudinal ultrasound scan shows a large multiseptate fluid collection due to the presence of a large abscess. The lesion is well-defined from the normal liver parenchyma (arrows).

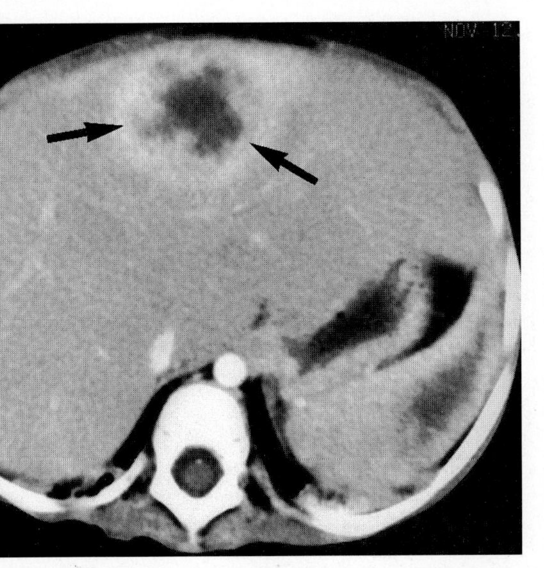

Fig. 5.20 Liver abscess on CT. CT scan after intravenous injection of contrast medium showing marked enhancement of the thick-walled liver abscess (arrows). A central non-enhancing area is due to purulent necrosis.

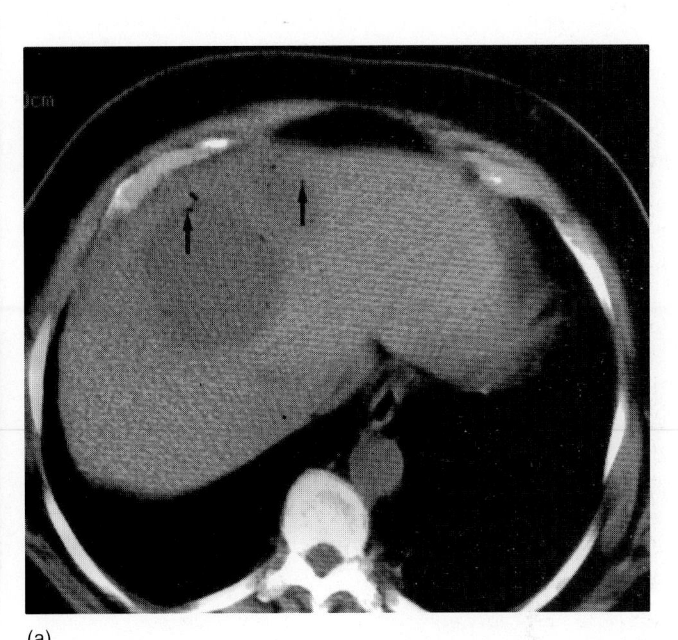

(a)

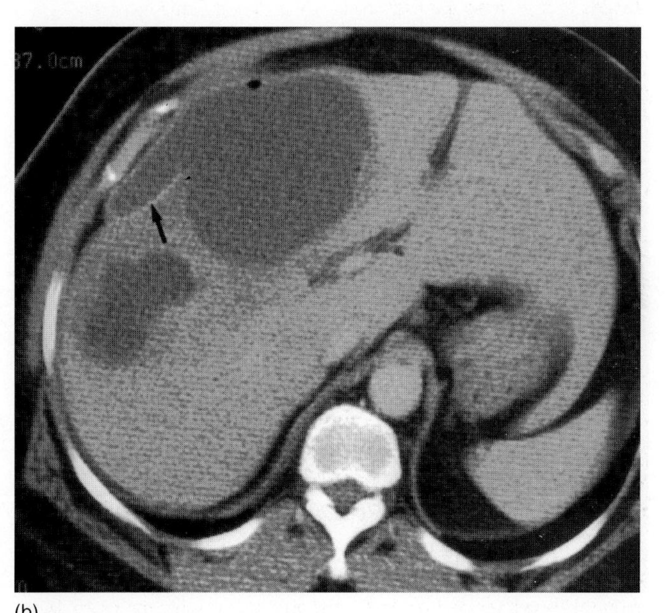

(b)

Fig. 5.21 (a) Multifocal liver abscess on non-contrast CT showing multiple pockets of air (arrows). (b) After contrast medium, an enhancing wall can be demonstrated (arrow).

liquefies to produce the typical irregular, cavitating lesion (Fig. 5.19). The central portion of such an abscess is purulent material which does not enhance on CT after intravenous injection of a bolus of contrast medium, but the periphery is frequently hypervascular and enhances strongly (Fig. 5.20). About a third of abscesses contain air (Fig. 5.21). In immunocompromised patients, infection with fungi such as *Candida* spp. typically produces multiple small abscesses. On ultrasound these may be seen as multiple minute areas of increased echogenicity (Fig. 5.22a) and on CT as areas of decreased density (Fig. 5.22b).

Hydatid disease

Echinococcus granulosus usually presents as a large cystic cavity, most often in the right lobe, whereas *E. alveolaris* frequently resembles an infiltrating tumour. The cysts are readily detected on ultrasound and CT, and in 50% of cases show the pathognomonic appearance of daughter cysts within the larger cyst (Fig. 5.23). Hydatid cysts are often indistinguishable from simple cysts. Debris within the cyst can be due to dead scolices or to superinfection. Calcification, present in 25% of cases, is most readily seen on CT, but can also be identified on plain radiographs and ultrasound.

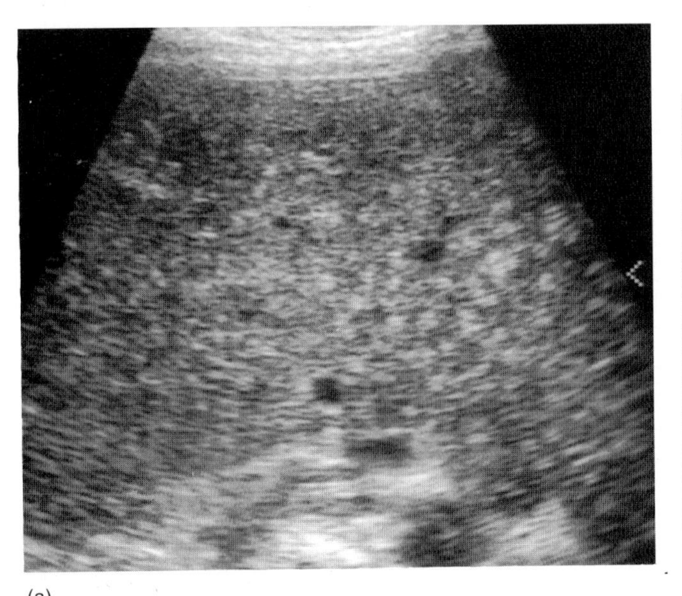

(a)

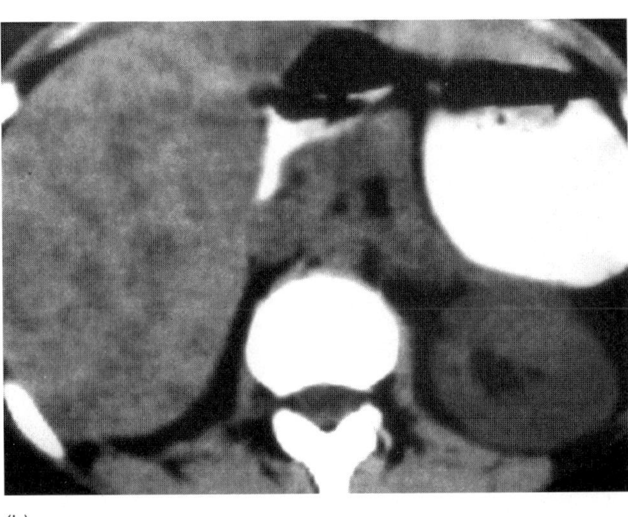

(b)

Fig. 5.22 Candida infection of the liver. (a) Transverse ultrasound scan of the liver showing multiple minute areas of increased echogenicity due to multiple minute Candida abscesses. (b) Non-contrast CT scan on the same patient as (a) showing multiple focal areas of decreased attenuation corresponding to the Candida abscesses.

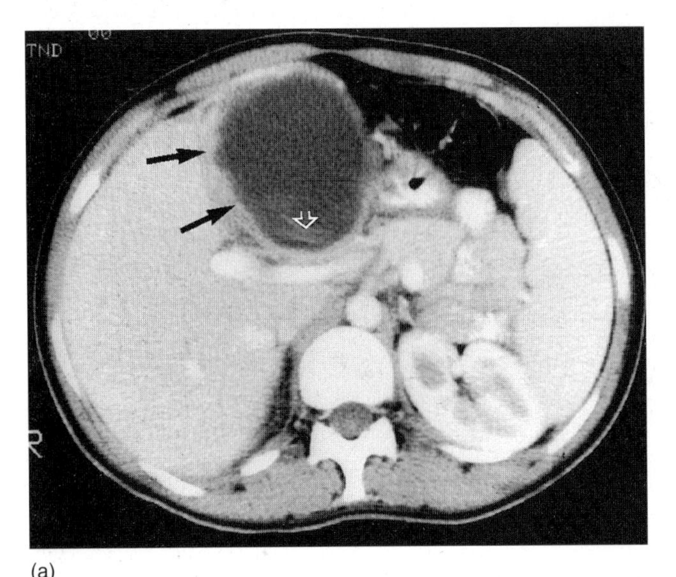

(a)

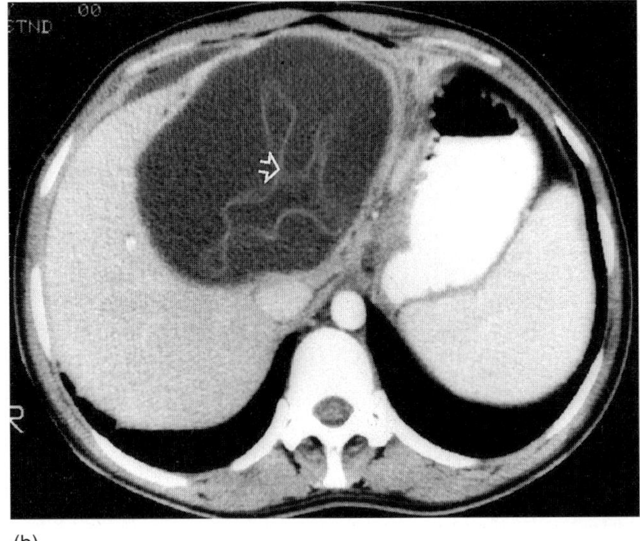

(b)

Fig. 5.23 (a) CT scan after intravenous injection of contrast medium showing a well-defined thick-walled fluid collection (arrows). (b) Obvious serpiginous enhancing strands within the cyst represent collapsed daughter cysts (open arrow). This was due to infection with *Echinococcus granulosus.*

HEPATIC TRAUMA

Plain radiographs provide a useful initial assessment of the patient with liver trauma by identifying right-sided rib fractures, local ileus in the right upper quadrant, elevation of the right hemidiaphragm and perhaps a right pleural effusion. However, trauma to the hepatic parenchyma is best assessed with CT.

Patients who are haemodynamically stable can be assessed by CT, but unstable patients, or those with severe penetrating injuries, may need to go directly to surgery or therapeutic angiography. Hepatic lacerations, intrahepatic and subcapsular haematomas and haemoperitoneum are all well demonstrated on CT (Fig. 5.24). The pelvis is always included because seemingly trivial lacerations with small amounts of blood in the upper abdomen may show surprisingly large amounts of blood in the pelvis.

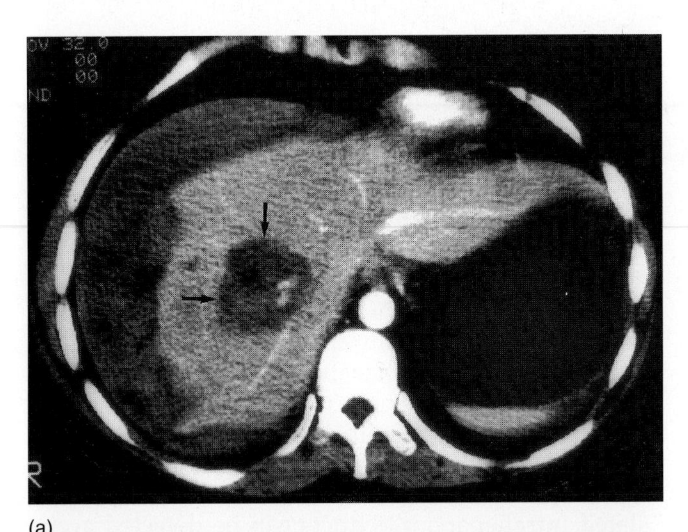

(a)

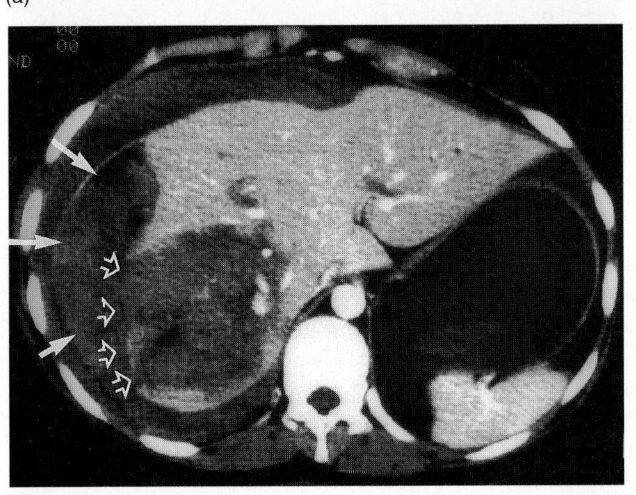

(b)

Fig. 5.24 Hepatic trauma. (a) CT after intravenous contrast medium showing an intrahepatic haematoma of low density, not enhancing with contrast medium (arrows). (b) A scan inferior to (a) showing a large subcapsular haematoma (arrows). Laceration of the margins of the liver can be identified (open arrows). Intraperitoneal blood is seen on both scans.

Hepatic lacerations are the most common hepatic injuries and are seen as linear, round or branching, poorly enhancing regions of low density. Intrahepatic haematomas are usually hypodense relative to the contrast enhanced parenchyma and may be seen in the absence of true lacerations. Subcapsular haematomas, usually associated with lacerations, are well-circumscribed, lenticular or oval fluid collections of low density that flatten or indent the underlying hepatic parenchyma.

BILIARY SYSTEM

IMAGING TECHNIQUES

ULTRASOUND

Ultrasound has revolutionized the approach to biliary tract disease and has replaced routine plain radiography, cholecystography and intravenous cholangiography. The gallbladder and biliary tree can be examined without the need for contrast media or ionizing radiation. There are no specific or relative contraindications to ultrasound and it should be the initial imaging approach for any gallbladder or biliary tree problem. Further investigations are largely determined by the ultrasound findings.

The common bile duct is usually readily identified on ultrasound (Fig. 5.25). The supraduodenal portion within the hepatoduodenal ligament is most frequently seen anterolateral to the portal vein. The

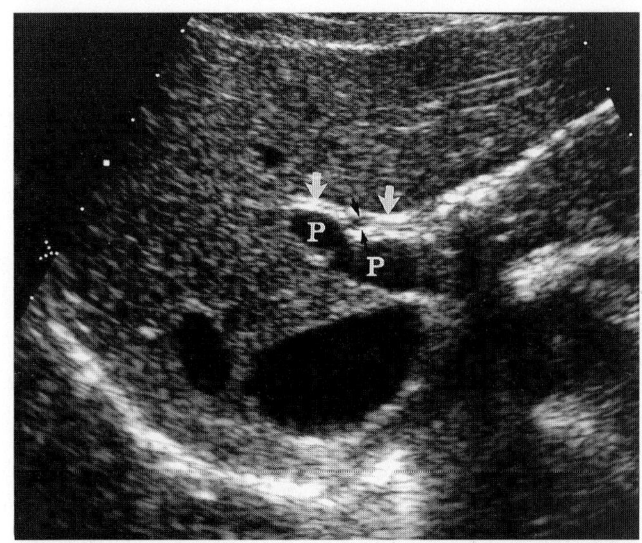

Fig. 5.25 Longitudinal ultrasound scan with the patient in the right anterior oblique position to show the normal common duct (arrowed) lying anterior to the portal vein (P). The right hepatic artery passing between the duct and the portal vein can also be demonstrated (arrowheads). The IVC is cut across in an oblique projection.

retroduodenal portion is less readily seen as it is obscured by gas within the duodenum. The upper limit of normal for the internal diameter of the common bile duct is 5–7 mm. As it is often not possible to identify the insertion of the cystic duct into the common hepatic duct, the common hepatic duct cannot be distinguished reliably from the common bile duct. Hence the term 'common duct' is applied to both structures. The cystic duct itself can be demonstrated sonographically in less than 50% of cases. Dilation of the intrahepatic and extrahepatic biliary system is reliably detected on ultrasound (Figs 5.26, 5.27). On ultrasound, the gallbladder

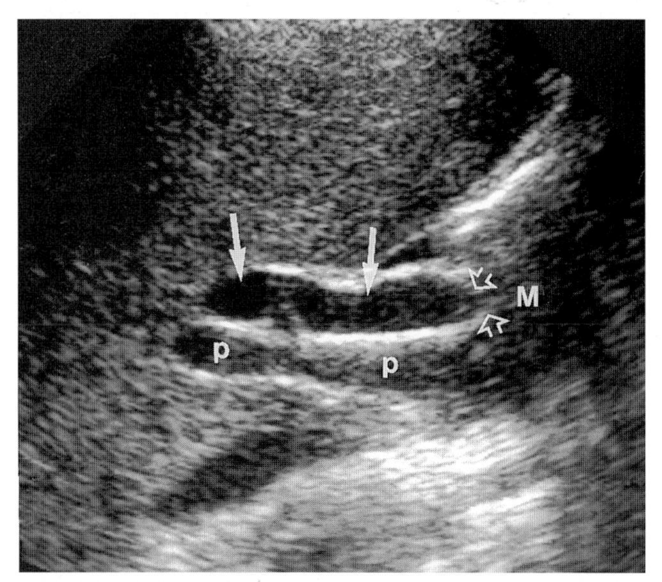

Fig. 5.26 Longitudinal ultrasound showing dilation of the common duct at the level of the porta hepatis (arrows). A normal portal vein is seen posteriorly (p). A mass in the head of the pancreas (M) can be seen narrowing the distal aspect of the dilated duct (open arrows).

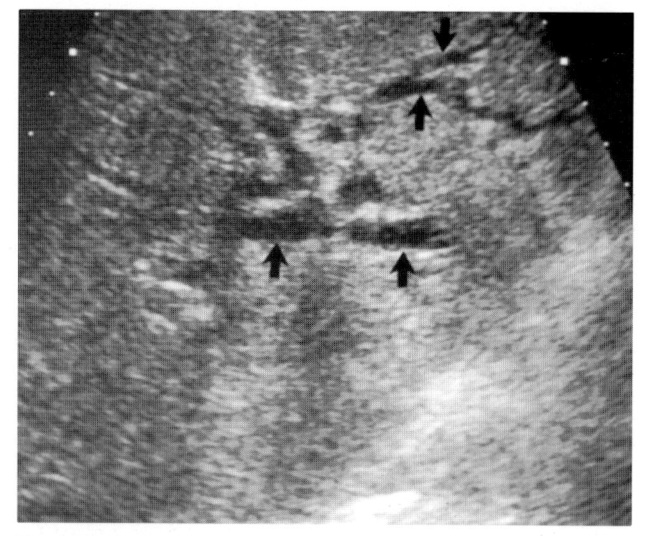

Fig. 5.27 Dilation of the intrahepatic biliary system demonstrated on a transverse scan through the liver. The dilated ducts (arrows) have a typical branched, stellate appearance and are distinguished from venous structures by their echogenic margins.

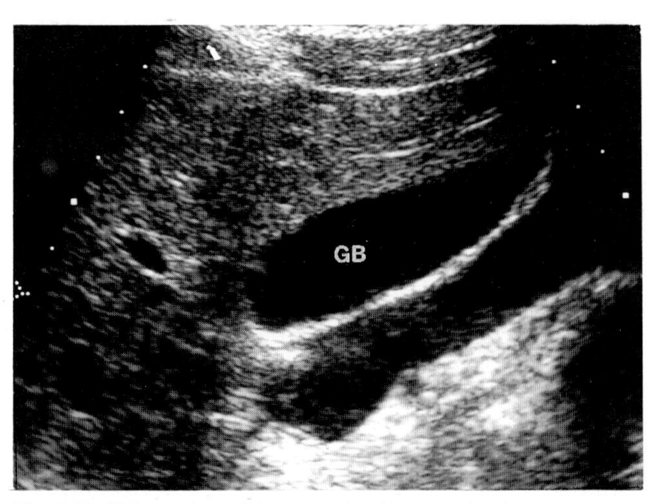

Fig. 5.28 Oblique view of the normal gallbladder (GB) on ultrasound lying anterior to the IVC.

appears as a sonolucent structure with increased through transmission. The normal thickness of the distended gallbladder wall is 2–3 mm (Fig. 5.28).

COMPUTED TOMOGRAPHY

CT is used infrequently as the primary approach to a biliary tract problem but is generally reserved for those patients in whom ultrasound proves inconclusive, particularly when bowel gas or obesity has prevented a satisfactory ultrasound examination. Demonstration of the gallbladder is less reliable than with ultrasound but the lower half of the common bile duct is shown more reliably than with ultrasound. Dilated intrahepatic bile ducts can be detected accurately (Fig. 5.29) and the distinction between medical and surgical causes of jaundice can be made in 90% of cases.

ENDOSCOPIC RETROGRADE CHOLANGIOPANCREATOGRAPHY (ERCP)

ERCP allows direct opacification of the biliary tree and the pancreatic ductal system. The indications include inconclusive ultrasound, for example where ultrasound has failed to reveal the cause of a dilated biliary system, or where ultrasound has shown normal calibre ducts in the presence of clinical and biochemical evidence of obstruction. ERCP also plays an important role in the management of choledocholithiasis as, although ultrasound is excellent for demonstrating stones within the gallbladder, it is less accurate for showing bile duct stones. ERCP is also indicated when bile duct stones are shown and sphincterotomy is indicated. Suspected sclerosing cholangitis is a further indication for ERCP. The

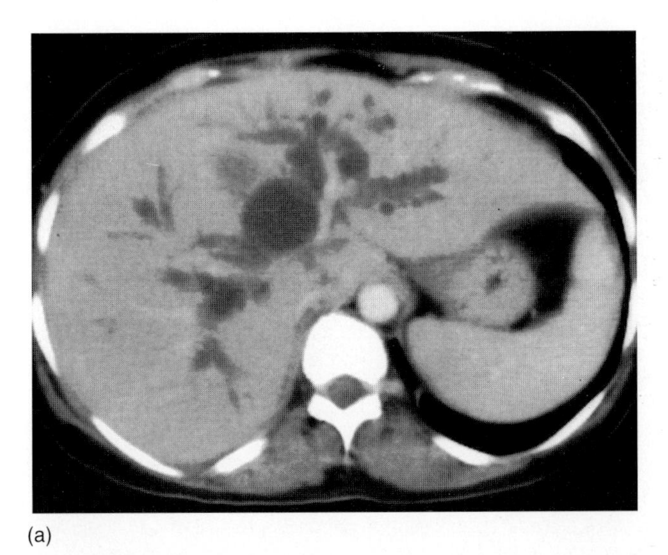

(a)

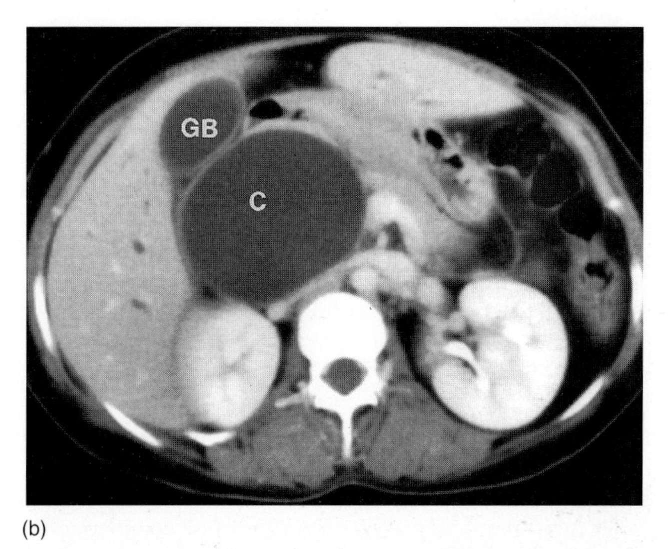

(b)

Fig. 5.29 Choledochal cyst. (a) CT scan after intravenous injection of contrast medium showing marked dilation of intrahepatic bile ducts. These have the typical low-density, tubular appearance. (b) Scan taken more inferiorly showing the cyst (C) lying along the course of the duct posterior to the normal gallbladder (GB).

major contraindication to ERCP is a recent attack of pancreatitis. Complications, notably post-ERCP pancreatitis, occur in 5% of procedures.

SCINTIGRAPHY

Hepatobiliary scintigraphy involves the use of radiopharmaceuticals which are excreted into the bile. Technetium-99m-labelled *N*-substituted iminodiacetic acid derivative (IDA) compounds are used, the most frequent being dimethyl IDA (or HIDA). Renal excretion increases with increasing hyperbilirubinaemia making HIDA an unsuitable agent in the presence of jaundice. On a normal scan taken 1 hour after injection, activity will be shown in the liver, major intrahepatic ducts, gall bladder, common bile duct and small intestine. Indications for bile scintigraphy include the diagnosis of acute cholecystitis, the detection of developmental anomalies of the biliary tree, assessing biliary dynamics and showing leaks following biliary duct trauma.

CONGENITAL ABNORMALITIES OF BILIARY TRACT

BILIARY ATRESIA

When investigating a child with biliary atresia, diagnostic imaging is aimed at demonstrating the anatomy and function of the liver and biliary tree, and distinguishing between neonatal hepatitis and biliary atresia. Ultrasonography and scintigraphy are the main imaging modalities. Sonography is used to exclude other causes of obstructive jaundice, e.g. a choledochal cyst; to evaluate the hepatic parenchyma and liver size. Hepatobiliary scintigraphy with HIDA will differentiate neonatal hepatitis from biliary atresia. In biliary atresia, no activity will be seen in the bowel on a HIDA scan. To improve the accuracy of the technique, the baby is pretreated with phenobarbitone for 3 days to increase biliary excretion.

CHOLEDOCHAL CYSTS

A choledochal cyst produces a soft-tissue mass in the right upper quadrant adjacent to the liver with inferior displacement of the duodenal loop and the right kidney. The cyst may be identifiable on plain film but ultrasound is the best imaging modality. Classic findings are a normal size extrahepatic bile duct entering a cystic mass. The cystic mass is usually adjacent to the gallbladder within the porta hepatis or within the pancreatic head. The intrahepatic ducts may be dilated. Biliary sludge or calculi may be detected within the cyst. As there is a greatly increased risk of gallbladder malignancy arising in choledochal cysts in adolescence or childhood, care should always be taken when a choledochal cyst contains debris because papillary neoplasms are often misinterpreted as debris.

CT is helpful for delineating the size and extent of both intrahepatic and extrahepatic choledochal cysts (Fig. 5.29) and for showing the relationship of the cyst to adjacent intraperitoneal and extraperitoneal structures.

A choledochocoele (Type II choledochal cyst) is a developmental dilatation of the intraduodenal portion of the distal common bile duct. This condition may be suspected first during a barium meal examination where a negative-filling defect is identified at the ampulla on the medial wall of the duodenum.

Intrahepatic biliary cysts (Caroli's disease or Type V choledochal cysts) may be demonstrated on ultrasonography as sonolucent intrahepatic tubular structures converging on the porta hepatis representing the grossly dilated biliary tree. Proving communication between these dilated structures is paramount in distinguishing Caroli's disease from cystic disease of the liver or multiple abscesses. This can best be achieved by ERCP.

GALLSTONES

High resolution, real-time ultrasound has an accuracy of greater than 95% in the detection of gallstones in the gallbladder. The false-negative rate is about 5% and most missed calculi are either <2 mm or are impacted in the neck of the gallbladder. Problems of interpretation arise at the neck because the valves of Heister characteristically appear strongly echogenic and may mimic gallstones. Ultrasound diagnosis of gallstones depends on several criteria: one or more echogenic foci within the gallbladder lumen; acoustic shadowing arising beyond an echogenic focus; and change in position of this focus with change in the patient's position (Fig. 5.30). With strict application of these criteria, a diagnostic accuracy of 100% can be reached.

The phenomenon of acoustic shadowing is due to a combination of reflection of the incident beam and absorption of sound by the stone, and is independent of calculus composition, shape and surface character-

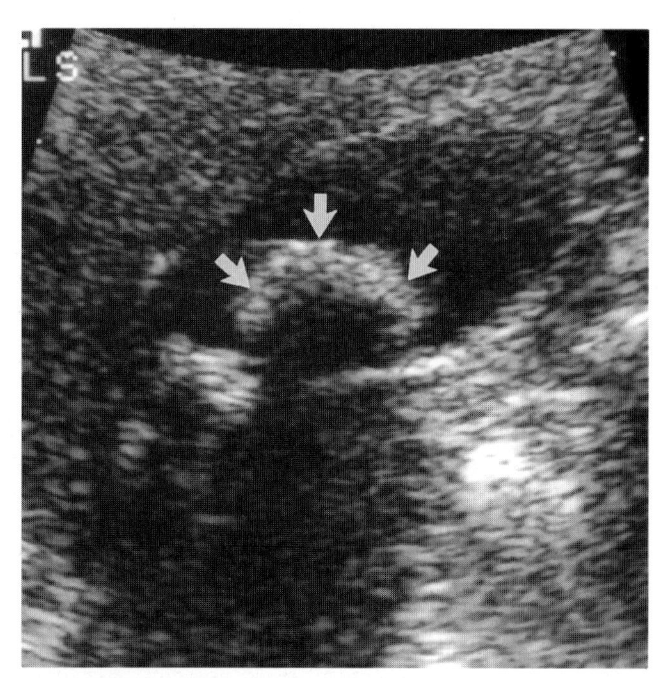

Fig. 5.30 Gallstone. A longitudinal ultrasound scan of the gallbladder containing an echogenic focus (arrows). An absence of echoes (acoustic shadow) is seen distal to the stone.

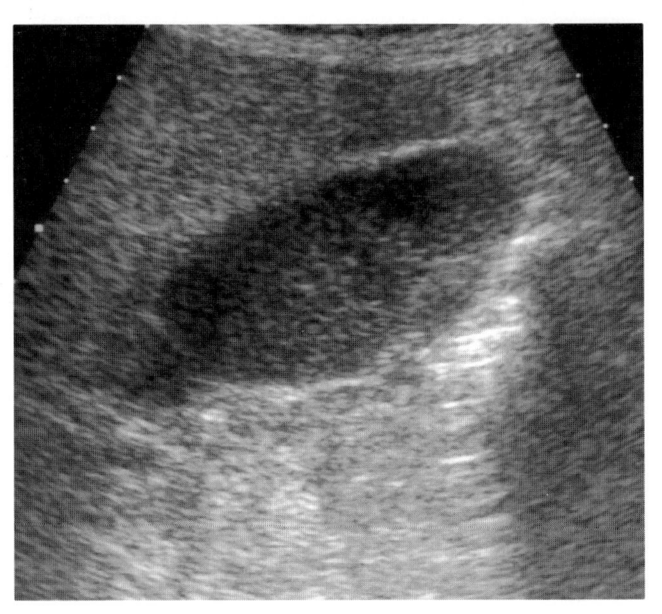

Fig. 5.31 Gallbladder sludge. A longitudinal ultrasound seen through the gallbladder showing echogenic material within it without casting an acoustic shadow.

istics. Most stones which do not cast acoustic shadows are <5 mm. Gallbladder 'sludge', which is due to a mixture of calcium bilirubinate and cholesterol, produces homogeneous low or mid-level echoes which form a dependent layer and slowly change position with gravity (Fig. 5.31). Sludge is seen in patients with biliary stasis on an obstructive or non-obstructive basis (such as prolonged fasting, hyperalimentation, haemolysis). However, the presence of sludge can make it difficult to distinguish between sludge and polypoid forms of gallbladder carcinoma. A repeat examination after resumption of eating, after which sludge should disappear, is usually required.

The sensitivity of ultrasound in detecting gallstones within the bile ducts is poor: only some 55–65% of stones will be found. This low rate of detection is partly accounted for by the fact that about one-third of patients with duct stones have normal calibre ducts, and partly because stones are usually impacted in the distal third of the common duct which is often obscured by intestinal gas (Fig. 5.32). If duct stones are thought likely clinically and ultrasound is not confirmatory, then direct cholangiography (Fig. 5.33) is required.

Duct stones are usually easily detected with ERCP which may show the common duct to be dilated or to be of normal calibre. An accepted rule of thumb is that complete obstruction of the common duct shown at ERCP is seldom due to calculi. The only exception is when a calculus becomes impacted at the ampulla. A major advantage of ERCP in the investigation of choledocholithiasis is the potential for endoscopic sphincterotomy. Most centres quote a success rate of 80%, complication rate of 8% and mortality rate of 1%,

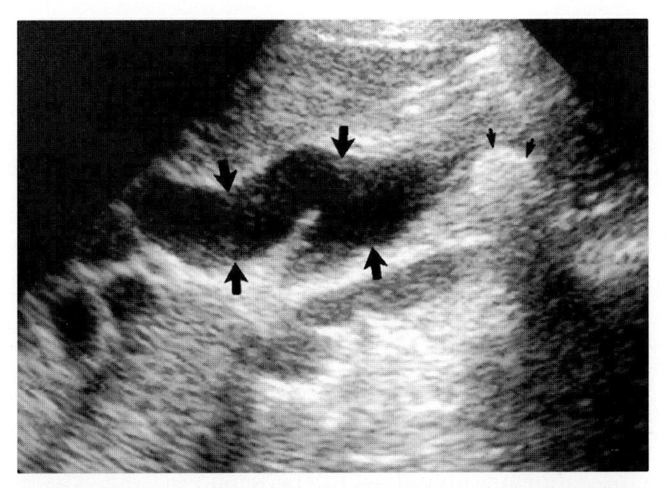

Fig. 5.32 Bile duct calculus. A longitudinal ultrasound scan through the common duct showing an extremely dilated common duct (arrowed) with an echogenic stone (arrowheads) impacted in the distal part of the duct and casting an acoustic shadow.

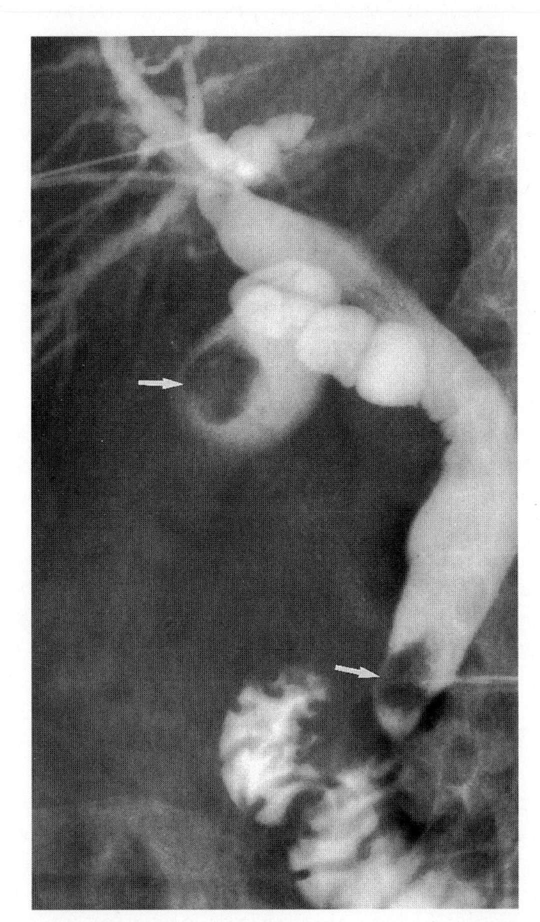

Fig. 5.33 A percutaneous transhepatic cholangiogram showing filling defects in the gallbladder and distal common bile duct due to gallstones (arrows).

the most common complications being perforation, cholangitis, haemorrhage and pancreatitis.

Ultrasound, ERCP and scintigraphy all play a role in the investigation of patients with persistent symptoms following cholecystectomy. In the immediate postoperative period, ultrasound or CT is able to identify haematomata and abscesses in the gallbladder bed, monitor their progression or resolution, and allow drainage under image guidance if necessary. ERCP will allow demonstration of the bile ducts and enable sphincterotomy. Scintigraphy can detect a bile leak and show its extent.

ACUTE CHOLECYSTITIS

ACUTE CALCULOUS CHOLECYSTITIS

Ultrasound and scintigraphy are both useful for 'emergency' diagnosis of acute cholecystitis. Factors such as the availability of the technique and the cost of the procedure must be taken into account before choosing which test to perform.

High sensitivities, in the range of 85–95%, are reported for both ultrasound and scintigraphy in the diagnosis of acute cholecystitis, but specificities are somewhat lower. The advantages of ultrasonography are speed, more consistent evaluation of adjacent structures, lack of dependence on hepatic excretory function and lower cost. In practice, ultrasound is more frequently requested for confirming a diagnosis of acute cholecystitis.

Ultrasound in acute cholecystitis

The demonstration of gallstones alone is not diagnostic of acute cholecystitis, as gallstones may be present in patients with right upper quadrant pain due to other causes. Other criteria must be demonstrated to make the diagnosis, including gallbladder wall thickening, gallbladder wall sonolucency, gallbladder distension and the sonographic Murphy's sign, where maximal tenderness is elicited over the gallbladder on palpation with the ultrasound transducer (Fig. 5.34). With the exception of focal gallbladder tenderness, there are many other causes for these secondary ultrasound signs. For example, gallbladder wall thickening can be seen in chronic cholecystitis, adenomyomatosis, renal failure, portal hypertension, pancreatitis and ascites. Similarly, a lucency within the gallbladder wall has a low positive predictive value for acute cholecystitis and gallbladder distension can occur in diabetes mellitus, hyperalimentation, narcotic analgesia and other non-obstructive causes of diminished gallbladder emptying. Using a combination of findings in an appropriate clinical setting gives a good positive predictive value for sonography. The more findings that are present, the higher the positive predictive value.

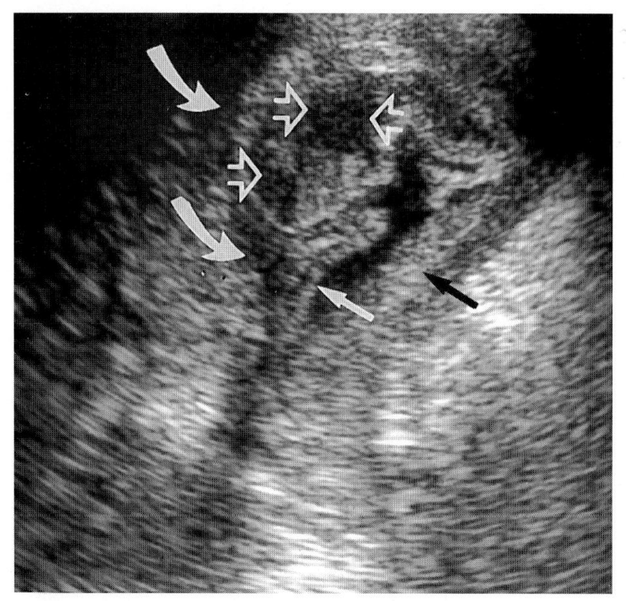

Fig. 5.34 Acute cholecystitis. Longitudinal ultrasound scan of the gallbladder showing markedly thickened walls (arrows), lucency within the thickened gallbladder wall (open arrows) and linear lucency adjacent to the gallbladder wall (curved arrows).

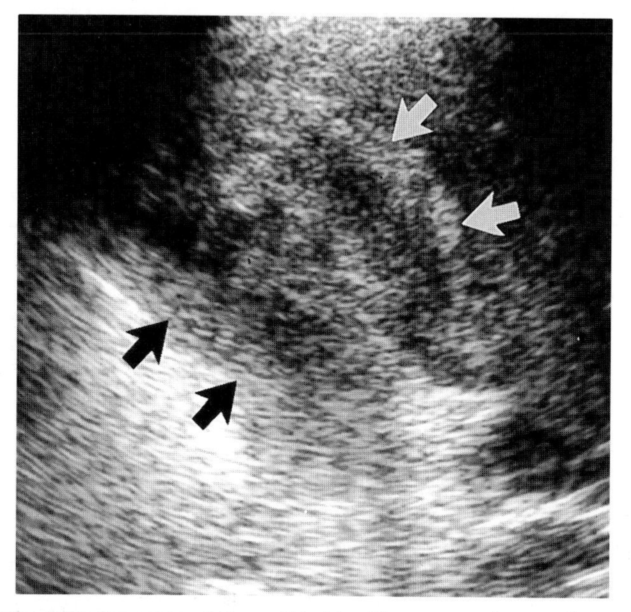

Fig. 5.35 Gangrene of the gallbladder. Transverse ultrasound scan showing irregular thickening of the gallbladder walls (arrows) which are poorly defined from the adjacent liver parenchyma. Echoes seen within the gallbladder lumen are due to desquamated mucosa.

Scintigraphy in acute cholecystitis

Cholescintigraphy, using ^{99m}Tc-IDA derivatives, is an accurate and efficacious means of evaluating patients suspected of having acute cholecystitis. When the cystic duct is patent, the gallbladder is visualized by 60 minutes following injection. Normal gallbladder visualization excludes acute cholecystitis with virtual certainty. Over 90% of patients with acute cholecystitis show an absence of gallbladder activity, about 7% show delayed gallbladder visualization and, very occasionally, an obstructive pattern with no activity in the gallbladder, common bile duct or small intestine despite satisfactory liver uptake. False-positive results occur in chronic cholecystitis, acute pancreatitis, alcoholic liver disease and hyperalimentation.

Computed tomography in acute cholecystitis

Although rarely performed with the intention of diagnosing acute cholecystitis, CT is capable of suggesting the diagnosis and occasionally the diagnosis is made with CT when unsuspected clinically (Fig. 5.36). Other than gallstones, the most common CT finding is gallbladder wall thickening, especially when focal or non-uniform. Low-density oedema in the space between the liver substance and the gallbladder is another feature; localized fluid collections adjacent to the gallbladder and in the subhepatic or subphrenic spaces suggest perforation.

Complications of acute cholecystitis

Acute **perforations** are associated with free spill of bile into the peritoneum and associated peritonitis. Subacute perforations are the most common, they tend to wall off and form pericholecystic abscesses. Chronic perforations are associated with fistulous communications with other organs. Ultrasound is best suited to demonstrating the free fluid associated with acute perforations and the irregular fluid collections which are seen in the hepatocholecystic space in subacute perforations.

Empyema of the gallbladder is suggested when findings of acute cholecystitis are accompanied by multiple highly reflective intraluminal echoes on ultrasound without shadowing, layering or gravity dependence. These echoes correspond to purulent exudate and debris within highly viscous bile and are indistinguishable from highly viscous sludge.

Gangrene of the gallbladder can be suggested in the appropriate clinical setting when ultrasound shows extremely shaggy, irregular and asymmetric walls. Intraluminal membranes corresponding to desquamated mucosa are common in gangrenous gallbladders. They are seen as irregular, non-shadowing echoes within the gallbladder lumen, close to and paralleling the wall.

ACUTE ACALCULOUS CHOLECYSTITIS

Sonography alone is often non-specific for diagnosing acalculous cholecystitis but when taken in conjunction with the clinical history, it may be diagnostic. The most suggestive sonographic findings are gallbladder wall thickening >4 mm (provided the gallbladder is distended to at least 5 cm in length), intraluminal membranes and pericholecystic fluid in

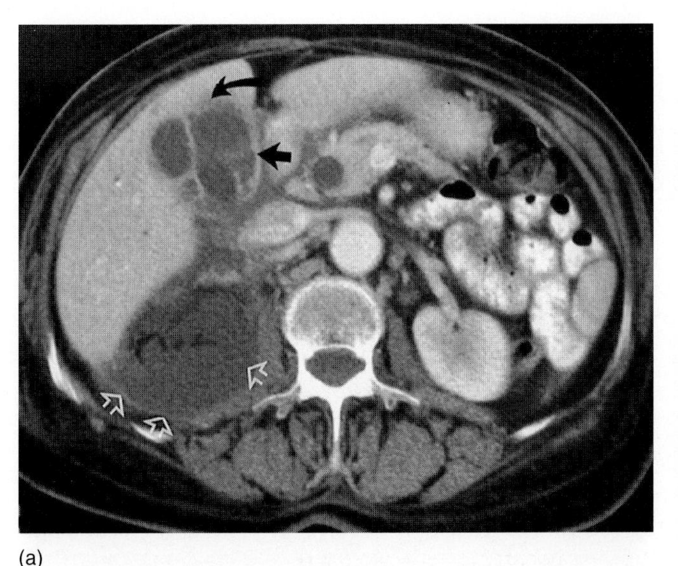

(a)

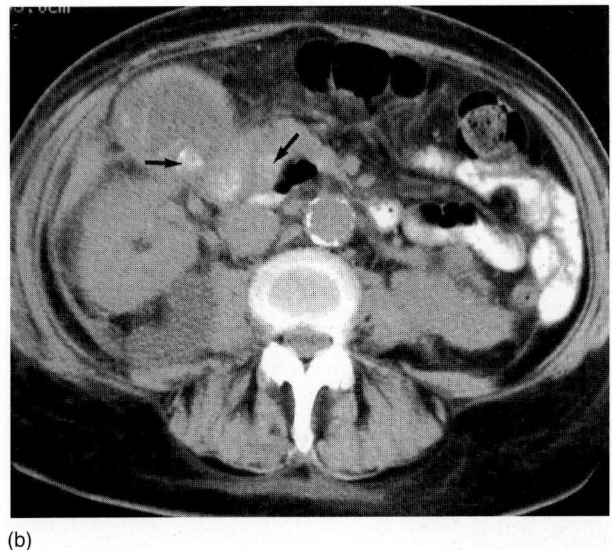

(b)

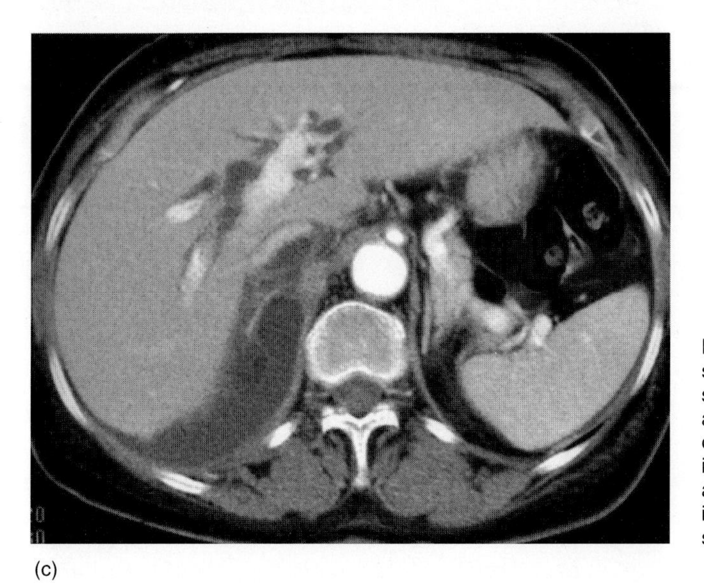

(c)

Fig. 5.36 Acute cholecystitis and perforation of gallbladder. (a) CT scan showing thickening of the gallbladder wall (straight arrow) with a small amount of fluid adjacent to the gallbladder (curved arrow). Bile is also present in the subhepatic space (open arrows) due to perforation of the gallbladder. The common duct is dilated. (b) A scan at a level inferior to (a) showing the presence of stones within the gallbladder and common duct (arrows). (c) A scan superior to (a) showing intrahepatic bile duct dilation and the extent of the bile leak into the subhepatic space.

the absence of ascites. Sludge or coarse echoes suggestive of pus within the gallbladder lumen and gallbladder distension (>8 cm in the long axis or >5 cm transversely) are abnormal but less specific findings. A normal ultrasound examination of the gallbladder does not exclude acalculous cholecystitis: the sensitivity of ultrasound in acalculous cholecystitis is significantly less than in calculous cholecystitis.

EMPHYSEMATOUS CHOLECYSTITIS

Plain film findings usually become visible only 24–48 hours after the onset of symptoms. Gas may be seen first in the gallbladder wall or lumen (Fig. 5.37). Intramural gas may be seen as a crescentic lucency, a

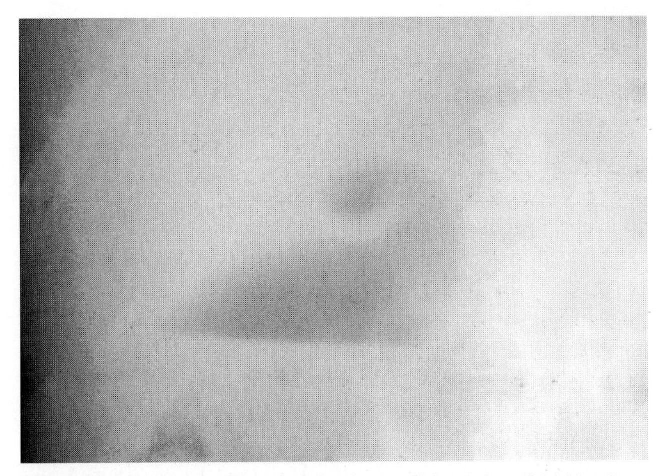

Fig. 5.37 Erect plain film showing gas within the gallbladder in a patient with emphysematous cholecystitis. (Courtesy of Dr J. E. Dacie).

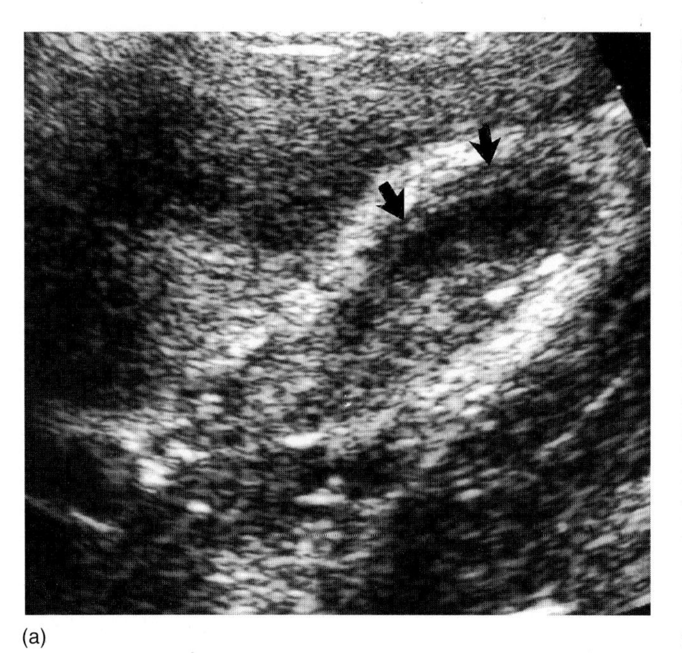

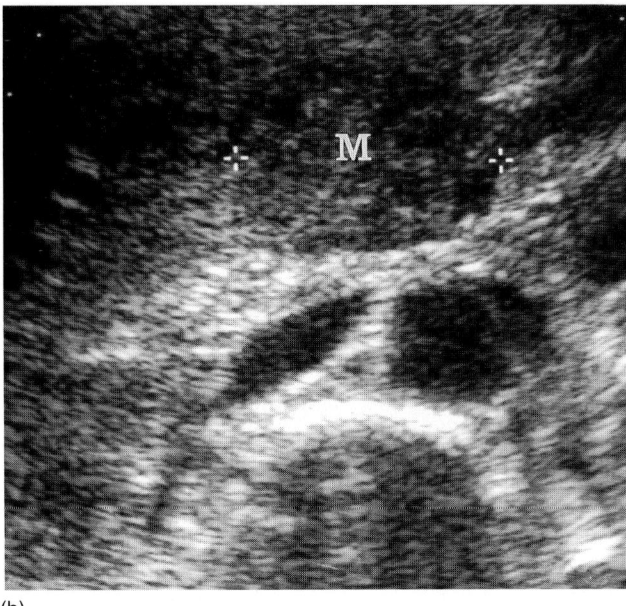

(a) (b)

Fig. 5.38 Gallbladder carcinoma. (a) Longitudinal ultrasound scan showing thickening of the gallbladder wall (arrows) containing an inhomogeneous echogenic mass due to neoplasia. (b) Transverse scan through the central portion of the mass (M) within the gallbladder.

lucent halo or a bubbly necklace around the gallbladder. Ultrasound can also diagnose emphysematous cholecystitis by demonstrating gas in the gallbladder wall or lumen.

COMPUTED TOMOGRAPHY IN COMPLICATIONS OF CHOLECYSTITIS

Although ultrasound is the study of choice, CT can detect complications of acute cholecystitis and is better at diagnosing perforations. This is because CT can depict small pericholecystic gas collections and differentiate them from bowel gas more easily than ultrasound and because CT is better at detecting a gallstone outside the gallbladder.

BILIARY TRACT NEOPLASIA

GALLBLADDER CARCINOMA

Primary carcinoma of the gallbladder is the fifth most common gastrointestinal tract malignancy and represents 1–3% of all malignancies at autopsy. The most common sonographic appearance, seen in 50% of patients, is replacement of the gallbladder by a complex mass (Fig. 5.38). In 20%, there is diffuse or focal irregular thickening of the gallbladder wall. Occasionally, there is an irregular, polypoid mass within the lumen. Ultrasound has a predictive accuracy of about 55–85% in the diagnosis of gallbladder cancer. Many of the false-positive results are due to misinterpretation of inflammatory changes. Ancillary findings are: gallstones within the gallbladder, seen in 50% of cases; biliary duct dilatation due to invasion of the porta hepatis; liver masses due to direct extension or metastases; and adenopathy in the peripancreatic region or in the porta hepatis.

Similar features are seen on computed tomography (Fig. 5.39). The most common finding is a mass in the region of the gallbladder fossa that replaces all or most

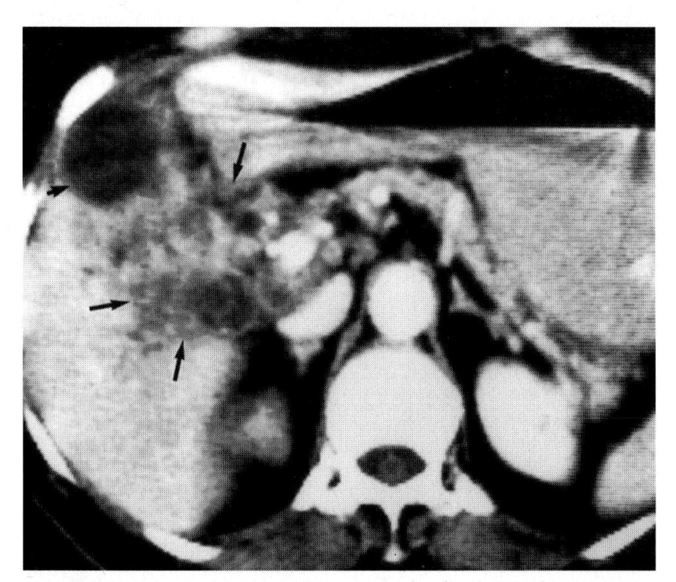

Fig. 5.39 Gallbladder carcinoma. A CT scan through the gallbladder fossa showing an inhomogeneous mass obliterating most of the gallbladder (arrows). A small remaining portion of the normal gallbladder can be demonstrated (arrowhead).

of the gallbladder. Direct extension into the adjacent liver is common. Less common appearances are irregular wall thickening or intraluminal masses. Ancillary findings include gallstones, wall calcification, dilated intra- or extrahepatic bile ducts, hepatic metastases and peripancreatic or para-aortic lymph node enlargement.

Adenocarcinomas account for 85% or more of gallbladder cancers. Other malignancies such as spindle cell sarcomas, carcinoids or oat cell carcinomas are radiologically indistinguishable from adenocarcinoma.

MALIGNANCY OF THE BILE DUCTS

Cholangiocarcinoma is an uncommon tumour accounting for only 0.3–0.5% of all malignancies. It originates in the larger bile ducts: about 10% arise in the intrahepatic ducts, 10–26% at the confluence of the hepatic ducts (Klatskin tumour), 15–30% in the proximal common duct and 30–36% arise in the distal common duct.

Percutaneous transhepatic cholangiography (Fig. 5.40) and ERCP are the best modalities for depicting bile duct neoplasms. Bile duct carcinoma can be classified cholangiographically as either obstructive, stenotic or protuberant. The obstructive type is the most frequent, occuring in about 70% of cholangiograms and appearing as a U- or V-shaped obstruction with a nipple, rat-tail, smooth or irregular termination. The stenotic type shows a strictured lumen with irregular margins and post-stenotic dilatation (Fig. 5.40). The length of stenosis may be long or short. The polypoid or protuberant type appears as an intraluminal filling defect with irregular margins, attached at one point to the wall.

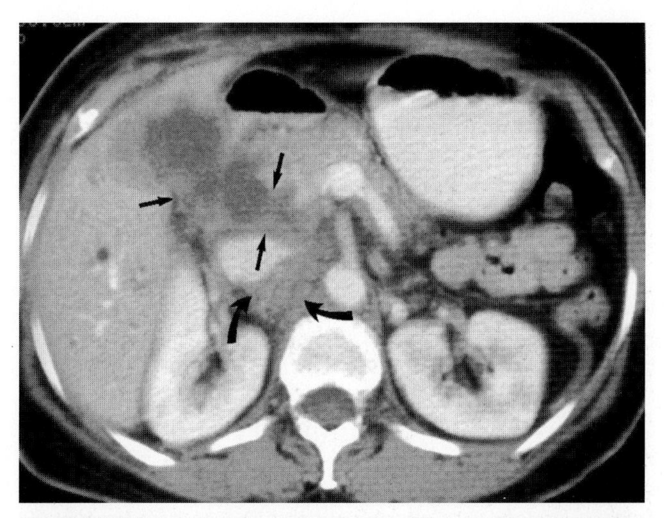

Fig. 5.41 Advanced cholangiocarcinoma. CT scan after intravenous injection of contrast medium showing an irregular low-density mass in the region of the head of the pancreas (arrows) due to a cholangiocarcinoma. Extension is seen with the gallbladder fossa. There is also enlargement of para-aortic lymph nodes (curved arrows).

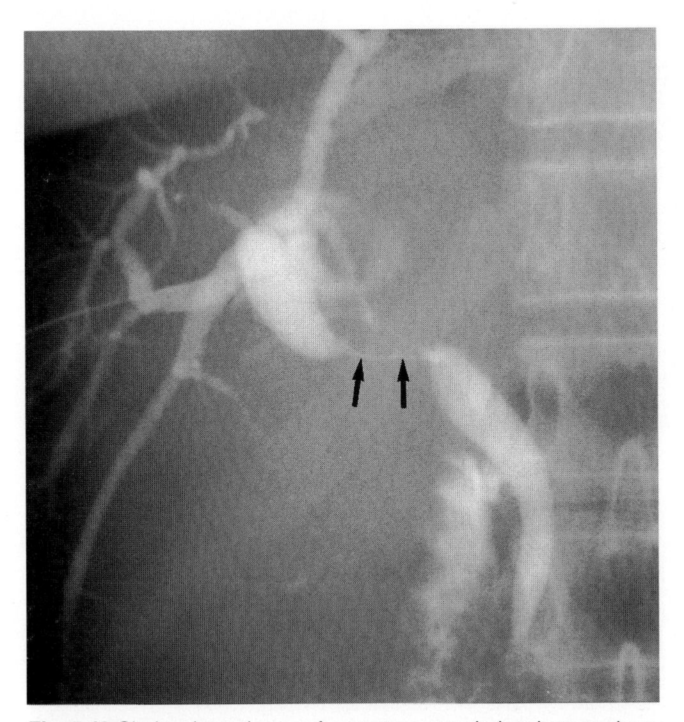

Fig. 5.40 Cholangiocarcinoma. A percutaneous cholangiogram showing an irregular narrowing of the common duct (arrows) with proximal dilation.

A specific diagnosis of biliary duct neoplasm can only rarely be made with ultrasound or CT. Ultrasound demonstrates dilation of the bile ducts proximal to the tumour in the vast majority of cases, but only occasionally can a mass be seen either within or surrounding the duct. The CT manifestations include biliary dilatation, metastatic disease and, least commonly, demonstration of the primary tumour itself. If the tumour is obstructive, the site of the tumour will determine the degree and distribution of bile duct dilatation, and whether the gallbladder is dilated. Local or distant metastatic disease may be seen. Proximal tumours invade the liver or gallbladder, whereas distal tumours may invade the duodenum and pancreas (Fig. 5.41). On both ultrasound and CT, an intrahepatic cholangiocarcinoma is usually indistinguishable from a **primary liver neoplasm**.

While bile duct carcinoma carries a poor prognosis, the outcome is better than for carcinoma of the pancreas. Preoperative imaging studies need to define the anatomical location and extent of the lesion. It may be evident at an early stage that the lesion is unresectable when ultrasound or CT shows extensive local spread, liver or lung metastases. ERCP or percutaneous cholangiography have a major role to play in the preoperative assessment because extension into second order branches of both lobes usually means that the tumour is unresectable.

BENIGN STRICTURES

It must be emphasized that there is great difficulty in radiologically differentiating between benign and malignant strictures of the biliary tree. The commonest causes of benign strictures are chronic pancreatitis and bile duct surgery. Other inflammatory conditions include tuberculosis and stone disease.

If ultrasound or CT indicate that the obstruction is low, then ERCP is the investigation of choice. It usually shows a long smooth stricture of the common bile duct. If it is known from ultrasound that the obstruction is high, then although ERCP may delineate the stricture, percutaneous transhepatic cholangiography should be performed as such strictures involve first- or second-order branches, and all separately obstructed segments need to be identified.

The secondary effects of long-standing biliary obstruction, such as fibrosis or cirrhosis with portal hypertension and varices, may also be seen on ultrasound or CT.

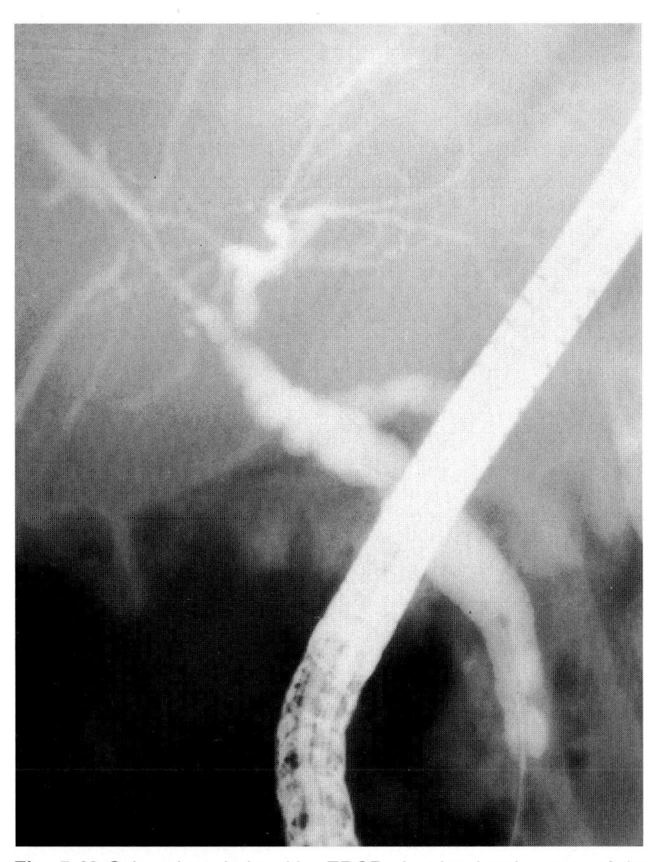
Fig. 5.42 Sclerosing cholangitis. ERCP showing involvement of the extra- and intrahepatic biliary tree with 'beading' of the common duct and irregular narrowing of ducts.

BILE DUCT INFLAMMATION

PRIMARY SCLEROSING CHOLANGITIS

The hallmark of primary sclerosing cholangitis, a disease of unknown aetiology, is involvement of all or some of the biliary tree by a chronic inflammatory process where any cause of secondary obstruction such as stones or infection has been excluded. The disease is associated with a variety of disorders of which ulcerative colitis is the most common, but which includes Crohn's disease, mediastinal and retroperitoneal fibrosis, pancreatitis, orbital pseudotumour and thyroiditis. Currently, the diagnosis is based on imaging findings in the majority of cases. Ultrasound is often normal or inconclusive, although non-specific bile duct wall thickening may be seen. CT may show mild duct dilatation with a distended irregular branching pattern. Characteristically, the ducts do not taper toward the periphery of the liver, as they typically do in other causes of duct obstruction. Direct cholangiography shows irregular, nodular, beaded narrowing of the extra- and intrahepatic biliary systems (Fig. 5.42). ERCP is the preferred approach to visualize the bile ducts as it provides a greater likelihood of success in the absence of intrahepatic duct dilatation. Although the findings are fairly characteristic, a rare multifocal cholangiocarcinoma can give an identical appearance.

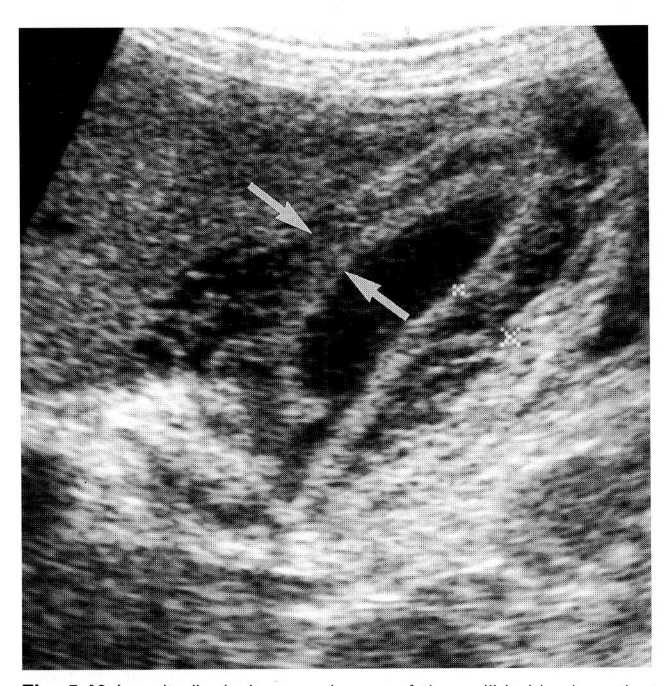
Fig. 5.43 Longitudinal ultrasound scan of the gallbladder in patient suffering from AIDS showing marked thickening of the gallbladder wall (arrows).

AIDS-ASSOCIATED CHOLANGITIS

Because opportunistic organisms such as cryptosporidium, cytomegalovirus and *Candida albicans* may be found in the bile of patients with AIDS, they are implicated in the biliary inflammation seen in some patients suffering from AIDS. Ultrasound often shows severe gallbladder wall thickening in the absence of gallstones and the common bile duct is dilated without any obvious cause (Fig. 5.43). Cholangiography may show findings similar to primary sclerosing cholangitis: intra- and extrahepatic ductal involvement with irregular strictures and mild dilatation. Papillary stenosis is frequently present and is sometimes considered the key feature. The liver may show an increase in periportal echoes.

ACUTE (ASCENDING) CHOLANGITIS

Usually, the role of imaging in acute cholangitis is to define the cause of obstruction and to confirm that no additional findings, such as abscesses, are present. Pus within dilated ducts may be seen at ultrasound as echogenic material or as filling defects on cholangiography.

RECURRENT PYOGENIC CHOLANGITIS (ORIENTAL CHOLANGITIS)

Plain films in recurrent pyogenic cholangitis may show gas in the biliary tree and occasionally may show intrahepatic calcifications, representing biliary stones. Nearly all patients show extrahepatic dilation on ultrasound and there is often dilatation of the intrahepatic ducts. The detection rate for stones by ultrasound is about 40%. CT readily shows the pattern of duct dilatation, the pneumobilia, stones and concomitant features such as extrahepatic fluid collections, pancreatitis and splenomegaly.

BILIARY PARASITES

In *Ascaris lumbricoides* infestation of the biliary system, intestinal worms are present in 90% of patients. Sonography is reliable for diagnosing the presence of the worm within the lumen of intrahepatic or extrahepatic common duct or gallbladder.

THE PANCREAS

NORMAL PANCREAS

On ultrasound, the normal pancreas displays a homogeneous echogenicity similar to liver in 50% of patients and greater echogenicity than liver in the other half. The pancreas is bounded by the higher echogenicity of the retroperitoneal fat and investing connective tissue (Fig. 5.44). As fat infiltration occurs,

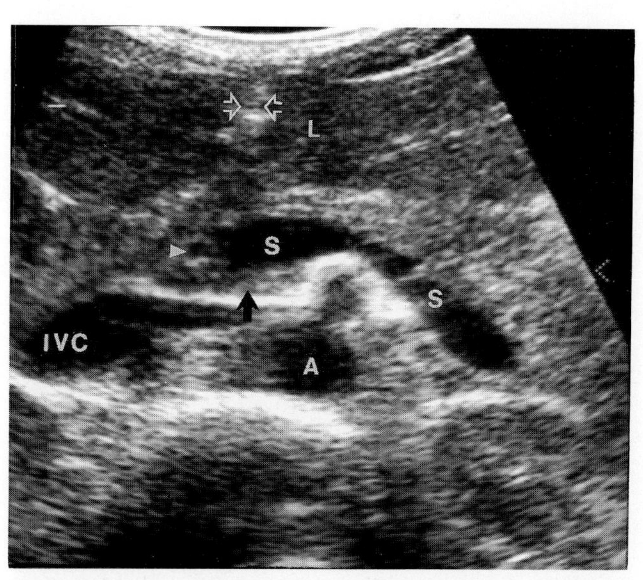

Fig. 5.44 Normal transverse ultrasound scan of the pancreas showing the pancreas lying anterior to the splenic vein (S), the common duct within the head of the pancreas (arrowhead), the uncinate process of the pancreas (arrow), the left lobe of the liver (L), and the falciform ligament (open arrows). Posteriorly lie the aorta (A) and the inferior vena cava (IVC) joined by the left renal vein.

the overall echogenicity of the pancreas increases, making identification of the pancreatic boundaries difficult. The major limitation of ultrasound is the inability to image the entire gland in 15–20% of cases.

On CT, the normal pancreas has an attenuation that is lower than liver or spleen, and similar to kidney, muscle and blood. It has a relatively homogeneous radiodensity except where it is infiltrated by fat in the obese and the elderly. Its borders are frequently lobulated but may be smooth. Evaluation of the pancreas with CT routinely requires intravenous administration of contrast medium because contrast-enhancement improves the rate of tumour detection and demonstrates the relationship of tumour to adjacent vessels. Peak enhancement of the pancreas occurs about 3 s after peak enhancement of the aorta and thus the best images of the pancreas are achieved by rapidly injecting a bolus of 100–150 ml of contrast medium and scanning rapidly either on 'dynamic' or 'spiral' mode. CT has become the leading technique for the evaluation of patients with known or suspected neoplastic and inflammatory disease. The high spatial and contrast resolution of current generation fast scanners permits visualization of pancreatic parenchyma in all patients.

The pancreas is visualized on MRI as a medium signal intensity structure surrounded by higher signal intensity fat on T1-weighted images (Fig. 6.1a, p. 166). On T2-weighted images, the retroperitoneal fat becomes iso-intense to the pancreas, making demonstration difficult. On fat-suppressed T1-weighted images, the pancreas appears very intense.

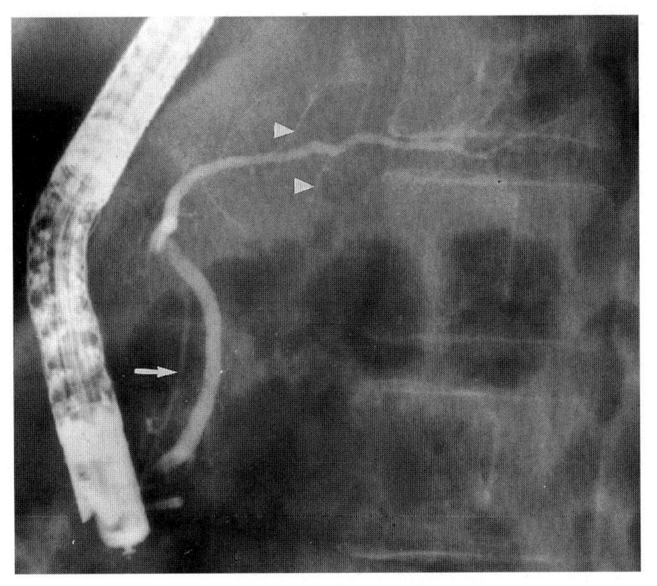

Fig. 5.45 Normal pancreatic duct on ERCP showing filling of intralobular ducts (arrowheads) and the accessory pancreatic duct (arrow).

Although evaluation of pancreatic size is important for recognizing pancreatic disease, it is difficult to assign precise measurements for normal pancreatic size, which varies with age, patient size, state of respiration, measurement site and measurement technique. Furthermore, various studies differ substantially in their estimates of the upper limit of normal.

The main pancreatic duct appears on ERCP as smooth-walled and tapers gradually from the head to the tail. Intralobular ducts enter at nearly right angles (Fig. 5.45). The normal main pancreatic duct measures up to 4 mm in internal diameter within the head, up to 3 mm within the body and 2 mm in the tail. On CT scans, the greatest normal internal duct diameter is 5 mm in the head and 3 mm in the tail. The main pancreatic duct tends to increase in size with age. The accessory pancreatic duct (of Santorini) drains the upper part of the pancreatic head and penetrates the anteromedial wall of the second part of the duodenum at the junction of its upper and distal thirds. In 10% of individuals, the accessory duct does not communicate with the duct of Wirsung (pancreas divisum).

PANCREATIC NEOPLASMS

PANCREATIC DUCT CELL ADENOCARCINOMA

Duct cell adenocarcinoma accounts for 75–85% of non-endocrine tumours of the pancreas. It is localized to the head in 70% of cases, the body in 10% and the tail in 5%. The entire gland is involved in the remaining 15% of cases.

Computed tomography

CT is the single best imaging modality for the detection and staging of pancreatic ductal adenocarcinoma in terms of overall accuracy, reliability and reproducibility. Modern CT scanners show a pancreatic abnormality in close to 99% of patients with cancer. Optimal use of intravenous and oral contrast medium improves evaluation. Thus, if abdominal symptoms are present, a normal CT strongly suggests that these symptoms are not due to duct cell carcinoma.

The most common CT finding is a focal non-calcified mass (Fig. 5.46), although non-focal enlargement has been reported in up to 15% of cases. As in the case of

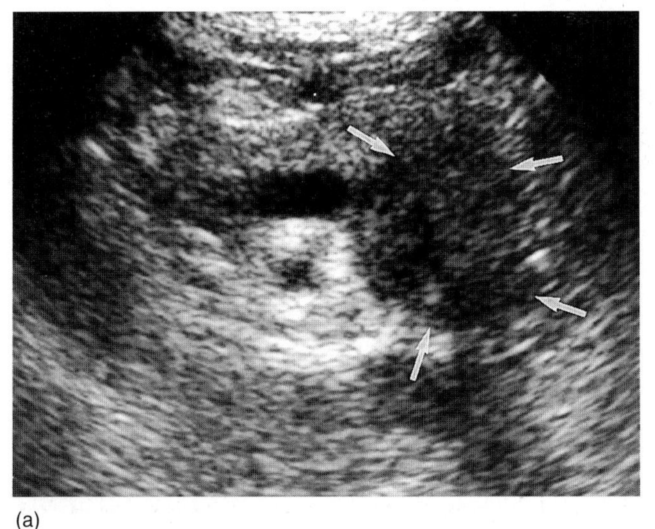

(a)

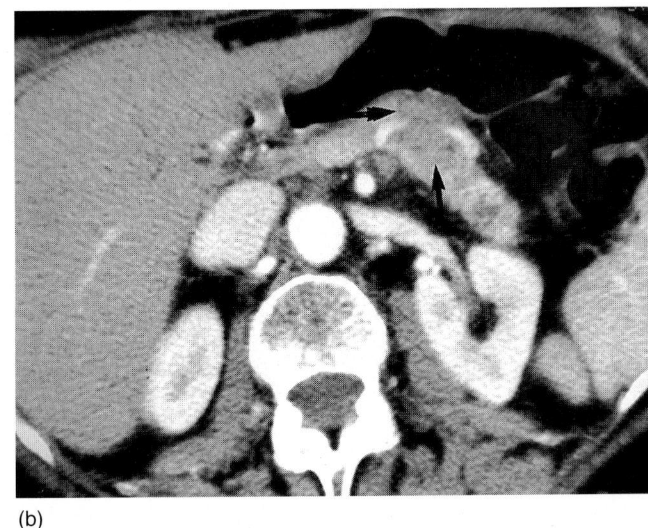

(b)

Fig. 5.46 Pancreatic carcinoma. (a) Transverse ultrasound scan showing a typical hypoechoic mass in the tail of the pancreas (arrows). The splenic vein is encased by the tumour. (b) CT scan in the same patient after intravenous injection of contrast medium showing a mass of lower density than the normally enhancing pancreas (arrows) encasing the splenic artery.

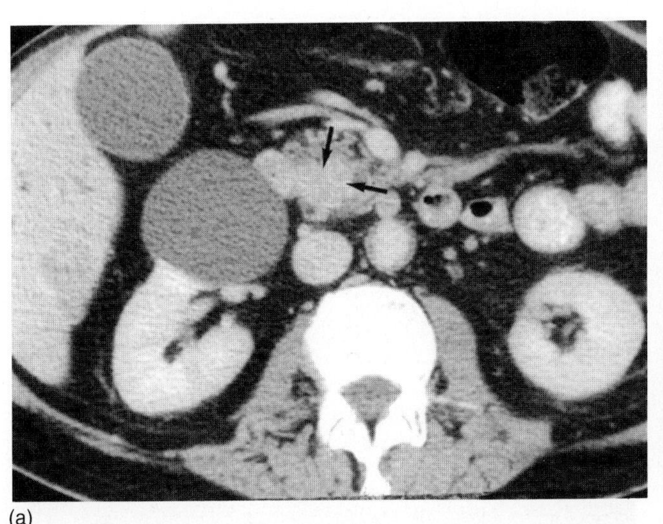

(a)

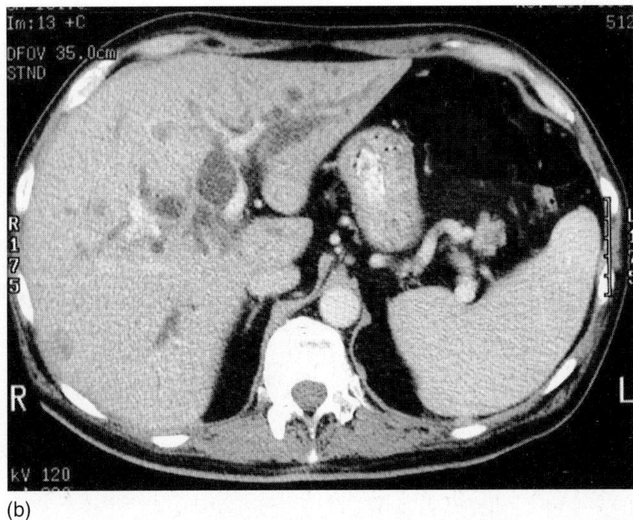

(b)

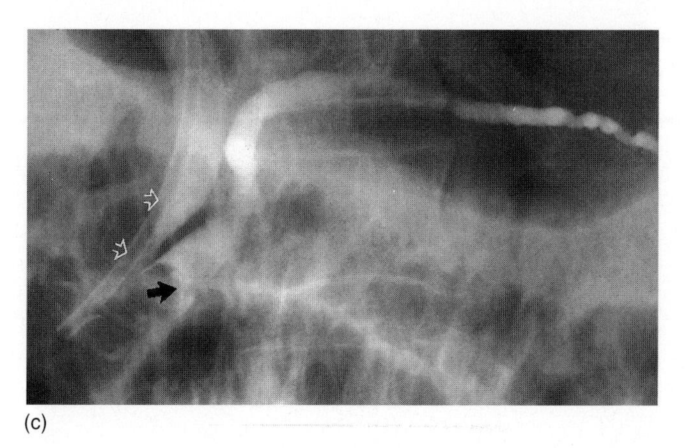

(c)

Fig. 5.47 (a) CT scan after intravenous injection of contrast medium with a small mass within the head of the pancreas (arrows) showing loss of the normal 'marbled' appearance of the pancreas. (b) Scan through the liver showing intrahepatic bile duct dilation. (c) ERCP showing the small mass demonstrated in (a) causing a filling defect within the distal pancreatic duct (arrow). A stent has been inserted into the dilated common duct (open arrows).

sonography, most duct cell carcinomas are not detected until they are at least 2 cm in size, large enough to alter the size and shape of the gland. Exceptions are small tumours in the head which present with bile or pancreatic duct dilation (Fig. 5.47). Most tumours will distort the contour of the gland, but some small masses may show more subtle features such as: 'rounding' of the usually wedge-shaped uncinate process (Fig. 5.48); a 'normal'-sized head in an otherwise atrophic gland, and focal loss of the normal 'marbling' of the gland usually seen in the elderly (Fig. 5.47). Almost all carcinomas enhance to a lesser extent than the surrounding pancreatic parenchyma after intravenous injection of a bolus of contrast medium (Fig. 5.49). Occasionally, lucent areas are seen within the mass which may be related to associated pancreatitis rather than to tumour necrosis.

Dilatation of the main pancreatic duct is detected in 50–75% of cases of pancreatic carcinoma (Fig. 5.49). This sign is particularly important in detecting a small duct cell carcinoma of the head of the pancreas or an

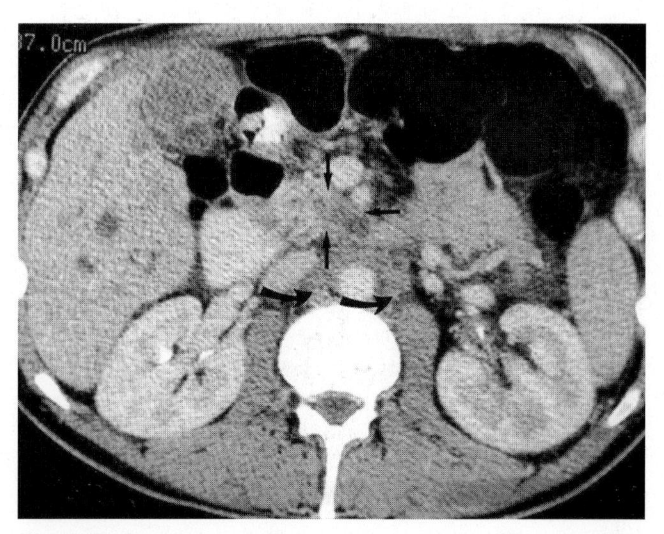

Fig. 5.48 Carcinoma of the uncinate process. CT scan after intravenous injection of contrast medium showing a small mass in the uncinate process (arrows). Retroperitoneal lymph node enlargement (curved arrows) and liver secondaries are noted.

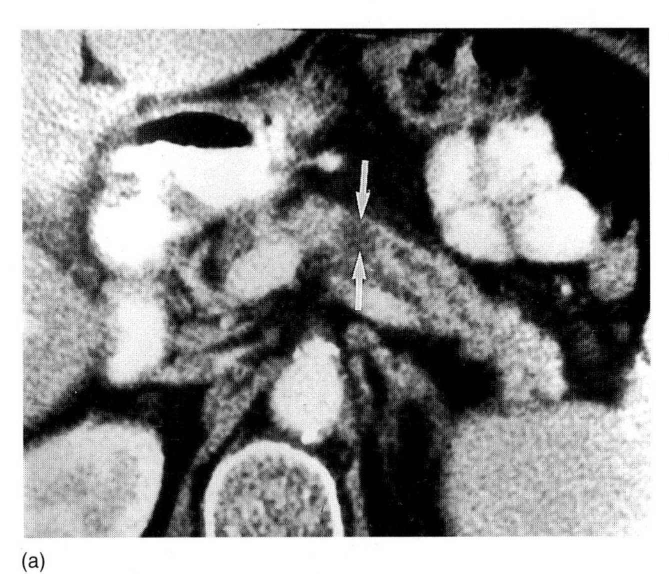

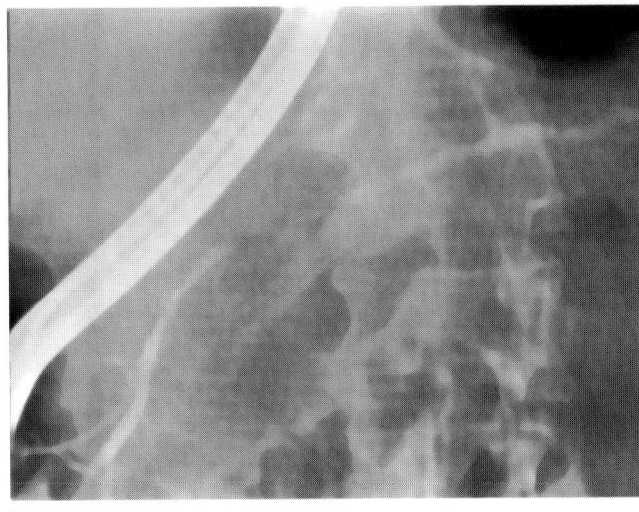

(a) (b)

Fig. 5.49 Small pancreatic carcinoma. (a) Small hypodense lesion is seen in the pancreatic body (arrows) which is not deforming the contour of the pancreas but causing dilation of the pancreatic duct. (b) Oblique view of ERCP corresponding to the CT showing an irregular stricture and duct dilation proximal to the tumour.

ampullary carcinoma, because pancreatic duct dilatation may be the only abnormality on CT. Parenchymal atrophy often accompanies duct dilatation.

Carcinoma of the head of the pancreas almost always results in biliary dilatation. Early or incomplete obstruction may be limited to the extrahepatic ducts. The gallbladder is often, but not always, distended, when the level of obstruction is distal to the cystic duct. Typically CT shows a dilated common duct down to the site of the tumour but, unlike benign disease, there is a sudden transition from a dilated duct to no visible duct at all within the tumour.

Ultrasound

In roughly 25% of patients delineation of the pancreas on ultrasound is inadequate, most commonly because of overlying bowel gas. Nevertheless, ultrasound is often the method most frequently used to investigate patients clinically suspected of having pancreatic cancer as it is relatively inexpensive, readily available and can accurately distinguish non-obstructive from obstructive jaundice – the presenting feature in 50% of patients. The fundamental ultrasound finding is a focal hypoechoic pancreatic mass (Figs 5.46, 5.50), although pancreatic carcinomas are occasionally isoechoic. Ultrasound may have the advantage of being able to distinguish changes in echogenicity which can make small tumours apparent before they cause a change in contour. A strong clinical probability of pancreatic neoplasm with a normal ultrasound always necessitates further investigation.

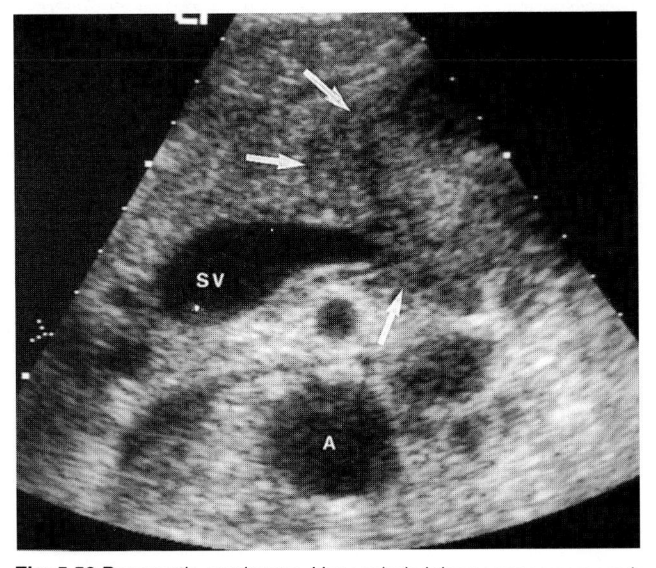

Fig. 5.50 Pancreatic carcinoma. Hypoechoic inhomogeneous mass in the body and tail of the pancreas (arrows) resulting in occlusion of the splenic vein (SV). Nodal enlargement is seen to the left of the aorta (A).

ERCP

Given the high accuracy of non-invasive studies, ERCP is used primarily as a technique to further assess patients with ambiguous CT findings or as part of the procedure of stenting. Obstruction of the main pancreatic duct is the most common pancreatographic finding in carcinoma. The obstruction may be difficult to differentiate from that caused by pancreatitis. In carcinoma the ducts distal to the obstruction may show post-stenotic dilatation but are otherwise usually normal, whereas changes consistent with pancreatitis are usually present in obstruction caused by pancreatitis. In carcinoma, the obstruction itself is usually irregular, nodular, rat-tailed or eccentric, and smooth or blunt in pancreatitis. Localized encasement of the main pancreatic duct is the next most common appearance after obstruction (Fig. 5.49). This encasement is generally 1–2 cm in length and is irregular. The distal duct is normal, the proximal (upstream) duct is dilated and the transition abrupt. Small side branches near the encasement are frequently compressed by tumour and do not fill. Occasionally a mass lesion can be seen within a dilated pancreatic duct (Fig. 5.47).

STAGING OF PANCREATIC CANCER

The aim of preoperative staging of pancreatic cancer is to identify potentially resectable tumours. Only about 10% of patients have resectable tumours. Conversely, as pancreaticoduodenectomy carries a high morbidity and mortality, imaging is also directed towards identifying those patients in whom the tumour has spread beyond the margins of the gland and is unresectable. The most generally accepted criteria of unresectability are the presence of liver metastases, adenopathy, tumour encasement of the coeliac or superior mesenteric arteries (not splenic artery), and obstruction or invasion of the portal and mesenteric veins.

Computed tomography

CT is the best imaging technique for staging patients with pancreatic cancer. Invasion of major adjacent arteries and veins is a contraindication to surgical resection. Involvement of the coeliac axis and its branches, the superior mesenteric artery or the major veins (portal, splenic, superior mesenteric) appears as a thickening of the wall of the vessel or as a soft-tissue mantle obscuring the normal sharp interface between the vessel and the renal and the perivascular fat (Fig. 5.51). Veins may be totally obliterated and venous obstruction may be recognized only by collateral vessels. Although the venous changes are generally

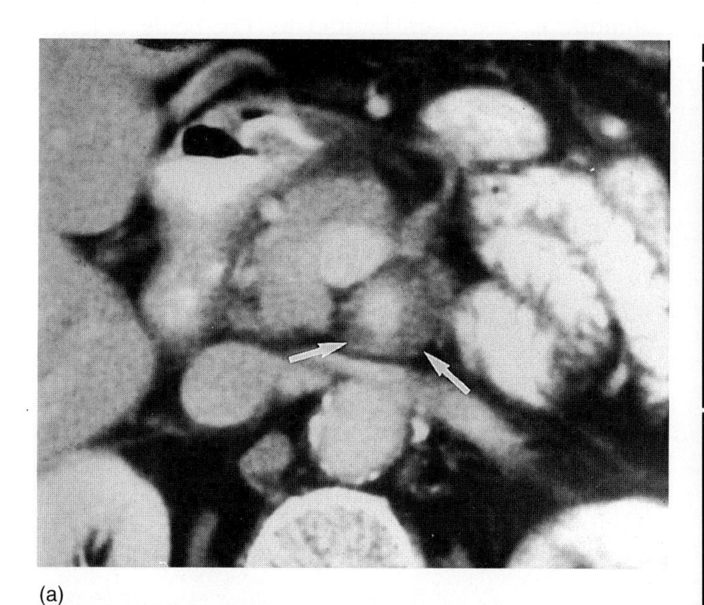

(a)

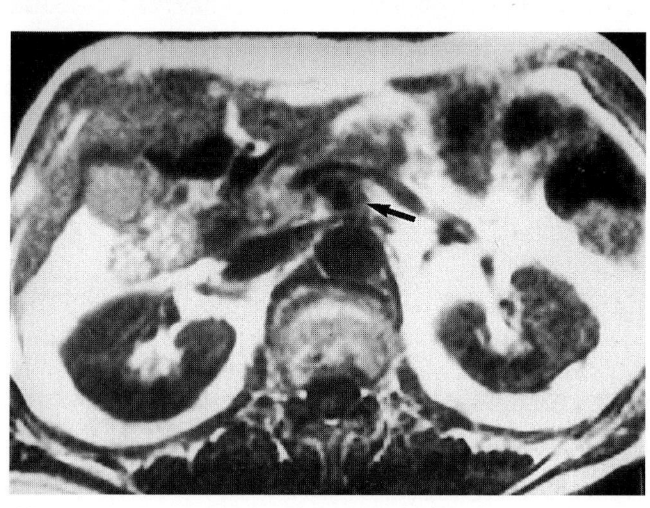

(b)

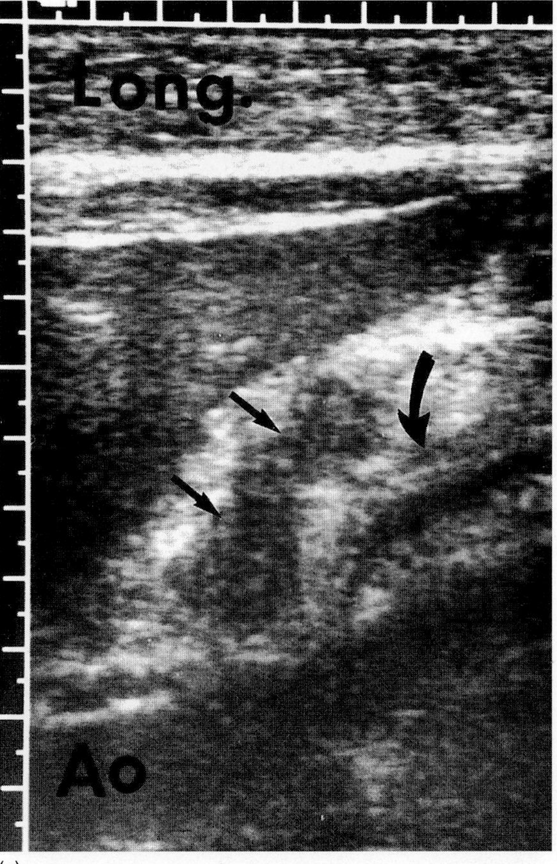

(c)

Fig. 5.51 Encasement of the superior mesenteric artery in pancreatic carcinoma. (a) CT scan after intravenous injection of contrast medium showing low density tumour encasing the superior mesenteric artery (arrows). (b) T1-weighted MRI scan showing the normal signal void encased by tissue of low signal intensity (arrow). (c) Longitudinal ultrasound scan showing encasement of the coeliac (arrows) and superior mesenteric arteries (curved arrow).

the result of invasion by a contiguous neoplasm, tumour growth in the perivascular lymphatics is responsible for periarterial 'cuffing'. Because of extrinsic intraparenchymal lymphatic connections, lesions anywhere in the gland can result in perivascular changes in any of the major arteries. As elsewhere in the body, CT can only demonstrate lymph node pathology by showing enlargement which may be the result either of malignant infiltration or of reactive hyperplasia (Fig. 5.48). Microscopic involvement of nodes without enlargement is fairly common in pancreatic cancer. Invasion of adjacent organs can best be diagnosed on CT when tumour tissue has entered the substance of the affected structure. In the absence of definite evidence of invasion, it may not be possible to decide whether the loss of intervening fat between the tumour and the adjacent organs is the result of invasion or mere contact between the mass and adjacent organs.

The positive predictive value of CT in predicting 'unresectability' of a pancreatic cancer is extremely high at between 90 and 100%; there are very few false-positive predictions of unresectability. The sensitivity of CT in detecting many of the features of unresectability is, however, lower. This is usually due to the failure of CT to detect lymph node metastases, small liver metastases and small peritoneal deposits. There is little difference between CT and angiography in detecting vascular involvement.

Ultrasound

Many of the vascular alterations that occur as a result of pancreatic carcinoma are demonstrable by ultrasonography. Encasement of the coeliac axis or superior mesenteric artery may be seen as thickening of the periarterial tissues, and venous involvement seen as abrupt change in the calibre of the affected vein (Figs 5.46, 5.51). Duplex Doppler may increase the sensitivity of ultrasound in detecting vascular involvement. Ultrasound is less sensitive than CT in detecting vascular involvement and lymphadenopathy.

Endoscopic ultrasound has proved extremely accurate in detecting local infiltration of the portal vein, adjacent arteries and lymph node infiltration. The technique is, however, limited by not being able to detect liver or peritoneal disease.

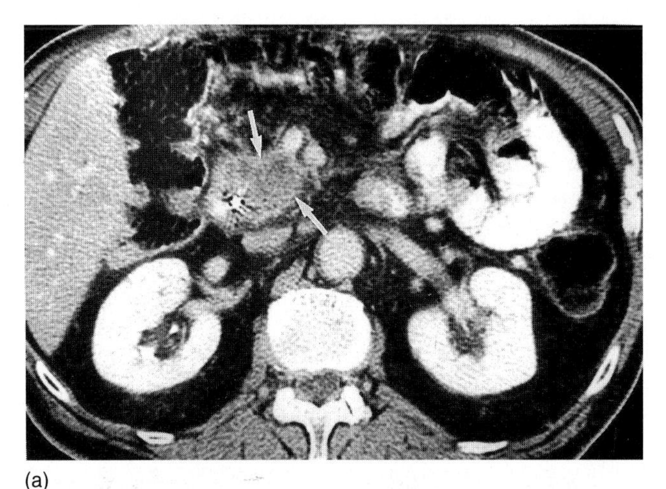
(a)

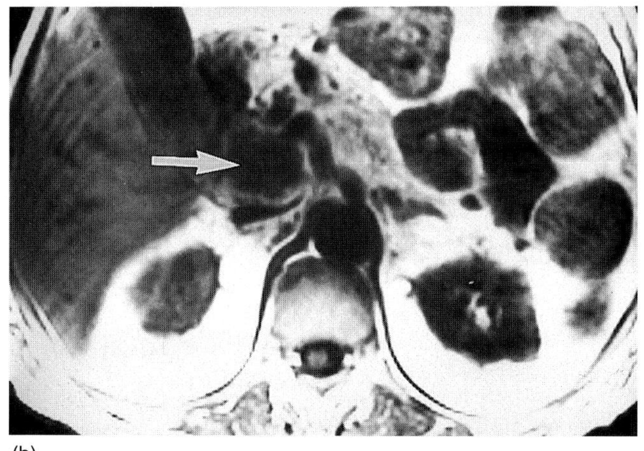
(b)

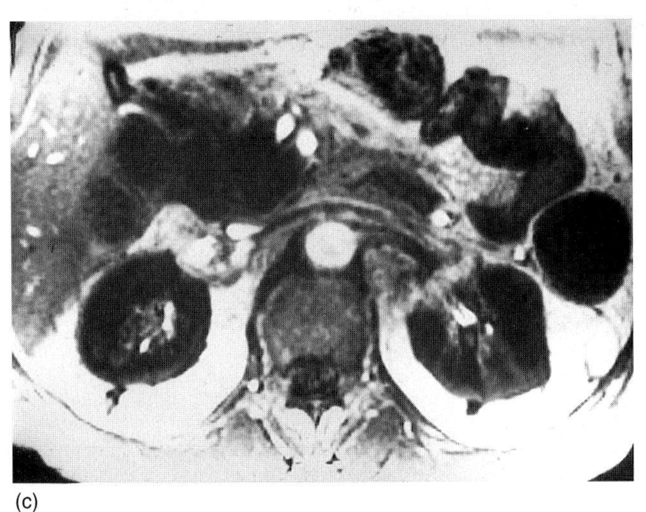
(c)

Fig. 5.52 Pancreatic carcinoma. (a) Low density mass (arrows) on contrast-enhanced CT lying within the head of the pancreas in close proximity to the superior mesenteric vessels. (b) T1-weighted MRI showing the typical appearance of a mass of low signal intensity (arrow). (c) Gradient echo MRI showing the mass encasing the superior mesenteric vessels.

MRI

The exact role of MRI in staging the local spread of pancreatic cancer has not yet been established. Pancreatic neoplasms, their retroperitoneal spread and venous patency are best evaluated using T1-weighted spin-echo sequences. On heavily T1-weighted images, pancreatic carcinoma typically appears as a mass with low signal intensity. Like CT, MRI is also capable of assessing arterial or venous involvement and lymph node enlargement (Figs 5.51, 5.52).

PRIMARY CYSTIC NEOPLASMS OF DUCT CELL ORIGIN

Primary cystic neoplasms of the pancreas, which represent 10–15% of pancreatic cysts in surgical series, are classified as either microcystic adenomas or mucinous cystic neoplasms. These are usually easily distinguished from each other by their imaging characteristics which correspond to their differing gross morphology.

Microcystic adenoma

The vast majority of these benign tumours occur in females over the age of 60 years. The tumour occupies the head, body or tail, but occasionally occupies the entire gland. Almost all the cysts are <2 cm in diameter and the CT appearance is usually a water density mass which sometimes contains solid elements. Individual cysts are too small to be identified on CT. Calcification occurs more frequently than in any other pancreatic tumour. The calcification is dystrophic in nature and is seen within a central fibrotic scar that may have a stellate appearance on CT. The tumour does not have a well-developed capsule on CT and is poorly demarcated from the normal gland. Contrast enhancement may be seen due to a rich network of capillaries within the tumour. On ultrasound, the most common pattern is a solid-appearing mild to moderately echogenic mass with or without small cystic areas, since almost all the cysts are <2 cm in diameter. Bright central echogenic foci with or without shadowing caused by calcification are sometimes visible. Septations are often better appreciated on sonography than on CT.

Mucinous cystic neoplasms

Like microcystic adenoma, this tumour occurs predominantly in females but unlike microcystic adenoma has a malignant potential, developing into a low-grade mucinous adenocarcinoma. On CT, the mass is a well-demarcated, round or oval thick-walled cyst. The mass is generally >5 cm in diameter (Fig. 5.53) and solid enhancing excrescences can occasionally be seen in the wall, particularly if the tumour is malignant. Dystrophic peripheral calcification is seen in about 15% of cases. The main differential diagnosis is a pancreatic pseudocyst.

ISLET-CELL TUMOURS

The term islet-cell tumour encompasses a range of rare neoplasms of neuroendocrine origin arising in or in close proximity to the pancreas. A small proportion are non-functioning but the majority, approximately 85%, secrete one or more biologically active peptides or amines normally found in the adult pancreas, or

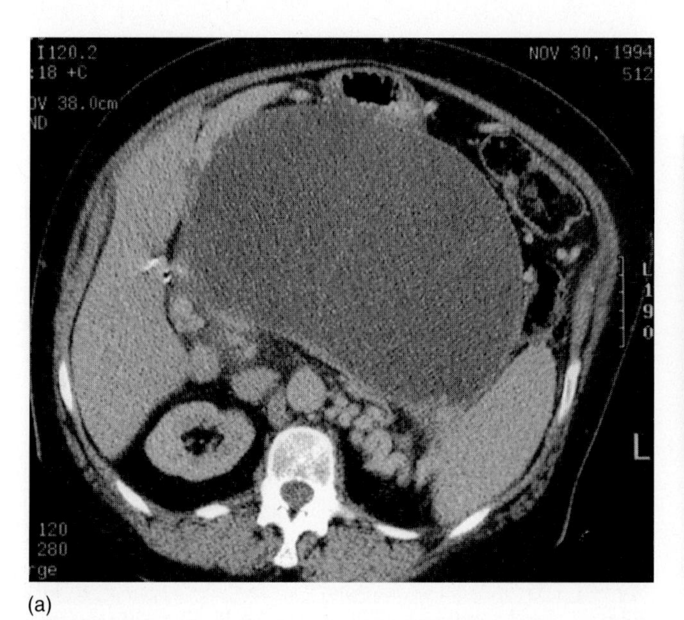

(a)

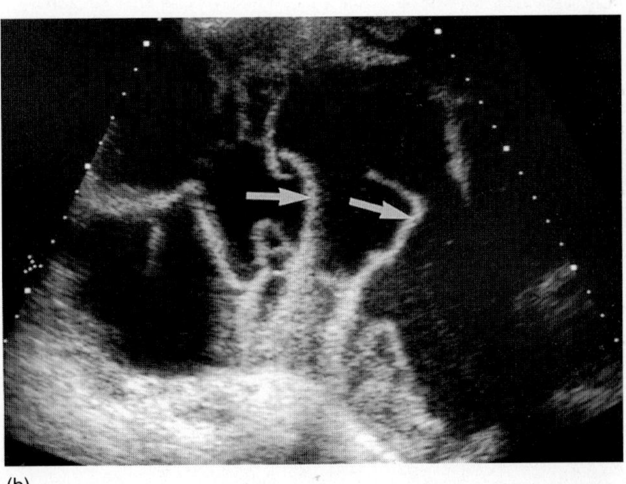

(b)

Fig. 5.53 Mucinous (macro) cystadenoma of the pancreas. (a) CT scan showing a typical large cystic mass replacing the body and tail of the pancreas. (b) Transverse ultrasound scan on the same patient showing a large fluid-filled mass. Echogenic septa (arrows) are more readily seen on ultrasound.

other substances not usually present in the pancreas such as gastrin. The role of imaging is to localize these tumours, usually prior to surgery, and to look for evidence of malignancy.

Insulinomas are the most frequent functioning pancreatic tumours accounting for 60% of all islet-cell tumours. They are usually very small: 90% are <2 cm, and are located with equal frequency in the head, body and tail of the pancreas; 10% are malignant. **Gastrinomas** account for about 20% of all islet-cell tumours, are found in the pancreas and in the proximal duodenal wall, and about 60% are malignant and often multiple. Other functioning islet-cell tumours such as glucagonomas, VIPomas, somatostatinomas and carcinoid tumours tend to be several centimetres in diameter at diagnosis and are frequently malignant.

Many imaging modalities are currently available for the investigation of patients with islet-cell tumours, including ultrasound, CT, MRI, arteriography, venous sampling and radionuclide imaging. None has established itself as clearly superior to the others.

Ultrasound is generally the first line of investigation and an islet-cell tumour is usually seen as a well-circumscribed mass of lower echogenicity than the normal pancreas (Fig. 5.54). Tumours as small as 7 mm have been detected. Liver metastases may be seen with malignant tumours and are most often hypoechoic. The sensitivity of transabdominal ultrasound is low, partly due to overlying bowel gas, but also because relatively poor resolution 3.5–5.0 MHz transducers are needed to obtain pictures from a structure positioned deep within the abdomen. **Endoscopic ultrasound** overcomes these problems by allowing the positioning of a high frequency (7.5–10 MHz) transducer in close proximity to the pancreas, obtaining high-resolution images. The early results are extremely encouraging. Intraoperative ultrasound also allows high-resolution examination of the pancreas and can be used as an adjunct to palpation during surgery.

The majority of islet-cell tumours are isodense on non-contrast-enhanced CT and cannot therefore be recognized. On postcontrast CT they are seen as rounded areas which enhance more than the surrounding pancreas (Fig. 5.55). Local nodal and liver deposits may also be seen, usually as enhancing masses. The sensitivity of CT for delineation of these tumours depends on size, but is usually about 65–75% for insulinomas and gastrinomas. Small tumours may also be seen on **MRI**, usually as round, low-signal lesions on T1-weighted images (Fig. 5.54), showing high signal on T2-weighted images.

Arteriography still has a role in localizing islet-cell tumours, particularly when this has not been achieved by less invasive techniques. Selective injections of contrast medium into the coeliac axis and superior mesenteric artery followed by superselective studies of the splenic, dorsal pancreatic, gastroduodenal and pancreaticoduodenal arteries are made. An islet-cell tumour typically appears as a round, well-circumscribed blush in the capillary phase and venous phases. Lesions may be missed on angiography because they are too small or too hypovascular, or because they are obscured by a blush of adjacent bowel or spleen.

Transhepatic portal venous sampling is the most sensitive but most invasive method of localizing functioning tumours, with a significant complication

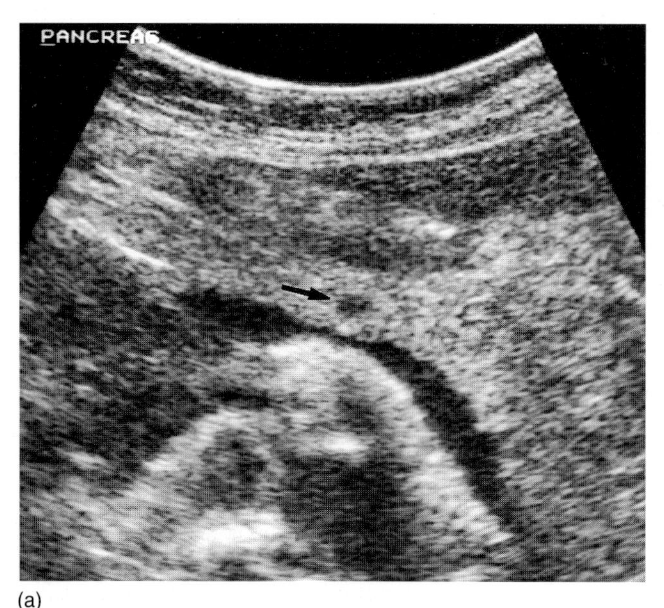

(a)

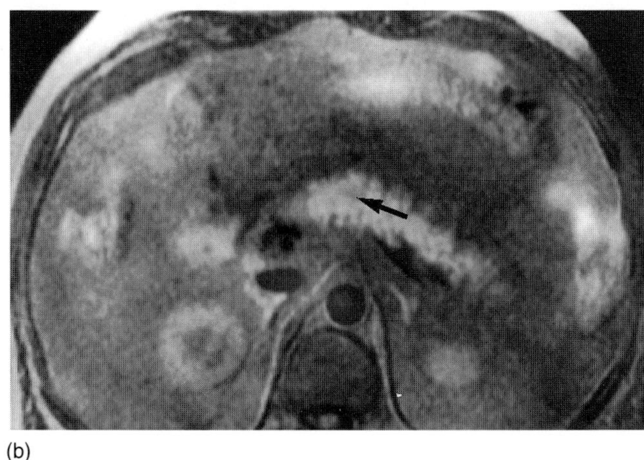

(b)

Fig. 5.54 Insulinoma. (a) Transverse ultrasound scan through the pancreas showing small islet-cell tumour (arrow). (b) T1-weighted MRI scan showing typical low signal intensity lesion (arrow) corresponding to the abnormality seen on ultrasound.

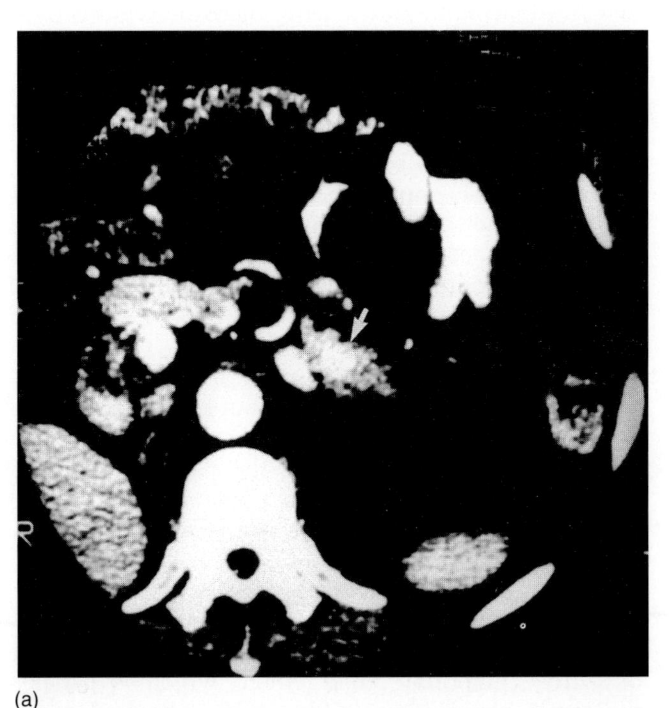

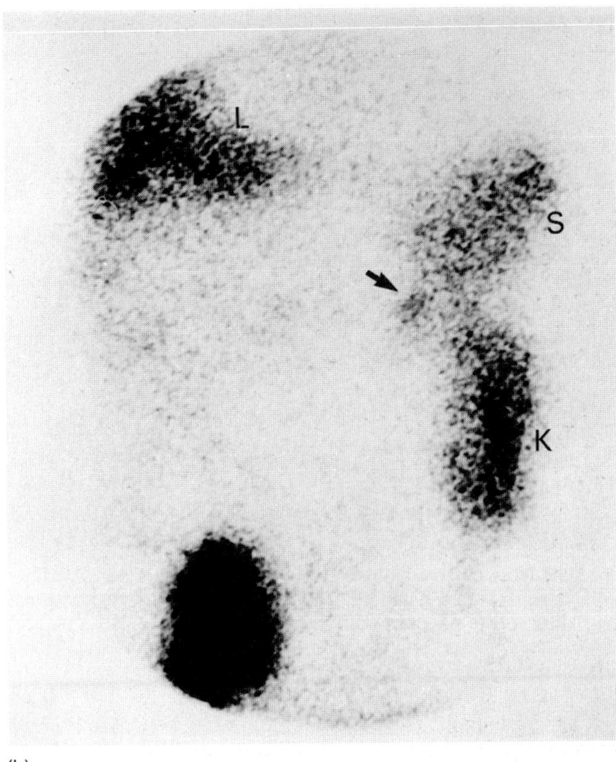

(a) (b)

Fig. 5.55 Insulinoma. (a) CT scan showing small enhancing lesion (arrowed) due to insulinoma. (b) Area of increased uptake (arrowed) in octreotide scan due to insulinoma corresponding to lesion seen on CT. The normal liver (L), spleen (S) and left kidney (K) are all demonstrated. The patient has a right pelvic kidney.

rate of close to 10%. The technique involves transhepatic catheterization of the splenic and portal veins with serial sampling of the splenic, superior mesenteric and portal veins. This technique cannot pinpoint a tumour in the same way as an imaging study but localizes it to a region of the pancreas.

A radiolabelled derivative of **octreotide**, ^{111}In-pentatreotide, a synthetic somatostatin analogue, can be used to localize pancreatic endocrine tumours if they express somatostatin receptors (Fig. 5.55).

In practice, in almost all cases, initial imaging is performed with a combination of transabdominal ultrasound and CT. When these tests are negative or equivocal, arteriography is the next line of investigation. Further investigation depends on local practice and suspected tumour type. Endoscopic ultrasound is rapidly emerging as a technique of high sensitivity. Transhepatic venous sampling and somatostatin receptor imaging have the advantage that they are not dependent on tumour size and are particularly applicable to difficult cases where other imaging modalities are negative.

PANCREATITIS

Pancreatic inflammatory disease can be classified by clinical or pathological criteria into acute or chronic forms. Acute pancreatitis is characterized clinically by the acute onset of abdominal pain and a rise of pancreatic enzymes in the blood. Most patients, although not all, recover without permanent morphological and functional changes in the gland. Chronic pancreatitis is characterized clinically by recurrent or persistent episodes of abdominal pain, usually with evidence of functional pancreatic insufficiency.

ACUTE PANCREATITIS

Imaging has four major roles in patients with acute pancreatitis:

- confirmation of the diagnosis;
- exclusion of other causes of pain where the clinical findings are equivocal;
- assessing the severity of the inflammation;
- the detection of complications.

Imaging

The **plain film** signs associated with acute pancreatitis are discussed on pp. 40–42 in Chapter 2.

CT is the most sensitive imaging modality for evaluating acute pancreatitis but in very mild cases the pancreas may appear normal. CT is better than ultrasound for detecting the presence of pancreatic

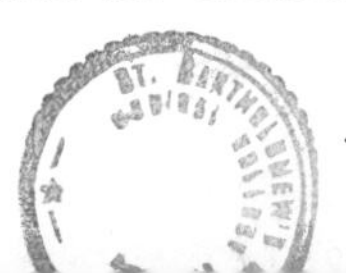

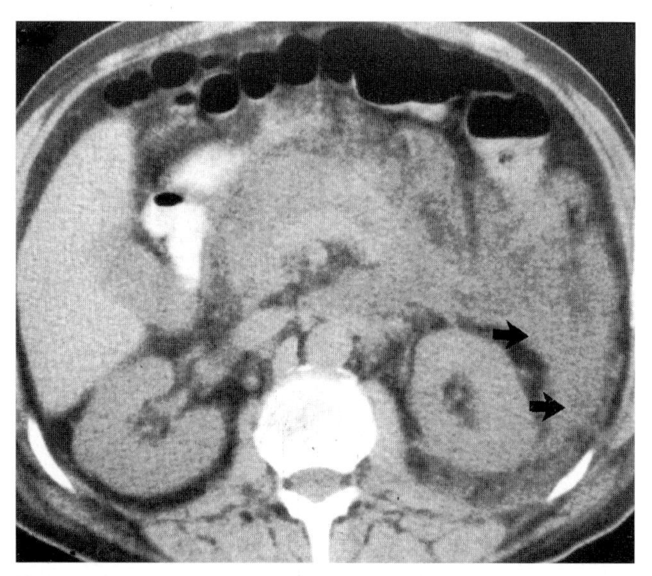

Fig. 5.56 Acute phlegmonous pancreatitis. Non-enhanced CT scan in a patient with acute pancreatitis showing swelling of the pancreas, loss of definition of the peripancreatic fat planes. There is extension of the inflammatory process into the left parerenal space (arrows).

necrosis and other complications, and is, therefore, better for predicting the outcome of acute pancreatitis. In most cases the gland is enlarged, the pancreatic contour is irregular and the parenchyma appears inhomogeneous. The peripancreatic fat is usually hazy and shows an increase in density accompanied by fascial thickening (Fig. 5.56). In more severe cases, fluid collections are seen within the gland and the peripancreatic exudate is more extensive (Fig. 5.57). Phlegmon, consisting of inflammatory exudate, necrotic tissue and blood, is seen on CT as poorly defined, irregularly contoured, solid and fluid elements in the peripancreatic regions (Fig. 5.57). Like transient fluid collections, these are seen first within the lesser sac and in the anterior pararenal space, particularly on the left side. Fluid collections or phlegmon may extend inferiorly along the pararenal spaces, bilaterally continuing inferiorly along the psoas muscle border into the pelvis, and rarely into the thigh. Mesenteric, mesocolic, posterior pararenal space and perirenal space involvement occurs less commonly. Direct mediastinal extension and involvement of the liver and spleen also occur occasionally.

Focal or segmental pancreatitis demonstrates findings similar to acute pancreatitis but is localized to the involved area of the gland, usually the head.

Ultrasound examination of the pancreas may be normal in mild cases of pancreatitis and even occasionally in more severe forms. Its usefulness early in the evaluation of pancreatitis is primarily to exclude other causes of abdominal pain and to identify choledocholithiasis or cholelithiasis. The ultrasound findings are similar to those seen on CT, namely focal or diffuse glandular enlargement which is usually uniformly hypoechoic (Fig. 5.58). Peripancreatic phlegmonous changes result in loss of definition of the pancreatic edge and thickening of the peripancreatic fascial planes. Extrapancreatic fluid collections develop usually within 2–4 weeks after earliest clinical symptoms. They may be anechoic or septate and most resolve within weeks or months. Secondary findings include dilatation of the pancreatic duct, ascites and thickening of the gall bladder and bowel walls.

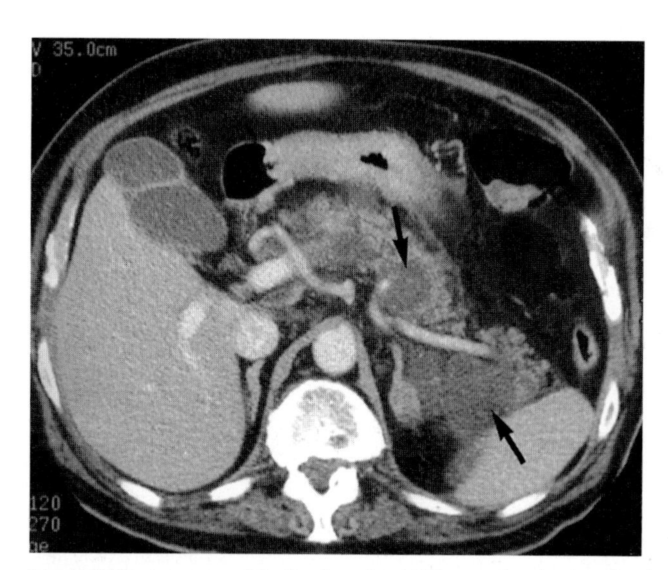

Fig. 5.57 Acute pancreatitis. Post-contrast CT scan showing localized fluid collections within the gland (arrows). Much of the normal gland parenchyma has been preserved.

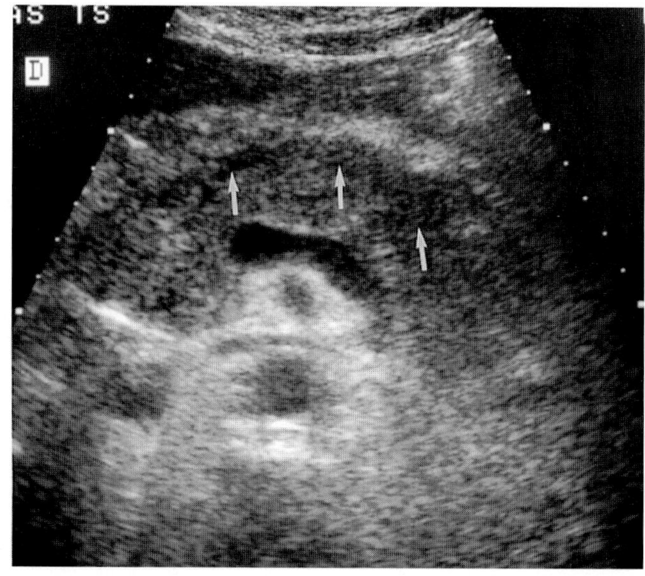

Fig. 5.58 Acute pancreatitis. Transverse ultrasound scan showing marked swelling of the gland which contains multiple hypoechoic areas due to necrosis (arrowed).

Complications of pancreatitis and grading of severity

CT has been shown to be extremely accurate in grading the severity of acute pancreatitis by detecting the most frequent and important complications which include gland necrosis, pancreatic abscess, fluid collections (including pseudocyst) and vascular, gastrointestinal or biliary tract involvement. The clinical severity of pancreatitis is usually best assessed with Ranson's criteria. Poor correlation exists between CT and Ranson's criteria, probably because CT primarily grades local complications whereas the Ranson classification evaluates systemic complications.

Pancreatic gland necrosis Necrotizing pancreatitis is a severe form of acute pancreatitis, occurring in 8–15% of patients, characterized by destruction of pancreatic parenchyma, peripancreatic tissues or both.

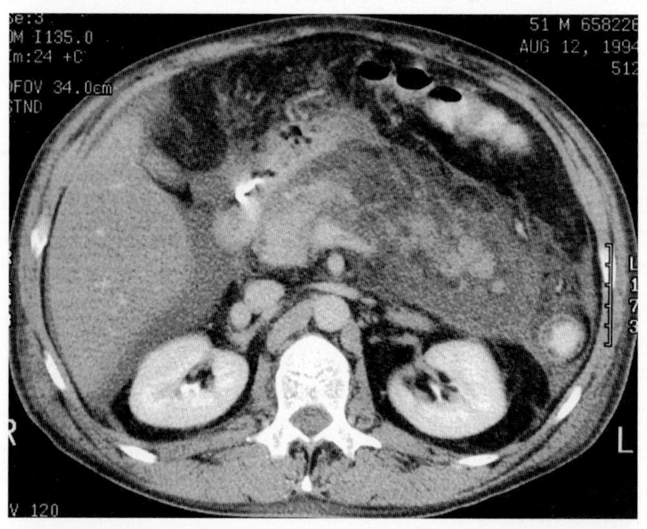

Fig. 5.59 Acute necrotizing pancreatitis. Contrast medium-enhanced CT scan showing areas of non-enhancing pancreatic parenchyma, with replacement of the pancreas by fluid and abnormal soft tissue.

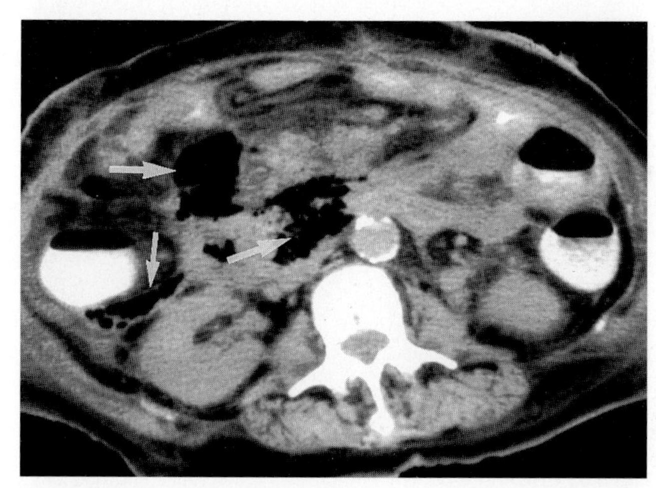

Fig. 5.60 Acute infection in necrotizing pancreatitis. CT scan showing multiple large pockets of gas within abnormal soft tissue (arrows) indicating infected necrosis.

Areas of pancreatic necrosis can be recognized on CT as areas of non-enhancing parenchyma after intravenous injection of a bolus of contrast medium (Fig. 5.59). Non-contrast CT cannot exclude pancreatic necrosis. Differentiating necrotizing from oedematous pancreatitis by ultrasound is not consistently possible. Pancreatic infection is a common complication, occurring in 40% of patients, and is often responsible for the high mortality in these patients. It may be recognized by the appearance of gas bubbles within the necrotic tissue (Fig. 5.60).

Peripancreatic fluid collections Peripancreatic fluid collections are common and usually develop early in the course of acute pancreatitis. They may be readily detected on ultrasound or CT. Many resolve spontaneously, usually within 6 weeks. Fluid collections which do not resolve within a few weeks tend to become encapsulated by fibrous connective tissue to form pseudocysts. Bacterial infection of a fluid collection will result in an abscess.

Pseudocysts Pancreatic pseudocysts can be found virtually anywhere in the abdomen and pelvis, and have even been reported extending into the mediastinum, neck, scrotum, groin or lower extremities. They complicate acute pancreatitis in less than 10% of patients and tend to occur in regions most likely to be affected by phlegmonous pancreatitis such as the lesser sac, perisplenic region and transverse mesocolon. Up to 30% resolve spontaneously, sometimes with spontaneous rupture into the pancreatic duct, stomach or peritoneal cavity. Spontaneous resolution of a cyst >5 cm or multiple lesions is unlikely.

Signs of pseudocyst formation are seldom seen on plain film as calcification is very unusual. Most pseudocysts of the head and body of the pancreas are

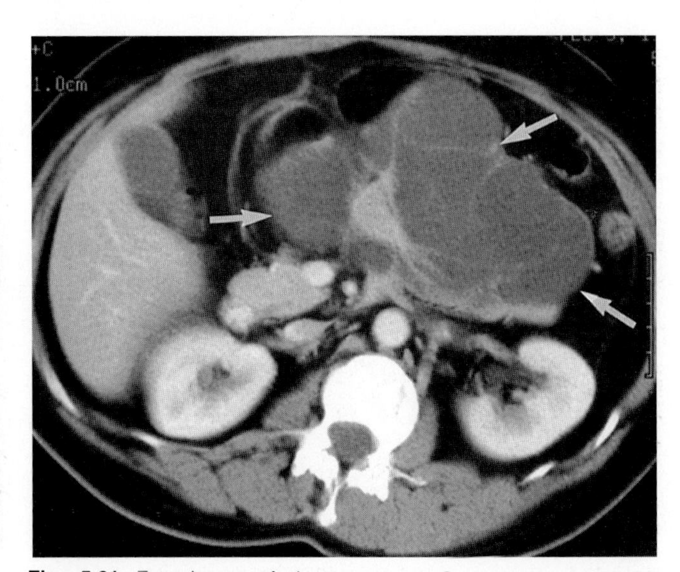

Fig. 5.61 Pseudocyst of the pancreas. Contrast-enhanced CT scan showing a septate fluid-filled pseudocyst of the pancreas (arrows).

readily seen on ultrasound. The wall is smooth and well-defined, and the fluid can be entirely echo-free or have internal echoes or debris. The CT number of the fluid is usually close to 0 HU, but can be as high as 25–30 HU; the wall is usually thin and smooth (Fig. 5.61). When the cyst wall is irregular, thickened and its contents echogenic, the possibility of superimposed haemorrhage or infection should always be considered. Overall, CT is better than ultrasound for depicting pseudocysts, especially those remote from the pancreas. Ultrasound often gives a better display of the internal architecture.

Pancreatic abscess Pancreatic abscess is a localized collection of pus confined by a wall or rind of inflammatory tissue (Fig. 5.62). It can usually be differentiated easily from infected necrosis on CT, where the inflammatory tissue is not confined (Fig. 5.60). Like other fluid collections, abscesses may be confined to the pancreatic bed or extend beyond the organ, even into the pelvis. The most obvious sign of an abscess is air within the inflammatory mass. This, however, does not constitute absolute evidence of pancreatic abscess as air within a fluid collection can be secondary to a fistula with the gastrointestinal lumen. Furthermore, a substantial proportion of pancreatic abscesses, probably the majority, do not contain gas.

Vascular complications Vascular complications of acute pancreatitis include occlusion or thrombosis of the splenic vein or other regional veins, direct arterial erosion or pseudoaneurysm formation. Pseudoaneurysms most commonly arise from the splenic artery, followed by the gastroduodenal artery. On CT, the demonstration of a homogeneously, brightly enhancing structure within or adjacent to a pseudocyst, or contiguous with a vascular structure after injection of contrast medium, is highly suggestive of a pseudoaneurysm. Ultrasound also demonstrates pseudoaneurysms as hypoechoic structures within a larger cystic structure. Turbulent and pulsatile flow is seen on duplex and colour-flow Doppler imaging.

Gastrointestinal complications Direct extension of inflammation from the pancreas can cause oedema, necrosis or perforation of the wall of the stomach or small bowel. Thrombosis of mesenteric vessels can cause similar changes. CT readily demonstrates these bowel wall changes. Pancreatico-enteric fistulae occur late in the course of pancreatitis, most commonly affecting the splenic flexure. These must be specifically suspected and sought with the use of gastrointestinal contrast studies. As many as 20% of fistulae may not be discovered before surgery. ERCP does not opacify all fistulae. A fistula can be recognized on CT by the presence of oral contrast material or gas within a pancreatic phlegmon.

Common bile duct obstruction Oedema in the head of the pancreas can cause transient compression of the common bile duct. This complication can be detected in about 6% of patients with acute pancreatitis on ultrasound, CT or ERCP.

CHRONIC PANCREATITIS

Chronic pancreatitis can be considered to have two main morphological forms. The most common type is **chronic calcific pancreatitis**. Less common is **chronic obstructive pancreatitis** resulting from any non-calculous obstructive lesion of the pancreas. The hallmark of chronic calcific pancreatitis on any imaging study is the identification of calculi in the

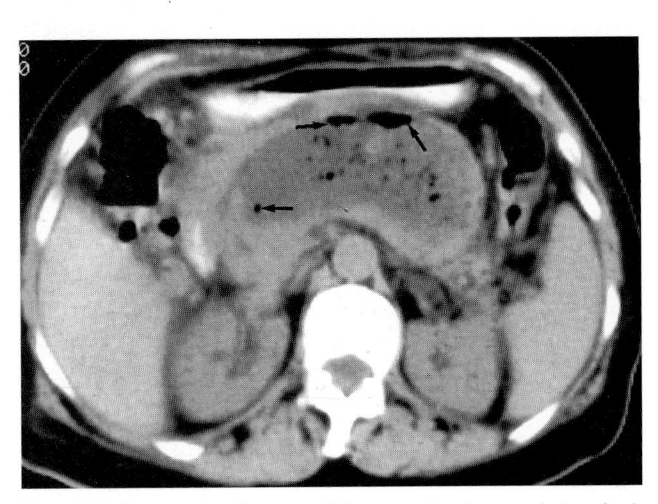

Fig. 5.62 Pancreatic abscess. CT scan showing pockets of air (arrows) within a thick-walled fluid collection within the body and tail of the pancreas due to infection of a pseudocyst.

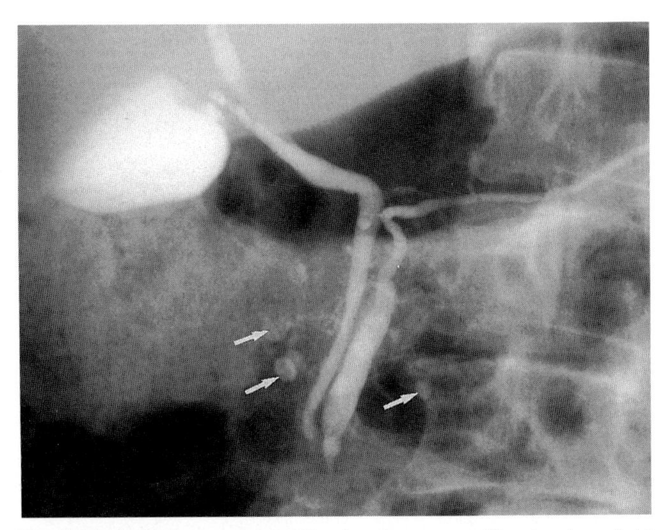

Fig. 5.63 ERCP in a patient with chronic pancreatitis showing slight dilation of the main pancreatic duct and impaired filling of the secondary ducts. Calcification of the pancreatic parenchyma (arrows) can also be seen.

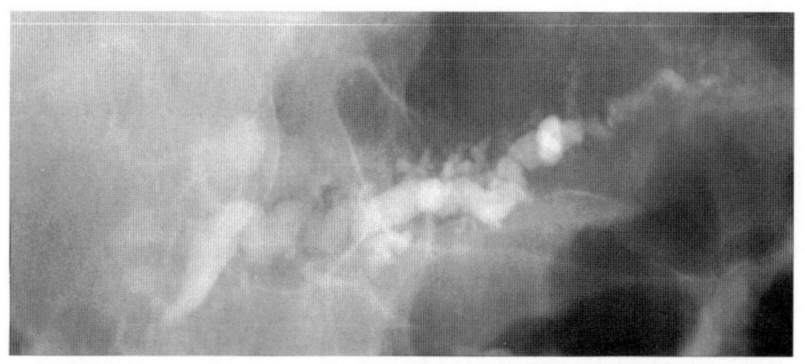

Fig. 5.64 ERCP in chronic pancreatitis showing marked 'beaded' dilation of the main pancreatic duct, marked dilation of several of the secondary ducts and non-filling of others.

pancreas. Pancreatic calcifications develop in close association with progressive pancreatic dysfunction and usually develop five years after onset of chronic pancreatitis in alcoholic chronic pancreatitis. Pancreatic calculi are almost always intraductal; true parenchymal calcification is unusual and may occur after haemorrhage or necrosis.

Demonstrating pancreatic calculi on abdominal radiography is the most cost-effective method for confirming chronic calcific pancreatitis as it will depict calculi in 90% of patients when compared with CT.

The three main indications for ERCP in chronic pancreatitis are to establish a diagnosis, to assess pancreatic anatomy and to perform endoscopic therapy. As many as 30% of patients with chronic pancreatitis have a normal pancreaticogram. The earliest identifiable changes are slight ectasia or clubbing of the side branches of the pancreatic duct. Side branch filling may be impaired. The main duct is usually minimally dilated and irregular (Fig. 5.63). Moderate chronic pancreatitis is characterized by dilation, tortuosity and stenosis within the main duct, with cystic dilation and obstruction of branch ducts (Fig. 5.64). Marked chronic pancreatitis is present when both pancreatic duct and side branches are severely involved by dilation, stenosis or obstruction. In most cases, the entire duct is involved and is usually beaded.

Signs on ultrasound include an enlarged main pancreatic duct (>4 mm), gland atrophy, echogenic foci within the parenchyma and an irregular contour to the gland, particularly focal enlargement (Fig. 5.65). The diagnostic accuracy of ultrasound is reported to vary between 60 and 80%.

Pancreatic duct dilatation, parenchymal atrophy and pancreatic calcifications are the most common CT manifestations of chronic pancreatitis (Fig. 5.65). Fluid collections, focal pancreatic enlargement and biliary duct dilatation also occur. Focal enlargement, which occurs in about 30% of cases of pancreatitis, can be difficult to distinguish from pancreatic malignancy unless calcification is present within the mass; calcifications are extremely uncommon in pancreatic adenocarcinoma. Cysts may also be found within the pancreas.

In the early stages of the disease, there is poor correlation between the radiological changes (as detected by ultrasound, CT and ERCP) and the degree of functional impairment. In the later stages, the correlation is good.

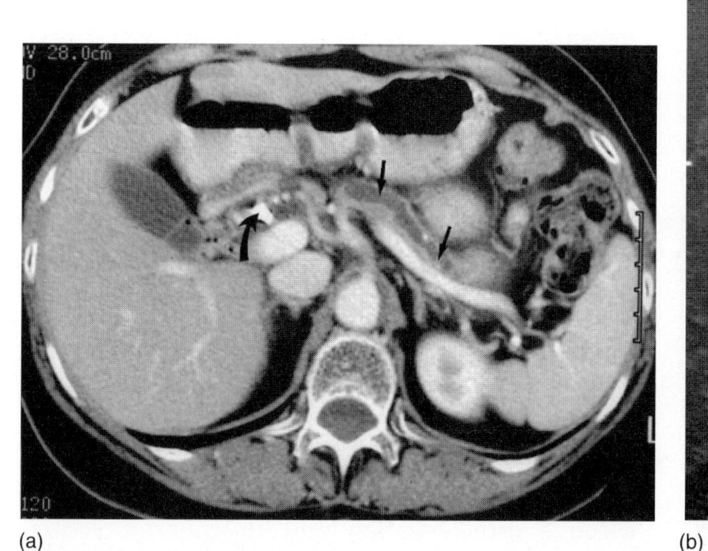

(a)

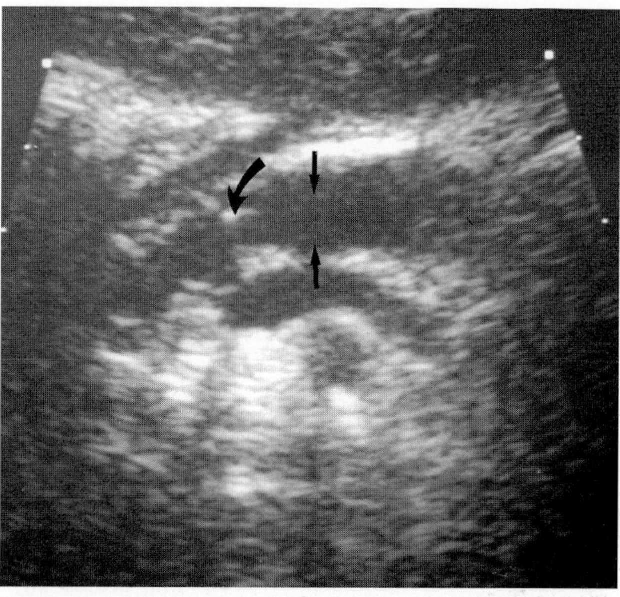

(b)

Fig. 5.65 Chronic pancreatitis. (a) CT scan showing marked dilation of the pancreatic duct (arrows) with calculi within the duct (curved arrow). There is also marked atrophy of the pancreatic parenchyma. (b) Ultrasound scan on the same patient showing dilation of the pancreatic duct (arrows) and parenchymal atrophy. An echogenic calculus can be seen within the duct (curved arrow).

PANCREATIC TRAUMA

Following pancreatic trauma, CT may demonstrate diffuse focal swelling of the gland with or without regional streaky inflammatory changes in the peripancreatic fat, anterior pararenal space, lesser sac or mesentery. A fracture may sometimes be identified. Trauma to the spleen, liver, gallbladder, bile ducts, duodenum and adrenal gland may be visible. Late sequelae of pancreatic trauma include pseudocysts, fistulae and abscesses. All of these findings can usually be demonstrated on CT. ERCP may be used on an emergency basis for the diagnosis of suspected pancreatic ductal rupture. It is more sensitive and specific for ductal rupture than combinations of CT, peritoneal lavage and serum amylase.

CONGENITAL ABNORMALITIES OF PANCREAS

A variety of congenital abnormalities of the pancreas can be demonstrated on imaging. CT may show the duodenum partially or completely encircled by an annular pancreas. An ERCP can be used to confirm the diagnosis by demonstrating a segment of pancreatic duct encircling the duodenum. Ectopic islands of pancreatic tissue are most commonly located in the wall of the stomach or duodenum. The diagnosis is usually made incidentally during barium examination which shows a smooth, submucosal nodule. In patients with autosomal dominant adult polycystic disease of the kidney, cysts may be demonstrated in the pancreas on ultrasound or CT. In von Hippel–Lindau disease cystic pancreatic neoplasms may be seen in the pancreas.

CYSTIC FIBROSIS OF THE PANCREAS

The pathological changes of fibrosis, fatty replacement, calcification and cyst formation in the pancreatic ductules are all reflected as an increased echogenicity of the pancreas that is usually markedly increased for age on ultrasound. The usual CT picture is fatty replacement depicted as a normal pancreatic contour with decreased attenuation values in the range of fat. Pancreatic cysts are occasionally seen.

SPLEEN

IMAGING TECHNIQUES

ULTRASOUND

The normal echo pattern of the spleen is evenly distributed echoes, similar but slightly greater than the liver. The size and shape of the spleen, the position of the hilum and its relationship to adjacent organs (diaphragm, stomach, pancreas, left kidney) can all be identified. Often the splenic vein can be identified in the hilum.

Ultrasound is useful for detecting and characterizing focal lesions within the spleen as cystic or solid, and can be used to estimate splenic size and volume. Colour Doppler ultrasound is useful for demonstrating the splenic artery and vein; this can be helpful in differentiating vascular structures, such as normal vessels or aneurysms, from non-vascular structures, such as pancreatic pseudocysts. Rapid measurements of splenic volume can be made, which is useful when following splenic size.

CT SCANNING

Computed tomography is exquisite in its ability to demonstrate the size, shape and location of the normal spleen, and in demonstrating focal intrasplenic abnormalities. Technical artefacts may result from motion or unusual enhancement. The density of the spleen on CT is usually close to that of liver and has a normal range of 35–55 HU. The splenic hilum and its relations are well visualized. The posterior surface of the spleen abutting the pleural space is called the 'bare area' and has a constant relation to Gerota's fascia. The significant variation in the size, shape and position of the spleen is well shown on CT. Enhancement with intravenous contrast medium is generally indicated when looking for splenic disease and results in dense enhancement of the normal spleen within 2 minutes after injection.

MAGNETIC RESONANCE IMAGING

MRI can equal, if not surpass, other modalities in the detection of focal splenic lesions, provided rapid scanning techniques combined with compensation for respiratory and cardiac motion (with or without contrast agents) are used.

RADIONUCLIDE IMAGING

^{99m}Tc-sulphur or tin colloid scanning of the spleen for the detection of focal abnormalities has largely been replaced by cross-sectional imaging such as ultrasound, CT and MRI. Gallium citrate scanning may be helpful in investigating inflammatory conditions.

ANGIOGRAPHY

Selective catheterization and injection of contrast medium into the coeliac axis or splenic artery provides excellent visualization of the arteries and delayed images show the splenic and portal veins. In many patients it is possible to show the main splenic artery and normal splenic and portal veins using **intravenous digital subtraction angiography**. **Splenoportography**, achieved by injecting contrast medium through a cannula or needle introduced percutaneously into the splenic pulp, has now become obsolete.

SPLENIC NEOPLASMS

BENIGN NEOPLASMS OF SPLEEN

Splenic haemangiomas

Haemangiomas are the most common benign splenic neoplasms and have similar appearances to liver haemangiomas. On ultrasound, they are usually hyperechoic and calcification may cause bright echoes with acoustic shadowing. On CT, the lesion is hypodense before contrast and then, like liver haemangioma, 'fills in' after intravenous contrast medium (Fig. 5.66). In patients presenting acutely with rupture of a splenic haemangioma, CT may show perisplenic or intraperitoneal blood.

Hamartoma (splenoma, splenoadenoma, nodular hyperplasia of the spleen)

To date the ultrasound and CT appearances do not allow differentiation from haemangiomata.

MALIGNANT NEOPLASMS OF SPLEEN

Lymphoma

Splenic lymphoma is usually a manifestation of generalized lymphoma and is the most common splenic malignancy. Primary splenic lymphoma is rare and comprises only 2% of all lymphoma. Laparotomy with splenectomy reveals splenic involvement at

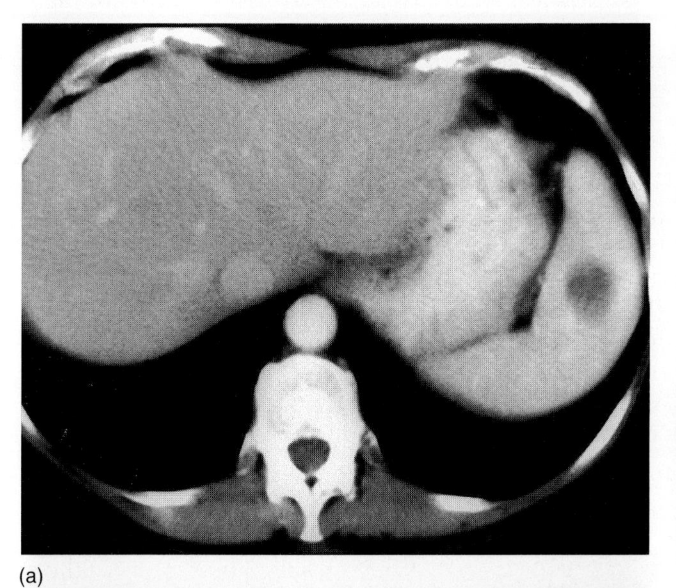

(a)

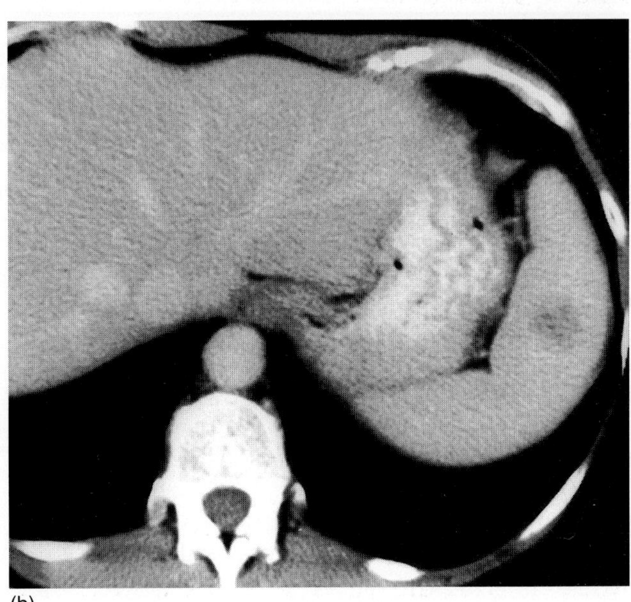

(b)

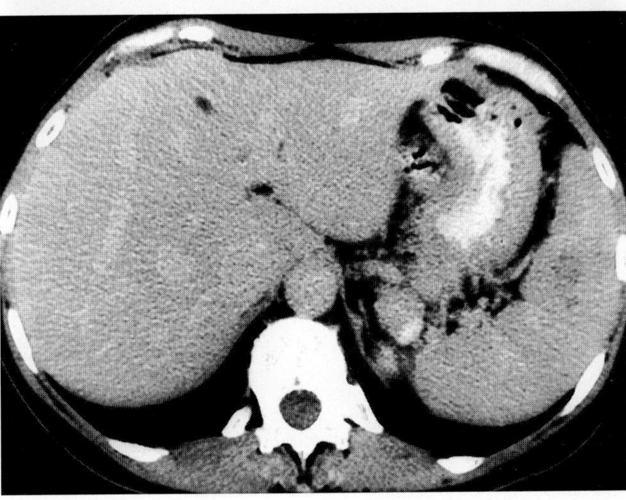

(c)

Fig. 5.66 Splenic haemangioma. (a) CT scan taken during intravenous injection of contrast medium showing a well-defined focal abnormality. (b) Scan taken after a delay of 3 minutes showing progressive enhancement of the margins of the lesion. (c) After 10 minutes further 'filling in' of the lesion is seen confirming the presence of a haemangioma.

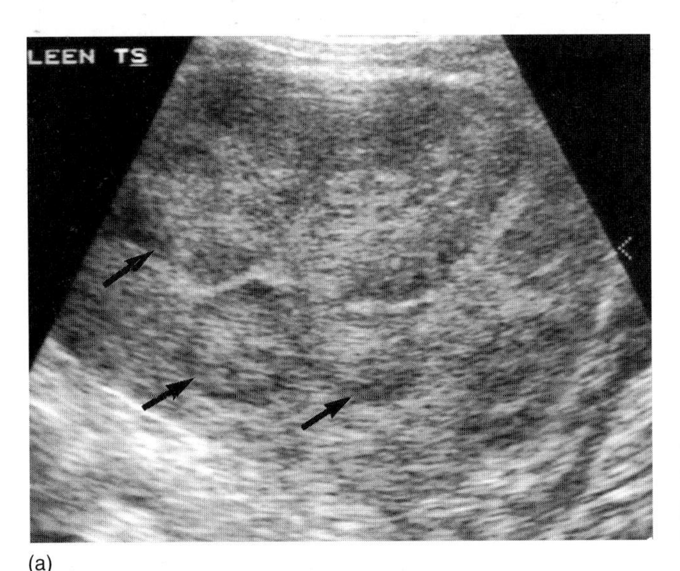

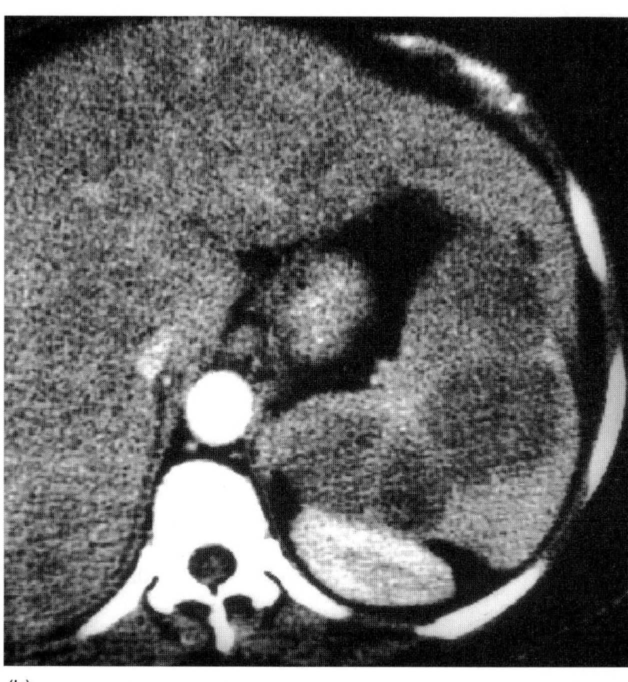

(a) (b)

Fig. 5.67 Non-Hodgkin's lymphoma of the spleen. (a) A longitudinal ultrasound scan of the liver showing multiple large inhomogeneous areas of abnormal echogenicity (arrows). (b) CT scan on the same patient showing the same focal abnormalities due to infiltration by non-Hodgkin's lymphoma.

presentation in 23–34% of patients with Hodgkin's disease and 30–40% of patients with non-Hodgkin's lymphoma. CT is the primary technique for diagnosing splenic lymphoma, evaluating the volume and extent of the tumour and monitoring response. However, CT is relatively insensitive for the detection of splenic involvement, partly because 45–70% of splenic tumours manifest with either diffuse tumour infiltration or tumour foci well under a centimetre in size.

The ultrasound, CT or MRI appearance of splenic lymphoma includes homogeneous enlargement without a discrete mass, a solitary mass, multifocal lesions, and diffuse infiltration. A poor correlation exists between the size of the spleen and the presence of splenic lymphoma. Splenomegaly does not always indicate involvement and a normal-sized spleen does not exclude disease. The majority of focal lesions are hypoechoic on ultrasound and of decreased density on CT before and after intravenous injection of contrast medium (Fig. 5.67). Diffuse infiltration may be seen as diffusely low echogenicity on ultrasound and diffusely low attenuation on CT before injection of contrast medium, and irregular enhancement after contrast medium. Infarction of the spleen is not uncommon and wedge-shaped peripheral areas of low CT attenuation may, therefore, be seen.

Non-lymphomatous tumours and metastases

The rare, primary, benign and malignant splenic tumours including angiosarcoma, lymphangioma, malignant fibrous histiocytoma, leiomyosarcoma and fibrosarcoma, all show a non-specific cystic, solid or complex mass.

Splenic metastases are found at autopsy in 7% of patients with malignancy but are seen relatively uncommonly on imaging. They occur most frequently from the breast, lung, ovary, stomach, cutaneous melanoma and prostate. The ultrasound

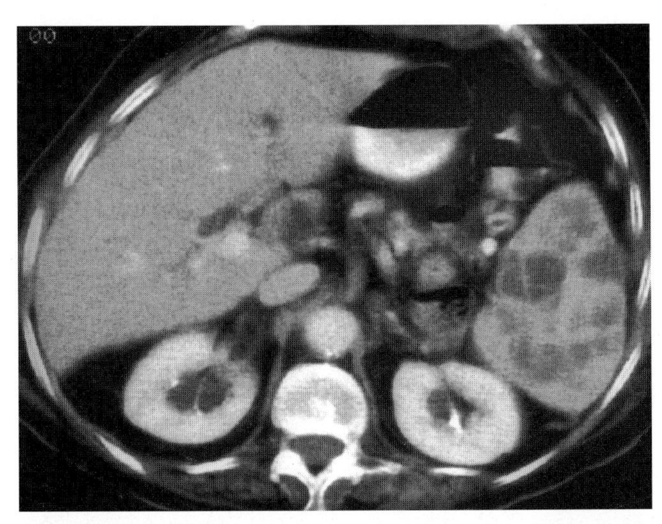

Fig. 5.68 Cystic splenic deposits. Contrast medium-enhanced CT scan showing multiple cystic lesions in the spleen in patient with disseminated malignant melanoma.

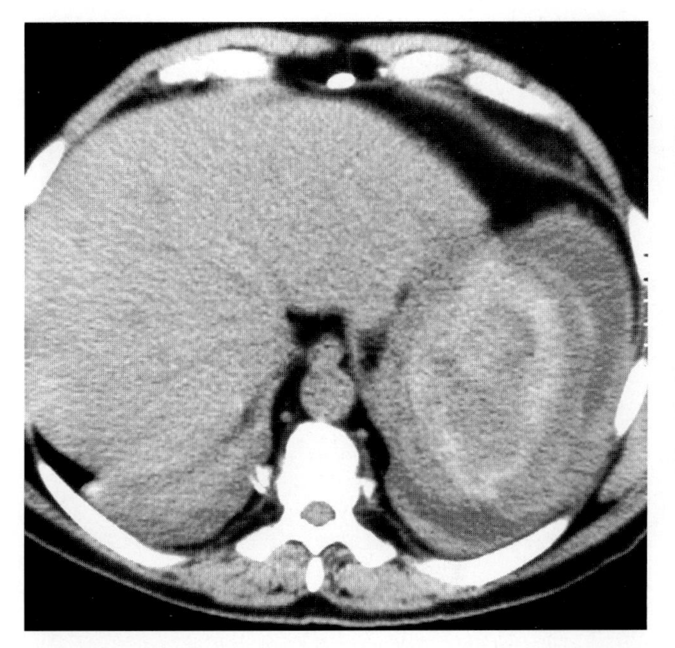

Fig. 5.69 Spontaneous rupture due to splenic deposit. Unenhanced CT scan showing high attenuation within the spleen due to a spontaneous bleed in a patient with disseminated breast cancer. Removal of the spleen revealed the presence of a deposit within it.

appearance of metastases varies greatly: they may be hypoechoic or hyperechoic. Cystic splenic metastases are seen typically in patients with melanoma, or primary tumours in the ovary, breast and endometrium (Fig. 5.68). Occasionally splenic metastases may present with a spontaneous splenic haemorrhage (Fig. 5.69). No correlation exists between the ultrasound features of metastases and the type of primary tumour. Lesions are more commonly multifocal than solitary. On CT, metastases are typically areas of slightly decreased attenuation in relation to normal spleen.

INFECTIONS OF SPLEEN

BACTERIAL ABSCESS

The frequency of splenic abscess has recently increased because of a rising number of immunocompromised people. Complications such as rupture and subsequent subphrenic abscess and peritonitis may result from delayed diagnosis. CT is currently the diagnostic method of choice because of its high sensitivity (up to 96%), non-invasiveness, applicability in unstable patients and value in allowing accurate localization of the lesion in relation to contiguous viscera. Bacterial abscess is frequently seen as a low-attenuation centre of fluid with peripheral contrast enhancement once a capsule has developed. The presence of gas within the fluid collection is

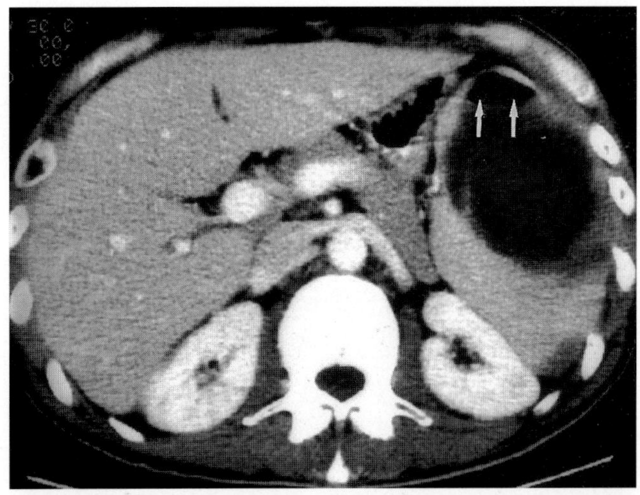

Fig. 5.70 Splenic abscess. CT scan performed after intravenous injection of contrast medium showing a large fluid-filled abscess with an air-fluid level anteriorly (arrows).

diagnostic of abscess, although the majority of splenic abscesses do not contain air (Fig. 5.70). A splenic abscess may contain septa of various thicknesses. Ultrasonography may be technically difficult because of an ileus, overlying ribs and perisplenic fluid, but has the advantage that it can be performed at the bedside if necessary. The ultrasound appearance depends on the stage of development. Initially there is an ill-defined mass of decreased echogenicity which may develop into a complex lesion with septations, debris and border nodularity. When a capsule has developed, the lesion is well-defined with a thick hyperechoic rim.

FUNGAL ABSCESSES

Fungal abscesses occur almost exclusively in immunocompromised individuals. Candida is the most frequent followed by Aspergillus and Cryptococcus. Because the lesions are often very small, fungal abscesses in neutropenic patients are not always detectable on imaging. On ultrasound they have a typical 'bull's-eye' appearance with bright central echogenic areas surrounded by a hyperechoic periphery (Fig. 5.71). On CT, typical lesions are smaller than 2 cm in diameter and are of relatively low attenuation (Fig. 5.71). Ring-like enhancement may be seen with contrast-enhanced CT on MR imaging. The appearance of *Pneumocystis carinii* infection can produce similar, multiple, small focal abnormalities early in the disease. With time, calcification may develop, often within a few months.

In patients with AIDS, the differential diagnosis of low-density lesions in the spleen includes fungal or mycobacterial infection, lymphoma or disseminated Kaposi's sarcoma.

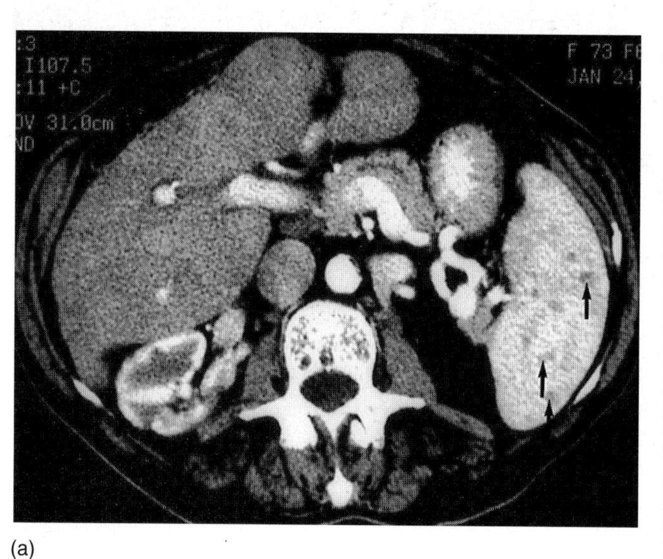

(a)

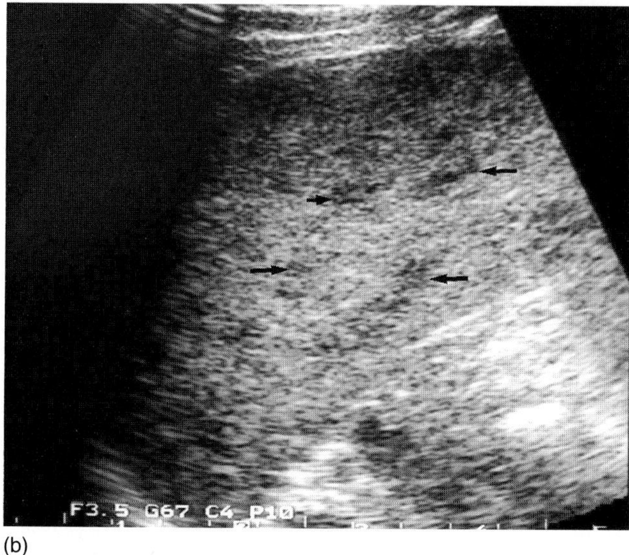

(b)

Fig. 5.71 Fungal abscesses within the spleen. (a) Contrast-enhanced scan in a patient with leukaemia showing multiple minute low-density foci within the spleen (arrows) due to candidal abscesses. (b) Longitudinal ultrasound of the spleen in the same patient showing multiple hypoechoic foci corresponding to the candidal abscesses (arrows).

SPLENIC TRAUMA

Splenic trauma may follow blunt or penetrating injuries and may be spontaneous or iatrogenic. In cases of blunt abdominal trauma, the spleen is the most commonly injured organ. Splenic injuries have been classified in a variety of ways, but a useful scheme is:

- contusion;
- subcapsular haematoma;
- parenchymal injury with small capsular tear;
- rupture with haemoperitoneum.

The need for imaging depends on the severity of the injury. Patients who are haemodynamically unstable are taken directly to laparotomy. Patients who are stable with suspected splenic injury should undergo CT as CT can be more than 95% accurate in identifying splenic injury. If CT is done after peritoneal lavage, it will be unclear whether the intraperitoneal fluid is from the initial trauma or the lavage. Thus if CT is to be used, peritoneal lavage should be delayed or omitted. Furthermore, haemoperitoneum can be diagnosed radiologically and the severity and extent of other organ injuries assessed.

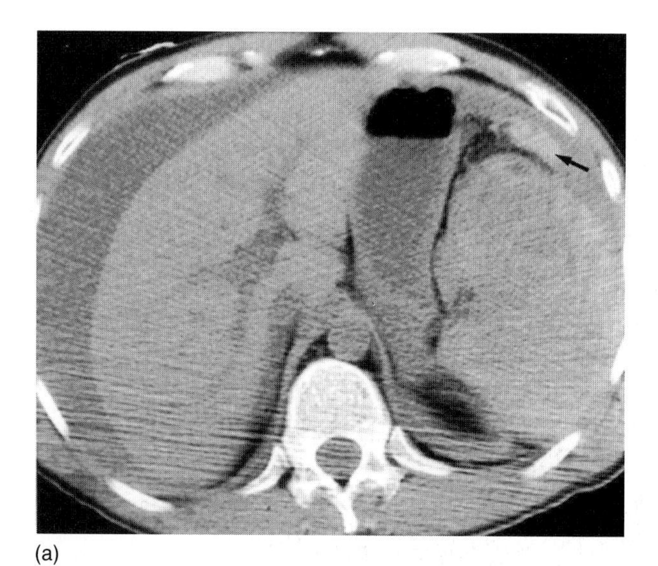

(a)

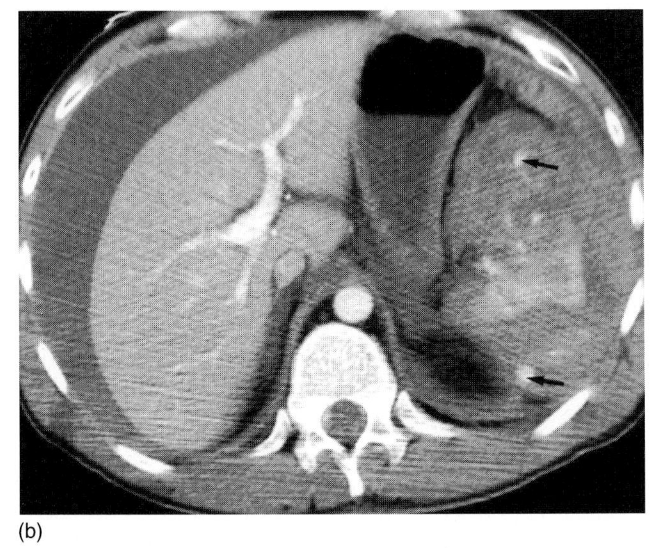

(b)

Fig. 5.72 Splenic trauma. (a) Precontrast CT scan showing high density soft tissue consistent with haematoma within the spleen, in the subcapsular region and in the extracapsular space (arrow). Ascites is also present around the liver. (b) After intravenous injection of contrast medium there is gross disruption of the splenic architecture with pools of contrast medium extravasating in the subcapsular haematoma (arrows). Non-enhancement of portions of the spleen are due to devascularization.

Plain film findings are necessary primarily to look for evidence of intraperitoneal or retroperitoneal air, pneumothorax and other injuries. When bleeding is confined to the parenchyma or subcapsular region, a plain film may show splenic enlargement with resultant displacement of the stomach. The presence of rib fracture(s), pleural effusion or severe gastric dilation should raise the possibility of significant splenic injury.

On **CT**, subcapsular haematomas are seen as peripheral low density lesions that flatten the contour of the spleen. Lacerations produce low-density bands across the splenic substance. Lacerations tend to involve the lateral aspect of the spleen and are associated with free intraperitoneal fluid. Splenic rupture may be seen as fragmentation of three or more sections of devascularized (non-enhanced) spleen (Fig. 5.72).

Although CT has now become established as the primary means of evaluating splenic trauma in the stable patient, it is not a useful predictor of outcome after splenic trauma, presumably because it fails to quantify active haemorrhage as opposed to inactive, old blood. Nevertheless, part of its value lies in the fact that a normal CT scan virtually excludes significant splenic injury.

SPLENIC CYSTS

Splenic cysts represent a heterogeneous group of lesions and include cystic neoplasms, parasitic cysts, 'true' and 'false' cysts. True cysts, also called primary, epithelial, epidermoid or congenital cysts, contain an epithelial lining, and false or pseudocysts are without an epithelial lining. False cysts are probably post-traumatic in origin and may be haemorrhagic or serous.

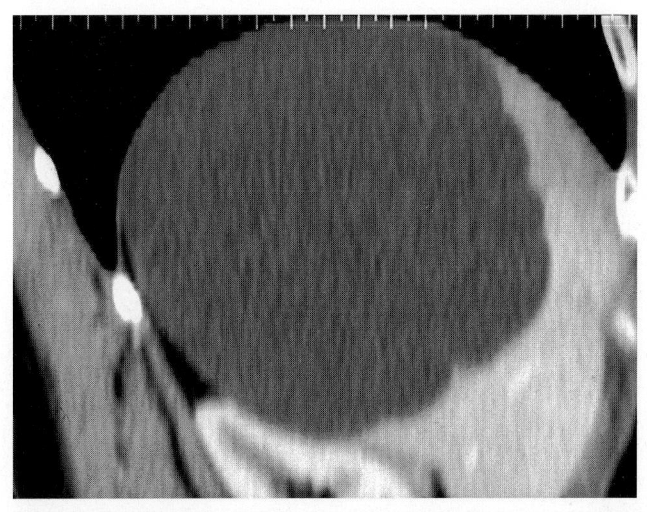

Fig. 5.73 Epitheloid ('true') cyst of the spleen. Longitudinal reconstruction of a contrast-enhanced CT scan showing a typically large epitheloid splenic cyst with scalloping of the splenic margin.

Plain films may show a left upper quadrant mass with elevation of the left hemidiaphragm with left lower lobe atelectasis. Curvilinear or plaque-like calcification may be present on plain abdominal films, more commonly in post-traumatic than true cysts. Ultrasound shows the usual features of a cyst. If haemorrhagic, ultrasound may demonstrate layering of two fluids within the cyst. Trabeculation may be seen. True cysts are well seen on CT (Fig. 5.73) and the differential diagnosis includes echinococcal cysts (which are usually multiseptated), large solitary abscess, haematoma, cystic neoplasm or an intrasplenic pancreatic pseudocyst.

CHAPTER 6

Adrenal glands

Rodney H. Reznek

IMAGING TECHNIQUES
NORMAL RADIOLOGICAL ANATOMY
IMAGING OF ADRENAL PATHOLOGY

IMAGING TECHNIQUES

COMPUTED TOMOGRAPHY

CT, because of its very high accuracy, has assumed the primary role in imaging the adrenal glands. A complete study of the adrenal gland involves narrow collimation (3 or 5 mm) scans through the adrenal gland both before and after intravenous injection of a bolus of contrast medium. Contrast medium will help to separate the adrenal glands from adjacent vessels and to assess the nature of an adrenal mass.

MAGNETIC RESONANCE IMAGING

MRI is now achieving adequate resolution, close to that of CT. With further experience in its use, MRI may well become the imaging investigation of choice in most cases of adrenal pathology.

ULTRASOUND

Ultrasound can demonstrate most adrenal masses >2 cm, but has far lower accuracy than CT or MRI, especially in obese patients.

RADIOPHARMACEUTICALS

Radiolabelled analogues of cholesterol such as ^{75}Se-6β-selenomethylnorcholesterol are used in the depiction and localization of adrenal cortical function. Appropriate imaging time intervals are dictated by the particular disease process under study and may require the addition of dexamethasone suppression studies of adrenal cortical function. Meta-iodobenzylguanidine (MIBG), an analogue of guanethidine, is concentrated in sympathoadrenal tissue. Studies with ^{131}I- and ^{123}I-MIBG take advantage of the ability to screen the whole body for sympathomedullary function. Imaging is performed 1 to 3 days following administration of the radiopharmaceuticals. Numerous drugs such as reserpine, tricyclic antidepressants and others interfere with the uptake of iodocholesterol into the adrenal cortex and MIBG into the sympathoadrenergic tissues, and must be avoided.

VENOUS SAMPLING

Venous sampling is extremely accurate in the preoperative localization of the source of abnormal hormone secretion. It is, however, an invasive procedure that is technically difficult to perform and necessitates long fluoroscopy times and consequently entails high radiation exposures. The technique usually requires hospitalization. Because of these disadvantages and the availability of less invasive procedures, venous sampling is best reserved for equivocal cases. Nevertheless, adrenal venous sampling is still used and is extremely accurate in the preoperative evaluation of primary aldosteronism. Whole body venous sampling is used in defining the source of ACTH-dependent Cushing's syndrome, ectopic sources of catecholamine excess and abnormal function in virilization syndromes.

PERCUTANEOUS BIOPSY

The accuracy of percutaneous adrenal biopsy ranges from 80 to 90%. Sonography can be used for imaging

Diagnostic and Interventional Radiology in Surgical Practice. Edited by P. Armstrong and M. L. Wastie. Published in 1997 by Chapman & Hall, London. ISBN 0 412 61960 1 (HB), 0 412 61970 9 (PB)

guidance if the adrenal mass and adjacent organs are sufficiently well demonstrated, but usually CT provides the best anatomical imaging for guidance. The most common complications are pneumothorax and haemorrhage. The major risk is biopsy of an unsuspected phaeochromocytoma, as a catecholamine storm following biopsy can be a life-threatening complication and is fatal in 50% of unsuspected phaeochromocytomas. The potential risk of this happening is high, since only 50% of patients with phaeochromocytomas have paroxysmal hypertensive episodes and 14% may have atypical or absent signs.

NORMAL RADIOLOGICAL ANATOMY

The adrenal glands are enclosed within the perinephric fascia and are usually surrounded by a sufficient amount of fat for identification on CT or MRI (Fig. 6.1). The right adrenal gland lies immediately posterior to the IVC, between the right crus of the diaphragm medially and the right lobe of the liver laterally. The left adrenal gland lies lateral to the aorta and the left crus of the diaphragm, anteromedial to the upper pole of the left kidney and posterior to the pancreas and splenic vessels. The adrenals normally extend over 2–4 cm in the craniocaudad direction. The shape of the adrenals can vary, depending on the orientation of the gland and the level of the image. The limbs of the adrenal gland have a uniform thickness and, on any cross-section, the normal thickness of these limbs, perpendicular to their long axes, does not exceed 4 mm, except at the apex of the gland where these limbs converge.

Demonstrating the normal adrenal glands and small adrenal lesions remains difficult on ultrasound, despite the introduction of high-resolution, real-time scanners. These small organs are high in location, deep within the rib cage, adjacent to the vertebrae, and are thus easily obscured by bone shadow and by stomach and bowel gas on ultrasound.

IMAGING OF ADRENAL PATHOLOGY

ADRENAL CORTICAL HYPERFUNCTION

Adrenal cortical hyperfunction includes primary hyperaldosteronism, Cushing's syndrome and androgen-producing lesions of the adrenal.

Conn's syndrome (primary hyperaldosteronism)
In 79% of cases, a benign cortical adenoma will be responsible for primary hyperaldosteronism; in 20%, the cause will be bilateral adrenal hyperplasia and very rarely an adrenocortical carcinoma will be responsible. As surgery should be considered for adenomas and bilateral hyperplasia is best treated medically, the distinction between these causes is extremely important. Imaging plays an important role in making this distinction.

Adrenal CT scanning is highly effective for the localization of small adrenocortical adenomas, which tend to be small, with an average size of approximately 1.6 cm, and of much lower density than the surrounding adrenal tissue (–18 HU to +13 HU), due to a high content of cytoplasmic lipid (Fig. 6.2a). These adenomas do not enhance significantly after intravenous injection of contrast medium and rarely calcify. As about 15–20% of aldosteronomas are

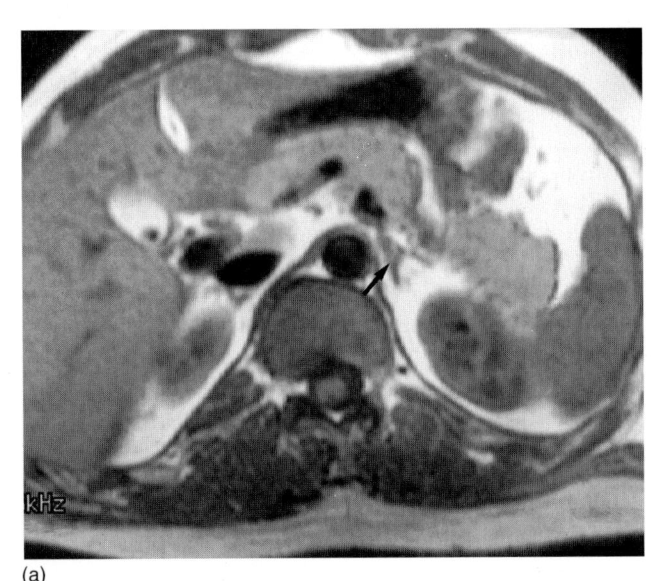

(a)

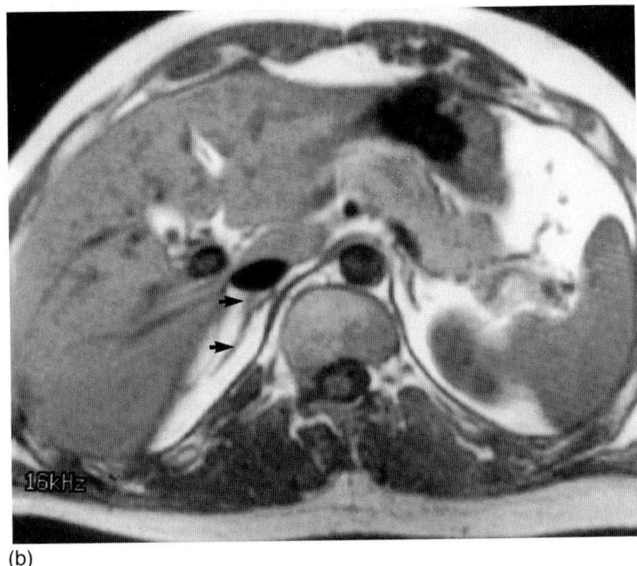

(b)

Fig. 6.1 (a) T1-weighted MRI scan showing normal left adrenal gland (arrow). (b) T1-weighted MRI scan showing normal right adrenal gland (arrows) lying posterior to the inferior vena cava.

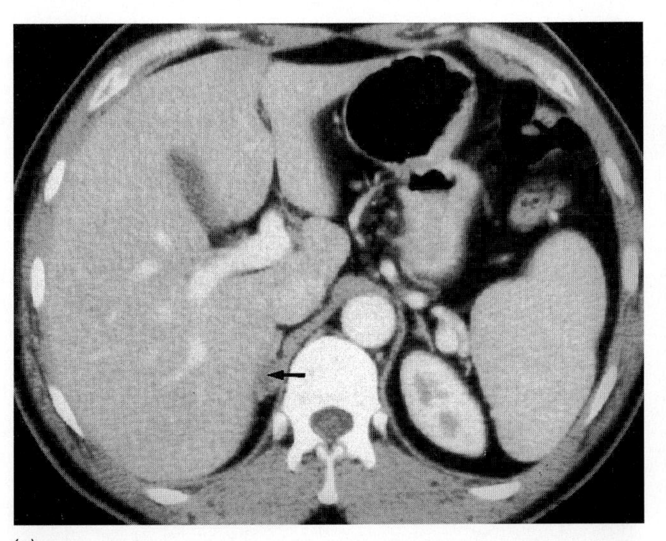

(a)

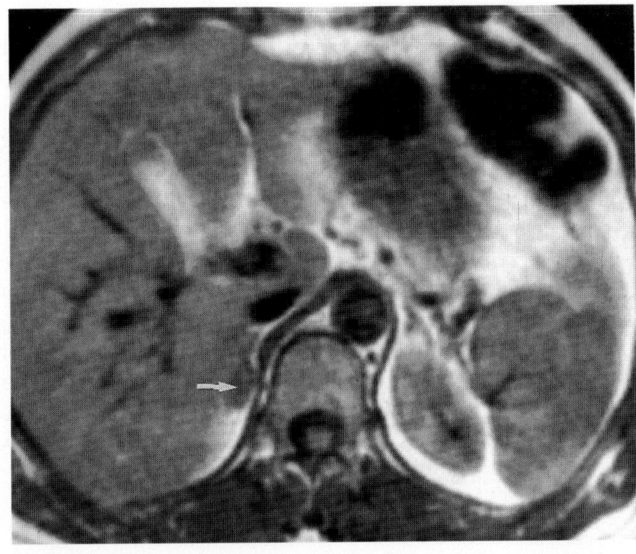

(b)

Fig. 6.2 Conn's tumour (a) CT scan after intravenous injection of contrast medium showing a small, low-density, non-enhancing mass in the right adrenal gland (arrow). (b) T1-weighted MRI scan showing the same small mass of low signal intensity (arrow).

micronodules, measuring <1 cm, meticulous examination technique is required to detect them, including very narrow collimation and magnification. The sensitivity of CT for detecting these small adenomas has improved markedly in recent years and currently about 90% of tumours will be detected. False-negative results arise when micronodules are missed. Conversely, CT cannot distinguish between aldosteronomas, macronodules in nodular hyperplasia and non-functioning adenomas, especially when the lesion is solitary. Nevertheless, false-positive results are infrequent, because the chance of a solitary adrenal mass in normal-sized glands, visualized by CT in the appropriate clinical and biochemical setting, being something other than an aldosteronoma, is extremely low. Similarly, although a macronodule in nodular hyperplasia can cause confusion, postural plasma aldosterone and 18-hydroxycorticosterone tests will provide an indication as to whether the patient has idiopathic hyperplasia or an adrenal adenoma.

At present, even with the use of surface coils, the sensitivity of MRI is slightly less than CT for detecting adrenal lesions < 1 cm in diameter. Most adenomas appear slightly hypointense or isointense relative to the liver on T1-weighted images (Figs 6.2b) and slightly hyperintense or isointense relative to hepatic parenchyma on T2 images. MRI has little advantage over CT in the evaluation of adrenal hyperplasia or in the identification of hyperfunctioning cortical adenomas which are best evaluated with thinly collimated CT sections.

The adrenal gland can be functionally characterized in primary aldosteronism using adrenal scintigraphy with a cholesterol-based radiopharmaceutical and dexamethasone suppression. This technique will distinguish between a unilateral adenoma and bilateral hyperplasia (Plate 3, opposite page 354). As with CT, the sensitivity of the technique is dependent partly on the size of the adenoma, and its accuracy compares unfavourably with that of CT. Because of this, and also because the procedure is time-consuming and expensive, it is seldom used as the initial investigation in patients with Conn's syndrome, except in cases considered equivocal on CT.

Venous sampling, when successful, is the most accurate means of localizing aldosteronomas. However, even in experienced hands, failure to catheterize the right adrenal vein occurs in 10–30% of cases. In those cases successfully catheterized, a sensitivity approaching 100% and a positive predictive value of 90% has been achieved. However, complications of the procedure are not infrequent and include adrenal infarction, adrenal vein thrombosis or perforation and intra-adrenal haemorrhage. Hypotensive crises and adrenal insufficiency may result.

In most institutions, in practice, CT is considered sufficiently accurate for localizing cortical adenomas to proceed to surgery without any further investigation, especially when the CT appearance is clear-cut and correlates with all the biochemistry. Venous sampling is reserved for those cases in which:

- the adrenal glands appear normal on CT (as a micronodule may be undetected);
- where there are bilateral nodules on CT scans which may be due to nodular hyperplasia or multiple adenomata;
- where there is disagreement between the CT findings and the biochemistry.

Cushing's syndrome

Biochemical studies, including determination of plasma ACTH levels and response to high-dose dexamethasone suppression, are used to distinguish between Cushing's disease, ectopic ACTH-producing tumours and cortisol-producing adrenal neoplasms. While these tests are usually successful in making this distinction, difficulties in interpretation can arise. The purpose of imaging is to localize or exclude an adrenal mass and, when the biochemical tests point to an ectopic source of ACTH, to identify the source. In 75% of cases, Cushing's syndrome results from an excess of ACTH production, of which about 80% is due to a pituitary abnormality (Cushing's disease) and the remainder is due to an ectopic source. In 25% of cases the syndrome is due to excess cortisol from an adrenal neoplasm, more commonly an adenoma than a carcinoma. Adrenal cortical adenomas resulting in Cushing's syndrome are usually >2.0 cm and are thus readily detected on any cross-sectional technique. On CT, these masses are of soft-tissue density, although occasionally they show lower density due to a high fat content. The mass may enhance after intravenous injection of contrast medium (Fig. 6.3).

Adenomas >2 cm may well be demonstrated on ultrasound (Fig 6.3). The ultrasound reflectivity of adenomas is low compared to the high reflectivity of the surrounding fat. A right adrenal mass typically compresses the inferior vena cava or displaces it forward, and may indent the inferior surface of the

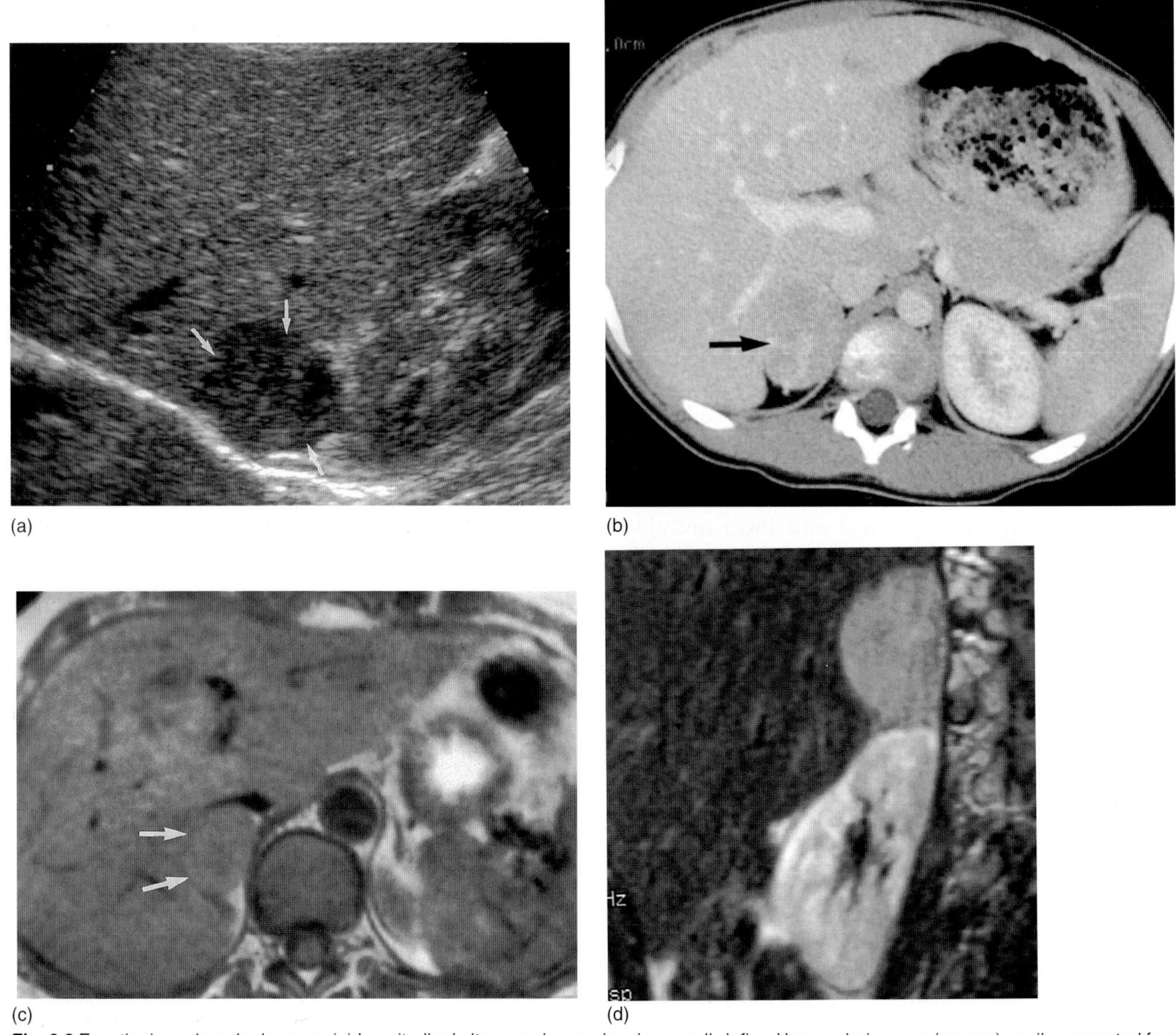

(a) (b) (c) (d)

Fig. 6.3 Functioning adrenal adenoma. (a) Longitudinal ultrasound scan showing a well-defined hypoechoic mass (arrows) easily separated from the upper pole of the right kidney. (b) CT scan after intravenous injection of contrast medium showing the right adrenal mass (arrow). (c) T1-weighted MRI scan showing the adrenal mass of low signal intensity (arrows). (d) Longitudinal T2-weighted MRI scan showing the adrenal mass of intermediate signal intensity.

liver. Whilst all tumours are usually homogeneous, heterogeneous reflectivity due to focal areas of necrosis or haemorrhage may be seen in larger masses.

MRI also readily identifies functioning adrenal adenomas and, because of their relatively large size, identifies them with similar sensitivity to CT. As with adenomas in Conn's syndrome, functioning adenomas are usually of low signal intensity relative to the liver on T1-weighted images and isointense or hyperintense relative to the liver on T2-weighted images (Fig. 6.3).

On all imaging techniques, the contralateral gland appears normal but, rarely, it may appear atrophic due to the suppression of ACTH.

Imaging with cholesterol-based radiopharmaceuticals is not usually performed except where the diagnosis is problematical. The usual pattern then is of unilateral activity in the functioning adenoma with virtual absence of uptake of the radiopharmaceutical in the contralateral gland.

Adrenal carcinomas account for 10–15% of cases of Cushing's syndrome (Fig. 6.4), almost always exceed 6 cm at the time of presentation and are readily detected on ultrasound, CT or MRI. Only about 15% of carcinomas are < 6 cm in diameter. Ultrasound can be extremely useful in distinguishing between a primary adrenal or renal mass because it is easy to scan in the longitudinal plane, (Figs 6.4a, b), the optimal plane for making this distinction. On CT, adrenal tumours are usually heterogeneous with areas of high and low density, which enhance patchily after intravenous enhancement of contrast medium (Fig. 6.4c). On MRI they are also usually inhomogeneous on T1- and T2-weighted images, showing areas of low and high signal intensity on both sequences (Figs 6.4d,e). Invasion of adjacent viscera such as the liver and venous structures is common. All three techniques can readily evaluate extension of thrombus into the inferior vena cava, although MRI most accurately predicts the true extent of the involvement of the entire inferior vena cava, including the intra- and infrahepatic portions. Direct involvement of the adjacent lymph nodes and extension into the liver and adjacent bones is equally well assessed on CT or MRI.

There is usually no uptake of cholesterol-based radiopharmaceutical by adrenal cortical carcinoma. Very rarely, a well differentiated carcinoma may show uptake, but in clinical practice, failure of uptake by a large adrenal mass in a patient with or without Cushing's disease is good evidence of a malignancy.

The differential diagnosis for an adrenal mass in a patient with Cushing's syndrome includes a functioning adenoma, a carcinoma, a metastasis from an ACTH-producing primary carcinoma elsewhere in the body, an incidental non-cortisol-producing adenoma, or even an ACTH-producing phaeochromocytoma.

The adrenals in ACTH-dependent Cushing's syndrome become hyperplastic pathologically. In about one-third of patients, hyperplastic adrenal glands look normal on CT or MRI. In some, the gland appears smoothly enlarged, with preservation of the normal contours of the gland. When there is nodular hyperplasia pathologically, a nodular configuration may be seen together with the diffuse enlargement on CT or MRI. Multiple nodules of varying size are usually seen but infrequently one of the nodules becomes dominant, reaching up to 4–5 cm in size and can be misdiagnosed as a unilateral adenoma, especially if the biochemical findings are equivocal.

There is a rare cause of Cushing's syndrome – primary, pigmented nodular cortical disease – in which multiple small nodules demonstrated on imaging, produce cortisol autonomously in the absence of elevated ACTH levels. This condition is indistinguishable on CT or MRI from secondary nodular hyperplasia.

Androgen-producing tumours of the adrenal gland

The role of imaging techniques in the evaluation of patients with virilism centres on the detection or exclusion of a tumour, or other surgically curable sources of androgen excess, in the adrenals, ovaries or testes. Androgen-producing tumours of the adrenals are rare; they are usually carcinomas, adenomas being less common. They usually exceed 2 cm in diameter and have the same characteristics described elsewhere for adenomas and carcinomas.

The commonest adrenal cause of excess androgens is congenital adrenocortical hyperplasia, usually the result of an inborn enzyme deficiency causing a partial block in adrenocortical steroids synthesis. The compensatory elevation of ACTH results in gross enlargement of the adrenals, easily recognizable on CT or MRI (Fig. 6.5). The adrenals, particularly when imaged in older patients, are likely to be so large as to simulate adrenal mass lesions.

CT has a limited role in the localization of extra-adrenal sources of virilizing syndromes because of the ionizing radiation dose to the gonads of patients who are often young. MRI is the best technique to image both the adrenal glands and the ovaries.

ADRENAL MEDULLARY TUMOURS

Neuroblastoma

Neuroblastoma is one of the most common tumours of childhood with 80% occurring in children under 5 years of age and a third under 2 years; 50–80% arise in the adrenal medulla, but the posterior mediastinum is the second most common site. Up to three-quarters have metastases at the time of presentation.

Ultrasound almost always demonstrates a mass which must be distinguished from other causes of abdominal masses such as a nephroblastoma. Neuroblastomas are typically heterogeneous on ultrasound

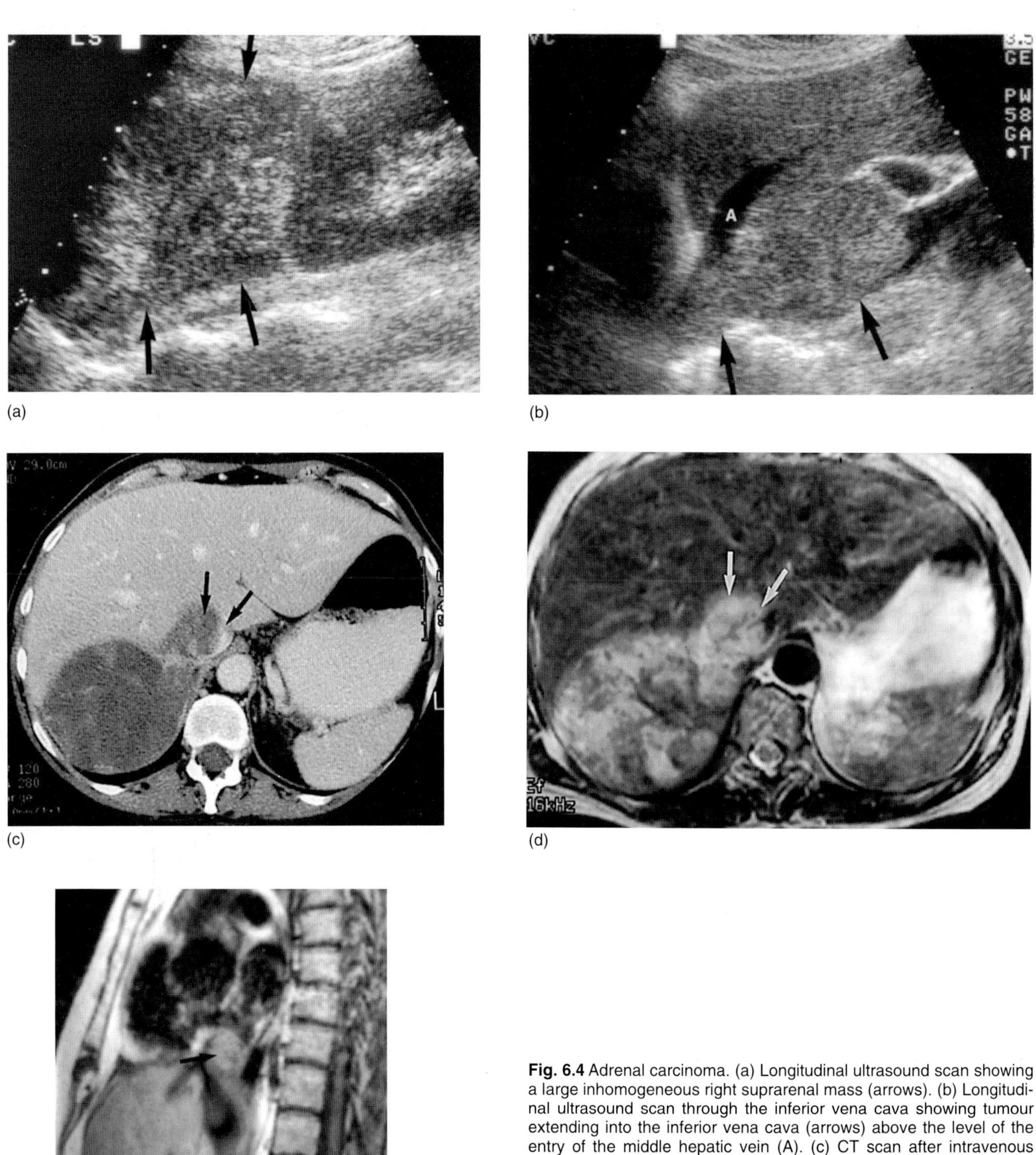

Fig. 6.4 Adrenal carcinoma. (a) Longitudinal ultrasound scan showing a large inhomogeneous right suprarenal mass (arrows). (b) Longitudinal ultrasound scan through the inferior vena cava showing tumour extending into the inferior vena cava (arrows) above the level of the entry of the middle hepatic vein (A). (c) CT scan after intravenous injection of contrast medium showing the right suprarenal mass extending into the inferior vena cava (arrows). (d) MRI axial T2-weighted image showing the suprarenal mass of mixed signal intensity extending into the inferior vena cava (arrows). (e) MRI longitudinal T1-weighted image showing thrombus within the IVC (arrows) extending above the level of the diaphragm into the right atrium.

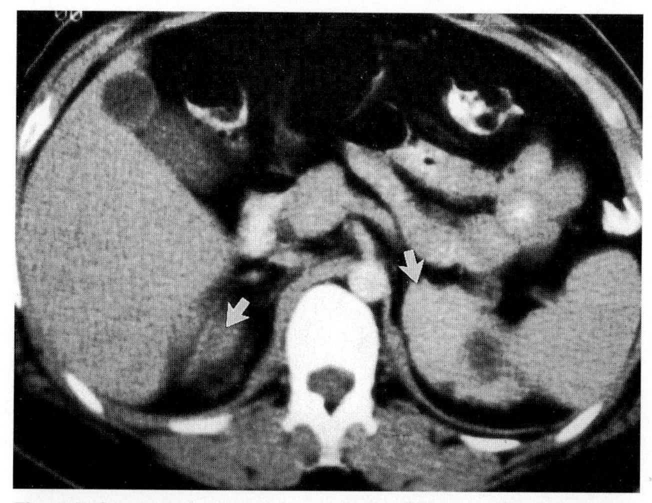

Fig. 6.5 Congenital adrenal hyperplasia. CT scan after intravenous injection of contrast medium showing massive bilateral adrenal enlargement (arrows).

with areas of high reflectivity which represent calcification. The margins of the tumour are usually ill-defined. Neuroblastomas often cross the midline and encase the coeliac and superior mesenteric vessels. Ultrasound is usually the first investigation but is often limited in showing the exact extent of the mass. It is, however, particularly valuable in monitoring the response of the tumour to chemotherapy.

On CT, the tumour is recognized as an irregular, pararenal soft-tissue mass which is lobulated, but has no definable rim or pseudocapsule (Fig. 6.6). On non-contrast enhanced scans, the mass usually has a density lower than that of surrounding tissues. Intravenous administration of contrast medium accentuates this difference. Calcification within the tumour,

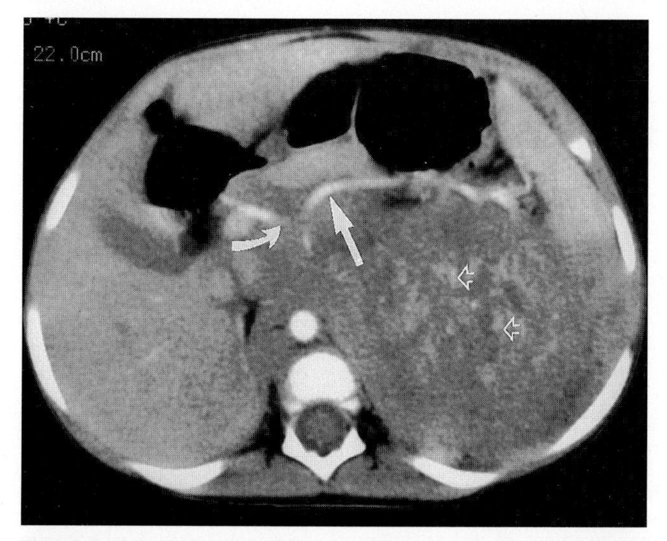

Fig. 6.6 Neuroblastoma. CT scan after intravenous injection of contrast medium showing a large inhomogeneous mass originating in the left adrenal, extending across the midline and encasing the splenic (arrow) and hepatic (curved arrow) arteries. Calcification is demonstrated (open arrows).

which can be coarse, mottled, solid or ring-shaped, can be observed in almost 85% of neuroblastomas on CT, whereas plain radiographs identify calcification in only 50% of patients. Prevertebral extension across the midline, which occurs in up to 60% of patients, is well demonstrated, as are encasement of the aorta and inferior vena cava, hepatic metastases and renal invasion.

On MRI, neuroblastoma has a low signal intensity relative to hepatic parenchyma on T1-weighted sequences, which increases relative to the liver on T2-weighting. Tumour heterogeneity is best demonstrated on T2-weighted sequences, and reflects calcification and necrosis. MRI is superior to CT in defining vascular encasement, hepatic metastases and particularly intraspinal extension through the intervertebral foramina, which occurs in 15% of patients (see Fig. 4.26 p. 117). MRI is thus currently the most accurate imaging method for staging the extent of the disease.

Neuroblastomas may also take up MIBG; in a small group of patients this can be shown to be more accurate than CT or MRI, usually by showing bony metastases.

Ganglioneuroblastoma and ganglioneuroma Ganglioneuroblastoma is a malignant tumour comprised of both primitive and differentiated cells; it may be totally or partially encapsulated. Ganglioneuroma is a benign tumour that is well circumscribed and consists entirely of ganglion cells. Both appear as soft-tissue masses with flecks of calcification. Differentiation of the various types of ganglion tumours requires tissue sampling.

Phaeochromocytoma

Phaeochromocytoma (also termed adrenal paraganglionoma) is a catecholamine-producing tumour which arises from the paraganglion cells. These cells are derived from the neural crest in close association with the autonomic ganglion cells, and paraganglionomas may thus arise anywhere from the neck to the bladder; 98%, however, originate in the abdomen and 90% arise in the adrenal medulla. Most extra-adrenal phaeochromocytomas arise in the paravertebral sympathetic ganglia, in the aortic bifurcation, and rarely in the bladder. Neuroectodermal disorders such as neurofibromatosis, tuberous sclerosis, von Hippel-Lindau syndrome or multiple endocrine neoplastic syndrome are associated with 10% of phaeochromocytomas. Multiplicity and malignancy, each of which occur in about 10% of cases, are more frequent when phaeochromocytomas occur in association with other diseases. Malignancy is also more frequent when the tumour is extra-adrenal. Tumours are more frequently non-functioning when extra-adrenal and when present as part of a systemic disorder. About 90% of adrenal medullary phaeochromocytomas are functional, whereas only 50% of sympathetic and 1% of parasympathetic tumours are functional.

On **ultrasound scanning** phaeochromocytomas are typically well-defined, round or ovoid masses with uniform reflectivity (Fig. 6.7a). Large tumours frequently undergo necrosis or haemorrhage with loss of homogeneity. The accuracy of ultrasound for detecting phaeochromocytomas is less than CT, MRI or MIBG scintigraphy, particularly for detecting small masses in the left adrenal gland or ectopic masses in the retroperitoneum where the ultrasound beam can be obscured by bowel gas.

On **CT**, in sporadic cases of phaeochromocytomas, unassociated with any syndrome, over 90% of masses will exceed 2 cm, with an average size of 5 cm. The lesions are often smaller when detected in patients with multiple endocrine abnormalities as they are often specifically sought. On unenhanced scans, these tumours are of similar density to surrounding soft-tissue structures. Calcification, usually speckled, occurs in about 12% of tumours. The hallmark of phaeochromocytomas is intense enhancement after intravenous injection of a bolus of contrast medium. Not infrequently, the tumours undergo marked necrosis so that the mass may have a fluid-filled centre (Fig. 6.7b). Nevertheless, marked enhancement of a

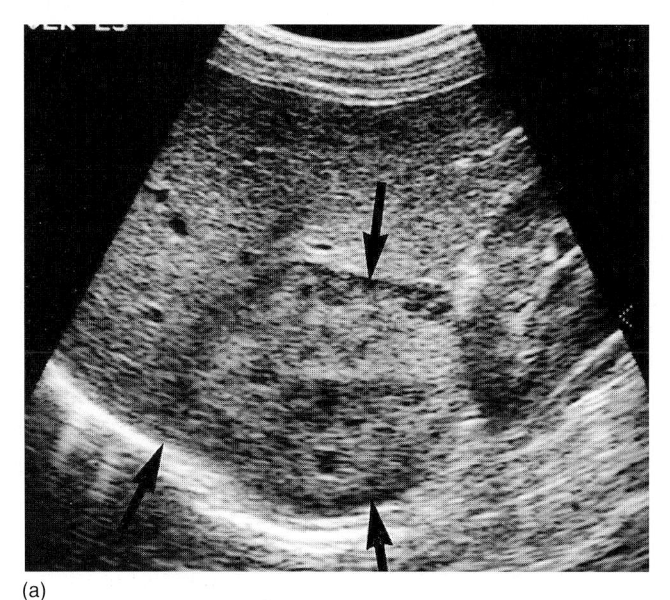

(a)

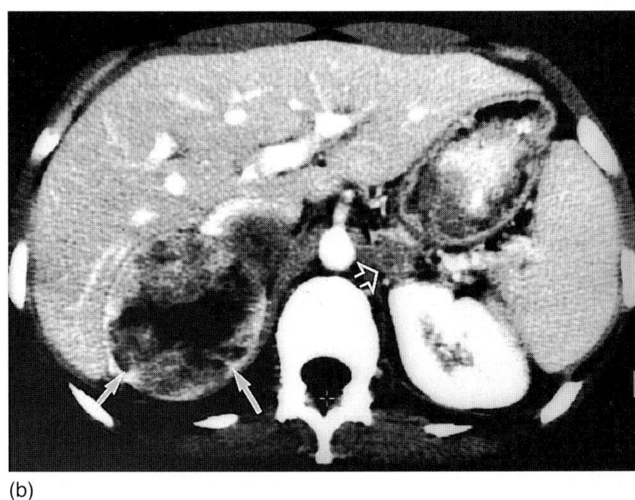

(b)

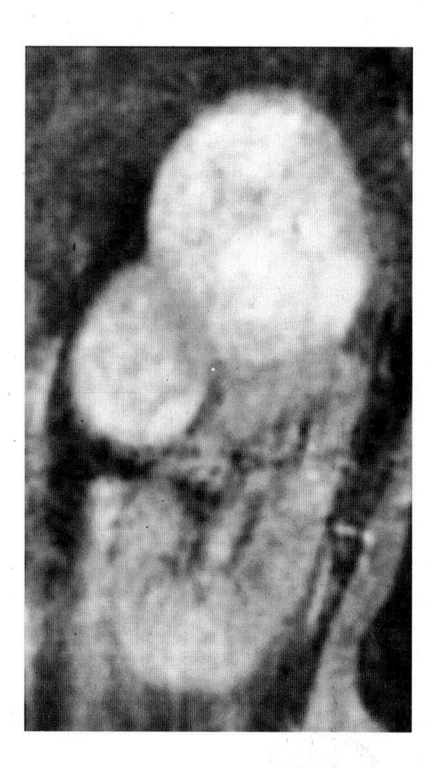

(c)

Fig. 6.7 Phaeochromocytoma. (a) Longitudinal ultrasound scan showing an inhomogeneous right-sided suprarenal mass (arrows). (b) CT scan after intravenous injection of contrast medium showing enhancement of the periphery of the lesion (arrows) with central necrosis. A small phaeochromocytoma is seen on the contralateral side (open arrow). (c) Longitudinal T2-weighted MRI scan showing typical high signal intensity in bilobed suprarenal mass.

peripheral soft-tissue part of the mass can usually be shown. As intravenous injection of contrast medium can precipitate a hypertensive crisis in some patients, α-adrenergic blockade is routine prior to performing the CT. The overall accuracy of CT for detecting adrenal phaeochromocytomas is very high with sensitivities ranging from 93 to 100%, and a positive predictive value exceeding 90%. This exceeds the accuracy of CT for detecting extra-adrenal paraganglionomas.

Meta-iodobenzylguanidine (MIBG) is an analogue of noradrenaline used for sympathoadrenal imaging. Paraganglionomas, including phaechromocytomas, are depicted as abnormal focal collections of activity. ^{123}I- or ^{131}I-MIBG scintigraphy is especially useful for the detection of ectopic phaechromocytomas and also for detecting metastatic or locally recurrent disease because, unlike ultrasound, CT or MRI, it is inherently a whole body imaging technique. The sensitivity of MIBG scintigraphy for detecting functioning phaeochromocytomas is slightly less than 90%; the specificity exceeds 90%. A positive MIBG always requires correlation with CT or MRI.

CT and MRI are equally accurate for identifying adrenal phaeochromocytomas. The multiplanar capability of **MRI** gives it the advantage of being slightly more accurate than CT for detecting extra-adrenal phaechromocytomas. On T1-weighted images, phaeochromocytomas show similar or slightly lower signal intensity than the liver, but most cases of phaeochromocytomas reported in the literature have been markedly hyperintense on T2-weighted images (Fig. 6.7c). This feature gives MRI a higher specificity than CT for differentiating between cortical adenomas and phaeochromocytomas when the biochemistry is equivocal.

The choice of initial investigation in a patient suspected of having a phaeochromocytoma depends on several factors other than accuracy, as CT, MRI and MIBG scintigraphy are of roughly equal sensitivity. MIBG has the advantage of allowing assessment of the whole body, but is not universally available, is very expensive and, because of poor spatial resolution, always requires supplementary imaging. Also, in patients with associated syndromes, MIBG scintigraphy will not demonstrate other associated tumours such as renal cell carcinoma, islet-cell tumours, neurofibromas or the other tumours which comprise the various multiple endocrine neoplastic syndromes. In time, CT may be replaced by MRI as the predominant imaging modality for adrenal phaeochromocytomas as it has the advantages of non-ionizing radiation, improved specificity and multiplanar display.

ADRENAL DISORDERS NOT RESULTING IN INCREASED HORMONAL ACTIVITY

Metastasis

Tumours of the lung, kidney, melanoma, breast and digestive tract are the most common primary sites to metastasize to the adrenal glands. The presence of an adrenal mass in a patient with a known malignancy does not necessarily indicate metastatic disease as 40–50% will turn out to be non-metastatic, representing adenomas rather than metastases.

On CT, metastases tend to be of soft-tissue density, inhomogeneous, with irregular margins; they enhance inhomogeneously after intravenous injection of contrast medium. They are more commonly unilateral than bilateral. On MRI, they are typically hypointense compared to the liver on T1-weighted imaging and relatively hyperintense on T2-weighted imaging. Features that favour malignancy include a size >3 cm, poorly defined margins, heterogenous internal architecture and no imaging evidence of fat contained within the mass.

Adenomas

Incidental, silent adenomas with a diameter of 1–3 cm are detected in 0.6–1.0% of upper abdominal CT examinations performed for indications other than for the detection of adrenal disease. On CT (Fig. 6.8a), they are characteristically round, well-defined in outline, homogeneous, without a perceptible wall, and usually are of low density due to relatively large amounts of lipid. They enhance only minimally after intravenous injection of contrast medium. These criteria usually allow a confident distinction between a metastasis and an adenoma. Cholesterol-based scintigraphy usually shows increased uptake in an adenoma compared with a normal gland. Distorted, absent or reduced uptake on the suspect side suggests pathology such as a carcinoma, metastasis or other space-occupying lesion.

Most adenomas appear either slightly hypointense or isointense relative to the liver on MRI T1-weighted images and slightly hyperintense or isointense relative to the hepatic parenchyma on T2-weighted images (Figs 6.8 b,c). As with adrenal metastasis, atypical adenomas exist that can be considerably hyperintense, relative to the liver on T2-weighted images.

Adrenal carcinoma

About 60% of adrenal carcinomas are non-functioning, the remainder can result in Cushing's syndrome, hyperaldosteronism, virilization or precocious puberty. The characteristic features on imaging are described earlier in this chapter.

Infection

Tuberculosis of the adrenal glands has increased in frequency recently, particularly in immunocompromised patients. The appearance of the gland on CT varies with the stage of infection. Involvement is usually bilateral and, if active, the glands are enlarged and inhomogeneous in density. Punctate calcification is a feature (Fig. 6.9). After intravenous injection of contrast medium, numerous small, non-enhancing

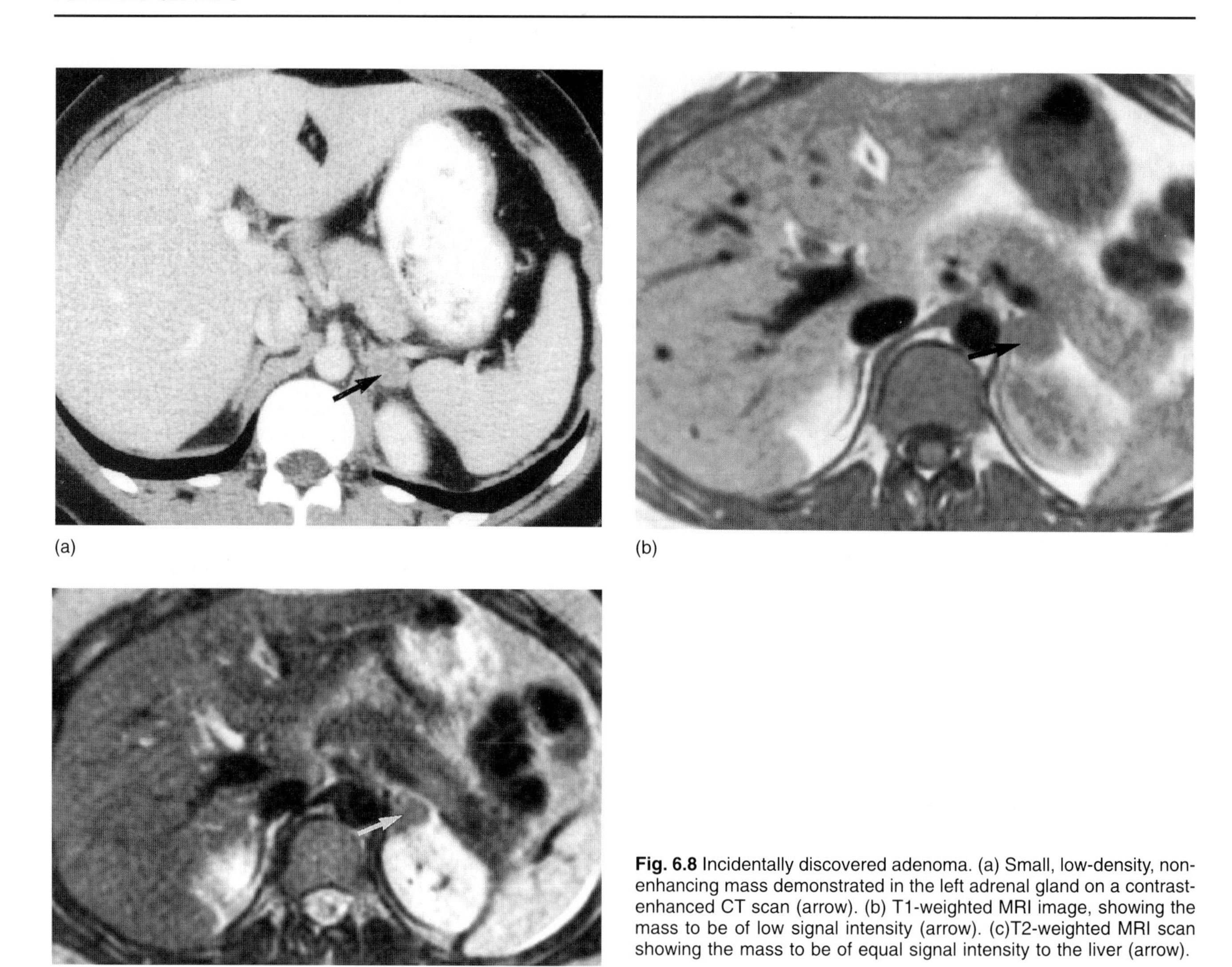

Fig. 6.8 Incidentally discovered adenoma. (a) Small, low-density, non-enhancing mass demonstrated in the left adrenal gland on a contrast-enhanced CT scan (arrow). (b) T1-weighted MRI image, showing the mass to be of low signal intensity (arrow). (c)T2-weighted MRI scan showing the mass to be of equal signal intensity to the liver (arrow).

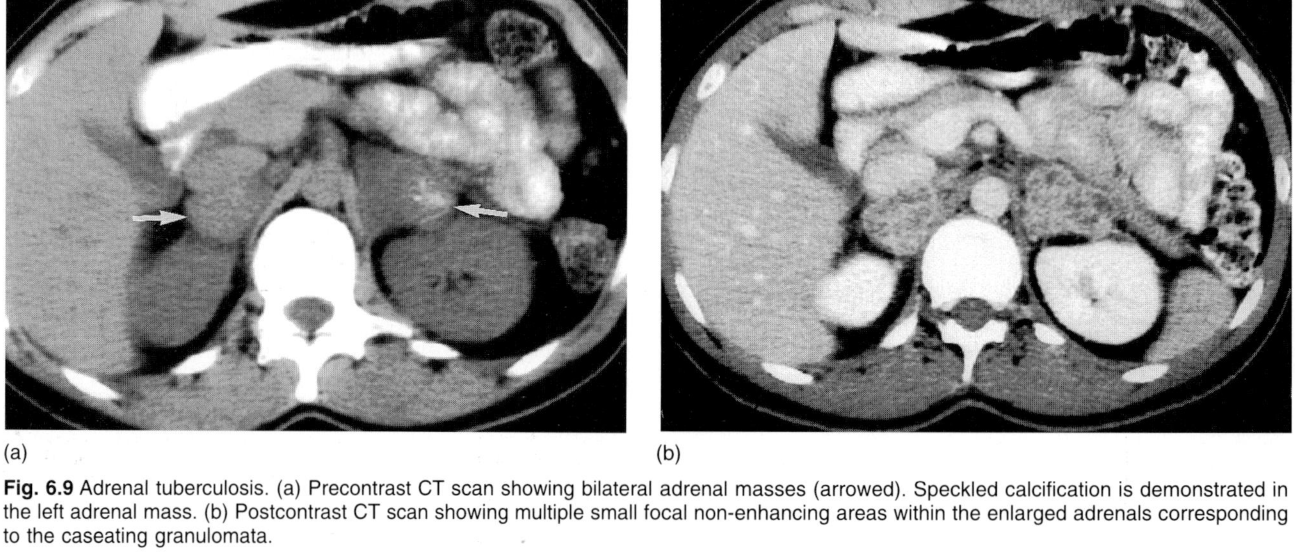

(a) (b)

Fig. 6.9 Adrenal tuberculosis. (a) Precontrast CT scan showing bilateral adrenal masses (arrowed). Speckled calcification is demonstrated in the left adrenal mass. (b) Postcontrast CT scan showing multiple small focal non-enhancing areas within the enlarged adrenals corresponding to the caseating granulomata.

areas representing caseous necrosis can often be identified. Long-standing tuberculosis results in atrophic glands.

Haemorrhage

Bilateral adrenal haemorrhage is usually associated with anticoagulant therapy (or other bleeding disorders) or with stress caused by surgery, burns and hypotension. Most cases of massive bilateral cortical haemorrhage in fulminant septicaemia occur in infants or children, but can occur in adults. On CT, the adrenals are usually bilaterally markedly enlarged and often mass-like (Fig. 6.10). If the adrenals are examined in the acute or subacute phase, the density of the enlarged adrenal is markedly increased and follow-up study shows a decrease in density. The increase in density of the centre of the gland is characteristic of adrenal haemorrhage.

Bilateral adrenal haemorrhage due to blunt abdominal trauma is very unusual. It is usually unilateral, results from injury to the right side of the abdomen, and is associated with ipsilateral visceral injury. It is seen in only 3% of children who have CT after blunt abdominal trauma.

Adrenal cysts

On CT, ultrasound and MRI, adrenal cysts have the same characteristics as cysts seen elsewhere in the body: fluid density, a clearly defined margin, a thin wall, and on CT and MRI, no enhancement after intravenous injection of contrast medium (Fig. 6.11). On CT, small adenomata, when they show uniform low density of their content, may simulate a cyst on CT, but unlike cysts, small adenomata usually enhance after intravenous injection of contrast medium. Endothelial cysts account for 45% of all adrenal cysts; the remainder being epithelial, parasitic or pseudocysts. They are almost always unilateral and detected incidentally. Pseudocysts are thought to represent the result of previous haemorrhage.

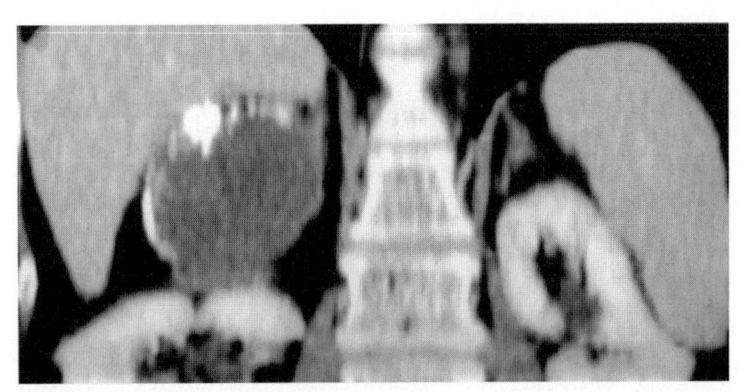

Fig. 6.11 Adrenal endothelial cyst. Coronal reconstruction on a spiral CT scan showing a benign right suprarenal cyst with calcification in the wall.

Lymphoma

Involvement of the adrenals in lymphoma is usually a part of widespread lymphoma, being detected in about 5% of cases of non-Hodgkin's lymphoma. Primary lymphoma is extremely rare. On CT, secondary adrenal lymphoma usually appears as solid homogeneous masses of soft-tissue density which enhance slightly after intravenous injection of contrast medium (Fig. 6.12).

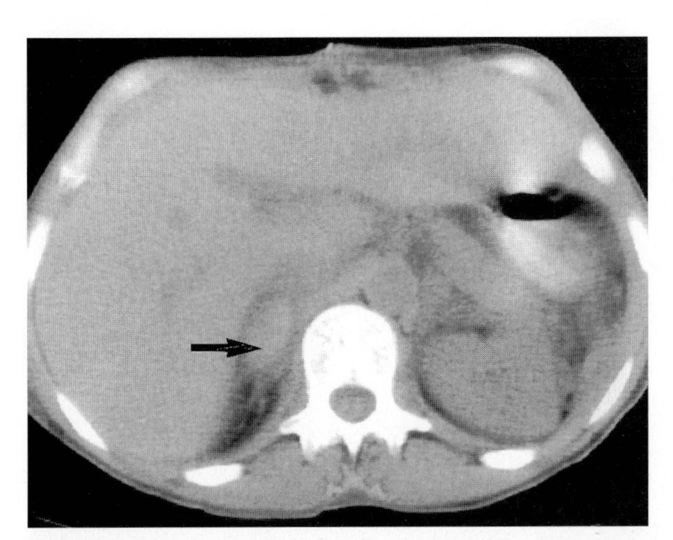

Fig. 6.10 Adrenal haemorrhage. Precontrast CT scan showing bilateral adrenal enlargement in a patient who had recently undergone a splenectomy for hypersplenism due to myelofibrosis. High-density haemorrhage is seen within the enlarged right adrenal gland (arrow).

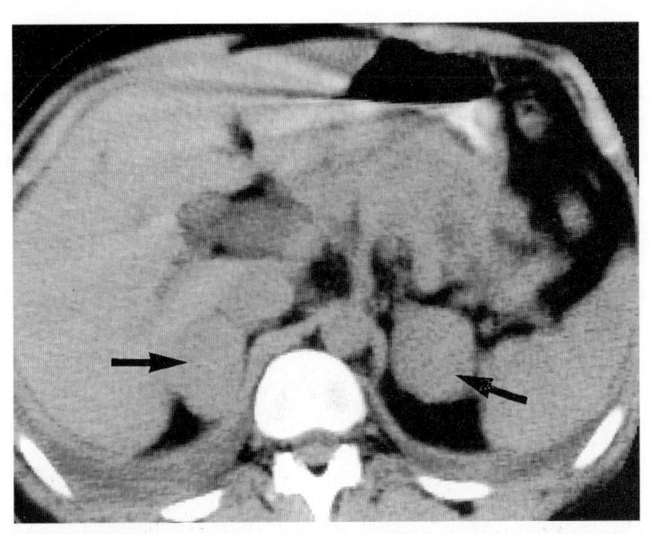

Fig. 6.12 Adrenal lymphoma. Bilateral adrenal masses demonstrated in both adrenal glands due to infiltration with high grade non-Hodgkin's lymphoma (arrows). A retroperitoneal mass due to lymph node infiltration is also seen.

Myelolipoma

Myelolipoma is a rare benign neoplasm composed of fat and bone marrow elements in varying proportions, and is usually incidentally discovered in asymptomatic patients. Occasionally, spontaneous haemorrhage may cause pain. The diagnosis is based on the demonstration of fat within an adrenal mass on ultrasound, CT or MRI. However, the proportion of fat may vary and those with only a small amount of fat may be difficult to differentiate from other adrenal masses.

HYPOADRENALISM

Imaging in patients with hypoadrenalism can be useful in identifying treatable causes. The usual cause in Western countries is primary idiopathic atrophy in which the adrenals appear extremely small and uncalcified, and may be difficult to identify. Calcification within small adrenals usually indicates tuberculosis, but can also be seen in amyloid, sarcoidosis, metastatic disease, haemochromatosis or fungal infection. In acute hypoadrenalism, CT can be useful in identifying haemorrhage.

CHAPTER 7

Urinary tract: imaging techniques, kidneys and ureters

Judith A. W. Webb

IMAGING TECHNIQUES AND NORMAL APPEARANCES

PLAIN FILMS

The principal role of plain films in the urinary tract is to identify urinary tract calcification. They are an important preliminary to intravenous urography.

Two films are usually necessary:

- full-length film, including the whole renal and bladder area, obtained on inspiration;
- coned renal area view obtained on expiration.

Calcifications which are intrarenal maintain their relationship to the renal poles on these two films. If there is still doubt about whether calcifications are intrarenal, oblique films or plain tomography will give a definite answer (Fig. 7.1). Plain tomography is also helpful when the renal areas are overlain by bowel which can obscure surprisingly large renal calculi. Although the renal outlines may be quite well seen on the plain film, measurement of the kidneys or diagnosis of abnormalities in their outline (e.g. scars,

Diagnostic and Interventional Radiology in Surgical Practice. Edited by P. Armstrong and M. L. Wastie. Published in 1997 by Chapman & Hall, London. ISBN 0412 61960 1 (HB), 0 412 61970 9 (PB)

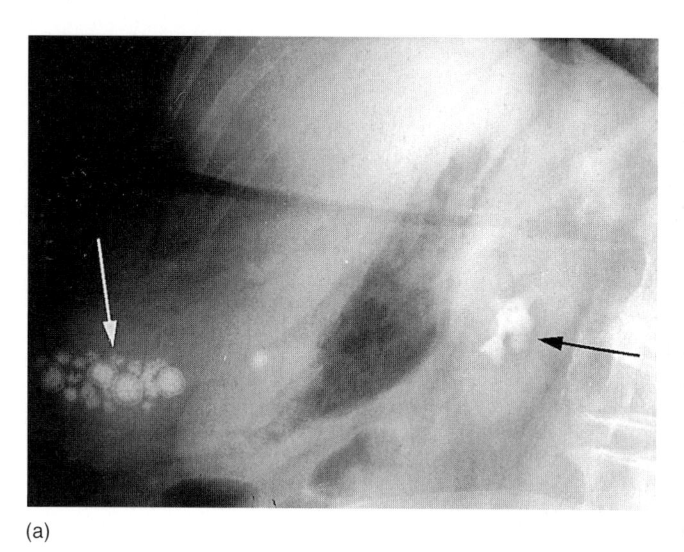

(a)

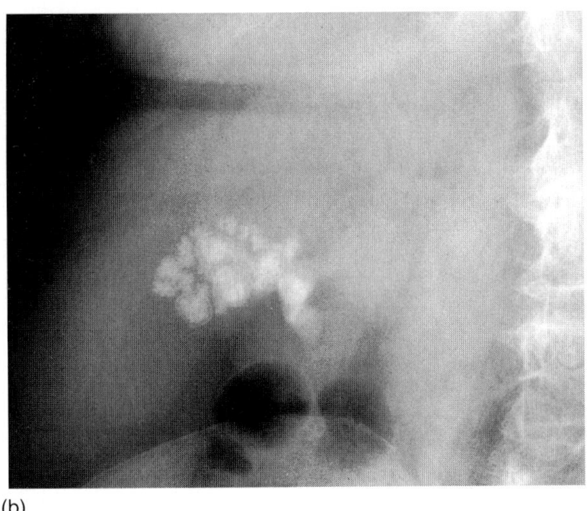

(b)

Fig. 7.1 Oblique plain film (a) showing calcification overlying right lower pole on AP film (b) is due to both a partial staghorn calculus (black arrow) and multiple gallstones (white arrow) which lie away from the kidney on the oblique film. (Reproduced with permission from W.R. Cattell, J.A.W. Webb and A.J.W. Hilson, *Clinical renal imaging*, published by John Wiley, Chichester, 1989).

masses) cannot be made sufficiently accurately from the plain film. These diagnoses should be obtained either from post contrast medium urogram films or from ultrasonography.

The course of the ureters is quite variable but the most common position is along a line crossing the tips of the transverse processes of the lumbar vertebrae and then curving medially into the pelvis. Calcifications along this line should be sought on the plain film. Decisions about whether or not such calcifications are ureteric, however, usually necessitate relating them to the contrast medium-filled ureter during urography. Bladder calculi may be suspected on the plain film, but precise anatomical localization of pelvic calcifications to the bladder requires either urography or ultrasonography. Prostatic calcifications may be seen superimposed on or just above the pubic symphysis.

INTRAVENOUS UROGRAPHY (IVU)

Intravenous urography gives an excellent rapid overview of urinary tract anatomy. It shows more detail of pelvicalyceal and ureteric anatomy than do the other imaging methods. It provides more limited information about the renal parenchyma and bladder than ultrasonography and computed tomography. Although production of the urogram depends on a functioning kidney which filters and concentrates the contrast medium, the functional information provided by urography is relatively limited.

INTRAVENOUS CONTRAST MEDIA

During the intravenous injection of contrast medium it is usual for the patient to feel a warm sensation and sometimes to notice a metallic taste or feel nauseated. None of these sensations constitute a 'contrast medium reaction'. Significant systemic side-effects which constitute a 'reaction' occur in about 5% with high osmolar contrast media and 1% with the newer low osmolar agents. The majority of reactions involve bronchospasm, urticaria, angioneurotic oedema or hypotension. Only a very small proportion of patients develop cardiac arrhythmias or cardiac arrest. The mortality following intravenous contrast media is of the order of 1:50 000 for high osmolar and 1:250 000 for low osmolar agents. The mechanism of these reactions is as yet poorly understood but they do seem to have an 'allergic' basis and are treated with steroids as well as symptomatic measures. Patients who give a history of previous contrast medium reaction or asthma should be given one of the low osmolar contrast media. Although the role of steroid premedication is controversial, the general consensus is that it should still be used as well. A suitable regime is prednisolone 20 mg tds for 48 hours, starting 24 hours before the contrast medium injection.

Although contrast media have no adverse effect on renal function in subjects with normal function, they can cause deterioration in function, usually temporary, in about 10% of patients with impaired renal function. To reduce the risk, such patients should always be well hydrated before they are given contrast medium, and care should be taken not to exceed the recommended contrast medium dose limits.

FILMS OBTAINED AND NORMAL APPEARANCES

Immediate (1-minute) films

A film of the renal area immediately after contrast medium injection shows the renal parenchyma (nephrogram) at its best. On this film the following features should be checked:

- The **renal length** should be the same length as the first three and a half lumbar vertebrae and their intervening discs, and should be more than 11 cm.
- The **renal axis** should be such that the upper pole lies medial to the lower.
- The **renal outline** should be examined for scars or masses.

5-minute renal film

Contrast medium should have entered the pelvicalyceal systems. If they appear normal, ureteric compression is usually applied with a tight band which compresses the ureters as they cross the pelvic brim. This band is left in place for 5 minutes.

10-minute renal film (Fig. 7.2)

The pelvicalyceal systems should be fully distended on this 'pyelogram' film obtained with ureteric compression in place. The film should be checked for:

- filling of all the calyces;
- filling defects in the pelvicalyceal system;
- contrast medium collections outside the pelvicalyceal system.

Full-length film

This is obtained following release of ureteric compression and shows the ureters and bladder filled with contrast medium (Fig. 7.3). A further full-length film is obtained after voiding to check bladder emptying and drainage of the upper tracts. These films should be checked for:

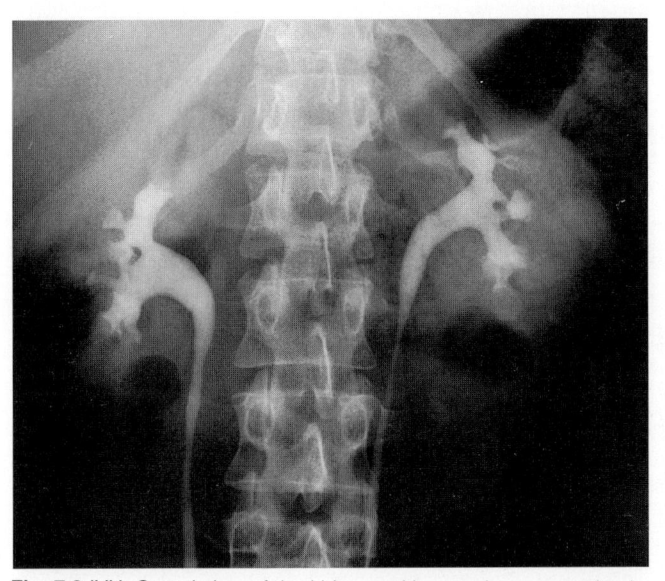

Fig. 7.2 IVU. Coned view of the kidneys with ureteric compression in place and good pelvicalyceal distension. (Reproduced with permission from W.R. Cattell, J.A.W. Webb and A.J.W. Hilson, *Clinical renal imaging*, published by John Wiley, Chichester, 1989.)

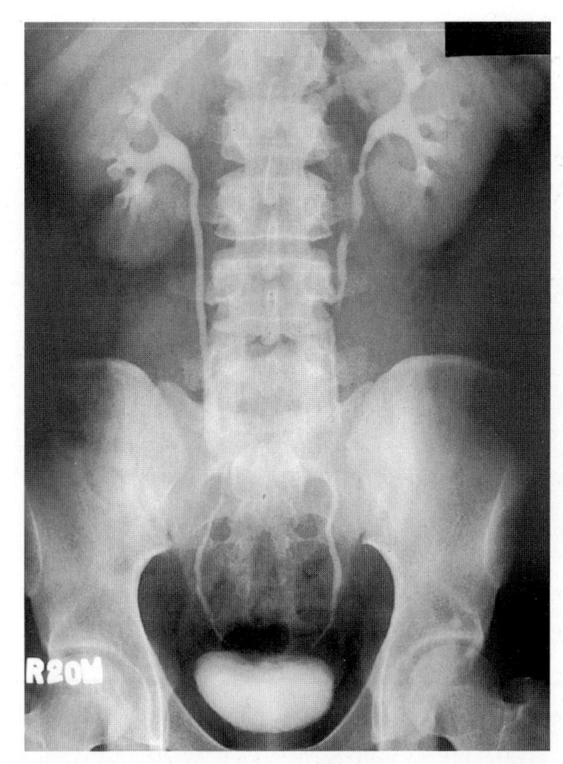

Fig. 7.3 IVU. Full-length film showing normal pelvicalyceal systems, ureters and bladder. (Reproduced with permission from H.N. Whitfield, W.F. Hendry, R.S. Kirby and J.W. Duckett, *Textbook of genitourinary surgery*, to be published by Blackwell, Oxford.)

- ureteric position, filling defects, strictures or calculi; normal ureteric peristalsis often makes it difficult to see the whole ureter filled with contrast medium at any one time;
- bladder position and size, filling defects, wall thickness and emptying.

Additional films such as oblique views, or tomograms, may be obtained by the radiologist to clarify the appearances. The techniques of emergency and frusemide urography are described on pages 188 and 191 respectively.

ULTRASONOGRAPHY

Ultrasonography provides predominantly structural information about the kidneys and bladder. It does not visualize the normal ureter which is obscured by overlying bowel, and in most instances does not show the normal pelvicalyceal system. However, it provides more detail about renal parenchymal structure and the perinephric space than the IVU and can characterize masses as cystic or solid. It also provides more information than urography about many intrinsic bladder abnormalities, such as tumours and calculi. Doppler techniques permit the detection of renal arterial and venous blood flow.

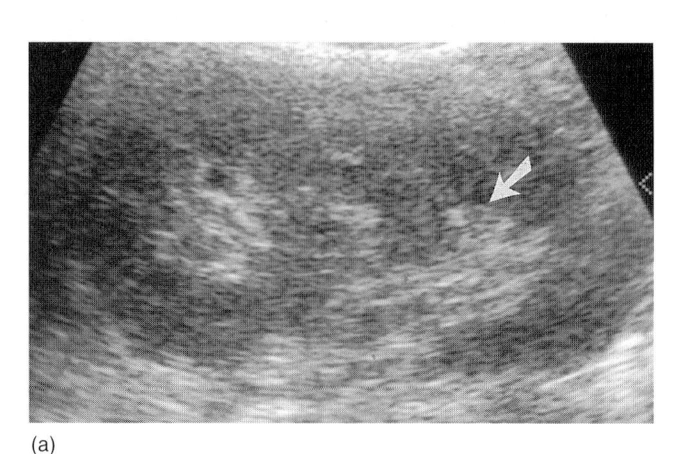

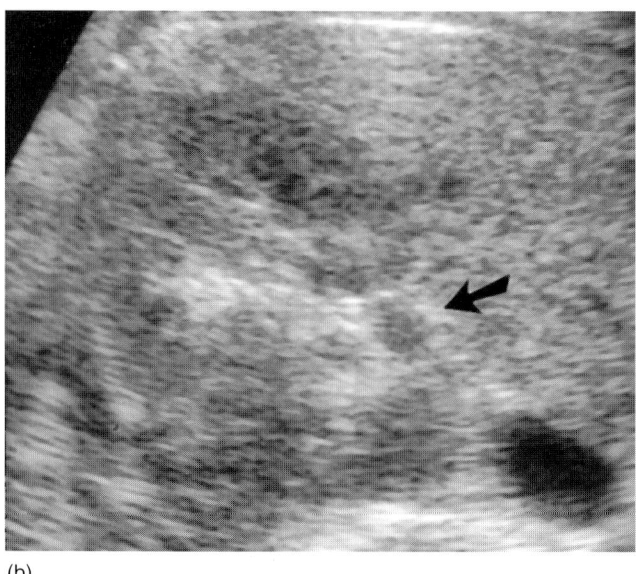

(a) (b)

Fig. 7.4 Normal renal ultrasound scans. (a) Longitudinal scan showing renal sinus echoes (arrowed); (b) transverse scan through hilum: note the sinus echoes extend to the renal margin (arrowed). (Reproduced with permission from R.W. Schrier and C.W. Gottschalk, *Diseases of the kidney*, 5th edn, published by Little, Brown & Co., Boston MA, 1993.)

TECHNIQUE AND NORMAL APPEARANCES

Scans of the kidneys (Fig. 7.4) are obtained in the longitudinal and transverse axes of the kidney by scanning through the flanks, usually with the patient lying on their side. The kidney is seen as an ovoid structure on the longitudinal scans and appears round on the transverse scans. It shows a central cluster of echoes – the sinus echoes – produced predominantly by fat in the renal sinus. On good quality parenchymal images, the pyramids are seen as triangular black structures arranged around the sinus, and surrounded by the more echogenic cortex. Renal length can be measured from the longitudinal scans. The examination must be done carefully to ensure that the distance between the upper and lower poles is measured, because oblique longitudinal measurements will underestimate length. A normal adult kidney measures 10–12 cm with 9 cm being the lower limit of normal. These measurements are less than the urographic measurements because the radiographic technique produces magnification.

The full **bladder** (Fig. 7.5) is seen as an ovoid, echo-free, fluid collection immediately superior to the pubic symphysis. The wall of the distended bladder should be less than 3 mm thick. From measurements of length, transverse and antero-posterior

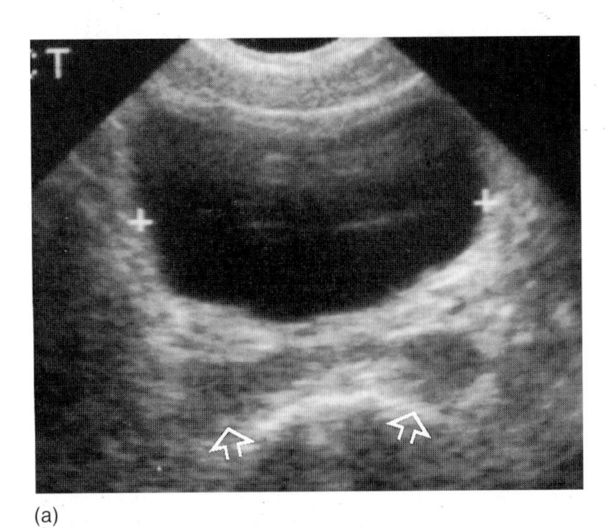

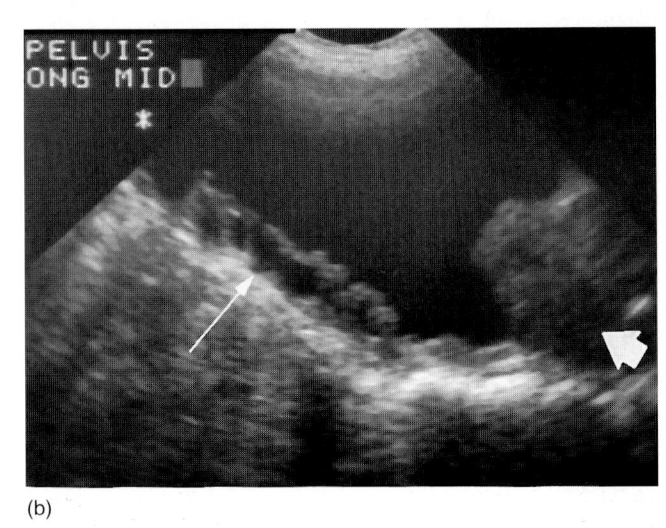

(a) (b)

Fig. 7.5 Bladder ultrasound. (a) Transverse scan: note seminal vesicles (arrowed); (b) longitudinal scan in another patient: note thick-walled bladder with sacculation (long arrow) and enlarged prostate (short arrow) at bladder base.

diameter, bladder volume before and after voiding can be estimated. A widely used formula is:

bladder volume =
0.7 × length × width × antero-posterior diameter.

COMPUTED TOMOGRAPHY

CT is used as a second-line investigation of the kidneys, ureters and bladder, giving predominantly anatomical information. Like ultrasonography it can characterize masses and show the perinephric space. It has the additional advantages of being a very sensitive detector of calculi, including 'lucent' calculi, of visualizing the ureter and retroperitoneum and of providing some limited functional information.

TECHNIQUES AND NORMAL FINDINGS

CT of kidneys and ureter

A full renal CT examination necessitates intravenous contrast medium. On the scans before contrast medium (Fig. 7.6a), the normal renal parenchyma is clearly outlined by the perinephric and sinus fat. The perinephric fascia is often seen. Scans immediately after intravenous contrast medium show the renal artery and vein with the renal pelvis lying posteriorly. Immediate scans show opacification of the renal cortex only (Fig. 7.6b). Subsequently, the medulla also opacifies giving a homogeneous nephrogram, and pelvicalyceal filling occurs by 2 to 3 minutes (Fig. 7.6c). The normal ureter can only be seen with certainty on postcontrast medium scans, but the water density of a dilated ureter can be seen without giving contrast medium.

CT of bladder (Fig. 7.7)

The bladder is seen as a rounded water density structure clearly outlined by perivesical fat. On scans after contrast medium, the bladder opacifies and the dense contrast medium often layers posteriorly. The seminal vesicles are seen as ovoid soft-tissue structures posterior to the bladder at its base, and inferior to the bladder base the prostate appears as a rounded soft tissue density.

URETHROGRAPHY

Urethrography in the male is used to diagnose urethral stricture and to evaluate the urethra after trauma. Female urethrography is technically difficult. The only indication is to check for urethral diverticulum and this can usually be demonstrated more

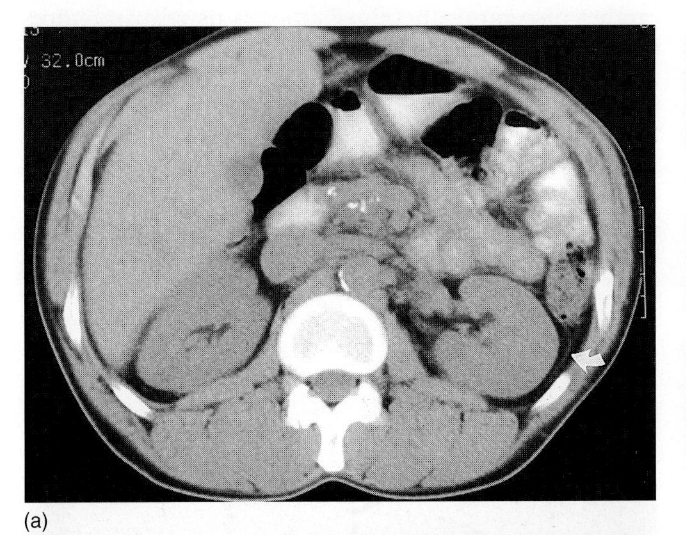

(a)

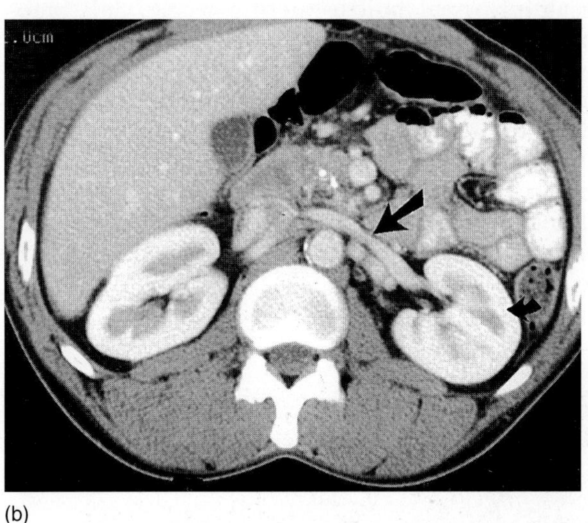

(b)

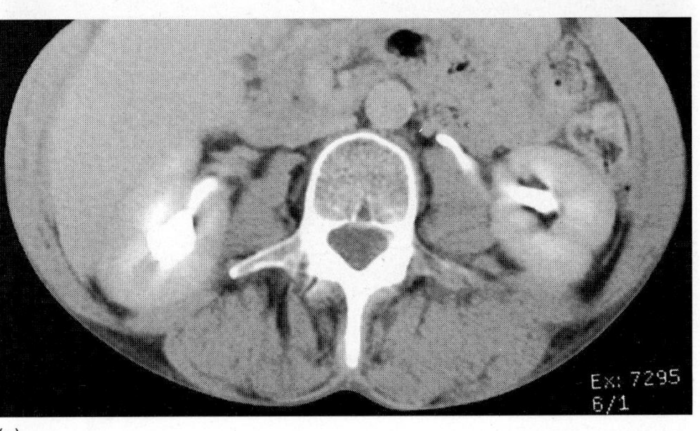

(c)

Fig. 7.6 Normal renal CT scans. (a) Precontrast medium scan. Arrow indicates renal fascia; (b) early postcontrast medium scan; note cortex (short arrow) defined from medulla, and left renal vein (long arrow) with renal artery posterior to it; (c) late postcontrast medium scan in another patient shows pelvicalyceal opacification.

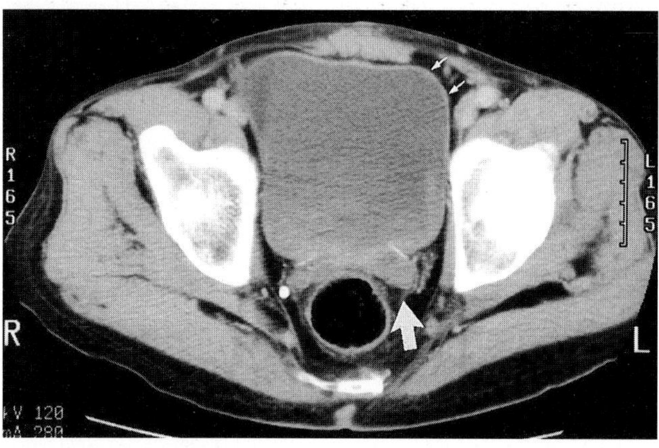

Fig. 7.7 Normal bladder CT scan. The bladder wall (small arrows) is outlined by unopacified urine and perivesical fat, and the seminal vesicles (large arrow) lie posterior to the bladder.

easily by micturating cystography or transvaginal ultrasonography.

In male urethrography the external meatus is occluded either by the nozzle of a specially designed clamp (e.g. Knutsson clamp) or by the balloon of a Foley catheter in the fossa navicularis. The penile and bulbar parts of the anterior urethra normally distend with the contrast medium to the level of the smoothly tapering proximal bulbar urethra (Fig. 7.8a). Since contrast medium is being injected against the external sphincter, there is usually incomplete distension of the posterior urethra. The bladder is usually filled after the anterior urethra has been visualized and a voiding study (micturating cystogram, see below) is then performed (Fig. 7.8b).

Recently, an ultrasonographic technique for urethrography has been described in which the urethra is distended by saline rather than contrast medium and longitudinal and transverse ultrasound images of the distended urethra are obtained. The advantage is that the periurethral tissues are visualized and may appear abnormal in inflammatory disease; the disadvantage is that only the anterior urethra is visualized.

MICTURATING CYSTOGRAPHY

This examination is performed alone relatively rarely in adults. It is not indicated in the routine evaluation of adult urinary tract infection. It may be performed following urethrography in the male to give a functional assessment of any obstructing lesion. It is also used in suspected bladder fistula, to check for vesicoureteric reflux, and occasionally to look for tumour in a bladder diverticulum or for a urethral diverticulum in females. Cystography alone is used in the assessment of bladder trauma.

The bladder is catheterized and filled with contrast medium. Intermittent fluoroscopy is used to check for bladder leaks in suspected trauma or fistula and for vesicoureteric reflux. For a micturating study, the catheter is removed when the bladder is full and the patient voids in the erect oblique position. In the normal male micturating cystogram, the prostatic urethra distends fully (Fig. 7.8b). It is usually indented posteriorly by an ovoid filling defect, the verumontanum. The membranous urethra extends from the lower verumontanum to the upper bulbar urethra. The anterior urethra is also visualized but, in the absence of obstruction, is less well distended than with anterior urethrography. In the female, the short urethra distends fully and may have a variable shape, usually being either ovoid or tubular.

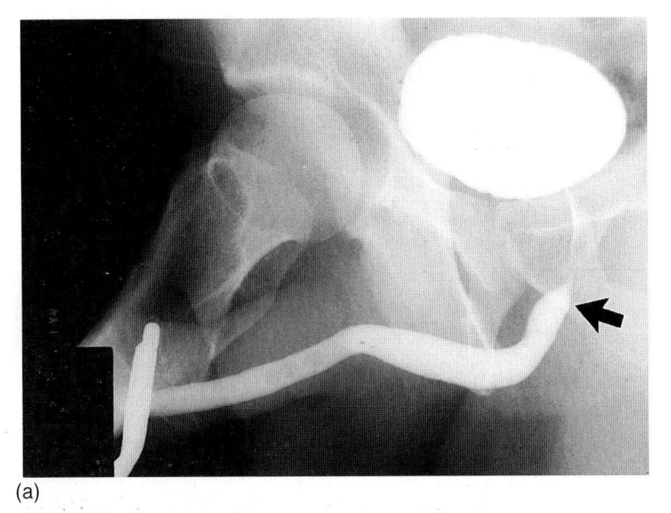

(a)

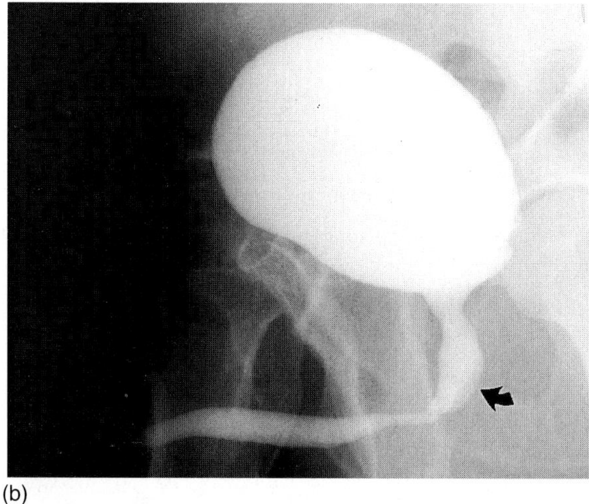

(b)

Fig. 7.8 (a) Normal male ascending urethrogram. Note smoothly tapered bulbar urethra (arrowed) and poor distension of posterior urethra superior to this. Rounded filling defects in the penile urethra are caused by air bubbles. (b) Normal male micturating cystogram. The posterior urethra is well distended and posteriorly is indented by the lucency of the verumontanum (arrowed). (Reproduced with permission from W.R. Cattell, J.A.W. Webb and A.J.W. Hilson, *Clinical renal imaging*, published by John Wiley, Chichester, 1989).

VIDEOURODYNAMICS

When functional bladder disturbance is suspected, e.g. bladder instability, neuropathic bladder or stress incontinence, videourodynamic evaluation is more helpful. Bladder and rectal pressure transducer lines are placed and bladder detrusor pressure is measured during bladder filling and emptying by subtracting rectal from bladder pressure. Video images of the bladder and urethra are also obtained so that both functional and anatomical assessment are performed.

NUCLEAR MEDICINE

Nuclear medicine studies are used to obtain information about renal function. There are two principal types of study; dynamic and static. In dynamic studies, radioactive tracers are attached to substances excreted by the kidneys so that serial images provide information about the excretion process. In a static study, the tracer is attached to a substance which is taken up and retained in functioning kidney tissue. Such uptake is proportional to renal function.

DYNAMIC STUDIES

The agents used for dynamic studies are ^{99m}Tc-labelled MAG-3 (mercaptoacetyl triglycine) which is excreted by glomerular filtration and tubular secretion, and ^{99m}Tc-labelled DTPA (diethylene triamine pentacetic acid) which is excreted by glomerular filtration only.

The hydrated patient is given an intravenous injection of the radioactive tracer and then lies on a couch above a gamma camera while data are collected. The information obtained may be presented as serial images which show the distribution of radioactivity in the patient. These images are viewed from the position of the gamma camera looking at the patient, so that the patient's right side is on the right side of the image. Alternatively, the information may be presented in the form of a plot of radioactivity over the kidney against time (renogram curve).

When the scintigram is studied, a series of phases may be appreciated (Fig. 7.9). The first 30 seconds represents the **perfusion or vascular phase** during which the tracer passes down the aorta into the kidney via the main renal artery. This is followed by the **uptake phase** in which the tracer enters the renal tubules and the activity of the renal parenchyma increases to a peak. There is then **parenchymal transit and clearance** as the tracer passes along the nephrons and enters the renal collecting system. In the **outflow phase** activity over the collecting system decreases as tracer passes to the bladder where a final **bladder phase** is seen. Bladder images before and after voiding are usually obtained.

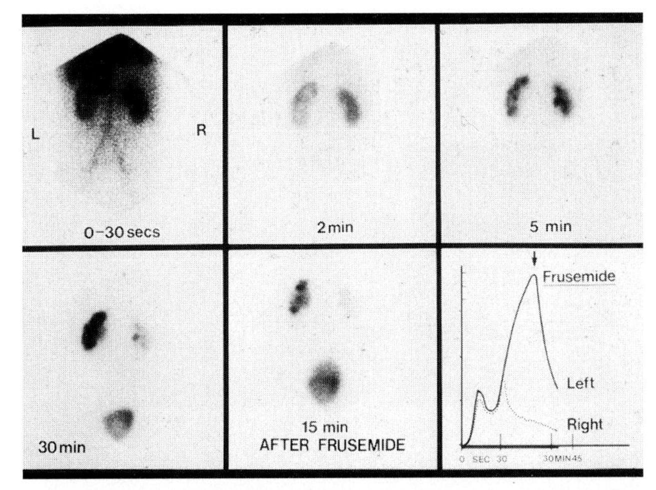

Fig. 7.9 ^{99m}Tc-labelled DTPA dynamic nuclear medicine scan images and renogram. The pelvicalyceal system in the left kidney is dilated but tracer clears rapidly after frusemide indicating that the kidney is not obstructed. (Reproduced by permission of Dr A. J. W. Hilson.)

A dynamic study may be used to evaluate:

- perfusion abnormalities, particularly renal artery stenosis;
- suspected obstruction (frusemide is often used to distinguish non-obstructed from obstructed dilated systems; if the pelvicalyceal system is dilated but not obstructed, tracer is rapidly washed out by frusemide (Fig. 7.9);
- glomerular filtration rate (DTPA only);
- relative uptake of the two kidneys (divided renal function).

STATIC STUDIES

The usual agent for static renal scanning is ^{99m}Tc-labelled DMSA (dimercaptosuccinic acid). Approximately 30% of the intravenously administered tracer is taken up and retained by the proximal tubular cells. Scans obtained 3 hours later can be used to estimate the relative function in each kidney. The images provide a sensitive method of detecting renal scars (Fig. 7.10) and are also helpful in showing whether bulges of the renal contour represent true masses or are 'pseudotumours' composed of normal functioning renal tissue which simulate masses.

ANTEGRADE AND RETROGRADE PYELOGRAPHY

In both antegrade and retrograde pyelography, contrast medium is directly introduced into the kidney or ureter. **Antegrade pyelography** (Fig. 7.28, page 194) is used to outline the pelvicalyceal and ureteric anatomy in patients with dilated obstructed pelvicalyceal systems. It involves injecting contrast medium into the

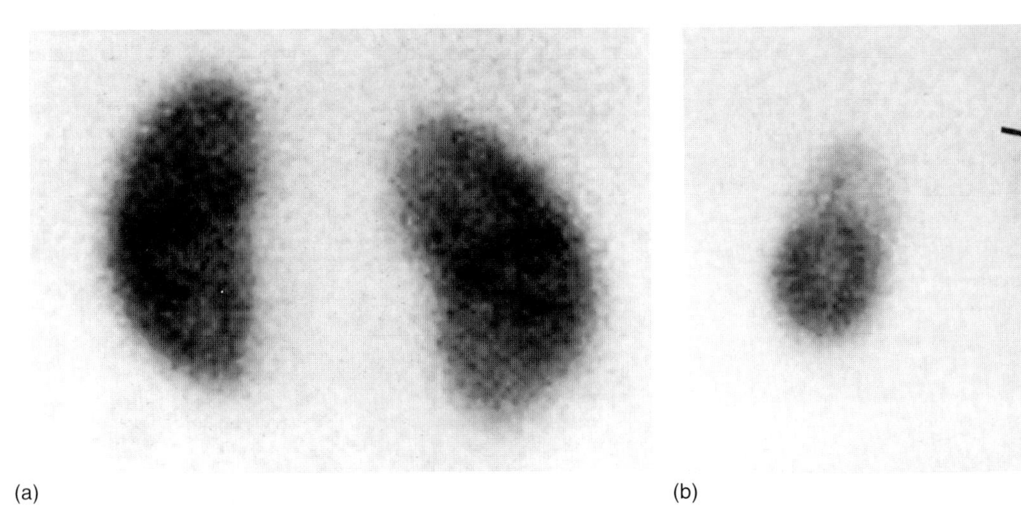

(a) (b)

Fig. 7.10 (a) Normal DMSA scan: equal homogeneous uptake of tracer by both kidneys. (b) DMSA scan in child with reflux nephropathy shows reduced uptake in the left kidney and multiple areas of reduced uptake (arrowed) at the sites of scars. (Reproduced by permission of Dr A. J. W. Hilson.)

pelvicalyceal system via a needle which has been introduced into the collecting system usually with ultrasonographic guidance. It is a preliminary to percutaneous nephrostomy (Chapter 10, p. 266). **Retrograde pyelography** (Fig. 7.29, p. 194) requires cystoscopy and the placement of a bulb tip catheter in the lower ureter through which contrast medium is injected to outline the pelvicalyceal system and ureter.

ANGIOGRAPHY

Angiography is no longer used in the characterization of renal masses. Its principal roles in the urinary tract relate to the diagnosis and treatment (angioplasty) of renal artery stenosis, and the diagnosis and, where appropriate, the treatment of haemorrhage by embolization. Occasionally it is used to provide an arterial 'road map' when partial resection of the kidney is planned.

An aortogram is performed first with the catheter in the aorta at renal artery level. This shows whether the renal arteries are single or multiple – an anomaly seen in about one-third of patients. Selective catheterization of the main renal arteries can then be used to provide more detailed images of the renal arterial tree.

UPPER URINARY TRACT

CONGENITAL ANOMALIES

ECTOPIC KIDNEY

During normal development the kidney ascends from the pelvis to its usual lumbar position. If this process is arrested, the ectopic kidney commonly lies in the pelvis (Fig. 7.11). Ectopic kidney should be suspected when a kidney is not found in the usual position on the early IVU films of the renal area. It can be readily diagnosed on a full-length film. With ultrasonography, when one kidney is not seen, the retroperitoneum should be checked and the pelvis should be examined through a full bladder. Pelvic ectopic kidneys should be seen easily with ultrasound but CT may be necessary to detect kidneys higher in the retroperitoneum. An alternative is to use DMSA scintigraphy to detect the ectopic functioning renal tissue.

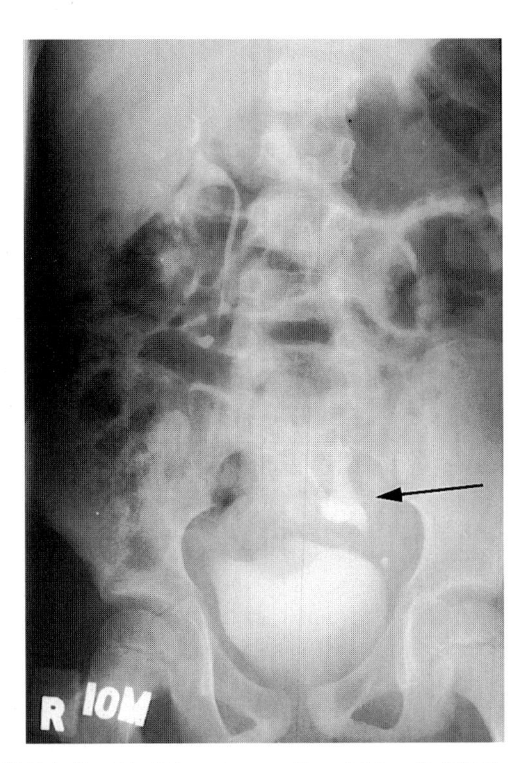

Fig. 7.11 Left pelvic kidney (arrowed) on full-length IVU film.

ABSENT KIDNEY

When only one kidney is seen in the lumbar area and an ectopic kidney is not shown with IVU or ultrasonography, unilateral renal agenesis may be suspected. CT is an excellent method to search for a shrunken abnormal kidney. If doubt persists, cystoscopy to check for a ureteric orifice on the affected side is more helpful than angiography, where it may be unclear whether there is a tiny thread-like artery supplying a shrunken kidney or no renal artery at all. If the single kidney is normal it shows compensatory hypertrophy.

DUPLEX KIDNEY

The normal ureteric bud divides in the kidney to produce the pelvicalyceal system. If division occurs outside the kidney, there is duplication of the pelvicalyceal system and ureter. **Partial duplication**, with a single ureter entering the bladder, is very common and usually has no pathological significance. **Complete duplication** is, however, associated with a number of other abnormalities. The ureter from the upper pole moiety inserts ectopically, either in the bladder distal to the normal ureteric orifice or into another structure. In females, insertion may be into the vagina or urethra, causing incontinence. In the male, insertion into the posterior urethra is usually not associated with incontinence, and insertion into the seminal vesicle or vas may occur. In addition to being ectopic, the upper pole moiety ureter often shows a ureterocoele, a markedly dilated terminal segment which prolapses into the organ in which it inserts. The ureterocoele is usually associated with ureteric obstruction. The lower pole moiety ureter inserts at the normal site but the insertion is commonly abnormal, predisposing to vesicoureteric reflux and the development of reflux nephropathy.

IVU is the best method for the investigation of duplication anomalies. The dilated pelvicalyceal system of an obstructed upper pole moiety may produce a mass effect at the upper pole with no or delayed filling of the dilated calyces and downward displacement of the lower moiety pelvicalyceal system ('drooping flower' appearance) (Fig. 7.12). The lower moiety ureter may be displaced laterally by the dilated non-opacified ureter from the upper pole and there may be a lucent filling defect in the bladder caused by the obstructed ureterocoele. There may be calyceal blunting with overlying parenchymal thinning at the lower pole if reflux nephropathy is present. Where the upper pole moiety is obstructed, ultrasonography may provide helpful further information by showing that the upper pole 'mass' is fluid-containing and by showing the dilated lower ureter and the ureterocoele in the bladder.

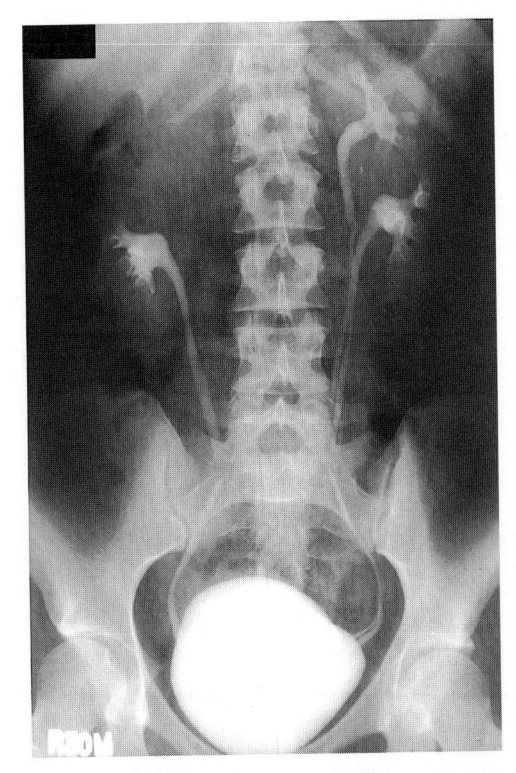

Fig. 7.12 Bilateral duplex kidneys on IVU. The right upper pole moiety is obstructed: the dilated pelvicalyceal system has not filled with contrast medium and is displacing the lower moiety pelvicalyceal system inferiorly ('drooping flower' appearance). (Reproduced with permission from W.R. Cattell, J.A.W. Webb and A.J.W. Hilson, *Clinical renal imaging*, published by John Wiley, Chichester, 1989.)

RENAL PSEUDOTUMOUR

One variety of renal pseudotumour, the hypertrophied column or septum of Bertin is often associated with duplex systems. In this anomaly, the cortices of two adjacent fused renal lobes in the mid-kidney are large with displacement of the adjacent pelvicalyceal system which simulates a tumour.

HORSESHOE KIDNEY

In horseshoe kidney the lower poles of the two kidneys fuse during their ascent. This gives rise to typical appearances at IVU (Fig. 7.13) with the two kidneys lying lower than usual, their long axes paralleling the spine. The isthmus joining the lower poles opacifies if it contains functioning renal tissue. The renal pelves usually face anteriorly and the lower pole calyces point medially because there is associated malrotation. It may be more difficult to make the diagnosis with ultrasound since the isthmus can be difficult to visualize when overlain by bowel gas. CT is an excellent method of examining horseshoe kidneys, including the isthmus, and is helpful when the presence of abnormalities such as tumours or stones are suspected.

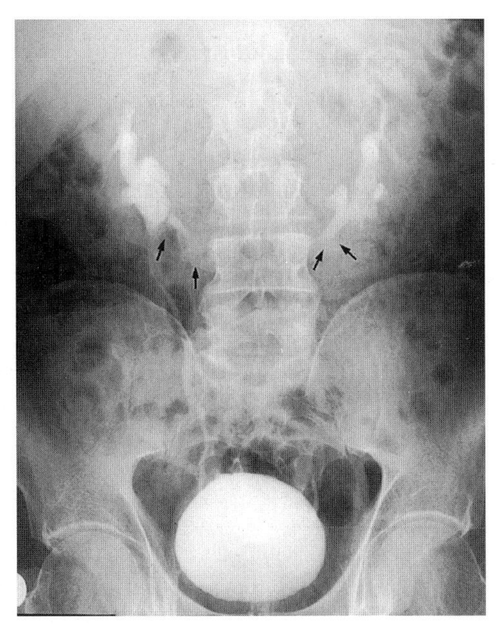

Fig. 7.13 Horseshoe kidney on IVU. Note the abnormal renal axes and medially pointing lower pole calyces (arrowed).

MEGACALYCES

Megacalyces is a congenital anomaly in which there is poor papillary development leading to non-obstructive dilation of the calyces. The pelvis and ureter are normal, distinguishing the condition from obstructive or postobstructive dilatation.

URETEROCOELE

A ureterocoele is a dilated segment of the distal ureter which prolapses into the bladder at its insertion. The dilated contrast medium-filled ureter is surrounded by a lucent margin consisting of the ureteric wall and overlying prolapsed bladder wall. This gives rise to the 'cobra-head' appearance at urography (Fig. 7.14). Simple ureterocoeles are common and of no pathological significance. When the ureteric orifice is stenotic, ureteric obstruction and stone formation within the ureterocoele may occur.

RETROCAVAL URETER

Retrocaval ureter occurs as a result of persistence of the right posterior cardinal vein during development of the inferior vena cava. This results in medial displacement of the right ureter which passes posteriorly to the inferior vena cava. The ureter may become obstructed at vena caval level, and may show a characteristic 'reversed J' appearance.

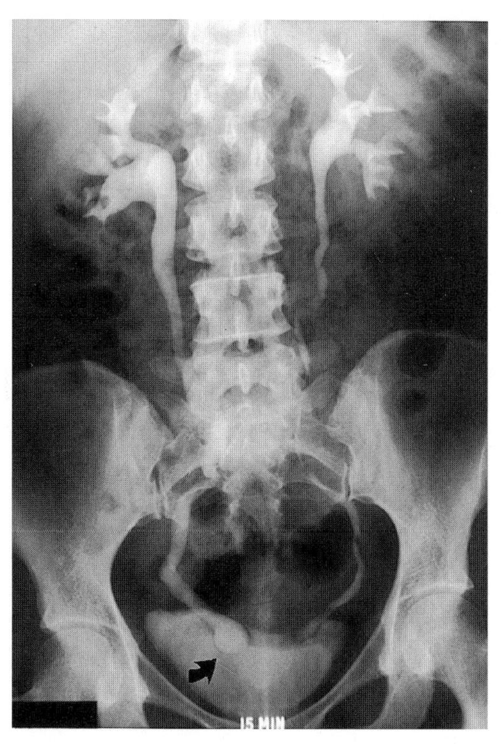

Fig. 7.14 Bilateral ureterocoeles on IVU. Note the typical 'cobra head' appearance and the mild ureteric hold-up caused by the right ureterocoele (arrowed).

STONE DISEASE, RENAL CALCIFICATION

A distinction must be made between renal stones and renal calcification. **Stones** lie in the lumen of the urinary tract: calyx, pelvis, ureter, bladder or urethra. The great majority of urinary tract stones (approximately 90%) appear opaque on plain films because they contain either calcium or cystine which is moderately radiopaque. So-called 'lucent' stones contain urate, xanthine or pure matrix and are readily detected by CT because of its high sensitivity to densities greater than that of soft tissue. They may also be demonstrated with ultrasound where they show the characteristic features described below.

Diffuse calcification in the renal parenchyma is described as **nephrocalcinosis**. Nephrocalcinosis is commonly medullary in distribution and is usually associated with medullary sponge kidney (Fig. 7.20, p. 190), renal tubular acidosis or hyperparathyroidism. More rarely it occurs in a variety of hypercalcaemic states. **Focal renal parenchymal calcification** is seen in tuberculosis (Fig. 7.47, p. 202), some adenocarcinomas (Fig. 7.35, p. 197) infarcts, haematomas and in the papillae in some patients with papillary necrosis.

Plain films, if necessary supplemented by plain tomography, readily demonstrate renal calcification. With the appropriate combination of plain films it should be possible to establish whether calcification is in the kidneys or is only projected over them (Fig. 7.1, p. 178). In most instances, further localization of the calcification requires urography, although the nature of large calculi which fill the pelvicalyceal system (**staghorn calculi**) may be recognized on plain films alone (Fig. 7.15).

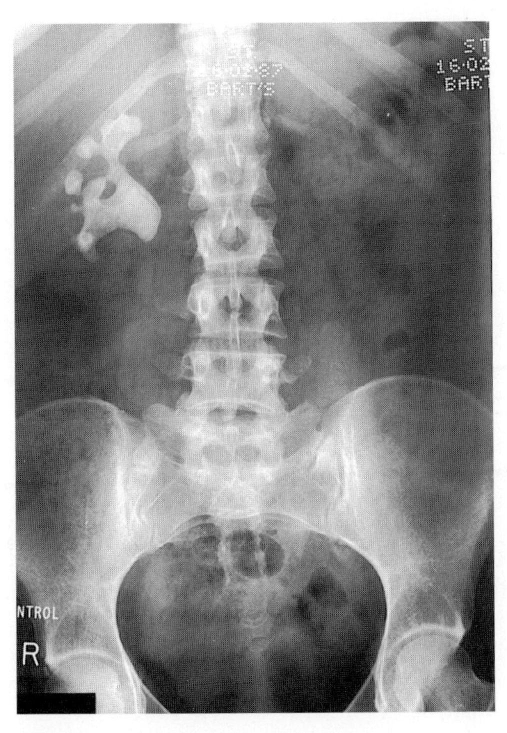

Fig. 7.15 Plain film showing right staghorn calculus.

Plain films are only moderately sensitive and specific for the detection of opaque ureteric stones. Small stones may be missed because of underlying bone (transverse processes, sacrum), or overlying bowel, or because their density is relatively low. Calcifications in the bony pelvis caused by phleboliths and arterial calcification are relatively common. **Phleboliths** may be suspected if the calcifications are rounded with lucent centres and lie below the level of the ischial spines, but from plain films alone it is impossible to be sure that they are not ureteric.

Intravenous urography remains the investigation of choice in the diagnosis and further evaluation of most urinary tract stone disease. With urography, opaque renal calculi can be distinguished from renal parenchymal calcification. Lucent renal calculi are seen as filling defects in the pelvicalyceal system. Treatment is chosen depending on the size and site of the stones, the anatomy of the pelvicalyceal system and ureter, and whether or not obstruction is present. Suitability for extracorporeal shockwave lithotripsy relates to stone size and demonstration of free drainage to the bladder for the stone particles. When percutaneous nephrolithotomy is planned, urography allows the pelvicalyceal puncture to be directed accurately to reach the stones which require treatment.

Urography allows accurate localization of calcifications which lie along the line of the ureter (Fig. 7.16). If they are within the ureter, they overlie the contrast medium-filled ureter whatever the projection used. Urography allows detection of lucent calculi as well as

(a)

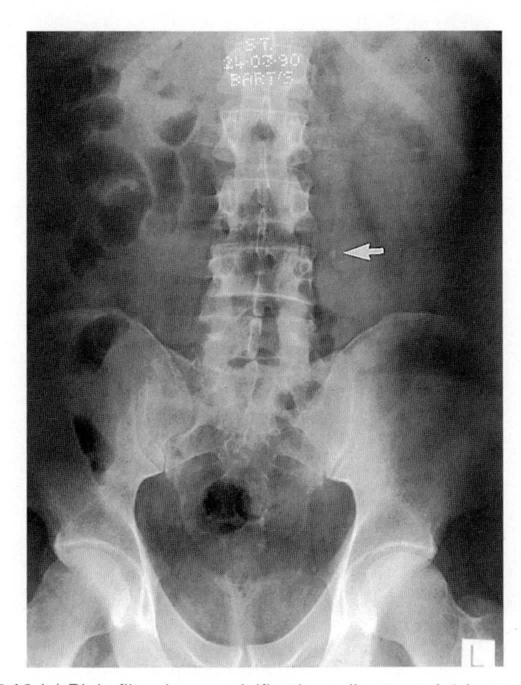

(b)

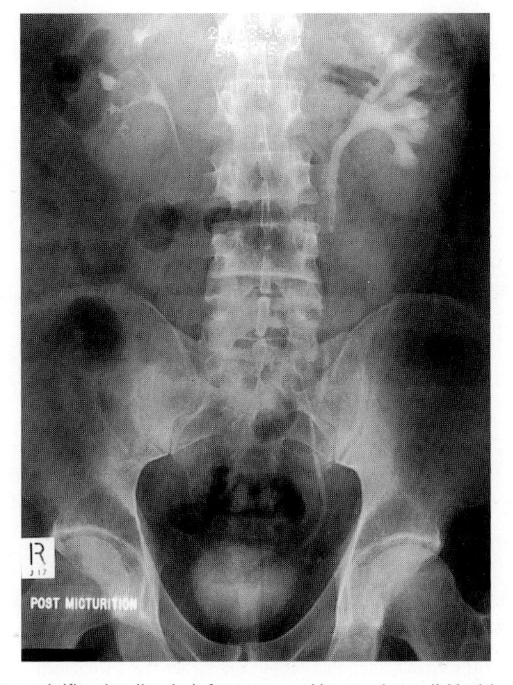

Fig. 7.16 (a) Plain film shows calcification adjacent to L4 (arrowed). (b) IVU shows calcification lies in left ureter and is causing mild hold-up.

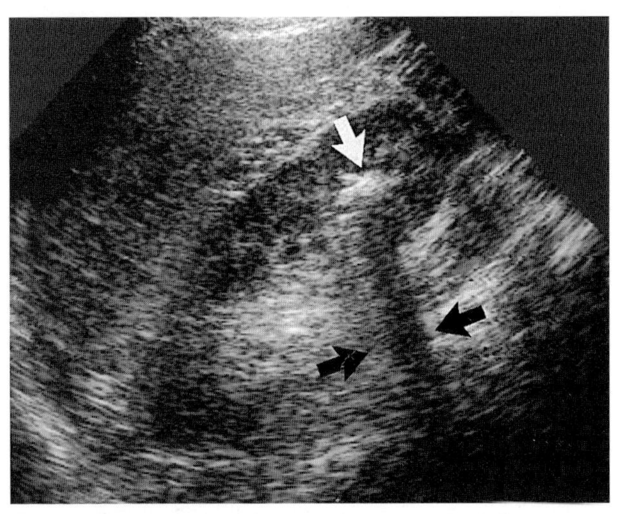

Fig. 7.17 Renal calculus (white arrow) on longitudinal ultrasound scan. Note the acoustic shadow (black arrows).

those calculi not readily detected on the plain film but which cause mild hold-up of contrast medium in the ureter.

At **ultrasonography**, a renal calculus appears as a brightly echogenic focus with a dark band-like acoustic shadow posterior to it (Fig. 7.17). This appearance is seen independent of the stone composition and occurs with radiographically lucent and opaque calculi. Ultrasound is recognized to be less sensitive than the combination of plain films and plain renal tomography for the detection of opaque calculi, which may get lost against the background of the inhomogeneous sinus echoes. There is also a significant incidence of false-positive stone diagnosis with ultrasound because acoustic shadows may arise from normal structures in the renal sinus and because an appearance identical to a stone can be produced by a catheter, other foreign body, or air in the pelvicalyceal system.

Because ultrasound does not visualize most of the ureter, it is an unsatisfactory method to check for ureteric stones. They may be shown if they lie in the upper few centimetres of a dilated ureter, or if they lie in the lower few centimetres of the ureter and can be seen through the full bladder.

CT is an excellent method for detecting urinary tract calculi. Its sensitivity to density differences means that calculi which appear lucent on plain films appear white on CT because they have high density values in relation to the soft tissues (Fig. 7.18). CT plays an important part in the differential diagnosis of a lucent filling defect in the pelvicalyceal system or ureter at urography. The demonstration of a dense opacity on CT allows differentiation of stone from transitional cell tumour or blood clot.

SUSPECTED URETERIC COLIC

Emergency urography is the investigation of choice for detecting calculi obstructing the ureter. A full-length abdominal film on inspiration and a coned renal view on expiration should be obtained and carefully examined for renal and ureteric calcifications. After intravenous contrast medium, only a very limited number of films is obtained, the first being a full-length film at 15 minutes.

In the presence of acute obstruction (Fig. 7.19) there is an immediate nephrogram on the affected side which persists and becomes denser with time because of continued reabsorption of salt and water from the renal tubules in which there is stasis. Filling of the pelvicalyceal system and ureter is delayed and there is usually mild dilation to the level of the obstructing

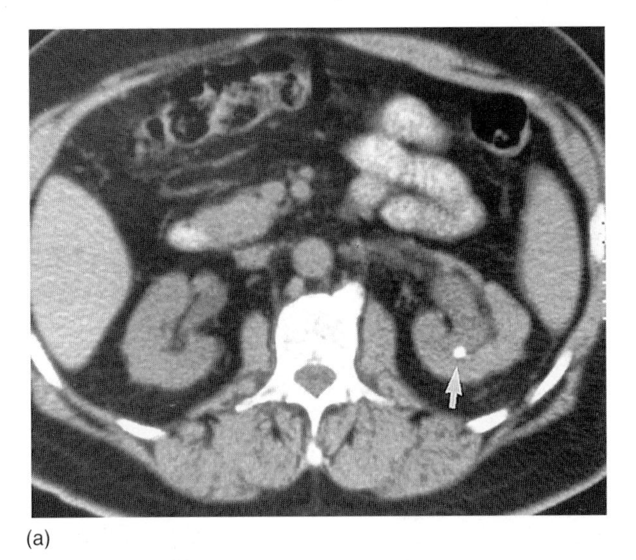

(a)

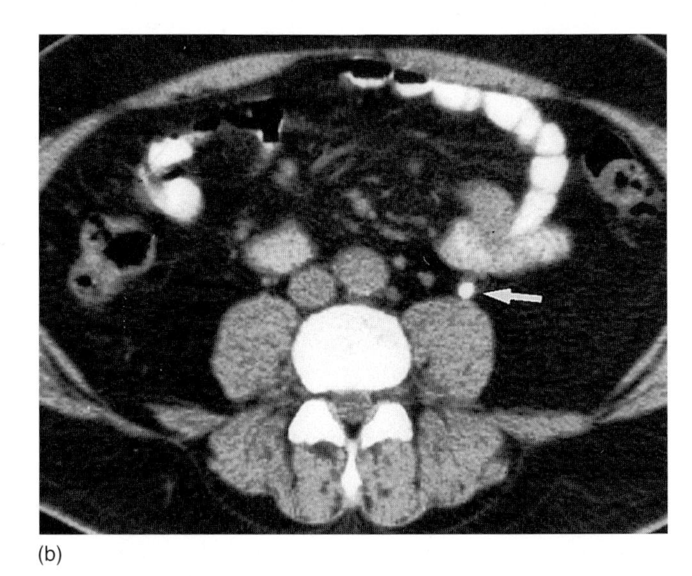

(b)

Fig. 7.18 (a) Renal CT shows small urate calculus (arrowed) in a dilated left pelvicalyceal system. (b) Left ureter is obstructed by a further urate calculus (arrowed). Note the high density of the calculi.

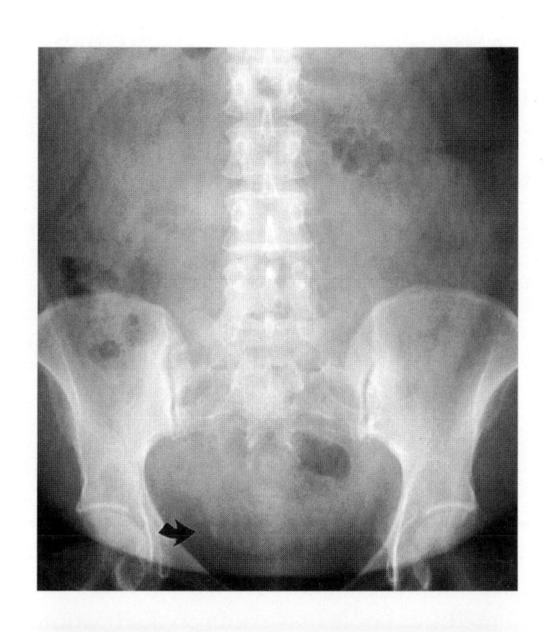

(a)

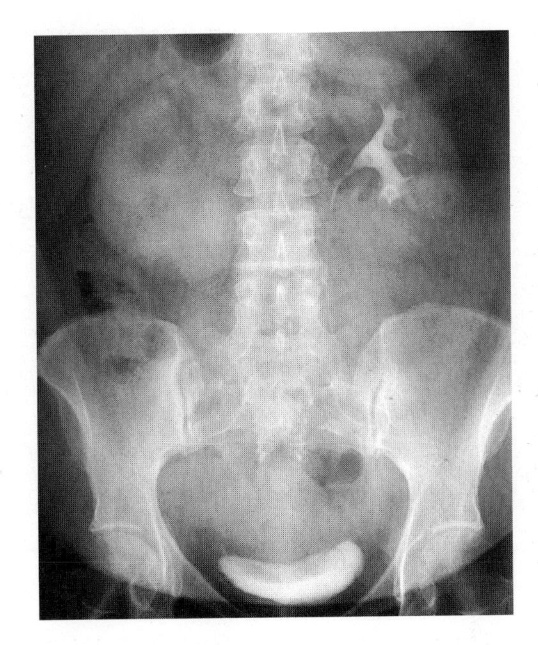

(b)

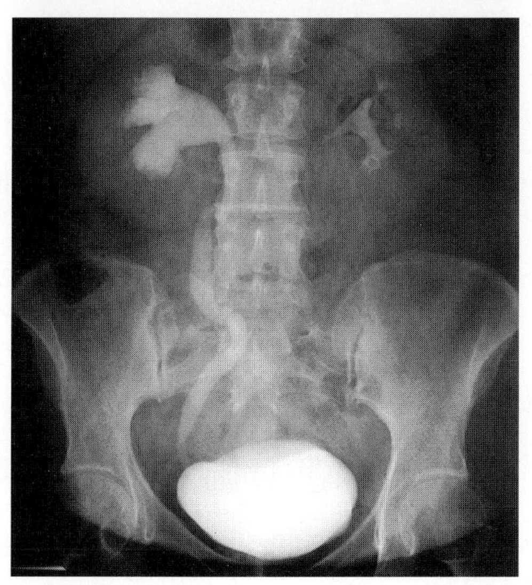

(c)

Fig. 7.19 Acute obstruction of the left ureter by a calculus at the vesicoureteric junction. Calculus (a) seen on the plain film (arrowed). Intravenous urogram: early after contrast medium shows dense right nephrogram (b). Delayed film (c) shows pelvicalyceal and ureteric dilatation to the level of the calculus.

stone. Delayed films (up to 24 hours) may be necessary to show ureteric filling to the level of the stone. When the obstruction is at the vesicoureteric junction, a full-length postmicturition film is helpful because it shows the pelvicalyceal system and ureter remaining full to the level of the calculus on the obstructed side, with normal drainage on the unaffected side. If obstruction is incomplete, the typical nephrogram pattern may not occur, but delay in pelvicalyceal filling and a dilated system to the level of the calculus will usually be shown.

As well as allowing a confident diagnosis of ureteric obstruction, the emergency urogram is also valuable if it is normal. A normal urogram at the time the patient has pain excludes ureteric colic.

Ultrasonography is a less satisfactory investigation than IVU in suspected ureteric colic. It may sometimes be preferred when urography is contraindicated. It should be combined with plain films to detect opaque ureteric stones and the patient should be hydrated (at least 500 ml fluid) before the examination to increase the likelihood that mild pelvicalyceal dilatation will be detected. Even with good hydration the minor pelvicalyceal dilation in some patients with ureteric obstruction may not be evident on ultrasonography. Conversely, the inability of the technique to see most of the ureter and its drainage make it impossible to assess the significance of minor degrees of dilation. Ultrasonography may, however, be a useful adjunct to urography in the detection of stones at the vesicoureteric

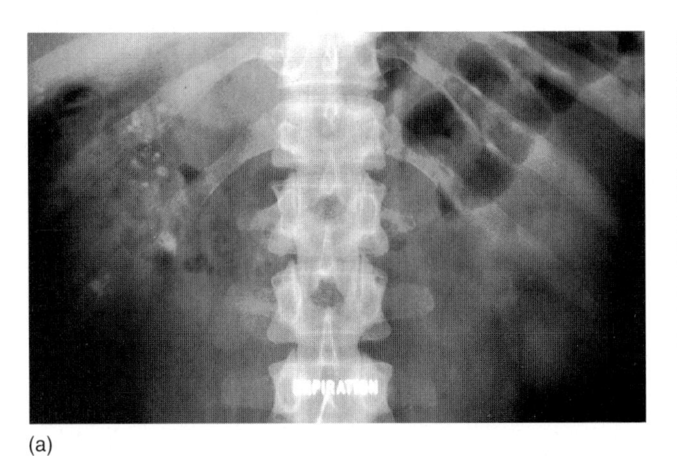

(a)

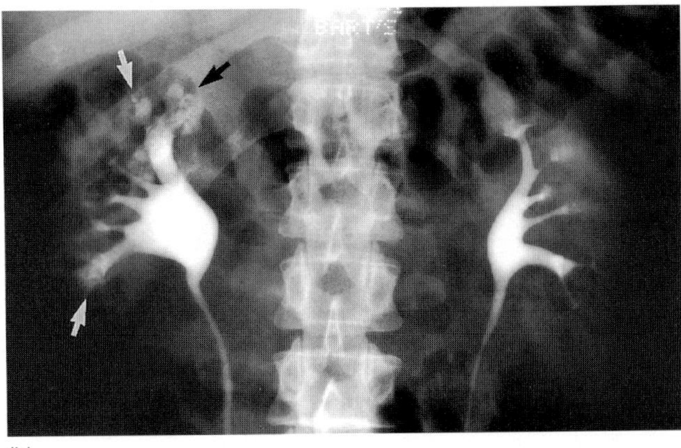

(b)

Fig. 7.20 Right medullary sponge kidney. (a) Plain film shows papillary clusters of calcification. (b) Postcontrast medium film shows contrast medium pools in the papillae (arrowed). (Reproduced with permission from W.R. Cattell, *Infections of the kidney and urinary tract*, published by Oxford University Press, Oxford, 1996.)

junction. IVU may show hold-up at this level but may not demonstrate a small low-density or non-opaque stone, while ultrasound can often show such distal obstructing ureteric calculi clearly through a full bladder.

MEDULLARY SPONGE KIDNEY

In medullary sponge kidney, there is fusiform and cystic dilation of the collecting ducts in the papillae leading to stasis which predisposes to stone formation. Part or all of one or both kidneys may be affected. Most patients are asymptomatic until they develop ureteric colic.

Plain films may show clusters of calcifications in the affected papillae (medullary nephrocalcinosis) (Fig. 7.20a). At urography, the abnormal collecting ducts are seen as linear streaks and pools of contrast medium within the papillae (Fig. 7.20b). This allows the condition to be differentiated from the other types of medullary nephrocalcinosis (p. 186). Some of the contrast medium pools may contain calcifications. The involved papillae or kidney may be enlarged.

Fig. 7.21 Steinstrasse (arrowed) in the distal right ureter on a plain film obtained after extracorporeal shockwave lithotripsy.

MONITORING OF TREATMENT

During the course of treatment, progress of calculi can be monitored by serial plain films. During extracorporeal shockwave lithotripsy, a characteristic appearance of an opaque column of stone fragments in the ureter ('Steinstrasse') (Fig. 7.21) may develop.

OBSTRUCTION

The imaging diagnosis of urinary tract obstruction is largely dependent on demonstrating the anatomical consequences of obstruction, i.e. the dilatation proximal to the obstructing lesion. Because IVU and CT involve contrast medium excretion, they both give some limited functional information, but scintigraphy is the only method which provides direct functional evidence of obstruction. The term 'hydronephrosis' is widely used to describe pelvicalyceal dilatation and is often used as if it were synonymous with obstruction. It cannot be overemphasized that **pelvicalyceal and ureteric dilatation do not necessarily indicate obstruction**. Dilatation may be seen in non-obstructed systems if there is vesicoureteric reflux, in a number of anatomical variants (e.g. extrarenal pelvis) and congenital anomalies (e.g. megacalyces). Also, the pelvicalyceal system and ureter may not return completely to normal and may still show mild dilatation following relief of obstruction.

Furthermore, when there is obstruction it is important to recognize that **the functional severity of the obstruction is unrelated to the degree of dilatation of**

the pelvicalyceal system and ureter. Thus mild dilatation is a recognized feature of severe obstruction with high intrarenal pressure in acute ureteric obstruction, for example by stone, and also in some cases of chronic obstruction, for example when caused by idiopathic retroperitoneal fibrosis (Fig. 7.25, p. 193) and by retroperitoneal malignancy.

ACUTE OBSTRUCTION

Urography is the method of choice when acute ureteric obstruction is suspected. The technique and findings have been described earlier (p. 188; Fig. 7.19, p. 189). Acute ureteric obstruction may also less commonly be caused by blood clot or a sloughed papilla, and idiopathic pelviureteric junction (PUJ) obstruction may present acutely. **Clot colic** occurs only in the presence of heavy haematuria. A lucent filling defect is seen and will usually have resolved if the IVU is repeated at 10–14 days. If the cause of bleeding was not evident on the original IVU, further investigation is essential once the haematuria has settled. A **sloughed papilla** is suspected when changes of papillary necrosis, particularly papillary tracks and pools of contrast and blunted calyces, are seen. With acute PUJ obstruction, the rounded soft-tissue density of the dilated pelvis may be seen on the plain film. The dilated pelvis should fill with contrast medium on delayed films and there is no ureteric filling.

Ultrasound is a less satisfactory method for the diagnosis of acute ureteric obstruction (p. 189).

CHRONIC OBSTRUCTION

The choice of investigation in suspected chronic obstruction depends on the clinical presentation. When there is pain, and stone disease or pelviureteric junction obstruction is possible, urography is best. In other settings, such as impaired renal function, prostatism or pelvic neoplasm, ultrasound combined with plain radiography is the method of choice. Scintigraphy is usually reserved until dilatation has been demonstrated, and can then be used to assess its functional significance.

On the IVU films obtained immediately after injection of contrast medium, the dilated pelvicalyceal system may be seen as a central lucency (negative pyelogram) surrounded by opacified parenchyma which may be thinned (rim nephrogram) (Fig. 7.22). The dilated pelvicalyceal system usually fills with contrast medium on delayed films but contrast-medium concentration is often poor and tomography may be necessary to show the calyces. If there is sufficient contrast-medium concentration, delayed films will also show the level of obstruction and may help define its cause.

When pelviureteric junction obstruction is suspected, the technique of **frusemide urography** is very helpful and usually permits the separation of patients with true obstruction from those with extrarenal pelves only. When a dilated pelvis is seen on the full-length film, 40 mg frusemide is given intravenously and another full-length film is obtained 15 minutes later (Fig. 7.23). In pelviureteric junction obstruction the frusemide-induced diuresis causes an increase in size of the pelvis and calyces with no ureteric filling, and the patient develops loin pain, whereas with an extrarenal pelvis the contrast medium will have washed out of the pelvis by this time.

Ultrasonography is a sensitive method of detecting pelvicalyceal dilatation in chronic obstruction. The dilated pelvicalyceal system is seen as a group of communicating, rounded fluid collections centrally in the renal sinus, representing the dilated pelvis surrounded by dilated calyces (Fig. 7.24). The upper and lower few centimetres of a dilated ureter may also be seen. In long-standing obstruction, thinning of the renal parenchyma due to obstructive atrophy will also be present.

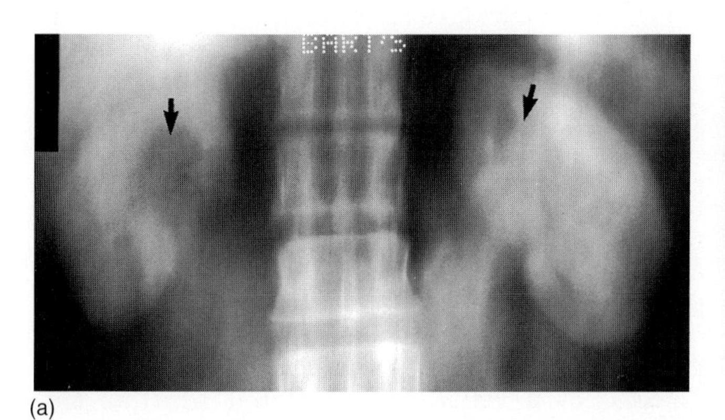
(a)

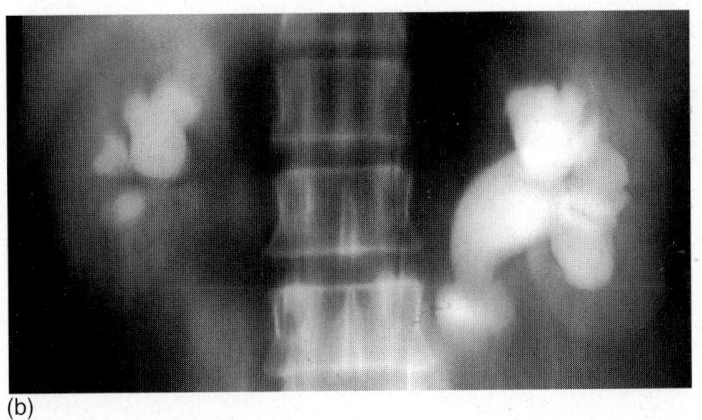
(b)

Fig. 7.22 IVU in chronic obstruction. (a) Film obtained immediately after contrast medium shows central negative pyelogram (arrowed). (b) Delayed film shows dilated calyces and pelvis in the position of the previous negative pyelogram. (Reproduced with permission from W.R. Cattell, J.A.W. Webb and A.J.W. Hilson, *Clinical renal imaging*, published by John Wiley, Chichester, 1989.)

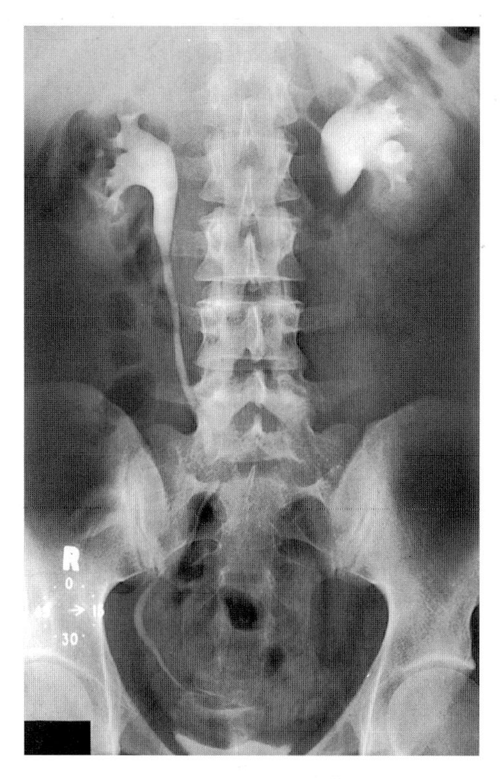

(a)

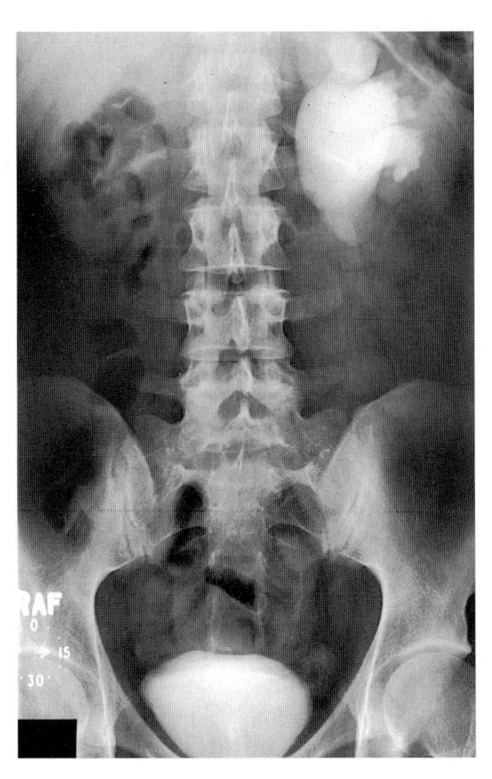

(b)

Fig. 7.23 Frusemide IVU in left pelviureteric junction obstruction. Note slight fullness of the left pelvis (a); 15 minutes after frusemide the left pelvicalyceal system has dilated further and the right has washed out (b). (Reproduced with permission from W.R. Cattell, J.A.W. Webb and A.J.W. Hilson, *Clinical renal imaging*, published by John Wiley, Chichester, 1989.)

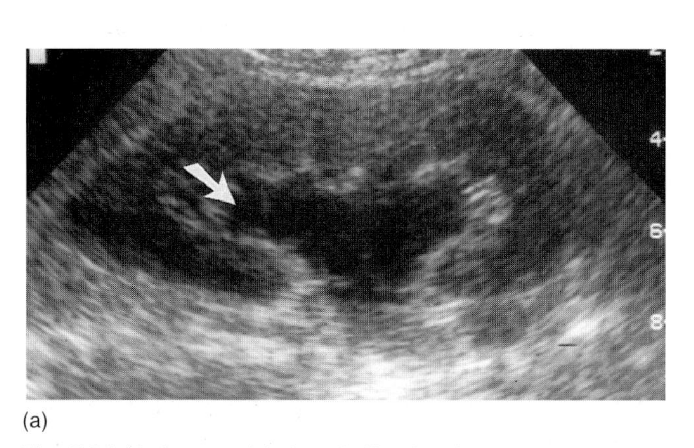

(a)

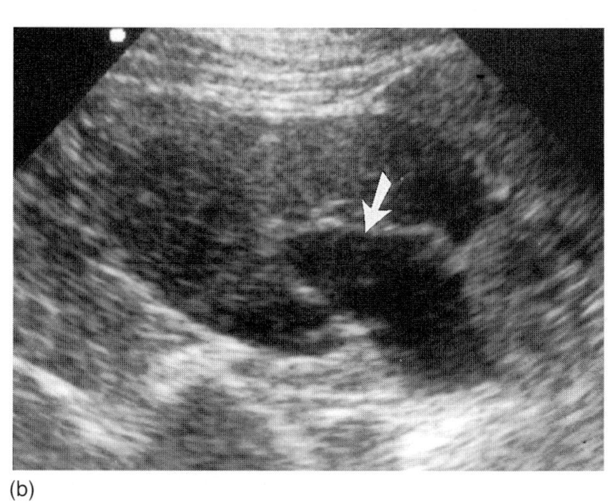

(b)

Fig. 7.24 Moderate pelvicalyceal dilatation (arrowed). Longitudinal (a) and transverse (b) renal ultrasound scans in renal obstruction. (Reproduced with permission from D. Cosgrove, H. Meire and, K. Dewbury, *Clinical ultrasound*, published by Churchill Livingstone, Edinburgh, 1993.)

Since minor dilatation can be associated with severe obstruction (Fig. 7.25), in a setting where obstruction is suspected, any degree of dilatation must be taken seriously and investigated further. This will, however, lead to a significant number of false-positive diagnoses. Ultrasound is more limited in this regard than IVU which, by virtue of its ability to show the ureter and to demonstrate drainage of the upper tracts, is associated with less false-positive diagnoses of obstruction.

On precontrast **CT scans** (Fig. 7.26) the dilated pelvicalyceal system of an obstructed kidney can be detected as a water density central structure surrounded laterally by dilated calyces. At CT a dilated intrarenal pelvis can be distinguished from an extrarenal pelvis, which is a normal variant. The intrarenal

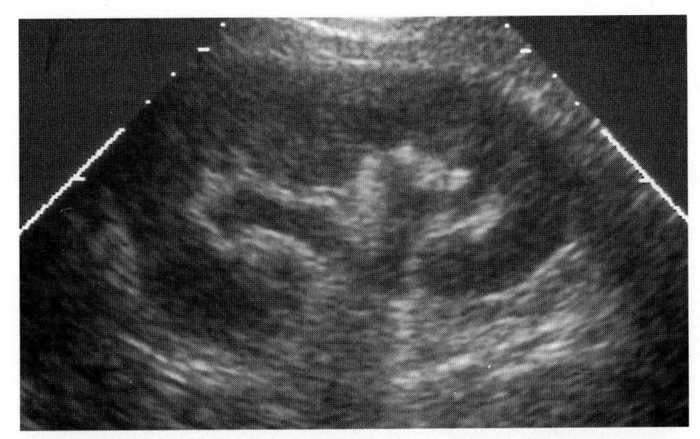

Fig. 7.25 Mild pelvicalyceal dilatation. Longitudinal ultrasound scan in severe renal obstruction caused by retroperitoneal fibrosis (both kidneys appeared similar). (Reproduced with permission from D. Cosgrove, H. Meire and K. Dewbury, *Clinical ultrasound*, published by Churchill Livingstone, Edinburgh, 1993.)

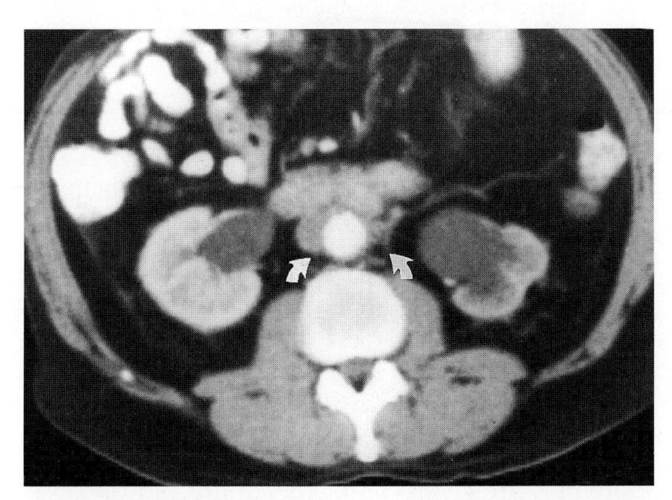

Fig. 7.26 CT scan in bilateral renal obstruction. Note bilateral pelvicalyceal dilatation, parenchymal thinning on the left and the periaortic soft-tissue mass (arrowed) of retroperitoneal fibrosis.

pelvis is defined as that part of the pelvis lying lateral to a line joining the hilar lips, the convexities of the parenchyma which border the renal sinus. Renal parenchymal thinning will be seen in long-standing obstruction. CT has the additional advantage over ultrasound that the water density of urine in a dilated ureter can be traced through the retroperitoneum to the level of the obstruction. Scans after contrast medium will show delayed filling of the dilated pelvicalyceal system and ureter which eventually opacify to the level of the obstruction.

MAG-3 or **DTPA scintigraphy** of an obstructed kidney shows delayed clearance of the parenchyma and delayed outflow from the collecting system. On the renogram, renal activity either rises to a plateau or keeps rising. A dilated extrarenal pelvis alone without obstruction may be associated with delayed outflow from the collecting system, but parenchymal clearance should be normal. Frusemide renography is very

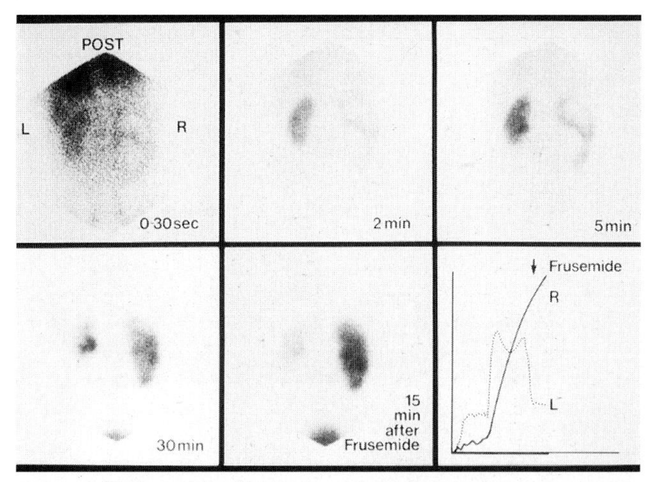

Fig. 7.27 ^{99m}Tc-labelled DTPA dynamic nuclear medicine scan images and renogram in a patient with a dilated, obstructed right pelvicalyceal system. Note that the obstructed system does not wash out after frusemide. (Reproduced by permission of Dr A. J. W. Hilson)

helpful. If frusemide is given after the postvoiding image is obtained, a subsequent image shows washout of a baggy, non-obstructed, extrarenal pelvis, but increase in size and retained activity in true pelviureteric junction obstruction (Fig. 7.27).

CAUSE OF OBSTRUCTION

Intravenous urography often shows the level and the cause of obstruction. Extrinsic ureteric obstruction is associated with smooth ureteric tapering, while an intrinsic lesion produces a filling defect in the lumen of the ureter.

When pelvicalyceal dilatation is shown by **ultrasound**, possible causes should be sought by examining the retroperitoneum and pelvis. It may be difficult to show by ultrasound retroperitoneal causes of obstruction but it can detect pelvic masses or the enlarged bladder of chronic retention. Where ultrasound shows pelvicalyceal dilatation in suspected obstruction, but not the cause of obstruction, either antegrade pyelography or CT is likely to be helpful.

Like urography, **antegrade pyelography** can usually distinguish intrinsic from extrinsic causes of obstruction (Fig. 7.28), but lesions of the ureteric wall such as transitional cell tumours may appear either intrinsic or extrinsic in origin. When polypoid they produce a filling defect and, if they lie in the wall, they produce smooth tapering which mimics an extrinsic obstruction. Antegrade pyelography is a usual preliminary to percutaneous drainage of the kidney.

CT is an excellent method for demonstrating masses such as enlarged nodes, tumours or retroperitoneal fibrosis causing extrinsic ureteric obstruction (Fig. 7.26). It can also distinguish stones (Fig. 7.18, p. 188), because of their high density, from other intraluminal

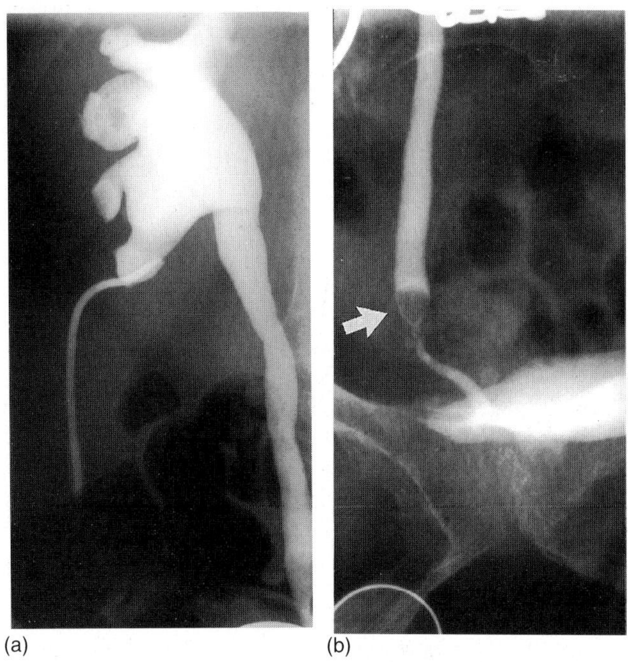

(a) (b)

Fig. 7.28 Antegrade pyelogram in partial ureteric obstruction caused by a urate calculus. (a) Nephrostomy catheter in the pelvicalyceal system; (b) lucent filling defect (arrowed) in the distal ureter.

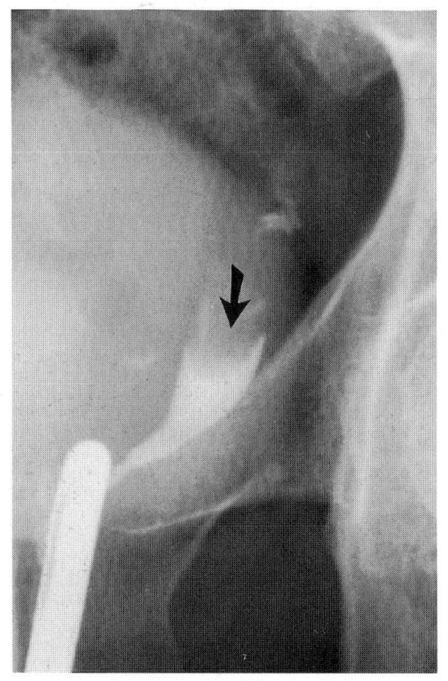

Fig. 7.29 Retrograde pyelogram. Note lucent filling defect (arrowed) of transitional cell carcinoma in the lower ureter. (Reproduced with permission from W.R. Cattell, J.A.W. Webb and A.J.W. Hilson, *Clinical renal imaging*, published by John Wiley, Chichester, 1989.)

filling defects such as transitional cell tumours or blood clots.

Retrograde pyelography is occasionally used to outline the lower end of an obstructed ureter if pelvicalyceal dilatation is mild and antegrade pyelography is likely to be difficult (Fig. 7.29). One of the reasons that the antegrade route is generally preferred is that the retrograde technique carries a risk of introducing infection into the obstructed system.

RENAL FAILURE

The main roles of imaging in a patient presenting with impaired renal function are to detect renal obstruction and to measure the kidneys, as normal or large kidneys indicate acute renal failure, while small kidneys indicate chronic irreversible failure. Ultrasound is the best initial imaging method since it is a sensitive detector of pelvicalyceal dilation in renal obstruction and can also measure the kidneys accurately. Ultrasound should always be combined with plain films to detect calculi. Once pelvicalyceal dilation has been shown, ultrasound should also be used to search for the possible cause of obstruction in the pelvis and retroperitoneum. Full evaluation of the cause of obstruction, however, often necessitates antegrade pyelography and/or CT. Rarely, retrograde pyelography may also be necessary. In cases where ultrasound examination of the kidneys is not diagnostic, CT without contrast medium is helpful, since it is also a sensitive detector of pelvicalyceal dilation. **High-dose urography**, using twice the normal contrast medium dose, may still be used in patients with mildly impaired renal function (serum creatinine 300 μmol/l or less) to demonstrate pelvicalyceal anatomy. There is potential for further deterioration in renal function after intravenous contrast medium. To minimize the risk, patients with impaired renal function must be well hydrated before they are given contrast medium, and the dose should be limited to the minimum consistent with a diagnostic result.

In patients with acute non-obstructive renal failure, ultrasound-guided renal biopsy is usually undertaken. In chronic renal failure the kidneys are reduced in size with thinning of the renal parenchyma. Further imaging evaluation is usually not warranted.

MASSES AND TUMOURS

A renal 'mass' detected by imaging most commonly represents a simple cyst, but a wide differential diagnosis must be considered, including benign and malignant tumours, inflammatory masses, pseudotumours, obstructed calyces, haematoma and aneurysm.

- Cysts
  - simple
  - complicated
    - septate
    - haemorrhagic
    - infected

- Tumours
  - benign
    - adenoma
    - angiomyolipoma
  - malignant: primary
    - adenocarcinoma
    - Wilms' tumour
    - invasive transitional cell tumour
  - malignant: secondary
    - metastasis
    - lymphoma
- Inflammatory
  - abscess
  - focal acute pyelonephritis
- Pseudotumour
  - hypertrophied column of Bertin
  - compensatory hypertrophy, e.g. in a scarred kidney in reflux nephropathy
- Obstructed calyces
  - obstructed upper pole moiety of duplex kidney
  - obstructed calyx, e.g. TB, stone, transitional cell tumour
- Haematoma
- Aneurysm, arteriovenous malformation

SIMPLE CYSTS

Simple renal cysts are common, occurring in more than 50% of individuals aged over 50. They may be multiple. With the widespread use of ultrasound and CT, simple cysts are now frequently detected.

At **IVU** a simple cyst is seen as a mass lesion which typically is lucent with a clear rounded margin. If the cyst protrudes from the kidney, smooth beaks of renal parenchyma are seen at its margins, and the part protruding from the kidney should not have a detectable wall (Fig. 7.30). If the cyst lies centrally in the kidney it may cause smooth displacement or compression of the pelvicalyceal system. However, the urographic criteria for diagnosing that a mass is cystic rather than solid are only correct in about 50% of cases. Detection of a renal mass always necessitates further investigation by ultrasound, even if the mass has features suggestive of a cyst at IVU.

Ultrasonography shows a renal cyst as a rounded echo-free mass with a sharply defined back wall and increased through transmission of sound, seen as a white band posterior to the cyst (Fig. 7.31). If these criteria are strictly observed the ultrasound diagnosis of a benign cyst is correct in over 95% of cases, and the majority require no further investigation.

CT shows a renal cyst as a rounded, well-defined, homogeneous mass of water density which has a smooth interface with the adjacent renal parenchyma, no detectable wall, and no enchancement after intravenous contrast medium (Fig. 7.32). If these criteria are strictly observed, the CT diagnosis of a simple cyst is virtually certain.

MRI shows a renal cyst as a rounded, well-defined, homogenous mass of lower signal intensity than adjacent normal parenchyma on T1-weighted images with no enhancement after gadolinium. On T2-weighted images the cyst is of high intensity compared to normal parenchyma (Fig. 7.33).

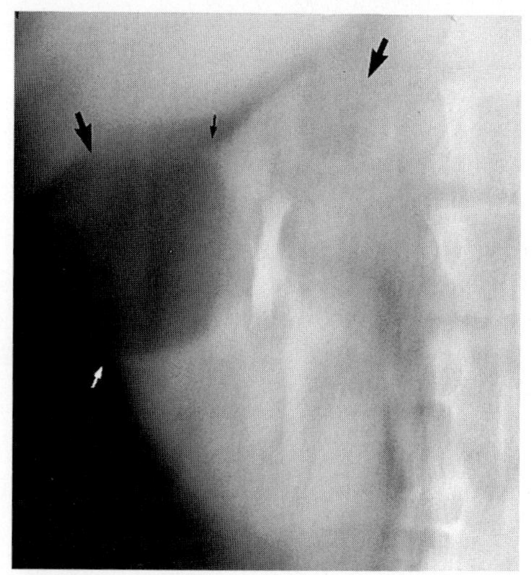

Fig. 7.30 Simple renal cysts. Tomogram from IVU shows two typical cysts (large arrows) in the upper kidney. Note the lucent masses are well defined and have 'beaks' (small arrows) at their margins. (Reproduced with permission from H.N. Whitfield, W.F. Hendry, R.S. Kirby and J.W. Duckett, *Textbook of genitourinary surgery*, to be published by Blackwell, Oxford.)

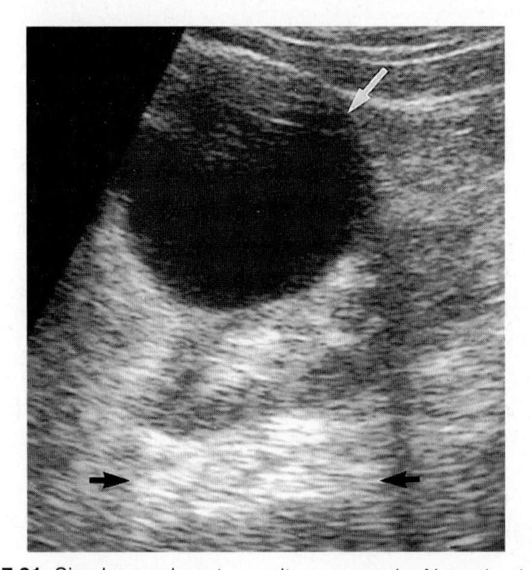

Fig. 7.31 Simple renal cyst on ultrasonograph. Note the band of increased through-transmission of sound (arrowed) posterior to the cyst (white arrow). (Reproduced with permission from R.W. Schrier and C.W. Gottschalk, *Diseases of the kidney*, 5th edn, published by Little, Brown, W., Boston MA, 1993.)

(a) 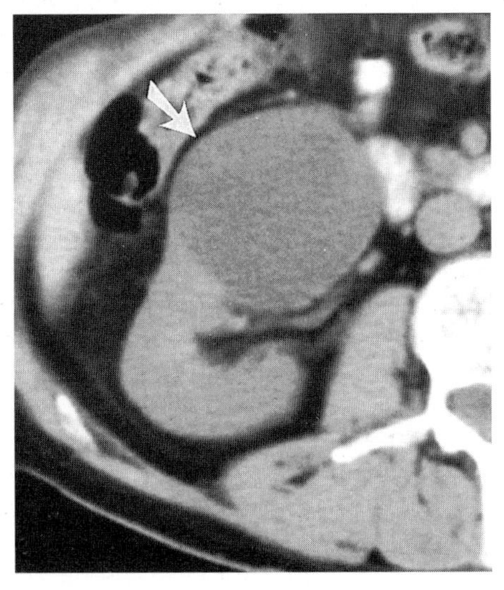

(b) 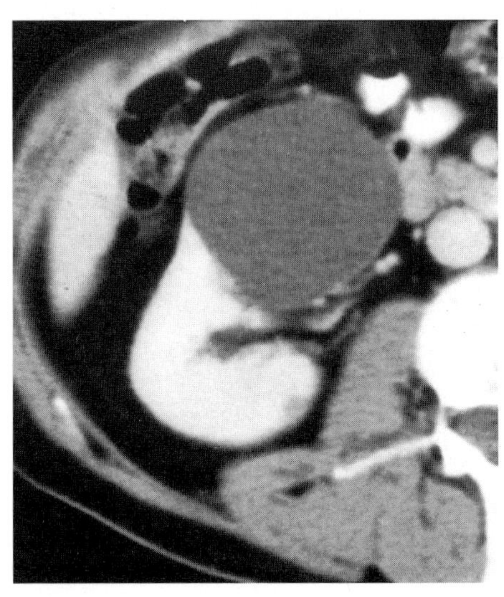

Fig. 7.32 Simple renal cyst on CT. Round water-density mass (arrowed) (a) with no enhancement after contrast medium (b). (Reproduced with permission from W.R. Cattell, J.A.W. Webb and A.J.W. Hilson, *Clinical renal imaging*, published by John Wiley, Chichester, 1989.)

(a) 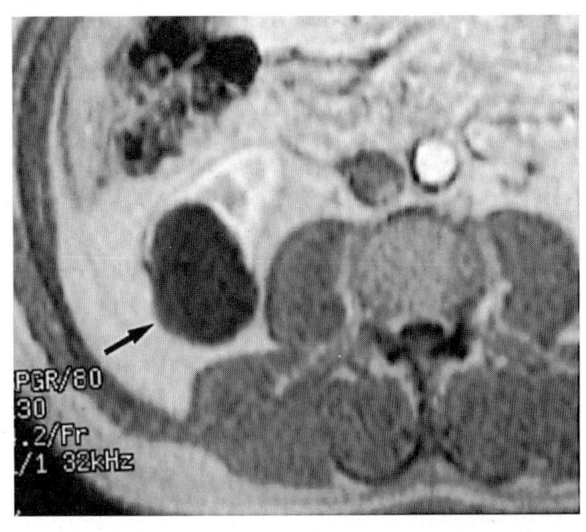

(b) 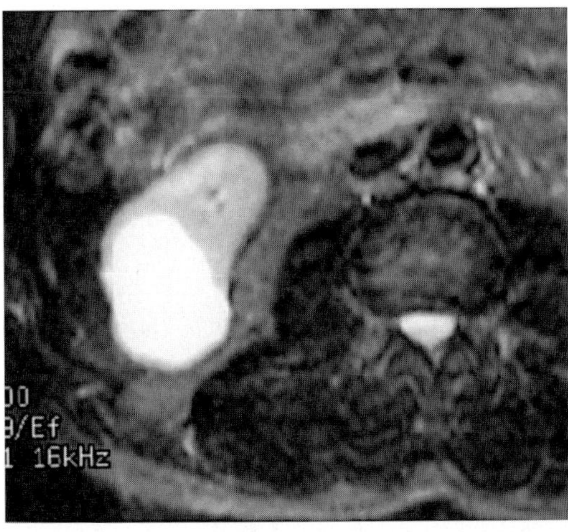

Fig. 7.33 Simple renal cyst on MR. (a) T1-weighted axial image after gadolinium. Note the low signal intensity of the cyst (arrowed) which has not enhanced, and the corticomedullary differentiation in the normal enhanced kidney. (b) T2-weighted axial image shows high signal intensity in the cyst.

ATYPICAL CYSTS

A number of features may lead to a cyst being classed as atypical at ultrasound or CT:

- calcification: some simple cysts have a pencil-thin rim of calcification in their wall, but such calcification may also occur in adenocarcinoma;
- septation (Fig. 7.34);
- echoes within the cyst at ultrasound;
- increased density or enhancement at CT.

These appearances raise the possibility of a variety of conditions including haemorrhagic cyst, infected cyst or abscess, necrotic tumour or haematoma. Further investigation is always indicated to confirm or exclude tumour. if the ultrasound features are atypical, CT or cyst puncture is performed. CT is preferred if the cyst is multiloculate or there are multiple cysts. If the CT features are atypical, ultrasound or cyst puncture may be helpful.

RENAL ADENOCARCINOMA (RENAL CELL CARCINOMA)

A proportion of renal adenocarcinomas calcify and typically the calcification is central and irregular. Peripheral calcification, however, does occur in adenocarcinoma and **any calcified renal mass should be considered malignant until proved otherwise**.

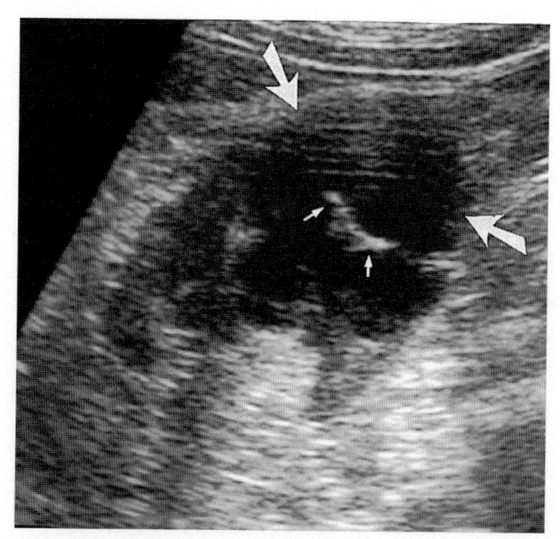

Fig. 7.34 Septate renal cyst (large arrows) on ultrasound scan. Note the central septum (small arrows). (Reproduced with permission from R.W. Schrier and C.W. Gottschalk, *Diseases of the kidney*, 5th edn, published by Little, Brown & Co., Boston MA, 1993.)

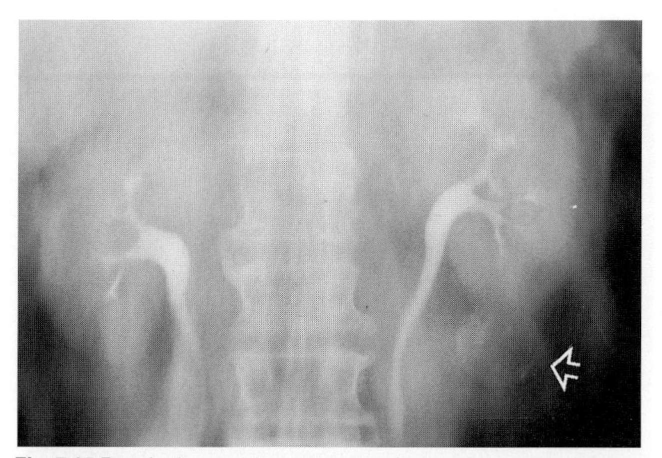

Fig. 7.35 Renal adenocarcinoma (arrowed) with peripheral and central calcification shows patchy opacification on IVU.

On **urography** the tumour usually opacifies in an irregular manner (Fig. 7.35) and is poorly defined from adjacent renal parenchyma. If it has a definable wall, the wall is thicker than 1 mm. If the tumour lies centrally within the kidney it may displace and compress the pelvicalyceal system and possibly invade it, producing irregular filling defects.

Renal adenocarcinoma is seen at **ultrasound** as a solid mass, typically slightly hypoechoic to adjacent renal parenchyma and commonly inhomogeneous (Fig. 7.36). It may, however, have similar or increased echogenicity compared to the parenchyma. If the tumour necroses it may show increased through-transmission of sound indicating the presence of fluid, but the fluid contains echoes and the wall is thickened. If the mass contains calcifications, bright echoes with associated acoustic shadowing are seen.

Renal adenocarcinoma typically has attenuation values close to or less than adjacent renal parenchyma on **CT** before contrast medium and may contain calcification. After contrast medium the mass enhances and has an irregular interface with renal parenchyma (Fig. 7.37). If it is necrotic and partly fluid-containing, the wall is thickened. The CT diagnosis of renal adenocarcinoma is sufficiently accurate that preoperative biopsy is not usually performed.

The most common pattern of renal adenocarcinoma on **MRI** is a mass of reduced signal intensity on T1-weighted images which enhances after gadolinium and shows inhomogenous higher signal intensity than normal kidney, but less than fluid on T2-weighted images.

Staging of renal adenocarcinoma

Currently CT is considered the best staging method for renal adenocarcinoma. It can define whether the

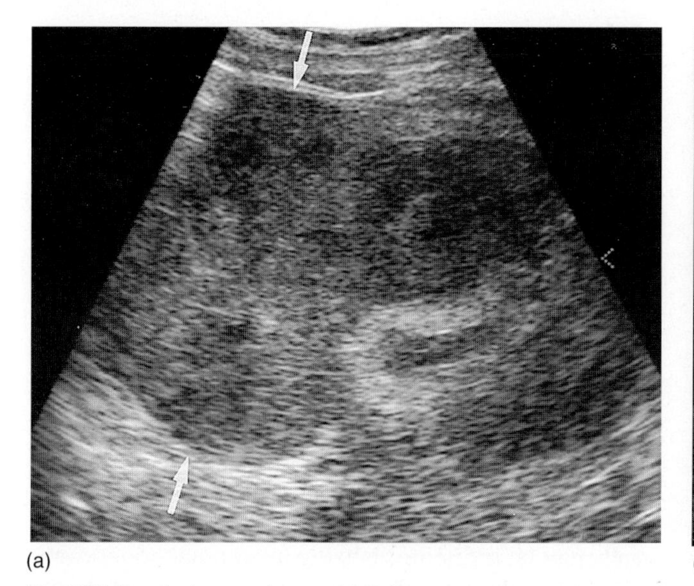

(a)

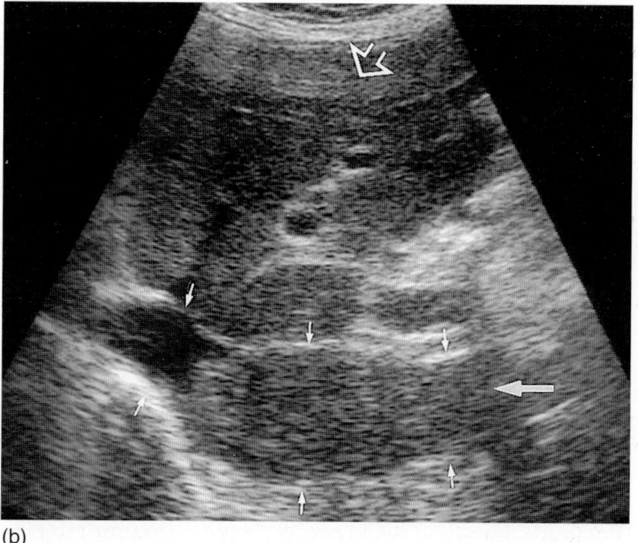

(b)

Fig. 7.36 Renal adenocarcinoma. (a) Solid upper pole mass (arrowed) on longitudinal ultrasound scan. (b) Tumour extension (large white arrow) into the vena cava (small arrows indicate caval walls) seen on longitudinal ultrasound scan (open arrow indicates left lobe of liver).

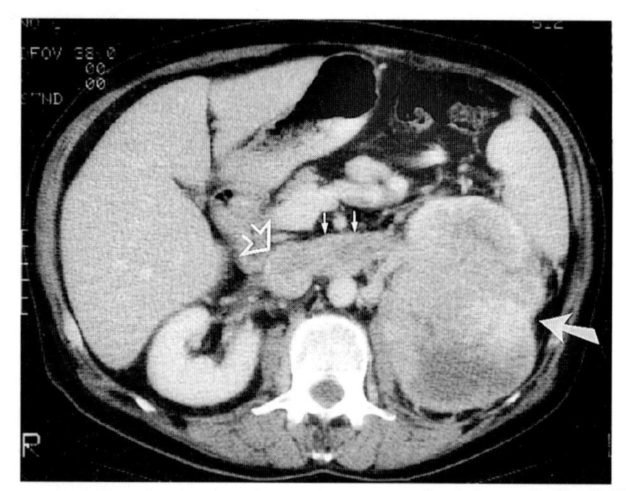

Fig. 7.37 Renal adenocarcinoma in same patient shown in fig. 7.36. CT scan after contrast medium shows inhomogeneously enhancing renal mass (solid arrow). There is tumour extension into an enlarged left renal vein (small arrows) and the vena cava (open arrow).

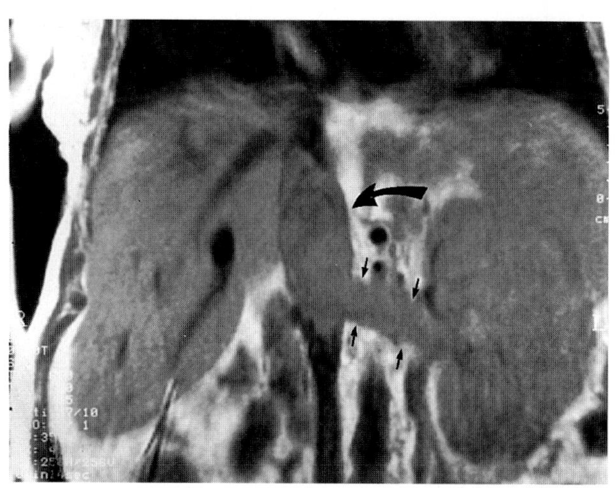

Fig. 7.38 Renal adenocarcinoma in same patient shown in fig. 7.36. Coronal T1-weighted MR scan shows tumour extension into left renal vein (short arrows) and vena cava (long arrow).

tumour breaches the capsule or the renal fascia, show venous extension and para-aortic lymphadenopathy, and detect liver metastases. Venous extension initially involves the renal vein and then may extend up the vena cava (Fig. 7.37) to the right atrium. The affected veins expand and the filling defect produced by the tumour can be defined on the scans obtained after contrast medium.

Ultrasound is also useful in detecting venous extension and can show tumour in the right renal vein, terminal portion of the left renal vein and vena cava (Fig. 7.36b, p. 197). It is particularly helpful in defining the relation of the upper end of the tumour to the diaphragm. Its limitations relate to the fact that bowel gas commonly obscures the proximal left renal vein and the infrahepatic vena cava. Liver metastases are well detected but perinephric extension is assessed less well than with CT.

Magnetic resonance imaging is particularly successful at defining venous extension of tumour which can be imaged in the coronal plane (Fig. 7.38). It can also demonstrate perinephric, nodal and liver involvement.

Angiography is no longer used in the diagnosis of renal adenocarcinoma but may occasionally be requested to demonstrate arterial anatomy if partial nephrectomy is planned.

ANGIOMYOLIPOMA

Angiomyolipoma is a benign tumour which contains fat. Solitary angiomyolipomas typically occur in middle-aged females and present with haemorrhage. Multiple angiomyolipomas occur in tuberous sclerosis. Small angiomyolipomas are frequently detected incidentally on ultrasound where they are seen as small, well-defined masses with markedly increased echogenicity, similar to that of sinus fat. While the tumour may be suspected from this sonographic appearance, the diagnostic test is CT which shows fat density within the mass (Fig. 7.39). Diagnosis may be difficult if haemorrhage obscures the fat.

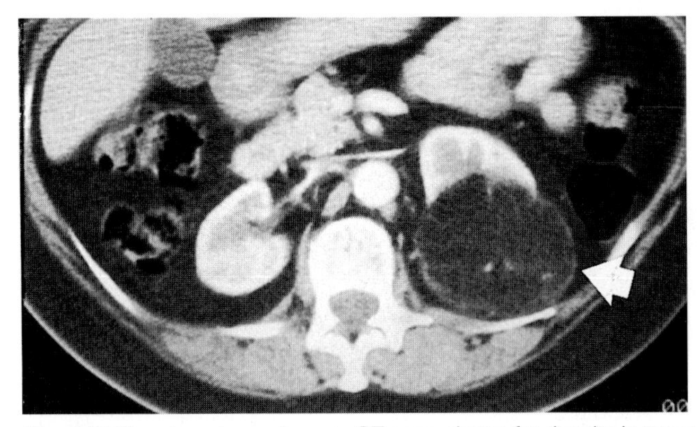

Fig. 7.39 Renal angiomyolipoma. CT scan shows fat density in mass (arrowed).

LYMPHOMA AND METASTASES

If solid renal masses are multiple and occur in a patient with a known primary tumour or with marked para-aortic lymphadenopathy, metastases or lymphoma should be considered. The imaging appearances may be indistinguishable from renal adenocarcinoma and if either metastases or lymphoma are suspected, biopsy is appropriate.

WILMS' TUMOUR

Wilms' tumour is predominantly a tumour of childhood but can occur in young adults. The diagnosis may be suggested by the patient's age, and by the appearance of the tumour which is typically large and contains areas of haemorrhage and necrosis.

TUMOURS OF THE COLLECTING SYSTEM AND URETER

The majority of tumours arising in the collecting system and ureter are transitional cell tumours. Squamous cell carcinomas are less common and are associated with stones or chronic infection. The tumours arise in the mucosa and urography is the best method to show them because it depicts detailed pelvicalyceal and ureteric anatomy.

Calcium salts may encrust the surface of transitional cell tumours and rarely will be seen as faint stippled calcification on the plain film. On **intravenous urography** the tumours are seen as either polypoid or plaque-like filling defects in the pelvicalyceal system and ureter, and may be multiple (Fig. 7.40). With growth they narrow the lumen and can produce obstruction of a calyx, the pelviureteric junction or the ureter (Fig. 7.29, p. 194). The ureteric stricture may be indistinguishable from that produced by an extrinsic mass. Renal transitional cell tumours may invade the renal parenchyma to produce a renal mass; differentiation from renal adenocarcinoma invading the pelvicalyceal system is then difficult.

Ultrasonography only detects large renal transitional cell tumours. Typically they are seen as hypoechoic solid masses centrally in the sinus displacing the normal bright echoes of the sinus.

Computed tomography also shows larger transitional cell tumours as masses of soft-tissue density or as thickening of the wall of the pelvis or ureter. CT is particularly helpful in the differential diagnosis of 'lucent' filling defects in the pelvicalyceal system, allowing calculi with their high CT density to be separated from tumour and blood clot.

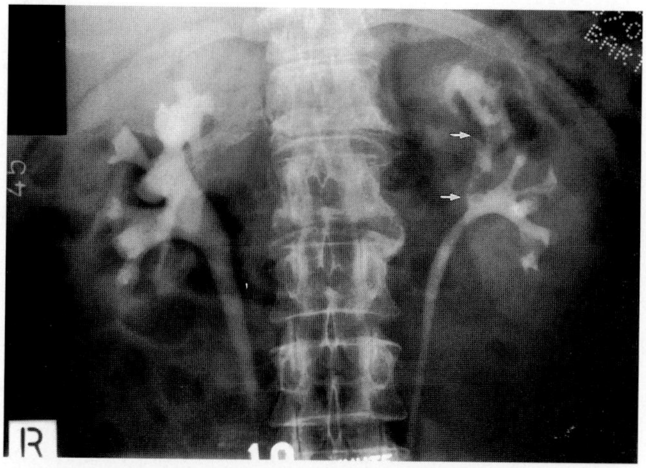

Fig. 7.40 Transitional cell carcinoma of the left upper pole calyces on IVU. Note the multiple small lucent filling defects (arrowed). (Reproduced with permission from H.N. Whitfield, W.F. Hendry, R.S. Kirby and J.W. Duckett, *Textbook of genitourinary* surgery, to be published by Blackwell, Oxford.)

RENAL CYSTIC DISEASE

Simple renal cysts are often multiple and their features are described on page 195. Renal anatomy may be distorted by the multiple cysts, but renal size is normal and the cysts are few enough to be counted.

AUTOSOMAL DOMINANT POLYCYSTIC KIDNEY DISEASE (ADULT POLYCYSTIC KIDNEY DISEASE)

Autosomal dominant polycystic kidney disease is always bilateral, although involvement may be asymmetric.

Ultrasonography is the diagnostic method of choice. The kidneys are enlarged. There is loss of the normal corticomedullary differentiation and of the normal pattern of sinus and parenchyma because the whole kidney is replaced by multiple cysts of varying sizes, too numerous to count (Fig. 7.41). This latter feature distinguishes the condition from multiple simple cysts.

Urography shows enlarged kidneys with lobulated outlines and multiple mass lesions. These produce rounded lucencies in the nephrogram with stretching and compression of the pelvicalyceal systems. Since these appearances can also be produced by multiple solid masses, ultrasound is necessary to confirm the diagnosis.

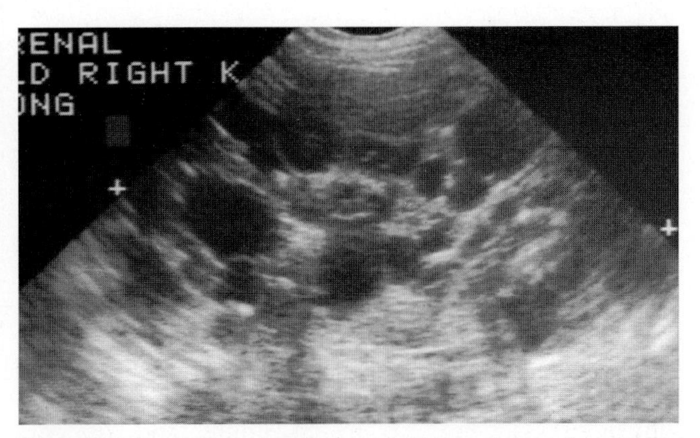

Fig. 7.41 Autosomal dominant polycystic kidney disease. Longitudinal ultrasound scan shows enlarged kidney (calipers mark poles) with normal internal structure replaced by multiple cysts.

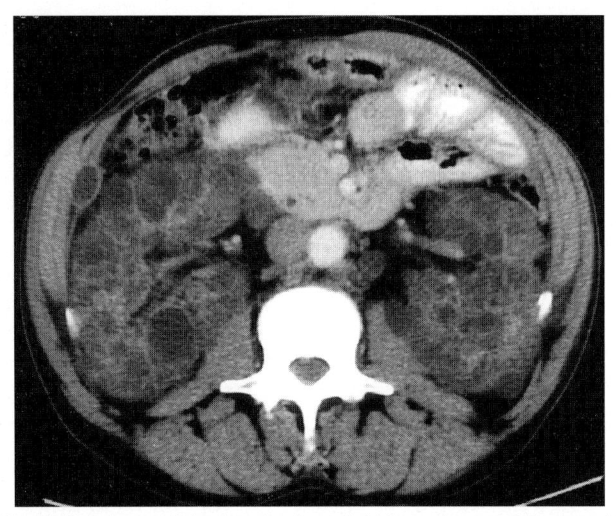

Fig. 7.42 Autosomal dominant polycystic kidney disease. CT scan with contrast medium enhancement shows enlarged kidneys containing multiple cysts.

Computed tomography also shows enlarged kidneys replaced by multiple cysts of varying sizes (Fig. 7.42).

About one-third of patients have liver cysts and 10% have pancreatic cysts detectable by ultrasound or CT. There may be haemorrhage into the renal cysts or they may become infected. Ultrasound or CT often then detects atypical features; contained echoes or increased density. Autosomal dominant polycystic kidney disease is not associated with an increased risk of renal malignancy.

Early disease may be detected before clinical presentation. Ultrasound is the method of choice for screening the relatives of affected individuals at age 18–20. In the early stages of the disease renal size is normal and a few small cysts only may be present.

AUTOSOMAL RECESSIVE POLYCYSTIC KIDNEY DISEASE (INFANTILE POLYCYSTIC KIDNEY DISEASE)

Autosomal recessive polycystic kidney disease is a rare inherited condition in which both the kidneys and the liver show cysts and fibrosis. The younger the presentation, the more severely the kidneys are affected, while liver involvement occurs in later childhood. Renal involvement is always bilateral and results in renal enlargement. At **ultrasonography** the cysts are commonly too small to be seen and the renal parenchyma shows diffuse increase in echogenicity caused by the walls of the multiple tiny cysts. Occasionally small discrete cysts are seen. **Urography** shows enlarged kidneys with a dense nephrogram which persists for up to 24 hours and appears streaky because of contrast medium in dilated tubules.

MULTICYSTIC DYSPLASTIC KIDNEY

Multicystic dysplastic kidney is a sporadic condition in which the kidney fails to develop normally and consists of a collection of non-functioning cysts and primitive tissues. In neonatal life, a large abdominal mass containing multiple cysts at ultrasound is the typical appearance. In older children and adults the dysplastic kidney is small. It may show curvilinear calcification peripherally. Faint enhancement only may be seen at urography with no pelvicalyceal filling. Ultrasound shows a collection of non-communicating cysts of varying sizes. If retrograde ureterography is performed, an atretic ureter may be shown. The contralateral kidney is usually hypertrophied and has an increased incidence of other congenital anomalies, especially pelviureteric junction obstruction.

ACQUIRED CYSTIC DISEASE

Acquired cystic disease occurs in many patients on long-term dialysis. The shrunken end-stage kidneys develop multiple, usually small cysts which may be detected by ultrasound or CT. Complications include haemorrhage into the cysts, which may lead to cyst rupture, and an increased incidence of malignancy. While ultrasound can reliably detect the cysts, CT is a better method to search for solid tumours in these shrunken abnormal kidneys.

UPPER URINARY TRACT INFECTION

ACUTE URINARY TRACT INFECTION

The diagnosis of acute urinary tract infection depends on the demonstration of significant bacteriuria, usually in association with typical clinical features. **The great majority of patients with acute urinary tract infection do not require imaging.**

Occasionally, if renal pain is severe, ureteric colic may be suspected and an IVU may be performed. In acute pyelonephritis the IVU may be normal. In about 25% of patients there may be swelling of the kidney, reduced nephrogram density and poor filling of the pelvicalyceal system which is compressed by the swollen parenchyma.

Imaging is indicated if the patient fails to respond normally to antibiotic treatment and if obstruction or focal sepsis is suspected. Ultrasonography is usually chosen and in acute pyelonephritis images may be normal or show diffuse or focal renal swelling. If computed tomography is performed, patients with severe pyelonephritis may show renal swelling on the precontrast medium scans. After intravenous contrast medium, these patients may show a distinctive pattern of enhancement with streaky and wedge-shaped areas of reduced enhancement within the parenchyma.

FOCAL ACUTE SEPSIS: RENAL AND PERINEPHRIC ABSCESS, PYONEPHROSIS

Renal abscess is seen at IVU as a mass with no specific features unless it contains air. Both on ultrasound and CT, a renal abscess may be seen as a simple fluid collection, or may show a thickened wall (Fig. 7.43); on ultrasound, it may be seen as contained echoes which may layer; on CT it may be seen as increased density of the contents. Air will be readily detected by CT and may be suspected on ultrasound if bright echoes with associated acoustic shadows are seen. Either ultrasound or CT may be used to guide needle puncture of an abscess for diagnostic purposes or for drainage.

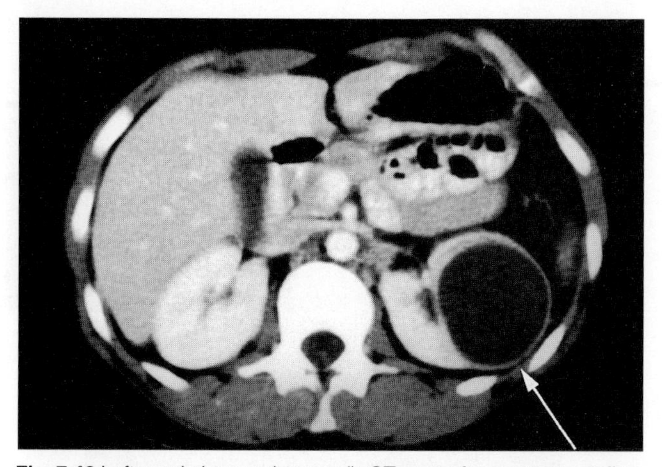

Fig. 7.43 Left renal abscess (arrowed). CT scan after contrast medium shows its thickened enhancing wall. (Reproduced with permission from W.R. Cattell, *Infections of the kidney and urinary tract*, published by Oxford University Press, Oxford, 1996.)

Perinephric abscesses are most often secondary to rupture of an obstructed infected collecting system, but can also arise from rupture of an intrarenal abscess. On plain films the psoas and renal outlines may be lost and at urography displacement of the kidney superiorly and anteriorly may be noted.

Ultrasound shows a fluid collection predominantly postero-inferior to the kidney which may appear simple or show contained echoes or features suggestive of air. Computed tomography provides an excellent demonstration of the extent of perinephric abscesses (Fig. 7.44) which may appear of water or increased density and may contain air. Either ultrasound or CT can be used to guide percutaneous drainage of a perinephric abscess.

In **pyonephrosis** an obstructed infected pelvicalyceal system may show features identical to a simple dilated collecting system or may show air or other findings indicating a complex fluid collection. At ultrasound, there may be contained echoes which may layer (Fig. 7.45), and at CT increased density may be shown. Usually no contrast medium excretion into the pelvicalyceal system is seen at CT.

CHRONIC SEPSIS: XANTHOGRANULOMATOUS PYELONEPHRITIS

Some patients with obstruction and infection develop the unusual chronic inflammatory condition of xanthogranulomatous pyelonephritis. This is characterized by macrophages which ingest fat ('foamy macrophages') within the chronic inflammatory tissue. The whole kidney is usually affected. Typically the renal pelvis is contracted,and contains a calculus. The ultrasonographic and CT findings are similar to those

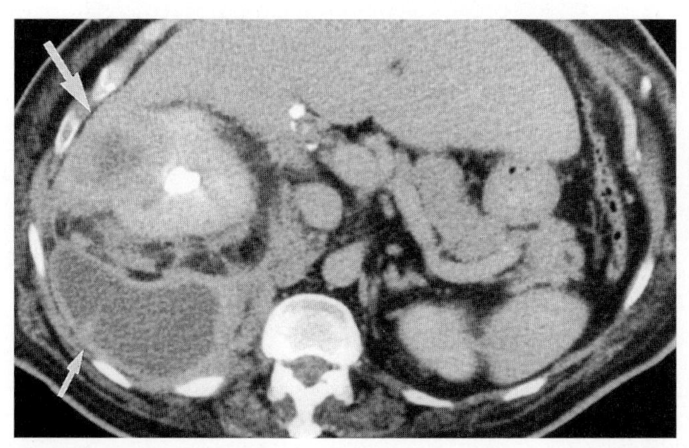

Fig. 7.44 Right perinephric abscess on CT scan. A lateral renal abscess has spread into the perinephric (large arrow) and paranephric (small arrow) spaces. (Reproduced with permission from W.R. Cattell, *Infections of the kidney and urinary tract*, published by Oxford University Press, Oxford, 1996.)

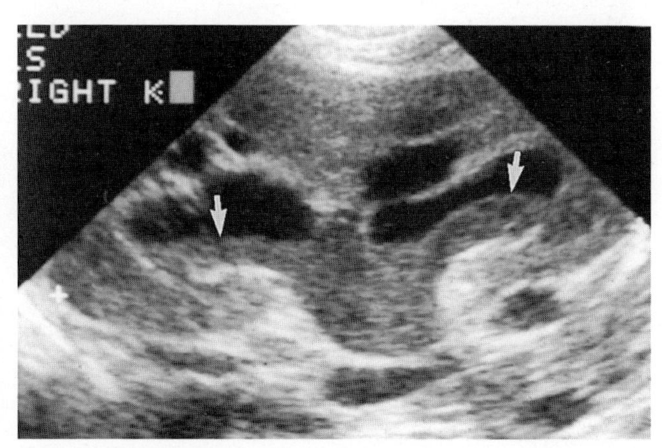

Fig. 7.45 Pyonephrosis. Longitudinal ultrasound scan of kidney shows dilated pelvicalyceal system with echoes layering posteriorly (arrowed). (Reproduced with permission from W.R. Cattell, *Infections of the kidney and urinary tract*, published by Oxford University Press, Oxford, 1996.)

in pyonephrosis, and there is commonly extension of the inflammatory process into the perinephric space or psoas muscle. The affected kidney enhances poorly after intravenous contrast medium and there is no pelvicalyceal filling. Despite the pathological findings, fat density is not detected at CT.

RECURRENT URINARY TRACT INFECTION

In patients with proven recurrent urinary tract infection, further imaging investigation may be warranted to check whether there are associated complicating factors which increase the risk of renal damage (such as stones, obstruction, reflux or papillary necrosis) or whether there are factors likely to predispose to relapse or reinfection (such as stasis, scars or poor bladder emptying). While some of these conditions may be detectable by ultrasound and plain films, the best investigation in the majority of instances is intravenous urography because of the detailed anatomical information it provides.

REFLUX NEPHROPATHY

The term reflux nephropathy is applied to the late sequelae of reflux of infected urine into the kidney, usually in early childhood. Occasionally it may develop later in life. The diagnosis usually requires urography. Typically the condition is focal and has a predominantly polar patchy distribution with areas of thinned parenchyma (scars) overlying blunted calyces (Fig. 7.46). Scarring at the poles is frequently associated with a smooth renal outline. The affected kidney often grows poorly and renal asymmetry is common. More rarely the condition is diffuse with generalized parenchymal loss and calyceal blunting, an appearance indistinguishable from the appearances following obstruction.

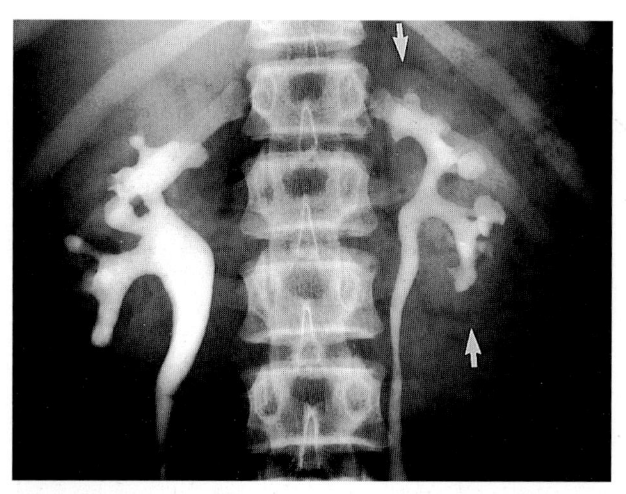

Fig. 7.46 Bilateral reflux nephropathy. Small left kidney (poles indicated by arrows) with diffuse calyceal blunting and irregularly scarred right kidney with multiple blunt calyces. (Reproduced with permission from W.R. Cattell, J.A.W. Webb and A.J.W. Hilson, *Clinical renal imaging*, published by John Wiley, Chichester, 1989.)

TUBERCULOSIS

Tuberculosis in the urinary tract is usually multifocal.

Urography is the best method to show the changes especially in early disease where detailed pelvicalyceal anatomy needs to be shown.

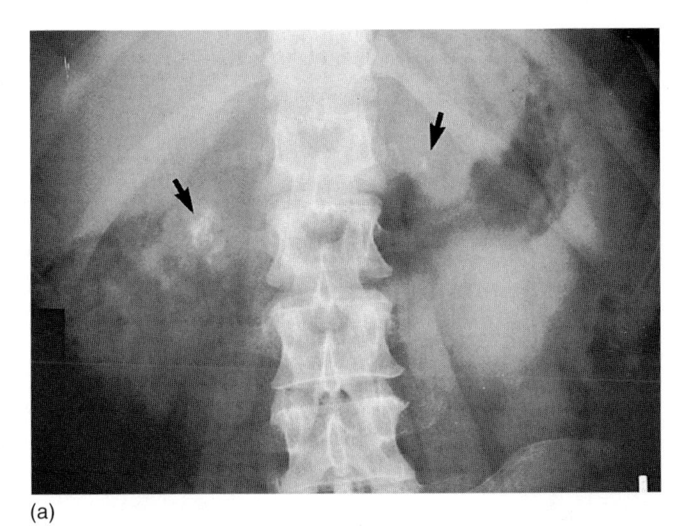

(a)

(b)

Fig. 7.47 Right renal and ureteric tuberculosis. (a) Plain film shows calcification (arrowed) at both upper poles. (b) IVU shows no calyceal filling at the right upper pole and dilation of the remaining right pelvicalyceal system and ureter to the level of a ureteric stricture at the pelvic brim.

Calcification is frequent. In the kidney it may be focal and speckled (Fig. 7.47) or more widespread and hazy. Late in the disease the whole pelvicalyceal system and ureter may be calcified: so-called tuberculous autonephrectomy. Calcification also occurs in the ureter, bladder, vas, seminal vesicles and prostate.

The earliest renal change is papillary with destruction of the papillary margins leading to poor definition of the calyces. Contrast medium density in the affected pelvicalyceal system is often poor. With progression cavities develop which communicate with the pelvicalyceal system. Healing occurs with fibrosis, and this causes stenosis of the calyceal infundibula with delayed or non-filling of dilated calyces proximal to the stenoses (Fig. 7.47). Pelviureteric junction obstruction may also develop by the same mechanism, and eventually the pelvicalyceal system filled with caseous material may calcify.

The ureters may develop smooth or irregular strictures. These may occur during treatment and a limited urogram is usually performed after the patient has been on chemotherapy for 3 months to check for ureteric strictures.

Ultrasound can show the calcification and pelvicalyceal dilatation associated with advanced disease but the appearances are usually non-specific. **Computed tomography** can also show the changes of advanced disease, particularly calcification, pelvicalyceal dilatation, ureteric strictures and extrarenal spread, but is less sensitive than urography in the detection of early renal and ureteric tuberculosis.

TRAUMA

RENAL TRAUMA

Most renal trauma is due to blunt injury. Less commonly injuries are penetrating or iatrogenic, for example following percutaneous nephrolithotomy or renal biopsy.

Plain films may show fractures of the lower ribs or transverse processes of the lumbar vertebrae. The renal and psoas outlines may no longer be seen if there is perinephric bleeding, and if the haematoma is large it may displace bowel.

Urography is usually performed first in localized blunt loin trauma in order to show:

- that the injured kidney is perfused, as evidenced by contrast medium excretion. (If there is injury to the renal pedicle, there will be no contrast medium excretion, and urgent intervention is then indicated.)
- any abnormality in the uninjured kidney which may affect decisions about nephrectomy if conservative management is unsuccessful.

These questions can be answered with a relatively limited IVU (Fig. 7.48). To define the renal injury fully a more detailed study with tomography is necessary. This will show abnormalities in the nephrogram, either local or diffuse reduction of the nephrogram or a wedge-shaped defect if there is laceration. The pelvicalyceal system may be compressed by haematoma and oedema, or may be disrupted with leak of contrast medium (Fig. 7.48). Clot in the pelvicalyceal system produces lucent filling defects.

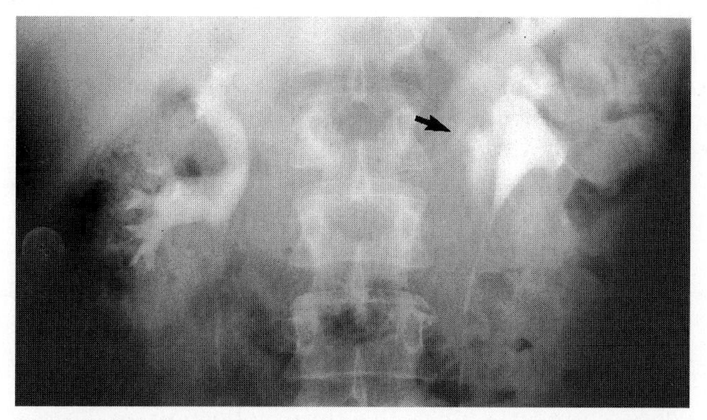

Fig. 7.48 Left renal trauma. IVU shows contrast medium extravasation (arrowed) from left pelvicalyceal system. (Reproduced with permission from W.R. Cattell, J.A.W. Webb and A.J.W. Hilson, *Clinical renal imaging*, published by John Wiley, Chichester, 1989.)

Computed tomography is used when the injury is more severe, when injury to multiple organs is suspected, or if there has been a penetrating injury. On the scans before contrast medium, high-density haematoma may be seen in the pelvicalyceal system, parenchyma or perinephric space. Following contrast medium, rapid sequence scans allow the renal vessels to be visualized. On the nephrogram phase lacerations can be detected as nephrogram defects. Contrast leak from the pelvicalyceal system will be shown and an excellent assessment of the size and extent of the perinephric haematoma can be made (Fig. 7.49). If

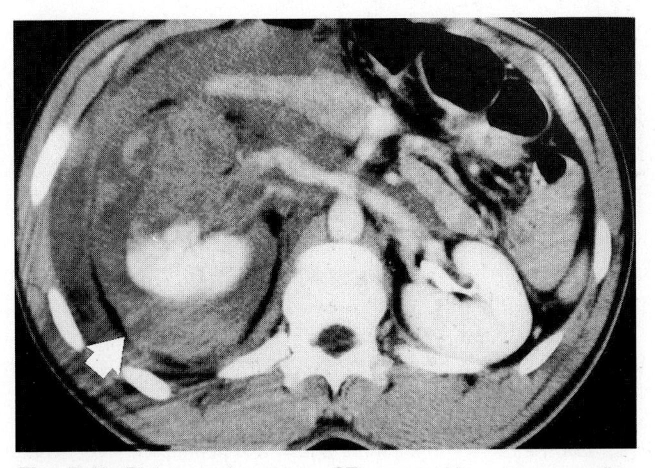

Fig. 7.49 Right renal trauma. CT scan with contrast medium enhancement shows large perinephric haematoma (arrowed) and disruption of the anterior renal parenchyma. (By permission of Dr S. E. Mirvis and Dr K. Shanmuganathan.)

there is injury to the renal artery resulting in occlusion, the renal artery shows abrupt cut-off and there is no renal excretion of contrast medium; however, there may be perfusion of a rim of cortex peripherally from collateral and capsular vessels.

Ultrasound may be used to assess the size of perinephric and intrarenal haematoma (Fig. 7.50). The use of ultrasonography is in part limited by the necessity to move the patient to obtain a good examination. This may not be practicable in severely injured patients. Initially haematomas have the same appearance as fluid, but with the development of clot, echoes appear within the fluid collection making it more difficult to visualize. Doppler ultrasound may be used to assess renal perfusion.

Angiography is no longer used in the diagnosis of renal injury, but may be employed if treatment of haemorrhage by embolization is planned.

Scintigraphy may be used to demonstrate renal perfusion and excretion but gives less anatomical information than the other methods.

Late effect of renal injury

When renal injury is managed conservatively the end result is often parenchymal loss with a relatively normal underlying pelvicalyceal system, appearances indistinguishable from a renal infarct.

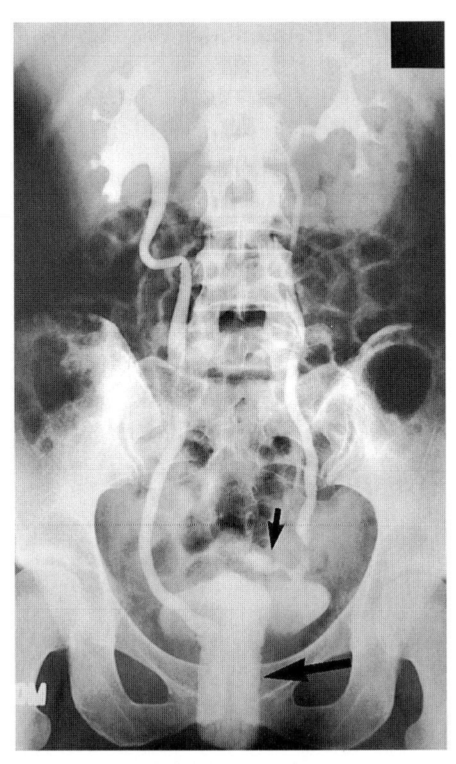

Fig. 7.51 Left ureterovaginal fistula following hysterectomy. IVU shows contrast medium leak from left ureter (small arrow) and contrast medium in the vagina (large arrow).

URETERIC TRAUMA

The ureter is mobile and relatively rarely damaged by blunt injury. It may be injured by penetrating or iatrogenic trauma, for example during bowel or gynaecological surgery.

Intravenous urography is the best method to show injury. Contrast medium leakage from the ureter may be seen, or there may be obstruction if there has been transection or ligation of the ureter. Following gynaecological surgery, there may be a ureterovaginal fistula with contrast medium entering the vagina (Fig. 7.51).

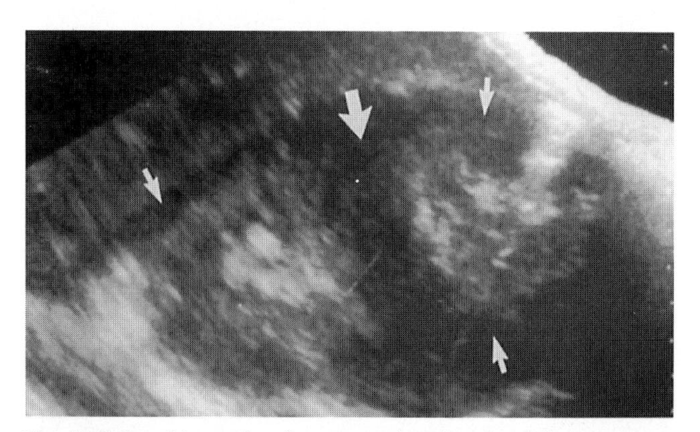

Fig. 7.50 Renal laceration (large arrow) and perinephric haematoma (small arrows) seen on longitudinal ultrasound scan. (Reproduced with permission from W.R. Cattell, J.A.W. Webb and A.J.W. Hilson, *Clinical renal imaging*, published by John Wiley, Chichester, 1989.)

HAEMATURIA

Haematuria, both macroscopic and microscopic, necessitates urinary tract imaging. Particular concerns include renal adenocarcinoma, transitional cell carcinoma of the bladder, pelvicalyceal system and ureter and calculus disease. Other imaging diagnoses which may be made include renal infarction, papillary necrosis and tuberculosis.

Traditionally, **intravenous urography** has been used as the method of choice to evaluate the kidneys and ureters for causes of haematuria, with cystoscopy being used to check the bladder because of the recognized poor sensitivity of urography in detecting bladder carcinoma. Many still consider that IVU combined with cystoscopy remain the best initial investigations in haematuria.

Ultrasound is a more sensitive detector of renal adenocarcinoma and bladder carcinoma than urography and has been recommended, combined with plain films, as the first imaging method of choice in haematuria. If this path is followed, the limitations of ultrasound in diagnosing calculi and the fact that detailed pelvicalyceal and ureteric anatomy are not shown must be borne in mind.

Where the ultrasonographic examination is negative and no cause for haematuria has been found, **IVU** is essential in order that many important causes of haematuria do not go undetected. Conversely, if IVU and cystoscopy are negative, ultrasonography or CT should be used to check for renal masses not detected by IVU.

CHAPTER 8

Lower urinary tract and male genital tract

Judith A. W. Webb

THE BLADDER

TRAUMA

Severe bladder trauma produces bladder rupture. This may be intraperitoneal, if the bladder is full at the time of injury, or extraperitoneal, usually in association with pelvic fracture. Lesser injury produces contusion without rupture and may be associated with bladder displacement by pelvic haematoma.

To image bladder trauma adequately, cystography is necessary. If there is possible urethral trauma, urethrography must be performed first (p. 181) before catheterization of the bladder for cystography. The bladder must be well distended to visualize rupture. Intraperitoneal rupture is seen as contrast medium outlining bowel loops and spreading into the flanks (Fig. 8.1a). In extraperitoneal rupture there is streaky extravasation into the perivesical tissues (Fig. 8.1b). The two may coexist.

Diagnostic and Interventional Radiology in Surgical Practice. Edited by P. Armstrong and M. L. Wastie. Published in 1997 by Chapman & Hall, London. ISBN 0 412 61960 1 (HB), 0 412 61970 9 (PB)

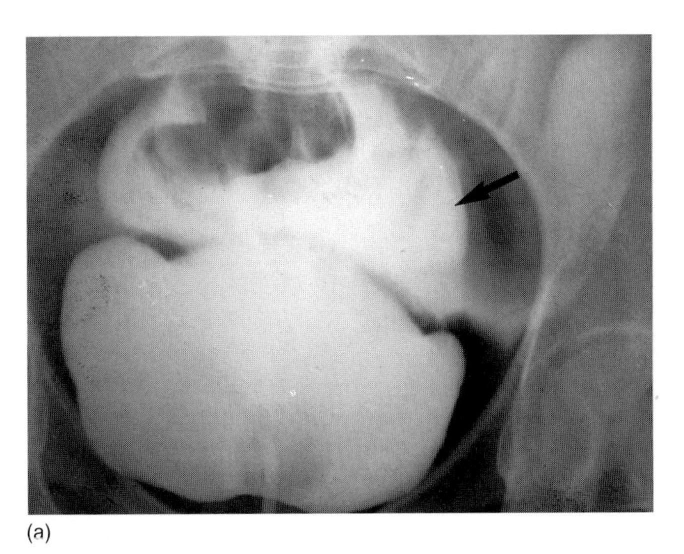

(a)

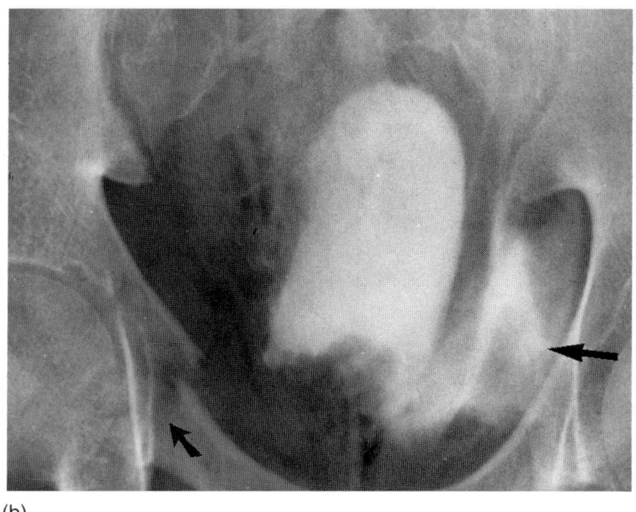

(b)

Fig. 8.1 Cystograms in bladder trauma. (a) Intraperitoneal rupture. The extravasated contrast medium (arrowed) outlines bowel and has a smooth lower margin. (b) Extraperitoneal rupture with associated pelvic fracture (short arrow). Contrast medium is tracking irregularly into the perivesical tissues (long arrow). (Reproduced by permission of Dr S. M. Goldman, in J. J. McCort and R. E. Mindelzun (eds) *Trauma radiology*, published by Churchill Livingstone, Edinburgh, London, 1990.)

CT can detect extravasation and shows its distribution very accurately. However, if intravenous contrast medium alone is used to distend the bladder, CT appears to be less sensitive than cystography. If CT is to be relied on to detect bladder rupture, the bladder should be distended with contrast medium installed through a catheter (CT cystography).

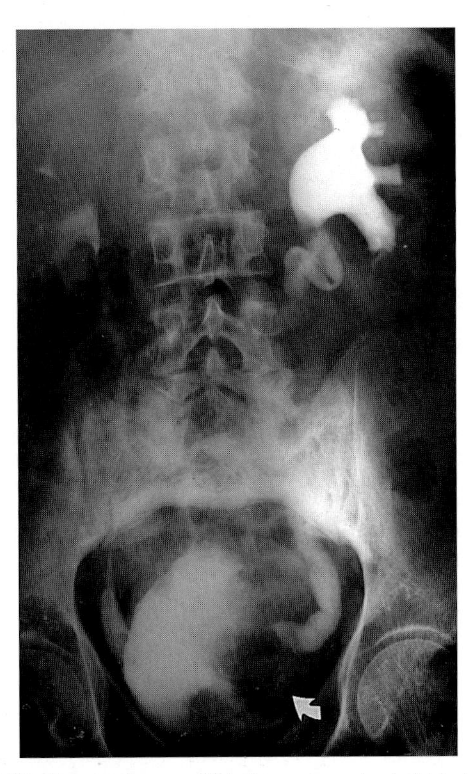

Fig. 8.2 Bladder carcinoma. IVU shows irregular left bladder mass (arrowed) causing ureteric obstruction.

NEOPLASM

The majority of bladder carcinoma is transitional cell in type. Squamous cell carcinoma is infrequent and associated with calculus and chronic infection. Adenocarcinoma is rare and arises in urachal remnants at the bladder fundus.

Calcification on the surface of the bladder tumour may be seen on plain films. On urography, the tumour may produce a polypoid or flattened filling defect (Fig. 8.2) or local bladder wall thickening. Oblique and postmicturition views may help to show whether an apparent filling defect is truly within the lumen rather than being caused by overlying bowel. **Urography is**

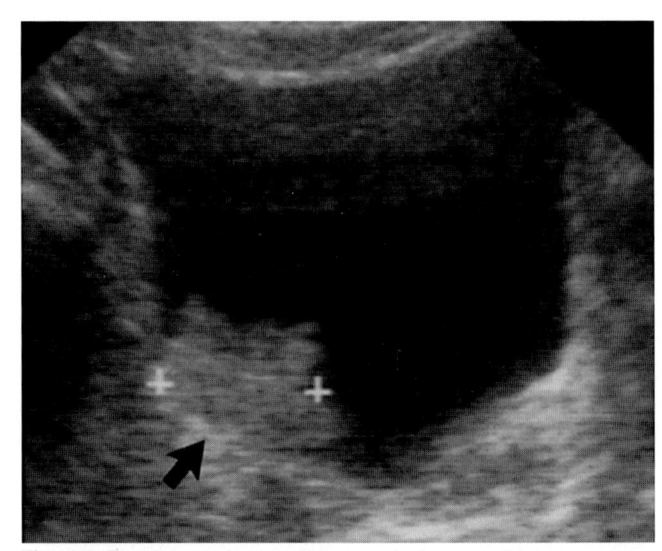

Fig. 8.3 Bladder carcinoma. Ultrasound shows solid tumour mass (arrowed) on the posterior right bladder wall.

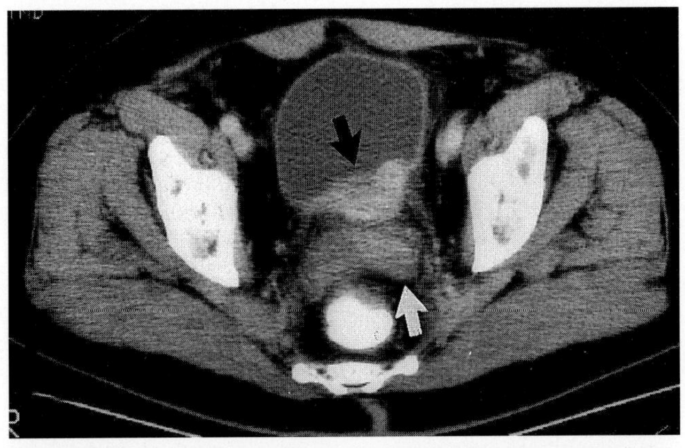

Fig. 8.4 Bladder carcinoma. CT shows posterior bladder tumour (black arrow). Note the clear plane between bladder and seminal vesicle. The white arrow indicates the left seminal vesicle.

relatively insensitive in the detection of bladder cancer. Even quite large tumours may be missed when the bladder is full of contrast medium. The post-micturition bladder film may be helpful in detecting smaller masses.

At **ultrasonography**, bladder tumours are seen as solid masses protruding into the urine-filled bladder (Fig. 8.3) or as localized bladder wall thickening. Ultrasound is more sensitive in the detection of bladder cancer than IVU.

Relatively small amounts of calcification on the tumour surface can be detected at **computed tomography**. The soft tissue density mass of the tumour may be outlined either by non-opacified water density urine (Fig. 8.4) or by contrast medium within the bladder. CT is used to stage bladder cancer. It can

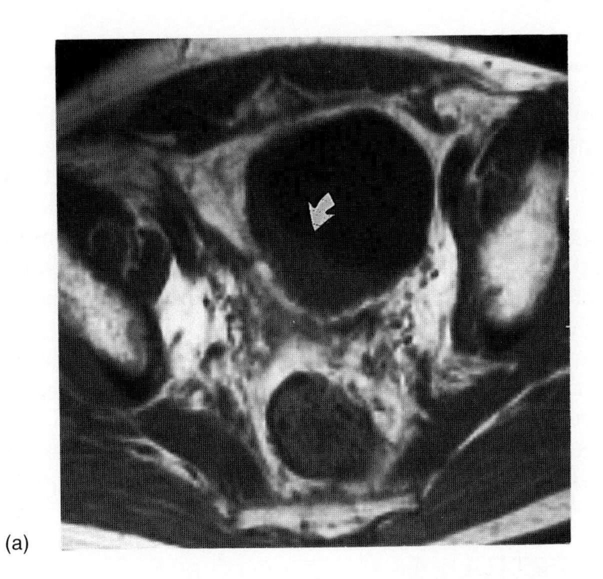

(a)

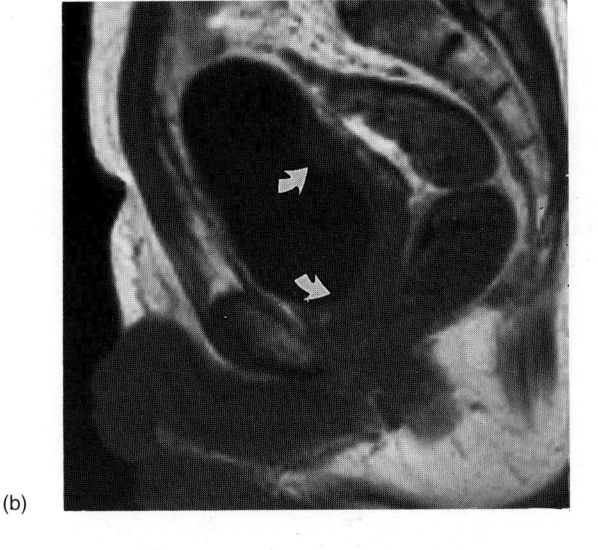

(b)

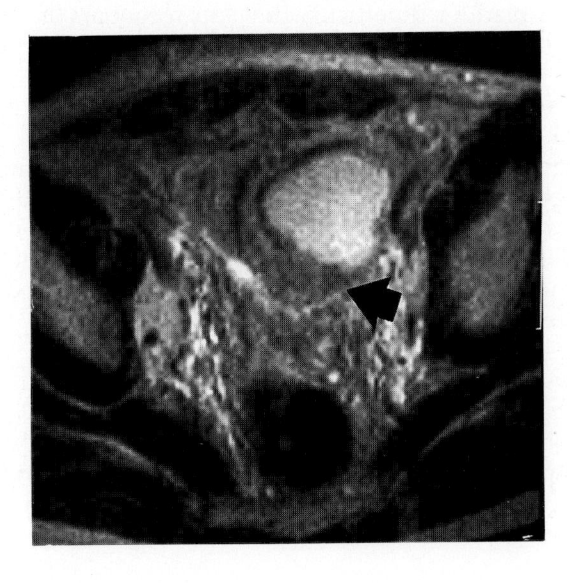

(c)

Fig. 8.5 Bladder carcinoma. Axial (a) and sagittal (b) images show the tumour (arrowed) on T1-weighted MR images Sagittal image clearly depicts involvement of the bladder base. (c) T2-weighted axial MR scan shows increased signal intensity in the tumour (arrowed). (By kind permission of Dr J. Husband.)

demonstrate extension into the perivesical fat and involvement of the adjacent structures – uterus, prostate, seminal vesicles and bowel – and can show whether there is a clear plane of separation between the tumour and the pelvic side wall (Fig. 8.4). CT can also detect pelvic and retroperitoneal nodal metastases. It is not able to show the depth of extension of the tumour within the muscle of the bladder wall.

On **magnetic resonance imaging**, bladder cancer is isointense with the bladder wall on T1-weighted images. The mass or wall thickening stands out well against the low signal intensity urine and the high signal intensity perivesical fat (Fig. 8.5a, 8.5b). On T2-weighted images the tumour usually has higher signal intensity than the wall (Fig. 8.5c). The degree of muscle infiltration can be assessed more accurately with T2-weighted MRI than with CT. The coronal and sagittal planes (Fig. 8.5b) are particularly helpful in demonstrating basal and fundal tumours. MRI, like CT, can demonstrate perivesical spread and lymph node involvement.

INFECTION

Bladder infection produces bladder wall thickening of non-specific appearance which can be demonstrated by IVU, ultrasound or CT. Calcification in the thickened bladder wall suggests tuberculosis or schistosomiasis, both of which produce a contracted bladder in their later stages.

CALCULI AND FILLING DEFECTS

Bladder calculi should be detected on plain films if they are opaque, but on the plain films alone the location of pelvic calcifications may be uncertain.

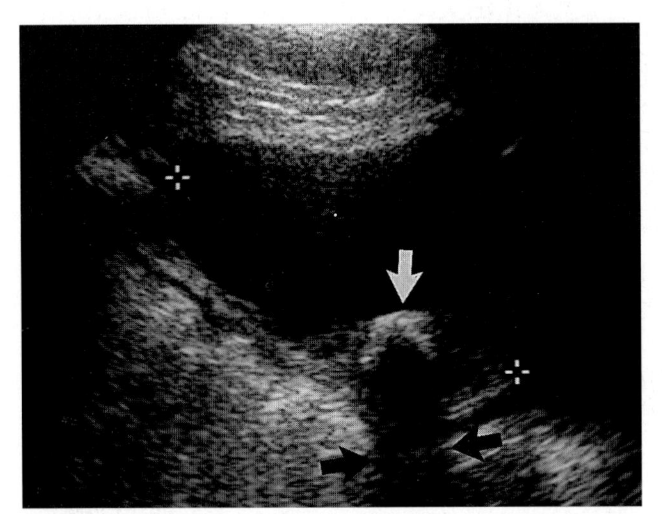

Fig. 8.6 Bladder calculus (white arrow) on longitudinal ultrasound scan. Note the acoustic shadow (black arrows).

Urography, with oblique or lateral views if necessary, demonstrates whether pelvic calcifications lie within the bladder. Bladder stones are well seen at ultrasound as mobile echogenic foci with associated acoustic shadows (Fig. 8.6). Ultrasound is more sensitive for the detection of small bladder stones than is IVU. On CT bladder calculi appear as high density mobile opacities within the bladder lumen.

A variety of other bladder filling defects are seen at urography and may need to be distinguished from calculi. Possible causes of a bladder filling defect are:

- calculus
  - lucent
  - opaque
- tumour
- blood clot
- sloughed papilla
- fungal ball
- foreign body
- ureterocoele
- enlarged prostate.

Lucent filling defects produced by tumour and blood clot may be indistinguishable, especially if clot is adherent to the bladder wall. These two entities also appear identical on sonography. The clinical setting may suggest the possibility of a fungal ball or sloughed papilla. A ureterocoele usually has a characteristic appearance (Chapter 7, p. 186). Prostatic enlargement is usually smooth and basal, producing elevation of the bladder base (see Fig. 8.16, p. 214), but a basal bladder carcinoma may be indistinguishable. Overlying bowel gas can usually be distinguished from a bladder abnormality with oblique films. The lucent bowel gas usually does not overlie the bladder in all positions of the patient.

DIVERTICULA

Most bladder diverticula develop secondary to bladder outflow obstruction; rarely, diverticula are congenital. In bladder outflow obstruction there is also bladder wall thickening and often evidence of prostatic enlargement. Most diverticula fill at urography (Fig. 8.7) and cystography. Their size is variable and if large they may cause displacement of the ureter or bladder. Diverticula may enlarge after voiding. Filling defects within them raise the possibility of calculus or tumour and ultrasound or CT may be used to differentiate these.

FISTULAE

Fistulae from bladder to bowel are usually secondary to diverticulitis or carcinoma of the colon; more rarely they may occur in other inflammatory disease, e.g.

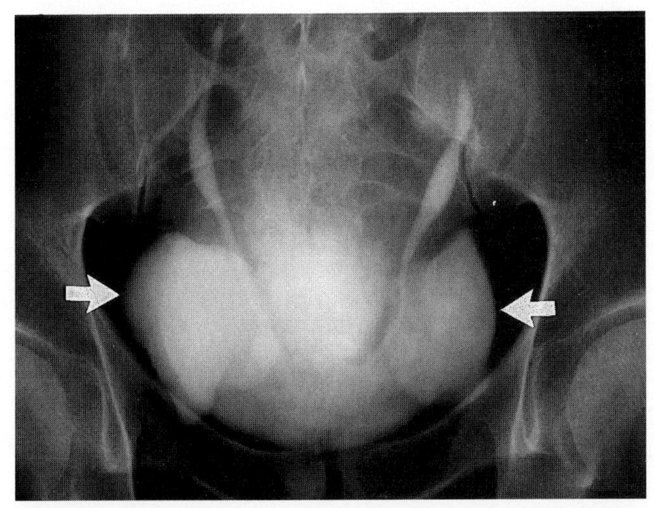

Fig. 8.7 Bladder diverticula. IVU shows bilateral diverticula (arrowed) causing medial deviation of the lower ureters.

Crohn's disease, or after trauma. Fistulae may be suspected if air is seen in the bladder on plain films or at CT. Air in the bladder can however also result from previous instrumentation including bladder catheterization or from infection with gas-forming organisms.

Demonstration of fistulae may be difficult and **cystography** is more likely to show the fistula than urography or barium studies (Fig. 8.8). **CT** is also helpful in detecting fistulae and shows air in the bladder, focal thickening of the bladder wall and adjacent adherent thickened bowel. As with cystography, contrast medium extravasation through the fistula is more difficult to demonstrate.

Fistulae from bladder to vagina usually result from radical pelvic surgery and/or radiotherapy for malignancy and less commonly from obstetric injury. They are usually relatively easy to demonstrate at cystography. Lateral views are helpful to show contrast medium in the vagina.

NEUROPATHIC BLADDER

Full assessment of bladder dysfunction in neuropathic bladder requires videourodynamics. Either IVU or cystography may demonstrate anatomic abnormality. Spinal cord lesions above the parasympathetic outflow cause detrusor hyperreflexia and detrusor–sphincter dyssynergia. These are associated with bladder wall thickening and trabeculation (Fig. 8.9) and in severe cases with an elongated bladder shape, the so-called 'Christmas tree' or 'pine cone' appearance. There may be secondary dilation of the ureters and pelvicalyceal systems caused by obstruction at bladder wall level and/or by vesicoureteric reflux. Bladder calculi are relatively common. Pelvic nerve injury is associated with an atonic bladder which is very large and has a smooth outline. Because of the low intravesical pressure, an atonic bladder may not be associated with dilatation of the pelvicalyceal systems and ureters.

URINARY DIVERSION

Ileal loop diversion may be assessed on an IVU but, to show the anatomy in full, **ileal loopography** is required, a procedure in which a Foley catheter is placed in the ileal loop with the balloon inflated just deep to the abdominal wall in order to occlude the stoma. Contrast medium injected to distend the loop normally refluxes freely into both ureters (Fig. 8.10). Failure to show reflux suggests obstruction at the

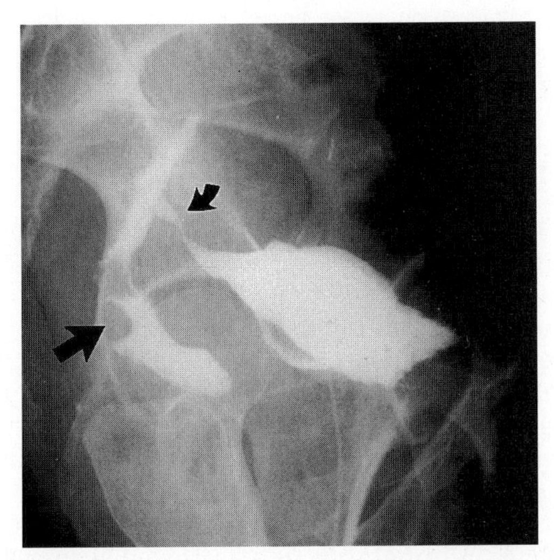

Fig. 8.8 Rectovesical fistula following radiotherapy for carcinoma of cervix. Lateral film shows contrast medium has entered the rectum (large arrow) through a fistula (small arrow) at the bladder fundus.

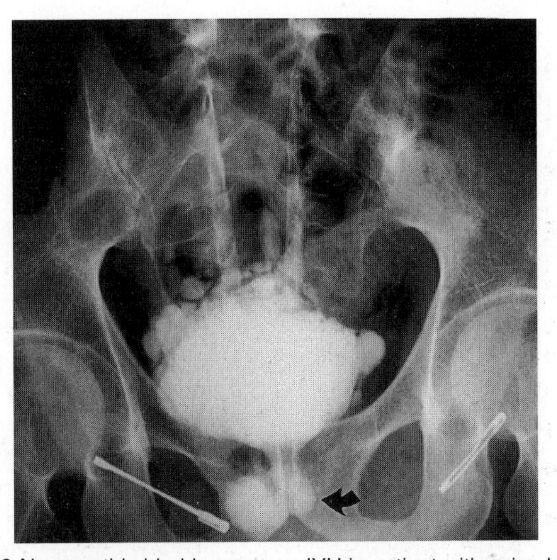

Fig. 8.9 Neuropathic bladder seen on IVU in patient with spina bifida. Note bladder wall thickening, multiple diverticula and contrast medium entering the urethra (arrowed).

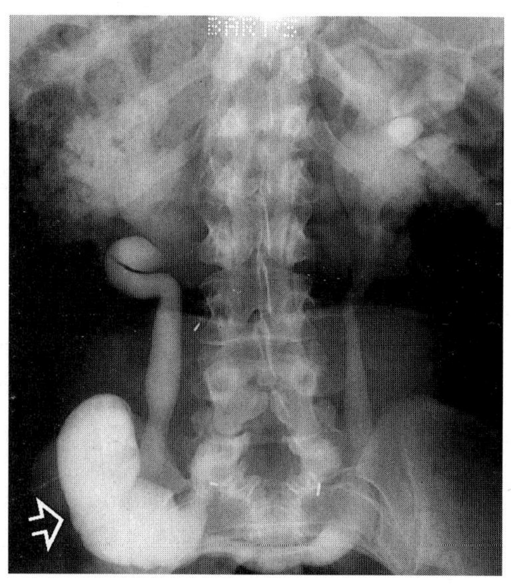

Fig. 8.10 Normal ileal loopogram. Arrow indicates ileal loop.

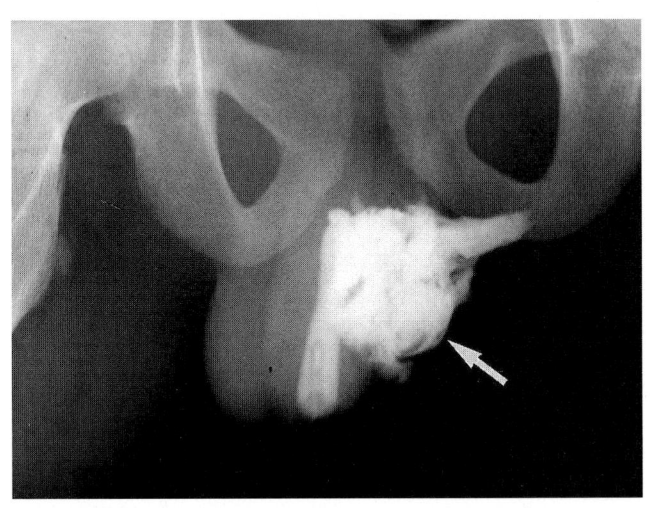

Fig. 8.11 Anterior urethral trauma. Urethrogram shows contrast medium (arrowed) tracking into the penile, scrotal and inguinal soft tissues. (By kind permission of Dr S. M. Goldman.)

uretero-ileal insertion. Other late complications such as ileal loop stenoses may also be demonstrated.

A variety of continent urinary diversions (e.g. Kock pouch, Mainz pouch) are now also undertaken and their anatomy can be demonstrated directly by contrast medium injection through a catheter placed in the pouch.

URETHRA

MALE URETHRA

TRAUMA

In any male patient where urethral trauma is possible, urethrography should be performed before bladder catheterization is attempted, as such attempts may further damage a partially ruptured urethra. Anterior urethral trauma is usually secondary to a straddle injury and contrast medium extravasates below the level of the membranous urethra into the soft tissues of the penis and scrotum (Fig. 8.11). Posterior urethral trauma is usually associated with pelvic fracture. The commonest pattern is a tear through the membranous urethra and urogenital diaphragm involving the prostatic and bulbar urethra (i.e. a combined anterior and posterior urethral injury). Contrast medium extravasation occurs both above and below the urogenital diaphragm. If the rupture is incomplete, some contrast medium may enter the bladder at urethrography (Fig. 8.12). Less commonly, there is stretching of the posterior urethra without rupture or rupture of the posterior urethra alone (Fig. 8.12).

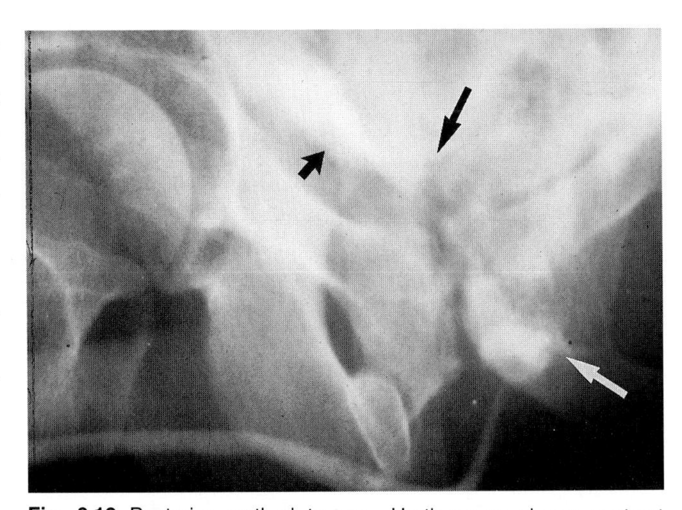

Fig. 8.12 Posterior urethral trauma. Urethrogram shows contrast medium extravasation (white arrow) from the posterior urethra, tracking into the perivesical tissues (short black arrow) around the bladder base (long black arrow). (By kind permission of Dr S. M. Goldman.)

STRICTURE

Stricture of the anterior urethra is usually either postinflammatory (penile and bulbar urethra), post-traumatic (straddle injury to the bulbar urethra) or iatrogenic (at the penoscrotal junction following catheterization or other instrumentation). Posterior urethral strictures are less common: they follow external trauma or may be iatrogenic, especially after transurethral prostate resection.

Anterior urethral stricture is demonstrated at ascending urethrography as a narrowed segment (Fig. 8.13a). In inflammatory stricture this may be irregular and may involve a long segment which fails to distend

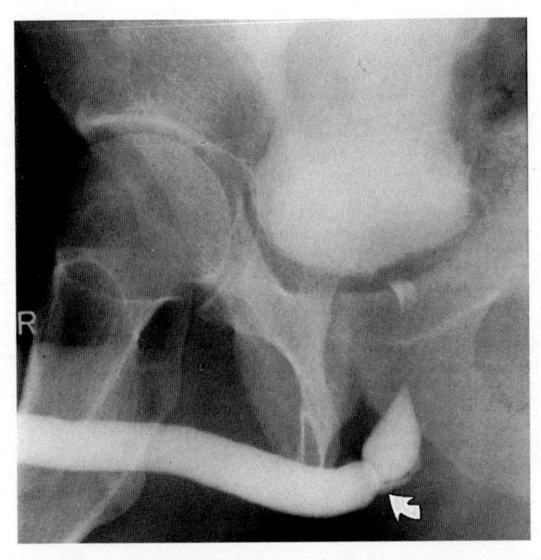

(a)

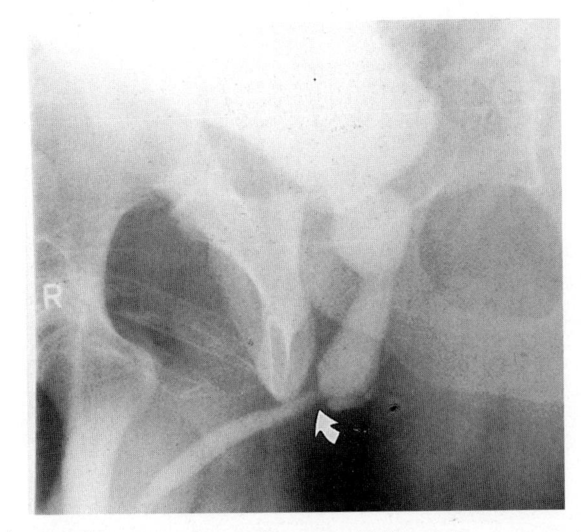

(b)

Fig. 8.13 Urethral stricture in a male. (a) Tight stricture of the bulbar urethra (arrowed) on ascending urethrogram. (b) Micturating cystography shows dilatation of the urethra to the level of the stricture (arrowed). (Reproduced with permission from H. N. Whitfield, W. F. Hendry, R. S. Kirby and J. W. Duckett, *Textbook of genitourinary surgery*, to be published by Blackwell, Oxford)

normally. With inflammatory stricture there may also be filling of Littre's glands, seen as small contrast medium pools alongside the penile urethra, and of Cowper's glands alongside the proximal bulbar urethra. A voiding study shows dilatation of the urethra to the level of the stricture (Fig. 8.13b). Where obstruction is marked, there may be filling of prostatic glands with contrast medium.

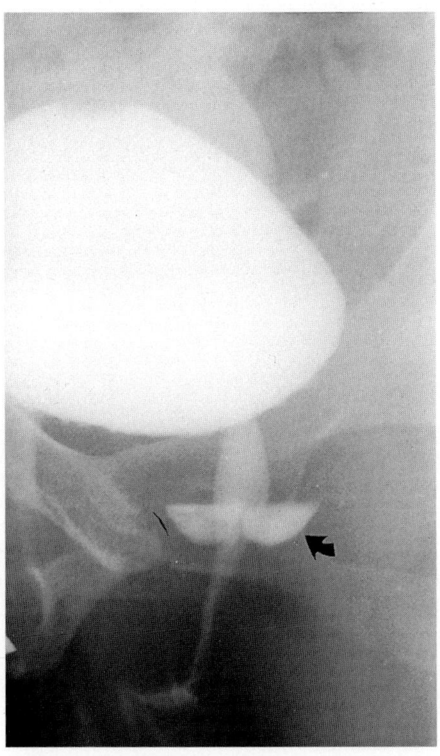

Fig. 8.14 Urethral diverticulum in a female. Biloculate diverticulum (arrowed) fills at micturating cystography.

FEMALE URETHRA

The short female urethra is injured much less frequently than the male urethra. **Urethral diverticula** are relatively uncommon. Many can be demonstrated as a small contrast medium pool inferior to the bladder on a postmicturition bladder film at IVU. The majority will be shown as a contrast medium pool posterior to the urethra at micturating cystography (Fig. 8.14). An alternative method of showing a diverticulum is by transvaginal ultrasonography. Female urethrography is cumbersome and unpleasant for the patient because of the difficulties in obtaining occlusion of the external meatus, and is now rarely used.

PROSTATE

NORMAL ANATOMY

Conventional urography and micturating cystography may show indirect evidence of prostatic enlargement, for example by bladder displacement or urethral compression. The prostate is directly visualized by ultrasound, used either transabdominally, scanning through the full bladder, or transrectally. With **transrectal ultrasound**, a high frequency transducer provides high resolution images, usually in the longitudinal and transverse planes. The zonal anatomy of the prostate and the seminal vesicles are seen (Fig. 8.15). The transition and central zones are usually not separable and appear of reduced echogenicity compared to the peripheral zone which occupies the posterolateral gland and gland apex.

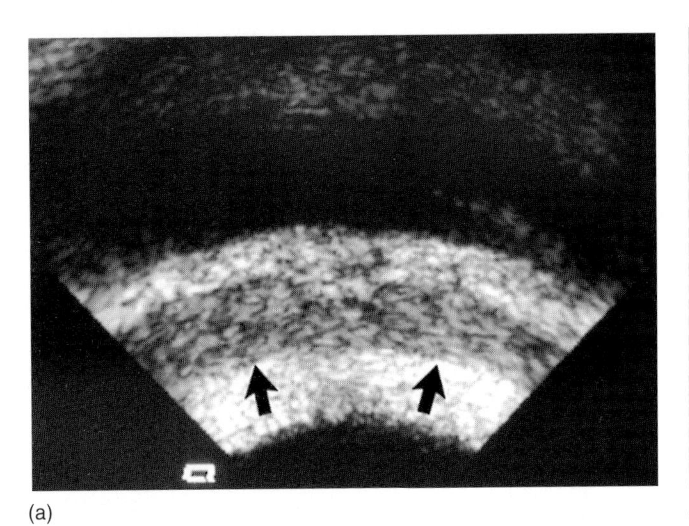

(a)

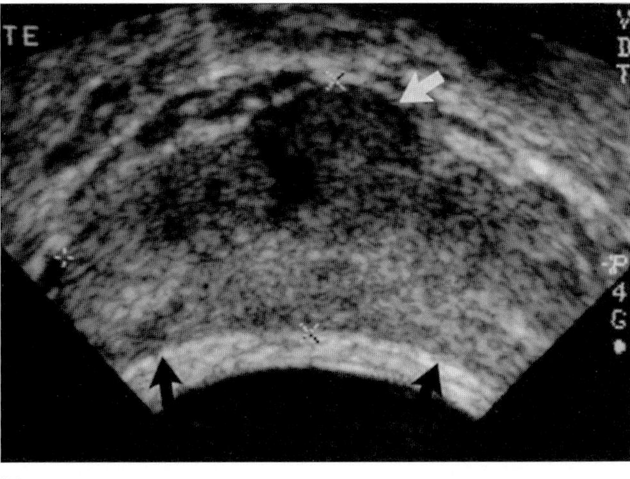

(b)

Fig. 8.15 Normal axial transrectal ultrasound scans. (a) Seminal vesicles (arrowed) lying posterior to the bladder base. (b) Periurethral hypoechoic transition zone (white arrow) and posterolateral peripheral zone (black arrows) on a scan inferior to (a).

CT provides relatively limited information about the prostate which is seen as a homogeneous rounded soft tissue density structure inferior to the bladder base.

MRI shows homogeneous signal intensity in the gland on T1-weighted images, but on T2-weighted images the high signal intensity peripheral zone can be identified separately from the lower intensity central and transition zones (see Fig. 8.19).

BENIGN PROSTATIC HYPERTROPHY

At **urography** the enlarged prostate of benign prostatic hypertrophy elevates the bladder base, commonly with a smooth lucent filling defect protruding into the bladder base (Fig. 8.16). Secondary effects of bladder outflow obstruction may be seen, with bladder wall thickening, trabeculation, diverticula, elevation of the distal ureters (so-called 'fish-hooking') and, in some patients, secondary pelvicalyceal and ureteric dilation. Bladder emptying is usually impaired.

On **transabdominal sonography**, the soft tissue mass of the enlarged prostate is seen protruding into the bladder base. On **transrectal ultrasound** it can be appreciated that the enlargement (Fig. 7.5b, p. 180) involves the central transition zone; this is globular in shape, of inhomogeneous reduced echogenicity and it may contain defined adenomatous nodules (Fig. 8.17). The enlarged transition zone compresses the higher echogenicity peripheral zone. Prostate volume can be calculated from measurements of the prostate in three planes.

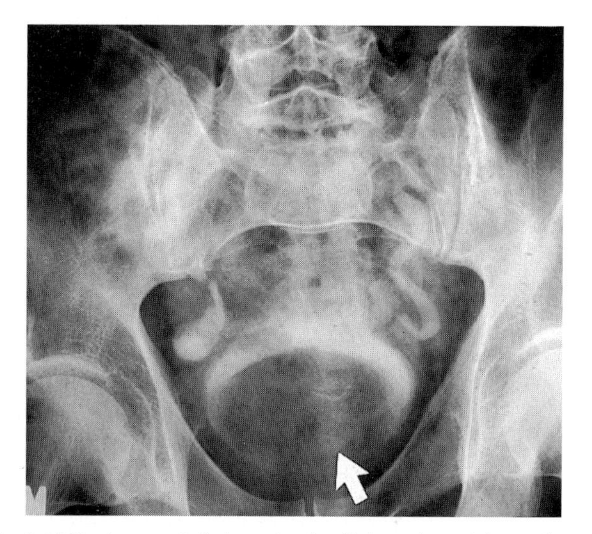

Fig. 8.16 Benign prostatic hypertrophy. Enlarged prostate produces a lucent filling defect (arrowed) at the bladder base and elevation of trigone causes 'fishhooking' of the distal ureters.

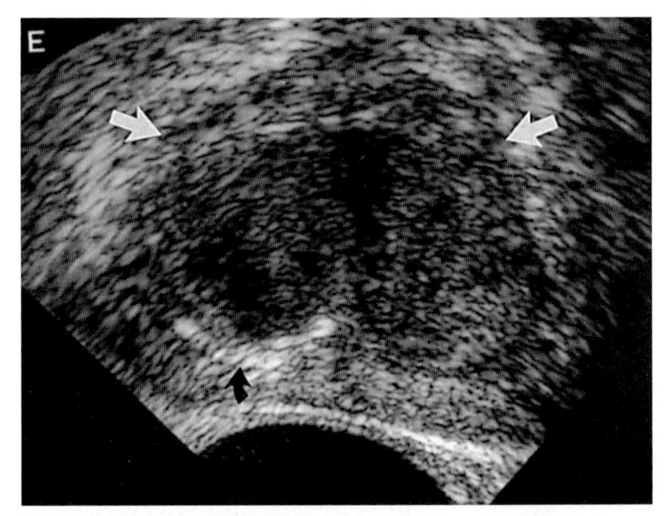

Fig. 8.17 Benign prostatic hypertrophy. Axial transrectal ultrasound scan shows the enlarged hypoechoic transition zone (white arrows). Note the calcification (small black arrow) in the 'surgical capsule' between transition and peripheral zones in the right lobe of prostate.

CARCINOMA

Approximately 70% of prostate cancer affects the peripheral zone. The classic **sonographic** finding in early prostate cancer is a nodule of reduced echogenicity in the peripheral gland. It should, however, be appreciated that hypoechoic nodules in the peripheral zone are often inflammatory rather than malignant. Also, about 25% of tumours have similar echogenicity to normal prostate. As the tumour grows, it spreads into the central and transition zones (Fig. 8.18). The minority of tumours which arise in the central and transition zones are much more difficult to detect with ultrasound, because most patients have some abnormality in this region caused by benign prostatic hypertrophy. Thus transrectal ultrasound of the prostate is associated with false-negative and false-positive scans for cancer.

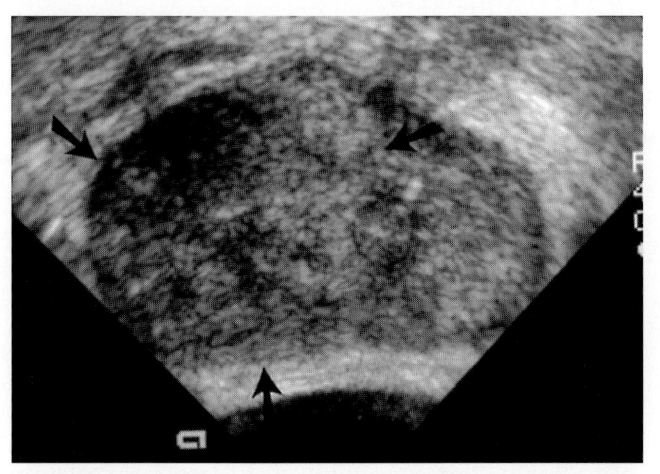

Fig. 8.18 Prostatic carcinoma. Irregular hypoechoic mass (arrowed) occupying the right peripheral and transition zones.

The best assessment in suspected prostate cancer involves combining the findings at digital rectal examination, transrectal ultrasound and the serum prostate specific antigen level. If any of these three methods raises the possibility of cancer, prostate biopsy can be performed either transperineally or transrectally using ultrasound guidance. The transrectal route is currently favoured because of the simplicity of obtaining multiple specimens and the ease with which guided biopsies of small abnormalities can be taken. It has the potential disadvantage of sepsis and antibiotic cover for transrectal prostate biopsy is, therefore, mandatory. Transrectal ultrasound may also be used for local staging of cancer, to see whether the gland capsule is intact and whether there is evidence of spread into the seminal vesicles.

On T2-weighted **MRI**, cancer in the peripheral zone is seen as an area of decreased signal within the high signal background of the normal peripheral gland (Fig. 8.19). T1-weighted images are best for assessing spread into the periprostatic fat, which is clearly seen as bright signal surrounding the lower signal intensity prostate. The major role of MRI in prostate cancer is for staging rather than detecting tumour. The use of endorectal coils to increase image resolution shows promise of being a more sensitive method than ultrasound in assessing capsular and seminal vesicle involvement.

Either MRI or CT may be used to assess whether there is spread into the perivesical fat or to lymph nodes.

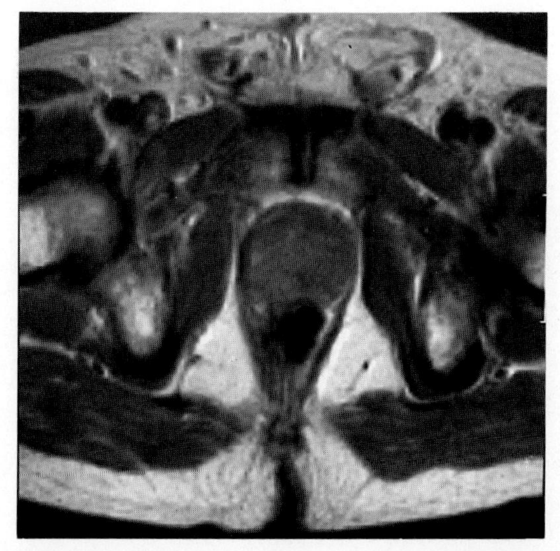

(a)

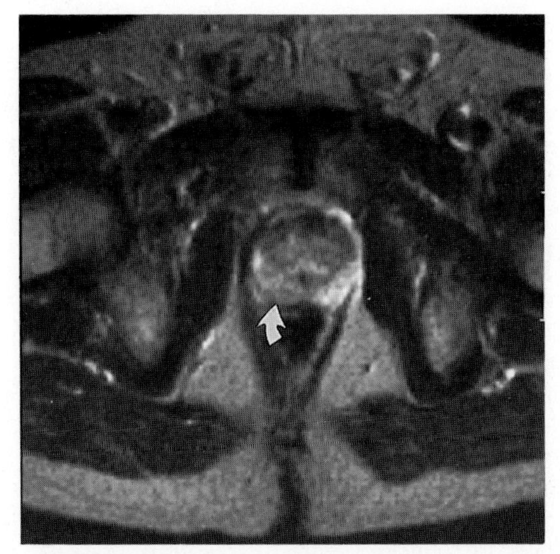

(b)

Fig. 8.19 Prostatic carcinoma. Axial magnetic resonance images. (a) T1-weighted image where tumour is difficult to detect. Bright signal of periprostatic fat outlines the gland clearly with no evidence of tumour spread. (b) T2-weighted image shows tumour (arrowed) as an area of reduced signal highlighted against the bright signal of the remaining peripheral zone. (By kind permission of Dr J. Husband)

PROSTATITIS

The findings on transrectal ultrasonography in prostatitis are non-specific. There may be abnormality in the central or peripheral gland, and the latter may be indistinguishable from carcinoma. Prostatic abscess may be diagnosed as a fluid collection by transrectal ultrasound, CT or MRI. Ultrasound may be used to guide transperineal drainage of an abscess.

SCROTUM

NORMAL ANATOMY

Ultrasonography is the most commonly used scrotal imaging method. The testis appears as an ovoid, clearly defined structure of homogeneous echogenicity with a linear band of increased echogenicity, the mediastinum testis, at one side of its long axis. The epididymis is seen as a separate elongated structure paralleling the testis and tapering from the head towards the tail which lies inferiorly. Doppler sonography can be used to detect blood flow in the epididymis and testis.

Scintigraphy is used to demonstrate testicular perfusion. ^{99m}Tc-labelled DTPA is used and dynamic and static images are usually obtained in suspected torsion to check whether there is normal testicular perfusion.

MRI is a secondary scrotal imaging method. Preliminary evaluation indicates that coronal T2-weighted images provide excellent depiction of scrotal anatomy. The wider field of view compared to ultrasound is helpful and MRI has been recommended as useful in patients in whom ultrasound does not give a clear diagnosis.

CT has no role in imaging normally sited testes. It is an important technique, however, in checking for retroperitoneal node enlargement in patients with testicular malignancy, and may be used to search for an undescended testis (p. 218).

INFECTION

In epididymitis the epididymis enlarges and often shows reduced echogenicity on ultrasound (Fig. 8.20). Enlargement may particularly affect the tail. If the inflammatory process spreads to the testis, the testis also may enlarge and become inhomogeneous. If the testicular abnormality is inflammatory it should resolve with antibiotic treatment. Resolution should always be checked with ultrasound because of the possibility that the abnormality could represent a testicular tumour. In epididymitis and orchitis there may be an associated hydrocoele and scrotal skin thickening. In primary orchitis ultrasound shows an enlarged testis which is usually of reduced echogenicity. Rarely, inflammation in either the epididymis or the testis may progress to abscess formation which then shows central fluid contents.

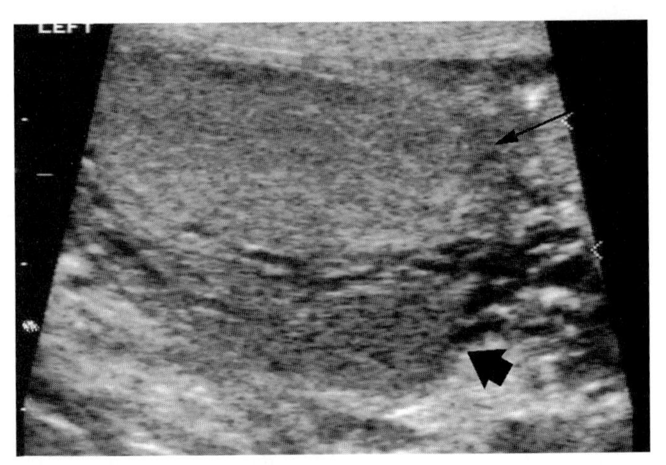

Fig. 8.20 Epididymitis. Longitudinal ultrasound scan of testis shows the enlarged hypoechoic epididymis (broad arrow) alongside the normal testis (long arrow).

TESTICULAR TUMOURS

Tumours of the testes are seen on ultrasound as intratesticular masses of reduced echogenicity. Seminoma is typically fairly homogeneous (Fig. 8.21), whereas teratomas and embryonal cell tumours are often inhomogeneous with cystic areas or calcifications. Differentiation of these appearances from a focal inflammatory process or infarct is not possible on ultrasound appearances alone. MRI may be helpful in delineating complex tumour masses (Fig. 8.22).

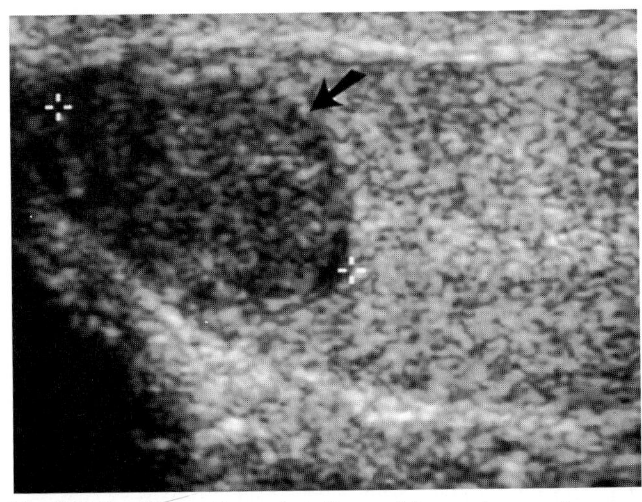

Fig. 8.21 Seminoma. Hypoechoic 2 cm solid mass (arrowed) seen at the upper pole of the testis on a longitudinal ultrasound scan.

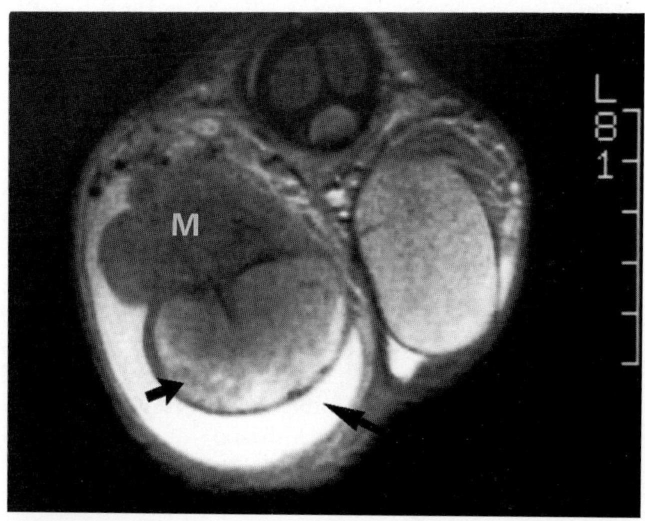

Fig. 8.22 Coronal T2-weighted image of the scrotum shows a low signal lymphomatous mass (M) arising in the right epididymis and infiltrating the right testis (small arrow). There is also a high signal hydrocoele (large arrow). (Reproduced by permission of Dr R. F. Mattrey and W. B. Saunders, in *Clinical magnetic resonance imaging*, (eds) R. R. Edelman, J. R. Hesselink, J. Newhouse and D. J. Sartoris published by W. B. Saunders, London, 1990.)

CYSTS AND FLUID-CONTAINING ABNORMALITIES

Benign testicular cysts are relatively common but should be carefully evaluated to check that they do not represent the cystic component of a tumour.

Epididymal cysts are common in any part of the epididymis (Fig. 8.23).

Spermatocoeles usually occur in the epididymal head and may be multiloculate.

Hydrocoele is readily detected by ultrasound as fluid surrounding the testis (Fig. 8.24). The underlying testis and epididymis may be difficult to palpate and ultrasound is helpful to check for underlying testicular neoplasm.

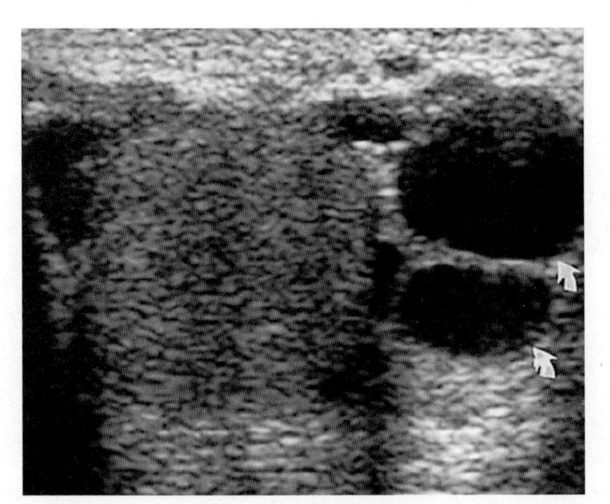

Fig. 8.23 Epididymal cysts. Transverse ultrasound scan through the upper testis shows two cysts (arrowed) in the epididymis lateral to the testis.

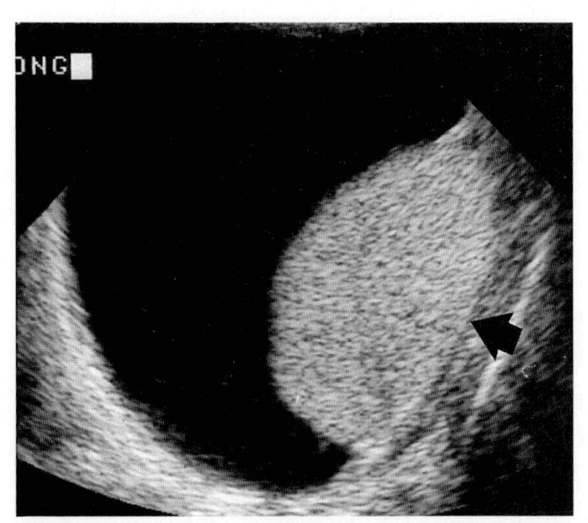

Fig. 8.24 Hydrocoele. Large fluid collection surrounds a normal testis (arrowed) on a longitudinal ultrasound scan.

Varicocoele is seen as a collection of dilated veins adjacent to the testis, which become more prominent when the patient stands or performs a Valsalva manoeuvre. Interventional radiological techniques may now be used to embolize the internal spermatic vein in patients with infertility and varicocoele.

TESTICULAR TORSION

Testicular torsion cannot be diagnosed by ultrasound imaging alone, because there is swelling of the testis and epididymis indistinguishable from the appearances in epididymitis or epididymo-orchitis. Doppler evaluation may be helpful by showing reduced epididymal and testicular blood flow compared to the normal side and scintigraphy may also show decreased perfusion. Since torsion may be intermittent and since neither method is infallible, early surgical exploration is vital if there is a strong clinical suspicion of torsion, even if Doppler ultrasound studies or scintigraphy do not confirm the diagnosis. Early studies with MRI indicate that it may provide helpful diagnostic information in torsion, especially subacute torsion (Fig. 8.25).

TRAUMA

Ultrasound is used following testicular trauma to check for testicular rupture. This may be seen as an interruption in the testicular contour or as a localized area of abnormal echogenicity within the testis caused by haemorrhage. Haemorrhage may also

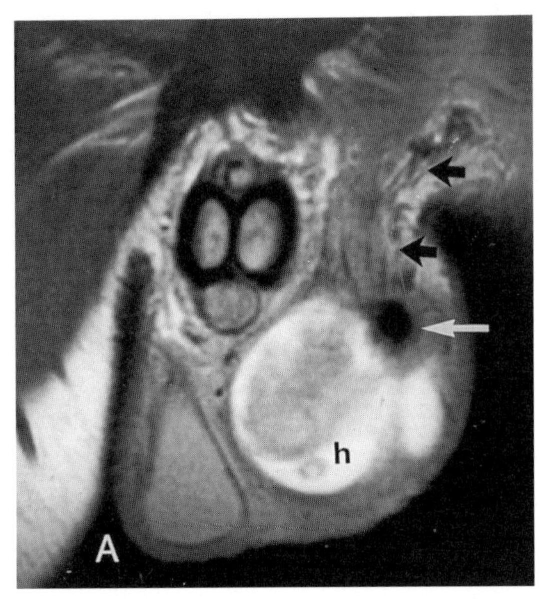

Fig. 8.25 Coronal proton density-weighted image of the scrotum in subacute left torsion. The thickened cord (black arrows) and knot (white arrow) are seen. There is a high signal haematocoele (h). (Reproduced by permission from Trambert, M. A., Mattrey, R. F., Levine, D. and Berthoty, D. P., *Radiology* 1990; **175**: 53–56.)

occur into the peritesticular tissues producing a haematocoele. This has the same distribution as a hydrocoele and shows contained echoes when blood clot develops.

UNDESCENDED TESTIS

The role of imaging in diagnosing the position of an undescended testis is controversial, and many consider that exploratory surgery is the best way to find an impalpable testis. When the undescended testis lies in the inguinal region, it can be readily shown by ultrasound. Identification of the mediastinum testis provides a helpful marker that the structure imaged is the testis and not an enlarged lymph node. Both CT and MRI have been used with moderate success to search for intra-abdominal undescended testes.

PENIS

There are relatively few indications for imaging the soft-tissue structures of the penis. In suspected **Peyronie's disease** ultrasound may be used to check for fibrous plaques, which may contain calcification. They are seen as plaques of increased echogenicity surrounding the corpora cavernosa in whole or in part.

In **impotence**, if a problem with either arterial inflow into or venous leak from the corpora cavernosa is suspected, penile Doppler ultrasound studies following intracavernosal injection of prostaglandin (Alprostadil) may be undertaken. In a normal subject there should be increased systolic inflow in the cavernosal arteries following prostaglandin, followed by cessation of venous flow with a decrease to zero in diastolic velocity in the cavernosal arteries when an erection develops. If systolic velocity does not increase normally, arterial inflow is impaired. Internal pudendal angiography may be carried out if the patient is a candidate for vascular surgery or angioplasty. If the diastolic velocity does not decrease normally, a venous leak from the corpora cavernosa may be suspected and this can be demonstrated by **cavernosography** in which contrast medium is infused into the corpora cavernosa (Fig. 8.26).

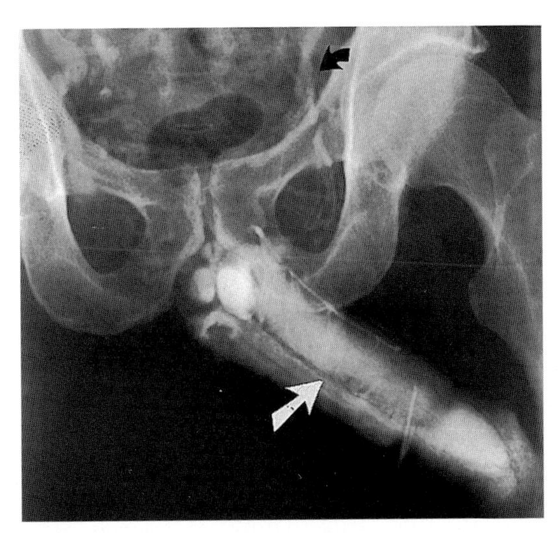

Fig. 8.26 Cavernosogram. Contrast medium in the corpora cavernosa (white arrow) with drainage into the pelvic veins (black arrow) indicating a venous leak.

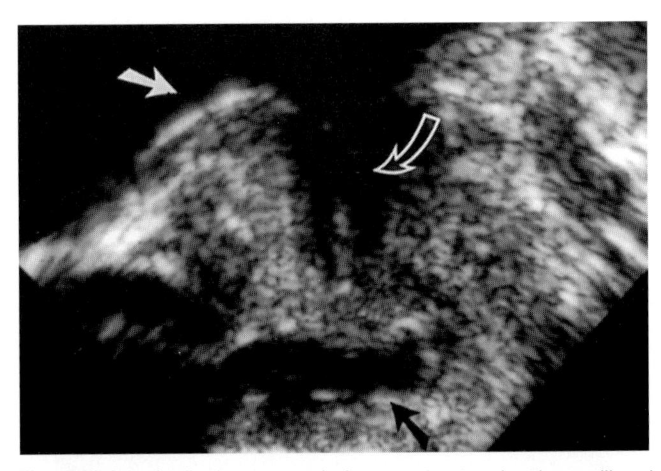

Fig. 8.27 Longitudinal transrectal ultrasound scan showing a dilated ejaculatory duct (black arrow) which is obstructed just above the verumontanum. White arrow indicates bladder base and open white arrow periurethral hypoechoic area.

MALE INFERTILITY

Imaging may be used to investigate the patency of the genital tract as a part of the investigation of infertility.

Vasography may be used to outline the ductal system. The vas is cannulated at surgery and contrast medium is injected to outline the vas, seminal vesicle and ejaculatory duct. Contrast medium should flow freely into the posterior urethra.

Transrectal ultrasonography may be used to visualize the ejaculatory ducts as they traverse the prostate. Obstructed ducts appear dilated (Fig. 8.27) and the obstructing lesion, a calculus or Müllerian duct cyst for example, may sometimes be demonstrated.

CHAPTER 9

Female pelvis

Jane M. Hawnaur

For most of the 100 years since X-rays were discovered by Wilhelm Röntgen, radiological diagnosis of pelvic conditions has relied on the plain film supplemented by X-ray contrast techniques such as intravenous urography, barium enema, hysterosalpingography, angiography and lymphangiography. Ultrasound and X-ray computed tomographic techniques, introduced in the 1970s, were technically refined and complemented by magnetic resonance imaging in the 1980s and 1990s. Modern pelvic imaging is largely based on these cross-sectional techniques which are capable of demonstrating pelvic pathology and providing detailed anatomical information non-invasively.

RADIOLOGICAL ANATOMY AND TECHNIQUES

RADIOGRAPHIC PROTECTION

Radiological techniques employed in the investigation of the female patient with symptoms referable to the urinary tract, bowel or pelvic musculoskeletal system are similar to those in males, with the proviso that techniques using ionizing radiation should only be used with full awareness of radiation protection guidelines. X-rays and radionuclides should not be used if the patient has missed a menstrual period and could be pregnant. The '10-day rule', where X-irradiation for non-urgent diagnostic purposes is only carried out in the 10 days following the onset of menstruation, continues to be applied in some centres to examinations such as pelvic CT or barium enema studies which involve direct irradiation of the female reproductive organs. Both the clinician and radiologist have a duty to protect the patient and unborn child from unnecessary X-irradiation with a consequently greater emphasis on the application of imaging techniques employing non-ionizing radiation in females of child-bearing age.

PLAIN RADIOGRAPHY

The bladder and uterus can be identified on a supine abdominopelvic radiograph as soft-tissue density masses outlined by relatively lucent pelvic fat. Bone metastases from female reproductive tract cancers are unusual except in advanced disease, but are relatively

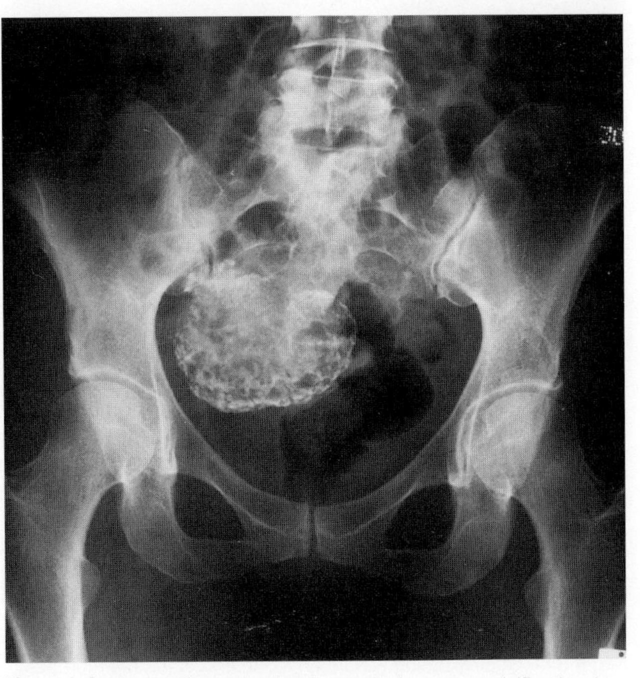

Fig. 9.1 Supine radiograph showing typical coarse calcification in a large uterine fibroid tumour.

Diagnostic and Interventional Radiology in Surgical Practice. Edited by P. Armstrong and M.L. Wastie. Published in 1997 by Chapman & Hall, London. ISBN 0 412 61960 1 (HB), 0 412 61970 9 (PB)

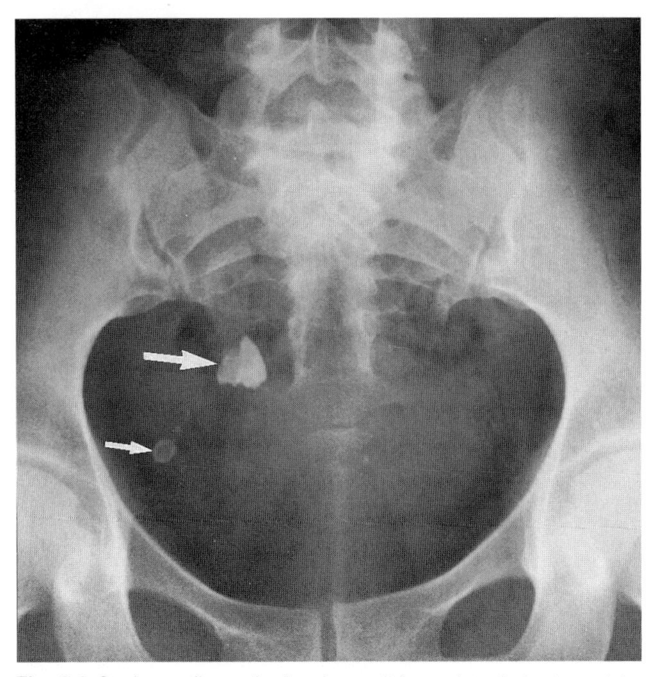

Fig. 9.2 Supine radiograph showing well-formed teeth in the pelvis, characteristic of a dermoid tumour arising in the ovary (large arrow). The adjacent round opacity has the typical appearance of a phlebolith (small arrow).

common from breast and bronchial carcinomas. Radiodense foreign bodies or devices such as tubal ligation clips or intrauterine contraceptive devices can be seen. Calcified thrombotic nodules in the pelvic veins (phleboliths) are common and more linear calcification may be visible in the pelvic arteries, especially in patients with renal failure or diabetes. Characteristic calcification in uterine leiomyomata (fibroids) or the combination of fat and teeth in an ovarian dermoid occasionally allow a specific diagnosis to be made from the plain radiograph (Figs. 9.1, 9.2). More typically, however, imaging with ultrasound, CT, MRI or contrast radiography is required to reach a diagnosis.

CONTRAST RADIOGRAPHY

Barium examination of the large or small bowel remains the best method for localizing adhesions, strictures and fistulae caused by pelvic inflammatory or malignant disease, and for demonstrating mucosal lesions. Large pelvic masses may present with altered bowel habit; a barium enema is then helpful to exclude colonic carcinoma and evaluate the effect of the pelvic mass on the large bowel (Fig. 9.3).

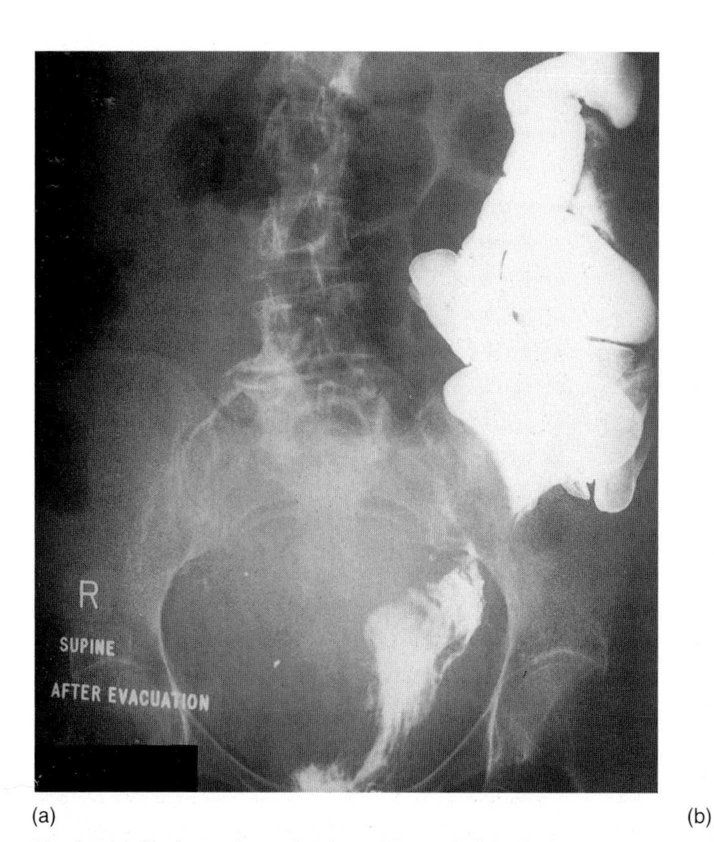

(a)

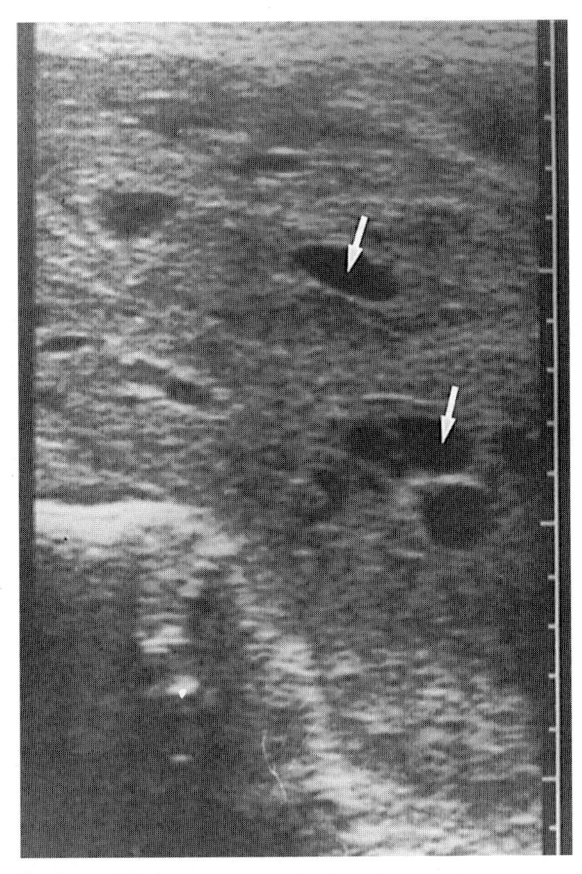

(b)

Fig. 9.3 (a) Supine radiograph taken at the end of the barium enema examination in an elderly woman complaining of altered bowel habit and pelvic fullness. The colon is displaced by a large abdominopelvic mass. (b) Ultrasound scan of the right iliac fossa shows the mass to be solid with multiple cystic areas (arrows): features consistent with ovarian carcinoma.

Intravenous urography can demonstrate ureteric obstruction due to a pelvic mass or malignant infiltration and is indicated for demonstration of iatrogenic damage to the ureters following surgery.

ANGIOGRAPHY AND LYMPHANGIOGRAPHY

Pelvic arteriography is now rarely performed except in the investigation of pelvic haemorrhage. Pelvic venography is undertaken to assess iliac vein compression or thrombosis. Demonstration of lymph node metastases by lymphangiography has largely been superseded by CT and MRI.

HYSTEROSALPINGOGRAPHY

Hysterosalpingography enables the shape of the uterine cavity and fallopian tubal patency to be assessed, and is often performed as part of the investigation of recurrent miscarriage or infertility. It is contraindicated in pregnancy and avoided in patients with pelvic infection or iodine sensitivity. Water-soluble iodinated contrast medium is injected into the endometrial cavity via a cannula in the cervical canal and radiographs are obtained. Contrast outlining the normal uterine cavity has a triangular shape and should pass rapidly along the slender fallopian tubes to spill into the peritoneal cavity. Abnormal findings include congenital abnormalities of the uterus, endometrial polyps and tubal occlusion or hydrosalpinx (Fig. 9.4, and see also Fig. 9.11, p. 227).

ULTRASOUND

Techniques

Transabdominal ultrasound is the imaging method for primary assessment of the uterus and related structures. It is used routinely for assessing the progress of normal pregnancy (Fig. 9.5). In the non-pregnant patient, a full bladder is vital for successful scanning, pushing the uterus upwards from behind the pubic symphysis, displacing small bowel and behaving as an acoustic window, improving transmission of the ultrasound beam. The transducers used are of relatively low frequency (3.5 MHz) resulting in relatively poor spatial resolution. Visualization of pelvic structures may be limited in obese patients.

Transvaginal ultrasound is used to monitor infertility treatment and to assess early pregnancy and its complications. It is the preferred technique for assessing pelvic inflammatory or malignant conditions, especially when the patient is obese or cannot achieve adequate bladder filling. With a transvaginal probe, the transducer is closer to the region of interest, there is less beam attenuation in superficial soft tissues and a higher ultrasound frequency (5–7.5 MHz) can be employed, increasing sensitivity and spatial resolution in the image. High-resolution ultrasound may also be performed by a transrectal route to assess local tumour spread in patients with carcinoma of the cervix.

Doppler ultrasound can provide useful additional information about vascular changes associated with physiological and pathological pelvic conditions. Ovarian vascularity fluctuates during the menstrual

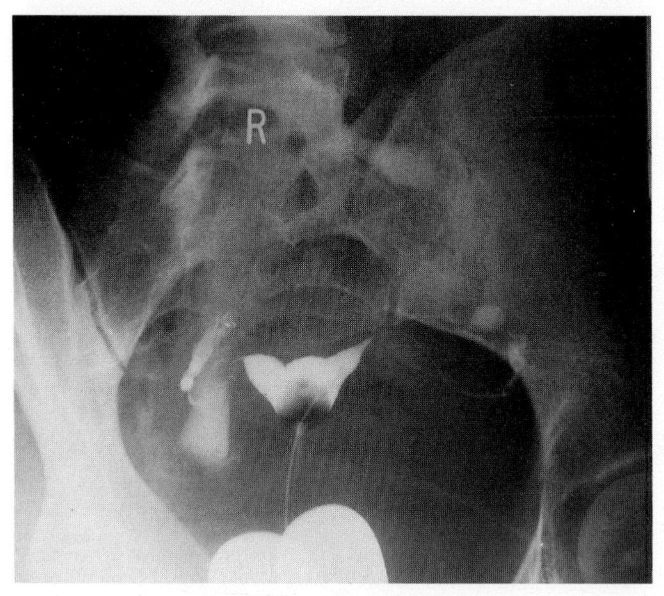

Fig. 9.4 Hysterosalpingogram performed in the investigation of infertility. The uterine cavity is of normal outline and the proximal tubes are of normal calibre. Saccular dilation of the distal fallopian tubes with lack of peritoneal spill indicates bilateral hydrosalpinges.

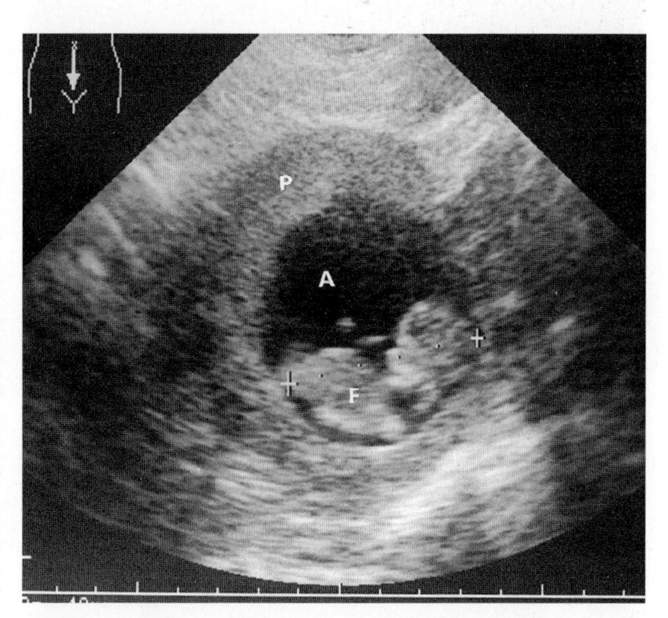

Fig. 9.5 Sagittal pelvic ultrasound scan obtained in early pregnancy. The fetal size indicates an 11-week gestation. The fetus (F), amniotic fluid (A) and placenta (P) can be identified.

cycle, low resistance to flow occurring in the presence of a functioning corpus luteum. Postmenopausal ovaries are relatively hypovascular, and the demonstration of abnormal vascularity by Doppler ultrasound examination is suggestive of a neoplastic process causing new vessel formation.

Normal ultrasound anatomy

In the reproductive period, the normal uterus measures about 7.5 × 5.0 × 2.5 cm, but is smaller in the prepubertal, postmenopausal or hypo-oestrogenized woman. Normal uterine stroma returns low-level, uniform echoes and the position of the endometrial and endocervical canals is indicated by linear echogenic stripes, representing the interfaces between mucus and mucosa (see Fig. 9.10, p. 227). The ovaries normally lie in the ovarian fossae with their long axes parallel to the internal iliac vessels and ureters posteriorly. Ovarian volume ranges from 4–10 cm^3 depending on hormonal status. Ovarian follicles appear as spherical echolucencies within the ovary and may reach a size of 2 cm in normal cycles. Normal fallopian tubes are not visible. A small amount of fluid in the pouch of Douglas is a normal finding, frequently seen at ovulation.

COMPUTED TOMOGRAPHY

Technique

CT is a second line investigation for pelvic disease in the female, particularly for patients of child-bearing age. It is often used for staging pelvic malignancy when, particularly in patients destined for radiotherapy, radiation protection considerations become irrelevant (Fig. 9.6, and see also 9.21 p. 235). In young women with benign disease CT should be reserved for patients with complex bowel-related, traumatic or

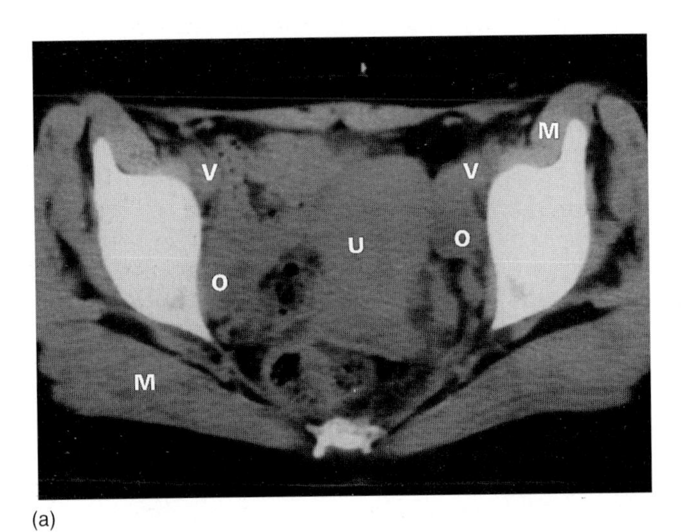

(a)

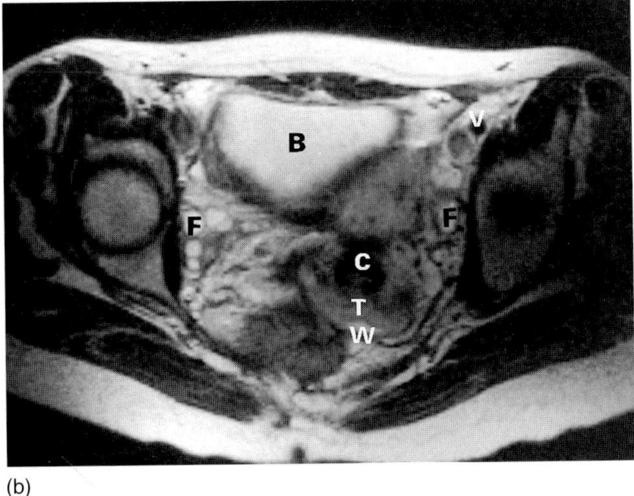

(b)

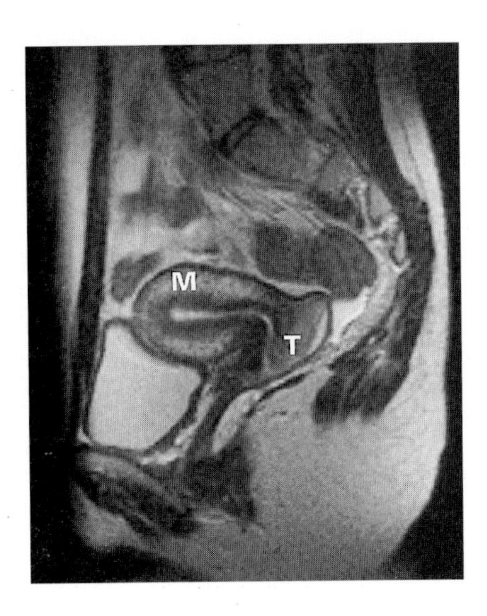

(c)

Fig. 9.6 (a) Axial CT section obtained for radiotherapy treatment planning in carcinoma of the cervix. Uterus (U), muscle (M), vessels (V) and ovaries (O) have similar soft-tissue density although follicles in the ovaries are visible because of lower density fluid content. (b) A T2-weighted MRI scan obtained at a similar level shows high signal from urine in the bladder (B) and fluid in ovarian follicles (F), medium signal from cervical tumour (T) and low signal from normal cervix (C), vaginal wall (W) and flowing blood (V). (c) Sagittal T2-weighted MRI scan demonstrates tumour (T) in the posterior cervical lip as medium signal intensity replacing the low signal of normal stroma. The zonal anatomy of the uterus is well shown, the outer two-thirds of myometrium (M) having medium signal intensity separated from hyperintense endometrium by a band of low signal representing the 'junctional' zone of myometrium.

osseous pathology in whom more basic radiographic or ultrasound techniques have not provided sufficient information for management decisions to be made. The technique involves a high radiation dose to the pelvic organs (around 25 mGy), with direct irradiation of the ovaries. Sections 10 mm thick are obtained from the pelvic brim to perineum. Opacification of the large and small bowel with oral contrast medium is important when looking for pelvic soft-tissue masses or fluid collections. Moderate distension of the bladder helps to improve demonstration of the bladder wall and lifts the uterus into a more vertical position. A tampon may be used to identify the position of the vagina in relation to the urethra and rectum. Repeated scanning after intravenous iodinated contrast medium may be necessary to identify the ureters, distinguish pelvic vessels from enlarged lymph nodes and assess the vascularity of any pelvic mass demonstrated. Faster, spiral (helical) CT scanning technology has recently been introduced, but its impact on pelvic imaging is still being evaluated.

Normal CT anatomy

The cervix is visualized as an ovoid soft-tissue density structure, which should not exceed 3 cm in diameter. The endocervical canal is not usually identifiable unless it contains gas, and the interface between cervix and vaginal fornix is usually unclear. Similar soft-tissue densities and partial volume effects between the uterus, bladder and rectum make the vesicouterine recess and the pouch of Douglas difficult to assess on CT. The orientation of the body of the uterus depends on the degree of filling of the urinary bladder and rectal distension. Consequently, axial CT sections are usually oblique in relation to the long axis of the uterus, so that measurements of the normal uterus or uterine masses are unreliable. The structure of the uterus is better shown after intravenous contrast medium, when the vascular endometrium enhances, leaving the uterine cavity visible as a relatively hypodense T-shaped structure. The broad ligament can sometimes be identified as a triangular density extending to the pelvic side wall. It encloses a layer of fibrous, vascular and fatty tissue lying lateral to the uterus called the parametrium. The round ligament may be visible as a tubular density extending from the uterine fundus towards the inguinal canal, but the parametrial vessels require enhancement with contrast for their identification within the parametrial soft tissues. The ovaries lie between the internal and external iliac arteries in the ovarian fossae, and have a density similar to other soft-tissue structures such as bowel, blood vessels and muscle (Fig. 9.6a). Their identification may be helped by opacification of the ureters, which run posterior to the ovaries. The ureter also has an important relationship to the cervix, running 1–2 cm lateral to the cervix before entering the bladder trigone anterior to the uterus.

MAGNETIC RESONANCE IMAGING

Technique

MRI uses non-ionizing radiation and has no known side-effects at diagnostic field strengths, provided that patients with ferromagnetic or electromagnetic implants are excluded. Image contrast can be manipulated extensively by altering sequence parameters, but in the pelvis the soft-tissue contrast of a combination of T1-weighted and T2-weighted spin-echo sequences is usually adequate for characterization of many tissues and is superior to that of ultrasound or CT. Sequences which suppress the signal from fat can also be useful in the pelvis. Bowel preparation using oral contrast material is not generally required, although agents which increase or decrease the signal intensity of the bowel lumen are commercially available. If obtrusive, gut peristalsis can be reduced with a short-acting smooth muscle relaxant given immediately before scanning. There are few specific indications for using intravenous paramagnetic MR contrast media in the female pelvis. Their administration is usually reserved for assessment of malignant disease, particularly if satisfactory T2-weighted sequences cannot be obtained.

Normal MRI anatomy

In the reproductive period, the uterus has distinctive zonal anatomy on T2-weighted MR images (Fig. 9.6c). The myometrium shows a medium intensity signal, separated from hyperintense endometrium by a band of low signal, representing the compact inner third of the myometrium. The cervical fibromuscular stroma is low in signal intensity. The ovaries show a low to medium signal on T1-weighted sequences, similar to that of adjacent vessels or bowel. Ovarian stroma has a medium to high signal intensity on T2-weighted sequences and the very high signal in developing follicles allows identification of the ovaries in the majority of women with normal ovarian function (Fig. 9.6b).

COMPLICATIONS OF PREGNANCY

ECTOPIC PREGNANCY

Ultrasound is indicated in women with clinical signs of ectopic pregnancy and raised human chorionic gonadotrophin levels. Identification of a normal gestation sac in the uterine cavity makes an ectopic gestation extremely unlikely, unless the patient has undergone ovarian stimulation. The ultrasound diagnosis of intrauterine pregnancy depends on demonstrating a gestation sac, yolk sac and an embryo with a beating heart. Transvaginal ultrasound is able to demonstrate these signs from 5 weeks' gestation, earlier than transabdominal ultrasound, and can also more easily identify an extrauterine gestation sac, without the need to wait for the patient's bladder to fill. The unequivocal ultrasound demonstration of an ectopic embryo with cardiac pulsation occurs in approximately 20% of patients (Fig. 9.7).

Trophoblastic reaction in the lining of the fallopian tube surrounding the ectopic gestation is the next most reliable sign seen in up to 70% of cases. Ultrasound demonstration of a corpus luteum cyst or haemorrhagic fluid containing low-level echoes in the pouch of Douglas are other confirmatory signs. Transvaginal Doppler ultrasound can be used to demonstrate increased blood flow associated with the gestational sac, although similar low resistance flow patterns may occur in other vascular adnexal masses. Transvaginal ultrasound can also be used to establish the presence and viability of the gestation sac in threatened abortion. Abdominal pregnancy, resulting from implantation of the embryo on the omental or mesenteric surface, may be difficult to diagnose on ultrasound and MRI may be useful to show the pregnancy outside the uterus.

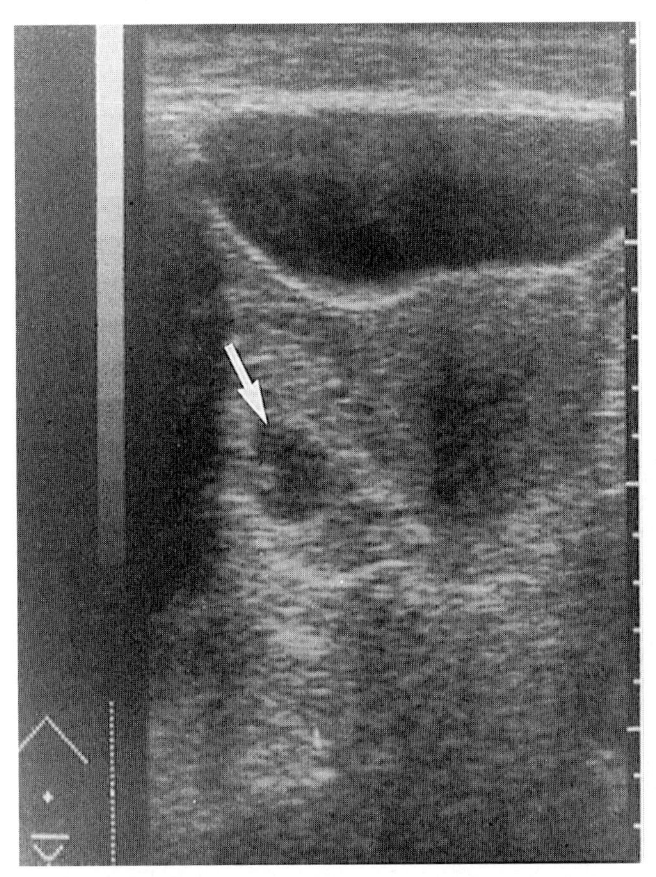

Fig. 9.7 Transaxial ultrasound scan in a woman with signs of ectopic pregnancy. No intrauterine pregnancy was identified but there is evidence of a gestation sac in the right adnexa (arrow).

GESTATIONAL TROPHOBLASTIC DISEASE

Hydatidiform mole occurs in 1 in 1500 pregnancies, when the embryo dies but fails to abort normally, and the chorionic villi proliferate to form multiple grape-like vesicles distending the uterine cavity. A partial mole contains fetal parts and in invasive mole there is penetration of uterine muscle by trophoblastic elements. Choriocarcinoma arises from malignant transformation of hydatidiform mole or from retained placenta after normal pregnancy or abortion. Signs include vaginal bleeding, high levels of beta human chorionic gonadotrophin and uterine enlargement greater than expected for the stage of pregnancy. On ultrasound, a complex multicystic/solid mass fills the uterine cavity and multiple theca lutein ovarian cysts may be seen (Fig. 9.8). Ultrasound cannot distinguish between complete hydatidiform mole, invasive forms and choriocarcinoma.

OVARIAN VEIN THROMBOSIS

Ovarian vein thrombosis may occur postpartum, due to sudden reduction in flow and venous stasis in the ovarian vein (usually the right). Symptoms and signs resemble those of appendicitis, patients often presenting with fever, pain and a tender, tubular mass in the iliac fossa. On ultrasound, the thrombosed vein can be appreciated as a tender mass with internal echoes and

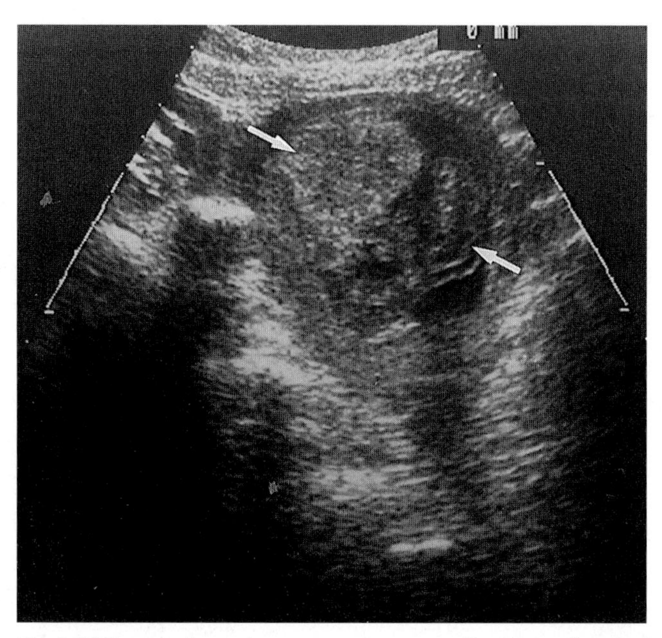

Fig. 9.8 Ultrasound scan in a pregnant woman with abnormal vaginal bleeding. The uterus is larger than expected for a 10-week pregnancy and contains no viable fetus, but is enlarged by a mass containing cystic and solid elements (arrows). A complete hydatidiform mole was subsequently evacuated.

no flow, and on CT or MR the enlarged ovarian vein can be followed proximally in the retroperitoneum to renal level.

APPENDICITIS IN PREGNANCY

Approximately 1 in 1500 pregnancies are complicated by appendicitis, the diagnosis of which is made more difficult by the high prevalence of nausea, vomiting and leucocytosis in normal pregnancies and the migration of the appendix towards the right iliac crest as the uterus enlarges. The decision to perform a laparotomy is made on clinical grounds and should not be unduly deferred to await imaging studies. Fetal loss is high if appendiceal perforation occurs. In the stable patient, ultrasound examination may be able to identify the inflamed appendix, or show other causes of a similar clinical picture such as biliary colic, ovarian lesions or urinary tract disease (Figs 9.9, 9.10).

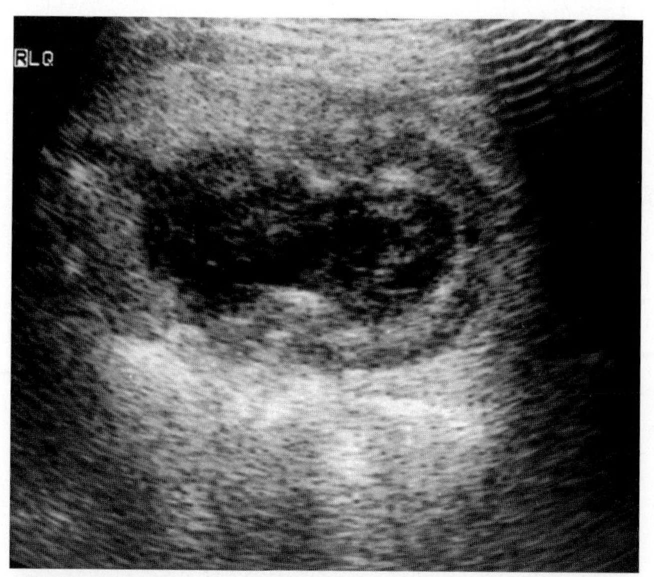

Fig. 9.9 Right iliac fossa ultrasound scan showing a thick-walled fusiform mass containing debris which was tender and contiguous with the caecal pole, indicating an inflamed appendix mass rather than a mass of adnexal origin.

IMAGING IN GYNAECOLOGY

CONGENITAL ANOMALIES

Duplication anomalies of the uterus and vagina are due to abnormal fusion of the Müllerian ducts in utero. Examples include double uterus (uterus didelphys), bicornuate and septate uterus, any of which may be associated with vaginal duplication (Fig. 9.11). There is an association with anorectal and urinary tract malformations.

Haemato(metro)colpos secondary to vaginal occlusion or imperforate hymen can present with a pelvic mass in an amenorrhoeic teenager. Diagnosis may be achieved by ultrasound, hysterosalpingography or MRI, but the best overall technique is probably MRI.

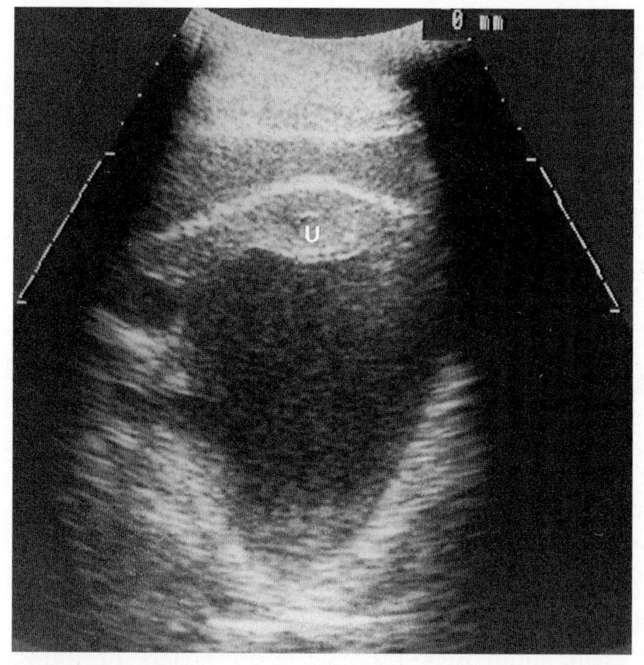

Fig. 9.10 Transverse pelvic ultrasound scan in a woman suspected of having pelvic inflammatory disease. There is a large fluid collection posterior to the uterus (U) secondary to appendicitis.

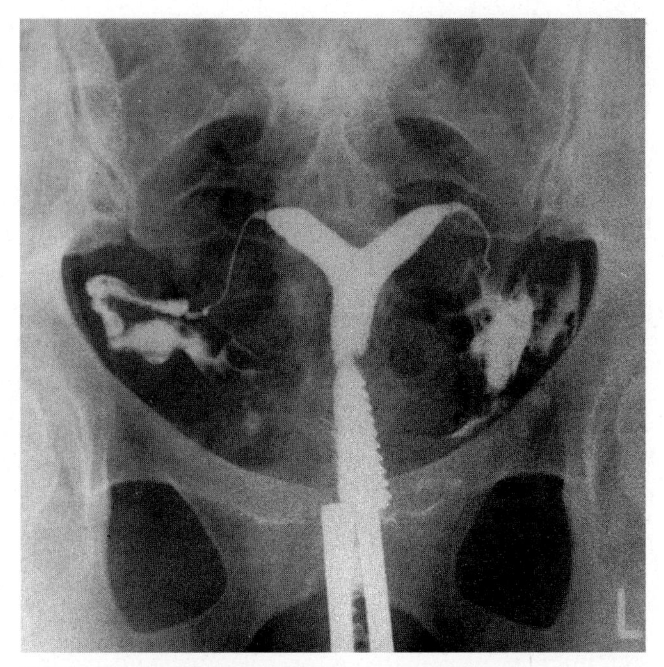

Fig. 9.11 Hysterosalpingography showing partial division of the uterine cavity due to congenital bicornuate uterus. The fallopian tubes are normal and there is peritoneal spill of contrast.

INFLAMMATORY CONDITIONS

Pelvic inflammatory disease
Sexually transmitted organisms are often responsible for pelvic inflammatory disease but adnexal inflammation may also be secondary to diverticulitis, appendicitis or inflammatory bowel disease. If an abdominal radiograph is performed, findings suggestive of pelvic inflammatory disease include obliteration of pelvic fat planes, local ileus and the presence of an intrauterine contraceptive device. Ultrasound, however, is the imaging investigation of first choice. The uterus may appear slightly swollen and hypoechoic with ill-defined margins and a prominent endometrial echo. There may be an inflammatory adnexal mass or ancillary signs of pelvic inflammatory disease such as free intraperitoneal fluid, loss of tissue interfaces or mild hydronephrosis. Normal pelvic ultrasound does not exclude the diagnosis. Once a clinical diagnosis of pelvic inflammatory disease is made, response of any inflammatory mass to conservative treatment with antibiotics can be monitored by ultrasound.

Hydrosalpinx
In acute salpingitis, the fallopian tubes may be visible on ultrasound as dilated tubular structures in the adnexae. In chronic pelvic inflammatory disease, hydrosalpinx is caused by secretions trapped in the tubal lumen by peritubal adhesions. Hysterosalpingography shows fusiform tubal dilatation with prolonged retention of contrast medium and no peritoneal spill (Fig. 9.4, p. 223). Demonstration of mucosal folds and continuity with the uterine cornua on ultrasound helps to differentiate hydrosalpinx from other cystic adnexal masses. Echogenic contents or layering of debris suggest the presence of blood or pus within the fallopian tubes. Haematosalpinx may occur in ruptured ectopic pregnancy.

Tubo-ovarian abscess
Acute salpingitis may be complicated by abscess formation, when pus from the fimbriated end of the fallopian tube becomes loculated between the tube and the adjacent ovary. The resultant tubo-ovarian abscess may involve adjacent bowel or bladder and, if rupture occurs, may be life-threatening.

Ultrasound demonstration of an irregular thick-walled cystic adnexal mass is not specific and may also occur in ectopic pregnancy, haemorrhagic or infected ovarian cyst, ovarian torsion, etc. Radionuclide scanning using gallium 67-citrate or indium 111-labelled leucocytes can be used to confirm the presence of infection and localize an abscess. CT and MRI are less commonly used, but may show a complex cystic mass incorporating the ovary, containing fluid of proteinaceous or haemorrhagic nature, and a thickened irregular wall enhancing after contrast.

Endometritis
Endometritis is a common cause of fever in the puerperium especially after Caesarian section or prolonged rupture of the membranes. Ultrasound demonstrates echogenic material within the endometrial canal in more advanced cases with fluid or gas in a distended endometrial cavity. The differential diagnosis includes retained products of conception and malignancy.

Pyometrium
Impaired drainage of the uterine cavity associated with cervical or endometrial carcinoma, previous uterine surgery, radiotherapy, benign tumours (such as fibroids) or inflammatory processes, may underlie the formation of a pyometrium (pus-filled endometrial cavity) or haematometrium (blood-filled). The presence of a dilated endometrial cavity can be confirmed by any cross-sectional imaging technique, but characterization of the contents is most accurate on ultrasound or MRI (Fig. 9.12).

BENIGN UTERINE TUMOURS

Uterine fibroids
Uterine fibroid tumours (leiomyomata) are common in women aged over 30 years. Submucosal or intramural tumours often cause heavy menstrual blood loss and anaemia. Subserosal fibroids may be asymptomatic until so bulky as to cause pressure symptoms. Pedunculated fibroids may also arise from the cervix or broad ligament. In about 30% of cases, the compact fibromuscular stroma of a fibroid becomes affected by haemorrhagic, mucinous or myxomatous degeneration. Sarcomatous degeneration is rare but cannot be distinguished from benign degeneration by diagnostic imaging methods.

In the UK, troublesome fibroids are often managed by hysterectomy in women who have completed their family. The surgical approaches to uterine leiomyomas with conservation of the uterus are hysteroscopic myomectomy for submucosal tumours or transabdominal myomectomy for intramural and serosal tumours.

MRI is the most accurate method for precise localization for planning such conservative surgery, but often fibroids can be equally well demonstrated by either ultrasound or MRI. On MRI, uncomplicated fibroids are well-circumscribed low signal intensity masses within the myometrium (Fig. 9.13). Degeneration of all types causes an increase in signal intensity, especially on T2-weighted sequences.

On ultrasound, fibroids appear as solid iso- or hypoechoic masses compared with normal myometrium. Degeneration may produce cystic spaces or fluid–debris levels on ultrasound, and calcific foci produce areas of echogenicity with acoustic shadowing. The

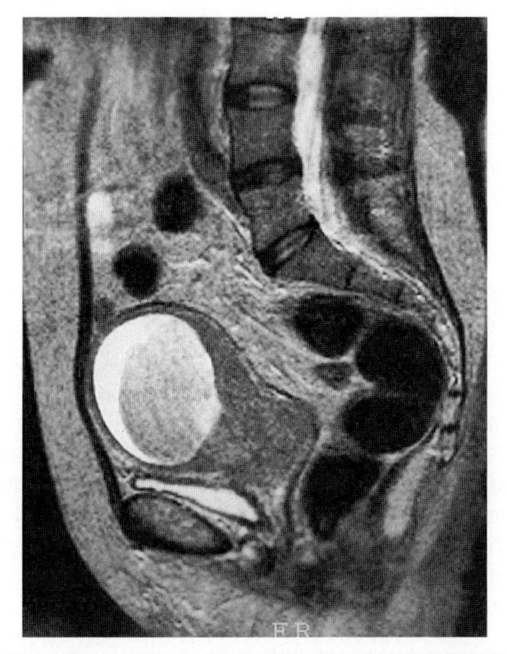

(a)

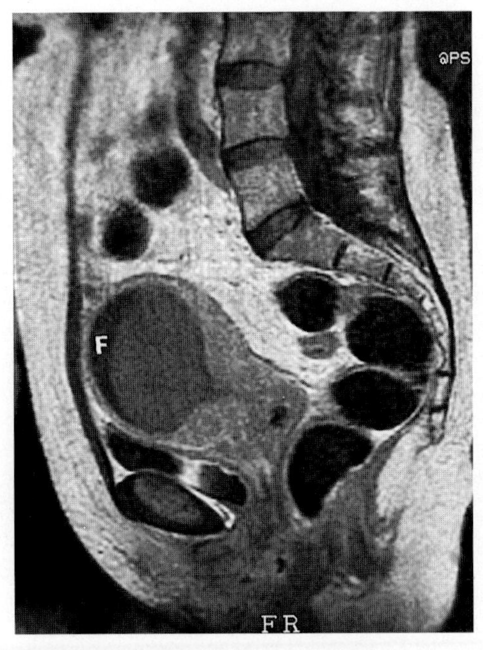

(b)

Fig. 9.12 (a) Sagittal T2-weighted MRI scan in an elderly woman with uterine cancer and canal stenosis showing distension of the endometrial cavity by hyperintense material. (b) A postcontrast T1-weighted MRI scan helps to identify the intrauterine masses as part fluid (F) with a non-enhancing mass, possibly blood clot in the obstructed uterine canal. Lack of enhancement effectively excludes viable tumour.

density of a simple fibroid is similar to that of normal myometrium on CT, but morphological distortion and the presence of coarse calcification within the mass suggest the diagnosis (see Fig. 9.18 p. 233). Degenerative changes cause increased tissue heterogeneity, with the appearance of hypodense areas or intralesional gas. Tumour margins may become more visible after bolus contrast administration.

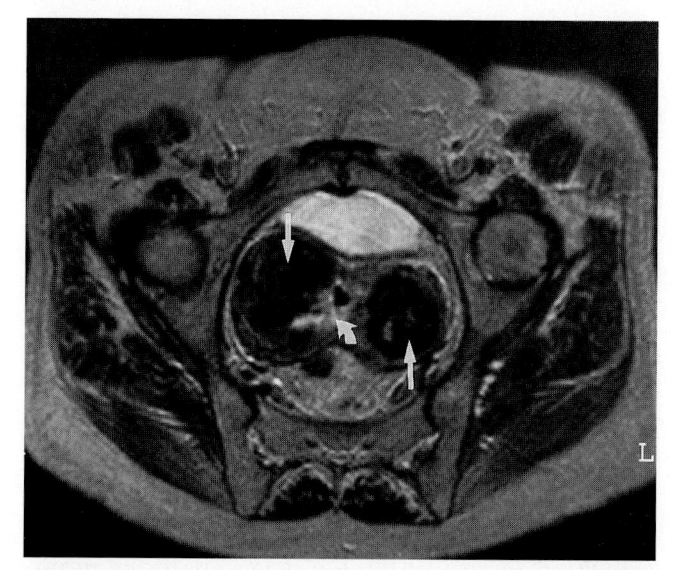

Fig. 9.13 Transaxial T2-weighted MRI scan showing multiple low-signal fibroids in the uterus (straight arrows). The irregular high signal centrally is due to carcinoma (curved arrow).

Adenomyosis

In adenomyosis, portions of the basal layer of the endometrium are ectopically deep within the myometrium, exciting reactive hyperplasia of the surrounding muscle. The condition may be asymptomatic, but dysmenorrhoea is common. Diffuse adenomyosis causes enlargement of the uterus whereas focal adenomyosis is difficult to distinguish from fibroids on CT and ultrasound. On T2-weighted MRI scans, diffuse adenomyosis results in uterine enlargement with thickening and loss of definition of the junctional zone extending into the outer myometrium. Focal adenomyosis appears as a low signal mass on T2-weighted sequences, similar to a fibroid, but with a more ovoid shape and less well-defined margins (Fig. 9.14).

MALIGNANT UTERINE TUMOURS

Endometrial carcinoma

Endometrial cancer is typically a well-differentiated adenocarcinoma with a slow rate of progression, manifesting with postmenopausal bleeding. At presentation, 75% of women have tumour confined to the endometrium (stage IA) for whom the 5-year survival rate is 80% following total hysterectomy. The International Federation of Obstetrics and Gynaecology (FIGO) committee recommends staging by total abdominal hysterectomy, bilateral salpingo-oophorectomy and lymphadenectomy, a counsel that is not

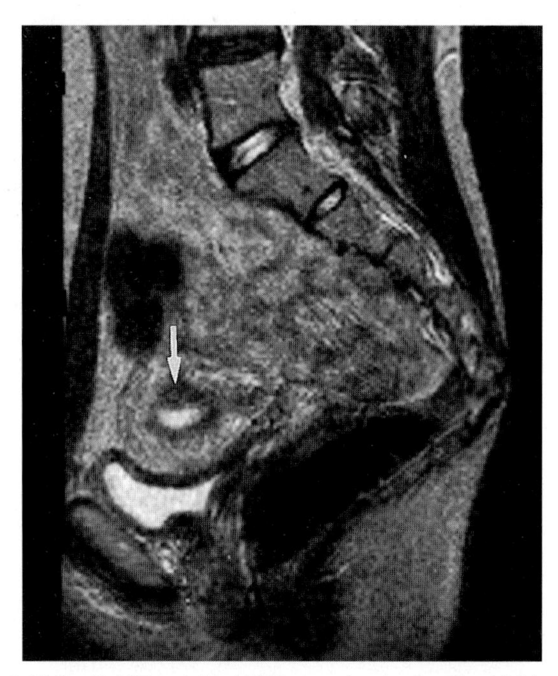

Fig. 9.14 Sagittal T2-weighted MRI scan showing localized thickening of the junctional zone due to focal adenomyosis (arrow).

achievable in all cases. Preoperative imaging may be helpful in assessing the depth of myometrial invasion, the presence or absence of cervical involvement and lymphadenopathy in patients in whom clinical examination is difficult or full staging laparotomy is inappropriate.

Transabdominal ultrasound can demonstrate uterine enlargement but does not adequately assess depth of myometrial invasion or lymph node enlargement. Transvaginal ultrasound gives a better assessment of the uterus but is insufficient to assess extrauterine spread.

On **CT** with intravenous contrast-enhancement, a large endometrial carcinoma may be visible as a hypodense mass deforming the uterus, often with eccentric spread within the myometrium and low density areas representing avascular tumour necrosis or retained secretions within the endometrial cavity.

Endometrial carcinoma is more easily shown by **MRI**, although early cancers may be difficult to detect because of similarity in signal intensity to endometrium on T2-weighted sequences. When tumours become large enough to distend or distort the uterine cavity, differentiation from benign tumour or blood clot may require intravenous paramagnetic contrast administration. Intravenous contrast also increases the accuracy of staging and allows assessment of the volume of viable tumour, since necrotic tumour, blood clot or other debris do not enhance (Fig. 9.12). When tumour invades the myometrium, there is loss of the normal low signal intensity of the junctional zone, although this may ordinarily be indistinct in postmenopausal women. Tumour invading less than half the myometrial depth is given a stage of IB, and greater than half, stage IC. Accuracy of staging of endometrial carcinoma by MRI is about 80%.

Uterine sarcoma

Leiomyosarcoma accounts for less than 1% of uterine malignancy. Although malignant transformation of uterine fibroids may occur, most leiomyosarcomas arise *de novo*. No imaging technique can reliably differentiate between benign degenerative fibroids and sarcoma.

Cervical carcinoma

In 60–70% of cases, cervical carcinoma is squamous in histological type, developing in the squamocolumnar junction, and potentially detectable in the preinvasive stages by the cervical smear population screening programme.

Adenocarcinomas tend to arise deeper in the endocervical canal and may remain occult until advanced. Diagnostic imaging is only appropriate in invasive cancer, the spatial resolution of currently available radiological techniques being insufficient to identify microinvasive disease. Clinical staging of invasive carcinoma of the cervix is inaccurate, particularly in women with disease extending beyond the uterus. Demonstration of lymph node enlargement by cross-sectional imaging may also modify treatment pathways, although no imaging method can reliably differentiate reactive from metastatic nodal enlargement. Although both ultrasound and CT have applications in cervical cancer staging, MRI is the most consistently useful modality in all tumour stages and is as accurate as contrast-enhanced CT for assessing lymph node status. It is the most suitable imaging method for staging women with carcinoma of the cervix during pregnancy (Fig. 9.15).

Transabdominal ultrasound does not contribute to staging the primary cervical tumour, but can show urinary tract obstruction, ascites or hepatic metastases in advanced disease. Transrectal ultrasound can demonstrate cervical enlargement and parametrial extension but because of a limited range of view, cannot evaluate the full extent of bulky tumours or screen the relevant lymph node regions.

On unenhanced **CT**, the density of cervical carcinoma is similar to normal cervix, but carcinoma can be inferred when there is eccentric enlargement of the cervix. An irregular or ill-defined interface with the parametrial soft tissues implies parametrial invasion, although a similar appearance may be seen following pelvic inflammatory disease or surgery. Obliteration of pelvic fat planes is well demonstrated by CT, enabling diagnosis of tumour extension to the pelvic side wall with a high degree of accuracy. Bolus administration of an intravenous contrast agent may

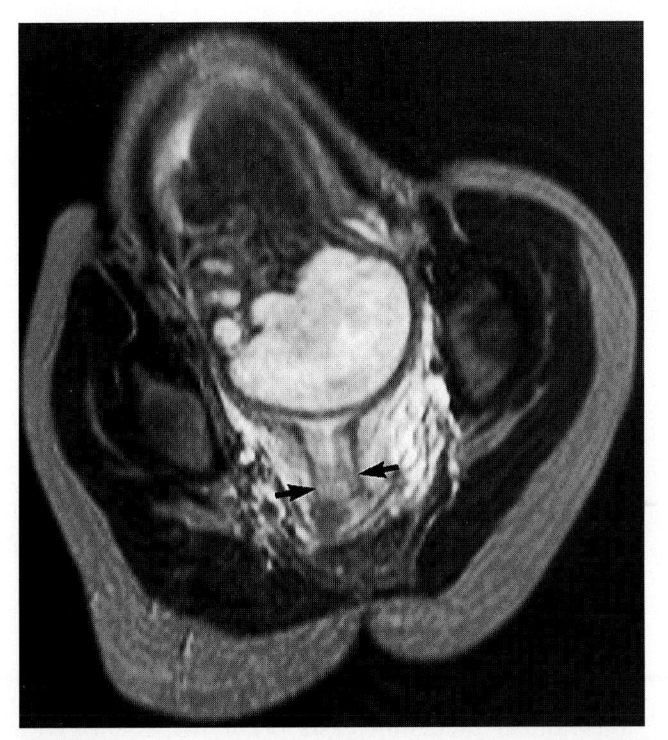

Fig. 9.15 Transverse T2-weighted MRI scan obtained to stage cervical carcinoma in a pregnant 23-year-old woman. Tumour was confined to the cervix (arrows). The fetal cranium lies in the lower uterine segment and the brain and orbit are seen as hyperintense structures.

demonstrate the primary tumour as an area of relative hypodensity in the enhanced cervix. It also facilitates identification of enlarged pelvic lymph nodes as nodular masses on the side wall of the pelvis, measuring greater than 1.0 cm in short axis or 1.5 cm in long axis; they do not enhance as much as blood vessels. In tumour staging, scanning must include the para-aortic lymph node areas up to renal artery level. Confident diagnosis of rectal or bladder wall invasion is extremely difficult due to the intrinsically poor separation of these structures by CT, even in normal subjects.

On **MRI**, carcinoma manifests as a hyperintense mass on T2-weighted sequences, replacing part or all of the low-signal cervical stroma (Figs. 9.6b,c, p. 224). A residual rim of low-signal stroma separating the tumour from the hyperintense parametrium is a reliable sign of tumour confined to the cervix. Detection of invasion of adjacent viscera is facilitated by the high soft-tissue contrast of MRI and the ability to image in any plane. T1-weighted sequences are useful to demonstrate the extent of parametrial invasion, giving the best contrast between tumour and fat, and are most sensitive for detection of lymph node enlargement (see Fig. 9.23, p. 236). With the use of the coronal plane, the retroperitoneum can be rapidly screened for lymphadenopathy and hydronephrosis.

ADNEXAL MASSES

Characterization of adnexal masses into solid, cystic or complex can be most easily achieved by ultrasound or MRI. Apart from consideration of the X-ray dose to the patient, successful CT requires a meticulous technique, with complete bowel opacification and thin section imaging. In addition to neoplastic and inflammatory lesions arising from the uterus, fallopian tube or ovary, inflammatory masses arising from bowel, such as an appendix or diverticular mass, can present as a complex adnexal mass (Fig. 9.9, p. 227). Sensitivity and specificity of diagnosis is similar for the different cross-sectional imaging techniques and choice depends largely on local availability and expertise.

Non-neoplastic ovarian masses

Non-neoplastic cysts of the ovary arise from the surface epithelium or follicles. Maturing follicles are visible as cysts measuring up to 2.5 cm in diameter which usually spontaneously regress within the month. Simple follicular cysts are also common, usually measuring between 2.5 cm and 5.0 cm, and not requiring surgical intervention unless persistent or symptomatic (Fig. 9.16). Criteria suggesting a benign lesion include size less than 4 cm, a smooth, well-defined wall less than 3 mm thick and homogeneous fluid content without thick septae, nodules or solid tissue areas.

Simple cysts are uniformly echo-free with a well-defined wall and enhanced transmission of the ultrasound beam. The contents are of water density on CT and on MRI they show the expected characteristics of fluid, namely homogeneously low signal intensity

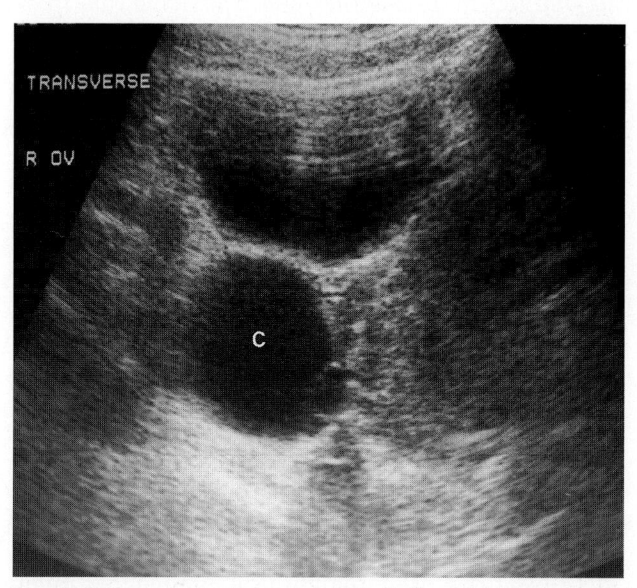

Fig. 9.16 Transverse ultrasound scan of the right adnexal region showing a well-defined echo-free mass (c) with posterior acoustic enhancement, consistent with a simple ovarian cyst.

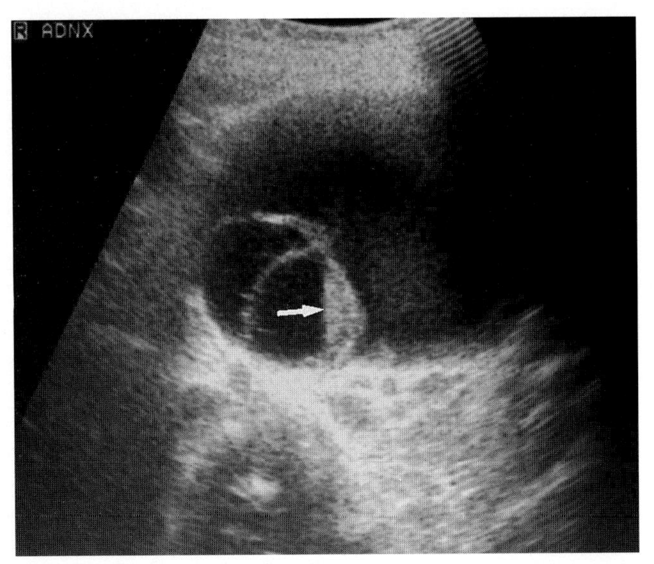

Fig. 9.17 Ultrasound scan of right adnexa showing a multiloculated cystic mass with septation and a fluid level (arrow). At subsequent surgery, an endometriotic cyst was removed from the right ovary.

on T1-weighted images and high signal intensity on T2-weighted images. Increased signal intensity on T1-weighted MR images implies the presence of protein, blood or cholesterol within the cyst fluid. Simple ovarian cysts may also occur in the post-menopausal woman, but may require laparoscopy to exclude malignancy if they do not resolve on follow-up ultrasound. Many types of benign cyst have a more heterogeneous appearance. Persistence of the corpus luteum results in a thick-walled cyst which may contain haemorrhage.

Complex cysts contain septae or other internal irregularities and haemorrhagic cysts have fine internal echoes on ultrasound, increased density on CT and increased signal intensity on T1-weighted MRI scans. Multiple haemorrhagic cysts with layering of blood products may occur in endometriosis (Fig. 9.17). Theca lutein cysts are observed when human chorionic gonadotrophin levels are high, as in hydatidiform mole.

Polycystic ovarian disease

Polycystic ovaries are characteristic of the Stein–Leventhal syndrome, in which infrequent or absent menstruation, obesity, hirsutism and infertility are due to overproduction of androgenic hormones. The diagnosis can be confirmed by ultrasound when the ovaries are of significantly greater volume than the normal 3–5 ml, because of hyperplasia of the ovarian stroma; they also have excessive numbers of subcapsular follicles measuring up to 5 mm in diameter. On T2-weighted MRI, the multiple high signal intensity cysts may appear to be arranged like a string of pearls around the periphery of the bulky ovary.

Ovarian torsion

Prompt diagnosis and treatment is required to prevent haemorrhagic infarction due to unrelieved occlusion of the twisted ovarian vascular pedicle. Ultrasound findings in the acute stage include enlargement of the ovary, often with multiple cystic areas and free fluid in the pelvis. Pre-existing ovarian abnormalities such as cysts or tumours predisposing to torsion may also be apparent. Because of the dual blood supply of the ovary, and in incomplete or intermittent torsion, findings on Doppler ultrasound may be minimal. The diagnostic advantages of CT or MRI over ultrasound have not been determined and these techniques are not appropriate unless immediately available in the emergency situation.

Other adnexal masses

Cysts of the broad ligament are usually derived from embryonic remnants and can reach a massive size. They can be complicated by infection, haemorrhage, torsion or rupture presenting as a surgical emergency. On imaging, broad ligament cysts are difficult to distinguish from ovarian or other adnexal cysts.

Peritoneal inclusion cysts occur in patients with pelvic adhesions from previous surgery or pelvic inflammatory disease. Fluid is trapped between thickened and adherent peritoneum and may be visualized on ultrasound as a cystic adnexal mass distorting the ovary.

On all imaging modalities, a **lymphocoele** is a unilocular thin-walled cyst on the pelvic side wall, containing watery or proteinaceous fluid.

Endometriosis

Functioning endometrial cells may implant on the ovary, broad ligament, uterine serosa or in the pouch of Douglas. The endometriotic tissue undergoes cyclical growth and bleeding in response to hormonal stimulation, forming haemorrhagic 'chocolate cysts'. Rupture causes intense serosal irritation and adhesions. Imaging techniques are generally unable to show small implants but may demonstrate secondary effects related to inflammation and scarring. Endometriotic adhesions can distort pelvic anatomy and cause conditions such as rectal tethering, hydrosalpinx and small bowel obstruction. Large implants are more likely to be detectable by ultrasound, CT or MRI.

Endometriotic cysts, or endometriomas, have variable morphology on imaging and can mimic other lesions which have a complex mixed cystic/solid appearance such as tubo-ovarian abscess, infected or haemorrhagic cysts and ovarian malignancy. The most characteristic appearance is multiloculated thin-walled cysts often with ill-defined margins. On ultrasound, internal echoes reflect the presence of blood products in the cyst fluid (Fig. 9.17). Endometriomas usually have increased density on CT and high signal intensity on MRI due to their haemorrhagic content. Signal intensity may vary in different parts of the cyst, especially on T2-weighted sequences, because of various stages of degradation of blood products; a low signal rim due to haemosiderin-laden macrophages or fibrosis may be visualized at the periphery of chronic endometriomas. The cysts often have angulated margins or show evidence of tethering. Implants occurring in unusual locations such as on bowel serosa or the liver are best investigated using ultrasound or CT scanning with full bowel preparation. MRI has a higher sensitivity and specificity than ultrasound or CT for the diagnosis of endometrioma. The definitive technique for staging endometriosis is, however, laparoscopy, at which the severity of endometriosis and the extent of pelvic adhesions is scored. Once diagnosed, the response of endometriomas to hormonal therapy can be assessed using ultrasound or MRI.

BENIGN OVARIAN TUMOURS

Tumours arising from the surface epithelium of the ovary include serous, mucinous, endometrioid, clear cell, Brenner and undifferentiated types, and account for 60% of ovarian tumours (Fig. 9.18). Cellular differentiation into benign and malignant types is not always clear-cut, up to one-third being classified as borderline malignancy on histological examination. The classification of ovarian masses by imaging is also imperfect. Benign tumours often have the appearance of simple cysts, while malignant tumours are more heterogeneous complex masses with a higher proportion of solid tissue. Any solid or complex pelvic mass demonstrated by imaging is therefore regarded with suspicion. Unfortunately, certain benign ovarian tumours such as fibromas and granulosa cell tumours (derived from ovarian stroma) and Brenner tumours are characteristically solid. Ovarian malignancy is also more likely to be associated with ascites.

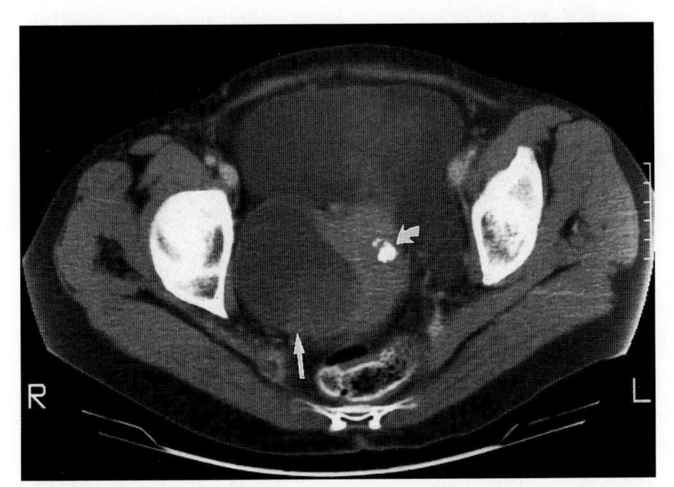

Fig. 9.18 Contrast-enhanced CT scan showing a cystic mass in the right adnexa, with poor definition and frond-like soft-tissue density posteriorly (straight arrow). A benign clear cell ovarian tumour was resected. Calcification is present in a uterine fibroid (curved arrow).

Ovarian cystadenoma

Serous cystadenomas account for 30% of benign ovarian neoplasms and are usually thin-walled unilocular or multilocular cysts, often bilateral, measuring 5–10 cm in diameter, with watery or minimally haemorrhagic contents. Fine calcification may occur in the cyst wall. Mucinous cystadenomas constitute 20% of benign ovarian tumours and are usually larger in size, more frequently multilocular and less often bilateral compared with the serous type. The wall is generally diffusely thickened and the cyst contents are mucinous. Cyst leakage into the peritoneal cavity can result in pseudomyxoma peritonei, with large gelatinous masses which may contain amorphous calcification filling the abdominal cavity.

Ovarian dermoids

Cystic ovarian teratomas, or dermoid tumours, account for 20% of ovarian tumours, and may be bilateral. Dermoid ovarian tumours classically contain a complex mixture of tissues in a multicompartmental, part cystic and part solid adnexal mass. The presence of fat, bone or teeth within the mass is characteristic (see Fig. 9.2, page 222).

Other possible constituents include proteinaceous or serous cysts, soft-tissue septa or nodules and rim calcification, which altogether may result in a complex and bizarre appearance on diagnostic imaging. Fat has a speckled hyperechoic appearance on ultrasound, a negative attenuation value on CT and a high signal intensity on both T1- and T2-weighted MR sequences (Fig. 9.19). Fat–fluid levels may be apparent on all imaging methods. On MRI, the chemical shift artefact which occurs at interfaces between lipid and water, or reduction in lesional signal on fat-suppression sequences may be useful corroborative evidence of the presence of fat within the tumour.

Calcification is identified as echo-bright areas with acoustic shadowing on ultrasound and as very high attenuation tissue on CT. MRI is relatively insensitive to calcification and will not identify fine mural calcification or focal calcification but can identify teeth and bone tissue if well-developed. Soft-tissue fronds, mural nodules and septa can be identified by all techniques. Differentiation between benign and malignant teratomas (2% of total), which also contain a mixture of mesodermal elements, is imprecise by all imaging techniques.

MALIGNANT OVARIAN TUMOURS

Ovarian cancer is a disease of postmenopausal women predominantly, most of whom present with advanced disease. After clinical examination, which may

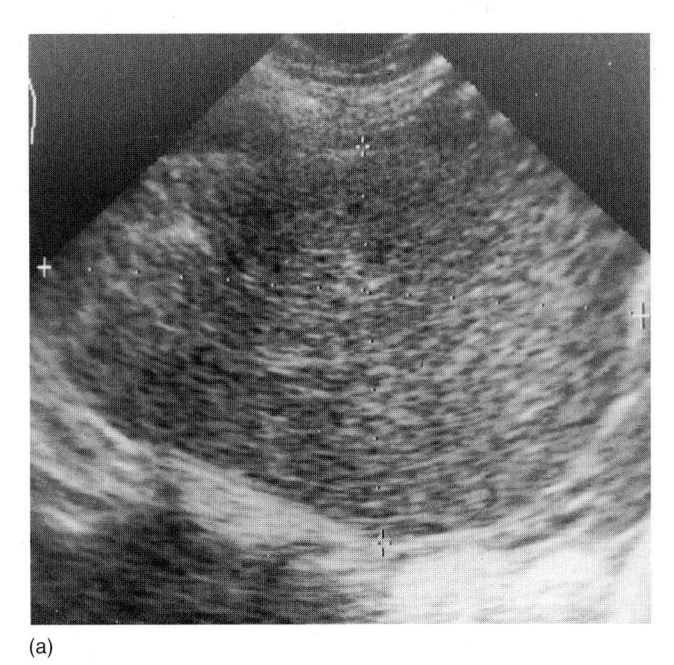

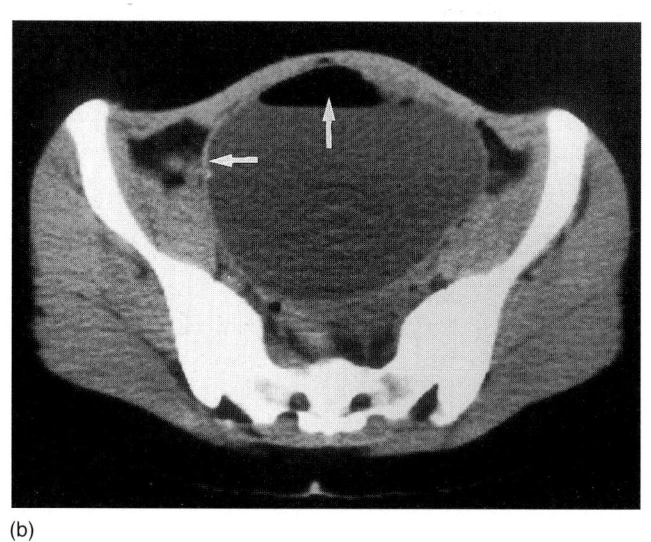

(a) (b)

Fig. 9.19 (a) Ultrasound scan, performed to assess an asymptomatic pelvic mass in a 21-year-old woman, demonstrates a uniformly echogenic mass arising centrally in the pelvis. A specific diagnosis could not be made from the ultrasound scan. (b) CT scan in the same patient shows a mass containing proteinaceous fluid (20 HU) with a fat–fluid level (vertical arrow) anteriorly and rim calcification (horizontal arrow). These features are typical of an ovarian dermoid cyst.

demonstrate a pelvic mass, ultrasound is the imaging investigation of first choice (see Fig. 9.3b, p. 222).

In postmenopausal women the ovaries are atrophic, measuring around 1–2 cm in maximum diameter, and can be difficult to visualize on ultrasound. Any solid or cystic ovarian enlargement has to be regarded as malignant until proven otherwise, and requires follow-up. A simple cyst of less than 4 cm in diameter in a postmenopausal woman is unlikely to be malignant and can be followed by ultrasound. Larger cysts,

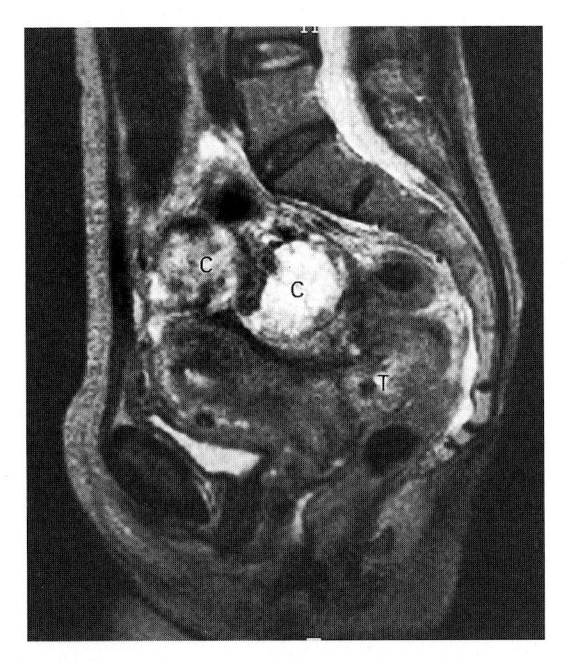

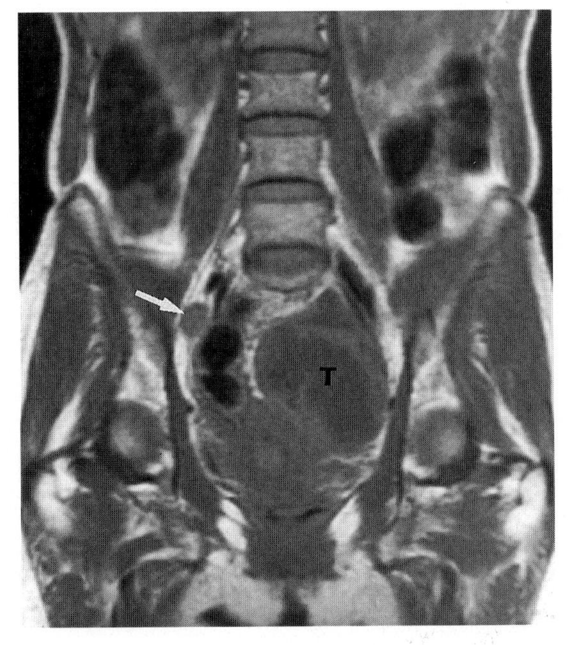

(a) (b)

Fig. 9.20 (a) Sagittal T2-weighted MRI scan in a 66-year-old woman with an ulcerating mass in the posterior vaginal fornix, thought clinically to be cervical in origin. In addition to tumour (T) in the pouch of Douglas invading the vagina and rectum, multiple complex cystic tumours (C) are present, consistent with ovarian carcinoma. Apart from a small fibroid in the anterior myometrium, the uterus is normal. (b) Coronal T1-weighted MRI scan demonstrates a cystic ovarian tumour (T) on the left, and right pelvic lymphadenopathy (arrow).

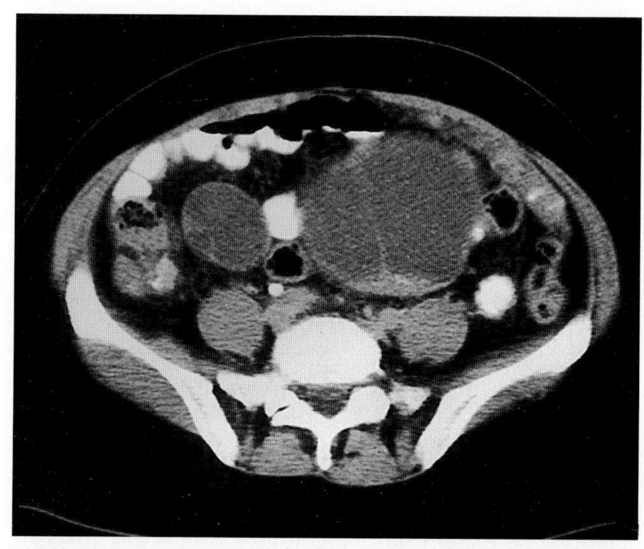

Fig. 9.21 CT scan showing complex cystic masses arising from the pelvis in a patient with bilateral ovarian serous cystadenocarcinoma.

especially those with a wall thickness of more than 3 mm, solid nodules, multiple irregular septa, prominent papillary excrescences or echogenic cyst contents, are more likely to be malignant. Benign cysts complicated by haemorrhage or infection can have an identical ultrasound appearance and although ultrasound demonstration of ascites or peritoneal masses favours underlying malignancy, the specific diagnosis may ultimately require laparoscopy.

Similarly, CT or MRI may confirm the clinical suspicion of an ovarian tumour using comparable features, but they do not provide a more specific diagnosis than ultrasound (Figs. 9.20, 9.21). Transvaginal ultrasound with colour flow Doppler has a higher sensitivity and specificity, tumour neovascularization being associated with a low impedance to blood flow through the ovarian vascular bed.

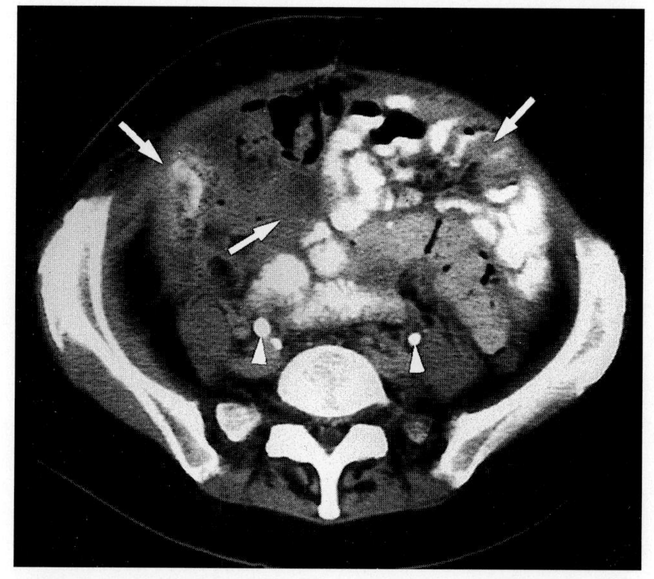

Fig. 9.22 Contrast-enhanced CT in a patient with advanced ovarian cancer. An 'omental cake' of metastatic ovarian tumour is present (arrows). The contrast-filled ureters can be seen posteriorly lying on the psoas major muscles (arrowheads).

Treatment of ovarian carcinoma is usually total hysterectomy, bilateral salpingo-oophorectomy and infracolic omentectomy, at which time formal laparoscopic staging is performed. Preoperative imaging can assist the surgeon when planning surgery and may be helpful postoperatively to assess the volume of residual disease and its subsequent response to chemotherapy. CT is particularly able to demonstrate peritoneal and omental tumour, hepatic metastases and lymphadenopathy (Fig. 9.22). Although MRI can stage the primary tumour and assess lymphadenopathy, it is less capable of demonstrating bowel and peritoneal involvement.

Ovarian cystadenocarcinoma

Two-thirds of ovarian cancers arise in the surface epithelium, producing serous or mucinous cystadenocarcinoma, endometrioid carcinoma, or more unusually, clear cell, Brenner, or undifferentiated types of carcinoma. Serous cystadenocarcinoma accounts for 40% of malignant ovarian tumours. Tumour cysts tend to be larger than 10 cm in diameter, with variable solid components, and are bilateral in 50% (Fig. 9.21). On CT and MRI, malignant soft-tissue nodules enhance after intravenous contrast medium. Psammomatous or dystrophic calcification may be apparent. Focal papillary projections disrupting the normally smooth outer margin indicate capsular invasion, associated with seeding of tumour cells into the peritoneal cavity.

Mucinous cystadenocarcinomas comprise 5–20% of malignant ovarian tumours; they are multicystic tumours containing mucinous material, haemorrhage, necrotic and solid tumour, and are bilateral in 15–25%. The rarer endometrioid tumour is a complex cystic or solid mass on imaging, affecting one or both ovaries or the fallopian tubes and spreading intraperitoneally.

Other ovarian malignancies

Malignant neoplasms may also arise from germ cell, sex cord stromal or mesenchymal cell lines in the ovary. These often appear on imaging as a solid soft-tissue mass, with or without lymphadenopathy. The ovaries are favoured sites of metastasis from primary gastrointestinal or breast adenocarcinoma producing so-called Krukenberg tumours, identical on imaging to primary ovarian carcinoma.

VAGINA AND VULVA

The vagina and external genitalia are readily accessible to clinical examination, and diagnostic imaging techniques are only used to assess deep invasion of vaginal or vulvar carcinoma and the presence of pelvic lymphadenopathy (Fig. 9.23). Imaging may also be helpful to confirm the presence of fistulae.

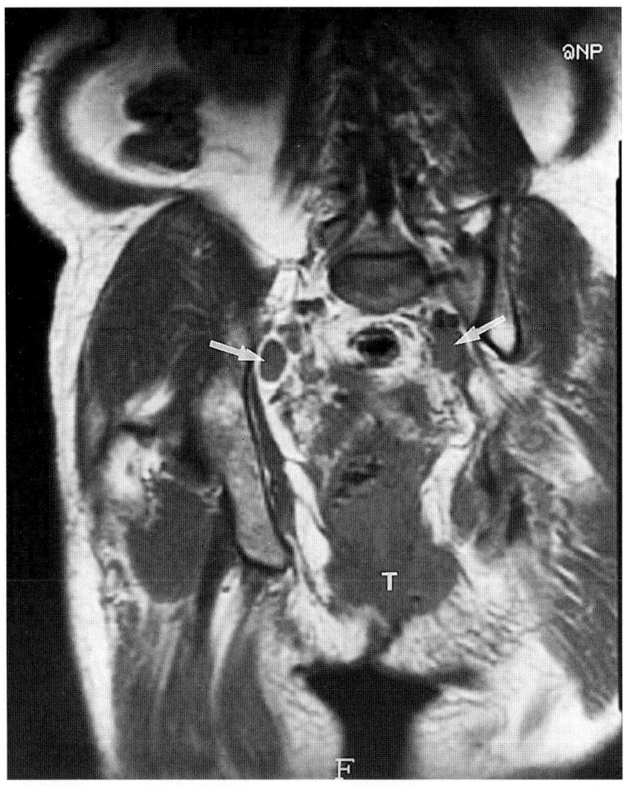

Fig. 9.23 T1-weighted MRI scan performed to stage carcinoma of the vulva in a 63-year-old woman. The primary tumour (T) was shown on other images to involve the anus, vagina, urethra and pubis. Bilateral pelvic lymphadenopathy is present (arrows).

TREATED PELVIC MALIGNANCY

Tumour recurrence

After hysterectomy for uterine malignancy, tumour recurrence usually occurs initially in the vaginal stump or on the pelvic side wall, with subsequent spread to the pelvic viscera and lymph nodes. Suitability for further treatment, e.g. pelvic exenteration, depends on the extent of local involvement and the absence of systemic dissemination. Pelvic imaging by CT or MRI can be very useful to demonstrate tumour extent, particularly when clinical pelvic examination is hindered by postoperative changes.

Postoperative changes

Postoperative changes can be easily demonstrated by cross-sectional imaging, with MRI being the most sensitive to inflammatory changes following surgery. This sensitivity and the lymph node enlargement which may follow even relatively localized surgery hinders the ability of all imaging methods to assess residual tumour in the first few weeks after operation.

Imaging is thus best delayed for a minimum of six weeks postoperatively, unless base-line scans are available for comparison or there is a case for urgent scanning. Over the period between six weeks and three months after uncomplicated surgery, vascular granulation tissue matures to a relatively avascular fibrous scar. Haematoma and oedema also tend to resolve. Three months after radical hysterectomy, CT should demonstrate the vaginal stump as a thin soft-tissue structure, the uterine bed being filled with fatty tissue containing only thin dense strands of fibrous scar.

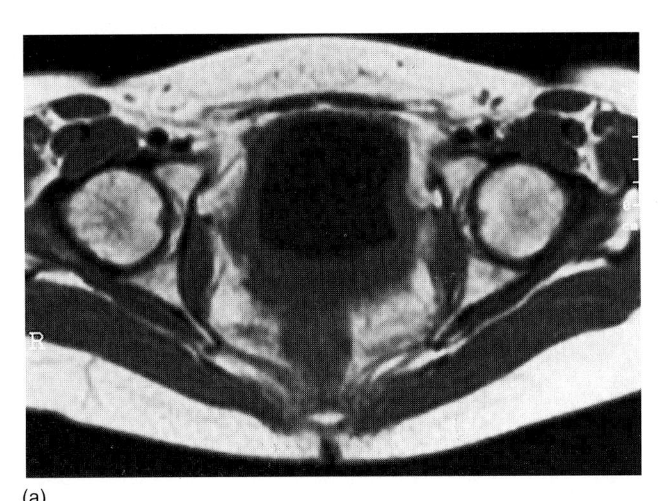

(a)

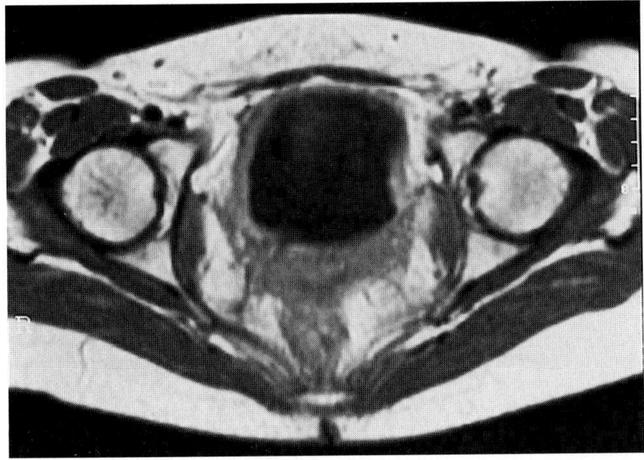

(b)

Fig. 9.24 Axial T1-weighted MRI scans pre- (a) and post-gadolinium-DTPA (b) in a patient with dysuria and bilateral hydronephrosis on ultrasound. Diffuse thickening of the bladder wall and rectum, enhancing after contrast, is secondary to inflammation rather than tumour recurrence. The patient received radical radiotherapy for cervical carcinoma 4 years previously.

The presence of nodular soft-tissue densities at the operative site or on the pelvic wall indicates tumour recurrence, especially if associated with enlargement of pelvic lymph nodes. Central low density due to necrosis may be apparent within recurrent tumour, but demonstration of a predominantly cystic mass with ring enhancement is more suggestive of abscess or organizing haematoma. If abnormal soft tissue is demonstrated on postoperative pelvic MRI, absence of high signal on T2-weighted sequences or lack of enhancement on T1-weighted sequences makes recurrent tumour very unlikely, although microscopic foci of tumour within scar or scirrhous cancers are causes of error. On CT, fibrous tissue tends to be more dense than other soft tissues but the differentiation is often unclear.

Postradiotherapy changes

Symptomatic acute cystitis and proctitis are frequent in women receiving intracavitary radiotherapy. Chronic radiation complications are less common and may involve the colon or small bowel, producing strictures or fistulae, or may involve the bladder or distal ureters, resulting in upper renal tract obstruction. The presence of hydronephrosis can be quickly ascertained by ultrasound, but the level and nature of the obstruction is best investigated by CT or MRI (Fig. 9.24).

Barium studies remain the most sensitive investigation for demonstrating bowel complications such as strictures, adhesions and fistulae. Asymptomatic thickening of bowel or bladder wall is a frequent incidental finding in patients imaged after radical pelvic radiotherapy. Changes are often diffuse, symmetrical and with little change on sequential scans, findings that help to differentiate postradiation inflammation from recurrent tumour. However, both diseases may present with a discrete enhancing pelvic mass on MRI and CT. Differential diagnosis may require image-guided biopsy or sequential scanning to assess change.

CHAPTER 10

Abdominal interventional radiology

Anthony F. Watkinson
and Andreas Adam

Interventional radiology has made a significant contribution to the management of many abdominal diseases. Technological advances are continuing to increase the success rate and minimize the complication rate of many procedures. In some instances, such as the control of haemorrhage, interventional radiology can replace conventional surgical methods, whereas in other situations it is a useful adjunct to surgery. The increasing complexity and sophistication of both surgery and interventional radiology demand careful joint planning for the choice of the optimum method of treatment.

Diagnostic and Interventional Radiology in Surgical Practice. Edited by P. Armstrong and M.L. Wastie. Published in 1997 by Chapman & Hall, London. ISBN 0 412 61960 1 (HB) 0 412 61970 9 (PB)

DILATATION OF BENIGN AND MALIGNANT LOWER OESOPHAGEAL STRICTURES

In patients with dysphagia the underlying cause must be investigated and fully evaluated. Benign causes of obstruction include achalasia or strictures secondary to reflux oesophagitis, postsurgical narrowing, radiation fibrosis, Crohn's disease, postvariceal sclerotherapy and caustic ingestion. Malignant obstruction in the lower third of the oesophagus is most likely to be due to squamous cell carcinoma or adenocarcinoma.

The dilatation of oesophageal lesions is not a new phenomenon: bougienage with whalebone dates back many centuries. Until recently, the treatment of benign lower oesophageal obstruction was by open surgical bypass or by unguided, transorally placed, soft mercury-weighted or rigid metal dilators. More recently, fluoroscopically guided dilatation using balloon catheters has been employed.

Balloon dilatation has the advantage of providing a controlled radial dilating force without producing the high longitudinal shear forces associated with bougie dilatation that are thought to predispose to oesophageal rupture. In addition the balloon inflation and oesophageal dilatation can be viewed in real time, the severity of the waist seen in the balloon indicating the degree of success.

Recent advances in self-expanding metallic stent technology has meant that malignant dysphagia can be treated effectively, with minimal hospital stay and a rapid return to a normal environment. These stents can create a normal-sized oesophageal lumen with some transmission of peristaltic waves and, in many instances, patients can resume a near normal diet. In addition, the newer stents have a variety of plastic covers to prevent tumour ingrowth. This design is also useful in dealing with oesophageal perforation or fistula formation.

ACHALASIA

Pneumatic dilatation is the initial treatment of choice for achalasia, with surgical myotomy being reserved for failure after several attempts of balloon dilatation. The aim is to purposely overdilate and traumatize the lower oesophagus in the region of the sphincter and cause sufficient tissue injury with rupture of the muscle layers, to eliminate the functional obstruction that exists in achalasia. The improvement in symptoms is immediate, the risks are low and the morbidity minimal when compared with surgery. Most cases can be performed with light intravenous sedation; however, general anaesthesia may be required in children or in patients unable to cooperate.

An initial contrast study is required to confirm the diagnosis, identify the level of obstruction and assess the amount of food residue in the dilated oesophagus (Fig. 10.1a). If significant food residue is identified, endoscopic washout prior to the procedure minimizes the risk of aspiration. Patients should receive antibiotic cover as bacteraemia is common during the dilatation. Light intravenous analgesia and sedation are used. Local anaesthetic e.g. lignocaine is applied to the oropharynx and a catheter introduced and passed into the stomach over a guidewire under fluoroscopic guidance. This ensures that the stricture is traversed with minimal trauma and that the risk of perforation is minimized.

The catheter is then withdrawn and successively larger diameter balloons used. In most cases the oesophagus is initially dilated to 20 mm progressing in 5 mm increments to a maximum diameter of 35 mm (Fig. 10.1b). At each stage it is hoped to achieve absence of waisting of the balloon. The procedure is terminated if the patient experiences significant pain or if there is blood on the balloon following withdrawal. Long-term symptomatic improvement is usually observed if dilatation of 30 mm or greater is achieved.

The radiographic result on a postdilatation contrast study (Fig. 10.1c) has been shown to correlate well with symptomatic relief. Overall, approximately 85–90% of patients are symptom free at 4–24 months.

BENIGN OESOPHAGEAL STRICTURES

There are many causes of benign strictures, the most common being reflux oesophagitis and postsurgical narrowing. A lumen of less than 12 mm almost always results in dysphagia and, if the lumen is greater than 20 mm, the vast majority of patients will be asymptomatic. Consequently, dilatation to a diameter of 20 mm is usually enough to relieve symptoms and enable the patient to eat a normal diet.

The technique is the same as for achalasia with the introduction of a balloon over a guidewire under fluoroscopic guidance. The initial balloon may be as small as 6 mm, the end point of the procedure being full dilatation of a 20 mm balloon with no residual waist. The procedure is terminated if the patient experiences significant pain or there is marked blood staining of the balloon. Even the tightest strictures can be traversed with a guidewire and subsequently dilated. Postradiation strictures tend to be more rigid and may require initial dilatation with small, high-pressure balloons before larger balloons are used.

MALIGNANT OESOPHAGEAL STRICTURES

Patients with lower oesophageal malignancy should be rigorously investigated and, if there is no evidence of metastatic disease or extensive local spread, offered surgical resection as a curative procedure. If the lesion is unresectable but the patient has few oesophageal symptoms, palliative radiotherapy or chemotherapy may be appropriate.

Patients with unresectable disease and symptoms of dysphagia, due to partial or complete oesophageal obstruction, are a difficult group. They have a limited life expectancy and therefore treatment should be minimally invasive, with the aim of returning patients to their home environment with good swallowing as quickly as possible. Surgery in these advanced cases now plays a minor role. Laser therapy, to reduce tumour volume within the oesophageal lumen and maintain patency, has been used extensively but requires numerous retreatments and also runs the risk of perforation.

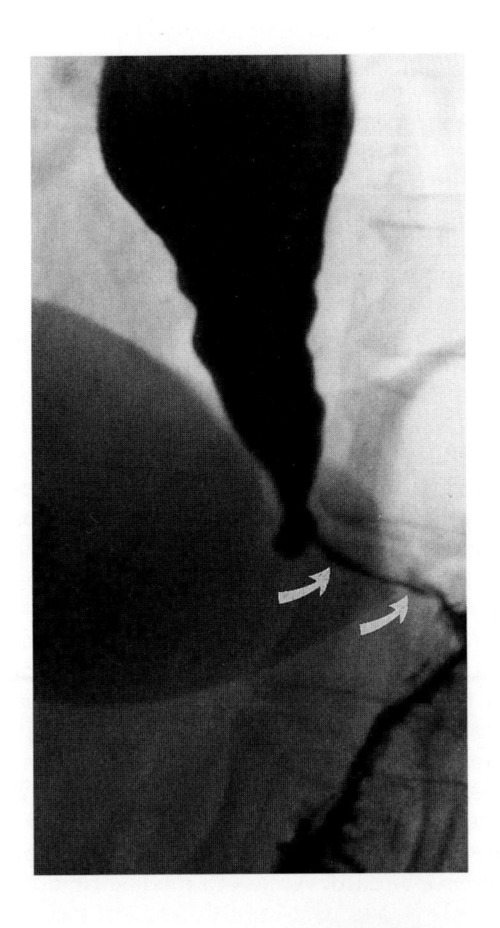
(a)

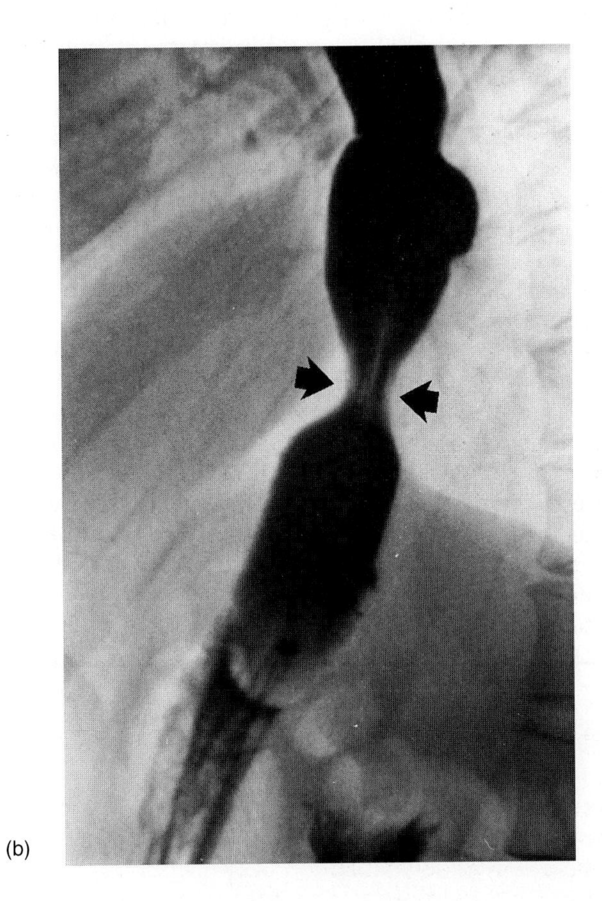
(b)

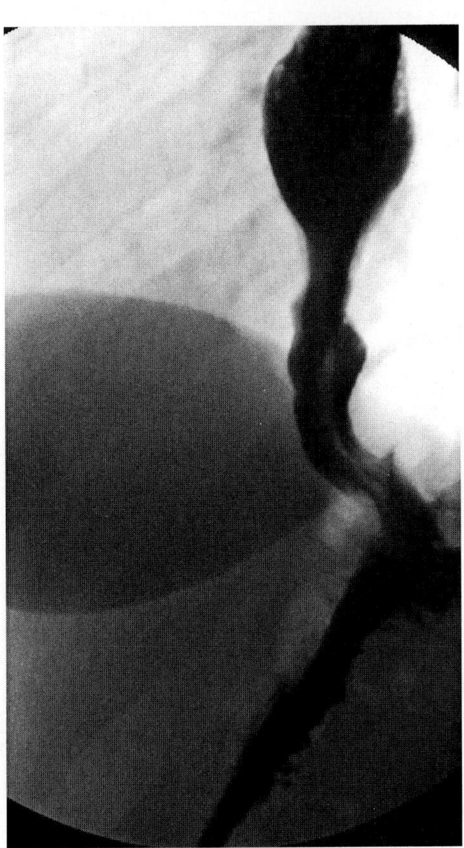
(c)

Fig. 10.1 Balloon dilatation of achalasia. (a) Barium swallow demonstrating dilated oesophagus above a smooth tight stricture in the lower oesophagus, typical of achalasia. (b) Dilatation of the lower oesophageal stricture using a 35 mm balloon. The balloon has been partially inflated with dilute contrast medium. Note the central waisting (arrows) at the site of the stricture. (c) Barium swallow after the procedure demonstrates satisfactory dilatation of the stricture.

The endoscopic placement of rigid plastic tubes, such as Celestin or Atkinson tubes, is gradually being superseded by self-expanding metal stents. Advantages include a wide lumen (up to 25 mm) and some flexibility which allows movement with peristalsis and thus near normal swallowing. Some of these stents are covered with plastic, minimizing tumour ingrowth and also sealing any associated perforation or fistulae. They relieve symptoms rapidly and the patient can return to a normal environment and tolerate a near normal diet.

A contrast swallow demonstrates the level of obstruction and any associated fistulae (Fig. 10.2a). Local anaesthesia to the oropharynx and intravenous analgesia and sedation are used. The stricture is traversed with a catheter and guidewire under fluoroscopic guidance. It is virtually always possible to traverse the stricture with the aid of hydrophilic guidewires. Serial balloon dilatation to a maximum diameter of 15 mm is performed under fluoroscopic guidance. In the presence of fistulae or perforation the dilatation is limited to 10 mm. The self-expanding metallic stent is then introduced over a guidewire and deployed across the stricture. If the postcontrast swallow (Fig. 10.2b) is satisfactory the patient can resume a near normal diet immediately.

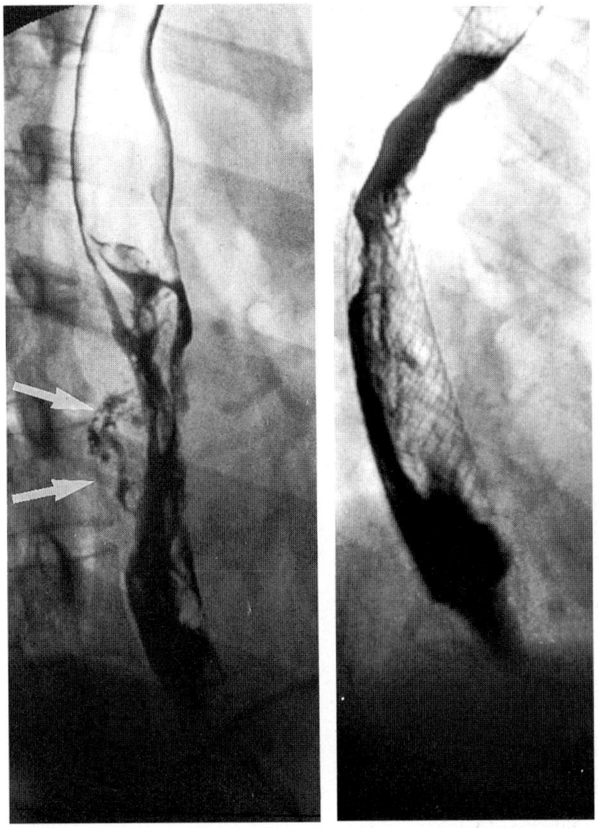

(a) (b)

Fig. 10.2 Metallic stents in malignant oesophageal obstruction. (a) A contrast swallow demonstrating a malignant stricture in the lower oesophagus with evidence of fistulation (arrows). b) A contrast swallow after placement of a self-expanding plastic-covered metal stent. There is rapid, free flow through the stent with no evidence of leakage. (Reproduced with permission from Watkinson *et al.* in *Radiology*, 1995, **195**, 821–827, published by the Radiological Society of North America)

MANAGEMENT OF ENTERIC STRICTURES

Traditionally, gastrointestinal strictures have been treated with surgical resection or bypass. Although surgical treatment is generally associated with a high success rate, it can be associated with significant morbidity and mortality, particularly in debilitated patients with multisystem disease. The radiological management of enteric strictures was first described in 1981 and since then many cases have been reported which document the ease of fluoroscopically guided balloon dilatation at many different sites along the gastrointestinal tract. This technique combines a high success rate with minimal morbidity. Any stricture which can be reached with a balloon catheter can be treated with balloon dilatation and it is worth trying this method before resorting to surgery.

Local anaesthesia is required at the mouth, anus or stoma site and intravenous analgesia and sedation may be helpful in certain circumstances. Extra long guidewires and catheters are required; otherwise the equipment is standard. Access to the gastric outlet or small bowel is via the mouth or an indwelling gastrostomy, if present. Progress through the small bowel requires gently curved catheters and soft guidewires. Rectal intubation is performed in the left lateral position and, with a combination of soft guidewires and gentle catheters, it is usually possible to reach the stricture site. Injection of water-soluble contrast agents will help to confirm the stricture location and define its contours and length. During manipulation in the upper gastrointestinal tract in patients with gastric stasis and in all manipulations in the lower gastrointestinal tract, mucosal disruption and bleeding can occur, which may lead to bacteraemia. Antibiotic cover in these patients is therefore advised.

GASTRIC OUTLET STRICTURES

Pyloric or antral scarring is usually the result of longstanding peptic disease, but occasionally results from ingestion of strongly acidic or caustic substances, or as a complication of pyloric surgery. Surgically created gastroenterostomies and surgical procedures that involve restriction of gastric volume or jejunal bypass for the treatment of morbid obesity are other settings which may lead to gastric outlet obstruction.

Relatively few studies of gastric, small bowel and large bowel stricture dilatations have been published.

However, sufficient information and experience have been obtained to identify factors which influence success, failure and complications.

PYLORIC STRICTURES

Pyloric canal or antral strictures are traversed using the catheter guidewire technique. Hydrophilic guidewires are often required due to the tightness of the stricture and the position of the pylorus. Once the stricture has been traversed the guidewire is replaced with a long, stiff exchange wire enabling a balloon catheter to be introduced. The goal of pyloric dilatation is to acheive full expansion of a 15 mm balloon, as this will usually relieve obstructive symptoms. Some pyloric strictures are very resistant and may require sequential dilation. The end-point of dilatation at any given session is determined by patient tolerance, because balloon inflation can be uncomfortable and significant discomfort is a reasonable end-point to use.

Technically, the most difficult part of any gastrointestinal stricture dilatation is the intubation of the stricture itself. Once this has been crossed, exchange for the balloon catheter and expansion of the balloon are straightforward in comparison. Strictures of the intact stomach, including those of the body, antrum and pylorus, present somewhat greater intubation problems than oesophageal strictures because of the increased length and angulation of the catheter path before the stricture is reached. However, the angles are fairly gentle and the anatomy predictable, so that the experienced interventionalist will succeed in crossing strictures in the intact stomach about 90% of the time compared to a near 100% success rate with oesophageal strictures. A success rate of about 90% would also be expected when strictures are intubated following horizontal and vertical restrictive gastroplasties.

In the small number of reported cases of dilatation for peptic disease, success rates of 67–80% have been reported. Such patients have, in general, been poor surgical candidates with a poor prognosis. The long-term evaluation of the success of pyloric stricture dilatation has, therefore been limited by this selection bias.

GASTROENTEROSTOMY STRICTURES

The most common gastric outlet obstruction treated with balloon dilatation is stricturing following surgical gastroenterostomy. Gastroenterostomies must be precisely constructed to allow adequate gastric emptying, but the size of the anastomoses must be small enough to prevent subsequent dumping syndrome. Anastomotic obstruction occurs in about 5% of patients with gastroenterostomies. Because of the many different surgical techniques involved, as well as differences in patient anatomy, gastroenterostomies are the most difficult strictures to cannulate. Pre-procedure review of available imaging studies, particularly barium studies and computed tomographic scans, can be invaluable in choosing the optimum patient orientation and which initial catheters and guidewires to use. In general, gastroenterostomies are constructed on the anterior wall of the stomach in a non-dependent location. If stenotic, the gastric remnant resembles a sphere with a pinhole and the difficult part of the procedure is locating the tightly strictured anastomosis somewhere on this otherwise featureless gastric wall. Once the gastroenterostomy has been located and traversed, the technique of balloon dilatation is as previously described, with a reasonable end-point of full inflation to 15 mm.

The failure rate of intubation is approximately 30%. However, many patients are referred only after endoscopic failure, creating a group of greater than average difficulty. In those that are successfully dilated, the procedure produces symptomatic relief in approximately 70% of patients over a 2-year period. Poor results appear to correlate with eccentric lesions and where a kink in the bowel exists rather than a true stricture.

Patients who have strictures following morbid obesity represent a special category. Many different operations are performed for obesity, of which some are simply restrictive procedures designed to reduce the volume of the gastric pouch, and others combine restriction of the gastric pouch with a bypass of some of the absorptive surface of the jejunum. Gastric pouch restriction is performed most commonly with either vertical or horizontal band gastroplasty. The bypass component, if used, is a gastrojejunal anastomosis. In cases of gastric outlet obstruction following gastroplasty, it is important not to overdilate the strictured channel, as this can defeat the purpose of the original operation. Close consultation with the referring surgeon is advised regarding the intended size of the channel. In general, the channel remaining after restrictive gastroplasty should not be dilated to more than 12 mm. Combining the advantages of fluoroscopy and endoscopy often increases the success rate in difficult cases. Endoscopy enables the stricture to be identified and a guidewire introduced, which can then be monitored fluoroscopically to ensure sufficient guidewire has passed beyond the stricture.

ENTEROENTERIC STRICTURES

The challenge when treating enteroenteric strictures is getting to the strictured site. In general the more distal the anatomical location of the stricture the less likely the fluoroscopically guided approach will succeed. This is another instance where combined fluoroscopy and endoscopy can be used to advantage. The balloon size is chosen to approximate, but not exceed, that of normal adjacent bowel. The optimal size is 15–20 mm.

COLORECTAL STRICTURES

The technique in reaching, cannulating and dilating strictures of the lower gastrointestinal tract is the same as for upper gastrointestinal strictures whether via the anus or via a stoma. If the stricture is at some distance from the entry site, a combined endoscopic and fluoroscopic approach is often successful. The main difference between treating strictures of the upper and lower gastrointestinal tract is the larger calibres required to produce a normal or near normal faecal stream through a colonic or rectal stricture. Balloon catheters of up to 40 mm may be necessary to achieve sufficient diameter to restore normal defaecation.

Fortunately, the majority of lower gastrointestinal strictures are distal and the distance from the anus is quite short. Technical success rates nearing 100% have been reported. For more proximal colonic lesions or small bowel-to-colon anastomoses, the path the catheter has to take can be long and tortuous and a combined endoscopic and fluoroscopic approach may lead to success where either technique alone has failed.

The goal of balloon dilatation in colonic and rectal strictures is to achieve a normal or near normal faecal stream and this can be achieved with a single dilatation in about 50% of patients with 2-year symptom-free periods being documented. In those requiring multiple dilatations, the symptom-free period has been shown to increase progressively. Because access is usually technically easy, multiple repeat dilatations represent a reasonable means of providing long-term symptomatic improvement.

PERCUTANEOUS MANAGEMENT OF GASTROINTESTINAL FISTULAE

Fistulae vary in complexity from a single track to multiple tracks with associated abscesses. In general, the simpler types are more likely to heal with conservative therapy whilst those associated with abscesses require intervention. Upper gastrointestinal fistulae are divided into low output and high output. Those with outputs of ≤200 ml/24 h are considered low output while those with >200 ml/24 h are defined as high output. Traditionally the volume of output has been inversely related to the likelihood of spontaneous closure without intervention. However, the recent aggressive use of total parenteral nutrition and pharmacological agents has made this distinction less valid. The location of the fistula along the gastrointestinal tract and the underlying aetiology are more important prognostic factors.

Abdominal surgery is the most common cause of gastrointestinal fistulae. Inadvertent enterostomy and leaking anastomoses are the major subgroups of surgically related fistula. Other causes include penetrating trauma, inflammatory diseases such as ulcers, diverticulitis, radiation enteritis and Crohn's disease as well as neoplasm.

The management of persisting fistula is to occlude the tract and prevent leakage as considerable fluid and electrolyte loss can occur. Also the bowel contents can be irritating, leading to skin ulceration. Sepsis and malnutrition frequently complicate management.

All patients presenting with gastrointestinal fistula should be evaluated with cross-sectional imaging, preferably CT scanning and contrast medium fistulography. The primary purpose of cross-sectional imaging is to detect abdominal abcesses associated with fistula which will need to be drained before healing can occur. Also, the underlying disease process may be identified, e.g. bowel wall thickening in Crohn's disease or a pericolic abscess associated with diverticulitis. If a soft-tissue mass suggestive of an abscess is seen, injection of dilute contrast medium along the fistulous tract whilst the patient is in the CT scanner, and re-imaging at this level, will demonstrate communication of the fistula with the abscess. If this is the case then contrast medium will outline the abscess cavity which can be drained, in most instances, under fluoroscopic guidance. If no contrast medium enters the abscess, then a separate puncture to localize the abscess should be done under CT guidance.

The purpose of fistulography is to determine the site of origin of the fistula, to establish whether there is distal obstruction and to show any abscess communicating with the tract. If there is neither then conservative management has a reasonable chance of success. Conservative management focuses on decreasing fistula output whilst treating infection, malnutrition and skin breakdown.

Enterocutaneous fistulae that are complicated by associated abscesses, fistulae which are discovered after initial drainage of abscesses, and simple fistulae not responding to conservative measures are all amenable to percutaneous therapy. The goals are:

- to place a tube or tubes precisely which will divert the bowel contents away from the site of the defect in the bowel wall,
- to drain thoroughly associated abscess collections.

CANNULATION OF ENTEROCUTANEOUS FISTULAE

An initial fistulogram is performed to define clearly the relationship between a sinus tract, the hole in the bowel and any abscesses. Subsequent cannulation of the sinus track is made with extreme caution to avoid dissection of the friable, often tortuous, pathways. Once the catheter has reached the lumen of the bowel, additional contrast is injected to evaluate the bowel distal to the fistula.

DIVERSION OF ENTERIC CONTENTS

Control of the effluent from the bowel can be achieved by placing a catheter just inside the bowel lumen thus diverting the bowel contents before they leak into the subcutaneous tissues. This is particularly advantageous when the leaking fluid is irritating such as from duodenal fistulae containing both hydrochloric acid and pancreatic enzymes. Alternatively, if the fistula is smaller, a drainage catheter can be positioned just outside the hole in the bowel to collect the contents as they leak and divert them from the subcutaneous tissues. Once the associated abscesses are resolved, all that then remains is a single fistula tract drain. When the volume of drainage falls below 100 ml/24 h, the tube is positioned several centimetres from the bowel wall. When drainage finally ceases a sinogram is performed to confirm closure of the fistula and the tube is removed incrementally.

DRAINAGE OF ASSOCIATED ABSCESSES

The second major focus of percutaneous therapy of enteric fistulae is drainage of associated abscesses. This may require multiple drainage tubes. The general principle is the same as for abscesses (see p. 255) not associated with fistula; however, a combination of fistula and abscess(es) tends to require more aggressive and longer term drainage. Once the fistula is controlled, the abscesses will heal with tube drainage. As with any drainage tubes, the drains must be kept patent by frequent flushing, typically with 10–20 ml saline tds. Repositioning and replacement are done in conjunction with repeat sinograms which monitor progress and direct optimal catheter position. When the sinogram demonstrates resolution of the abscess cavities, the drainage tubes are backed out incrementally and removed.

Gastrointestinal fistulae related to pancreatic inflammatory disease are particularly challenging with abnormal communications to the pancreatic duct and biliary tree. They most commonly occur after pancreatic surgery or drainage of pancreatic abscesses. Catheter diversion of both pancreatic and biliary output is sometimes necessary to allow healing. Prolonged healing is routinely required in this setting. However, the principles applied are the same as for other gastroenteric fistulae with the initial focus being resolution of the abscesses followed by closure of any fistulae.

RESULTS

Before the aggressive use of total parenteral nutrition, the spontaneous closure rate of gastroenteric fistulae was reported to be as low as 25%. Parenteral nutrition has doubled this closure rate, but about 50% of fistulae will require intervention. Complete closure can be achieved in approximately 60–80% with the use of percutaneous techniques. The success rate depends on a number of factors.

- It was previously thought that low output fistulae resolved in a higher proportion of cases, however, with aggressive use of total parenteral nutrition and pharmacological manipulation of the effluent, the initial output volume appears to be less important.
- Location appears to be important. Gastric and proximal duodenal fistulae are very difficult to treat percutaneously with approximately 75% eventually requiring surgery. Distal duodenal and other small bowel fistulae tend to close on average between 60–80% of the time.
- If the underlying bowel at the site of the fistula is diseased, the likelihood of cure is small. Crohn's disease is a good example: a spontaneous fistula to bowel involved by Crohn's will close with percutaneous drainage in only 20% of cases. However, if the fistula occurs postoperatively following removal of a diseased segment of Crohn's disease then it will close in approximately 80% of cases with percutaneous management.
- The success rate of percutaneous management of colonic fistulae is dependent on the underlying disease. Fistulae secondary to diverticulitis or appendicitis appear to respond well to tube drainage. However, in cases secondary to abnormal segments of bowel affected by radiation enteritis or colitis, successful closure with percutaneous management is unlikely.

PERCUTANEOUS GASTROSTOMY AND GASTROJEJUNOSTOMY

Patients unable to maintain nutrition with oral intake require either enteral or parenteral feeding. The most common indications are inabilty to swallow due to cerebrovascular accident or upper gastrointestinal malignancy. Other indications include chronic neurological disorders (multiple sclerosis, senile dementia, Alzheimer's and Parkinson's disease), severe burns, chronic pancreatitis, Crohn's disease and radiation enteritis. Enteral feeding is preferable, if possible, as it is more physiological and cost-effective. This form of feeding has traditionally been via surgical gastrostomy or nasogastric feeding tube. Surgical gastrostomy has the disadvantage of high cost with a higher morbidity and mortality. Long-term nasogastric tube feeding is cheap but poorly tolerated and can lead to gastro-oesophageal reflux, peptic oesophagitis and stricture formation.

Recent advances for placement of gastrostomy feeding tubes using endoscopy and fluoroscopy with the Seldinger technique have rendered surgical gastrostomy almost obsolete. The choice between endoscopic and fluoroscopic placement depends on local expertise, although the fluoroscopically guided method does have several advantages: apart from reduced cost there is a decreased risk of wound infection and aspiration. In addition, the fluoroscopic placement of a gastrojejunostomy tube, in patients who require jejunal infusional feeding, is a relatively simple extension of the basic technique. Although endoscopic placement of the catheter into the jejunum is possible, the procedure is more tedious to perform and catheters are difficult to exchange. The complications associated with endoscopic placement have been as high as 80% with catheter dysfunction in more than 50%. The decision to perform gastrostomy or gastrojejunostomy depends on the underlying pathology and the general condition of the patient. If the patient is ambulatory and can tolerate a single large feed two to three times daily, without risk of reflux, a gastrostomy tube is indicated. In addition, a small group of patients with advanced abdominopelvic malignancy requires gastrostomy tube placement for palliative bowel decompression. If the patient is bed-bound with a decreased level of conciousness, a gastrojejunostomy tube with a slow infusion feed is placed to reduce the risk of reflux.

TECHNIQUE

An abdominal ultrasound scan is performed prior to the procedure to map out the position and so avoid puncture of the left lobe of the liver. Following placement of a nasogastric tube the stomach is inflated with carbon dioxide or air in order to increase the size of the stomach and make it an easier target. It also causes the anterior wall to lie subcutaneously just beneath the abdominal wall. If passage of a nasogastric tube is not possible, direct percutaneous puncture of the collapsed gastric antrum is possible (with ultrasound or CT guidance) with direct inflation of the stomach with carbon dioxide down the needle lumen.

Antero-posterior and lateral fluoroscopy is then performed to ensure that the stomach lies subcutaneously with no interposing small bowel and that the transverse colon has been deflected inferiorly. The procedure is performed under local anaesthesia, intravenous analgesia and sedation.

Under fluoroscopic guidance an appropriate puncture site is selected overlying the body of the stomach near the antrum clear of the liver and transverse colon. A 22-gauge fine bore needle is introduced such that the tip lies within the insufflated stomach angled towards the fundus for a gastrostomy tube or the pylorus for a gastrojejunostomy tube. If a gastrostomy is required, various guidewires and dilators are used coaxially and a 12F loop catheter is positioned with its retention loop in the stomach.

If a gastrojejunostomy is required, a catheter-guidewire combination is manipulated across the pylorus into the duodenum and onward beyond the ligament of Treitz; the catheter is then removed leaving the guidewire in place. A 12F gastrojejunostomy catheter can then be introduced over the guidewire such that the tip is in the jejunum and the retention loop lies in the stomach (Fig. 10.3a,b). There is a variety of catheters on the market but most have 20 side holes in the last 15 cm. The catheter can be left *in situ* for up to 6 months before exchange is required.

The technique has a success rate which approaches 100% with low morbidity (5–8%) and mortality (< 1%). Minor complications include wound infection and tube dislodgement. The main major complication is peritonitis, which some authors have attempted to minimize by performing gastropexy. Others argue that the incidence of gastric leakage and peritonitis is no higher with the percutaneous endoscopic approach and no higher than following surgical gastrostomy. With careful selection of patients for gastrostomy and gastrojejunostomy tubes, the incidence of chronic aspiration is extremely low.

PERCUTANEOUS MANAGEMENT OF BENIGN AND MALIGNANT BILIARY STRICTURES

In patients with obstructive jaundice good imaging is required with computed tomography (CT) or ultrasound to identify the level of obstruction and the cause. It still may not be possible to make a diagnosis and direct cholangiography is often required. The least invasive approach is via endoscopy; however, this is not always successful, does not always demonstrate the intrahepatic radicles completely and depends on local expertise. Percutaneous transhepatic cholangiography provides excellent delineation of the intra- and extrahepatic biliary tree and is the initiating step in percutaneous access and treatment of biliary strictures.

Good clotting function is essential with a platelet count of more than 80 000 and a prothrombin time of no more than 4 s greater than control. All patients should receive prophylactic broad-spectrum antibiotic therapy during the procedure. The initial diagnostic study is carried out using a 22-gauge needle from a

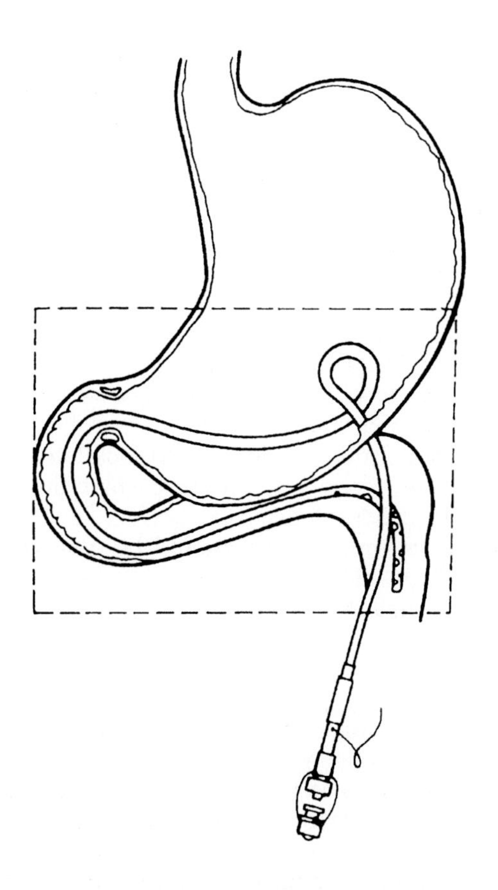

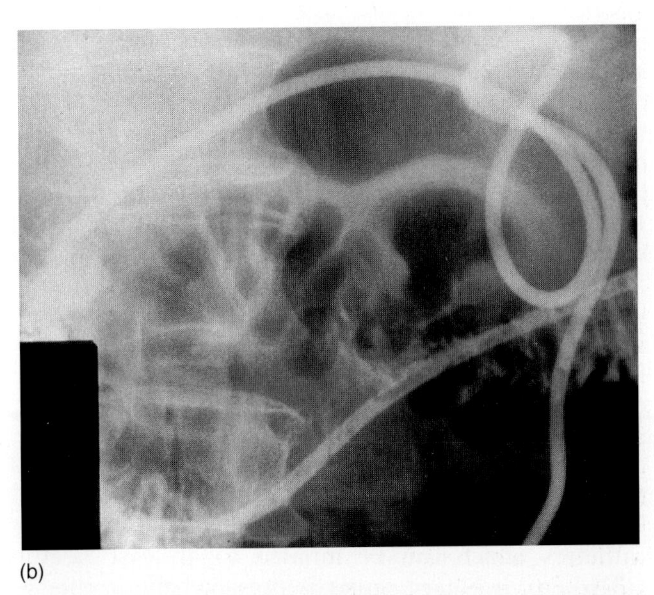

(a) (b)

Fig. 10.3 Gastrojejunostomy tube insertion. (a) and (b) A 12F gastrojejunostomy tube is seen with the retention loop in the stomach and the tip of the tube beyond the ligament of Treitz. (Reproduced with permission from Watkinson *et al.* in *European Radiology*, 1995, **5**, 13–18, published by Springer Verlag, Berlin)

right intercostal approach. Although easier to perform if the intrahepatic biliary tree is dilated, it is still successful in most instances if the biliary tree is only minimally dilated; however, more needle passes may be required. Once a duct has been punctured it is important to aspirate bile so that contrast can be introduced in equal aliquots and not further distend the biliary tree, which would increase the risk of endotoxic shock or cholangitis. Good images are then obtained (Fig. 10.4) which, when combined with the clinical history, ultrasound or CT, should indicate the diagnosis, though a fine-needle aspiration biopsy may be necessary for final confirmation.

If a decision is made to proceed to drainage, a suitable duct for access is selected. This should have a direct line of approach toward the common hepatic duct. In most instances a peripheral duct on the right is chosen in both benign and malignant disease. Initial puncture is once again performed with a 22-gauge needle and access to the intrahepatic ducts is obtained using the Seldinger technique. Further manipulation in the biliary tree is performed with specially designed catheters and guidewires. Teflon-coated hydrophilic guidewires are particularly useful in traversing even the tightest strictures.

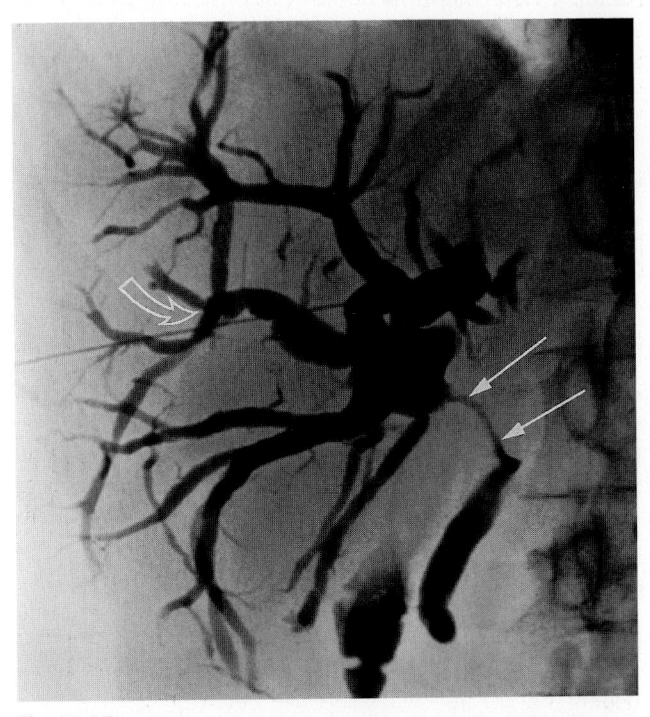

Fig. 10.4 Percutaneous transhepatic cholangiography (PTC). There is a tight stricture (arrows) of the common hepatic duct caused by cholangiocarcinoma, with intrahepatic biliary dilatation above the stricture. If it is decided to proceed to percutaneous drainage a second puncture should be performed via a suitable duct (curved arrow).

BENIGN BILIARY STRICTURES

About 95% of biliary strictures are postoperative secondary to surgery. Other causes include sclerosing cholangitis and chronic pancreatitis (Fig. 10.5), or are secondary to biliary calculi. Postoperative strictures usually occur at the site of a hepaticojejunostomy following bile duct excision (Fig. 10.6a) or at the site of insertion of the cystic duct postcholecystectomy. Recurrent strictures cause intermittent bouts of cholangitis associated with pain and jaundice. The traditional method of treatment is surgical repair; however, the recurrence rate is between 10–40% with an operative mortality of 2–4%. Balloon dilatation through a percutaneous tract was first described in 1978 and since then has become a well established technique.

Technique

If the stricture can be traversed using standard catheter-guidewire techniques then a balloon catheter can be introduced coaxially over the guidewire after catheter withdrawal. Subsequent balloon inflation can then be performed to dilate the stricture (Fig. 10.6b). This is usually performed using 8–10 mm balloon catheters which can be inflated to at least 12 atm (1216 kPa). If biliary sepsis is present balloon dilatation should not be performed until this has settled during a period of external drainage and antibiotic therapy. After balloon dilatation an access catheter is sometimes left in place to facilitate repeat dilatation should early recurrence occur. The catheter is removed following check cholangiography 3–4 weeks later, provided the patient is asymptomatic and the anastomosis fully patent (Fig. 10.6c).

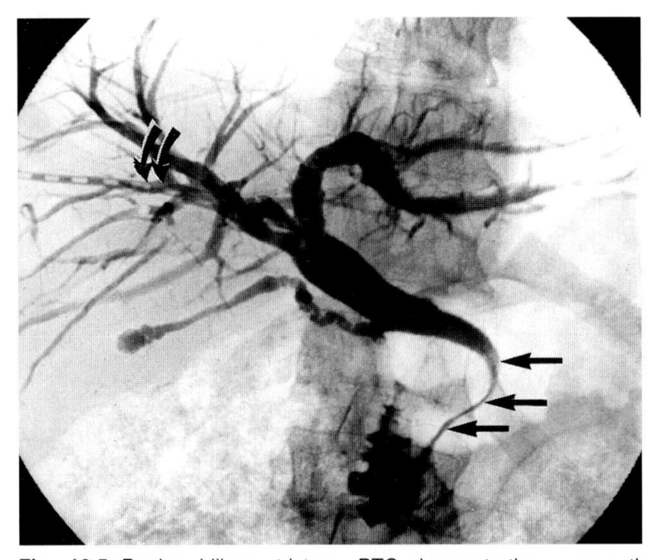

Fig. 10.5 Benign biliary stricture. PTC demonstrating a smooth tapered stricture of the lower common bile duct secondary to pancreatitis (straight arrows). Note the catheter is entering the biliary tree via a duct providing good access for percutaneous intervention (curved arrows).

Results

The success rate is approximately 80% after 30 months, falling to 55% after 5 years. The results of balloon dilatation are, however, poor in patients with sclerosing cholangitis.

Good surgical practice demands that all patients undergoing hepaticojejunostomy should have a Hutson loop formed (Fig. 10.7). This should be marked with a radiopaque circular ring to facilitate repeated percutaneous access for stricture dilatation in the event of future problems.

Expandable metal stents should be used only as a last resort in benign disease when strictures are resistant to balloon dilatation or if the patients are unfit for surgery.

MALIGNANT BILIARY STRICTURES

Biliary drainage is usually a palliative procedure in patients with biliary tract obstruction due to unresectable malignancy. The most common neoplasm producing extrahepatic biliary obstruction is carcinoma of the pancreas which, if inoperable, has a mean survival time of approximately six months. Percutaneous relief of this obstruction is an accepted mode of treatment; however, the recent advances in endoscopically placed stents have meant the role of percutaneous drainage in pancreatic carcinoma is usually limited to endoscopic failures. The choice of treatment varies according to local expertise.

Primary bile duct tumours are more difficult to manage endoscopically, particularly when located at the hilum of the liver (Klatskin tumours) or extending into the intrahepatic ducts. In non-surgical candidates these lesions are readily treated by percutaneous techniques. Transhepatic biliary drainage may also provide palliation for patients with metastases or other tumours at the hilum of the liver. However, in patients with multiple peripheral intrahepatic metastases associated with biliary tract obstruction, drainage should be avoided as it is generally ineffective in relieving jaundice. Usually, it is sufficient to drain only one side of the obstructed biliary tree as drainage of 30% or greater of the liver parenchyma will relieve the obstructive symptoms.

The initial technique is identical to the approach in benign biliary strictures with diagnostic cholangiography as the initial step. The anatomy of the biliary tree and the level of obstruction determine the choice of appropriate duct for drainage (Fig. 10.8). Biliary drainage on the left side may be necessary in cases of extensive tumour invasion, via an anterior subcostal

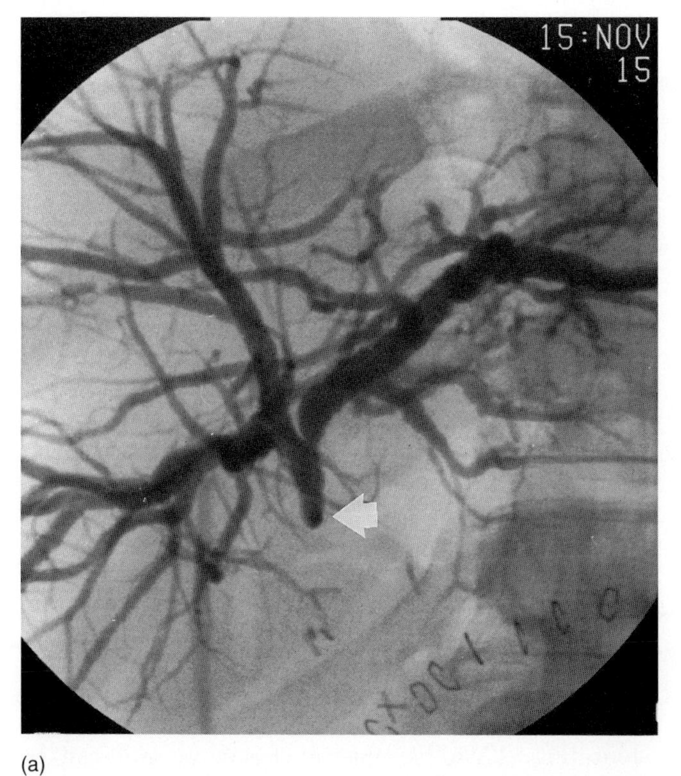

(a)

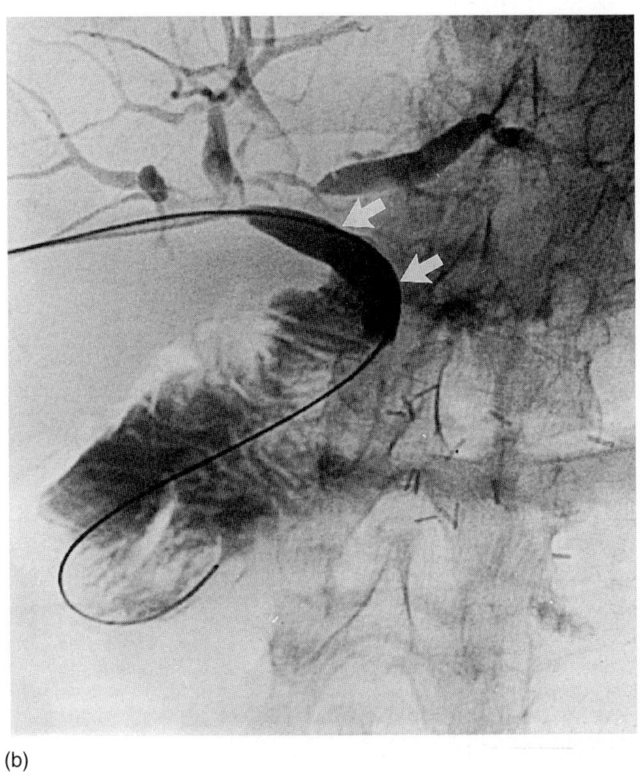
(b)

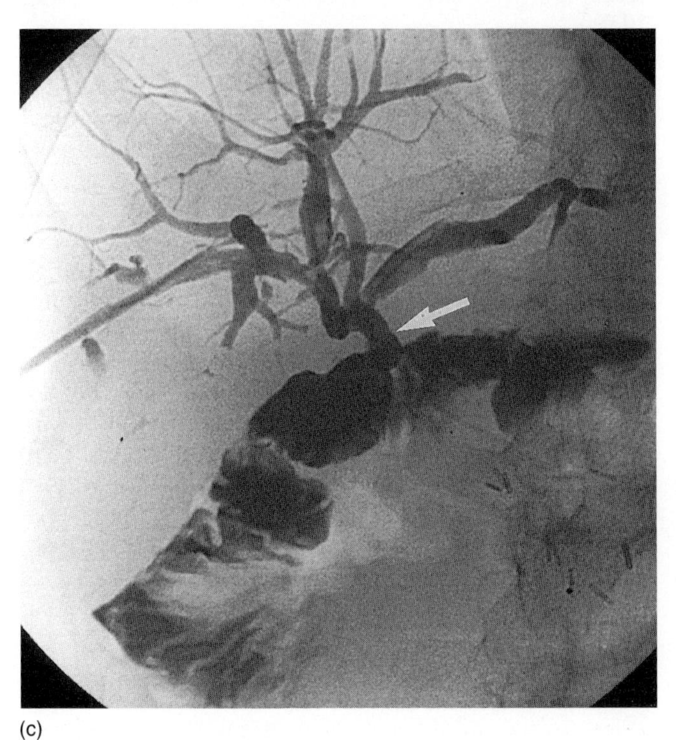
(c)

Fig. 10.6 Dilatation of benign biliary stricture. (a) PTC demonstrating complete obstruction of the common hepatic duct (arrow) after construction of a hepaticojejunostomy. (b) The obstructed hepaticojejunostomy has been traversed and a balloon dilatation catheter introduced along the percutaneous tract. This has been inflated (arrows) across the strictured segment. (c) A cholangiogram performed via a percutaneous catheter with the tip in the left main hepatic duct. The hepaticojejunostomy is now widely patent (arrow) and the catheter can be removed. (Reproduced with permission from Watkinson A.F. and Adam A. (1996) *Interventional radiology: a practical guide*, published by Radcliffe Medical Press, Oxford)

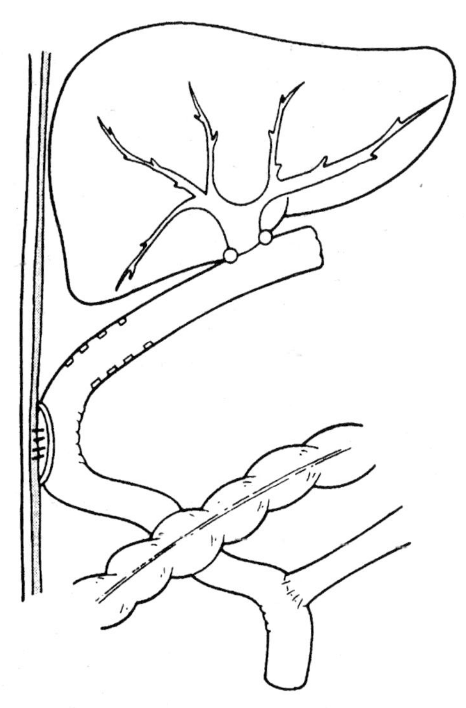

Fig. 10.7 Diagramatic representation of a Hutson loop. An end-to-side hepaticojejunostomy has been constructed and the jejunal loop attached to the abdominal wall with a radiopaque metal ring marker to facilitate future percutaneous access. (Adapted from Watkinson A.F. and Adam A. (1996) *Interventional radiology: a practical guide*, published by Radcliffe Medical Press, Oxford)

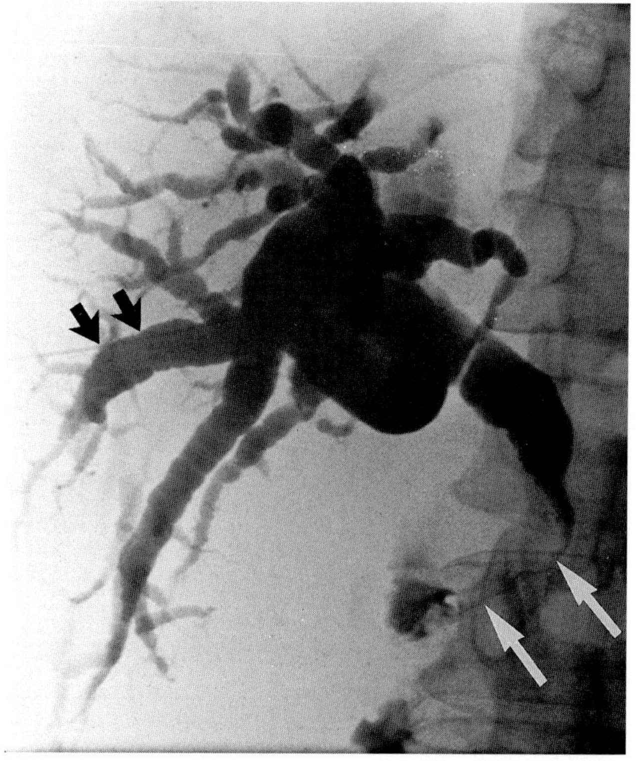

Fig. 10.8 Malignant biliary stricture. PTC demonstrating a markedly dilated intra- and extrahepatic biliary tree. There is an irregular stricture in the lower common bile duct secondary to carcinoma of the pancreas (white arrows). The ideal duct for percutaneous access has been punctured (black arrows).

approach. A combination of specifically designed catheters and hydrophilic guidewires ensures that even the tightest strictures can usually be traversed; if not, a period of external drainage for two to three days usually opens up the stricture to allow the guidewire through. The stricture is then dilated with a balloon catheter prior to stent placement.

Choice of endoprosthesis: plastic or metal?

Plastic endoprostheses require a percutaneous tract of 12F or greater with associated increased morbidity and patient discomfort. The recent introduction of self-expanding metallic endoprostheses means that a smaller percutaneous tract is sufficient and that the stent can often be inserted at one sitting without a period of external drainage. The disadvantage of cost is overcome by a reduced reintervention rate because of the decreased rate of occlusion of metallic stents compared with conventional devices. This factor is important in the treatment of cholangiocarcinoma, which grows more slowly than pancreatic lesions and, with adequate decompression, patients can achieve a 1-year survival of approximately 50%.

Metallic endoprotheses, which are self-expanding, are introduced over a guidewire across the predilated stricture. Once the stent has been released across the stricture a small safety catheter can be left within the stent (Fig. 10.9a) so that a cholangiogram can be performed the following day to check patency of the endoprosthesis prior to removal of the catheter (Fig. 10.9b).

Stent occlusion is usually the result of bile encrustation, tumour ingrowth or overgrowth. The problem of bile encrustation is reduced by the use of metallic stents. Tumour ingrowth is a problem and several companies are working on the development of plastic-covered stents to minimize its occurrence. Tumour growth above or below the endoprosthesis can be reduced by the placement of long stents extending from the intrahepatic radicles to the duodenum just beyond the ampulla of Vater.

The perfect biliary stent would be a removable endoprosthesis that is safe to insert along a narrow tract associated with a low rate of complications, in particular recurrent jaundice, cholangitis and stent occlusion. Metallic stents have gone a long way to solving some of these problems; however, new developments are awaited to further improve the design and reduce the initial cost.

MANAGEMENT OF PROBLEMATIC BILIARY CALCULI

Stones in the common bile duct are found in approximately 10% of patients undergoing cholecystectomy, rising to over 30% in those over 80 years of age. Since the advent of endoscopic sphincterotomy in 1974, the

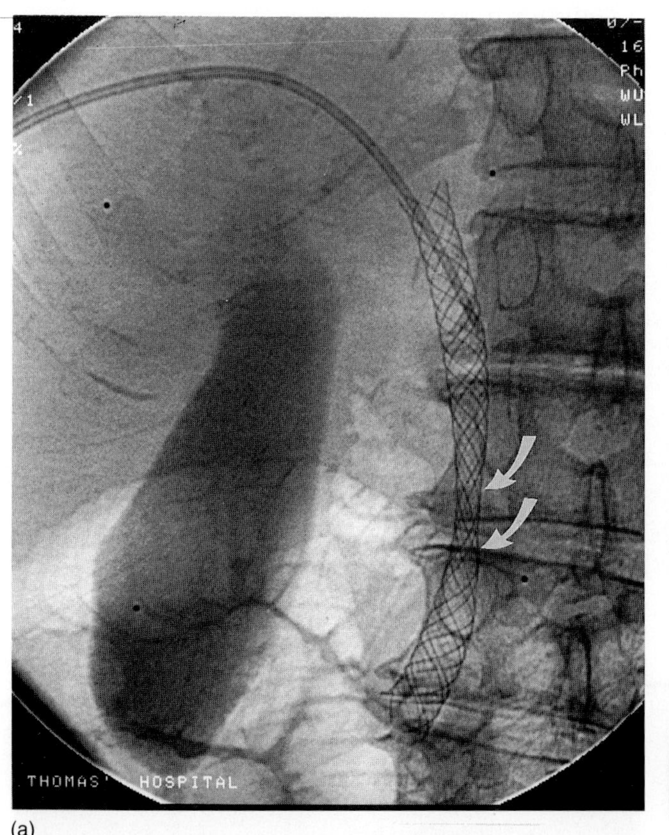

(a)

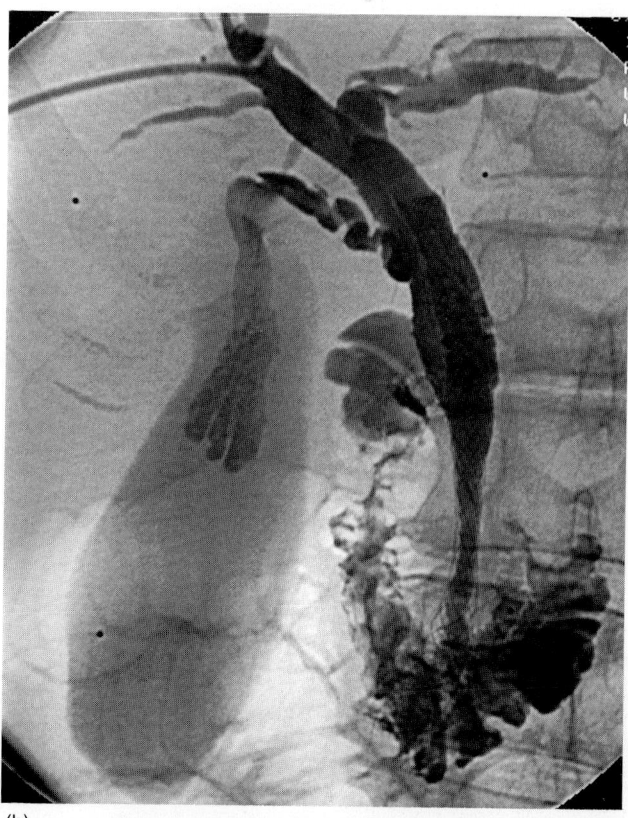

(b)

Fig. 10.9 Malignant biliary stricture. (a) A self-expanding metallic stent has been positioned across a malignant stricture in the lower common bile duct secondary to carcinoma of the head of the pancreas. The narrowing (arrows) of the stent represents the site of the stricture. A safety catheter has been left within the stent. (b) A cholangiogram via the safety catheter 24 hours after stent placement demonstrates free flow into the duodenum with a satisfactory radiological result. The safety catheter can now be withdrawn. (Reproduced with permission from Watkinson A.F. and Adam A. (1996) *Interventional radiology: a practical guide*, published by Radcliffe Medical Press, Oxford)

approach to treating common bile duct calculi has changed fundamentally. The overall success rate of endoscopic sphincterotomy in clearing these stones is 85–90% with a lower morbidity and mortality than surgery. This procedure is, therefore the technique of choice in the majority of cases for removal of common bile duct calculi. An exception is in patients who have a T-tube *in situ*; here, percutaneous removal under fluoroscopic guidance, with a steerable catheter and basket (as popularized by Burhenne who performed this technique on the Shah of Iran in 1979), has a high success rate with very low morbidity. The disadvantage is that the T-tube tract must be left to mature for 5–6 weeks. T-tubes are not usually left in place after laparoscopic cholecystectomy; any retained stones are usually removed postoperatively via an endoscopic sphincterotomy.

Problematical biliary calculi are ductal or intrahepatic stones that are not amenable to treatment with endoscopic sphincterotomy or removal via a T-tube tract using basket techniques. Patients with these stones usually have one of the following:

- **Inaccessible biliary tree**. Because of altered anatomy, secondary to either gastric surgery or the presence of a duodenal diverticulum, it may not be possible to cannulate the ampulla of Vater.
- **Bile duct stricture**. With bile stasis calculi often form proximal to strictures and even with endoscopic papillotomy and dilatation the calculi are often difficult to clear.
- **Large and impacted stones**. Stones >1.5 cm in diameter are often difficult to remove and can become impacted. Intrahepatic stones can be remote from the ampulla and difficult to reach with the basket.

TECHNIQUE OF PERCUTANEOUS BILIARY STONE REMOVAL

Percutaneous cholangiography, as described on page 246, is performed through the right or left intrahepatic bile ducts depending on the location of the stones. If the stones are in the extrahepatic biliary tree then a relatively horizontal approach to the right main duct allows access to the common bile duct. Once drainage has been performed, the tract is allowed to mature for 1–2 days, in order to enable sheath systems of up to 18F to be introduced with minimal discomfort

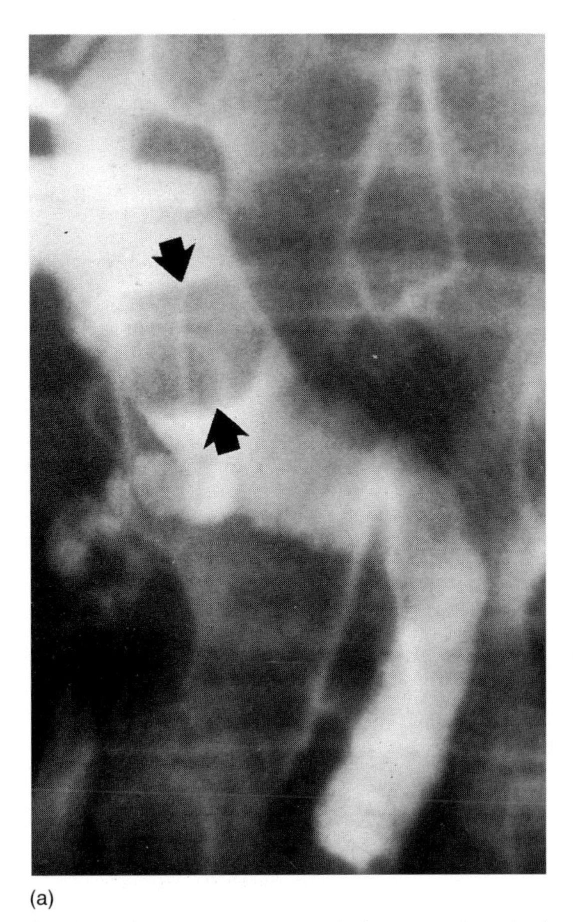

(a)

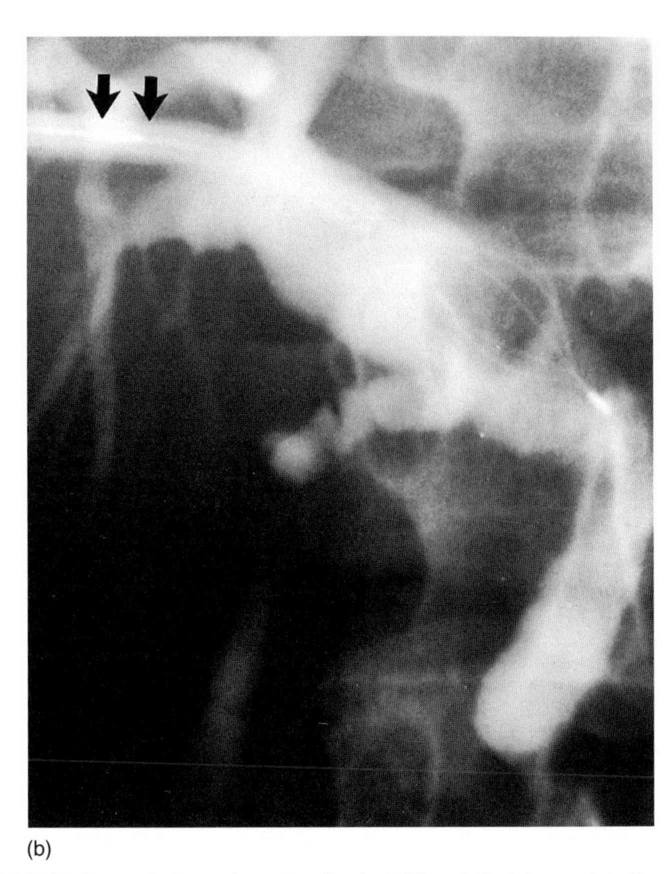

(b)

Fig. 10.10 Percutaneous removal of common hepatic duct calculi. (a) PTC demonstrates a large intraluminal filling defect (arrows) in the common hepatic duct. (b) A basket introduced coaxially (arrows) has captured the calculus; this can now be fragmented and pushed into the duodenum or removed percutaneously.

(Fig. 10.10a,b). With a percutaneous access route, various methods can be used to fragment, flush and dissolve the stones. Direct fragmentation with baskets (Fig. 10.10b) and electrohydraulic lithotripsy are the most commonly used techniques. Chemical dissolution has not been widely adopted and is unlikely to become so, because only cholesterol-containing stones are amenable, dissolution may take a prolonged period and the agents used (methyl *tert*-butyl ether [MTBE] and mono-octanoin) have potentially significant side-effects and complications. Stone fragments are usually removed by antegrade passage through the ampulla although retrograde removal through the larger sheaths is possible. A prior endoscopic or transhepatic sphincterotomy or balloon dilatation of the ampulla is usually required (Fig. 10.11a–c).

An alternative is the combined radiological endoscopic approach. The intial percutaneous puncture is performed as previously desribed and, following access to the biliary tree with a standard catheter-guidewire technique, a guidewire is manipulated into the duodenum (or jejunum if the patient has had a Roux loop formed). An experienced endoscopist can then locate the wire and use this to guide retrograde access to the ampulla of Vater and common bile duct, thus overcoming the problems of abnormal anatomy.

If endoscopic cannulation of the ampulla is possible, but the stones are too large or too many for removal even after sphincterotomy and basket fragmentation, then alternative techniques are necessary. These include chemical dissolution through a nasobiliary tube, extracorporeal shockwave lithotripsy and intracorporeal lithotripsy devices introduced via the endoscope.

INTERVENTIONAL RADIOLOGY OF THE GALLBLADDER

Interventional radiology and surgery of the gallbladder have gone through dramatic changes in recent years and, although the overwhelming success of laparoscopic techniques now means that the radiologist no longer offers alternatives to elective surgery, gallbladder puncture and catheterization techniques remain useful in the management of complicated gallbladder disease.

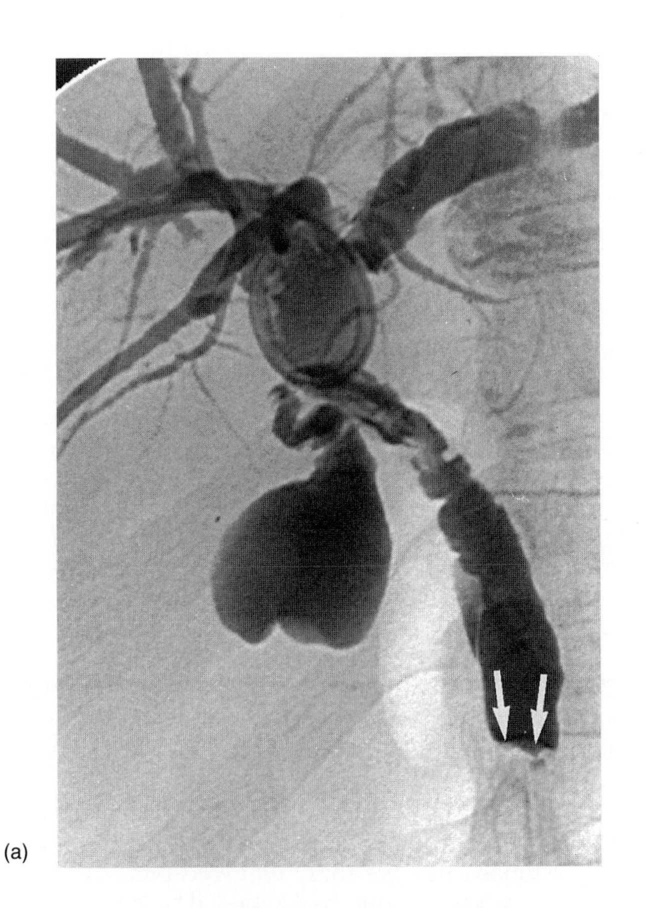

(a)

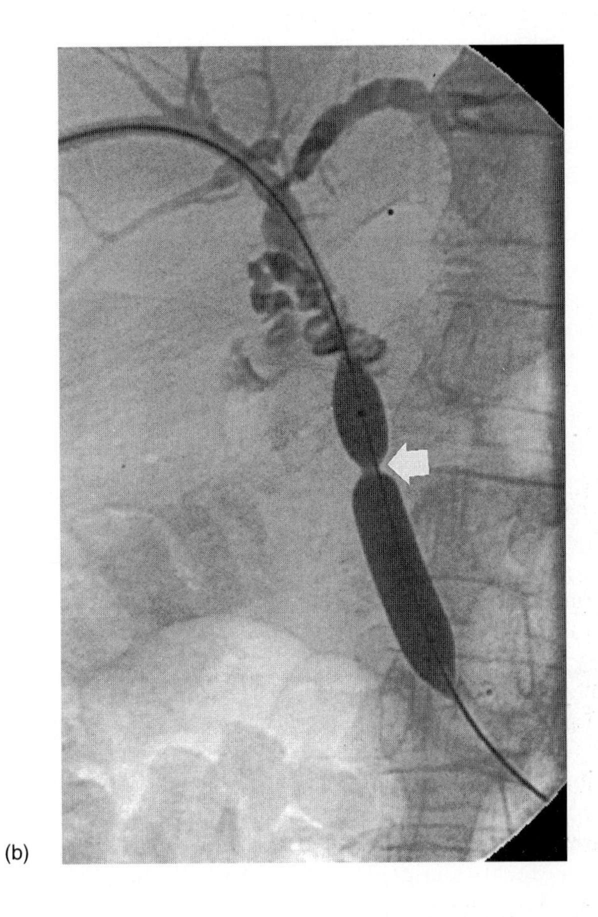

(b)

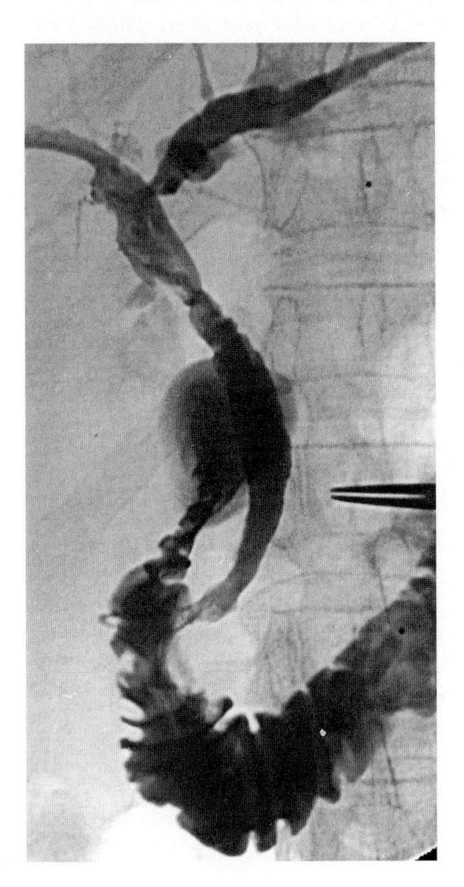

(c)

Fig. 10.11 Percutaneous sphincteroplasty of the ampulla of Vater. (a) PTC demonstrates obstruction of the lower end of the common bile duct, with a curved meniscus (arrows), caused by an impacted common duct calculus. (b) A balloon catheter has been introduced percutaneously and inflated across the ampulla of Vater (arrow) to perform sphincteroplasty. (c) A cholangiogram after sphincteroplasty demonstrates free flow into the duodenum. The calculus has passed spontaneously through the dilated ampulla of Vater. (Reproduced with permission from Watkinson A.F. and Adam A. (1996) *Interventional radiology: a practical guide*, published by Radcliffe Medical Press, Oxford)

FINE NEEDLE ASPIRATION

Fine needle aspiration of the gall bladder is a relatively safe procedure and is usually performed under ultrasound guidance via the transhepatic or transperitoneal approach. The aspirate can be sent for cytology and culture; however, patients are often on intravenous antibiotics and the infective agent can only be determined in approximately 60% of cases. Consequently, the decision to proceed to percutaneous drainage is often made on clinical grounds rather than the bacteriological results.

PERCUTANEOUS CHOLECYSTOSTOMY

The current indications for performing percutaneous cholecystostomy are:

- decompression and drainage in acute cholecystitis and empyema;
- to develop an access tract for stone removal (which may follow the above);
- access for biliary drainage.

Technique when treating acute cholecystitis and empyema

Percutaneous cholecystostomy is usually performed under local analgesia with intravenous sedation. Anaesthetic assistance may, however, be requested as these patients are frequently unfit for major surgery. The traditional approach has been the transhepatic route under ultrasound guidance. The aim is to puncture the bare area of the liver and thus minimize the risk of bile leak into the peritoneal cavity. The incidence of peritonitis via the transperitoneal approach appears to be no different and, therefore, either method is acceptable. The gallbladder can be punctured directly with a sheathed needle or a fine-needle introduction set, the aim being to leave a self-retaining catheter, with a locking loop at the tip, within the gallbladder lumen. The single-stick technique is frequently used in patients with an empyema and profound sepsis, as the gallbladder is usually distended in an immediately subcutaneous position. Recovery in such circumstances can be dramatic and catheter drainage can be performed for 2–3 weeks prior to definitive cholecystectomy. The technique does not preclude laparoscopic cholecystectomy. If the cholecystitis is secondary to malignant obstruction of the biliary tree then long-term drainage can be carried out with repeated catheter exchange although, if possible, internal drainage via an endoprosthesis should be used following recovery from the initial episode.

There is increasing evidence to support performing percutaneous cholecystostomy in patients in intensive therapy units who are septic without traceable cause. Culture of the bile is usually unhelpful in diagnosing bile infection, because these patients are usually recieving a wide range of antibiotics. The ultrasound features of acalculous cholecystitis are thickening of the gallbladder wall and pericholecystic fluid. Sludge, a non-specific finding, is usually present within the bile. Approximately half the patients in this clinico-radiological setting will improve following percutaneous cholecystostomy.

STONE EXTRACTION AND DISSOLUTION

The traditional technique for treatment of gallstones has been open cholecystectomy since Langebuch first performed the operation in 1884. In the 1980s, prior to the introduction of laparoscopic cholecystectomy, there was great interest and development in the fields of lithotripsy and various mechanical devices to crush and fragment the stones if a percutaneous tract existed. Nowadays, the combination of laparoscopic surgery and endoscopic sphincterotomy manages the vast majority of gallbladder and common duct calculi, but there is still a small group of patients who require alternative methods of treatment for a variety of reasons.

Patients who have had percutaneous cholecystostomy performed for acute cholecystitis secondary to gallstones can have these removed percutaneously when the acute episode has settled. The tract is left to mature for 4–6 weeks and then dilated up to 12–14F gauge. Using a variety of baskets or forceps the stones can then be extracted. Alternatively rotary lithotrite devices can be introduced to emulsify the stones. For very large or impacted stones it may be neccessary to deal with these stones using a rigid nephroscope via the original tract dilated to 28–30F under general anaesthesia.

If a percutaneous catheter is in the gallbladder lumen, and the gallstones consist predominantly of cholesterol, they can be successfully dissolved using methyl *tert*-butyl ether or mono-octanoin via manual instillation. This technique has proved to be unpopular due to the toxicity of the dissolution agents, the time involved to carry out the procedure and the high stone recurrence rate as residual calcium carbonate fragments act as future nidi for gallstone formation. Extracorporeal shockwave lithotripsy is still appropriate in patients who decide they do not want surgery, either laparoscopic or open. Modern units can usually fragment most gallstones up to 3 cm although more than one session may be required. This technique is carried out under local anaesthesia on an out-patient basis and the patient is usually started on oral urso-deoxycholic acid as a dissolution agent. If the gallbladder is functioning and the cystic duct is patent (assessed on ultrasound pre- and post-fatty meal) clearance of stones will be achieved in greater than 70% of cases at 1 year. However if the gallbladder is left *in situ* there is a significant risk of stone recurrence.

If there is no contraindication to surgery, and the patient gives informed consent, the best treatment for symptomatic gallstones is laparoscopic cholecystectomy by a surgeon experienced in the technique.

BILIARY DRAINAGE

In the acute setting in a jaundiced, septic patient with a distended gallbladder a rapid percutaneous cholecystostomy under ultrasound guidance (which can be performed at the bedside) can dramatically improve the patients condition. More formal assessment of the biliary tree with subsequent intervention can be delayed until more clinically appropriate.

PERCUTANEOUS INTRA-ABDOMINAL BIOPSY AND ABSCESS DRAINAGE

IMAGE-GUIDED BIOPSY

Percutaneous biopsy can provide information about the presence, nature and extent of intra-abdominal disease and almost any radiologically detected abnormality is technically amenable to needle biopsy or aspiration.

Patients with a prothrombin time >4–5 s above control or a platelet count <80 000/ml should have these parameters corrected if possible prior to biopsy. Patients who have severe, uncorrectable coagulopathies and require liver biopsy should be considered for a percutaneous biopsy with plugging of the tract or biopsy via the transvenous route (transjugular or transfemoral). If there is gross ascites this should be drained prior to biopsy.

Antibiotic prophylaxis should be considered in immunocompromised patients or if there is a high probability of traversing a contaminated field (e.g. transcolonic biopsy). All patients should have an intravenous line inserted prior to the procedure in case analgesia or resuscitation is required. Most percutaneous biopsies can be performed on an outpatient basis. Patients should be observed for at least 2 hours afterwards and if vital signs remain stable they can be discharged.

Choice of needle

The choice of needle type and size often depends on personal preference and the suspected underlying pathology. In patients with suspected malignancy, immediate cytological analysis of a cellular aspirate obtained through a fine needle (19 gauge or smaller) is often sufficient to make the diagnosis. If after two or three passes a diagnostic specimen has not been obtained a core biopsy is taken with an 18-gauge cutting needle (manual or spring-loaded) and sent for histological examination. In patients with benign parenchymal disease affecting the liver or kidney, where architectural information is important, an 18-gauge core biopsy with a cutting needle is usually required. If larger needles are used the complication rate appears to increase.

Choice of imaging modality

Generally the shortest route from the skin to the lesion is chosen, providing no vital structures (e.g. the spleen or lung) are interposed. The size and location of the lesion combined with operator preference determine the optimum imaging modality. When the target is visible on conventional radiography, fluoroscopy is suitable for biopsy guidance. In the abdomen, contrast examinations are often needed (e.g. abnormal lymph node seen on lymphangiography or bile duct stricture with an indwelling biliary stent [Fig. 10.12]).

Most biopsies, however, are performed using CT or ultrasound guidance. Targets affected by respiratory motion are often biopsied more readily using ultrasound because real time imaging can be used. Similarly, because of the multiple scan planes possible with ultrasound, angled approaches (e.g. craniocaudal angulation) are easier. Other advantages include low cost, rapid scan time and no radiation dose. CT should be used for small lesions, especially in areas which cannot be imaged satisfactorily with ultrasound, such

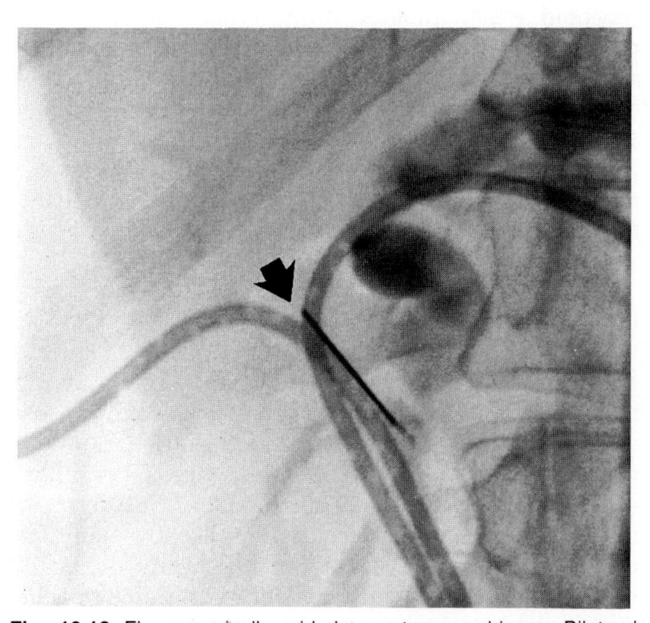

Fig. 10.12 Fluoroscopically-guided percutaneous biopsy. Bilateral indwelling biliary internal-external drainage catheters have been positioned across a stricture at the confluence of the right and left main hepatic ducts (arrow). A 21-gauge needle has been introduced percutaneously, under fluoroscopic guidance, to biopsy the hilar lesion.

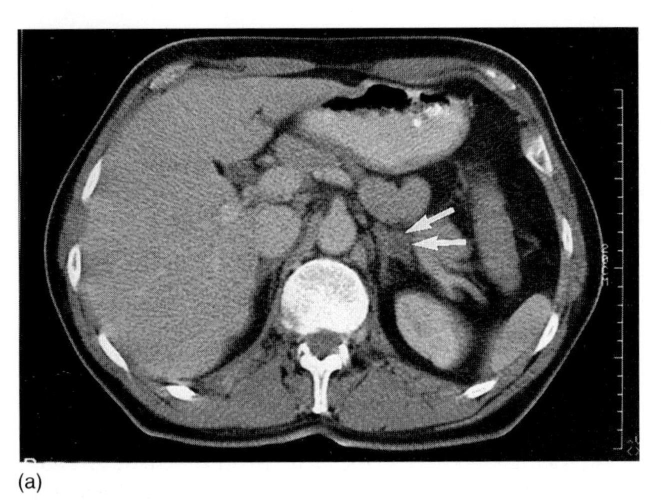
(a)

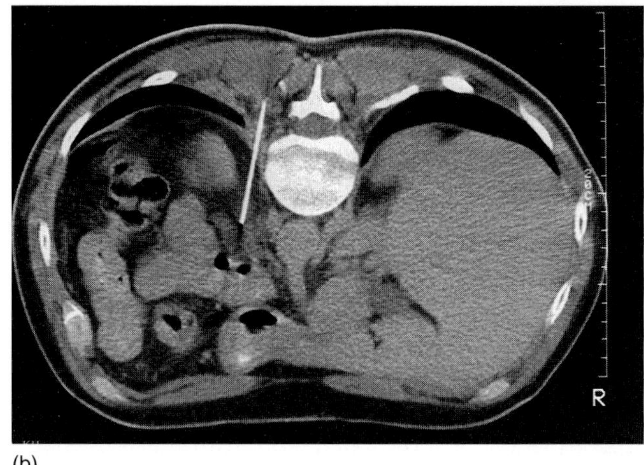

(b)

Fig. 10.13 CT-guided biopsy. (a) A CT scan at the level of the mid-abdomen demonstrating a 2 cm mass on the lateral limb of the left adrenal gland (arrows). (b) A prone CT scan in the same patient demonstrating a needle with its tip in the adrenal lesion. Note how CT guidance has enabled puncture of the lung to be avoided.

as masses in the retroperitoneum (Fig. 10.13a, b) or bone. CT is also useful for biopsying partially necrotic lesions, when intravenous contrast enhancement allows targeting of the viable part of the tumour.

Results and complication

Overall accuracy rates of most percutaneous abdominal biopsies exceed 80%. False-negative biopsies may be due to an off-target biopsy or sampling of the necrotic or fibrous portion of a tumour (e.g. pancreatic carcinoma) or the reactive hyperplasia accompanying many tumours. Thus, a negative biopsy should be repeated when there is strong clinical suspicion of malignancy. Complication rates from percutaneous abdominal biopsy are extremely low (<1.5%), especially when fine gauge needles are used (smaller than 19 gauge). If peripheral liver lesions are biopsied it is important to traverse normal parenchyma first as the normal tissue will help to tamponade any haemorrhage.

IMAGE-GUIDED DRAINAGE

Percutaneous drainage has replaced surgery as the treatment of choice for most intra-abdominal abscesses and collections. Almost any intra-abdominal fluid collection demonstrated by either CT or ultrasound may be considered for drainage. This not only includes simple, unilocular fluid collections but also more complicated collections such as necrotic tumour, haematomas and phlegmonous masses. Percutaneous drainage may not always totally eradicate these complex collections; however, the procedure allows improvement in the patient's general state of health so that definitive surgical drainage and debridement can be performed.

There are few contraindications to percutaneous drainage and most are relative. Any clotting abnormality should be corrected and the access route should avoid bowel or lung. A retroperitoneal, as opposed to a transperitoneal, approach is preferable to reduce the risk of intraperitoneal spillage of infected material. Except for simple cysts and loculated ascites, an intravenous line is mandatory and patients not already receiving antibiotics should be given broad-spectrum cover before and after percutaneous drainage.

Choice of imaging modality

The image guidance techniques are the same as for percutaneous biopsy. Percutaneous drainage of intra-abdominal collections is most often performed using ultrasound guidance; however, CT either alone or with fluoroscopy can also be used. Ultrasound is particularly useful in the drainage of superficial collections and those requiring an angled approach (e.g. subphrenic, high hepatic and splenic abscesses). Deep abdominal and pelvic collections are poorly visualized by ultrasound, and CT guidance is preferred. However, CT-guided drainage is not real time and the guidewire, tract dilators and drainage catheter are inserted by feel alone. Therefore, extra care is required to avoid misplacement of the catheter, and combination with fluoroscopy can be helpful in difficult cases.

Technique

The CT and ultrasound appearances of intra-abdominal fluid collections cannot reliably differentiate between abscess, sterile collections and organizing haematomas. When the decision to drain a collection depends on its nature or the presence of infection, diagnostic fine needle aspiration may be performed before drainage (Fig. 10.14). If the fluid is not obviously purulent, immediate microscopy should be performed. Biochemical analysis may also help to characterize the fluid (e.g. identification of a bile leak after a cholecystectomy or injury to the pancreas after splenectomy).

Subsequent catheter insertion uses the Seldinger guidewire exchange technique or a single-step trocar drainage catheter system, depending on personal preference. The trocar technique is more appropriate for large, superficial collections when there is little risk of misdirection. The pigtail catheter should end up in a coiled position within in the abscess cavity. Multiple adjacent abscess cavities may require several drainage catheters for adequate treatment. The choice of catheter depends on the viscosity of the fluid. The catheter should be large enough for steady drainage and usually 8–10F is adequate for bilomas and loculated ascites. If the material aspirated is thick or particulate, larger bore catheters, 12–18F in diameter, are required. The cavity should be evacuated as completely as possible; however, aspiration should be stopped if the patient experiences sudden pain or the aspirate becomes bloody. Sudden decompression of large collections may be extremely uncomfortable and can precipitate haemorrhage from the abscess wall. Gentle irrigation with saline may help to decrease the viscocity of the contents and encourage drainage.

Good care following catheter placement is essential. Regular saline irrigation (10–20 ml tds) is important to maintain patency during the postdrainage days. The patient's condition usually improves noticeably within 24–48 hours after successful drainage. Failure to improve usually means drainage is inadequate, the collection is loculated or the catheter side-holes are incorrectly positioned. Repositioning of the catheter may be required. Continued drainage of 50 ml/day or more several days after the procedure often suggests a fistulous communication (e.g. with bowel, bile duct or pancreas), which can be confirmed by a contrast study. As long as the normal internal flow is unobstructed, these fistulae will close although drainage may continue for four to six weeks or more. The catheter should not be removed until drainage has ceased and ultrasound or CT and a contrast study through the catheter confirm that the cavity has been obliterated.

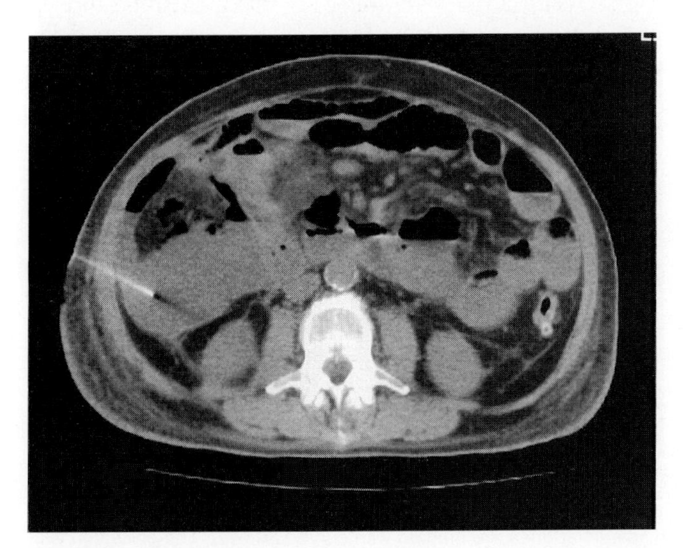

Fig. 10.14 CT-guided aspiration. A needle is seen within a right paracolic collection for diagnostic aspiration.

Results and complications

With good technique and meticulous catheter care the overall success rate should be approximately 80% and approach 100% for unilocular collections. Success rates are lower for patients with complex collections (multiloculations, inflammatory masses and enteric or biliary fistula). The major complications include sepsis, haemorrhage and injury to adjacent structures. Minor complications include skin infection, catheter blockage and displacement. Careful planning of the approach to the collection should minimize the risk of inadvertent puncture of bowel, vascular structures and pleura.

PANCREATIC COLLECTIONS

The radiological management of pancreatic collections deserves special mention and depends on the type.

Pseudocysts

Pseudocysts are walled-off collections of pancreatic secretions within or adjacent to the pancreas. They most commonly occur in the lesser sac region and usually form 4–6 weeks after acute pancreatitis. Although pseudocysts frequently resolve spontaneously, those >5 cm in diameter often require intervention. Endoscopic retrograde pancreatography may be useful prior to drainage to demonstrate any communication with the duct system. Drainage in patients with pseudocysts with persisting communication with the duct system is less successful and usually takes longer. In these cases a transgastric approach is advised (see below). An uninfected pseudocyst with no communication to the duct system should be drained electively when the wall has become well-defined and acute pancreatitic inflammation has subsided (usually at least 4 weeks after the acute episode). Earlier drainage may be contemplated if the patient's symptoms (abdominal pain and upper gastrointestinal obstruction) are worsening or the pseudocyst is enlarging. Infected pseudocysts should be drained more urgently. The reported success rate of percutaneous pseudocyst drainage ranges between 60–90%.

Technique A transgastric approach is attempted after distending the stomach with air. Puncture of the cyst is through the anterior abdominal wall and the anterior and posterior walls of the stomach. The procedure is best performed under CT guidance, although fluoroscopy or ultrasound may be used. Drainage via a direct percutaneous approach is acceptable, if the transgastric route is not feasible, but there is at least a theoretical risk of development of a persistent cutaneous pancreatic fistula.

The catheter is removed after CT once catheter contrast medium injection has confirmed complete resolution of the collection with no residual loculated areas, and drainage volumes have decreased to below 10 ml/day. Persistent drainage suggests communication with a pancreatic duct and in this case the catheter should be left in place until an established tract has formed between the cyst and the stomach. Alternatively a double pigtail stent may be used to establish communication between the pseudocyst and stomach to ensure internal drainage. The stent may be removed endoscopically later.

Pancreatic phlegmon, abscess and necrosis

The success rate of percutaneous drainage of pancreatic phlegmon, abscesses and necrosis is less successful than for other intra-abdominal abscesses. Contrast enhanced CT should be performed (Fig. 10.15a). If a definite fluid collection is identified, with an attenuation value higher than simple fluid and consistent with pus, then percutaneous drainage, as previously described, should be performed with large bore catheters (Fig. 10.15b). Even if the abscess does not resolve this can serve as an interim measure to improve the condition of a critically ill patient before surgical debridement and drainage. However, if the CT scan reveals an enlarged, oedematous pancreas with areas of non-perfusion consistent with necrosis but no identifiable collection, percutaneous drainage will probably be of no value and intervention, when required, should be primarily surgical.

LIVER BIOPSY IN PATIENTS WITH ABNORMAL COAGULATION

Percutaneous liver biopsy is an established procedure with a very low morbidity and mortality in patients with normal coagulation. Image-guidance with ultrasound or CT is advised, even in the presence of diffuse disease, as there is a risk of pneumothorax, puncture of the bowel and damage to large vascular structures within the liver parenchyma. In many patients with diffuse liver disease, such as cirrhosis or widespread malignant infiltration, there are abnormalities of blood coagulation which significantly increase the risk of bleeding after a biopsy. This can be minimized by performing percutaneous biopsy with subsequent plugging of the tract or the use of a transvenous approach via the femoral or jugular veins.

In patients with abnormal clotting (prothrombin time 4–5 s greater than control or a platelet count < 80 000/ml) every effort should be made to correct the abnormality with vitamin K, fresh frozen plasma or platelet transfusions. If the clotting abnormalities cannot be corrected then the biopsy technique must be modified.

In patients with a moderate coagulopathy with an INR (International Normalized Ratio) of 1.4–2.0, or a platelet count of 50 000–80 000/ml, plugging of a percutaneous tract is a safe procedure with good results and minimal complications. However, in

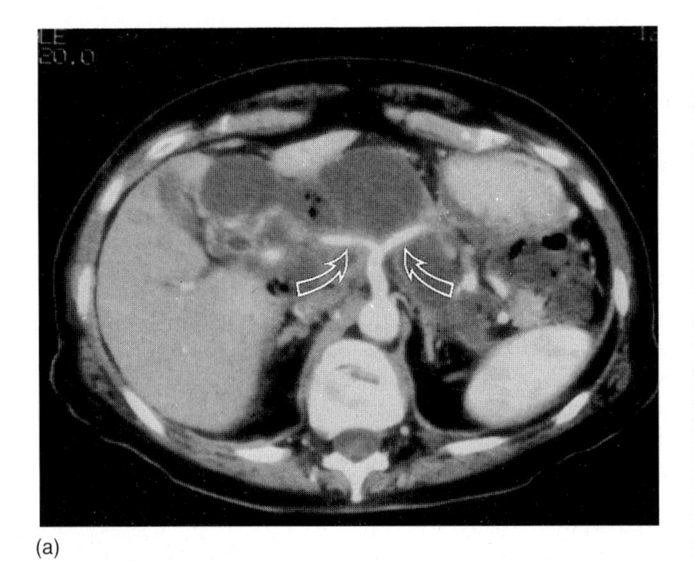

(a)

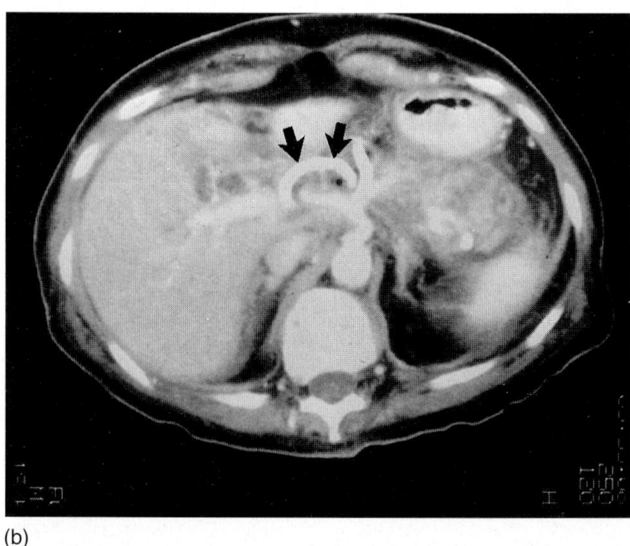

(b)

Fig. 10.15 Percutaneous pancreatic abscess drainage. (a) Contrast-enhanced CT scan demonstrating a large pancreatic collection of relatively low attenuation, surrounding the origin of the coeliac axis (the hepatic and splenic arteries are marked with curved arrows). The collection is of higher attenuation than water and is consistent with pus. (b) A 12F catheter has been inserted into the collection and after 72 hours a repeat CT scan shows considerable resolution. The catheter is seen coiled within the pancreatic bed (arrows).

patients with an INR >2.0 or a platelet count of <50 000 the percutaneous approach is not advised as, although tract plugging can occlude the bleeding site in the liver, small subcutaneous or subcapsular veins cannot be occluded and can cause catastrophic haemorrhage. A transvenous approach is advised in patients with an INR >2.0 or a platelet count <50 000 which will not correct with vitamin K, fresh frozen plasma or platelet transfusions).

PLUGGED LIVER BIOPSY

There are various versions of this technique but the basic principle is biopsy through a sheath followed by embolization of the tract with steel coils or particulate material. The appropriate needle is usually of the 'Tru-cut' type which consistently produces satisfactory specimens.

Technique

An intravenous line is established and the patient given platelets or coagulation factors as required. The biopsy is performed under fluoroscopic guidance. Preliminary screening helps to identify the position of the liver and any adjacent bowel gas. The needle is introduced inside a covering sheath in the mid-axillary line parallel to the table top. The biopsy is taken and the needle withdrawn. Contrast medium is injected to demonstrate the point of communication between the tract and the vessel responsible for the bleeding, usually a hepatic or portal vein branch. The embolic material is deposited within the tract, adjacent to the bleeding vessel. The sheath is then withdrawn and more embolic material deposited within the tract (Fig. 10.16). Particular care is taken to place a coil close to the liver capsule to prevent extracapsular leakage.

Various modifications of this technique have been described using differing needles and embolic agents, including gelfoam and other haemostatic agents, depending on personal preference. The use of a covering plastic sheath, rather than direct deposition of embolic material through the needle cannula minimizes damage to the liver capsule during respiratory movement of the liver. We prefer steel coils because other haemostatic agents are not suitable for stopping massive bleeding, as may occur from a transected artery or large portal vein radicle. In addition the embolic fragments may be swept out of the tract by the force of blood flow.

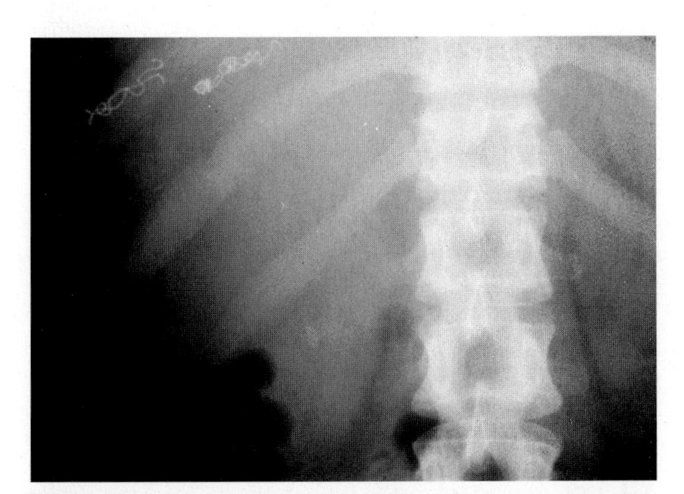

Fig. 10.16 Percutaneous liver biopsy with embolization of the tract. Steel coils can be seen in the right upper quadrant following embolization of the biopsy track. (Reproduced with permission from Watkinson A.F. and Adam A. in *Seminars in Interventional Radiology* 1994, **11**, (3) 254–266, published by Thieme Medical Publishers, NY)

TRANSJUGULAR LIVER BIOPSY

This form of biopsy is performed within the liver parenchyma via the hepatic veins thus avoiding external bleeding. The procedure is performed under fluoroscopic guidance with an intravenous line in place and a pulse oximeter monitoring oxygen saturation. In the supine position the internal jugular vein is punctured and a sheath positioned in the right or middle hepatic vein. The biopsy needle is then advanced until it lies at the tip of the sheath (Fig. 10.17) and then advanced into the liver substance whilst continuous suction with a syringe is maintained.

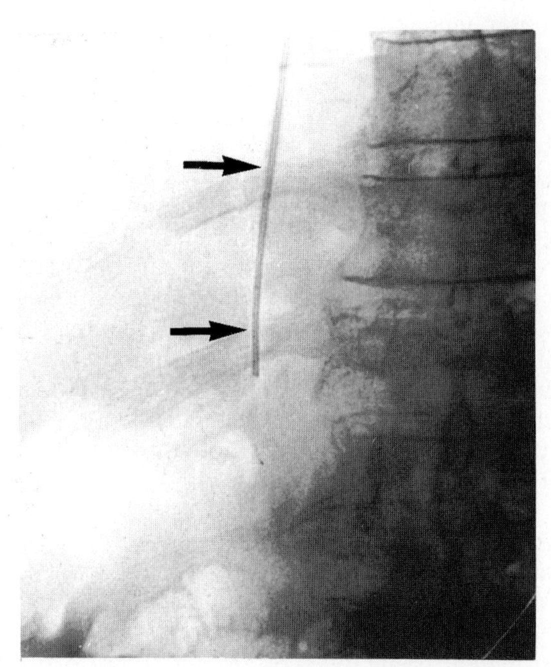

Fig. 10.17 Transjugular liver biopsy. A biopsy needle is seen positioned in the middle hepatic vein (arrows). This can now be advanced into the liver parenchyma to aquire a biopsy specimen.

Complications

The main complication is perforation of the liver capsule leading to intraperitoneal bleeding. Capsular perforation is seen in approximately 3.9% of patients, but usually there are no clinical sequelae, significant intraperitoneal haemorrhage occurring in only 0.35% of patients. The mortality rate is approximately 0.13%. Other complications mostly relate to the puncture site and access route. These include haematoma, puncture of the carotid artery, transient hoarseness, Horner's syndrome, cardiac arrhythmias, pneumothorax and interference with indwelling central lines. In addition patients often find the procedure frightening due to the proximity of such a large needle to the face.

Results

It is possible to pass the needle into the liver in 90% of cases, but the success rate is lower in patients with small livers or when the diaphragm has been elevated by ascites. In 15–20% of cases the specimen is uninterpretable, because usually the specimen is too small or too fragmented to allow accurate pathological diagnosis. Probably the most important factor in the success of transjugular liver biopsy is the presence of a highly trained pathologist able to make an accurate diagnosis from a relatively minute particle of tissue.

The recent introduction of a core biopsy needle is likely to improve these results and make the transjugular route the transvenous approach of choice.

TRANSFEMORAL LIVER BIOPSY

A transfemoral approach is more familiar to most angiographers and also overcomes many of the local complications described for the transjugular approach.

Technique

As for the transjugular approach the procedure is performed under fluoroscopic guidance with intravenous access and pulse oximeter assessment of the oxygen saturation. The femoral vein is punctured and the right or middle hepatic vein is cannulated by means of a catheter guidewire technique. A specially designed curved sheath is then introduced such that the tip lies within the cannulated hepatic vein and biopsy forceps are introduced (Fig. 10.18) to obtain the sample. An effective 'Tru-cut' type needle that will traverse corners and obtain an adequate core sample would be the ideal solution; such needles are currently being evaluated.

Results and complications

A biopsy specimen sufficient to give an accurate histological diagnosis is obtained in approximately 90% of cases. Technical failures tend to be associated with small atrophic livers or are due to acute angulation of the hepatic veins and inferior vena cava, or hard, cirrhotic livers which make it difficult to obtain sufficient material. The technical success in such cases increases with experience.

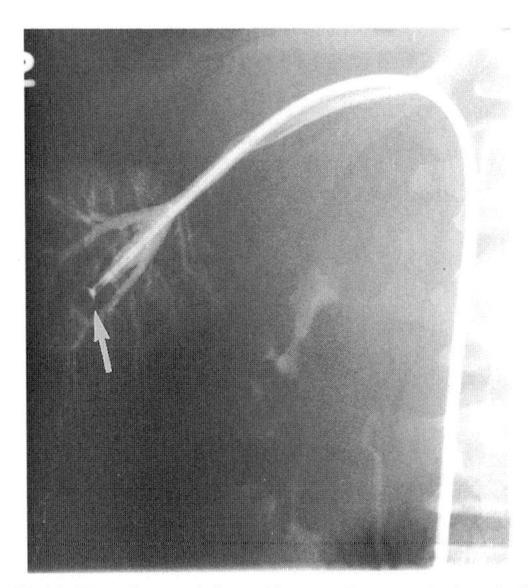

Fig. 10.18 Transfemoral liver biopsy. A curved sheath has been positioned in the hepatic venous system. Crocodile biopsy forceps have been introduced (arrow) to aquire biopsy specimens.

The major complication is perforation of the liver capsule. When perforation is demonstrated on a postbiopsy venogram the tract should be embolized with steel coils. This problem can be minimized by the use of lateral screening to ensure that the biopsy forceps remain within the liver parenchyma well away from the liver capsule.

EMBOLIZATION OF THE LIVER, PANCREAS AND GASTROINTESTINAL TRACT

Embolization or, more precisely, transcatheter vascular occlusion therapy of visceral structures makes a significant contribution to the treatment of abdominal inflammatory disease, blunt or iatrogenic abdominal trauma and both benign and malignant tumours. It may have a curative role for a variety of conditions such as intractable bleeding or vascular malformations or may have a palliative role in the alleviation of symptoms caused by malignant disease.

Before visceral artery intervention it is important to perform coeliac and superior mesenteric arteriography to identify the abnormality and to demonstrate any variants of vascular anatomy. Some lesions need to be treated by superselective catheterization with the catheter tip as peripheral as possible; others should be treated more centrally.

No single embolic material is suitable for all purposes and in each clinical situation certain substances are more appropriate than others (as discussed in Chapter 23, p. 537).

LIVER

Embolization is indicated in a variety of benign and malignant conditions. Pre-existing occlusion of the portal vein is a contraindication to embolization of the hepatic artery unless it is performed at a subsegmental level to avoid major parenchymal loss. Sepsis and decreased liver function from any cause are relative contraindications.

Indications

Benign disease In general, haemorrhage from blunt abdominal trauma is managed either conservatively or surgically in the first instance. The main indication for embolization is the identification of a circumscribed intrahepatic vascular lesion:

- a pseudoaneurysm, not accessible to surgery and causing significant blood loss;
- haemorrhage following a liver biopsy, when the bleeding site is usually focal;
- the relatively rare arteriovenous malformation which causes pain or has led to right heart failure;
- on occasion, benign liver tumours such as ruptured adenomas that may cause life-threatening haemorrhage, or giant haemangiomas to reduce the volume of the lesion and the risk of haemorrhage.

Malignant disease Unresectable liver tumours, especially hepatocellular carcinoma, represent the

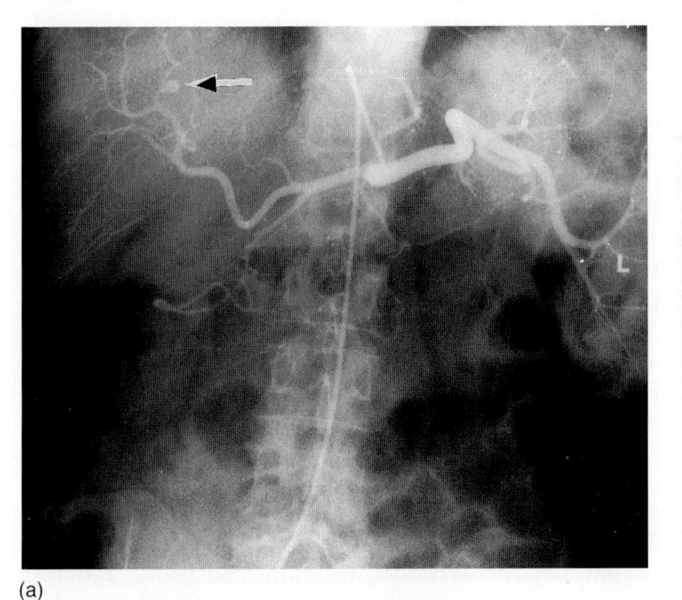

(a)

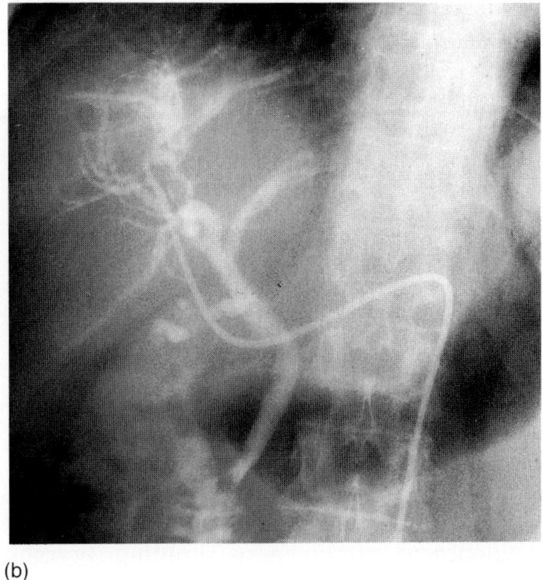

(b)

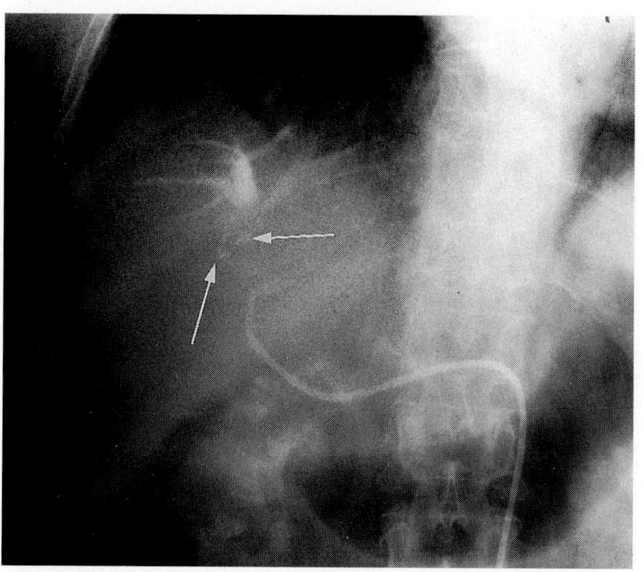

(c)

Fig. 10.19 Embolization of hepatic artery–bile duct fistula following percutaneous biopsy. (a) A coeliac axis arteriogram demonstrates a focal bleeding site in the right lobe of the liver (arrow). (b) The catheter has been advanced selectively within the right hepatic artery. A delayed phase arteriogram demonstrates opacification of the intra- and extrahepatic biliary tree and flow into the duodenum. (c) Selective embolization of the arteriobiliary fistula with a steel coil (arrows) has effectively sealed the leak.

most frequent indication for liver embolization. The procedure is usually performed for palliation of abdominal pain and ascites; however, in some patients with unresectable tumours in the liver, chemoembolization may prolong life expectancy.

The effectiveness of therapeutic embolization depends partly on the histological characteristics of the tumour. Colorectal primary neoplasms are the most frequent source of liver metastases; such deposits usually cause no symptoms and therapeutic embolization is unnecessary in most patients. Hypervascular metastases from malignant endocrine pancreatic or other intestinal tumours (apudomas) may produce clinical symptoms early in the course of the disease. For example, carcinoid syndrome is characterized by episodes of flushing, vomiting and diarrhoea. In addition hypervascular liver metastases tend to be more painful than colorectal metastases and embolization may provide useful palliation.

Technique

Pseudoaneurysms should be treated as selectively as possible; steel microcoils are preferred with a microembolization catheter introduced coaxially and advanced to the site of the pseudoaneurysm, ideally within the neck of the lesion. If this is not possible then the coil should be positioned in the feeding vessel as close to the lesion as possible. The same technique is used to occlude a focal bleeding site following trauma or percutaneous liver biopsy (Fig. 10.19a–c). If the source of bleeding or a pseudoaneurysm can be reached subselectively then the success rate is near 100% and the complication rate is very low.

Embolization of benign liver tumours also requires a subsegmental approach and a coaxial catheter technique. In giant haemangioma or bleeding adenoma without evidence of arteriovenous shunting, peripheral embolization with non-resorbable particulate matter is most appropriate. In arteriovenous malformations a different approach is neccessary: whilst embolization at a subsegmental level is still required, special attention must be paid to arteriovenous shunts. The safest and quickest method is to deploy coils in the feeder artery because particulate matter may reach the pulmonary circulation via arteriovenous shunts.

Focal malignant lesions (Fig. 10.20a), fed by distinct subsegmental arteries, may be treated using selective chemoperfusion with *cis*-platinum, often combined with lipiodol as a CT contrast agent, followed by occlusion of the feeding artery with particulate matter. Within a period of 24–72 hours a CT scan will establish the extent of tumour embolization, which is reflected in the lipiodol distribution around the tumour (Fig. 10.20b). A CT examination at 1 month demonstrates the effectiveness of the embolization and if unsatisfactory the procedure can be repeated. Primary occlusion of the hepatic artery should be avoided in order to maintain access for further embolization procedures. Various percutaneous techniques, such as injection of alcohol or laser photocoagulation under ultrasound guidance, are also being used in an attempt to reduce tumour volume, treat symptoms and improve survival. However, it remains to be seen which combination will achieve these aims most effectively.

In patients with metastatic deposits the approach is slightly different. The metastases most suitable for embolization are hypervascular lesions such as those arising from neuroendocrine tumours or renal carcinoma. The hypervascularity of the deposit is used to flow-direct the embolization material which makes subsegmental positioning of the catheter unnecessary. The tip of the catheter can be placed in either the right or left hepatic arteries and non-resorbable material

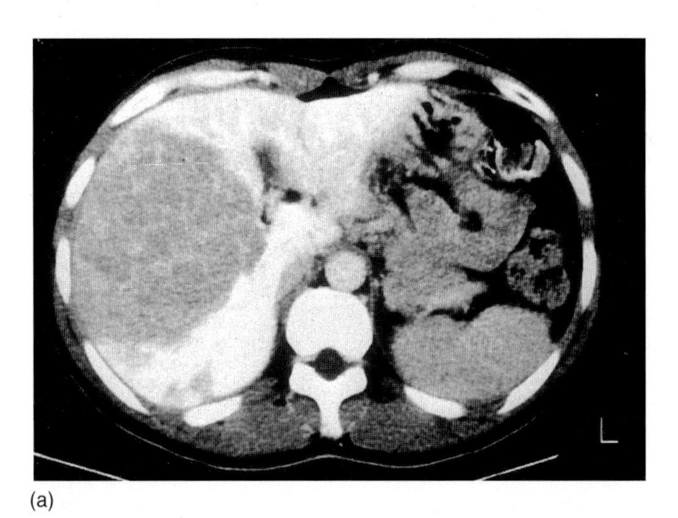

(a)

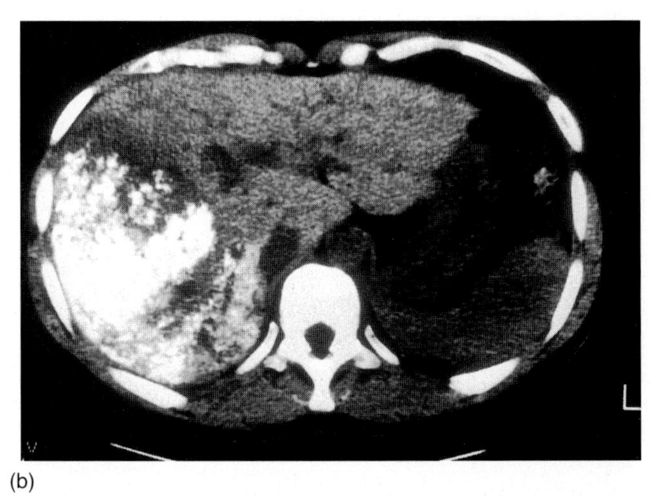

(b)

Fig. 10.20 Chemo-embolization of hepatocellular carcinoma. (a) A CT arterioportogram (CTAP) following selective catheterization of the superior mesenteric artery. This demonstrates a large non-enhancing lesion in the right lobe of the liver, with several small satellite nodules, consistent with hepatocellular carcinoma. (b) A delayed CT scan at 72 hours after selective chemoperfusion with *cis*-platinum and lipiodol followed by particulate embolization of the feeding artery.

infused until peripheral stasis appears. Embolization tends to be effective in relieving severe clinical symptoms and improving survival in patients with hypervascular endocrine tumours. In patients with colorectal carcinoma the procedure usually results in relief of symptoms but does not prolong survival in most cases.

Complications

The most common complication is vascular damage caused by catheter introduction, which may cause severe vasospasm, intimal tears or dissection. The incidence of this type of complication has decreased since the introduction of coaxial catheters. Reflux and inadvertent transport of embolic material to inappropriate areas is a dangerous complication which may occur with any embolic substance. When coils lodge elsewhere in the liver there are usually no serious clinical sequelae because of the presence of a good collateral supply in most instances. When liquid embolization substances are used, the danger from reflux is much more significant, particularly when the reflux occurs into the cystic and gastroduodenal arteries. Therefore, whenever substances are injected that are toxic to mucosa, the catheter tip must be well beyond the origins of these arterial branches.

PANCREAS

In general, the indications for embolization of the pancreas are less frequent and less well defined than those for liver embolization. Also the multiple arterial supply of the pancreas may reduce the effectiveness of therapeutic embolization.

Embolization in benign disease is usually employed in the control of haemorrhage from pseudoaneurysms caused by chronic pancreatitis. The technical success rate of embolization of pseudoaneurysms approaches 100% but the clinical success depends on the initial condition of the patient. Patients may die when the time gap between the onset of symptoms and treatment is too long and multiorgan failure develops; 30-day mortality often approaches 20%.

Embolotherapy has no role in the palliation of the commonest forms of carcinoma, but in recurrent hypervascular tumours, such as malignant apudomas (carcinoid tumours, gastrinomas), superselective embolization may have a role in the management of intractable pain or other severe tumour-related symptoms. The success rate in the embolization of recurrent endocrine tumours is high, with clinical regression of the tumour being observed in most cases.

Technique and complications

Most false aneurysms have a number of feeding vessels and the technique is aimed at direct occlusion of the aneurysm with coaxial superselective catheters and microcoils. If the false aneurysm cannot be reached, all feeding vessels should be occluded with coils. In recurrent pancreatic apudomas it is best to use particulate material in order to preserve access for repeat embolization.

When steel coils in the pancreas are being used, complications are uncommon because of the multiple arterial supply. An exception is misdirection of the coils down the main trunk of the superior mesenteric artery with subsequent bowel necrosis. Particulate matter may backflow after overembolization.

SPLEEN

Elucidation of the role of the spleen in the immune response has increased the interest in splenic salvage for patients who have suffered blunt abdominal trauma. The outcome of conservative treatment in patients who have splenic damage demonstrated on CT is poor, approximately 70% having recurrent or persistent bleeding requiring delayed laparotomy. However, in certain cases timely therapeutic embolization of the splenic artery can obviate the need for splenectomy.

Haemodynamically unstable patients who have suffered blunt abdominal trauma should have diagnostic peritoneal lavage and if this is positive the patient should undergo exploratory laparotomy. If the patient is haemodynamically stable but diagnostic peritoneal lavage is positive, CT should be performed. If damage to the spleen is seen, the patient should be further evaluated with arteriography and, if extravasation of contrast material is seen, embolization of the proximal splenic artery can be carried out with steel coils; these can be delivered by coaxial catheters in the proximal splenic artery. Embolization of specific bleeding intrasplenic arteries prior to main splenic artery occlusion should only be attempted when it is safe and technically possible to advance the catheter into the spleen. Experience is currently limited. As interest increases, the technique may become more widely adopted. In haemodynamically stable patients with evidence of contrast extravasation on CT and angiography, splenic salvage and avoidance of laparotomy is achieved in >95% of cases.

Complications specific to splenic embolization are the theoretical risks of infarction due to incorrect coil positioning or perforation of the damaged splenic capsule from catheter manipulation within the splenic substance.

GASTROINTESTINAL TRACT

Indications

The indications for gastrointestinal embolization depend on the section of bowel affected by the disease and on the feasibility of surgical or endoscopic methods of management. Hence embolization procedures in the stomach or rectum are rare whilst embolotherapy is performed more frequently for duodenal, small bowel and proximal large bowel lesions. Attention to technical detail is vital for the achievement of satisfactory results and avoidance of complications. Capillary embolization should be avoided because of the risk of bowel gangrene, but delivery of emboli into large, proximal vessels is ineffective.

A frequent problem is the difficulty of demonstrating the source of bleeding. Direct angiographic visualization of intestinal haemorrhage requires a substantial rate of blood loss at the time of the procedure (>1–2 ml/min). Unfortunately, by the time most patients are brought to the angiographic table, the bleeding has either stopped or fallen below the level necessary for angiographic visualization.

In patients with gastric haemorrhage, embolization is only indicated if both endoscopy and an aggressive haemostatic drug regimen have failed to control active bleeding. Indications include:

- inoperable tumours;
- bleeding caused by chemotherapeutic agents, particularly in lymphoma;
- anastomotic bleeding after gastric surgery, particularly in septic patients;
- ruptured pseudoaneurysms.

Duodenal embolization, too, is only considered as second line therapy after failure of endoscopy. The incidence of acute bleeding from duodenal ulcers has decreased with the advent of effective medication for the treatment of early ulcer disease. Consequently, the commonest source of duodenal haemorrhage is a pseudoaneurysm of the gastroduodenal arteries or one of its major branches. These can occur as a result of atherosclerotic disease or as a rare, late complication of pancreatitis. Duodenal haemorrhage may also occur following gastrectomy or papillotomy.

Small or large bowel embolization is a rare procedure performed in carefully selected cases. There is a significant risk of infarction (in contrast to embolization in the liver, stomach or duodenum) because of the end-artery character of the vascular supply to the bowel. For satisfactory results a careful embolization technique, involving superselective catheterization combined with a detailed knowledge of the arterial supply of the bowel, is required. Colonoscopy of the large bowel should always precede angiography and attempted embolization in an attempt to identify the bleeding site and arrest haemorrhage. If a bleeding site is identified which is not correctable at endoscopy then surgery is the treatment of choice in most instances. If several unsuccessful attempts have been made to localize the source at open surgery, or patients are not fit for general anaesthesia or have religious objections to surgery, embolization may be considered. Indications include vascular malformations, telangiectasia, postanastomotic haemorrhage and bleeding diverticula.

Technical success is defined as complete occlusion of the lesion and no recanalization during the 30-day post-treatment period; when the lesion can be selectively accessed, success this should approach 100%. However, the clinical results are often influenced by the generally poor state of the patient at the time of the procedure; the outcome is often determined by renal or multiorgan failure if the patient has experienced prolonged periods of hypotension.

Technique and complications

The femoral artery approach is most commonly used with selective catheterization of the appropriate mesenteric vessel. The approach to the lesion should be as superselective as possible. The main limitation of the technique is difficulty of access to the bleeding site in certain instances; for example, the left gastric artery is often technically demanding to cannulate. When gastric or duodenal embolization is performed, coils are the embolic material of choice, although particulate matter is used in certain cases. Considerable caution should be exercized in small and large bowel embolization if bowel necrosis is to be avoided. Coils are the preferred embolic material and should be placed as close to the lesion as possible. Particulate or liquid embolic agents are not usually employed as they can occlude capillaries and lead to bowel necrosis. Mere reduction of flow by the insertion of a few coils combined with correction of any coagulation defects may be clinically sufficient. The exception is mesenteric telangiectasia where complete obstruction of the feeding vessels often requires a combination of coils and particulate material.

The main risk of embolization of gastrointestinal lesions is bowel necrosis from occlusion of the superior or inferior mesenteric arteries or their branches. The use of coils rather than particulate matter or liquid agents is often sufficient to reduce the bleeding significantly but not compromise the immediate adjacent bowel. Pancreatitis can also result from ischaemia secondary to embolic infarction.

TRANSJUGULAR INTRAHEPATIC PORTOSYSTEMIC SHUNT (TIPS)

The percutaneous creation of a communication between the portal and hepatic venous systems for the relief of portal hypertension was first attempted in patients with the use of repeated balloon dilatation in the early 1980s. However, it was not until the introduction of expandable metal stents that the problem of progressive shunt occlusion was resolved. The first successful procedure was performed by Richter in Germany in 1988 and since then the technique has become well established worldwide. As clinical and technical experience has increased the clinical indications have become better defined. However, longer term follow-up, particularly on stent occlusion, and reintervention rates will help to outline a treatment strategy accurately. The advantages of TIPS include:

- avoidance of open surgery that may be difficult because of the large varices;
- an entirely intrahepatic shunt (avoiding adhesions which may interfere with subsequent liver transplantation);
- ability to measure and adjust the degree of shunting.

INDICATIONS

Current indications for TIPS include:

- chronically recurring variceal bleeding despite continuing sclerotherapy or endoscopic banding;
- recurring variceal bleeding and severe ulcerative or erosive disease from repeat sclerotherapy;
- repeat bleeding episodes from major gastric varices inaccessible for sclerotherapy or endoscopic banding;
- recurring variceal bleeding from occluded surgical shunts.

Patients may be considered for TIPS because the risks associated with surgery are unacceptable in certain cases. For this particular subset of patients no therapeutic choice other than TIPS exists. For patients fit for surgery with Child's stage A or B liver disease, the traditional surgical option has been a distal splenorenal shunt. In this group of patients TIPS competes with surgery and more information is required on outcome (patency rates, encephalopathy, morbidity and mortality) to decide on appropriate treatment strategies.

One area where TIPS has emerged as the treatment of choice is in patients already enrolled on a liver transplantation programme who are at high risk of bleeding. In these patients the shunt relieves the portal hypertension leaving the main vascular structures untouched. It is not clear yet whether TIPS is indicated in intractable ascites. Early results indicate a role in rapid onset ascites with a high portosystemic gradient. However, in patients with a long history of cirrhosis, small liver and only a moderate portosystemic pressure gradient, TIPS may precipitate rapid liver failure from deprivation of portal blood nutrition.

CONTRAINDICATIONS

Absolute contraindications include:

- right heart failure or other cardiopulmonary factors contributing to substantial elevation of right ventricular pressure;
- presence of pulmonary or ascitic sepsis;
- significant acute liver failure not attributable to active bleeding;
- presence of extensive malignancy (hepatocellular carcinoma or metastatic disease) compressing or infiltrating the hepatic vessels or liver parenchyma in the proposed shunt tract.

Relative contraindications include portal vein occlusion or a peripheral, small hepatocellular carcinoma in a patient unfit for surgical resection.

TECHNIQUE

The procedure is performed in the supine position with a fluoroscopic machine. Intravenous access is obtained and analgesia and sedation administered via this route. ECG and pulse oximetry are mandatory. Usually, acutely bleeding patients in whom medical treatment has failed to control variceal haemorrhage present in a poor or critical clinical state, resulting from substantial blood loss and coagulopathy, often with hepatic encephalopathy. Consequently anaesthetic assistance is required to maintain clinical stability.

The internal jugular vein is punctured with a standard Seldinger technique and a 9F catheter positioned in the proximal right or middle hepatic vein. The hepatic vein pressure is then recorded. A modified Colapinto needle is introduced through the catheter and under ultrasound guidance it is advanced into one of the main portal branches. The correct position can be confirmed by a direct portal venogram through the puncture needle (Fig. 10.21a). As experience is gained it is possible to puncture the portal branches without ultrasound guidance. The portal vein pressure is then recorded. With the use of standard catheter-guidewire-angioplasty techniques, the track is then predilated to a diameter of 8–10 mm and an expandable metallic stent positioned to create the portosystemic shunt (Fig. 10.21b). The stent diameter is chosen to reduce the portosystemic gradient to within the range of 10–15 mmHg. This lowers the gradient sufficiently to reduce variceal bleeding but does not create a high-volume shunt with subsequent increase in the incidence of postprocedural encephalopathy. If bleeding gastric varices are present they can be embolized with steel coils prior to catheter withdrawal.

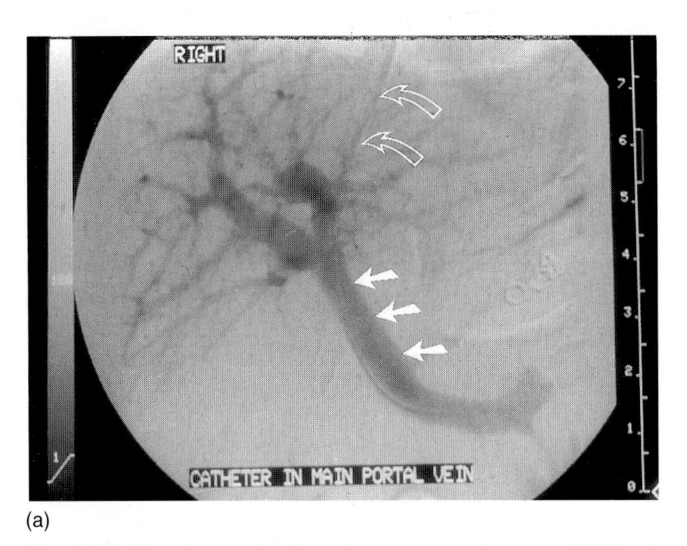

(a)

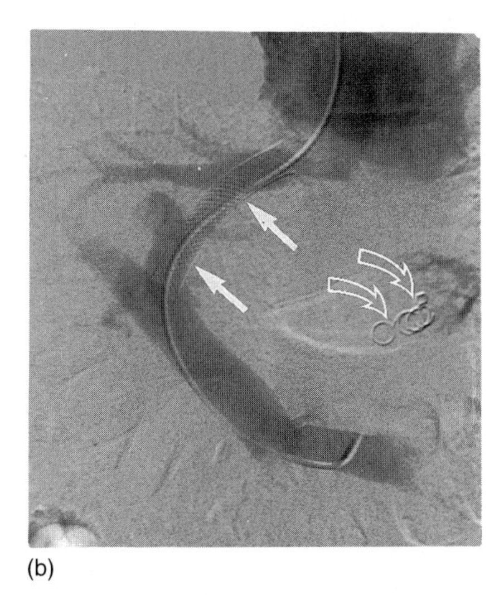

(b)

Fig. 10.21 Transjugular intrahepatic portosystemic shunt (TIPS). (a) A catheter (curved arrows) has been introduced through the liver parenchyma from the middle hepatic vein into the portal vein. A venogram demonstrates the portal vein (straight arrows) and its tributaries (b) A self-expanding metal stent (arrows) has created a shunt between the left branch of the portal vein and the hepatic venous system. Embolization coils (curved arrows) have been used to occlude gastric varices. (Reproduced with permission from Watkinson A.F. and Adam A. (1996) *Interventional radiology: a practical guide*, published by Radcliffe Medical Press, Oxford)

RESULTS AND COMPLICATIONS

The technical success rates of TIPS is >90% and the average procedure time is between 1–2 hours. Procedural mortality is uncommon (1–4%) and usually relates to inadvertent puncture of the extracapsular portal vein or septic complications. Postprocedural morbidity includes puncture site haematomas, transient elevation of liver enzymes and complications related to the sedatives used.

The clinical success after 30 days is >90% with rebleeding ocurring in less than 10% of patients. Hepatic encephalopathy can occur after the procedure and is highest in patients where the gradient is reduced to <10 mmHg. In many patients with hepatic encephalopathy prior to shunting the symptoms do not seem to worsen after the procedure, probably because the hepatic encephalopathy is caused by severe acute bleeding and significant intestinal protein uptake, which decreases once the shunt is established. The most common late complication is shunt occlusion, usually due to intimal hyperplasia. This appears to be more common than initially thought with reintervention rates (involving balloon dilatation or second stent insertion) approaching 50% in patients surviving ≥12 months.

As currently performed, TIPS is a safe, non-invasive and efficient method for the treatment of variceal haemorrhage. It is particularly indicated in patients awaiting liver transplantation both in the emergency stage and also possibly at an earlier stage of the underlying liver disease. If transplantation is performed within 6–12 months, then the problems of late shunt occlusion and intimal hyperplasia should not happen. Further research is required to investigate haemodynamically significant intimal hyperplasia which appears to be responsible for late shunt occlusion, rebleeding and reintervention rates.

RENAL INTERVENTION

The specialty of urology has undergone many changes in recent years with advances in minimally invasive therapy in the treatment of diseases of the kidney, ureter, bladder and prostate. The application of the Seldinger technique to percutaneous catheterization of the renal pelvis has enabled techniques such as percutaneous nephrostomy, percutaneous nephrolithotomy, antegrade ureteric stent placement and ureteric balloon dilatation to be performed without resorting to open surgery.

PERCUTANEOUS NEPHROSTOMY

Percutaneous nephrostomy can be both diagnostic and therapeutic. Diagnostic indications include:

- accurate delineation of the anatomy of the collecting system in cases of filling defects or outflow obstruction (in most cases this is combined with a drainage procedure);
- aspiration of urine for microscopy, culture and sensitivity;
- evaluation of suspicious lesions in the urinary tract with cytology of brush biopsy specimens;
- a Whitaker test to quantitate the significance of pelviureteric or ureteric obstruction.

Therapeutic indications include:

- relief of urinary tract obstruction which may be secondary to calculus, stricture, tumour or pyonephrosis;
- percutaneous nephrolithotomy in patients not suitable for lithotripsy;
- urinary diversion in patients with fistula;
- abscess drainage and relief of urinoma.

Technique and results

Patient preparation is extremely important to minimize the risk of sepsis and haemorrhage. A complete blood count, coagulation profile, serum electrolytes and urine culture are mandatory. Intravenous access is established and the procedure is performed in the prone position with appropriate antibiotic cover, analgesia and sedation. An initial ultrasound examination determines the location and depth of the kidney as well as the degree of hydronephrosis.

The preferred entry site is just medial to the posterior axillary line inferior to the twelfth rib. Under ultrasound guidance a fine needle is guided into an appropriate renal calyx. In most circumstances the preferred angle of approach is via a posterior middle calyx as this gives a direct line of access to the renal pelvis and ureter. If the procedure is the initiating step for percutaneous nephrolithotomy then the needle should be directed towards the stone-containing calyx or the posterior calyx nearest to the stone. Aspiration of urine confirms that the needle is within the collecting system and a catheter can be introduced coaxially. Instillation of dilute contrast delineates the anatomy of the collecting system often giving information on the level and cause of obstruction (Fig. 10.22).

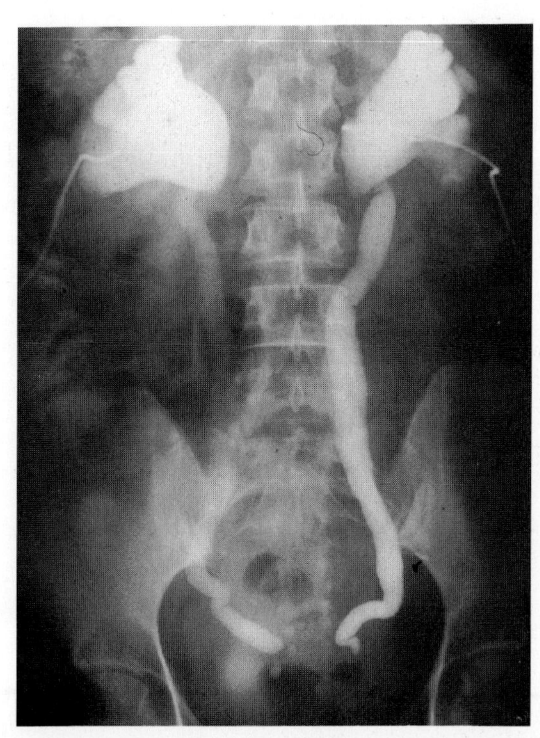

Fig. 10.22 Bilateral nephrostomies are seen inserted via the lower pole calyx on both sides. Nephrostograms demonstrate bilateral hydronephrosis and hydroureter to the level of the vesicoureteric junctions. Obstruction is caused by extensive carcinoma of the cervix.

The refinement of interventional guidewires and catheters ensures that an appropriate nephrostomy catheter (usually 8 or 10F) with a self-locking loop can then be introduced with the minimum of trauma and discomfort. The self-locking catheters have reduced the risk of catheter dislodgement; however, the catheter should still be firmly attached to the skin with sutures or one of the many available specific devices. The technique, with ultrasound guidance, should ideally gain access to the collecting system after a single pass, thus minimizing the incidence of haemorrhage and septic shock due to urinary leakage into the renal substance and renal vessels. If long-term drainage is required, the catheter should be exchanged every two to three months. However, long-term drainage is best achieved by a double-J pigtail stent inserted antegradely thus dispensing with the need for a external catheter (see below).

If the procedure is the initiating step for percutaneous nephrolithotomy, the puncture is directly onto the calculus. The tract is then sequentially dilated to an appropriate diameter (usually 24–28F) and the largest diameter sheath left *in situ* for endoscopic access and forceps removal of the stone. A safety wire is usually left in the upper ureter in case of sheath dislodgement.

If there is more than a mild hydronephrosis the technical success of the procedure approaches 100%. If the pelvicalyceal system is not dilated then the correct positioning of a nephrostomy can be extremely difficult, with success being directly proportional to experience. This problem can occur if there is a leak of the renal pelvis or ureter decompressing into the retroperitoneum, or in acute calculous obstruction of the collecting system where the system has not had time to dilate. There is normally good renal function in these instances and an intravenous pyelogram usually helps to delineate the pelvicalyceal system to assist successful puncture.

Complications

The incidence of complications is low compared to open surgical nephrostomy, which has a perioperative mortality rate as high as 10% and a morbidity rate of over 30%. Minor complications include catheter dislodgement or occlusion. The introduction of self-locking catheters has reduced dislodgment; however, ward staff must be made aware of this technical modification and asked not to attempt removal of the

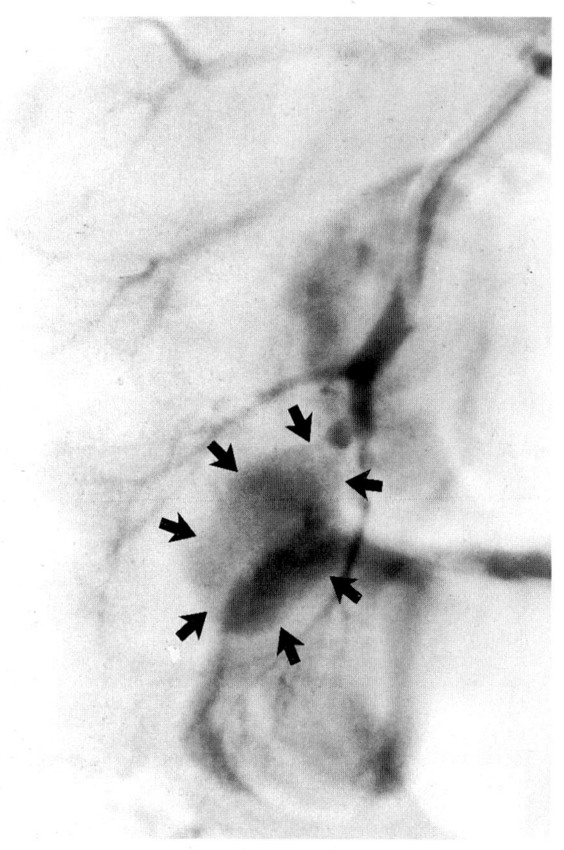
(a)

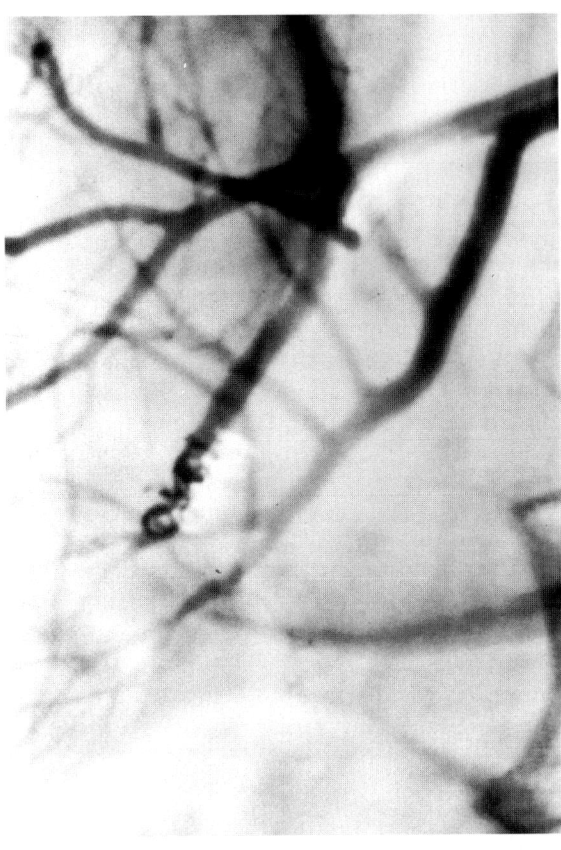
(b)

Fig. 10.23 Embolization of a false aneurysm of a segmental renal artery. (a) Digital subtraction arteriography of a lower pole artery of the right kidney after percutaneous liver biopsy. This demonstrates a large false aneurysm (arrows). (b) The feeding artery has been embolized with steel coils occluding the aneurysmal sac. (We are grateful to Dr J. Reidy for donating these illustrations.) (Reproduced with permission from Watkinson A.F. and Adam A. in *Seminars in interventional radiology* 1994, **11**, (3) 254–266, published by Thieme Medical Publishers, NY)

catheter. Catheter occlusion can lead to hydronephrosis, pyonephrosis, septicaemia and urinoma. If signs of obstruction are present a new catheter should be inserted. This is usually a straightforward procedure with the placement of a guidewire down the mature tract.

Clinically significant haemorrhage occurs in 1–2% of cases and can lead to massive intrarenal bleeding with haematuria as well as expanding pararenal haematomas. Usually the haematuria decreases after 1–2 days and the nephrostomy can be kept patent with frequent saline flushes. If the haematuria continues or there is a significant drop in haemoglobin then arteriography is advised. If a bleeding point, arteriovenous fistula or false aneurysm is identified then they should be embolized with coils, as selectively as possible (Figs 10.23).

The incidence of septic complications varies between 1–2%. These are potentially fatal and every precaution should be taken to minimize their occurence including antibiotic cover and minimal catheter-guidewire manipulation. Urinomas and infected perirenal haematomas usually resolve with appropriate antibiotic cover and a functioning nephrostomy.

ANTEGRADE STENT PLACEMENT

If double-J pigtail stent insertion is required to relieve ureteric obstruction, the initial approach should be retrogradely via cystoscopy. Only when unsuccessful, or if the patient already has an indwelling nephrostomy, should the stent be positioned antegradely.

Indications

Antegrade stent placement allows urine to flow from the pelvicalyceal system to the bladder in ureteric obstruction or perforation thus obviating the need for long-term nephrostomy. It is indicated in a number of clinical situations including:

- relief of ureteric obstruction secondary to calculi, which can be due to a single large obstructing calculus or post-extracorporeal shock wave lithotripsy with many small fragments;
- healing of ureteric perforations or rupture;
- relief of ureteric obstruction secondary to benign or malignant strictures; in both instances associated balloon dilatation assists in passage of the

stent. In benign disease stenting is temporary but in malignant disease it is usually permanent; if necessary stent change can be performed retrogradely at 3–4 monthly intervals.

Technique

In most instances a percutaneous nephrostomy tube is already *in situ*. If not, one should be inserted as described above. An initial nephrostogram is used to define the anatomy and level of obstruction or leakage. The nephrostomy tube, if present, is then withdrawn over a guidewire and the guidewire with specially shaped catheters is manipulated into the ureter, advanced to the level of obstruction and, if possible, pushed through the strictured segment into the bladder. Most strictures can be traversed with the aid of low-friction, hydrophilic guidewires. If it is not possible to traverse the stricture during the initial session, a period of external drainage, via a nephrostomy, usually allows reduction of oedema and passage of a guidewire. The hydrophilic guidewire is then exchanged for a stiff exchange wire and a protective peel-away sheath inserted through the renal parenchyma into the ureter; this prevents buckling at the level of the kidney, allows easy introduction of a balloon catheter to dilate the stricture (Fig. 10.24) and aids insertion of the double-J pigtail stent (Fig. 10.25). It is important to choose the correct length of stent to ensure that the upper and lower pigtails are in the renal pelvis and bladder respectively.

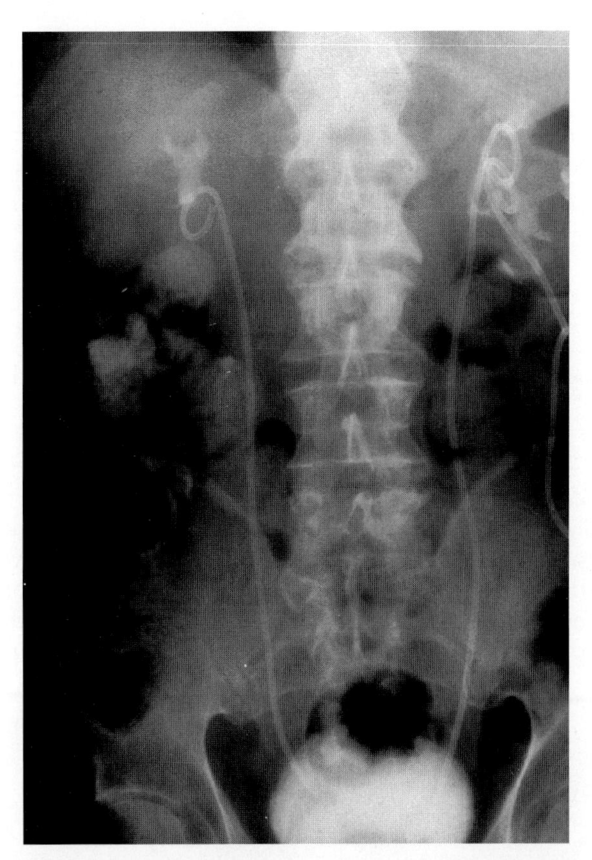

Fig. 10.25 Antegrade ureteric stent placement. Bilateral double-J pigtail stents have been positioned satisfactorily with the upper ends in the pelvicalyceal systems and the lower ends in the bladder. A safety nephrostomy catheter is seen within the left collecting system.

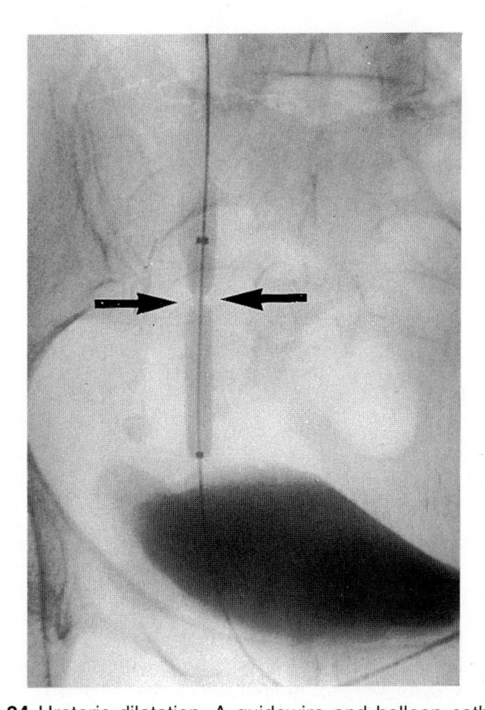

Fig. 10.24 Ureteric dilatation. A guidewire and balloon catheter are seen traversing the right ureter, with the tip of the guidewire in a partially filled bladder. The balloon is partially inflated showing waisting (arrows) at the site of a tight ureteric stricture.

Results

The technical success rate exceeds 95% and the complications are the same as for percutaneous nephrostomy, with the added risk of ureteric perforation during balloon dilatation or passage of the guidewire. If this occurs then the patient should be given antibiotics and placed on external drainage via a nephrostomy; antibiotics should be given until healing occurs. The stent will eventually occlude from encrustation and should be replaced via the retrograde approach every 3–4 months or earlier if required.

RENAL ARTERY ANGIOPLASTY AND STENT PLACEMENT

As equipment and techniques have advanced, interest in the use of angioplasty for the treatment of renovascular hypertension and improvement, or maintenance, of renal function has increased. The evaluation of the significance of renal artery narrowing is most effectively performed during intra-arterial angiography. Intravenous digital studies frequently do not provide sufficient information and intravenous sampling for renin is expensive and unreliable. Lesions that are resistant to balloon dilatation, such as ostial stenoses, may benefit from placement of metallic endoprostheses.

Indications

Indications for this procedure include:

- renovascular hypertension (blood pressure >140/95), from either atherosclerosis or fibromuscular dysplasia, which is poorly controlled on medical therapy and where a lesion is seen on arteriography;
- impaired or deteriorating renal function with a proven lesion on arteriography;
- renal transplant arterial stenosis.

Technique and results

The femoral approach is used preferentially for both native and transplant kidneys. In patients with severe atherosclerosis, with associated abdominal aortic aneurysms or atheromatous pelvic vessels, a brachial approach may be necessary. Abdominal aortography prior to cannulation of the renal artery confirms the presence of the lesion (Fig. 10.26a). The renal artery is engaged with a catheter specially shaped to cannulate the orifice, and 5000 units of heparin are given intra-arterially. The lesion is then traversed gently with a hydrophilic guidewire and the catheter advanced. A stiff guidewire is introduced enabling the catheter to be withdrawn and the angioplasty balloon to be introduced over the wire to straddle the lesion. On balloon inflation a waist will appear at the site of the lesion (Fig. 10.26b); this disappears at full distension of the balloon. A postangioplasty flush aortogram will show if the procedure has been technically successful (Fig. 10.26c). If the lesion does not dilate or recurs within a short time period then a metal stent may be indicated. Balloon-expandable endoprostheses are preferable as accurate placement is easier to achieve with these than with self-expandable devices.

Renal angioplasty has a technical success rate of approximately 90%. Patients with hypertension due to fibromuscular disease show improvement of their

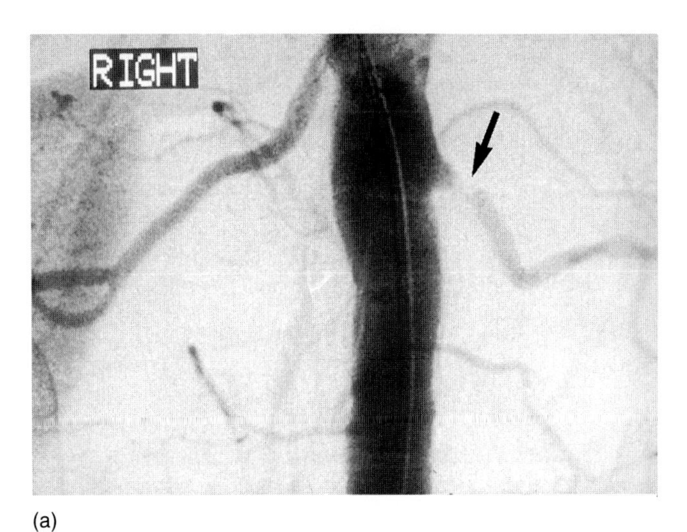

(a)

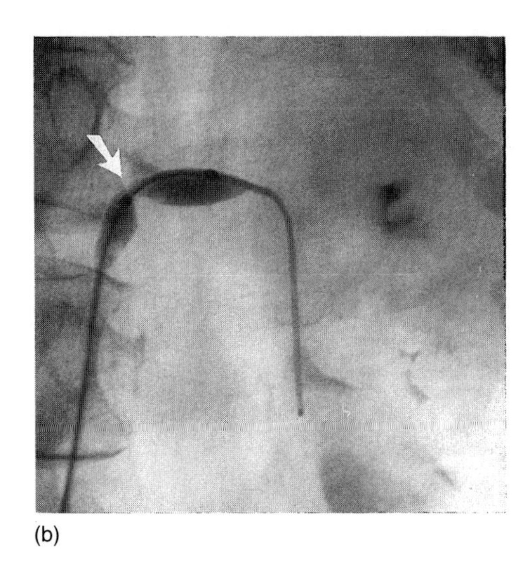

(b)

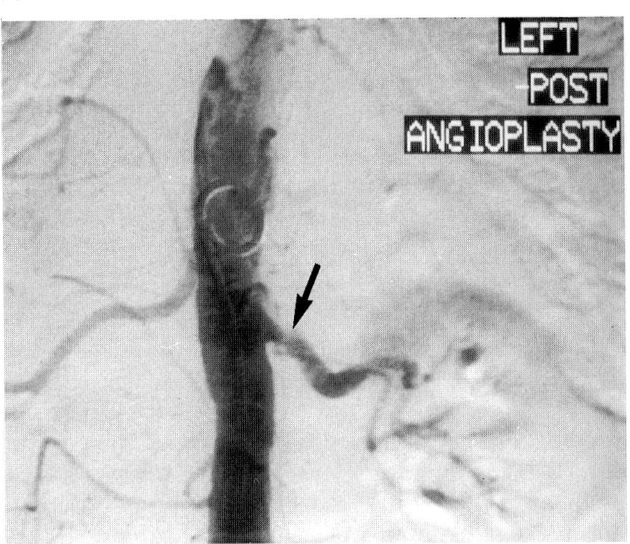

(c)

Fig. 10.26 Renal artery angioplasty. (a) Digital subtraction flush aortography at the level of the renal arteries. There is a tight stenosis of the proximal left renal artery (arrow). There is poor opacification of the vessel beyond this narrowing as only a small amount of contrast has managed to pass through this tight stenosis. (b) A partially inflated balloon catheter is positioned across the renal artery stenosis. Waisting is seen (arrow) at the site of the stenosis. (c) Digital subtraction flush aortography after balloon dilatation demonstrating a satisfactory radiological result. There is some irregularity at the site of angioplasty (arrow), however, there is good flow to the distal vessel.

hypertension in 80–90% of cases. In patients with unilateral atherosclerotic stenoses away from the renal ostium there is usually an improvement in only 60–70% of cases. Ostial stenoses are difficult to treat; they result from large atheromatous plaques in the aorta which partially occlude the origin of the renal artery. In these patients primary success from angioplasty may be as low as 20–30% and metallic stenting may be the most appropriate management. Angioplasty in patients with deteriorating renal function is less successful with improvement or stabilization of biochemistry in approximately 50% of cases.

Complications

The complications of the procedure can threaten the viability of the kidney and a vascular surgeon should be aware of all renal angioplasty and stent cases so that intervention can be undertaken if required. The most common complication, occuring in approximately 5% of cases, is deteriorating renal function. Occlusion of the renal artery, which can occur from thrombosis or a dissection flap, has an incidence of approximately 3–4%. If a clot occludes the artery, thrombolysis using tissue plasminogen activator may recanalize the vessel. However, if the dissection flap is significant a metallic stent may be required to re-establish patency of the vessel. The renal artery ruptures in approximately 1% of cases, in which case the angioplasty balloon should be re-advanced, over a guidewire, across the ruptured segment and re-inflated. The vascular surgeon should then be contacted urgently. Prompt action can minimize the blood loss, thus decreasing the warm ischaemic time preventing loss of the kidney.

general, fractures involving a single column (e.g. wedge compression fractures) may be considered to be stable. Disruption of two or more columns, especially the middle and posterior columns, is associated with a high risk of instability. The most unstable injuries include facet joint fractures and/or dislocation and major translational injuries where there is *en bloc* displacement of the spine in the lateral or anteroposterior plane.

Flexion injuries

Flexion injuries occur at sites of maximum spinal mobility, typically the lower cervical spine and the cervicothoracic and thoracolumbar junctional zones. Vertebral body compression or wedging is the predominant feature. More significant forces disrupt the posterior ligamentous column, resulting in facet joint luxation and transient or fixed vertebral displacement (Fig. 11.2). The addition of rotational forces increases the risk of facet joint distraction and ligamentous injury.

Extension injuries

Hyperextension injury occurs most commonly in the cervical region. Fractures involve the spinal canal ring and, particularly, the facet joints. Stability is particularly compromised if the anterior column complex is disrupted.

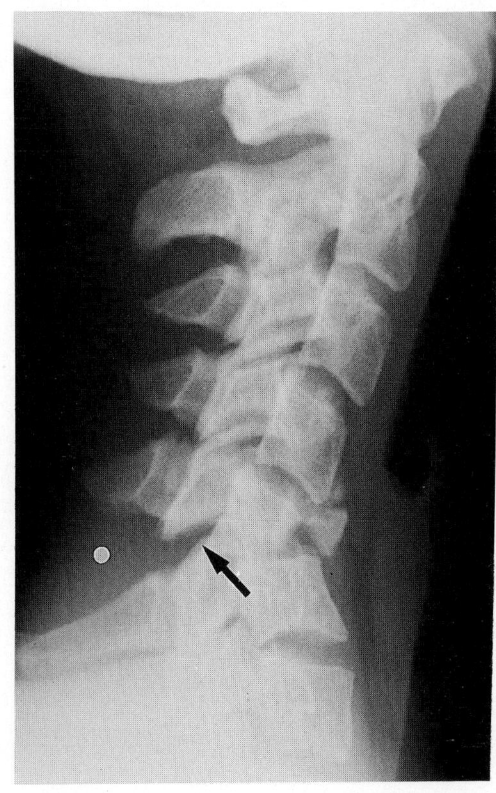

Fig. 11.2 Hyperflexion injury with fracture dislocation at C5/6. Note widened interspinous gap (circle) and subluxed articular facet joints (arrow).

Axial (burst) compression injuries

Vertical transmission of forces results in splaying or bursting of the vertebral body and posterior elements, particularly the pedicles or lateral masses. Common sites of involvement include C1 and the lower cervical, thoracolumbar and upper lumbar regions. Retropulsion of bony elements into the spinal canal may compress neural structures, with a high incidence of major irreversible cord damage in cervical injuries. CT not infrequently demonstrates involvement of both the middle and posterior columns indicating potentially unstable injuries.

Rotation–translation injuries

A combination of factors including hyperflexion and hyperextension which, when combined with lateral or rotational forces, result in major spinal disruption or instability. The cervical, upper and lower thorcacic regions are the most common sites for this type of injury.

Acute spinal injury may be considered according to the three spinal regions.

Cervical injuries

Upper cervical injuries are often unstable with a high incidence of associated severe neurological compromise or death and usually result from a major head injury. However, because the spinal canal is relatively capacious (and if further instability is prevented) the late outcome may often be good. Injuries to the atlas include axial compression bursting injuries (**Jefferson fractures**), in which cord damage is rare. CT clearly demonstrates the disruption of the anterior and posterior arches of C1. Atlanto-occipital dislocation, usually fatal, is recognized by widening of the gap between the tip of the odontoid peg and the basion (anterior lip of the foramen magnum) to above 12.5 mm. Atlanto-axial dislocation usually occurs in association with fractures of the upper cervical spine and disruption of the transverse ligament.

Fractures of the axis (C2) may either involve the odontoid process or the lateral masses (**hangman's fracture**). Odontoid fractures are common and are classified into type I (tip), type II (base of dens) and type III (C2 body). Type II are the most common, being seen as a horizontal lucency at the base of the dens on the open mouth projection or cortical disruption on a lateral view. Non-union can occur in up to 72% of cases with an increased risk of atlanto-axial instability. A hangman's fracture represents a traumatic spondylolysthesis with fractures through the pars interarticularis produced by a hyperextension injury. The neural arch becomes separated from the body, which subluxes anteriorly. Although this fracture is responsible for death in judicial hanging, in clinical practice neurological damage is uncommon as the spinal canal becomes effectively widened.

From C3 to C7 the injuries are flexion, extension and axial compression. Flexion injuries which leave the middle and posterior columns intact result in simple wedge fractures. More severe flexion forces, as occur in contact sports or diving accidents where the neck becomes flexed whilst the head is relatively fixed, lead to disruption of the posterior longitudinal ligament and posterior column osteoligamentous complex with a significantly increased risk of anterior subluxation or dislocation (Fig. 11.3). The posterior disc space and interspinous distance at the affected level become widened. Uni- or bilateral facet joint fracture–dislocation may also occur with this type of injury. Oblique views are useful but CT is more effective in demonstrating the full extent of the injury. The risk of cord injury is high with cord contusion and/or compression.

Extension injuries range from whiplash soft-tissue injuries without disruption of the spinal column to more significant trauma in which the anterior ligamentous complex is disrupted and there may be avulsion fractures of the anterior vertebral bodies or compression fractures of the posterior arch. The disc space becomes widened anteriorly and there is often an associated prevertebral soft-tissue swelling. Severe hyperextension 'sprain' injuries may result in transient subluxation with resulting cord impaction and a central cord syndrome, in the absence of overt malalignment. These injuries are, however, unstable in extension. Axial loading compression fractures (e.g. falls onto the vertex in diving accidents) result in major disruption of the vertebral body with bursting and cleavage of the vertebral body (Fig. 11.4). Retropulsion of vertebral body bony elements posteriorly into the cervical spinal canal often results in major cord damage (Fig. 11.5).

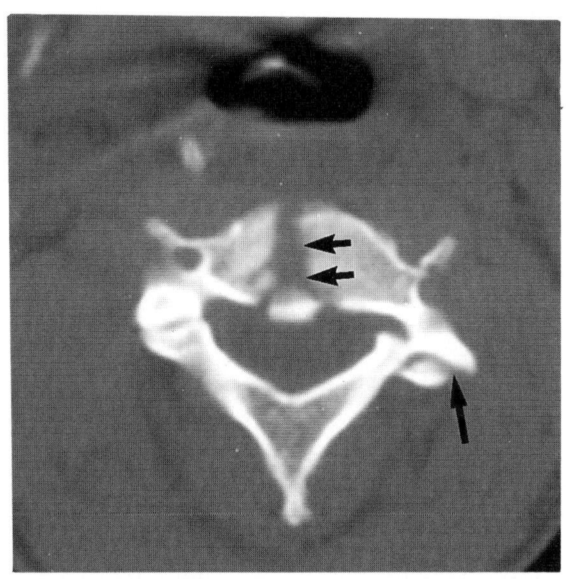

Fig. 11.4 Cervical axial burst fracture at C3 with vertebral body cleavage (small arrows) and left-sided facet joint fracture dislocation (arrow).

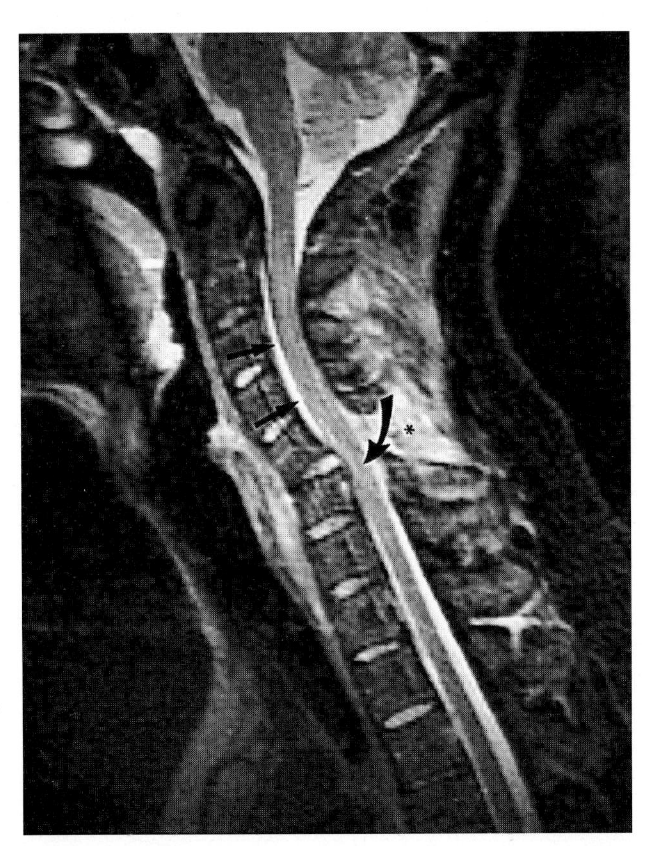

Fig. 11.3 T2-weighted sagittal MRI of an acute hyperflexion injury. Disruption of the C5/6 posterior annulus and posterior ligamentous complex (✱) is present along with some cord contusion (curved arrow), seen as ill-defined high signal in the cord. There is an anterior extradural haematoma (arrows).

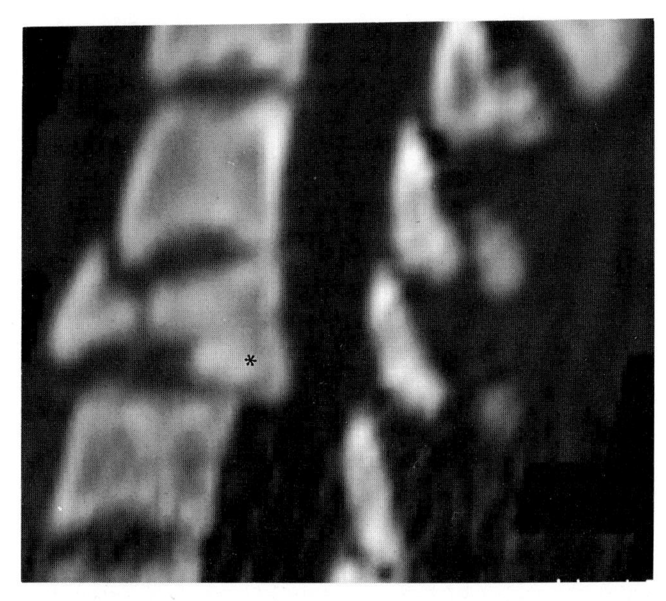

Fig. 11.5 Sagittal CT reconstruction in the midline showing a retropulsed vertebral body fragment (✱) narrowing the spinal canal by 50%. MRI demonstrated cord compression and contusion.

Thoracic injuries

Fractures in the thoracic spine are less common than in the cervical and thoracolumbar regions. Axial loading compression injuries may result in burst fractures. With major trauma the sternum and/or ribs are often fractured and there is an increased incidence of translational injuries with anterior displacement and acute angulation of the spine. Major cord disruption not infrequently accompanies these injuries.

Thoracolumbar injuries

Injuries in this region account for approximately a third of all spinal trauma, L1 being the most commonly affected. Flexion injuries occur most commonly, often accompanied by compressive forces. Loss of vertebral height anteriorly and increased kyphosis are seen on lateral radiographs. As the middle and posterior columns are usually intact, these are stable injuries. Axial compression forces result in herniation of disc through the end-plate with subsequent bursting of the vertebral body. Lateral splaying of the pedicles, with or without a vertical fracture through the vertebral body, is seen on the frontal views with loss of height of the posterior part of the vertebral body on the lateral views. CT scanning is most valuable in demonstrating comminuted bone fragments which are most often derived from the posterosuperior part of the vertebral body, spinal canal narrowing and integrity of the posterior neural arch. CT demonstrates the frequent involvement of both the middle and posterior columns and thus the inherently unstable nature of these lesions (Fig. 11.6). Involvement of the conus accounts for the not infrequently associated paraplegia.

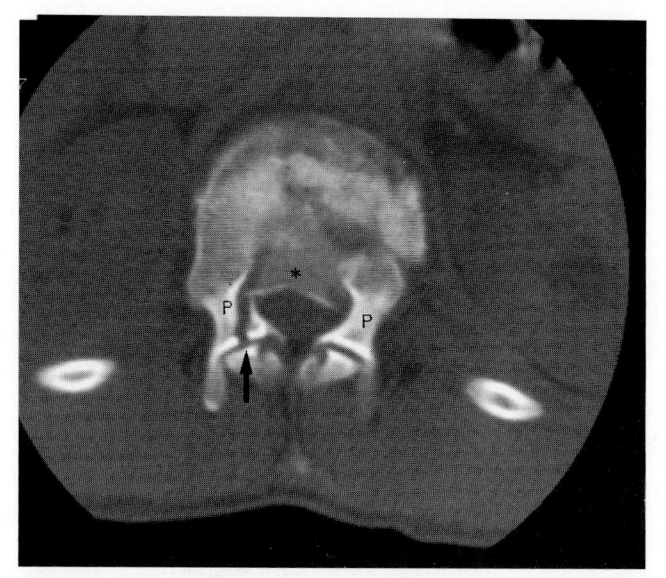

Fig. 11.6 L1 burst fracture with splaying of the pedicles (P), right-sided facet joint fracture dislocation (arrow) and 60% narrowing of the spinal canal by a large retropulsed fragment of the vertebral body(✱) compressing the conus.

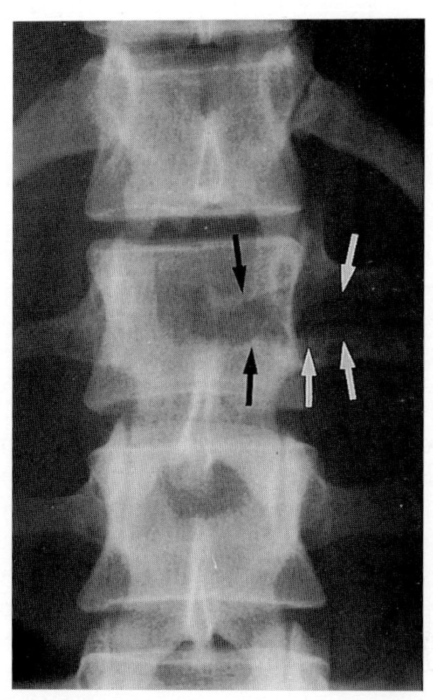

Fig. 11.7 Plain radiograph of a 'Chance' fracture, a horizontally orientated fracture through the body of L1 extending into the left transverse process (arrows).

Flexion–distraction forces may result in disruption of the middle and posterior columns with annular tears resulting in vertebral body subluxation and the frequently associated neurological deficits. Hyperflexion forces result in horizontal slicing injury which may extend through the vertebral body and posterior neural arch and/or ligaments or may pass through the disc space. This type of injury, known as a **Chance or 'seat belt' fracture dislocation**, is uncommon but is important to recognize because of the high incidence of associated major visceral damage. Neurological deficits are, however, uncommon. Plain radiographs or conventional tomography may define the horizontally orientated fracture through the vertebral body or posterior neural arch (Fig. 11.7). The orientation of these fractures may lead to difficulty in interpretation with CT unless multiplanar reconstructions are made.

Flexion–rotation and shearing fracture–dislocation injuries are uncommon, highly unstable injuries which involve all three spinal columns and are usually accompanied by paraplegia. There may be varying degrees of AP or lateral vertebral body displacement and locking. CT best demonstrates the degree of spinal canal involvement and the presence of facet joint dislocation.

SOFT TISSUE INJURIES

Cord and root injury

Injury to the spinal cord may result from:

- stretching of the cord at the time of hyperextension injury;
- focal cord compression or laceration of the cord as it is trapped between the neural arch posteriorly and vertebral body elements anteriorly, particularly in association with a dislocation;
- from direct impact of a disc protrusion or bony fragment upon the cord.

Neurological evidence of spinal cord injury when there is incomplete loss of or recovering motor or sensory function, or a neurological deficit in the absence of obvious bony injury, merits further investigation by MRI. Both haemorrhagic and non-haemorrhagic contusional injury may be readily identified as may cord compression by vertebral elements or disc protrusion. Reversible cord injury can arise from cord concussion and oedema and carries a more favourable prognosis than a haemorrhagic contusional injury. With non-haemorrhagic contusion the cord appears isointense on T1-weighted images; it may appear swollen and on T2-weighted images demonstrates focal hyperintensity (Fig. 11.3). Haemorrhagic contusion may show high signal on both T1- and T2-weighted images. There is less indication for MR imaging in completed spinal injuries; however, major cord disruption or transection may be confirmed and identifying any remediable pathology above the site of injury may prevent ascending neurological damage.

Traumatic brachial plexus injuries may be detected with equal accuracy (approximately 60–70%) by myelography and MRI. Root avulsion is most easily identified if there is an accompanying meningocoele or an enlarged empty root sleeve (Fig. 11.8). Brachial plexus injuries frequently involve more than one root.

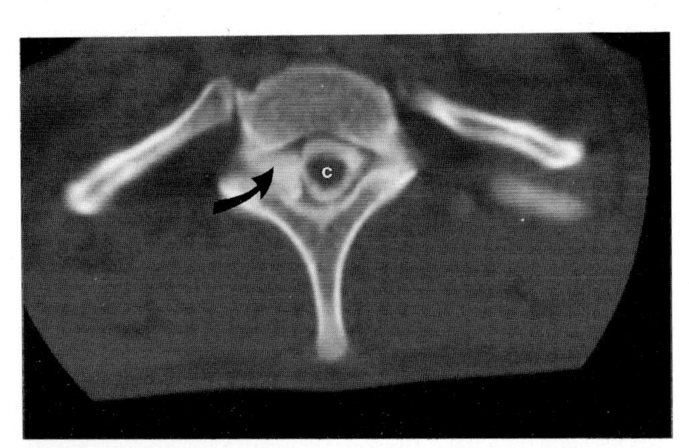

Fig. 11.8 Nerve root avulsion. CT myelogram demonstrating a right-sided post-traumatic meningocoele (arrow) with no identifiable nerve root within it; C=spinal cord.

Traumatic disc protrusion and intraspinal haematoma

Both these injuries may occur in the absence of associated vertebral fractures and are best demonstrated with MRI. The herniated disc may be of high signal intensity due to the presence of blood products and oedema. Acute spinal haemorrhage may demonstrate variable signal characteristics depending on the age, size and compartment into which the haemorrhage has occured. Acute haemorrhage may be difficult to demonstrate on MRI. Subacute haemorrhage (>48 h) may be of high or mixed high and low signal intensity on both T1- and T2-weighted images due to the presence of blood degradation products at differing stages of evolution. Extrinsic compression of the spinal cord by a sub- or extradural haematoma is readily identified.

Extraspinal soft tissue injury

Disruption of the anterior and posterior ligamentous complexes may accompany major spinal injury or occur in isolation, such as occurs with whiplash injuries of the neck.

CHRONIC SPINAL INJURY

Assessment of the late sequelae of spinal trauma is required when there is late or evolving neurological deterioration and/or a progressive spinal deformity. MRI can detect early cord damage such as cystic myelomalacia which may progress to frank cord cavitation (post-traumatic hydrosyringomyelia), accounting for an ascending pattern of neurological dysfunction (Fig. 11.9).

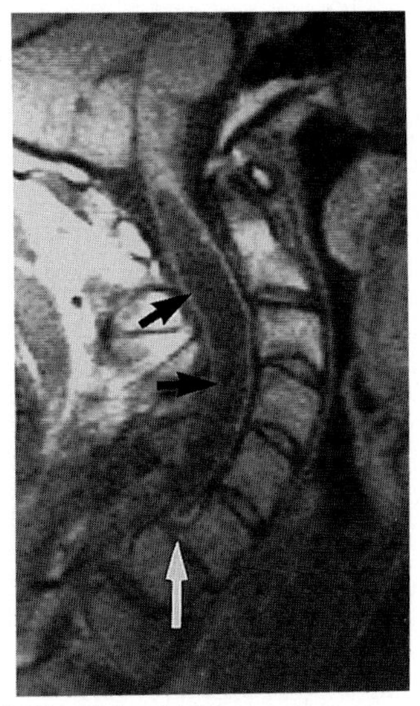

Fig. 11.9 Sagittal T1-weighted MRI showing a large cervical hydrosyrinx (small arrows) above an old C6/7 fracture dislocation (long arrow).

Progressive spinal deformity may occur either in isolation or associated with cord cavitation. Plain radiographs can be used to monitor the spinal deformity.

TUMOURS

Neoplastic diseases of the spine and spinal cord are traditionally classified by location into:

- extradural
- intradural extramedullary
- intramedullary (Fig. 11.10).

Imaging of these lesions has been transformed by MRI, which can clearly define the relationship of the lesion to the spinal cord and assess the extent of the tumour. Plain radiographs supplemented by conventional tomography, radionuclide studies and plain CT may be useful in certain osseous tumours.

EXTRADURAL TUMOURS

These tumours may be benign or malignant. Metastases to the spine are the most common malignant spinal tumours.

Benign tumours

One of the commonest benign tumours is the vertebral body **haemangioma**, increasingly seen as an incidental finding on MRI, with a reported incidence of 11% in autopsy cases. Haemangiomas occur with

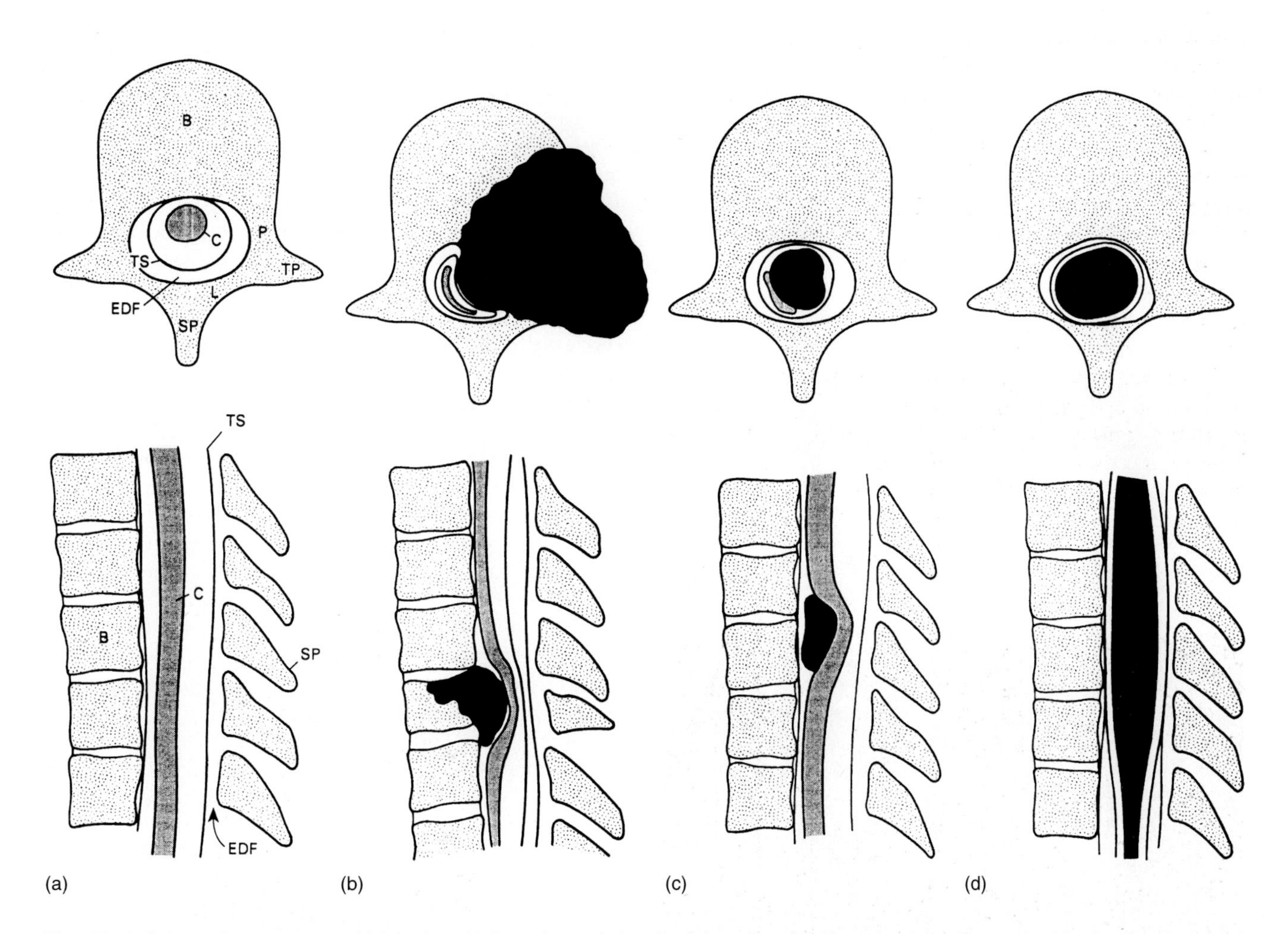

Fig. 11.10 Schematic transverse axial and sagittal sections of the thoracic spine. (a) Normal, where B=vertebral body; C=spinal cord; EDF=extradural fat; TS=thecal sac; L=lamina; P=pedicle; TP=transverse process; SP=spinous process. (b) Extradural metastatic tumour. Extrinsic compression of the thecal sac and spinal cord, which are compressed to an ellipse and displaced away from the tumour. (c) Intradural extramedullary tumour. The tumour is contained within the undisplaced thecal sac but compresses and displaces the spinal cord. (d) Intradural intramedullary spinal cord tumour. The spinal cord is expanded but undisplaced. There is little or no visualization of the cerebrospinal fluid in the thecal sac around the spinal cord.

increasing frequency from middle age. All or part of the vertebra is affected and any part of the spine may be affected, particularly the lower thoracic region. Plain radiographs demonstrate a coarse trabeculated pattern whilst small punctate densities within a discrete area of reduced attenuation may be seen with CT. On MRI fibroadipose stroma within these vascular hamartomatous lesions leads to heterogenous high signal intensity on both T1- and T2-weighted images (Fig. 11.11). Less commonly extraosseous extension into the neuroforaminal or spinal canal may lead to compression of neural tissue.

Tumours in younger patients, usually in their second and third decades, include **osteoid osteomas**, which occur particularly in the posterior neural arch. Although an osteoid osteoma may be difficult to appreciate on plain films, the tumour shows a focal area of intense increased uptake on a radionuclide scan. CT demonstrates a small radiolucency within an area of dense sclerosis and corresponding low signal intensity on MRI.

Osteoblastomas also tend to involve selectively the posterior neural arch, appearing as well-defined expanded lucent lesions.

Osteochondromas occur most commonly in the cervical spine, particularly C2, arising from the spinous or transverse processes. Although rarely producing neurological symptoms, they can grow into the spinal canal and compress the cord. Osteochondromas appear as sessile or pedunculated masses. The cartilaginous cap may exhibit punctate calcifications on CT and heterogenous signal characteristics on both T1- and T2-weighted images (Fig. 11.12).

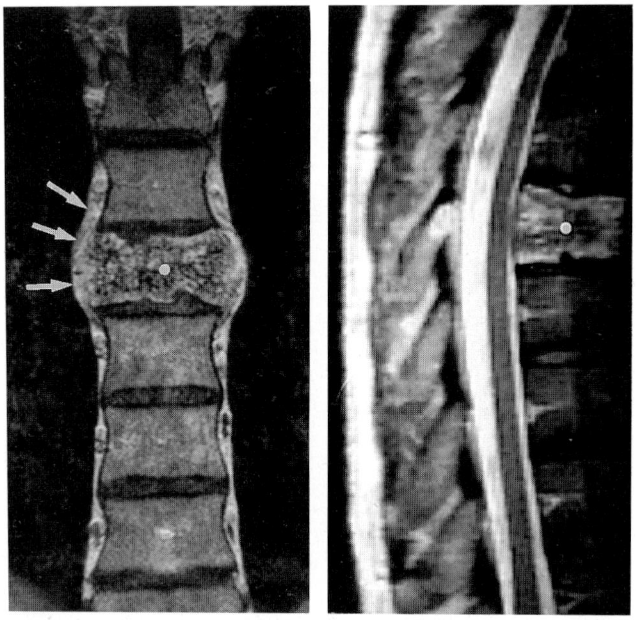

Aneurysmal bone cysts are non-neoplastic expansile lobulated soft-tissue mass lesions with a highly vascular stroma, occuring most often in the second and third decades. The posterior elements are usually involved but extension into the vertebral body, across adjacent disc spaces or into the spinal canal may occur. MRI demonstrates altered blood products resulting in high signal intensity on both T1- and T2-weighted images, internal septations and fluid levels with a low signal intensity rim.

(a) (b)

Fig. 11.11 T6 vertebral body haemangioma. (a) Coronal T1-weighted and (b) sagittal T2-weighted MRI showing heterogeneous high signal intensity on both sequences, a coarse trabeculated internal structure (circles) and paravertebral soft tissue involvement (arrows).

Malignant tumours

Metastases, particularly from carcinoma of the breast, lung and prostate, are the most common extradural tumours. The posterior part of the vertebral body is most frequently affected. Extension into the adjacent paraspinal soft tissues, the neuroforaminal canals and the spinal canal is commonly seen. Plain radiographs may demonstrate lytic foci or collapse of one or more vertebral bodies, pedicular destruction or a paraspinal soft-tissue mass. However, metastases from carcinoma of the prostate or breast, particularly following treatment of breast cancer may appear as sclerotic or mixed lytic and sclerotic lesions.

Whilst 40–50% of the affected bone mass must be destroyed before changes become evident on the radiograph, radionuclide bone scanning is sensitive to a much smaller degree of bone destruction (approximately 10%) and is thus commonly employed as the screening method of choice for the detection of metastases. MRI employing specific pathology-sensitive sequences such as STIR is an even more sensitive alternative for the detection of metastases. MRI has the additional advantage of being able to assess the spinal canal and location of any intraspinal tumour (Fig. 11.13). Metastases from other primary tumours, such as Hodgkin's and non-Hodgkins lymphoma may arise within the paraspinal and extradural soft tissues and secondarily involve the vertebral bodies. In children spinal metastases most commonly arise from a neuroblastoma.

The vertebrae are frequently involved in **multiple myeloma**, with peak incidence in the fifth to seventh decades. Focal or diffuse lytic lesions with vertebral collapse may be seen on plain films. The MRI features are multiple lesions which show heterogeneous signal characteristics (Fig. 11.14). Fat-suppressed sequences are helpful in distinguishing between myeloma and patchy fatty marrow replacement, a phenomenon which is increasingly prevalent with advancing age. Myeloma is also accompanied by vertebral body collapse.

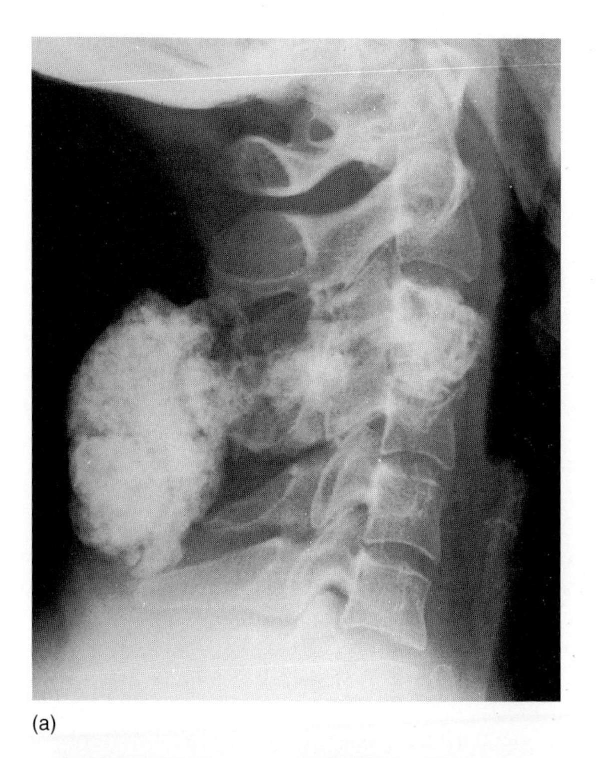

(a)

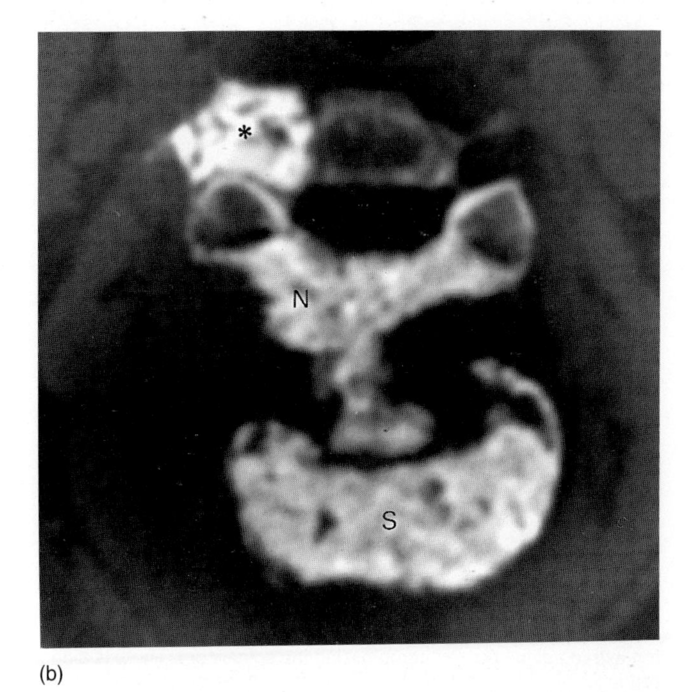

(b)

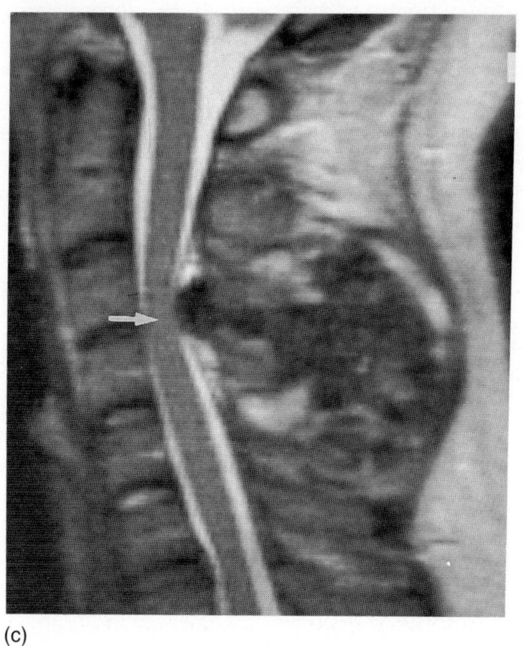

(c)

Fig. 11.12 Osteochondroma of C3. (a) Plain radiograph showing primary involvement of the spinous process. (b) CT more clearly defines the extent of the tumour in the spinous process (S), posterior neural arch (N) and region of the right foramen transversarium (*). (c) T2-weighted sagittal MRI scan shows posterior cord compression and early cord signal alteration (arrow).

Other malignant tumours include **chordomas**, which arise from intraosseous notochordal remnants. Over 50% of chordomas occur in the sacrococcygeal region, 35% at the skull base and 15% in vertebral bodies, mainly in the upper cervical region; they appear on CT as expansile lytic masses containing punctate calcifications. Chordomas are typically hypointense on T1-weighted sequences and hyperintense on T2-weighted images, demonstrating internal septations and strong contrast enhancement.

INTRADURAL EXTRAMEDULLARY TUMOURS

The most common intraspinal mass lesions are extramedullary intradural tumours, of which meningiomas and nerve sheath tumours account for 80–90%. Other benign tumours and cystic masses are relatively uncommon and are largely represented by developmental tumours, e.g. dermoid cysts, lipomas, neurenteric cysts, teratomas and arachnoid cysts, often associated with spinal dysraphism. Intrathecal

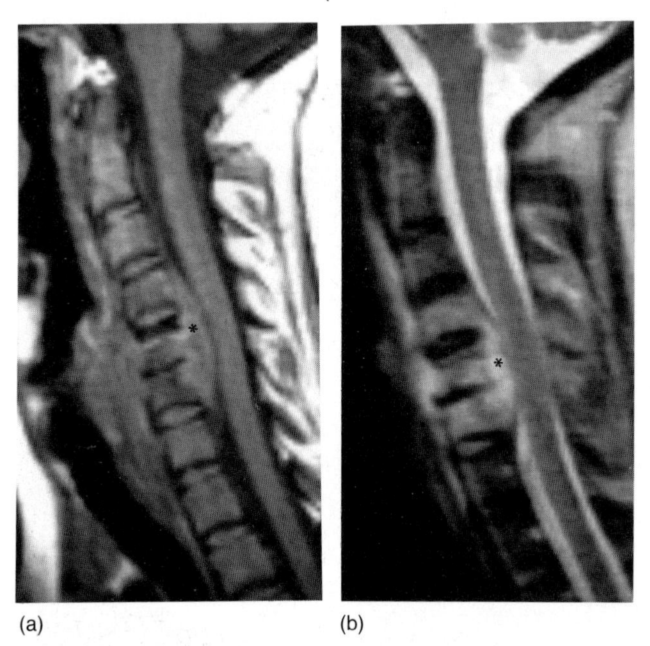

Fig. 11.13 Renal cell carcinoma metastasis of the C4–6 vertebral bodies. (a) Sagittal T1-weighted and (b) T2-weighted MRI demonstrating extradural tumour (✻) compressing the spinal cord. There is signal reduction in the vertebral bodies on the T1-weighted images and corresponding high signal on the T2-weighted images.

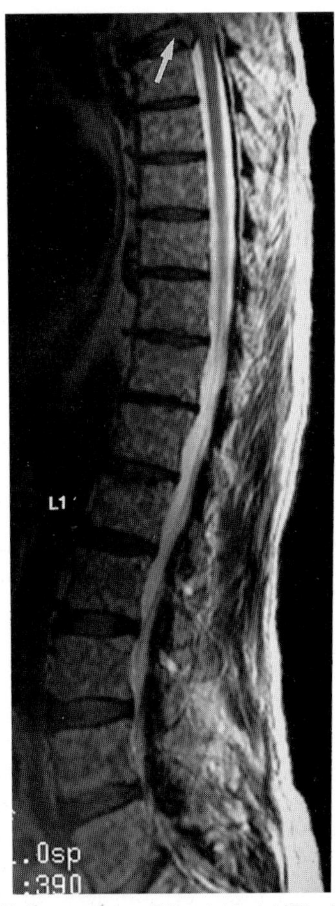

Fig. 11.14 Multiple myeloma. T2-weighted MRI showing extensive patchy destructive changes with heterogeneous signal from the vertebral bodies. There is partial collapse of L1 and collapse of T5 (arrow) with spinal cord compression.

malignant tumours occur as a result of metastatic dissemination of tumour cells shed into the CSF, usually from an intracranial malignant mass in direct contact with the ventricular system or subarachnoid spaces.

Benign tumours

Nerve sheath tumours such as **schwannomas** and **neurofibromas** are the most common benign tumours. They present usually in the third to fifth decades and occur anywhere in the spine, most often the thoracic region. Although usually solitary, multiple lesions may occur particularly in association with neurofibromatosis type I. Approximately 75% of the tumours are intradural in location, 15% are both intra- and extradural ('dumbell') and 10% may be entirely extradural. Pedicular erosion, posterior vertebral body scalloping (which may be localized in relation to tumour) or generalized (due to dural ectasia), kyphoscoliotic deformities and paraspinal soft tissue masses may be seen on plain radiographs, particularly in neurofibromatosis. Malignant degeneration occurs in 5–10% of neurofibromas.

MRI is particularly useful in the assessment of neurofibromas, being ideally suited to demonstrate the intra- and extraspinal components, multiple lesions and any secondary cord changes, e.g. hydrosyringomyelia. The tumours appear as isointense well-circumscribed masses on T1-weighted images and corresponding high signal intensity on T2-weighted images. Strong enhancement with contrast is an almost constant feature.

Meningiomas typically arise in the thoracic spine with a 4:1 female to male preponderance, usually after the fifth decade. Over 90% of the tumours are intradural, the remainder being either 'dumbell' or entirely extradural in nature. As plain films are usually unremarkable, MRI is the most useful imaging technique. These lesions usually appear relatively isointense on both T1- and T2-weighted sequences (Fig. 11.15). Modest contrast enhancement is seen with contrast.

Malignant tumours

This group is largely represented by CSF spread of deposits from bronchogenic or breast carcinoma and non-Hodgkins lymphoma. In children, dissemination occurs from primary neuraxial, especially posterior fossa, tumours such as primitive neurectodermal tumours (PNETs), ependymomas, glioblastoma multiforme and germ cell tumours. The lesions may appear either as nodular masses on the surface of the cord and/or nerve roots, particularly in the region of the cauda equina, or as sheet-like masses over the surface of the cord. Myelography has been superseded by MRI which is more sensitive and much safer, particularly in the presence of intracranial disease. Whilst T2-weighted sequences may provide an excellent

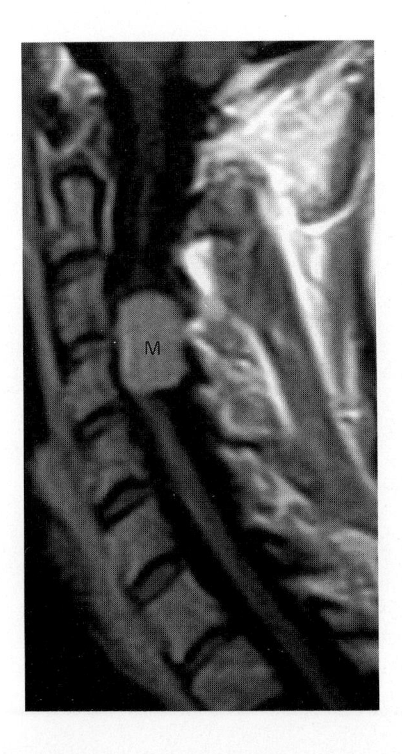

(a)

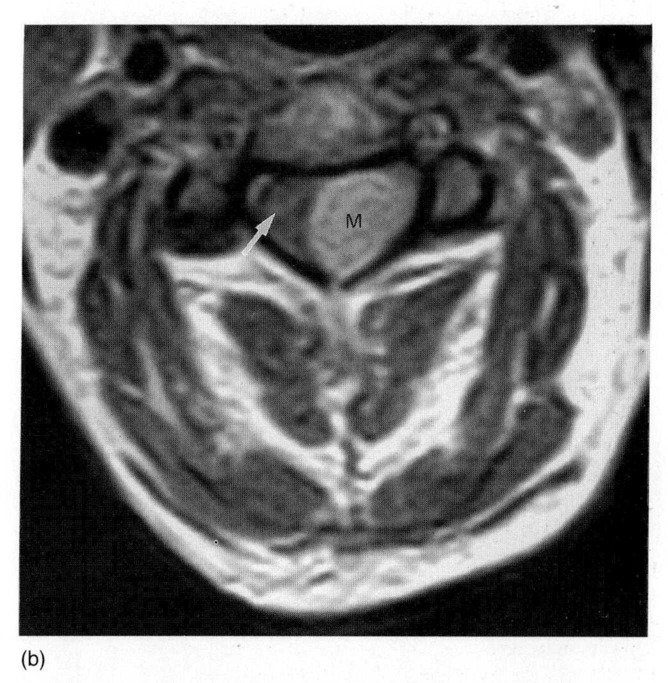

(b)

Fig. 11.15 Left-sided C3/4 meningioma (M) showing mild enhancement on (a) parasagittal and (b) axial T1-weighted MRI. The spinal cord (arrow) is tightly compressed by the tumour.

'myelographic' effect, which may be diagnostic, contrast-enhanced T1-weighted images are more sensitive for the detection of these lesions, particularly the extensive sheet-like lesions coating the cord and nerve roots (Fig. 11.16) which may not be appreciated on T2-weighted images.

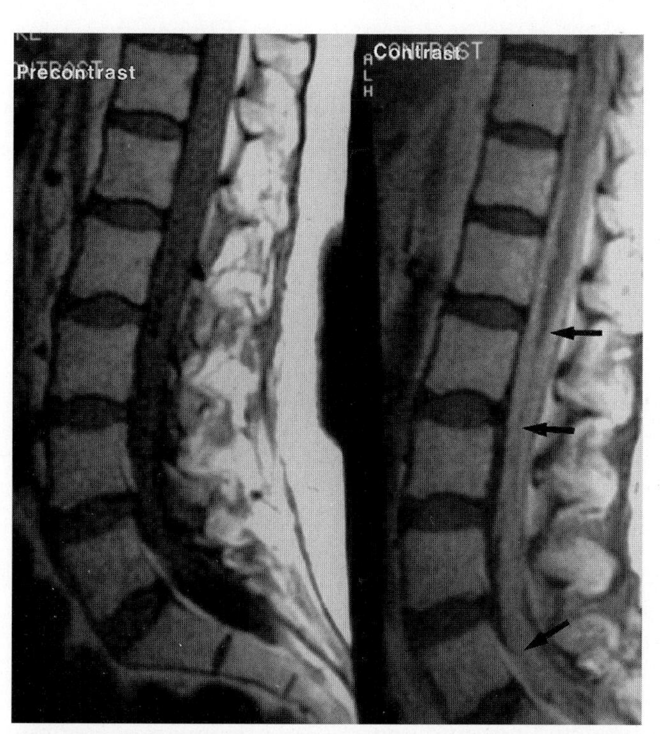

Fig. 11.16 Leptomeningeal metastases. Pre- and postcontrast T1-weighted sagittal MR showing flowing enhancement over the cauda equina (arrows).

INTRAMEDULLARY TUMOURS

Spinal cord gliomas are by far the commonest intramedullary tumours, representing over 90% of this group. Haemangioblastomas and metastases make up most of the remainder. MRI is the imaging modality of choice, demonstrating these lesions with a high degree of sensitivity.

Astrocytomas occur most frequently in children; they are low-grade lesions often extending over many vertebral body segments. The cord is often diffusely expanded, showing hypo- or isointensity on T1-weighted images, hyperintensity on T2-weighted sequences and variable heterogeneous enhancement with contrast. Tumour-related cysts are common. Extension into the brain stem and cerebellar hemispheres is not uncommon in cervical lesions (Fig. 11.17).

Spinal **ependymomas** are the commonest lesions in adults, accounting for 90% of tumours arising in the region of the conus medullaris and filum terminale. As these lesions are slow-growing, focal expansion of the spinal canal may be seen with posterior vertebral body scalloping on plain films. MRI demonstrates a discrete mass related to the conus, isointense with the cord on a T1-weighted sequence and showing marked enhancement on images after contrast. T2-weighted

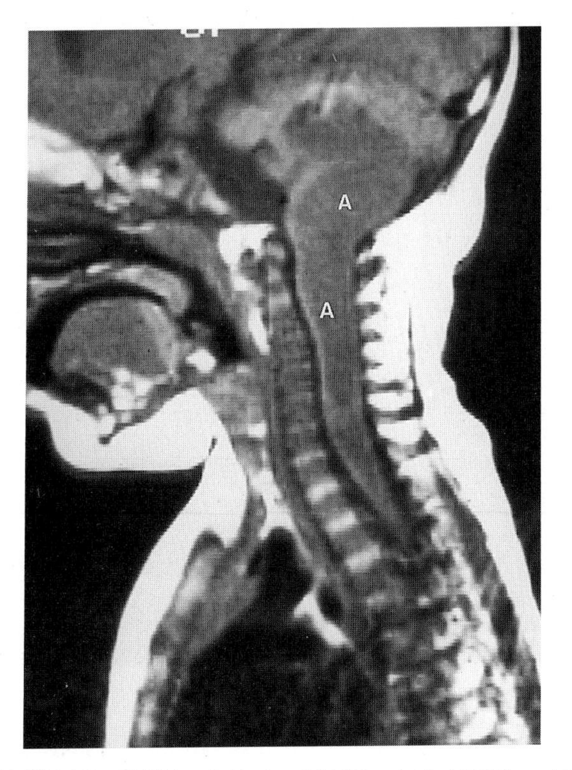

(a)

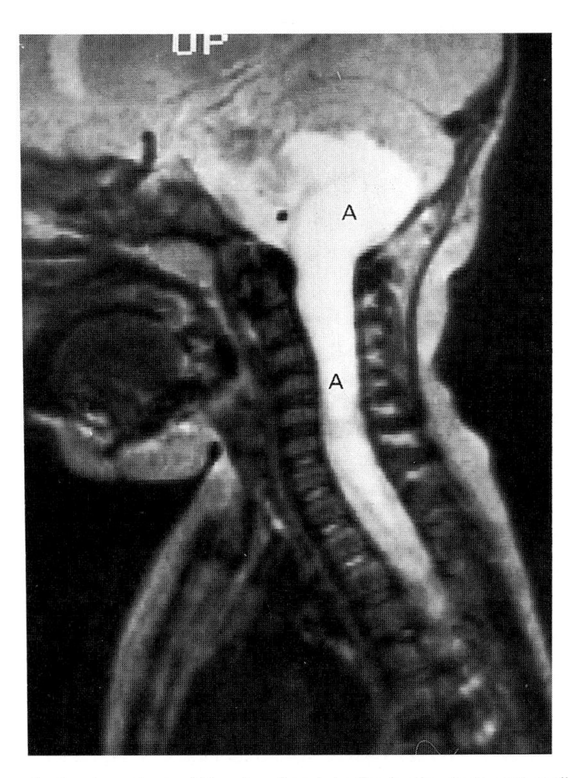

(b)

Fig. 11.17 (a) Sagittal T1-weighted and (b) T2-weighted MRI in a child with a cervical astrocytoma (A) extending into the brain stem, expanding the spinal cord and canal.

(a) (b)

Fig. 11.18 Conus ependymoma. (a) T1-weighted MRI shows the tumour (T). (b) After gadolinium the tumour enhances strongly (arrows) and reveals a cystic component (C) within the tumour.

images often demonstrate stongly hyperintense foci indicating intratumoral cyst formation or haemorrhage (Fig. 11.18).

DEGENERATIVE DISORDERS

Degenerative spinal disorders are the commonest cause of chronic pain and loss of working days in most developed countries. Approximately 60–80% of the adult population will develop low back pain at some point in their lives, although in over 90% of cases it is a self-limiting process, resolving without medical intervention. The effective diagnosis and management of these patients presents a major undertaking with far reaching socioeconomic implications.

Degenerative changes can be recognized on plain films as disc-space narrowing, end-plate sclerosis and osteophyte formation. Although frequently requested, plain films add very little to diagnosis and management as disc protrusion cannot be detected and there is little correlation between the plain film findings and the patient's symptoms. Prior to the era of CT scanning, myelography was the diagnostic mainstay. CT extended diagnostic accuracy,

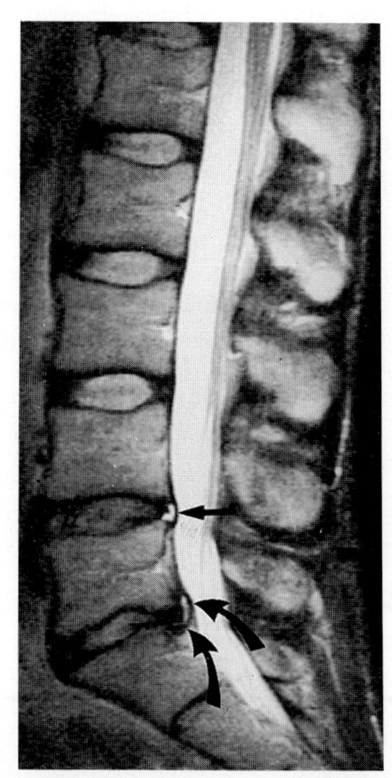

Fig. 11.19 L4/5 and L5/S1 disc degeneration with a posterior annular tear seen as a focal hyperintensity on a sagittal T2-weighted MRI at L4/5 (straight arrow) and a small subligamentous posterior protrusion at L5/S1 (curved arrows).

particularly when used in combination with myelography, and also offered a non-invasive alternative for the assessment of suspected disc herniation and spondylosis in the lumbar region. MRI provides increased sensitivity in the study of degenerative disc disease, in associated thoracic and cervical cord compromise and in the postoperative 'failed back' syndrome.

DISC DEGENERATION AND PROTRUSION

There is a well-recognized age-related pattern of normal disc dehydration and degeneration that commences over the age of 20 years. This is associated with a reduced water-binding capacity of the disc, a reduction of large molecular proteoglycans and progressive disc fibrosis. These changes are best seen with MRI as signal reduction in the disc on T2-weighted images. There may be an accompanying loss of disc height. Lengthening of annular fibres results in diffuse disc bulging. Focal radially orientated tears in the annulus, recognized as small hyperintensities on T2-weighted images (Fig. 11.19) or foci of enhancement on T1-weighted scans, may result in disc herniation. Discal herniations may be contained by the posterior longitudinal ligament (subligamentous) or rupture through the ligament to enter the spinal canal.

Disc protrusions vary from minimal focal disruptions of the posterior annulus to larger posterior, posterolateral or far lateral herniation of disc material (Fig. 11.20). The protruded disc can migrate a considerable distance and become detached (sequestrated) from the parent disc. The vast majority of disc protrusions in the lumbar spine occur at the L4/5 and L5/S1 levels (Fig. 11.21). The region of the conus and lower thoracic spine should, however, be inspected carefully as compressive lesions in this region may

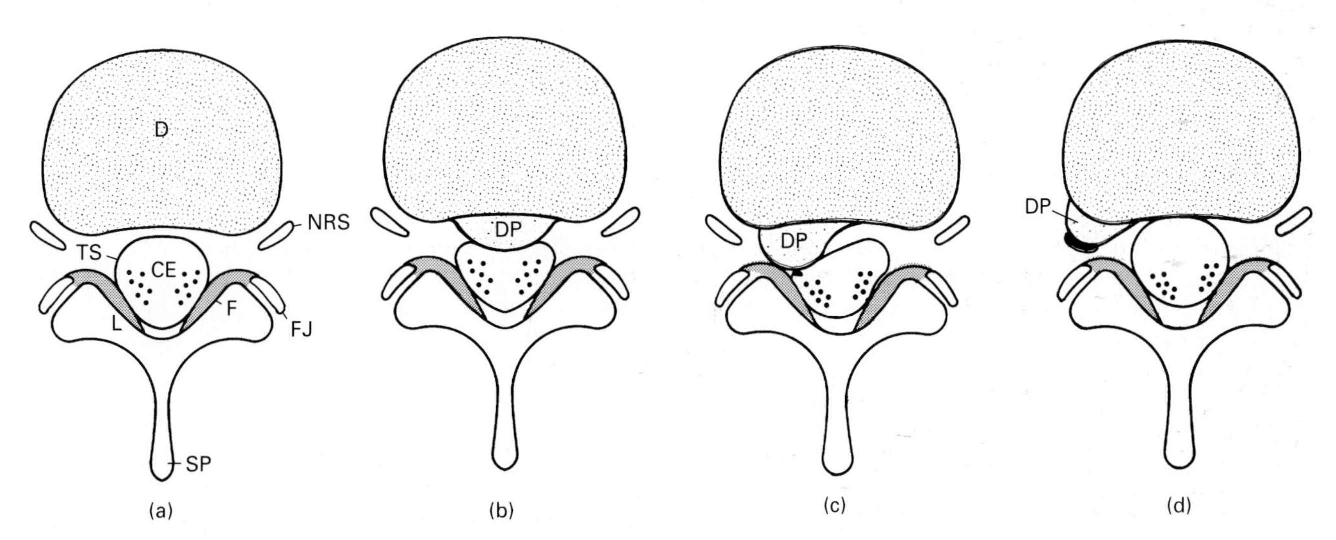

Fig. 11.20 Schematic transverse axial sections taken at the disc space level. (a) Normal where CE=cauda equina; D=intervertebral disc; F=flaval ligament; FJ=facet joint; L=lamina; NRS=nerve root sleeve; SP=spinous process; TS=thecal sac. (b) Central posterior disc protrusion (DP). Disc material indents the thecal sac, however, there is no root compression. (c) Paracentral disc protrusion (DP) compressing the thecal sac and the exiting nerve root just before it enters the nerve root sleeve. (d) Lateral disc protrusion (DP) compressing the nerve root sleeve within the neuroforaminal canal.

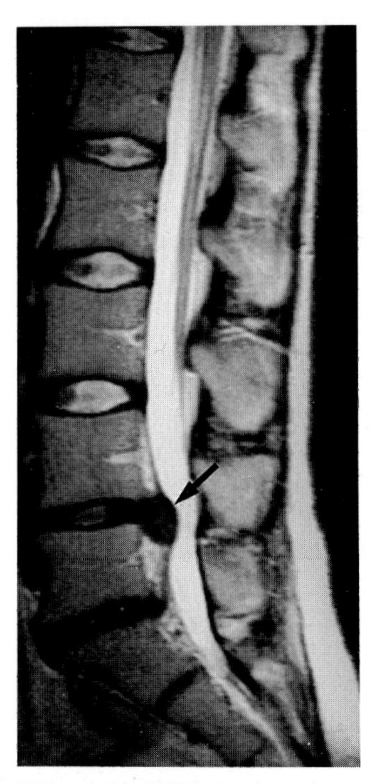

Fig. 11.21 Sagittal T2-weighted MRI showing a large central posterior disc protrusion at L4/5 rupturing through the posterior longitudinal ligament, compressing the thecal sac (arrow). The L5/S1 disc is degenerate and narrowed.

present initially as low back pain. Intraspinal fat encases the thecal sac and exiting nerve root sheaths. Loss of visualization of the fat is a helpful sign in the recognition of subtle or far lateral disc protrusions in the neuroforaminal canal. These lesions cannot be assessed by myelography and are far more sensitively detected by CT or MRI. Over 60% of lumbar disc herniations involve the posterolateral margin of the disc and tend to compress the exiting nerve root. However, it should be noted that disc protrusions are often asymptomatic, particularly when the patient is over 50 years.

Disc protrusions in the thoracic spine are now often identified incidentally during MRI of the spine, particularly in the lower thoracic spine. Whilst most disc protrusions in the thoracolumbar region are degenerative in nature, there is also a significant relationship to trauma.

In the cervical region the intervertebral discs are smaller and assessment of disc status is more difficult. CT-assisted myelography has been regarded as the 'gold standard'; however, improved MR pulse sequences, surface coil design and the ability to obtain thinner slices has increased the sensitivity of MRI. In many centres MRI alone is now considered sufficient for preoperative assessment. Plain films retain a role in correlating osteophytes projecting into the spinal and neuroforaminal canals with the abnormalities demonstrated on MRI, since small bony abnormalities can be difficult to assess with MRI. Plain films are also of value for confirming the vertebral level prior to surgery and assessing the position of metallic fixation devices or bone grafts following surgery. If the MR study is equivocal the patient should be referred for CT or CT-assisted myelography.

Over 90% of protrusions occur at the lower three cervical disc space levels. Central posterior protrusions are readily identified on MRI, indenting the anterior thecal sac and cord. Laterally situated disc protrusions can be more difficult to detect. Associated findings are asymmetrical appearances of the epidural fat and CSF in the lateral part of the spinal canal and in the neuroforaminal canal.

END-PLATE CHANGES

Striking end-plate changes may be seen on MRI in association with disc degeneration, probably resulting from fissuring of the end-plate regions with subsequent ingrowth of granulation tissue (Fig. 11.22). A classification (Modic) has been proposed based upon the MR appearances of the end-plates (Table 11.1).

SPONDYLOSIS AND FACET JOINT ARTHROPATHY

These two conditions are also associated with low back pain. The facet joints are richly innervated and

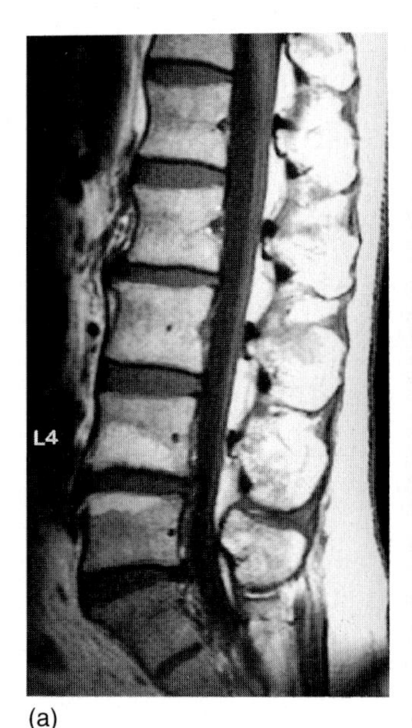

(a)

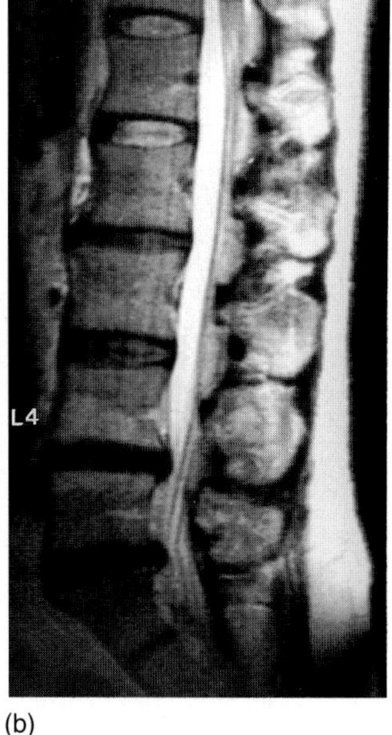

(b)

Fig. 11.22 Type 2 end-plate and marrow changes at L4/5 with (a) high signal on T1-weighted images and (b) mild hyperintensity on T2-weighted MRI. Note the associated disc degeneration, also present in the adjacent discs.

Table 11.1 Modic classification of end plate changes in degenerative disease

Type	*Pathology*	*T1 signal*	*T2 signal*	*Disc signal*	*Enhancement*
Type I	Granulation tissue deposited in end-plates	Low	High	Low	Mild/moderate
Type 2	Granulation tissue replaced by fat	High	Mildly increased	Low	Mild
Type 3	End-plate/marrow sclerosis	Low	Low	Low	None

may give rise to pain when associated with inflammation. There may also be direct compression of the exiting nerve root sheath in the exit canal as a result of facet joint hypertrophy or osteophyte formation. Juxta-articular synovial cysts may occasionally project into the spinal or neuroforaminal exit canal compromising the thecal sac or exiting nerve root. Increased facet joint laxity may lead to degenerative spondylolisthesis, resulting in spinal or exit canal narrowing.

Cervical spondylosis occurs as a consequence of disc degeneration. Posteriorly directed vertebral body osteophytes, often associated with reversal of the normal spinal curvature, impinge upon and compress the spinal cord, resulting in focal hyperintensities on T2-weighted MRI, probably as a consequence of chronic repetitive microtrauma and ischaemic damage (Fig. 11.23). Osteophytes arising from the uncal processes encroach upon the neuroforaminal canal and may compress the exiting nerve root. The degree of compromise of the nerve root may be difficult to assess by MRI. Axial gradient-echo sequences are usually employed but may overestimate the extent of narrowing of the exit canal. Oblique thin slice images may help to assess the exit canals more effectively.

SPINAL CANAL STENOSIS

Acquired or degenerative spinal stenosis is usually caused by a combination of spondylosis, disc bulge/herniation, facet joint and flaval ligament hypertrophy. There is often an underlying predisposition due to constitutional narrowing of the central spinal canal and the lateral recesses. The AP and lateral dimensions of the spinal canal are reduced and the thecal sac is concentrically compressed. CT scanning is particularly well suited to defining the canal dimensions and precise contribution of any associated spondylosis (Fig. 11.24), whereas MRI best defines the

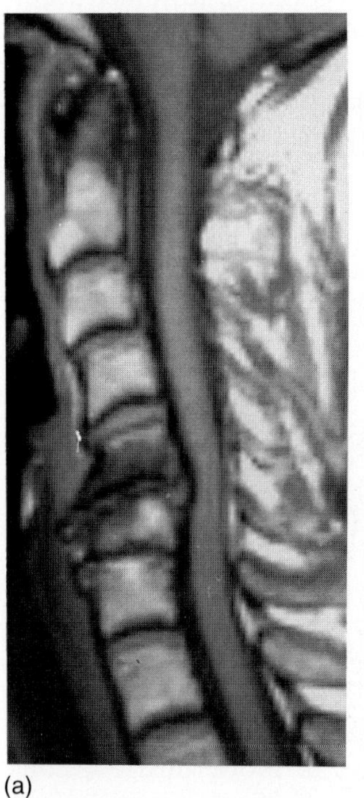
(a)

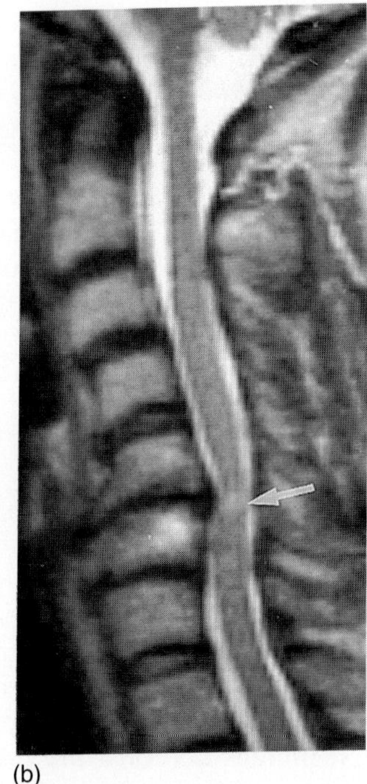
(b)

Fig. 11.23 Cervical spondylosis with localized curvature reversal, osteophytic cord impingement at C5/6 better seen on (a) the T1-weighted MR scan, and focal cord compression and hyperintensity (arrow) indicative of gliosis on (b) the T2-weighted MRI.

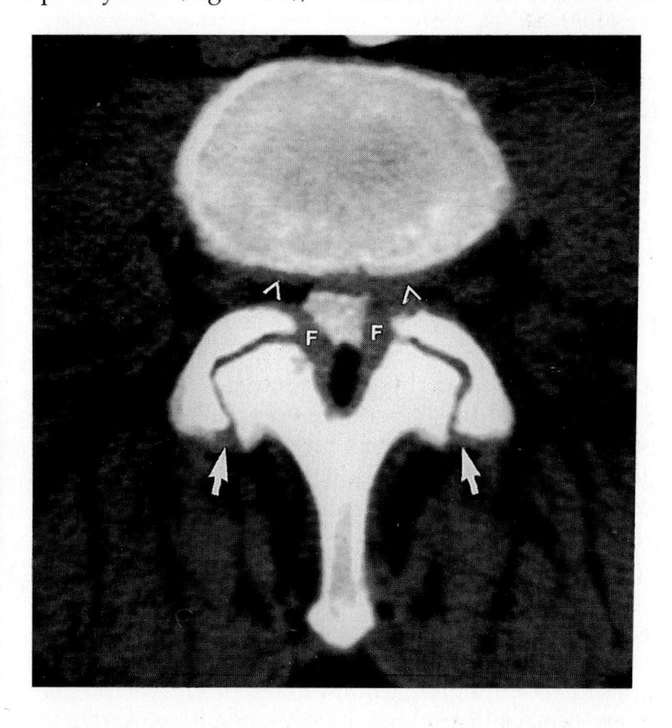

Fig. 11.24 Axial CT following myelography. Focal canal stenosis with large degenerate facet joints (arrows), thickened ligamenta flava (F) and posterior annular disc bulge (arrowheads) compressing the opacified thecal sac.

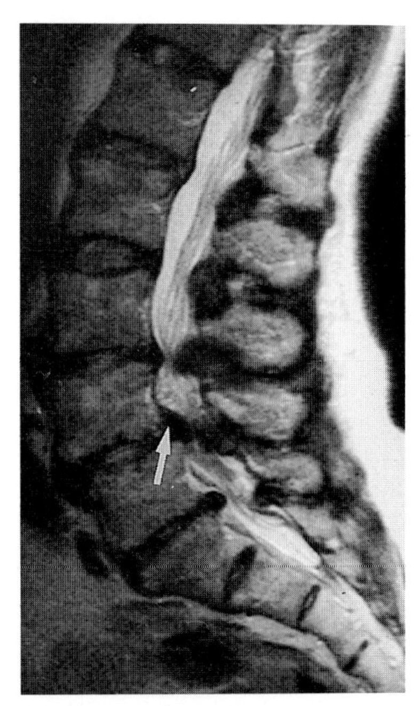

Fig. 11.25 Lower lumbar canal stenosis associated with a degenerative spondylolisthesis at L4/5 (arrow). Sagittal T2-weighted MRI showing anterior and posterior compression of the thecal sac and poor visualization of the CSF.

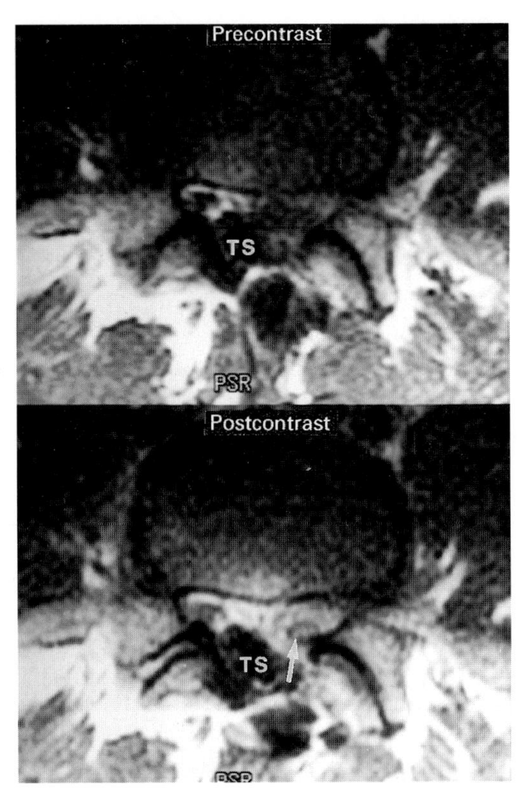

Fig. 11.26 Pre- and postcontrast T1-weighted axial MRI at L4/5 demonstrating enhancing postoperative scar tissue surrounding the proximal left L5 root sheath (arrow). Note some compression of the thecal sac (TS) has occurred.

degree of cord or thecal sac compression and the number of disc space levels involved (Fig. 11.25). In the cervical spine, ossification of the posterior longitudinal ligament may contribute towards the overall degree of spinal canal narrowing.

Spinal canal stenosis in the thoracic region is relatively uncommon; however, when present, it is not infrequently associated with calcification or ossification of the ligamenta flava and/or hypertrophy of the articular facet joints. These changes are particularly well demonstrated by CT-assisted myelography. MRI now offers a more acceptable non-invasive alternative.

FAILED BACK SYNDROME

Recurrent signs or symptoms following spinal surgery constitute a difficult diagnostic and therapeutic dilemma. Common causes are recurrent disc protrusion at the operative level or another disc space, extradural fibrosis and scarring which may involve a nerve root sheath, nerve root inflammation, arachnoiditis, spinal canal stenosis, facet joint arthropathy, discitis or extradural abscess. In the first few weeks following surgery, soft-tissue swelling, extradural haematoma and residual disc fragments or protrusions are commonly encountered. In the subacute and chronic phase the principal differential diagnosis to be made is between residual/recurrent disc protrusion and postsurgical scarring. MRI can be of great help particularly when T1-weighted images are employed before and after intravenous contrast administration. Protruded disc material tends to show some mass effect and variable degrees of rim enhancement. Scar tissue may or may not produce mass effect but enhancement following contrast administration is often intense (Fig. 11.26).

End-plate changes are not usually seen following uncomplicated disc surgery. High signal intensity on T2-weighted or STIR sequences with corresponding signal loss on T1-weighted images should alert the physician to the possibility of infection, particularly if enhancement is seen following contrast administration.

INFLAMMATION AND INFECTION

INFLAMMATION

Inflammatory processes affecting the spinal cord are mostly due to multiple sclerosis, transverse myelitis and neurosarcoidosis. In multiple sclerosis T2-weighted images demonstrate focal or more diffuse lesions of high signal intensity (Fig. 11.27). Solitary lesions presenting acutely may simulate a cord tumour; however, lesion multiplicity is more common. Demonstration of further lesions in the brain helps to confirm

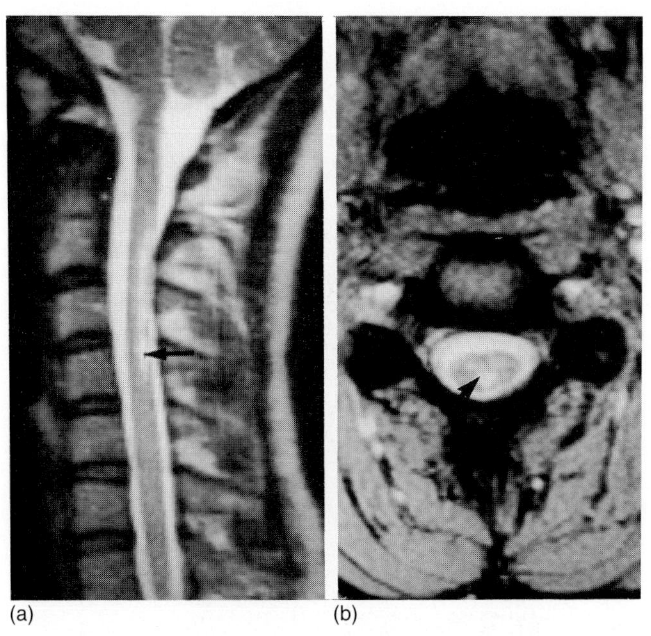

Fig. 11.27 Demyelinating plaque in the upper cervical cord shown on (a) sagittal and (b) axial T2-weighted MRI. The high signal intensity plaque (arrow) is situated centrally in the dorsal aspect of the cord.

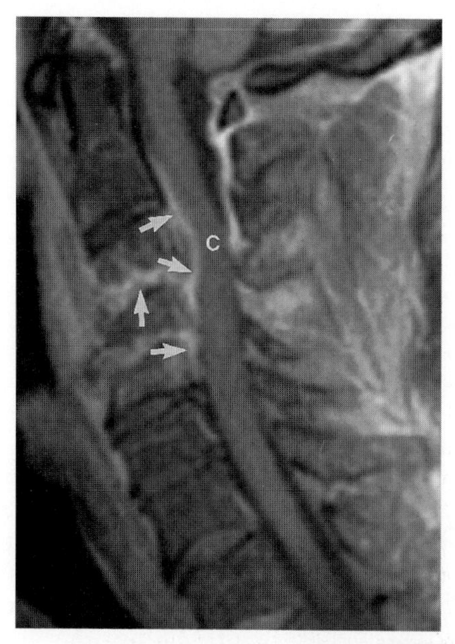

Fig. 11.28 Vertebral osteomyelitis and discitis. Postcontrast T1-weighted MRI showing infected tissue which is enhancing (arrows), extending into the anterior epidural compartment and compressing the spinal cord (C).

the diagnosis of multiple sclerosis. Acute transverse myelitis is usually identified by more diffuse cord expansion extending over several vertebral body segments. There may be moderate to marked enhancement with contrast making differentiation from tumour difficult. Cord atrophy is invariably a late feature.

Leptomeningeal thickening and enhancement is seen with sarcoidosis or malignant pachymeningitis. Cord involvement with peripheral enhancing cord lesions may also be seen with sarcoidosis.

INFECTION

Infection may involve the vertebral bodies, discovertebral complexes, epidural space, leptomeninges or spinal cord.

Infection of the vertebral bodies (**spondylitis** or **vertebral osteomyelitis**) often coexists with discal infection. In children infection usually commences in the richly vascular disc and then spreads to the vertebral body. The subchondral portion of the vertebral body is more typically affected in the adult with subsequent infection of the rest of the vertebral body and the adjacent disc. The course of discitis is more benign in children than in adults. A wide variety of pathogens may be involved, with *Staphylococcus aureus*, Enterobacteriaceae and *Escherichia coli* being most common. Plain radiographs are frequently normal in the acute phase; disc space narrowing and end-plate irregularities occuring after 1–2 weeks. Radionuclide scanning previously had an important role in the diagnosis of these lesions. However, MRI is considerably more sensitive and demonstrates the disease at a very early stage. The narrowed disc appears hyperintense on T2-weighted images as does the adjacent vertebral body. Contrast administration may demonstrate subligamentous or epidural spread (Fig. 11.28). Tuberculous spondylitis is characterized by greater bony destruction, more frequent involvement of the posterior vertebral body elements, large paraspinal soft-tissue masses (which frequently calcify late in the disease), severe end-stage kyphoscoliotic deformities and relative sparing of the intervertebral disc. All these features can be recognized on plain films. The onset and subsequent progress of the disease is more insidious than that of pyogenic spondylitis.

Epidural abscesses are uncommon, occurring by haematogenous spread or following spinal puncture or penetrating injuries. *Staphylococcus aureus* is the most common pathogen. The abscess may involve several vertebral body segements and is frequently associated with discitis or vertebral body osteomyelitis. MRI shows a mass compressing the thecal sac and cord. T2-weighted images show variable hyperintensity depending on the degree of liquefaction and pus formation as well as any vertebral body/disc involvement.

Leptomeningeal infection most frequently occurs as a consequence of pyogenic cerebral meningitis or secondary to infected spinal dysraphic lesions such as dermal sinuses. Postcontrast T1-weighted MRI may show enhancement over the surface of the cord and nerve roots particularly in the cauda equina or enhancing nodular filling defects.

VASCULAR LESIONS

Vascular lesions affecting the spine are relatively uncommon. The two main pathologies are vascular malformations and spinal cord ischaemia/infarction.

VASCULAR MALFORMATIONS

Most spinal vascular malformations are intradural arteriovenous malformations, of which 40% occur within the cord, or arteriovenous fistulae, which are predominantly dural in location. They occur most frequently in the thoracic region. Myelography has been the basis for the detection of these lesions; however, MRI is now considered to be superior, not only for their diagnosis but also for the assessment of any associated cord damage. MRI identifies serpiginous filling defects representing the tortuous arterialized draining veins as flow voids or as enhancing structures following contrast administration. MRI demonstrates the secondary effects of vascular steal or chronic venous hypertension which may appear as cord swelling or atrophy (Fig. 11.29). Spinal angiography is definitive and mandatory for operative or endovascular treatment (Fig. 11.30). An extensive search for all the feeding arteries is required as well as identification of the normal spinal arterial anatomy, specifically the artery of Adamkiewicz in the thoracic region.

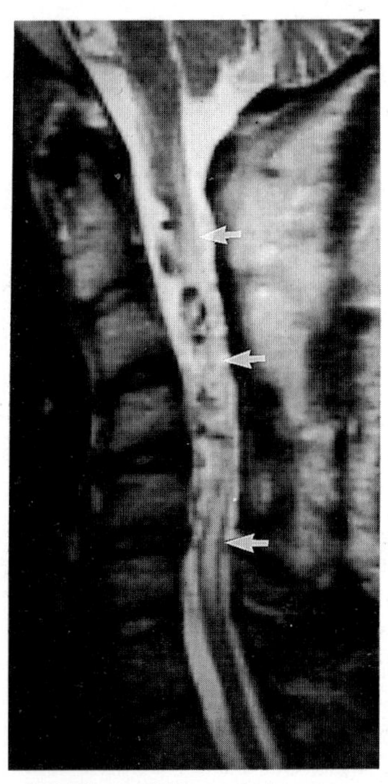

Fig. 11.29 Cervical intramedullary arteriovenous malformation. Sagittal T2-weighted MRI defines serpiginous signal voids indicative of vessels. The spinal cord is atrophic and demonstrates extensive high signal (arrows) representing chronic ischaemic damage and congestive myelopathy.

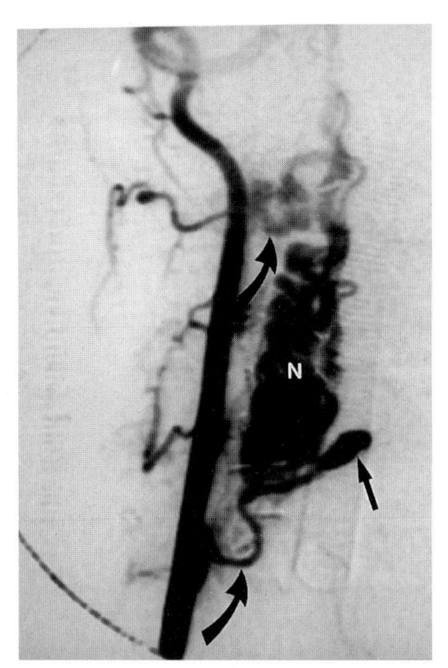

Fig. 11.30 Arteriovenous malformation of cervical cord. Selective vertebral angiography shows a compact nidus (N) fed by several branch arteries (curved arrows) with a small flow related aneurysm (arrow).

The increased use of MRI has resulted in the detection of cavernous haemangiomas, which cannot be demonstrated by angiography. Cavernous haemangiomas account for approximately 30% of all spinal vascular malformations and may be asymptomatic incidental findings, particularly when associated with multiple lesions in the brain. However, they may present with progressive painful cord dysfunction particularly if there has been haemorrhage into the lesion.

CORD ISCHAEMIA AND INFARCTION

Severe atherosclerotic disease, aortic dissection and aortic or spinal surgery are usually responsible for cord ischaemia or infarction. Clinical presentation is often acute with para- or tetraparesis, with or without accompanying pain. Vascular watershed areas between the major arterial territories are most frequently affected, specifically the cervicothoracic junction and lower thoracic cord. MRI may demonstrate focal cord expansion and hyperintensity on T2-weighted images with subsequent progression to late cord atrophy. Chronic venous ischaemia occurs not infrequently with vascular malformations; however, acute venous infarction may follow partial or complete spontaneous thrombosis of an underlying vascular malformation with vascular flow voids accompanying a swollen cord.

CONGENITAL DISORDERS

Developmental abnormalities of the spine are generically known as spinal dysraphism. The basic defect is abnormal formation or fusion of neural (myeloschisis) and mesenchymal (spina bifida) elements in early gestation. The majority of these abnormalities occur in the lumbosacral region. MRI has now become the imaging modality of choice for this group of lesions, but spinal ultrasound in the first few months of life may be a useful screening tool and CT-assisted myelography may be of use in certain cases. There are three major types of lesions: spina bifida aperta, cystica and occulta.

OPEN SPINAL DYSRAPHISM (SPINA BIFIDA APERTA)

This group is represented by the incomplete closure of the neural tube with exposure of neural tissue which may lie flush to the skin (**myelocoele**) or is elevated by an underlying herniating CSF sac (**myelomeningocoele**). Both are associated with wide defects in the posterior neural arches of contiguous vertebrae. Varying degrees of kyphoscoliosis are often seen. Presentation at birth is with an exposed lesion which usually requires primary repair. Secondary dysraphic lesions are not uncommon, particularly diastematomyelia (see below) with an almost invariable presence of a Chiari II malformation and various congenital intracranial abnormalites. Hydrocephalus frequently develops following closure of the defect.

CLOSED SKIN COVERED CYSTIC MASS (SPINA BIFIDA CYSTICA)

The commonest lesion in this group is the **lipomyelomeningocoele** in which there is a large lipomatous mass continuous with the subcutaneous fat. This is associated with herniation of a CSF sac, containing spinal cord, into which the lipomatous mass enters and merges. Multiple posterior neural arch defects are present and in 30–50% of cases a distal cord hydrosyrinx develops.

OCCULT SPINAL DYSRAPHISM (SPINA BIFIDA OCCULTA)

This group contains a wide spectrum of abnormalities and represents the most commonly encountered lesions. The skin is intact but there may be cutaneous stigmata such as a hairy patch, haemangioma or deep skin pit. In many cases there is little or no neurological deficit or associated spinal deformity and these patients often escape detection during life. Symptomatic patients tend to present in late childhood or

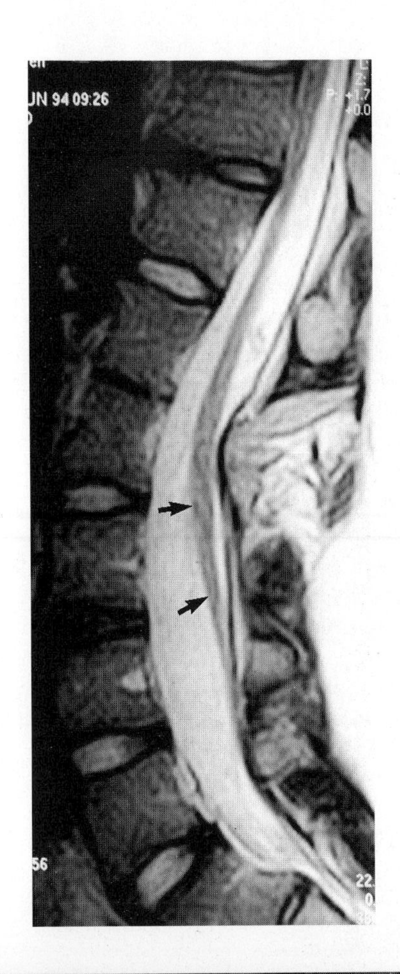

(a)

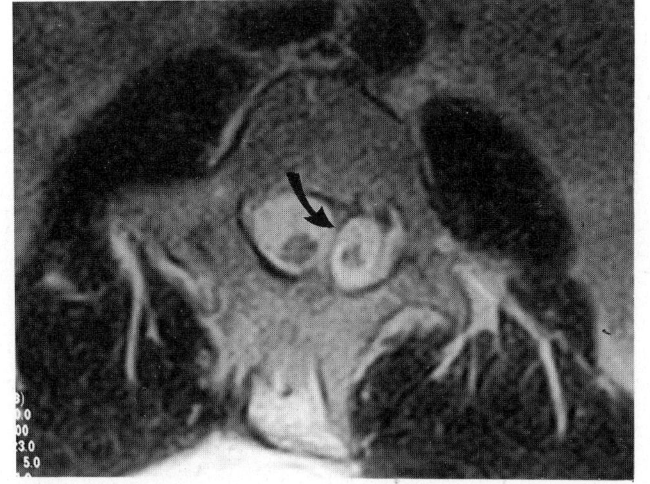

(b)

Fig. 11.31 Dual arachnoid-dural sac diastematomyelia demonstrated on (a) sagittal and (b) axial T2-weighted MRI. The spinal cord extends down to the lower border of L3 (arrows) with a complex posterior neural arch defect at L2. Note the bony spur interposed between the two sacs and hemicords (curved arrow).

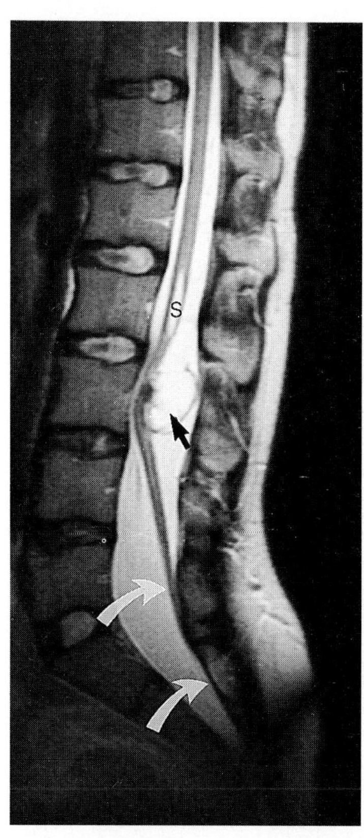

Fig. 11.32 Sagittal T2-weighted MRI showing a low spinal cord tethered by a thickened filum terminale (curved arrows). An intraspinal dermoid cyst (arrow) is also present and there is a slender high signal syrinx (S) in the cord.

early adulthood with a wide range of problems including pes cavus, leg length inequality, lower limb and sphincter dysfunction or progressive spinal deformity. **Diastematomyelia** is the partial or complete splitting of the spinal cord and associated clefting abnormalities of the vertebral bodies and posterior neural arches. The pial lined split 'hemicords' may be contained within a single arachnoid-dural tube or each hemicord may lie within its own arachnoid-dural envelope (Fig. 11.31). The latter type has a fibrous or bony spur interposed between the two hemicords and is more frequently symptomatic. The cord is tethered and secondary hydrosyringomyelia develops in over 50% of the cases. A thickened filum terminale is often present, further tethering the cord distally.

Other lesions include a simple thickened filum terminale (which may contain a lipoma) often tethering a low lying spinal cord (Fig. 11.32); dorsal dermal sinus (an epithelial lined tract that extends from the skin surface to the spinal column, thecal sac or into the sac to merge with a low spinal cord) and intraspinal lipoma (a fatty mass intimately related to the dorsal aspect of the cord and tethering the cord to the thecal sac).

In all these conditions imaging attempts to demonstrate the defect prior to possible surgery and to define any features such as tethering of the spinal cord, cord cavitation or intraspinal sepsis due to communication with the skin or bowel.

CHAPTER 12

Skeletal trauma

Sarah Burnett
and Asif Saifuddin

Rather than give an exhaustive description of all fractures, we provide general principles of skeletal trauma, followed by a section devoted to specific fractures. We attempt to illustrate these principles with examples of classic fractures. (Spinal trauma is covered in Chapter 11).

An X-ray is not the most important aspect of the evaluation of a case of trauma. A carefully performed physical examination and the taking of a precise history to determine the mechanism of injury should precede any decision to image. It is essential to understand the common patterns of injury and their associations. Successful treatment starts with an accurate diagnosis and an X-ray must be well performed and accurately interpreted. Therefore, the patient should be stablized and possible fractures splinted in order to reduce morbidity and ease patient handling. Radiographs should, where possible, be performed in two planes and include the bone ends. Most fractures are readily identified on the plain film, but subtle evidence may be overlooked and serious injuries may even occur in the absence of radiographic findings. A search for specific signs on the film will be more accurate than a general viewing and soft-tissue clues can point to the site of injury. Direct searching will lead to easier recognition, confident interpretation and a correct diagnosis.

The location, nature and number of fractures is dependent on the age of the individual and the nature and severity of trauma. The skeleton is weak when immature, increases in strength in adulthood, and is again weakened by age and underlying disease, both local and systemic. Hence the same mechanism of injury will produce different fractures at different ages. For example, the fall on an outstretched hand in a child may produce a greenstick fracture of the radius, in an adult a fractured scaphoid, and in an elderly or osteopenic patient may result in a Colles' fracture.

CLASSIFICATION OF FRACTURES

Fractures are described and classified by the extent, direction, position, number of fracture lines and integrity of the overlying skin. In a long bone, the precise position within the bone should be described.

Diagnostic and Interventional Radiology in Surgical Practice. Edited by P. Armstrong and M. L. Wastie. Published in 1997 by Chapman & Hall, London. ISBN 0 412 61960 1 (HB), 0 412 61970 9 (PB)

A **complete** fracture implies discontinuity between two or more fragments of bone. Where part of the cortex remains intact the fracture is described as **incomplete**. The latter is more common in children, where the cortex bends, and is termed a **greenstick** fracture. If the overlying skin is intact the fracture is **closed**; if there is a skin breach then it is **open** or **compound**. This may occasionally be identified radiologically by bone protruding through the skin, or the presence of air in the adjacent soft tissues on the immediate postinjury film.

Direction is determined in relation to the long axis of the bone, and the location is stated in terms of its anatomical relationship. The shafts of long bones are conventionally divided into thirds. **Transverse** fractures may occur because of a direct blow, but are uncommon and are likely to be pathological. **Oblique** fractures result from a compressive force, with or without angulation, and are very common. A **spiral** fracture results from torque around the shaft of a long bone, and is usually associated with some compression, resulting in the ends of the fracture being more obliquely orientated. **Vertical** fractures occur from vertical loading and are rare but may occur as a component of a comminuted fracture. A **comminuted** fracture refers to more than two fragments. **Avulsion** fractures occur when a fragment of bone is pulled away from its origin by a ligament or tendon, and is defined by the site of insertion. Sharpey's fibres are sufficiently strong that the bone may yield before the soft tissue, particularly in children. Avulsion injury results from an indirectly applied force and is often a marker for more serious soft-tissue injury.

A fracture involving the end of the bone often extends into the joint or is limited to the joint surface, in which case it is termed an **intra-articular** fracture. It can be oblique, resulting from excessive angulation, and oblique views may be necessary to demonstrate this extension. A comminuted intra-articular fracture becomes impacted, and an **osteochondral fracture** results when shearing or rotational forces are applied. The osteochondral fragment is often entirely cartilaginous and cannot therefore be identified on plain films. It can subsequently cause problems as a loose body and, if radiolucent, can be identified with MRI. Injury may involve the joint capsule, internal structure, ligaments or tendons, without bony abnormality.

Displacement of one bone relative to the apposing bone at a joint is termed dislocation, subluxation or diastasis, and is defined by the movement of the distal bone relative to the proximal. **Dislocation** is defined as complete loss of continuity at a joint surface, while **subluxation** is partial loss of continuity. **Diastasis** is displacement of bone in relation to the apposing bone in a normally minimally mobile joint. This separation may involve either a fibrous or cartilaginous joint and is sometimes associated with fracture of one of the involved bones.

Stress fractures happen in otherwise normal bone due to repeated activities. There is usually no history of an acute injury and X-rays may be normal initially. A radionuclide bone scan (Fig. 12.1) may however be positive at this stage, and may reveal an occult contralateral fracture. At 10 days to 3 weeks a transverse or oblique radiolucency can be identified on the plain films. Other changes include a periosteal reaction (Fig. 12.2) and endosteal sclerosis, and the differential diagnosis includes an osteoid osteoma, osteomalacia, Paget's disease, osteomyelitis or a malignant neoplasm. A history of repeated physical activity and occurrence in a characteristic site should lead to the correct diagnosis. It is important to diagnose a stress fracture as continued athletic activity can result in conversion to a frank fracture. If clinical suspicion remains high and the plain film or bone scan findings are confusing, then a CT may demonstrate the characteristic linear appearance of the fracture line.

Stress fractures are particularly common in runners; occurring in the second or third metatarsals; the so called **march** fracture is the most common stress fracture (Fig. 12.2). It is undisplaced and not visible until 7–10 days when early callus formation or periosteal reaction is seen. In the distal fibula a stress fracture will occur 3–7 cm from the tip of the fibula and, rarely, fractures of the junction of the pubis and

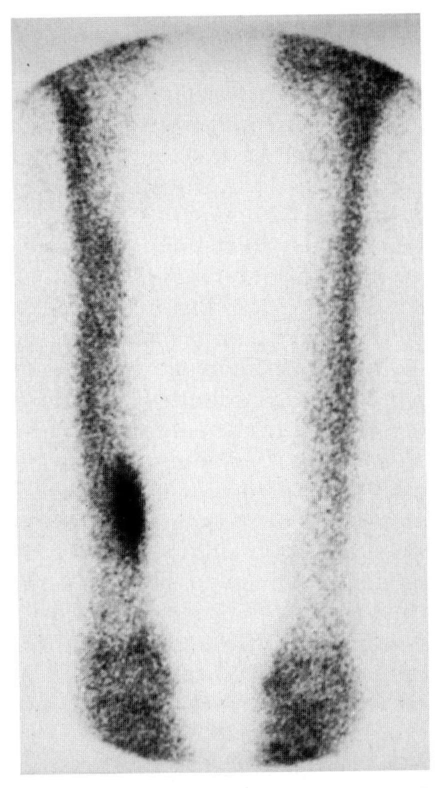

Fig. 12.1 ^{99m}Tc-MDP bone scan. A stress fracture is indicated by the area of increased uptake in the distal right tibia.

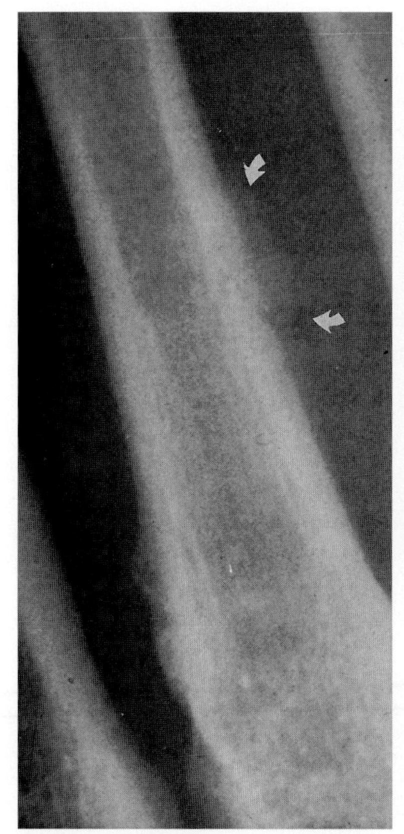

Fig. 12.2 AP view of the metatarsal. The curved arrows indicate a localized area of fluffy periosteal reaction around a march fracture in the third toe metatarsal.

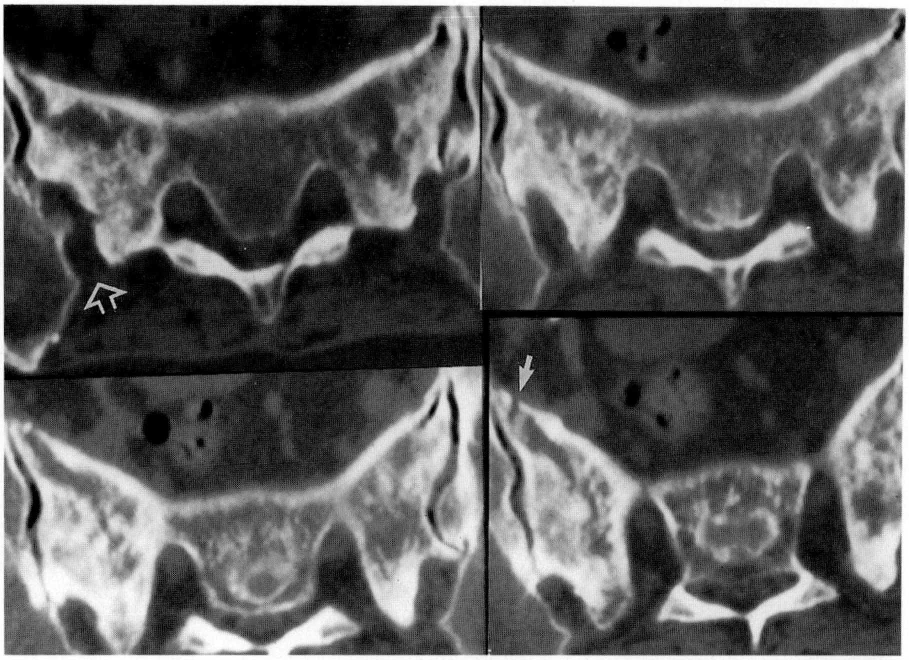

Fig. 12.3 CT scan of sacrum. An insufficiency fracture is present in the right sacral ala of this elderly woman. The open arrow demonstrates an area of sacroiliac joint diastasis posteriorly and the closed arrow shows the position where the fracture breaches the anterior sacral cortex.

ischium can be seen in female marathon runners. Horizontal stress fractures of the navicula and vertical stress fractures of the calcaneum are seen in joggers. Another common site for a stress fracture is the proximal tibial shaft; in runners, gymnasts and dancers, they occur in the posterior or anterior cortex and can be seen as a dense periosteal reaction.

An **insufficiency** fracture is the result of normal activity in a weakened bone, commonly from osteoporosis or osteomalacia, or in the elderly. It can also be the result of trivial trauma. Common sites are the tibia, fibula, femoral neck, sacrum (Fig. 12.3), and again march fractures are seen.

Insufficiency fractures occur characteristically in the sacrum due to osteoporosis, and are usually vertical. They are seen as a dense line, parallel to the sacroiliac joint. They are difficult to see and thus frequently missed, although they are readily evident on bone scan or CT. Insufficiency fractures of the pubic rami are also common. In the presence of marked osteoporosis, the fracture line may expand and resemble infection or neoplasm. Pubic rami fractures may mimic the clinical findings of a fractured neck of femur.

In the ribs, insufficiency fractures may result from coughing. These may, on occasion, produce confusion on bone scans performed for the evaluation of diffuse metastatic disease, but with insufficiency fractures, like conventional traumatic rib fractures, the hot spots characteristically occur in a vertical line running across several ribs.

A **pathological** fracture is a fracture occurring at a site of abnormal bone. It can be due to either a focal or generalized process, e.g. rheumatoid arthritis. Both lytic and sclerotic bone abnormalities can fracture; distorted trabecular anatomy will weaken even dense bone. Outside the spine, the most common cause of a pathological fracture is a metastasis (Fig. 12.4), and clues to the presence of an underlying lesion are thinning of the cortex, expansion, bone destruction and the presence of a transverse fracture line. Common primary sites for metastases are breast, responsible for more than half of all metastatic pathological fractures, prostate, lung, kidney and thyroid, and the proximal axial skeleton is predominantly affected. The most frequent primary bone lesion to produce a pathological fracture is myeloma. The presence of a pathological fracture does not imply that a neoplastic process is malignant, as fractures occur from many benign lesions.

Other causes of pathological fracture include osteoporosis, osteomalacia, neuropathy, Paget's disease and osteogenesis imperfecta.

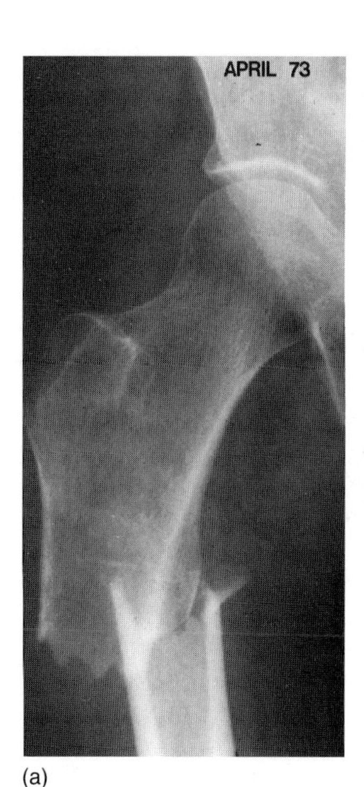

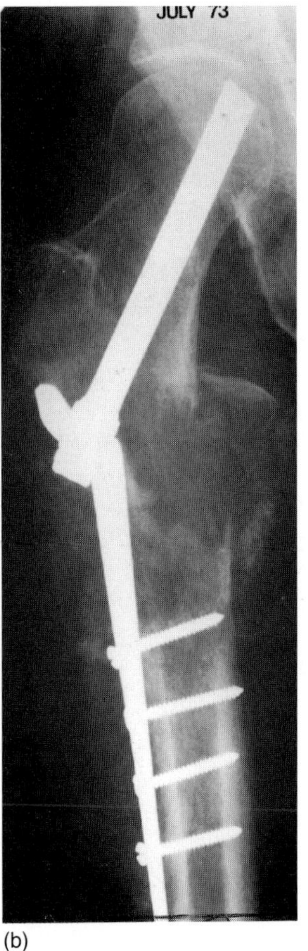

(a) (b)

Fig. 12.4 (a) AP view of right hip. A transverse fracture is seen of the proximal femoral shaft. There is some ill-defined lucency in the proximal fragment but the suspicious nature of the fracture cannot be identified with certainty. (b) Three months later, following internal fixation, a large lytic lesion is now evident at the site of the previous fracture. The patient had a primary renal carcinoma.

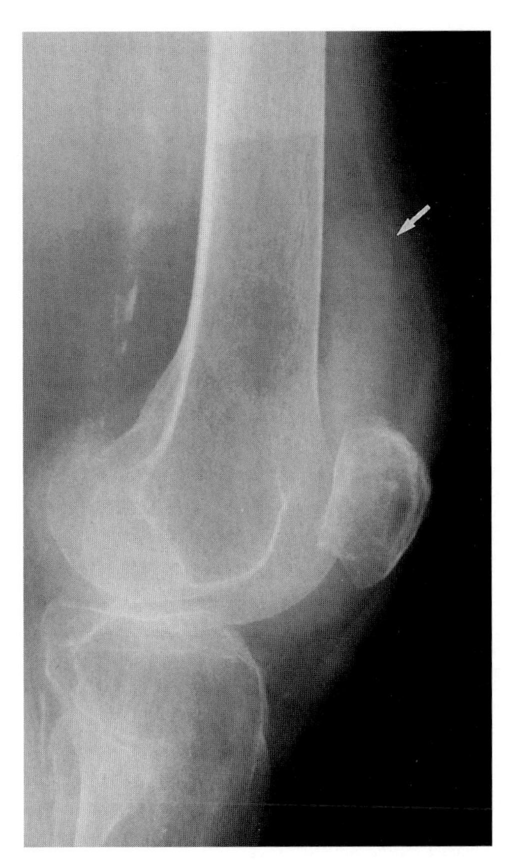

Fig. 12.5 Horizontal beam film of knee. Although the tibial plateau fracture is not identifiable on this lateral film, the fat–fluid level in the suprapatellar pouch is clearly seen (arrow).

SIGNS OF FRACTURE

A fracture is a discontinuity in bone. On X-rays this is shown as an **abnormal line of radiolucency**, the width of which is dependent on the degree of displacement. The clarity of the line is dependent on the alignment of the beam, and therefore two views in orthogonal planes (at 90° to each other) are mandatory, whenever practical. Most commonly these views will be antero-posterior and lateral; 90% of fractures are identified on both views, while 5% will be visible on one view alone, and a further 5% only identified on special views or further imaging techniques. A fracture may also be evidenced by **irregularity of the cortex** or an angular projection or distortion in the flare of the metaphysis, for example the torus fracture (p. 298) in children. An abnormal line of radiopacity may be seen where fracture fragments over-ride each other. There may be disruption of certain anatomical lines or angles as described in more detail later in this chapter.

The soft tissues may provide clues to the presence of a fracture. Oedema or haemorrhage can lead to displacement or effacement of fascial planes or the presence of an effusion. These lucent lines are due to the fat in normal fascial planes. In the chest, a pleural effusion, pneumothorax or lung contusion can result from a rib fracture; indeed exclusion of these complications is the main purpose of performing a chest film in cases of suspected rib fracture. Free intraperitoneal air or fluid may result from perforation of a viscus by a fracture fragment. When there has been an intra-articular fracture medullary fat can enter the joint creating a fat–fluid level seen on a horizontal beam X-ray; the finding of such a lipohaemarthrosis should lead to renewed vigour in searching the film for a fracture (Fig. 12.5).

NORMAL VARIANTS MIMICKING FRACTURE

A number of normal variants and radiographic phenomena can occur which may mimic a fracture. The lucent component of a joint may be projected through an adjacent bone and look like a fracture site. The **'Mach' effect** occurs where two bones overlap, a line of lucency closely parallels the periphery of the cortex of one of the bones. This is, effectively, an optical illusion as the eye tends to enhance the inherent contrast between the radiographic densities. It is seen commonly in the ankle and the wrist and may be mistaken for an undisplaced fracture. Further views, possibly including an oblique view, should confirm or refute the presence of genuine pathology.

Unfused ossicles and **apophyses** are seen in many sites, classically around the foot and ankle; for example, the os trigonum is often seen posterior to the talus, the os peroneum by the cuboid, and the os tibiale externum adjacent to the navicula. These may be confused with fracture fragments but are more rounded, have a distinct cortical margin and may often be symmetrical. They occur in characteristic positions and are therefore readily recognizable. Serious clinical confusion arises when the diagnosis of a fracture has important clinical consequences, such as the os odontoideum, an unfused ossicle at the tip of the odontoid peg. A further site that may cause confusion with a fracture is the unfused apophysis at the base of the fifth metatarsal (Fig. 12.6); the apophysis shows a vertical plane of cleavage, whilst a fracture line is horizontal. The patella and sesamoid bones may be bipartite or multipartite. If doubt persists, a reference text of normal variants, such as Theodore Keats' *Atlas of Normal Roentgen Variants that may Simulate Disease* (6th edn, 1996, Year Book Medical Publ., St Louis, Missouri), should be consulted.

SPECIAL CONSIDERATIONS IN CHILDREN

The young, although accident-prone, are both more agile and more flexible and therefore less likely to injure themselves. The forces generated in an accident are not as great because children and infants weigh less and their shorter stature reduces leverage. The skeleton of the young individual is less brittle because it contains a higher percentage of water. Also the periosteum is thicker and more elastic; therefore, it is more likely to remain attached to the fragments and act as a hinge, which helps considerably in both the reduction and stabilization of the fracture. Non-union is rare.

Complete fractures are the most common fractures seen in children but several types of incomplete fractures are also seen.

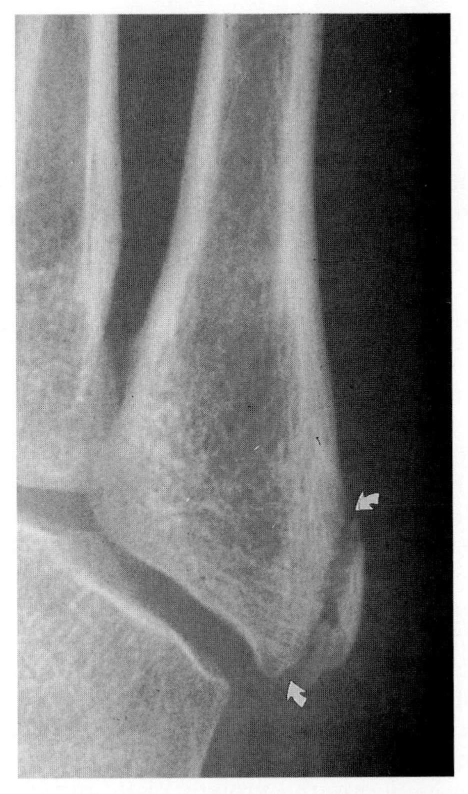
(a)

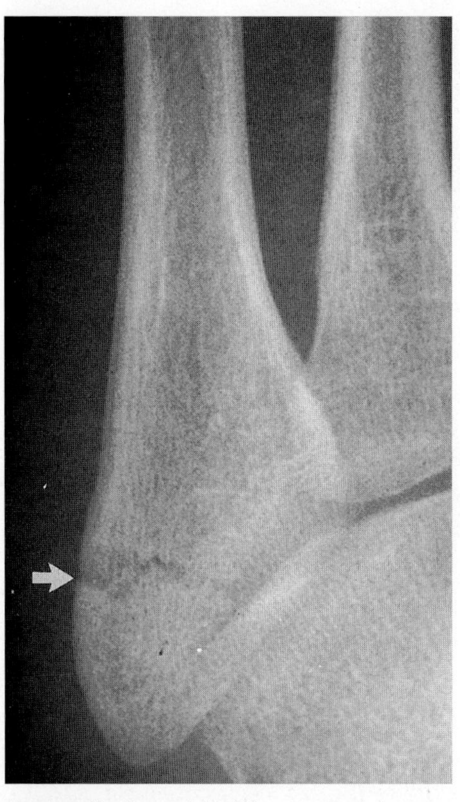
(b)

Fig. 12.6 (a) AP view of base of fifth toe metatarsal in an adult. The unfused apophysis at the base of the fifth metatarsal shows a vertical line of cleavage (curved arrows). (b) The same view in a different patient. The Jones' fracture of the base of the fifth metatarsal demonstrates the fracture line in a horizontal plane (arrow).

The classic **greenstick** fracture is an incomplete transverse fracture of one cortex (Fig. 12.7). There may be a longitudinal component; the opposite cortex remains bent or bowed but is intact. It most commonly occurs in the radius, ulna and clavicle. In hyperextension injuries of the fingers, greenstick fractures may occur at the diametaphysis of the proximal phalanx, and these fractures are often overlooked in the emergency situation.

A **torus** fracture is a buckling of the cortex due to compression perpendicular to the long axis (Fig. 12.8); the buckling is subtle and may be missed. They occur at metaphyses, which normally should be gently flared. Even minor changes, if they correspond to the site of tenderness, should be viewed with suspicion. Impaction at the fracture site may produce a fine line of increased density. **Bowing** fractures are due to a series of microfractures leading to curvature of the affected bone, usually a slender long bone. As the associated clues to the presence of a fracture are usually absent, this entity may be overlooked unless the observer is aware of its existence. It is most common in the radius or ulna, followed by the fibula. In paired bones, both may be bowed, or one actually fractured. Callus will develop subsequently and a permanent, worsening deformity may result; this may also interfere with the correct alignment of an associated fracture. Successful treatment may depend on converting the bowing into a complete fracture.

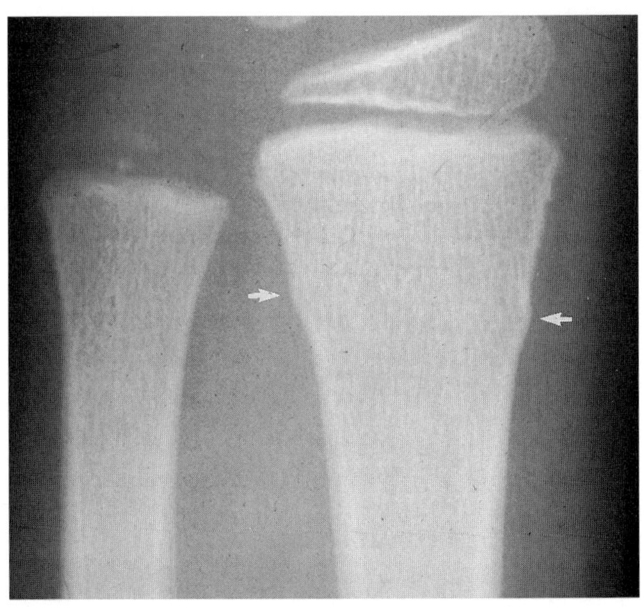

Fig. 12.8 AP film of the wrist in a child showing a concentric buckling of the cortex of the distal radius (arrows).

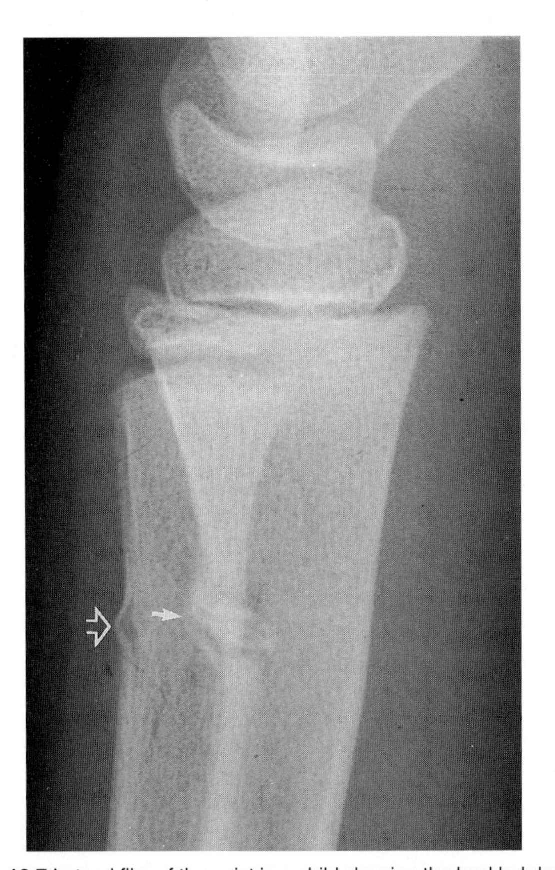

Fig. 12.7 Lateral film of the wrist in a child showing the buckled dorsal cortex of both the radius (arrow) and ulna (open arrow).

SALTER–HARRIS FRACTURES

The **epiphyseal complex** (epiphysis, physis (or growth plate) and metaphysis) is involved in 6–15% of fractures of the long bones in a child. Growth disturbances such as deformities and shortening commonly result as the integrity of the complex is responsible for normal growth and contour.

TYPE I

Epiphyseal separation was first described by Poland in 1898, and can be thought of as the analogue of dislocation or ligamentous injury in the adult. There is no involvement of the metaphysis or epiphyseal ossification centre. It is relatively uncommon and is seen at a younger age. The only plain film evidence is displacement of the ossification centre, or a residual widening of the physis if there has been spontaneous reduction (Fig. 12.9(I) and 12.10). An identical injury occurs at an apophysis, where there is a bony projection for musculotendinous insertion. Violent contraction of the muscle may thus avulse the apophysis. The prognosis is generally favourable unless callus forms across the growth plate anchoring the epiphysis to the metaphysis leading to a cessation of growth.

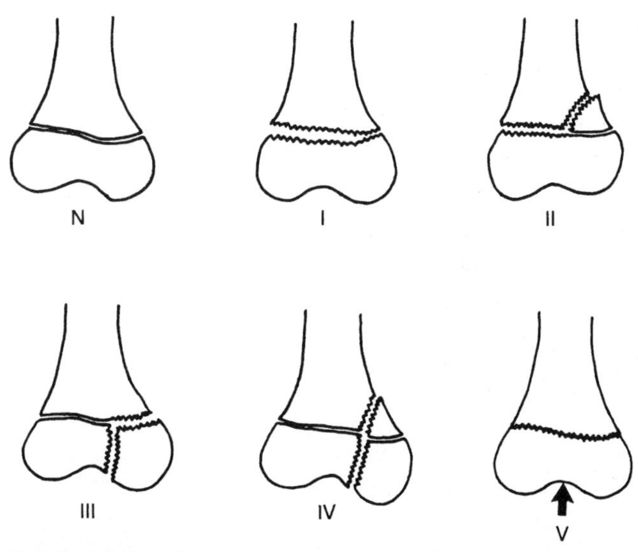

Fig. 12.9 Salter–Harris classification. N = Normal appearance of epiphyseal complex; I = the physis is widened; II = a fragment from the metaphysis accompanies the displaced epiphysis; III = only a fragment of the epiphysis is detached; IV = the fracture extends across the metaphysis, physis and epiphysis; V = the arrow denotes the direction of force; the physis is compressed between the epiphysis and metaphysis.

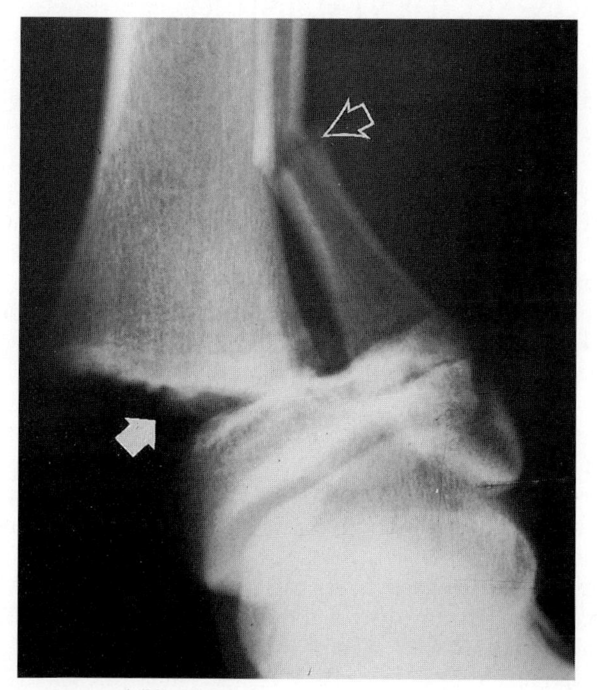

Fig. 12.10 AP view of the ankle in a child with a Salter–Harris Type I fracture. The entire tibial epiphysis has been displaced laterally (closed arrow). Note also the fracture through the distal fibular shaft (open arrow).

TYPE II

Type II is the most common type, accounting for 75% of Salter–Harris fractures. A fragment from the metaphysis accompanies the displaced epiphysis; thus a triangular fragment of metaphysis may be identified, and oblique views may aid detection (Fig 12.9(II) and 12.11). The prognosis is favourable.

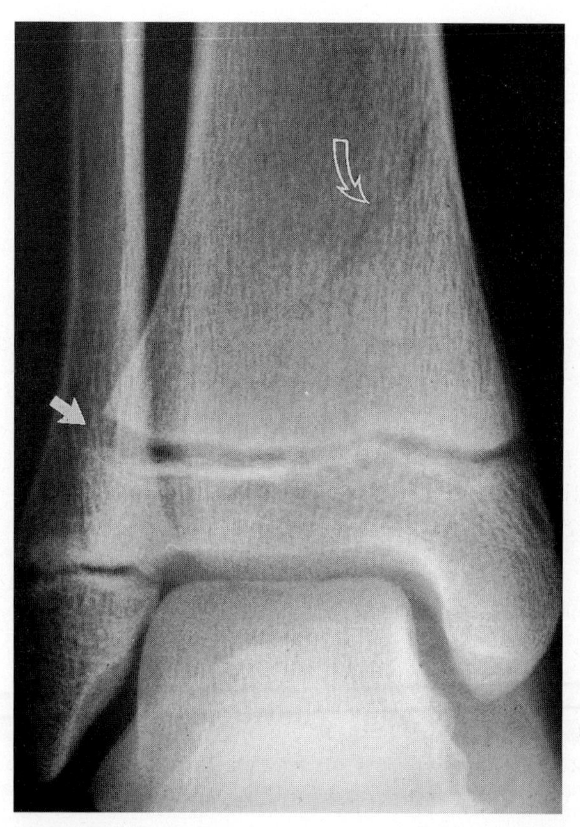

Fig. 12.11 AP view of the ankle in a child with a Salter–Harris Type II fracture showing widening of the lateral aspect of the physis (arrow) in association with an obliquely placed fracture line through the metaphysis (curved open arrow).

TYPE III

An intra-articular shearing force results in a fracture line running vertically through the epiphysis and growth plate and then turning horizontally, through the growth plate, to the periphery. On the X-rays a portion of the epiphysis is detached with minimal displacement (Fig. 12.9 and 12.12). The most common site for this injury is the distal tibia and the prognosis is generally good provided that the fragment can be accurately replaced.

TYPE IV

A fracture extends across the epiphysis, growth plate and metaphysis, fragments of part of both the epiphysis and metaphysis are seen on the films (Fig. 12.9(IV) and 12.13). Growth arrest and joint deformities are a distinct possibility although the chances are reduced by proper reduction and fixation.

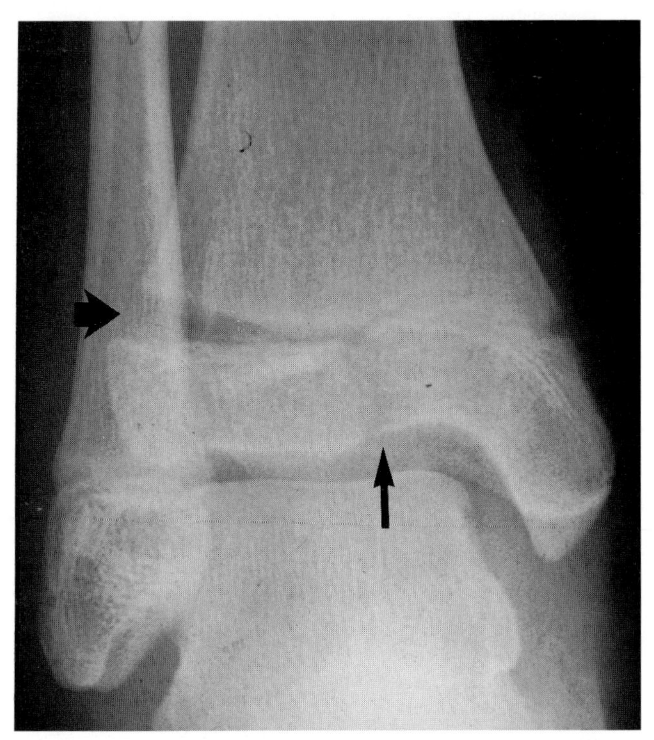

Fig. 12.12 AP view of the ankle in a child with a Salter–Harris Type III fracture through the lateral aspect of the tibial growth plate (large arrow) and through the middle part of the epiphysis (long arrow).

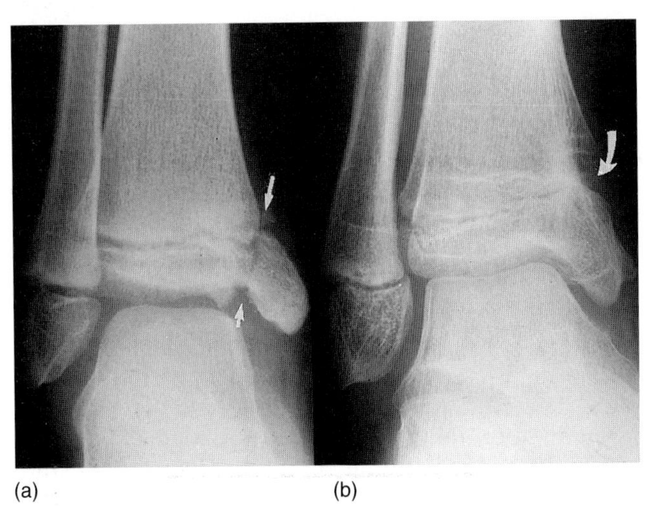

(a) (b)

Fig. 12.13 (a) AP view of the ankle in a child with a Salter–Harris Type IV fracture through the medial malleolus extending through the epiphysis and metaphysis (short arrows). (b) The same view 18 months later. The fracture has resulted in premature fusion of the growth plate (curved arrow) and attendant growth deformities.

TYPE V

Type V injuries constitute 10% of Salter–Harris fractures and result from a pure crush injury. There is usually no immediate radiographic evidence and they very commonly lead to shortening and deformity (Fig. 12.9).

The majority of injuries are Types I and II and are manifest by displacement of the shaft relative to the ossification centre and widening of the growth plate. Changes may be minimal, necessitating additional or comparative views. In Type II the metaphyseal fragment is easily seen if it is caught in profile on the X-ray, but *en face* may be mistaken for buckling of an incomplete fracture or indeed overlooked. Subtle widening of the growth plate should be looked for and oblique views should be considered. Spontaneous reduction may occur, leaving only the metaphyseal fragment visible.

Apophyseal separations are seen when the apophysis is at a distance from the underlying bone. They may heal by callus bridging the entire gap or a fibrous union may form. Rarely a deformity may result from overgrowth. In fractures that result in deformities, a variable time may elapse between the injury and cessation or relative retardation of growth. Two years must elapse before one can confidently exclude shortening or deformity; therefore, clinical review with repeat X-rays should happen at 3–6 month intervals.

NON-ACCIDENTAL INJURY

The clinical condition of non-accidental injury, specifically the association of long bone fractures with subdural haematomas, was first described by Caffey in 1946. Most victims are below the age of 3 years, and 50% of injuries occur in children younger than 1 year of age. Conversely, accidental fractures are rare below the age of 1 year. It is a very important diagnosis to make, because failure to remove the child from the environment of abuse may at least result in long-term physical and psychological damage, and tragically, in some cases, death.

There are both clinical and radiological manifestations of repeated injury. The child may show evidence of burns and bruises, be withdrawn and underweight, and the history given for the injuries is often inconsistent or bizarre. There may be delay or failure to seek medical advice.

The cardinal radiological sign is the presence of multiple fractures at different stages of healing. The following sites of fracture are considered to have a high specificity for child abuse: metaphyses, ribs, scapula, outer end of the clavicle, spine, bilateral fractures, complex skull fractures, and finger injuries in non-ambulant children.

The metaphyseal fractures of child abuse are usually very close to the growth plate (unlike accidental metaphyseal fractures which are normally at the diametaphysis) and of the torus type. The fractures occur through the most immature part of the metaphysis and an ossified ring of metaphysis is avulsed with physis giving the characteristic **'corner' fracture**

(Fig. 12.14). A less well-known variant of metaphyseal injury is a lucency in the immediate subphyseal region; these have been proven to be true fractures by histological studies. Metaphyseal fractures are most common in the tibia, femur and proximal humerus. The significance of metaphyseal injuries is that they are often caused by shaking the infant or child and are therefore associated with brain damage due to subdural haematoma. Even when recent, these fractures may be undetectable clinically as they do not commonly cause pain. The only evidence for them is radiological, thus a skeletal survey is indicated. Even in the absence of a skull fracture, shaking may result in haemorrhage leading to raised intracranial pressure and widened sutures. A head CT scan may be indicated to exclude subdural haemorrhage, as may MRI to search for damaged or ischaemic tissue.

Metaphyseal fractures, although said to be specific for child abuse, are in fact much less common than diaphyseal fractures. With the exception of supracondylar fractures, all fractures of the humerus in children under the age of 3 years are strongly suggestive of abuse, and femoral fractures occurring under the age of 1 year are, more often than not, due to abuse. Long bone fractures are often associated with a florid subperiosteal reaction (Fig. 12.15), mimicking metabolic disease or dysplasia. This generally indicates repeated trauma, as do breaches in the outer layer of new bone.

Salter–Harris type epiphyseal injuries may on occasion result from child abuse but are rare. Rib fractures are virtually diagnostic of child abuse, being rarely seen even in severe accidental trauma, such as road traffic accidents. They are more frequent in the posterior and axillary parts of the ribs and are frequently multiple and bilateral. Posterior and neck fractures may be difficult to identify on plain films and may be more readily detected by isotope bone scanning. However, although scintigraphy may be useful to detect some occult injuries, skull fractures may not show increased uptake.

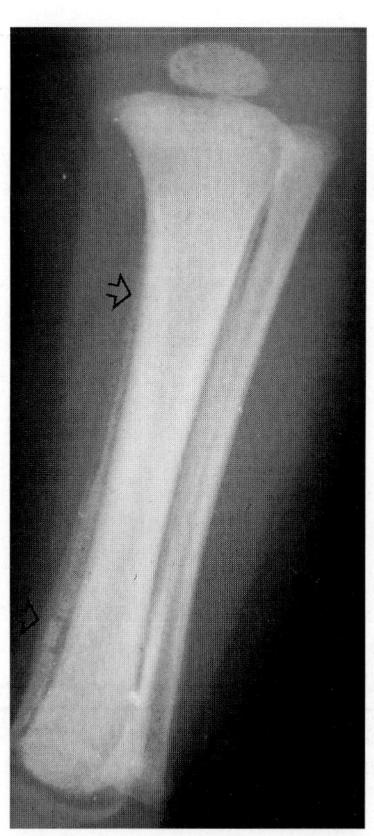

Fig. 12.15 AP view of the tibia and fibula in an infant. A multilayered periosteal reaction is seen surrounding both the tibia and the fibula in this battered baby (open arrows).

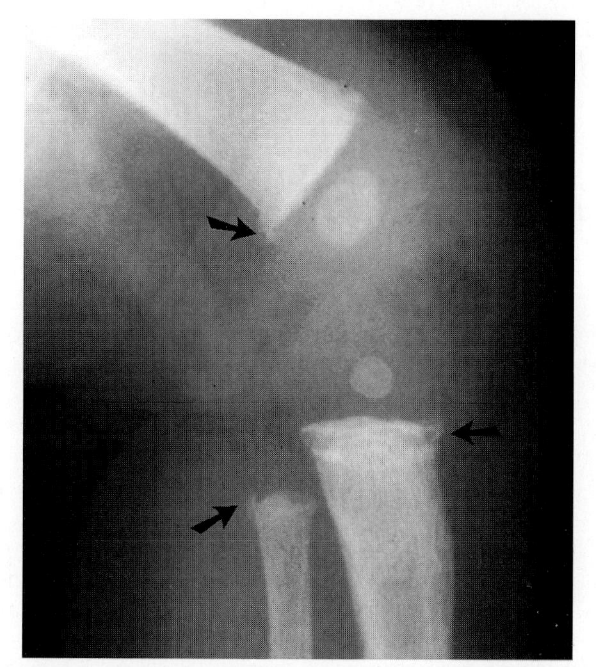

Fig. 12.14 Lateral view of the knee in a toddler. Metaphyseal corner fractures are seen at the distal femur, proximal tibia and proximal fibula (arrowed).

The main differential diagnoses are metabolic bone disease and osteogenesis imperfecta. Rickets and scurvy are readily eliminated by blood tests, and copper deficiency is extremely rare. In osteogenesis imperfecta the severe forms do not cause a diagnostic problem, and the milder manifestations rarely result in fractures until the child is ambulant.

NORMAL FRACTURE HEALING

Fracture healing may be divided into three phases: inflammatory, reparative and remodelling, although there is overlap in the temporal sequence of events. It should be remembered also that in addition to the injured bone there will be an associated soft-tissue injury with haematoma formation. Shortly after the injury the periosteum begins to proliferate and haematoma is transformed into granulation tissue by ingrowth of fibroblasts and capillaries. Metaplasia of the fibrous tissue into cartilage occurs and a layer of woven bone cements itself to the outer layers of the fracture fragments. The cartilage adjacent to bone then becomes ossified and is eventually remodelled into mature bone.

Not all fractures heal at the same rate, or with the same amount of **callus**. More callus is seen in the long bones, in the diaphysis and where distraction is greater. Thus less callus is seen with internal fixation, indeed the formation of significant amounts of callus may suggest either excessive movement or infection. There is also a paucity of callus in bones such as the scaphoid, where the cortex is thin and healing occurs via endosteal or medullary callus formation. The same phenomenon is seen in other intra-articular fractures. Fracture healing may be slow in the elderly, where vascularity is compromised, or where the fragments are widely separated or inadequately immobilized. Corticosteroids will slow healing, but increase the amount of callus seen.

The earliest plain film finding of repair is widening and blurring of the fracture line due to resorption of the underlying bone. This is seen by 10–14 days. The next manifestation is the appearance of fluffy and amorphous calcified callus around the fracture site, found initially at the periphery of the haematoma, so it may not be adjacent to the fracture site. As mentioned previously, endosteal or medullary callus is difficult to identify radiologically. Gradually the callus fills in, increasing in both density and quantity, until eventually it becomes mature callus with the texture of bone. It is rare for callus to develop at an equal rate around the circumference of the fracture site, due to variable amounts of periosteal stripping, apposition and so forth. Ultimately the fracture line is entirely obliterated (Fig. 12.16).

Disuse osteopenia is commonly seen following a fracture and is due to immobility and inactivity. There is acute and rapid resorption of both medullary and cortical bone distal to the fracture site in the affected extremity. It can be distinguished from other forms of osteopenia because of the focal nature of the process, the pronounced subcortical linear lucencies from endosteal resorption and the 'spotty' nature of the osteopenia. The changes reverse spontaneously once the patient resumes normal activity. Persistence, or even worsening, of the appearances following removal of a cast may suggest the development of a reflex sympathetic syndrome (**Sudeck's atrophy**). In the elderly, the combination of disuse osteopenia on a background of senile osteoporosis may result in an insufficiency fracture.

Clinical **union** occurs before radiographic union. The latter is evidenced by a continuous external bridge of callus uniting the fracture fragments. The callus should be uniformly ossified with a density approaching that of normal bone. The findings should be present on views taken at right angles to each other, as overlapping fragments may mimic union in one projection. In assessing the healing process it is important to compare the current findings with the previous films. If there is a question about the solidity of a union then stress films may be of value.

Malunion is the healing of a fracture with the fragments in a faulty position, with excessive angulation or rotation. In all except the very young, surgical intervention may be required to correct the deformity. An angular malunion is readily identified on plain films but a rotational abnormality may be harder to define. CT scanning, sometimes with three-dimensional reconstruction, may help in the anatomical definition of a malunion.

Delayed union is the term used to describe a fracture which fails to unite within a normal time scale for a given site taking the age of the patient into account. There is persistent movement at the fracture site and bridging callus is not complete.

Once the healing process has stopped completely and the fragments are not united then **non-union** has

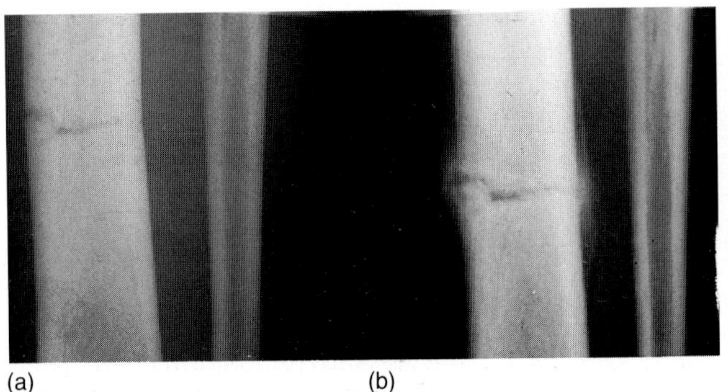

(a) (b)

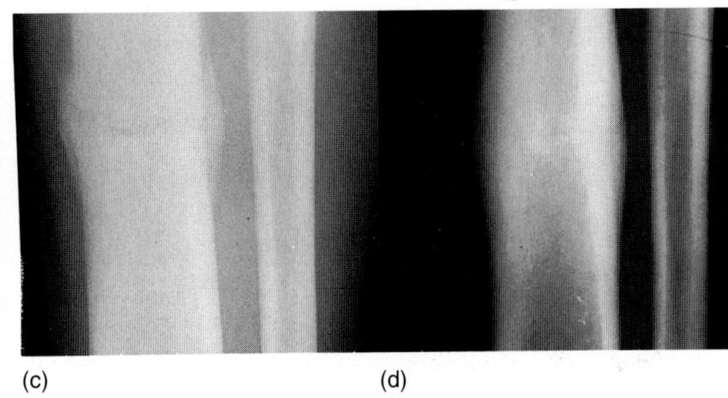

(c) (d)

Fig. 12.16 Series of films of the midshaft of the tibia and fibula. (a) A transverse fracture is seen through the tibia. (b) The edges of the fracture line have become slightly blurred and early callus formation is seen together with a periosteal reaction, predominantly on the lateral aspect. (c) More mature callus is seen to surround the fracture, although the fracture line itself remains visible. (d) The callus has largely remodelled and the fracture line can no longer be identified with certainty.

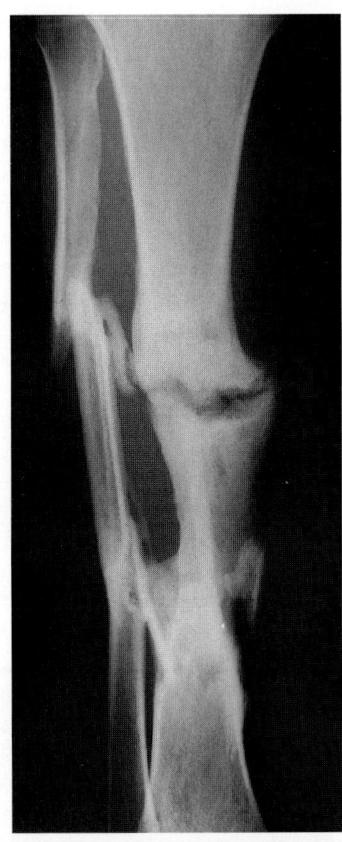

Fig. 12.17 AP view of the tibia and fibula. Following a motorcycle accident, this patient, with extensive compound trauma of the tibia and fibula, has developed a hypertrophic non-union.

occurred. Non-union is rare in children. In hypertrophic non-union the margins of the fracture are well defined, smooth and sclerotic (Fig. 12.17). No callus crosses the fracture site and a pseudarthrosis, or false joint, may form. In the much less common atrophic form there is only a fine sclerotic line across the medullary canals of the apposing fragments. An established non-union requires operative intervention with a combination of resection of the fracture line, internal fixation and bone grafting. Small fragments of bone from intra-articular fractures may not unite with the bulk of the fracture and cause later complications by remaining free in the joint as loose bodies.

POST-TREATMENT RADIOGRAPHY

The aim of fracture treatment is to produce a united fracture without residual deformity or other complications. In practice, this means reducing the fracture, by open or closed manipulation, and then fixing it by external or internal means. Postreduction films, again in two planes, are therefore important to check for apposition and reasonable alignment, bearing in mind that some remodelling will occur during treatment. It is important to make a careful comparison of the pre- and postreduction films. In cases of dislocation, review films following relocation may reveal fracture fragments that were not evident on the initial films. Separation of the fragments may indicate either interposed soft tissue, or excessive traction, from either fixation devices or muscular spasm.

Following internal or external fixation, the entire length of the appliance must be imaged. Intramedullary nails may fracture through the distal cortex of a long bone and, therefore, the distal joint must also be included. Subsequent films are necessary both to check fracture healing, and also to look for complications of fixation, such as migration of metal work, or infection around pin and screw sites, as evidenced by increasing areas of lucency. Shortening should be checked for, if a butterfly fragment was treated with an intramedullary rod. Rotation may be seen where the rod occupies the entire canal of the fractured segments; this can be prevented by the use of an interlocking nail.

COMPLICATIONS OF FRACTURES

Vascular injuries may be due to either blunt or penetrating injury, the latter often from direct transection or laceration by a bony fragment. The sites of predilection for vascular involvement are where the artery lies close to the bone, or where it is tethered on either side of a joint. A tear of an adjacent artery and vein may lead eventually to pseudoaneurysm formation. If there is clinical suspicion of vascular injury, then arteriography may help to confirm the diagnosis prior to surgery. In trauma associated with catastrophic haemorrhage, such as pelvic fractures, percutaneous embolization may reduce or stop the bleeding.

Soft tissue infection may occur following a compound fracture. Although plain films are likely to be normal, ultrasound, CT or MRI scanning may show an abscess cavity. With soft-tissue ischaemia or gross contamination of the wound, there is a risk of gas gangrene or other anaerobic infection. This may be seen on plain films if air bubbles are identified in the tissues; often there are linear lucencies tracking along fascial planes. However, small, rounded, pockets of gas may be seen as a normal finding in the early post-traumatic or postsurgical period.

Fat embolism was first described by Bergmann in 1873, and pathological studies suggest that subclinical emboli occur very frequently. Only a small percentage of patients sustaining fractures of the long bones show clinical or radiological manifestations of fat embolism. Symptoms, such as respiratory insufficiency associated with marked desaturation, confusion, pyrexia, petechiae and haemoptysis, normally occur some 48 hours after the injury and are most common in patients with multiple sites of fracture. Radiographic findings are somewhat non-specific and lag a little behind the clinical features. On the chest radiograph, a diffuse mixed alveolar and interstitial pattern is seen, which may worsen until a 'white out', with some sparing of the apices, is present bilaterally. Pleural effusions are normally absent. The appearance may be impossible to distinguish from adult respiratory distress syndrome, but in the uncomplicated case spontaneous clearing should occur in 7–10 days.

Bone infection is potentially one of the worst complications of bone trauma, resulting in delayed healing at best, and at worst necessitating amputation or even ending in death. Post-traumatic osteomyelitis is normally due to a focus of infection introduced either at the time of a compound injury, or during open reduction and internal fixation. Very rarely it may be associated with a closed fracture, usually in children with intercurrent sepsis. The dominant symptom of osteomyelitis is an increase in the degree of pain experienced by the patient. From the time the infective process begins, 10–14 days must elapse before the plain film changes are evident. There may be soft-tissue swelling, periosteal new bone formation, and bone destruction with lytic areas, all of which may also be seen with non-infected fractures. Where internal fixation is in place, these lytic areas may occur around the pin or screw sites (Fig. 12.18), a finding which suggests infection. Periosteal reaction is unusual in the presence of non-infected internal fixation devices and, when it does occur, it is almost never layered.

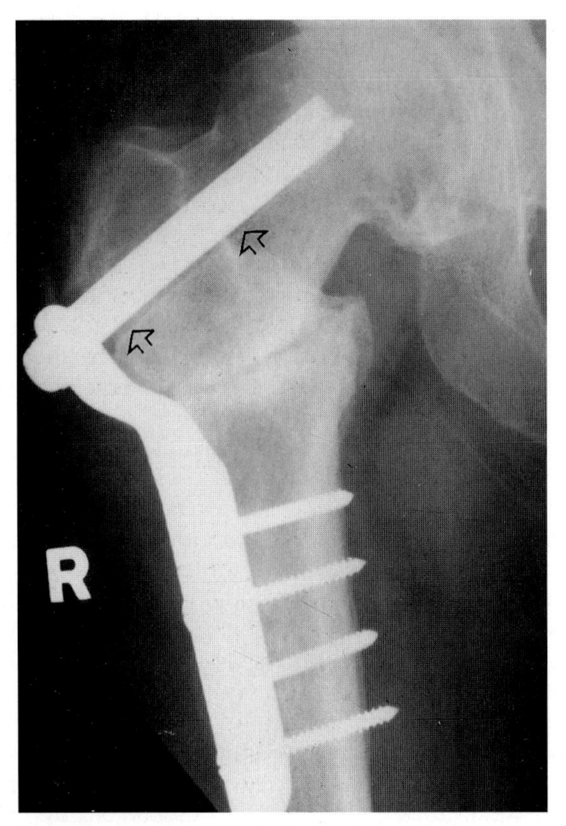

Fig. 12.18 AP view of right hip. Following internal fixation, the patient presented with pain in the hip. A zone of lucency (open arrows) is seen around the pin in the femoral neck, indicating infection around the pin site.

Other imaging modalities may assist in the detection of infection. Ultrasound may show a subperiosteal abscess; this may be aspirated under ultrasound guidance, confirming the diagnosis and providing microbiological evidence of the cause. MRI may also be useful for showing areas of high signal on the T2-weighted scans, although in the presence of metalwork there may be significant artefact obscuring the site of interest.

Sclerosis, excessive callus formation and the presence of sequestra, or small fragments of dead bone, indicate chronicity. Replacement or complete removal of metalwork may be necessary to effect a cure. Antibiotic beads, particularly gentamicin, are sometimes inserted to deliver a local effect. They are seen on plain radiographs as multiple rounded opacities.

Post-traumatic reflex dystrophy is a poorly understood condition and is difficult to diagnose. It was first described by Sudeck following a penetrating injury, but is most commonly seen following closed, and often trivial, fracture of the extremity. The limb is affected distal to the site of the injury. A variant of the syndrome occurs as a result of repetition injury, often associated with the patient's occupation, and on occasion leads to litigation. Although the precise mechanism is not known, the process is mediated through the sympathetic nervous system and treatment is aimed at abolishing the sympathetic response. The diagnosis is essentially clinical, based on increasing pain and oedema after the injury. The skin is classically red, hot and shiny. Plain films may show only marked osteopenia, due to the hyperaemia, often starting in a periarticular distribution, although soft-tissue swelling may be evident. The appearances may progress until there are small erosions and cortical breaks. The only other imaging modality of value is the three-phase radionuclide bone scan, where the affected extremity may show increased uptake on dynamic, blood pool and static images.

Avascular necrosis is the result of compromise of the blood supply to part of the fracture. The affected bone shows a pattern of mixed sclerosis and lysis and may eventually collapse. Where it is the result of repeated minor trauma, a number of eponymous syndromes are described, e.g. **Freiberg's** disease of the second metatarsal head (Fig. 12.19).

Osteochondritis dissecans is common in adolescents and young adults. It is probably due to repeated minor trauma although the aetiology is uncertain; the patient may present with a history of pain but no definite previous injury. The most frequently affected site is the lateral surface of the medial femoral condyle, and a small, dense fragment of bone is seen lying in a shallow cavity. MRI can be used to demonstrate whether the

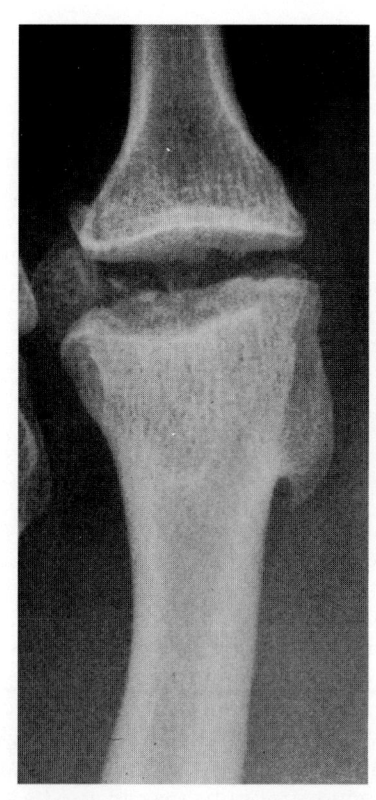

Fig. 12.19 AP view of the second toe metatarsophalangeal joint in a patient with the classic appearance of Freiberg's disease. Fragmentation, flattening and sclerosis is noted of the second metatarsal head in this young ballet dancer. The spur seen on the lateral aspect of the metatarsal head is almost certainly due to secondary degenerative change.

overlying cartilage is intact and whether the bony fragment is viable. In early stages, arthroscopic pinning may be used to secure the fragment. Occasionally, the fragment may become a loose body. Loose bodies may also result from an osteochondral fragment of bone being separated acutely at the time of injury.

Deep venous thrombosis is relatively common in patients who are immobile following trauma. The imaging of venous thrombosis is discussed on p. 560.

OCCULT FRACTURES

On occasion, there may be a high clinical index of suspicion while plain films do not show any sign of a fracture despite supplemental plain radiographic views. Treatment may be decided on the basis of clinical findings alone but it may be necessary to define a fracture more clearly. At some sites, such as the scaphoid, a delayed film after 10–14 days may show sclerosis or a clearly defined lucency which were not seen at the time of presentation. The patient may be treated symptomatically in a plaster cast until that time.

A useful procedure in selected cases is the **radionuclide bone scan**. A radionuclide bone scanning agent is injected into a peripheral vein, and once incorporated into bone some 3–4 hours later, images are taken using a gamma camera. This highly sensitive technique detects fractures at a very early stage and is useful for confirming injury in equivocal cases. It can also be used to confirm stress fractures which may be difficult to identify on the plain films at presentation. The drawback of the technique is that it is entirely non-specific, giving positive results in any bone pathology. It is therefore of limited use in answering whether pain is due to fracture or another pathology, although in cases of stress fracture a characteristic linear pattern of uptake is sometimes seen.

Plain films may suggest that a fracture is present; for example a lipohaemarthrosis in the knee indicates that a fracture must have occurred in order to allow marrow fat into the joint space. Plain tomography is a method of imaging at different depths through the bone by bringing individual planes into focus. The whole of the affected area can be covered and this method is used to demonstrate tibial plateau fractures.

Because of the ability to scan in the axial plane and excellent anatomical resolution for bone, **CT** is extremely useful in confirming and defining fractures, particularly in the spine, pelvis and foot. Reconstructions in multiple planes and three-dimensional reconstructions aid the surgeon in planning his approach.

Ultrasound is of limited value in the diagnosis of bony injuries although it may demonstrate an effusion and therefore lend support to the suspicion of a fracture. Rarely a fracture fragment may be identified in the soft tissues.

MRI was initially thought to be of limited value in the evaluation of bony trauma because cortical bone does not contain mobile hydrogen and therefore appears as an area of signal void (blackness) on the scan, but recent studies have suggested that it can be used to detect a fracture line, seen as a dark line across the normal, bright signal of marrow fat. MRI has been shown to be more sensitive than radionuclide scanning in the detection of occult fractures of the femoral neck.

FOREIGN BODIES

A careful history from the patient should indicate whether there is a risk of a foreign body and the presence or absence of a foreign body following penetrating injury can usually be imaged. Radiographs should be taken in two planes with a marker to show the site of skin puncture: even tiny metal density fragments are easily seen as they are extremely dense. Glass fragments are variably dense but fragments over a couple of millimetres in size can usually be found. Wood and thorn splinters are not radiopaque and plain films are not, therefore, of value, but ultrasound is sensitive in locating such foreign bodies. Appropriate imaging should be repeated following removal of fragments to confirm that no significant residual foreign bodies remain.

MUSCLE TEARS

A muscle tear is frequently the result of sports injury and cannot usually be identified on plain films. Ultrasound, performed using a 7.5 MHz linear array probe, gives excellent resolution of muscle fibres. The appearances can be graded, from minor separation of the muscle fibres, to a tear along the fascial attachment, and complete rupture of the muscle substance (Fig. 12.20). The latter is normally associated with a significant haematoma, seen as a hypoechoic region within the muscle bulk and disruption of the normal anatomy. A haematoma lying in the subcutaneous soft tissues has a similar appearance. MRI can also be used to demonstrate muscle tears but is more expensive, less readily available and less sensitive to the different types of tear.

A soft-tissue haematoma may heal with calcific and eventually ossific changes, and is then called **myositis ossificans** (Fig. 12.21). After 2–3 weeks amorphous calcifications are seen within a soft tissue mass. The mass may appear attached to the underlying bone and a periosteal reaction can be seen. This combination of findings may resemble a malignant neoplasm. Often the history of antecedent trauma is forgotten and a tentative diagnosis of tumour is made. The characteristic finding of post-traumatic myositis is that the new bone becomes more mature, a feature that can be demonstrated on subsequent films from 6 to 8 weeks following the injury. In contrast to parosteal osteosarcoma there is also mature bone on the inner aspect of the lesion. Full

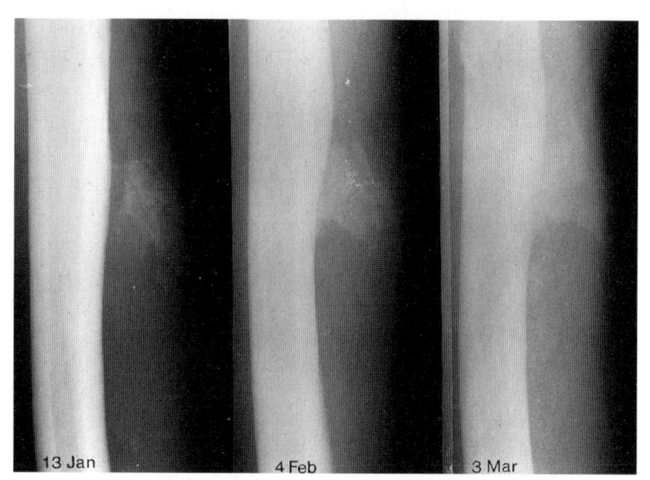

Fig. 12.21 A series of X-rays taken over a 2-month period show an area of maturing ossification in the posterior aspect of the thigh in this patient who had suffered soft-tissue trauma.

radiological maturity occurs at 5–6 months when there may be some shrinkage and separation from the underlying bone. It is important to recognize the condition as post-traumatic in nature as the histology can also appear malignant and early resection may lead to a recurrence. Myositis ossificans can also be seen in association with burns and around the hips in approximately one third of paraplegic patients.

TENDON INJURIES

Tendon injuries are often the result of sporting endeavour, from a repetition injury or occurring as an acute rupture. The Achilles tendon and patellar

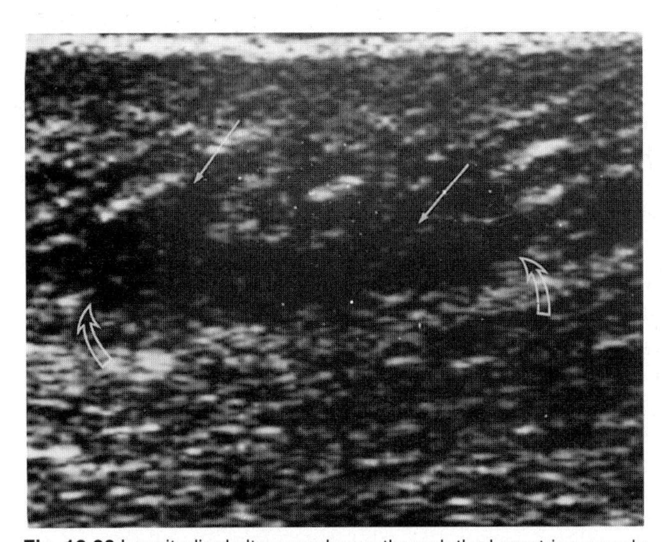

Fig. 12.20 Longitudinal ultrasound scan through the hamstring muscle in a middle-aged cricketer. The normal muscle fibres are shown as multiple longitudinal and obliquely positioned striations. A haematoma cavity is identified (curved open arrows) and some torn muscle fibres are identified superficial to this (fine arrows).

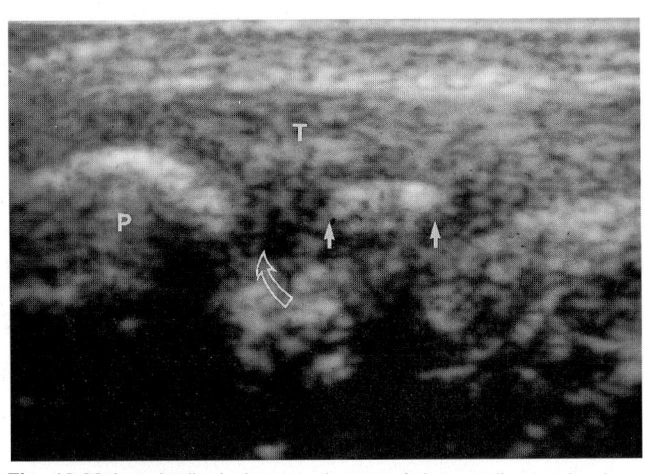

Fig. 12.22 Longitudinal ultrasound scan of the patellar tendon in a 24-year-old professional footballer who complained of pain at the interior patellar pole. P = patella; T=tendon. There is an area of highly reflective material (arrows) contained within a more diffusely hypoechoic area (open arrow) in the proximal patellar tendon representing calcific, and therefore moderate to severe, tendinitis.

tendon are most commonly affected. Ultrasound is able to show the integrity of ligaments and the changes of tendonitis: the normal tendon is relatively hyperechoic with the internal fibrillary structure well shown provided a 7.5 MHz probe is used. Features of tendonitis are: a hypoechoic area at the bony insertion of the tendon; fusiform thickening of the tendon; and a peritendinous effusion indicating a tenovaginitis. Calcific deposits may form in severe cases (Fig. 12.22). A full thickness rupture is readily identified. Again the changes are visible on MRI but grading the severity of the lesion may be difficult.

SPECIFIC REGIONAL INJURIES

HAND

Avulsion fractures are common in the hand, are easily missed and are functionally important. The **mallet finger** results from forcible flexion of the extended finger and the common extensor tendon is avulsed. There is, therefore, a fracture of the dorsal aspect of the base of the distal phalanx. A **volar plate** fracture results from a hyperextension injury and displaces a fragment from the palmar aspect of the base of the middle phalanx (Fig. 12.23). Collateral ligaments are found at all the small joints; the most common injury is the avulsion of the ulnar collateral ligament of the metacarpophalangeal joint of the thumb, or **skier's thumb** (**gamekeeper's thumb** being a chronic instability). This fracture may cause an intra-articular fragment at the base of the proximal phalanx on the ulnar side. Otherwise stress views may be required to demonstrate the lesion. A commonly missed fracture in children is a greenstick fracture of the diametaphysis of the proximal phalanx after a hyperextension injury. A sudden angulation in the cortex indicates its presence.

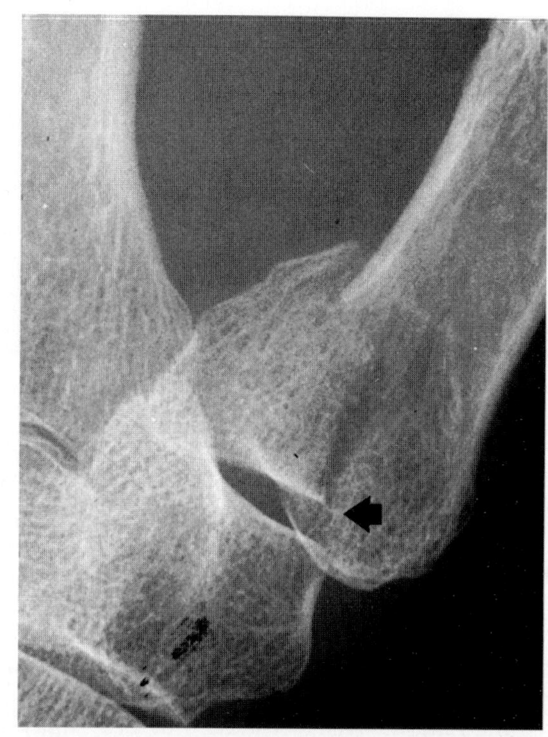

Fig. 12.24 AP view of carpometacarpal joint of thumb in Bennett's fracture. The fracture line runs obliquely through the base of the thumb disrupting the proximal, intra-articular cortex (arrow).

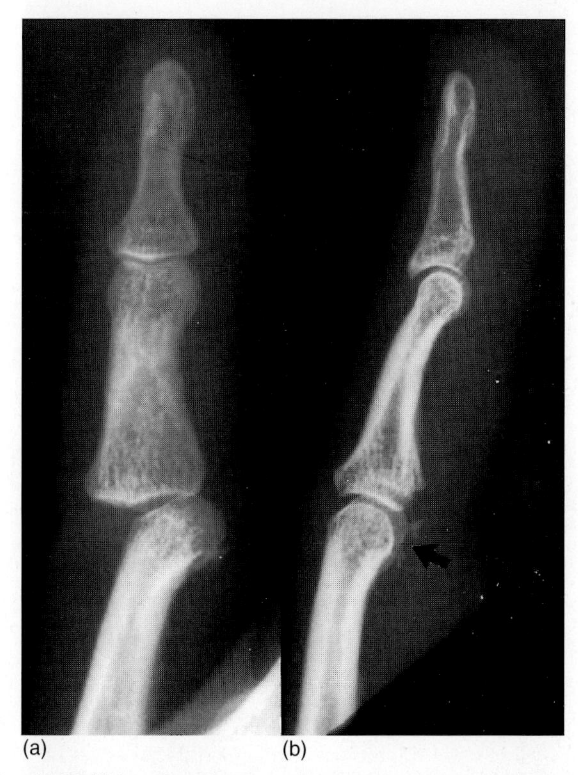

(a) (b)

Fig. 12.23 Volar plate fracture. (a) Lateral view of middle finger showing a dorsal dislocation at the proximal interphalangeal joint of the middle finger. (b) On the postreduction film, bone fragments are identified deep to the head of the proximal phalanx with a small defect at the base of the middle phalanx (arrow).

It is important to differentiate between intra- and extra-articular fractures of the thumb as the former require open reduction. **Bennett's fracture** forms 30% of thumb metacarpal fractures; it is a fracture dislocation with an oblique intra-articular fracture at the base of the metacarpal and dorsal dislocation of the large fragment of metacarpal (Fig. 12.24). Bennett's fractures usually require treatment by open reduction and internal fixation. Less common is the **Rolando** fracture, a markedly comminuted but impacted fracture with a separate dorsal fragment. Fixation is generally not of value in the presence of such marked impaction.

WRIST

A fall on the outstretched hand results in different injuries depending on the age of the patient: greenstick or torus fractures of both bones in a young child; a Salter–Harris II fracture of the distal radius in an

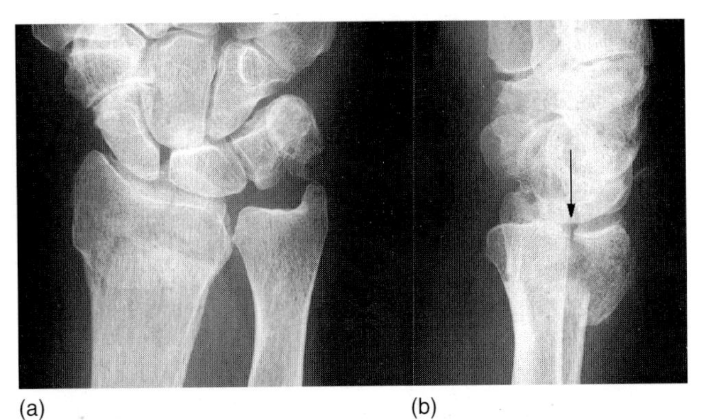

Fig. 12.25 Barton's fracture. (a) AP and (b) lateral view of the wrist. In addition to the slight posterior displacement of the distal fragments, there is clearly an intra-articular fracture of the distal radius (arrow), thus distinguishing this from an ordinary Colles' fracture.

older child; scaphoid fracture in a young adult and fractures of the distal radius, commonly **Colles' fracture**, in the elderly. The Colles' fracture is a fracture of the distal 2–3 cm of the radius with dorsal angulation. A **Smith's fracture**, on the other hand, has volar angulation. Distal radial fractures may be radiographically occult, and a clue may be the presence of the pronator quadratus sign, in which the fat pad in front of the pronator muscle is displaced in a palmar direction.

Distal radioulnar dislocation may be suggested by an abnormal position of the head of the ulna in the ulnar notch. This may be seen as part of a **Galeazzi fracture**, in which the radius is also fractured. A **Barton's fracture** is an intra-articular fracture of the dorsal lip of the radius, with the carpus following the dorsal fragment (Fig. 12.25). As this is an unstable fracture, frequently requiring internal fixation, it is important to differentiate from a Colles' fracture, where there is a fracture of the distal radius with volar angulation producing the classic 'dinner-fork' clinical deformity.

Wrist injuries are ten times more common than carpal injuries; the latter are rare in children under the age of 12. Fractures of the scaphoid form 60–70% of injuries, 10% are dislocations or fracture dislocations, and 10% are dorsal chip fractures, the vast majority being from the triquetral, and these are only identified on the lateral view. On the PA view the width of the intercarpal joints should be about 2 mm; three parallel arcs have been described to assist in evaluating the alignment (Fig. 12.26).

- along the proximal articular margins of the proximal carpal row;
- along the distal articular margins of the proximal carpal row;
- along the proximal articular margins of the distal carpal row.

The lunate is trapezoidal in shape on the PA film; if

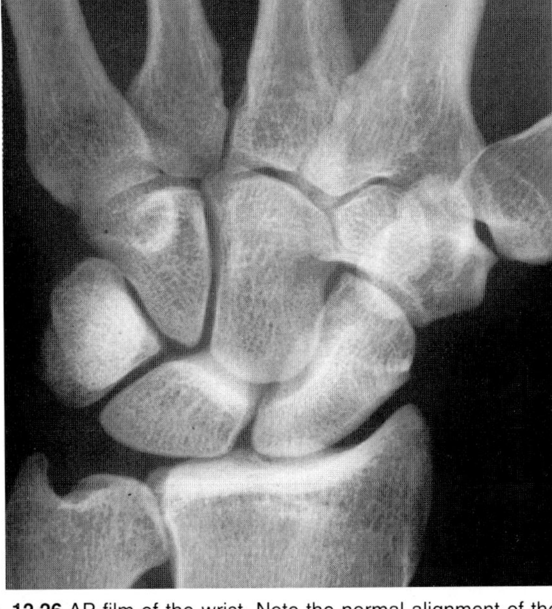

Fig. 12.26 AP film of the wrist. Note the normal alignment of the two rows of the carpal bones.

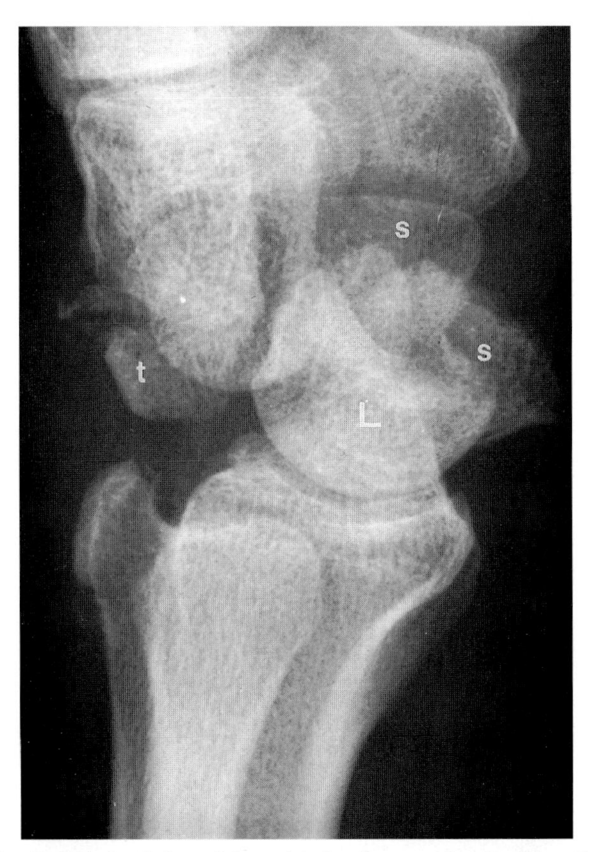

Fig. 12.27 Lateral view of the wrist showing a perilunate dislocation. The lunate (L) lies in its normal position with respect to the radius. The scaphoid is in two fragments (s) and there is also a fracture of the triquetral (t). This is, therefore, a trans-scaphoperilunate fracture.

it appears triangular then it is abnormally rotated. On the lateral view there should be a co-axial arrangement of the articular surfaces of the radius, lunate, capitate and third metacarpal.

Up to 70% of scaphoid fractures are at the waist and undisplaced. As the blood supply to the proximal pole enters at the waist, these fractures are at risk of delayed or non-union and of avascular necrosis. It may take up to 2 years for radiographic union to occur. Lunate fractures are difficult to identify, but again there is a risk of avascular necrosis; findings of mixed sclerosis and lysis, with cortical collapse (**Keinbock's disease**), are thought to be due to previous trauma.

Carpal dislocations can be identified by disruption of the normal anatomical arcs described above, and loss of the co-axial appearance on the lateral. Fracture dislocations are more common than pure dislocations so the films should be carefully examined for a fracture line. In a **perilunate dislocation** (Fig. 12.27), the capitate articular surface is dorsally dislocated from the lunate, while the lunate maintains its normal articulation with the radius. In a **mid-carpal dislocation** the lunate tilts in a volar direction but is not dislocated from the radius. The capitate is dislocated from the lunate, but is not placed as posteriorly as above. In a **lunate dislocation** (Fig. 12.28), there is loss of the lunate articulation with both the capitate and the radius and it is displaced volarly with a 90° angulation. The capitate remains in alignment with the radius but drops down towards it.

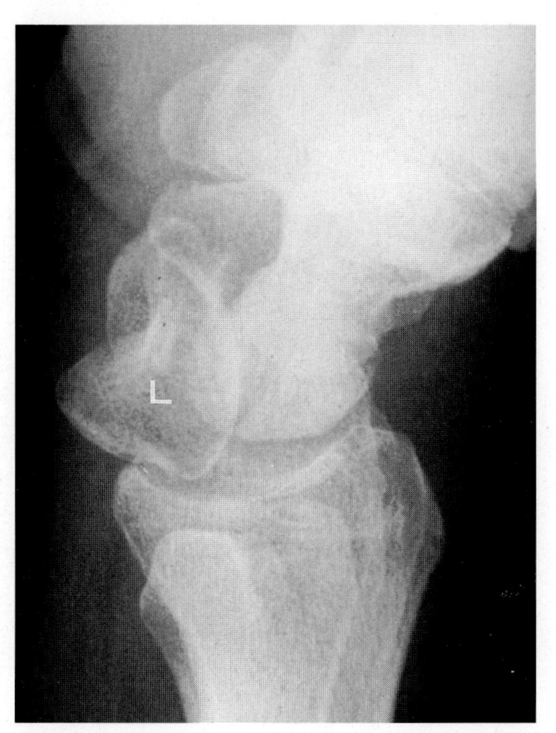

Fig. 12.28 Lateral view of the wrist showing lunate dislocation. Unlike the previous film, the lunate (L) has been displaced anteriorly and has lost its normal articulation with the radius.

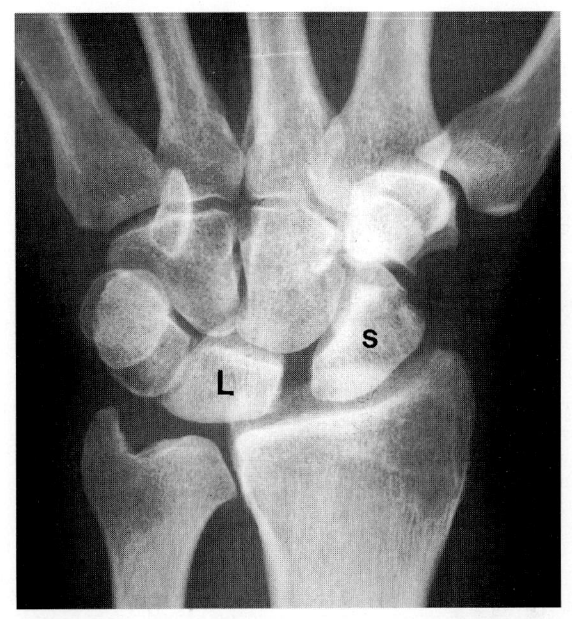

Fig. 12.29 AP view of wrist showing the 'Terry Thomas' sign. Note the wide space in between the scaphoid (S) and lunate (L) indicating disruption of the scapholunate ligament.

Ligamentous injury can cause instability without a frank dislocation. The PA film should be examined for >2 mm diastasis at the scapholunate joint and lunate tilt: the **Terry-Thomas sign** (Fig. 12.29), which indicates scapholunate dissociation and may be associated with rotatory subluxation of the scaphoid. Other forms of instability are complex and may only be identified at fluoroscopy with either ulnar or radial stresses or distraction applied. Wrist arthrography may be necessary to identify a ruptured triangular fibrocartilage complex or interosseous ligaments. Contrast injected in between the scaphoid and radius should normally be contained within the radiocarpal compartment. Contrast entering the distal radioulnar joint indicates a triangular fibrocartilage complex tear; if contrast enters the mid-carpal joint there is a rupture of one of the interosseous ligaments. Degeneration of these ligaments and the triangular fibrocartilage complex is a normal ageing phenomenon and renders evaluation by MRI prone to false positives. If surgery is contemplated then arthrography is the recommended method of evaluation.

ELBOW

In the normal patient the radius articulates with the capitellum and the ulna articulates with the trochlea. On a true lateral film a line, the anterior humeral line, drawn along the anterior humeral cortex, should intersect the capitellum in its middle third. With the elbow in any position a line, the radiocapitellar line

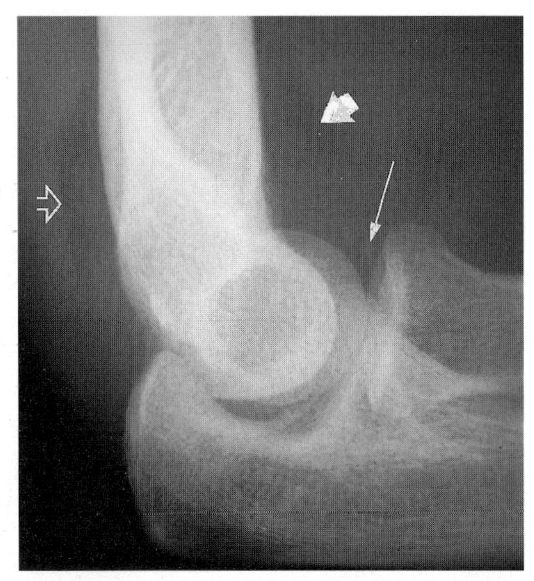

Fig. 12.30 Lateral view of the elbow showing a radial head fracture. Both anterior (arrow) and posterior (open arrow) fat pad signs are identified around the distal humerus. In addition, the fragments from the radial head can be seen lying in the anterior joint space (fine arrow).

bisecting the proximal radial shaft, intersects the capitellum; if not, there is a radial head dislocation. The anterior fat pad should normally be identified in the coronoid fossa on the lateral film and the posterior fat pad is not seen. In the presence of an effusion, the anterior fat pad is convex and the posterior fat pad can be identified. Multiple views may be necessary to identify an associated fracture.

In children 60% of elbow fractures are supracondylar; almost all have posterior displacement of the condyles and an abnormal anterior humeral line. In adults 50% of elbow fractures are of the radial head and this is the commonest cause of a positive fat pad sign in an adult (Fig. 12.30). Of elbow dislocations, 80–90% are postero-lateral and are often associated with fractures of the coronoid process or radial head. An isolated dislocated radial head is rare in adults and there may be an associated ulnar fracture (**Monteggia fracture**).

SHOULDER AND STERNOCLAVICULAR JOINT

The normal clavicular articular surface extends above the manubrium so the sternoclavicular articulation has an unusual and confusing appearance, but it should be symmetrical. Anterior dislocation at the sternoclavicular joint is more common than posterior, but the latter may compress the great vessels and therefore necessitate surgery; thus accurate diagnosis is mandatory. A limited CT scan of the area is probably the most accurate method of diagnosis.

Acromioclavicular joint separation may involve the acromioclavicular joint itself, with a tear of the acromioclavicular ligament as well as the coracoclavicular ligaments. The acromioclavicular joints are both X-rayed, with and without hand weights. The width of the acromioclavicular joint is normally 3–5 mm but may be up to 8 mm; the disparity between the two sides should be no greater than 3 mm. The length of the coracoclavicular ligament is 11–13 mm, with no greater than 5 mm difference between sides.

Shoulder dislocations are common due to the shallow joint; 95% are anterior or subcoracoid. The posterolateral portion of the humeral head may impact on the antero-inferior part of the glenoid. Particularly after repeated dislocations, this may produce a wedge-shaped **Hill–Sach's defect** of the humeral head, seen best on the Stryker view (Fig. 12.31). The corresponding chip fracture of the glenoid is called the **Bankart lesion**. If only the labrum is involved, it is best seen on double-contrast CT arthrography, although some may be seen on MRI which also allows accurate evaluation of the anterior glenohumeral ligament. It is important to identify these lesions as they may be associated with instability.

Posterior dislocations are usually secondary to fits or electroconvulsive therapy. The humeral head is usually locked in internal rotation, and this gives the **light bulb** appearance where the humeral head is seen as symmetrical and round (Fig. 12.32). The congruity of the joint space is lost. These are, however, relatively subtle signs and many posterior dislocations are missed. The abnormality is obvious on an axial view of the shoulder, or if this cannot be obtained, a 'Y' view of the scapula will show the dislocation. A

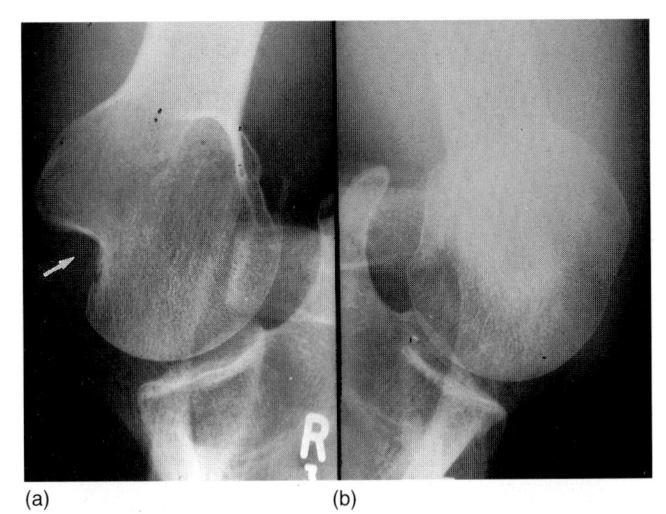

(a) (b)

Fig. 12.31 Bilateral Stryker's views of the shoulders. (a) The right shoulder shows a large Hill–Sach's defect of the humeral head (arrowed). The glenoid cavity is however normal. (b) The left humeral head is normal.

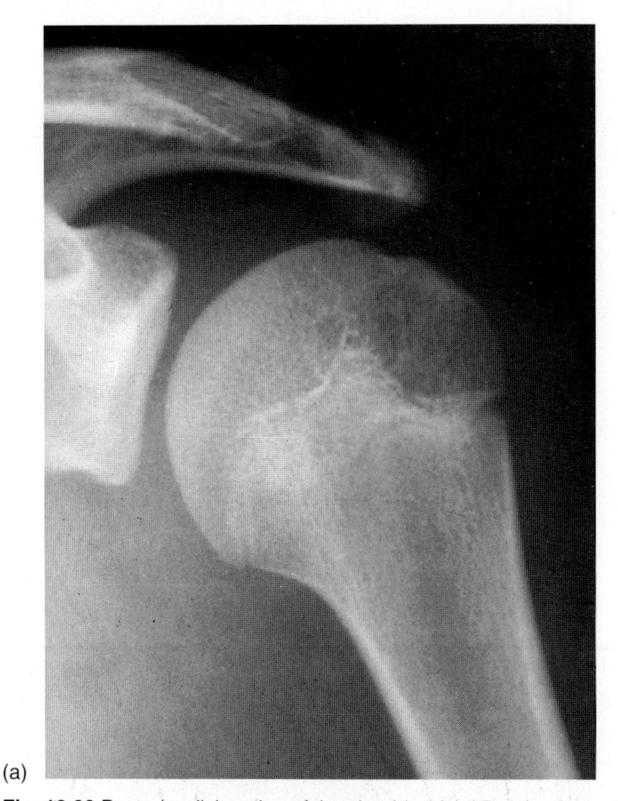

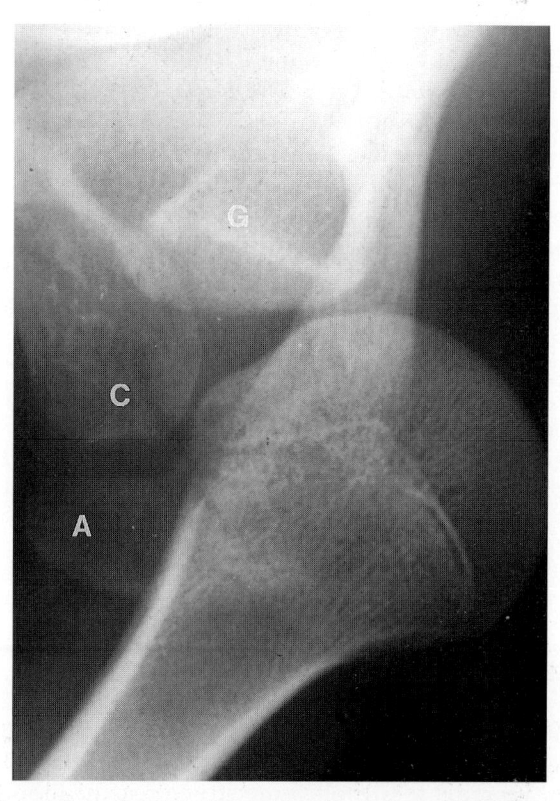

(a) (b)

Fig. 12.32 Posterior dislocation of the shoulder. (a) AP view of the shoulder. The configuration of the humeral head is more rounded than on the normal AP view. (b) However, the abnormal position of the humerus, displaced posteriorly with respect to the acromion (A), clavicle (C) and glenoid (G) is more evident on the axial view.

reverse Hill–Sach's, and/or reverse Bankart lesion may be seen. The rare inferior dislocation results in the articular surface being dislocated inferiorly to the glenoid with fixed abduction of the shaft.

The rotator cuff consists of the supraspinatus, infraspinatus and teres minor muscles which insert on the greater tuberosity, and the subscapularis muscle which inserts on the lesser tuberosity. The supraspinatus muscle and subacromial bursa occupy the space between the humeral head and the acromion; thus it is the supraspinatus tendon that is most commonly torn. Tears of the rotator cuff can be acute or chronic. In the latter, plain films may show a reduction in the subacromial space, sometimes with erosion of the inferior surface of the acromion from mechanical forces; however, in the acute tear, radiographs are normal. The diagnosis is frequently made on MRI where a disruption of the normal black signal of the supraspinatus tendon is seen in association with an effusion and retraction of the belly of the supraspinatus muscle (Fig. 12.33). Ultrasound is also used to make the diagnosis and both of these techniques have superseded the use of arthrography. Clinical signs suggestive of a rotator cuff tear, painful and limited abduction in acute trauma, may be due to an avulsion

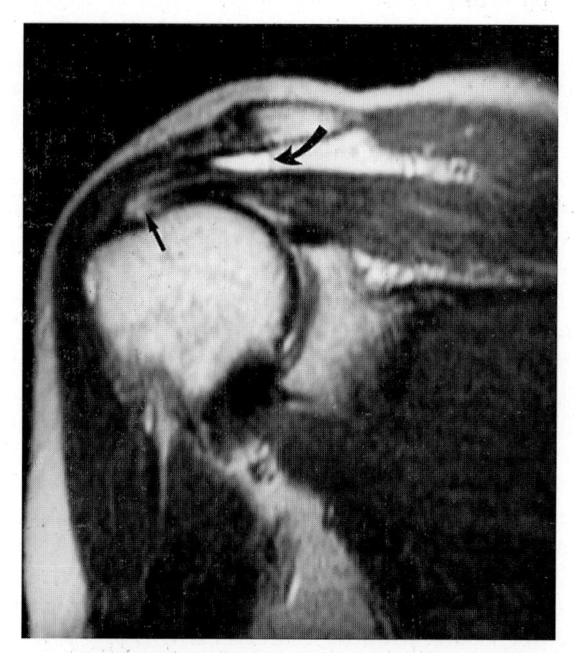

Fig. 12.33 T2-weighted paracoronal MRI through the right shoulder. A small area of bright signal under the acromioclavicular joint represents an effusion in the subacromial bursa (curved arrow). The high signal defect in the distal supraspinatus tendon is also readily identified (arrow).

of the greater trochanter. Avulsion of the lesser trochanter by the subscapularis tendon is rare and difficult to see on plain films, and diagnosis may be aided by ultrasound.

Proximal humeral fractures are common, especially in osteoporotic bone. **Neer's four segment classification** helps in guiding treatment and suggesting prognosis. The four segments are: humeral head, humeral shaft, greater and lesser trochanters. If any of the segments is displaced by >1 cm or 45° then it is significantly displaced; if none of the fragments is displaced then it is undisplaced, irrespective of the degree of comminution. A lateral film must be obtained since anterior angulation is relatively common and is not identified on the other views. If one segment is displaced it is a two-part fracture; if two are displaced it is three-part, etc. Pseudosubluxation may occur due to haemarthrosis or weakness of the deltoid and rotator cuff muscles.

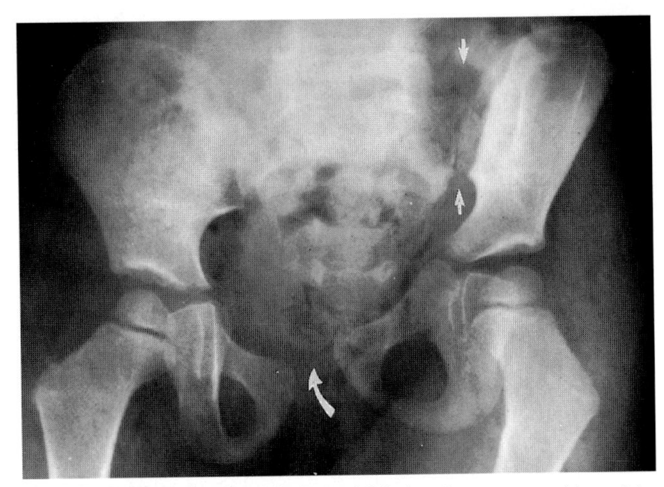

Fig. 12.34 AP view of pelvis in a child showing an unstable pelvic fracture. The pubic symphysis is diastased (curved arrow). In addition, there is disruption of the left sacroiliac joint (arrows). The double break in the pelvic ring indicates that the fracture is unstable.

PELVIS

Pelvic fractures and dislocations may be difficult to diagnose. The films should be evaluated with particular attention to the following structures: the iliopubic and ilio-ischial lines should be intact, as should both anterior and posterior acetabular rims. **Judet**, or 45° oblique, views of the acetabulum are very useful: the posterior oblique view shows the posterior column and anterior acetabular rim, while the anterior view shows the anterior column and posterior rim. Femoral head subluxation and dislocation can be checked, as can disruption in the dome of the acetabulum, with medial migration of the femoral head, **protrusio acetabuli**. Sacral fractures and sacroiliac joint disruptions are particularly hard to identify on the plain films. An apparent single break in the pelvic ring, or a fracture of the transverse process of L5 should alert one to the possibility of sacral or sacroiliac joint injury. The symphysis pubis and sacroiliac joints should not be diastased. The former may be up to 10 mm in children but not >5 mm in adults, and the sacroiliac joints should be 2–4 mm wide in adults.

Two thirds of pelvic fractures are stable and are single breaks along the peripheral margins: avulsion, iliac wing fracture, sacral fracture, or pubic rami fracture. Pelvic disruption in two or more places constitutes an unstable pelvic fracture (Fig. 12.34). The most common is the vertical shear, or **Malgaigne fracture**; this is usually a sacral fracture with ipsilateral inferior and superior pubic rami fractures. Another is the **straddle fracture**, involving both the superior and inferior pubic rami bilaterally. These unstable fractures are associated with a significant risk of haemorrhage and visceral damage, and often require internal fixation.

CT is unnecessary in routine evaluation of stable pelvic fractures but is useful for unstable injuries, sacral and sacroiliac joint fractures. CT may show more extensive disruption to the posterior ring than is seen on the plain films. CT is also of value in searching for intra-articular loose bodies which may prevent adequate reduction following hip dislocation.

Isolated traumatic sacral fractures are usually transverse and result from a direct blow; when seen in conjunction with complex pelvic trauma they are usually vertical and disrupt the sacral foramina and neural arches.

Apophyseal avulsion injuries are common in adolescents around the pelvis. The anterior superior iliac spine is the origin of the sartorius muscle, the anterior inferior iliac spine the origin of the rectus femoris, the ischial tuberosity is the origin of the hamstring muscles (Fig. 12.35), and the inferior pubic ramus, at the symphysis, is the site of origin of the adductor muscles. In the early stages, apophyseal avulsion injuries may be difficult to diagnose, and amorphous new bone formation may be confused with an osteogenic tumour. Occurrence at characteristic sites, together with an appropriate history, and gradually maturing bone, should lead to the correct diagnosis.

HIP

The AP film should show the hip in slight internal rotation. The neck of the femur is thus elongated, the greater trochanter is seen in profile and the lesser trochanter is partly hidden. A true lateral view can be difficult to obtain but may be important in order to confirm a subtle fracture line. Comment is sometimes made about the fat planes surrounding the hip, but

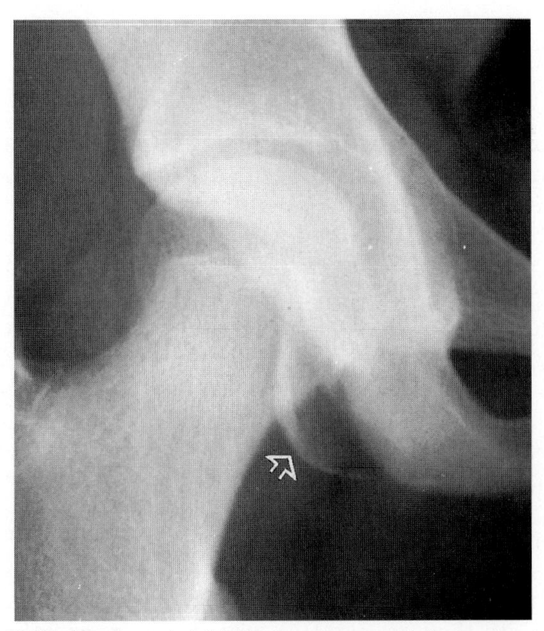

Fig. 12.35 AP view of right hip in a young adult showing ischial tuberosity avulsion. A fragment of bone has separated from the ischial tuberosity and is pulled laterally and inferiorly by the attached hamstring muscles (open arrow).

displacement of these lines is not useful in confirming the presence of an effusion.

Hip fractures are rare in the young and middle-aged, unless there has been severe trauma. Because of senile osteoporosis, however, they are extremely common in the elderly, and subcapital fractures are twice as common as intertrochanteric fractures. The subcapital fracture may be obvious as a change in angulation or as disrupted or angulated trabeculae or, if impacted, it may be seen as a line of increased density, or an irregularity at the outer cortex at the junction of the head and neck. A ring of osteophytes on the superior border of the greater trochanter may be mistaken for an impacted fracture. The blood supply to the femoral head enters through the neck in an adult, and therefore the blood supply is easily compromised in the presence of a subcapital fracture, leading to avascular necrosis in up to 30%. Subcapital fractures are thus commonly treated by hemiprosthetic replacement, although on occasion, if there is significant acetabular degenerative change, the surgeon may elect to perform a total hip replacement.

Intertrochanteric fractures occur in a slightly older age group than subcapital fractures; they may be two, three or four part, depending on the involvement of the trochanters. The oblique fracture usually runs from the greater trochanter superiorly to the lesser trochanter inferiorly, with the greatest amount of comminution seen posteriorly. The fractures are normally internally fixed with a dynamic hip screw. This allows some settling and impaction, and shortening of the screw maintains tension across the fracture. In a severely osteoporotic patient there is a risk of the screw cutting out the femoral head and neck, so the tip of the screw should be placed as posteriorly and inferiorly as possible. Avascular necrosis is rare in intertrochanteric injury.

Avulsion fracture of the lesser trochanter is not an uncommon injury in children and adolescents. If the fragment is pulled up over the pelvis it may not be seen, and the lesser trochanter may just seem to have 'disappeared'. If found as an isolated fracture in an adult then it is usually pathological and metastatic in nature.

Hip dislocation is the occasional result of severe trauma and is most often posterior. The head is located superiorly and there may be an associated acetabular rim fracture. It may be difficult to recognize, although lack of congruity of the joint surfaces and a smaller femoral head on the affected side may be seen. The femoral head can often be palpated in the buttock. Early diagnosis is imperative as the risk of avascular necrosis increases with time: 50% after 24 hours.

Slipped capital femoral epiphysis is seen in 10–16-year-olds. Male, overweight or black patients are more commonly affected; 20% are bilateral, but they are rarely synchronous. Slipped capital femoral epiphysis occurs at the age of rapid growth during which the alignment of the femoral neck changes from valgus to varus, thus producing a factor of shear stress in the growth plate. The slip may, therefore, be precipitated by minor trauma, but it is also more common in the presence of infection, congenital hip dislocation or metabolic bone disease. On the AP film the epiphyseal plate appears wider with indistinct margins, and the epiphysis appears shorter (Fig. 12.36). A line drawn along the lateral aspect of the femoral neck intersects no more than a small portion of the femoral head. The frog-leg lateral will confirm the findings. The treatment is to pin the slip *in situ*. Avascular necrosis develops in 10%, and this complication is more often seen in severe slip and where open reduction has been attempted.

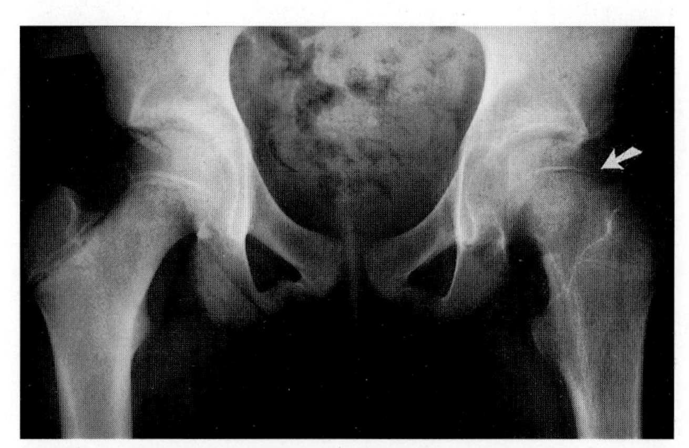

Fig. 12.36 AP view of pelvis in an adolescent showing slipped capital femoral epiphysis. The left capital femoral epiphysis is displaced medially and posteriorly as compared with the right (arrowed).

KNEE

Most knee injuries involve only the soft tissues, to which the only clue may be the presence of an effusion. The lateral view is sensitive to the presence of an effusion. In the normal knee, the fat pad posterior to the quadriceps tendon is divided in two by a line of soft-tissue density, the suprapatellar bursa, which should be no more than 5 mm wide. An anterior cruciate ligament avulsion may, however, be associated with an avulsion injury of the anterior tibial spine, an injury more commonly seen in children and adolescents than adults, because at this age the ligaments are stronger than the bony attachments. Avulsion of the posterior cruciate ligament may result in avulsion of a sliver of bone from the posterior tibia.

The most sensitive imaging method for detecting an internal derangement is MRI, although on occasion it may still be necessary to perform arthrography on a patient who is unable to undergo MRI. Cruciate ligament tears, collateral ligament tears, extensor mechanism pathology and meniscal tears are all readily identified. The normal tendons, ligaments and menisci give low signal (black) on MRI, and tears may seen as linear high signal (white) extending through these structures (Fig. 12.37). The popliteal tendon runs obliquely along the posterior part of the lateral meniscus and may be confused with a tear. The normal menisci are 'bow-tie' shaped in sagittal images, and the medial is thicker posteriorly than anteriorly; a discoid meniscus, usually the lateral, is uniformly thick throughout, and is associated with pain, tears and locking. Meniscal cysts often occur peripherally in the meniscus and are readily identified.

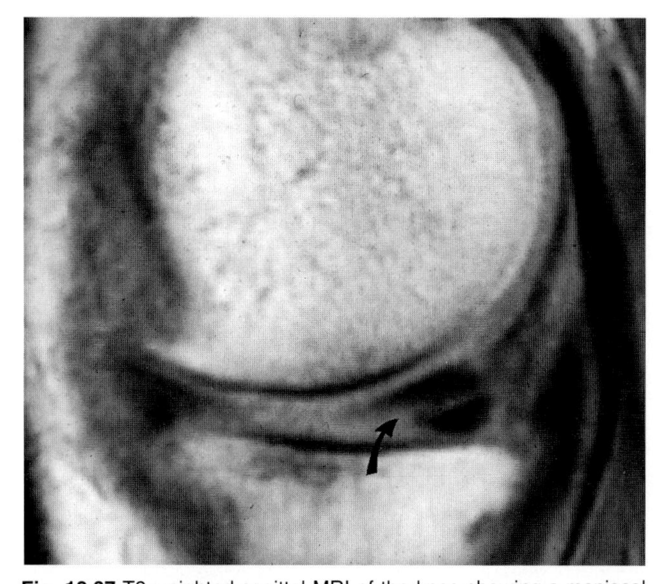

Fig. 12.37 T2-weighted sagittal MRI of the knee showing a meniscal tear. The normal triangular shape of the posterior horn of the medial meniscus is disrupted by a line of high signal running through it (curved arrow).

Many surgeons proceed directly to arthroscopy if there are strong clinical indications of an internal derangement, but the equivocally abnormal knee, following previous surgery, discoid meniscus, or persistent symptoms following an apparently normal arthroscopy, may all be indications for an MRI to be performed first. Bone bruises and other subchondral pathologies can be seen at MRI but not at arthroscopy, while ultrasound is useful for delineating a **Baker's cyst**, showing a large, fluid-filled posterior lesion, and may show the site of a connection with the joint space.

Epiphyseal injuries around the knee are rare, but complications are frequent; 70% are Salter–Harris Type II, and 15% type III. The latter usually involve the medial condyle and are due to valgus stress. They are often undisplaced and therefore occult. The knee is the most common site of Salter–Harris Type V fractures; they are usually seen in the proximal tibia and are associated with tibial shaft fractures. As the rate of growth plate disturbances is so high, prognosis should be guarded, and a careful search maintained for early diagnosis of bony bridging across the physis.

Tibial plateau fractures are common in road traffic accidents involving pedestrians, as the tibial plateau is at the level of a car bumper: 80% are confined to the lateral plateau as they are the result of valgus stress. They may be subtle but it is important to establish the extent of tibial plateau depression as a >1 cm depression or a widely separated (5 mm) vertical split will probably need internal fixation.

Sixty per cent of **patellar fractures** are transverse from indirect force, such as a violent contraction of the quadriceps tendon. The majority of the remainder are stellate due to a direct blow. Beware the bipartite or multipartite patella: the separate fragments are commonly seen on the superolateral aspect of the patella and have well corticated margins. The pattern may be symmetrical. Patellar dislocation is usually lateral, a tendency dictated by the presence of the following anatomical variants: patellar tilt, lateral patellar displacement and patella alta (the ratio of the normal length of the patellar tendon to the length of the patella should be between 0.8 and 1.2).

ANKLE

The lateral margin of the tibia has a fibular notch into which the fibula should fit snugly. If the fibula is shortened after a fracture, the more bulbous distal part of the fibula does not articulate properly with this notch. This in turn leads to lateral shift of the talus, reducing the congruity of the joint, and early degenerative change. Therefore, only 2–3 mm of fibular shortening is acceptable. The joint space should be even across the entire ankle mortise; over 2 mm widening at any point is abnormal. In stress views, valgus and varus force is applied to the calcaneus. There is a wide range of normal ankle laxity, with talar tilt of up to 20° in exceptionally lax ankles, so on occasion comparison views may be necessary. MRI may be helpful to delineate ligamentous injury.

The **Weber classification** is used as it correlates well with treatment and prognosis. It uses the level of the fibular fracture to deduce the injury to the tibiofibular ligaments. The Weber A is a transverse avulsion fracture of the lateral malleolus at, or distal to, the tibiofibular joint and thus does not involve the tibiofibular ligament complex. It may be associated with an oblique fracture of the medial malleolus. The Weber B is a spiral fracture of the lateral malleolus beginning at the level of the ankle joint. This leads to a partial disruption of the tibiofibular ligament complex and so the diastasis of the mortise depends on the severity of the injury. It may be associated with a transverse or slightly oblique fracture of the medial malleolus below the ankle joint or with a deltoid ligament rupture. The Weber C is a fibular fracture proximal to the ankle joint which invariably tears the tibiofibular ligament complex and leads to lateral talar instability. The medial malleolus is avulsed just below the level of the ankle joint, or the deltoid ligament may be torn (Fig. 12.38). Exact anatomic, stable reconstruction of the mortise is essential to prevent post-traumatic arthritis.

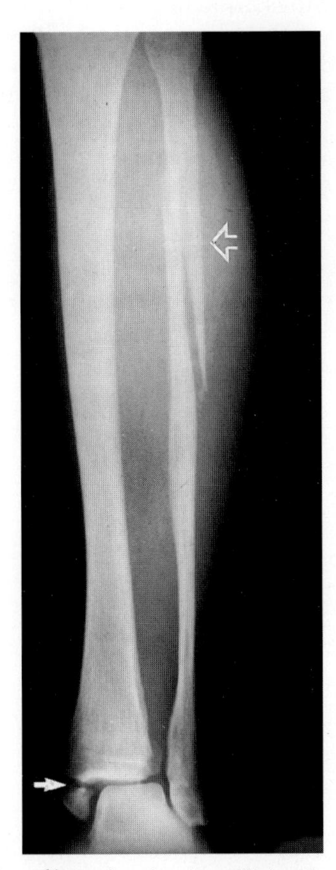

Fig. 12.38 AP view of lower leg showing a Weber C ankle fracture. The fibula is fractured in the proximal to mid-shaft (open arrow). There has been an avulsion of the medial malleolus (closed arrow) and therefore there is lateral talar instability.

Osteochondral fractures of the lateral or medial dome of the talus can occur during ankle trauma and may not be evident on the plain films at the time of injury. There is a high incidence of avascular necrosis, and plain film, CT or MRI may aid diagnosis. With any fracture resulting in widening of the mortise, there may be an associated tear of the proximal tibiofibular ligament and fracture of the proximal fibula, the **Maisonneuve fracture**. The entire fibula should therefore be X-rayed under these circumstances.

Fusion of the distal tibial epiphysis starts at 12–13 years of age; it begins centrally and proceeds medially and then laterally. The unfused portion is often confused with a fracture. The **juvenile Tillaux** fracture may be seen during this pattern of fusion. This injury is a Salter–Harris Type III fracture of the lateral portion of the distal tibial epiphysis which occurs after fusion of the medial part. The **triplane fracture** also occurs in children; it involves the lateral half of the distal tibial epiphysis and a posterior triangular metaphyseal fragment.

The base of the fifth metatarsal should be included on the lateral ankle film as a fracture at this site (**Jones' fracture**) may be mistaken clinically for an ankle injury as they both may follow inversion injury.

FOOT

Several normal appearances can be confused with trauma: notably, the calcaneal apophysis and the navicular may appear dense and fragmented in the normal growing skeleton and the proximal epiphysis of the proximal phalanx of the great toe may be bifid.

The articulations of the tarsals and metatarsals may seem confusing, but normal alignment is important to exclude mid-foot dislocations, which may quickly compromise the vascular supply to the forefoot.

On the AP film:

- the lateral border of the first metatarsal should align with the lateral border of the medial cuneiform;
- the medial border of the second metatarsal should align with the medial border of the middle cuneiform.

On the lateral oblique film:

- the lateral border of the third metatarsal should align with the lateral border of the lateral cuneiform;

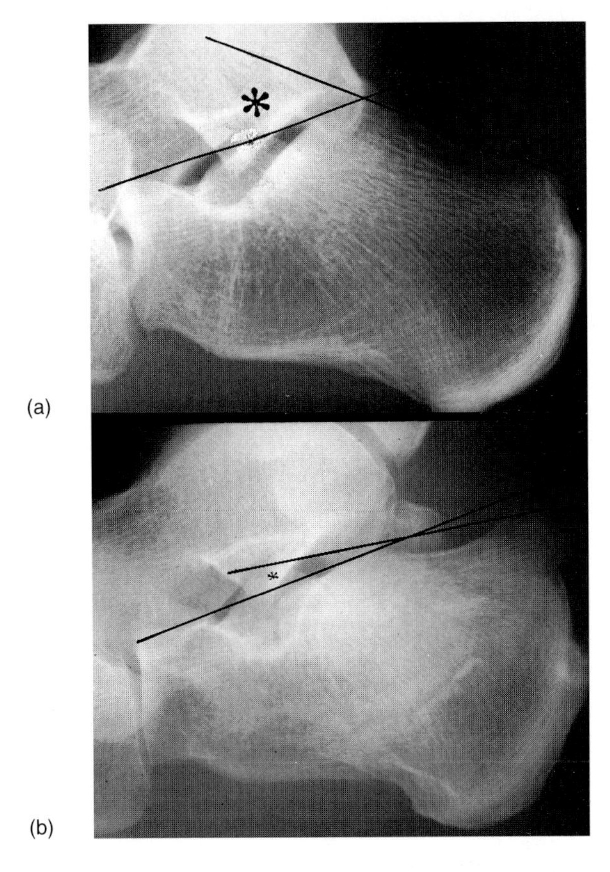

Fig. 12.39 (a) Normal lateral view of the calcaneum illustrating Bohler's angle (large asterisk). The normal range is from 28–40°. (b) The patient has an intra-articular fracture of the calcaneum and Bohler's angle is markedly reduced (small asterisk).

- the medial border of the fourth metatarsal aligns with the medial border of the cuboid;
- the base of the fifth metatarsal articulates with the cuboid but extends lateral to the lateral border of the cuboid.

The base of the second metatarsal is recessed between the medial and lateral cuneiform in a lock and key configuration.

Fractures of the calcaneus may be seen best on the axial, or Harris view. They are classified as either intra- or extra-articular. The presence of an intra-articular, crush, fracture is denoted by a decrease in **Bohler's angle** (Fig. 12.39): 10% are bilateral and 10% are associated with thoracolumbar fractures, the **Don Juan** fracture, so called because the common mechanism is a fall from a height, such as hurrying through a window! A talar fracture may occur through the neck and may be associated with a talar dislocation.

The **Lisfranc fracture dislocation** is a dorsal dislocation at the tarsometatarsal joints with a fracture of the base of the second metatarsal. It is either homolateral, with lateral dislocation or neutral position of the great toe metatarsal, or divergent, with medial subluxation of the great toe metatarsal. Continued weight-bearing leads to progressive displacement. The injury is frequently a manifestation of a neuropathic foot. Early changes may be subtle and require CT for diagnosis

The nail bed of the great toe is attached to the periosteum at the level of the proximal metaphysis, and in a child a stubbed toe may result in a Salter–Harris Type I or II fracture and/or osteomyelitis.

CHAPTER 13

Bones, joints and soft tissues

Asif Saifuddin
and Sarah Burnett

This chapter covers the major acquired diseases of bone, joints and soft-tissues, excluding skeletal trauma; congenital or developmental syndromes are beyond the scope of this book.

DISEASES OF BONE

INFECTIONS

ACUTE PYOGENIC OSTEOMYELITIS

Acute osteomyelitis is typically a disease of childhood and most commonly due to haematogenous spread of *Staphylococcus aureus* from a distant focus. Other less common organisms include salmonella spp., particularly in patients with sickle-cell anaemia, and pseudomonas spp. in drug abusers. Less commonly, infection is due to direct spread from soft-tissue infection or follows penetrating injury (traumatic or iatrogenic).

The site of infection within a bone depends on age. Acute haematogenous osteomyelitis in childhood typically involves the metaphysis of a long bone, because here the blood flow is sluggish and the metaphyseal vessels do not cross the growth plate. Therefore, involvement of the epiphysis and joint is rare. The femur and tibia are involved in 65–75% of cases. Up to 1 year of age, the metaphyseal vessels penetrate the growth plate and therefore epiphyseal and joint involvement may accompany metaphyseal osteomyelitis in the infant. This may result in slipped epiphysis, dislocation and growth deformity. Multifocal osteomyelitis is also relatively common in neonates. In adults, the growth plate is closed and terminal metaphyseal vessels anastomose with epiphyseal vessels. Joint infection is, therefore, relatively

Diagnostic and Interventional Radiology in Surgical Practice. Edited by P. Armstrong and M. L. Wastie. Published in 1997 by Chapman & Hall, London. ISBN 0 412 61960 1 (HB), 0 412 61970 9 (PB)

common in association with metaphyseal osteomyelitis although in adults the spine and small bones are the commonest sites of involvement.

Initially there is inflammation and pus formation in the medulla with associated vascular thrombosis. Infection then spreads through the adjacent cortex resulting in subperiosteal abscess formation and periosteal elevation. Necrosis of cortical bone may result, producing a sequestrum, while subperiosteal bone formation results in development of an involucrum. Extension of the infective process may occur subperiosteally, both along and around the shaft of the bone. If pus escapes through the periosteum (resulting in cloaca formation), soft-tissue abscesses may develop.

Initial plain film findings include soft-tissue swelling with loss of fat planes within the first week. Bone changes are not seen until 10–14 days and consist of osteopenia and poorly defined lytic areas in the metaphysis together with, typically, a single layer of periosteal reaction (Fig. 13.1). This usually develops by 2 weeks after the initial symptoms. Areas of cortical destruction and multilayered periosteal reaction may also be seen.

Involvement of the epiphysis may result in diminished size or absence of the epiphysis. Sequestrum formation is identified as one or more areas of dense, necrotic cortical bone, while soft-tissue abscesses may be manifest as gas in the soft tissues and soft-tissue swelling.

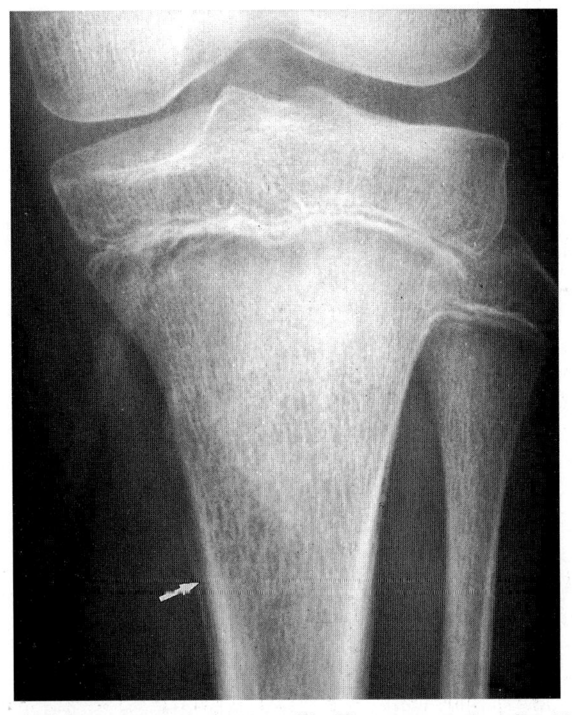

Fig. 13.1 Acute pyogenic osteomyelitis. There are poorly defined lytic and sclerotic areas in the proximal tibial metaphysis and a single layer of periosteal reaction (arrow).

Subperiosteal pus collections can be identified with ultrasound well before plain film bone changes occur and ultrasound can be used to guide aspiration/biopsy.

Bone scintigraphy with ^{99m}Tc-methylene diphosphonate (MDP) can demonstrate abnormality in bone within hours to days. Within the first 3 days, there may be a 'cold' area due to vascular thrombosis in the medulla, but this progresses to increased activity. Scintigraphy is the method of choice for identifying multifocal osteomyelitis. Gallium-citrate scans and labelled WBC scans are more specific for osteomyelitis than ^{99m}Tc-MDP bones scans.

MRI is also abnormal early and is very sensitive, demonstrating bone oedema as areas of reduced signal on T1-weighted scans and increased signal on STIR and T2-weighted scans. Ultrasound, CT and MRI are all of value in identifying soft-tissue abscess formation.

Acute osteomyelitis secondary to soft-tissue infection may result in focal, poorly defined bone destruction and periosteal reaction. If plain films are normal, three-phase bone scintigraphy can help to differentiate osteomyelitis from cellulitis, since the latter will show minimal or no uptake in bone on the delayed (static) images. MRI will also be able to differentiate cellulitis from osteomyelitis.

CHRONIC OSTEOMYELITIS

If treatment of acute osteomyelitis is delayed or inadequate, chronic osteomyelitis may develop. This is characterized pathologically by a prominent involucrum, sequestra and cloaca with sinus formation to the skin. It is the presence of infected dead bone which results in recurrent infection.

Typical radiographic findings include thick sclerotic periosteal reaction and the demonstration of a sequestrum which appears as relatively dense bone that may lie within the medullary cavity (Fig. 13.2).

Additional imaging is aimed at demonstrating a sequestrum as a source of recurrent infection, and at identifying active infection. A sequestrum, if not identified on plain films, is best demonstrated with thin-section CT. Demonstrating activity is more difficult. Increased uptake on ^{99m}Tc-MDP bone scanning is non-specific. However, if ^{99m}Tc-MDP scanning is combined with ^{67}Ga-citrate scanning, infection is likely to be present if the uptake on the gallium scan exceeds that on the MDP scan. MRI may also be useful in assessing activity by identifying medullary inflammation. Sinography, CT and MRI are all useful for identifying sinus tracts.

Complications of chronic osteomyelitis include amyloidosis and malignant transformation in a chronic draining sinus tract, usually 10–20 years after the initial infection.

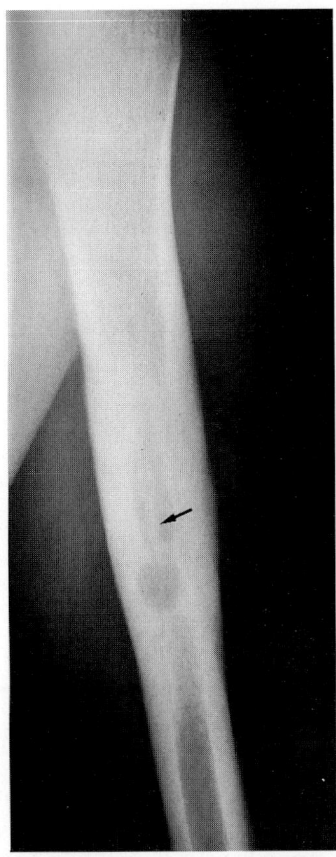

Fig. 13.2 Chronic osteomyelitis of the humerus. There is concentric thickening of the cortex. A sequestrum is identified within the medullary cavity (arrow).

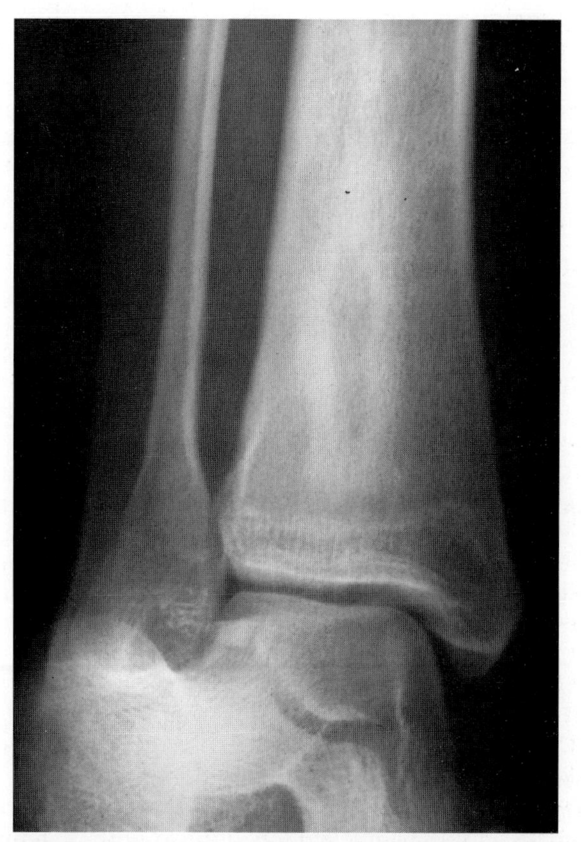

Fig. 13.3 Brodie's abscess of the tibia appearing as an oval lytic area in the metaphysis with surrounding sclerosis.

BRODIE'S ABSCESS

The term 'Brodie's abscess' refers to a particular form of chronic osteomyelitis in which the infection is closely contained resulting in a chronic medullary abscess composed of pus or jelly-like granulation tissue. Radiographs demonstrate a well-defined lytic lesion in the medulla with variable surrounding sclerosis and periosteal reaction (Fig. 13.3). The lesion usually occurs in children in the metaphysis of a long bone. Occasionally, a Brodie's abscess arises within the cortex, where it may elicit a marked sclerotic reaction, mimicking osteoid osteoma.

TUBERCULOUS OSTEOMYELITIS

Bone and joint tuberculosis usually results from haematogenous spread from lung infection. However, in up to 50% of cases no radiological evidence of active or healed pulmonary tuberculosis is found. The incidence of tuberculous osteomyelitis is relatively high in patients of African and Asian origin and in those with AIDS.

Tuberculosis results in a much more indolent infection than pyogenic osteomyelitis so that, even

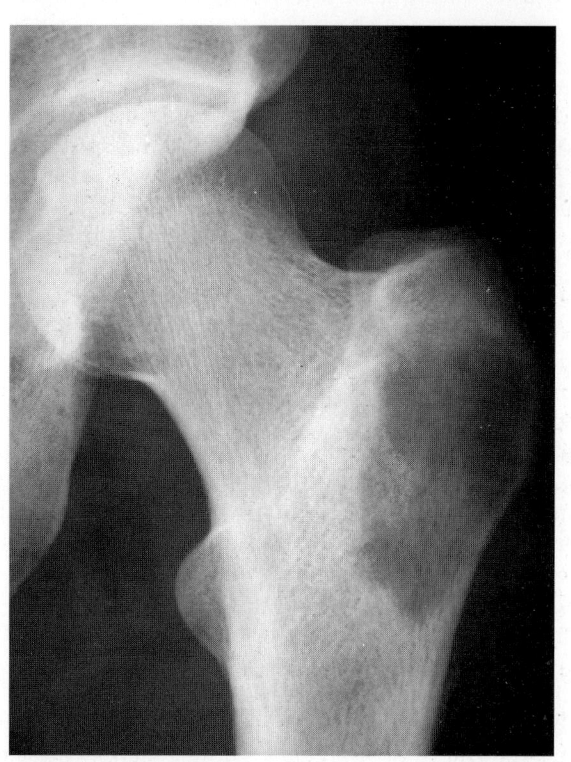

Fig. 13.4 Tuberculous osteomyelitis of the left proximal femur appearing as a well-defined lytic lesion without marginal sclerosis or periosteal reaction. The location adjacent to a tuberosity is characteristic.

though symptoms are much less severe, there is usually obvious radiological abnormality at the time of presentation.

Infection is most common in the spine, following by the large joints. Other sites include the metaphyseal regions of long bones and, rarely, diaphyseal lesions or involvement of bones such as the sternum, calcaneus, rib and skull. Soft-tissue infection may also result in bursitis or tenosynovitis.

The typical radiological features of tuberculous bone infection include irregular, destructive lesions in the metaphysis without marginal sclerosis and little, if any, periosteal reaction (Fig. 13.4). Involvement of the epiphysis is relatively common. Sclerosis occurs as healing takes place.

Rarer forms of tuberculous osteomyelitis include **dactylitis**, resulting in expansion and thinning of the metacarpals or metatarsals (spina ventosa), and cystic tuberculosis resulting in multiple well-defined lytic lesions in the shafts of long bones and in flat bones.

MISCELLANEOUS INFECTIONS

Chronic recurrent multifocal osteomyelitis

This is a rare condition of unknown aetiology occurring in children and young adults, with a female predominance. It typically presents with episodes of pain and swelling at affected sites with or without low-grade fever. The clinical course of exacerbations and remissions has been reported to last up to 15 years. There is an association with pustulosis palmaris and plantaris. Bone biopsy demonstrates a non-specific subacute or chronic osteomyelitis and culture of biopsy material is invariably negative. There is a predilection for the metaphyseal ends of long bones, particularly the tibia and femur. Other common sites include the clavicle, particularly the medial end, fibula, radius and humerus, but many other sites of involvement have been reported.

The initial radiographic finding is a lytic area in the metaphysis, adjacent to a growth plate, associated with periosteal reaction which may become very thick and dense. Lesions may be symmetrical. The multifocal nature of the condition is well demonstrated by bone scintigraphy. CT or MRI will exclude the presence of an associated soft-tissue mass.

Diabetic foot

Osteomyelitis in the diabetic foot is often difficult to diagnose because of the common coexistence of cellulitis, vascular insufficiency and neuropathy.

Bone infection usually occurs secondary to cellulitis. Plain radiographs may not show osteoporosis and periosteal reaction (the classical findings in acute haematogenous osteomyelitis). Also, bone destruction may be a consequence of neuropathy, making the diagnosis even more difficult. ^{99m}Tc bone scanning will show increased activity in both neuropathy and infection, but a negative bone scan virtually excludes the possibility of osteomyelitis. Increased specificity for osteomyelitis may be obtained with labelled-leucocyte scans and, possibly, MRI.

Syphilis and yaws

Syphilis is now so rare that yaws lesions of bone are more common, particularly in patients from Africa, South America and the Far East. Syphilis may be congenital or acquired, but congenital transmission of yaws does not occur.

The bone changes in congenital syphilis consist of a periostitis and an osteitis, which are usually symmetrical. The periosteal reaction is initially laminated, then consolidates to new bone. The commonest site is the tibia, resulting in a 'sabre tibia'.

The osteitis is due to intraosseous granulomata, usually in the metaphysis. This may be associated with widening of the growth plate and metaphyseal lucent bands. The upper tibia and humerus are common sites. Granulomas may also be found in the skull and digits, the latter causing a dactylitis that resembles tuberculosis.

In acquired syphylis, the periostitis may be either laminated or more local and hypertrophic. The osteitis results in a mixed sclerotic/lytic change, usually within the diaphysis of a bone, associated with periosteal reaction.

The bone lesions of yaws are virtually identical to those of acquired syphilis. Once again, common sites include the long bones, skull and digits.

Leprosy

Leprosy is relatively common in Africa, Central and South America, the Indian subcontinent and the Far East. Bone disease may be either due to direct infection or, more commonly, due to neuropathy.

Lepromatous osteitis results initially in osteoporosis. Destructive lesions usually affect the small bones of the hands and feet, and are accompanied by periosteal reaction.

Neuropathic changes manifest as bone resorption, usually from the distal ends of the phalanges and metatarsals. The tips of the resorbed ends may be sharply pointed. Superadded infection results in osteoporosis and bone destruction, with periosteal reaction. Calcification of the peripheral nerves is a rare, but pathognomonic finding.

Fungal infections

There are many fungi which may affect bone, either by direct spread from soft-tissue lesions or from disseminated disease, in which case infection arises in the marrow cavity, resulting in areas of permeative bone destruction, periosteal reaction and variable sclerosis. Sequestrum formation tends not to be a feature.

Recognized causes of fungal osteomyelitis include actinomycosis, streptomyces, histoplasmosis, blastomycosis, coccidioidomycosis and cryptococcosis. They all tend to occur in the Tropics and some areas of North America.

Hydatid disease

Hydatid disease is classically associated with sheep farming. Less than 30% of infected individuals develop bone infection, most commonly in the long bones, pelvis and spine. The intraosseous cyst causes pressure atrophy from within the bone as it enlarges.

Radiographs therefore show a well-defined lytic lesion that expands the bone. Lesions may be multiple and, when long-standing, can develop a sclerotic rim and provoke some cortical thickening.

BONE TUMOURS

GENERAL ASPECTS

Bone tumours commonly present with localized pain and swelling or pathological fracture. Following initial clinical evaluation, a plain radiograph is likely to be obtained. Various radiographic features of the lesion need to be considered and, when combined, may produce a specific diagnosis or a good indication of whether the lesion is or is not aggressive.

When a specific radiological diagnosis, such as simple bone cyst or non-ossifying fibroma, can be made, no further action may be necessary. Similarly, a specific diagnosis of osteoid osteoma can allow definitive treatment to be instituted. In most cases, however, biopsy is required for an unequivocal diagnosis.

Radiological assessment of bone tumours

Clinical and radiographic features that must be considered in the assessment of a bone lesion include the following:

Age Age is one of the most important factors in the evaluation of a solitary bone lesion and is considered in detail under individual tumours.

Site Both the site within the skeleton and the site within the individual bone are important. These, again, are dealt with in detail under individual tumours.

Pattern of bone destruction This may be described as either geographic, moth-eaten or permeative:

- A **geographic pattern** of bone destruction appears as a lytic area with well-defined, sharp margins. Such an appearance indicates a slow rate of growth and is commonly seen with benign tumours and tumour-like conditions. Some malignant lesions, notably myeloma, may produce this pattern of destruction. Other malignancies rarely appear so well-defined.
- A **'moth-eaten' pattern** of destruction implies a more aggressive process. The term refers to multiple, small, lytic areas of varying sizes with intervening normal cancellous bone. The lesion has a poorly defined margin and the medullary involvement by tumour is always more extensive than that indicated by the radiograph. Most malignant tumours can produce this type of destruction, along with some benign conditions such as osteomyelitis and eosinophilic granuloma.
- A **permeative pattern** of bone destruction is the most aggressive pattern. It appears as multiple, tiny, lytic areas throughout the bone and may sometimes be difficult to appreciate. The extent of medullary involvement is poorly determined on the plain film. Most malignant lesions can produce this appearance, as can osteomyelitis and eosinophilic granuloma.

Margin of lesion The appearance of the margin of the lesion gives an indication of its rate of growth. The presence of a sclerotic rim indicates a relatively slow rate of growth, since the surrounding bone has had time to react. The thicker the margin of sclerosis, the slower the growth rate. Faster growing lesions may have a well-defined border but no sclerosis, whereas lesions with the most rapid rate of growth will have poorly defined, non-sclerotic margins.

Matrix The matrix of a lesion is the cellular material produced by the tumour cells. It may be either osteoid, chondroid, collagenous or myxomatous and is only radiographically visible when calcified. Osseous matrix appears cloud-like or hazy and is seen in bone-forming tumours (e.g. osteosarcoma). Cartilaginous matrix may show punctate calcification or rings and arcs of calcification.

Periosteal reaction The presence and type of periosteal reaction can give clues to the nature and aggressiveness of the associated underlying lesion. A single layer of periosteal reaction may be seen with osteomyelitis, eosinophilic granuloma, Ewing's sarcoma and osteosarcoma. These same conditions can produce multilayered (onion-skin) periosteal reaction.

Solid periosteal reaction indicates a slow process and is almost always associated with benign lesions. However, periosteal reaction may become solid in malignant tumours that have responded to treatment.

A spiculated periosteal reaction may be of either the perpendicular ('hair-on-end') type or the 'sunburst' type. The former is commonest with Ewing's sarcoma whereas the latter is usually seen in osteosarcoma. Both may be seen with metastasis.

A **Codman's triangle** refers to the radiographic appearance of elevated periosteum at the junction with the cortex. It indicates the extraosseous margin of a lesion and can be seen in any benign or malignant process that elevates the periosteum.

It should be noted that the periosteum is only visible radiographically due to mineralization of its deep layer, which usually takes 10–21 days from the onset of the initial insult, whether infection, trauma or tumour. Some tumours may be so aggressive that they do not allow time for this mineralization to occur, and therefore periosteal reaction is not identified radiographically.

FURTHER IMAGING OF PRIMARY BONE TUMOURS

As a rule, plain radiography is the most specific technique for establishing a prebiopsy diagnosis of a focal bone lesion using the signs described above. Many benign lesions require no further imaging for adequate treatment. However, in the case of a malignant tumour, the plain film does not indicate accurately the extent of intramedullary spread, the size of extraosseous mass or its relationship to surrounding structures, and the presence or absence of bony or pulmonary metastases. The major role of further imaging is therefore in the local and distant staging of a malignant bone lesion.

MRI is the most accurate technique for local staging of a tumour (Fig. 13.5). T1-weighted scans clearly indicate the intramedullary extent since tumour tissue has low signal intensity which contrasts well with the high signal of adjacent medullary fat. T2-weighted scans are ideal for assessing the extraosseous component, since tumour tissue is generally hyperintense compared to surrounding muscle. The relationship to adjacent neurovascular bundles can also be assessed. MRI is relatively poor at demonstrating subtle cortical erosion and small calcifications. These are better identified by CT. Following chemotherapy, MRI can be used to define the extent of residual tumour.

^{99m}Tc-MDP bone scanning is used to identify bone metastases at presentation. These are reported to occur in approximately 10% of Ewing's sarcomas and 2% of osteosarcomas. In the latter case, pulmonary metastases may also be identified if large enough. It is important to realize that the bone scan is generally of

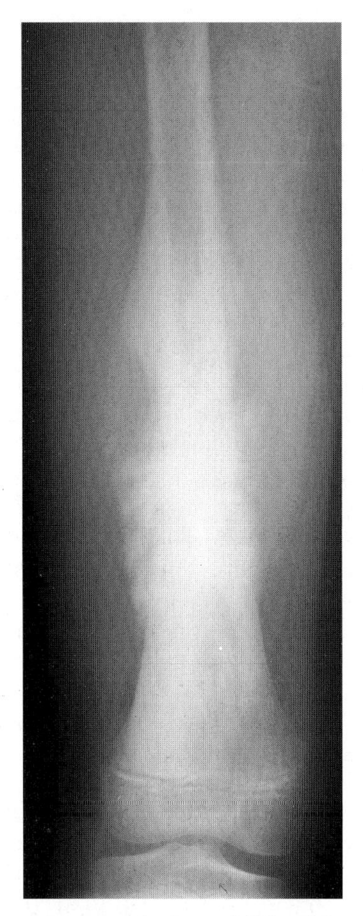

(a)

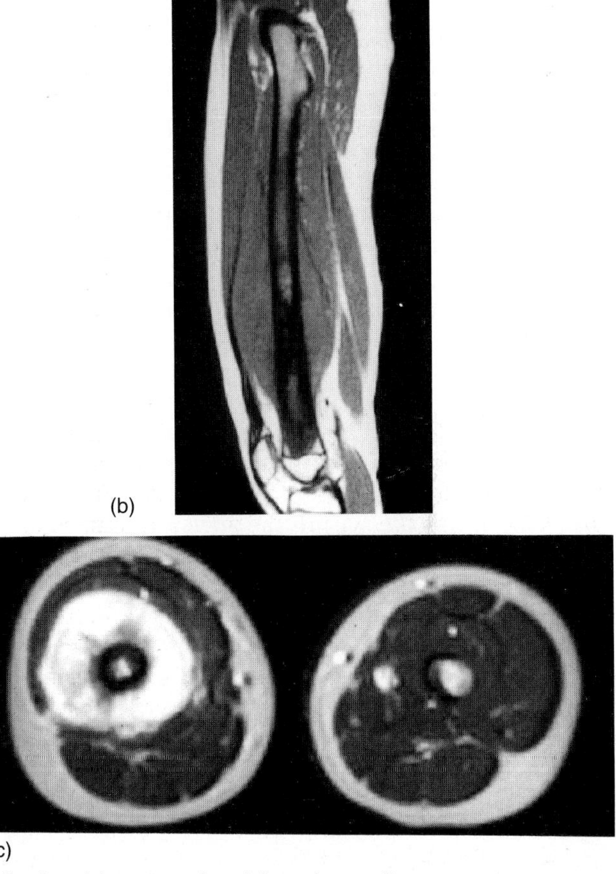

(b)

(c)

Fig. 13.5 Osteosarcoma of the femur. (a) The plain radiograph gives little indication of the extent of medullary abnormality or extraosseous mass. (b) Sagittal T1-weighted MRI scan showing the intraosseous tumour as a region of low signal intensity compared to the normal high signal of the marrow. (c) Axial T2-weighted MRI scan clearly demonstrates the extent of extraosseous tumour as a high signal intensity region. The normal left side is shown for comparison.

limited value in the assessment of the primary lesion, since it cannot differentiate accurately between neoplastic and non-neoplastic conditions, or between benign and malignant neoplastic lesions.

The major role of **CT** is in the identification of pulmonary, pleural and mediastinal metastases, since CT is much more sensitive than the plain chest radiograph. CT may also be useful for biopsy guidance in areas such as the pelvis and spine.

The preoperative investigation of a primary malignant bone tumour should therefore include plain radiography and MRI of the primary lesion, whole body bone scintigraphy, chest radiography, and CT of the thorax.

BENIGN BONE TUMOURS AND TUMOUR-LIKE CONDITIONS

Osseous lesions

Osteoma and enostosis (bone island) Osteomas and bone islands are hamartomatous conditions producing well-defined, purely sclerotic lesions. Both lesions are non-aggressive. Osteomas usually arise from the outer table of the skull or paranasal sinuses. Multiple osteomas are associated with familial polyposis coli (**Gardner's syndrome**). Bone islands occur within the medullary cavity and any bone may be affected. They must be differentiated from sclerotic metastases.

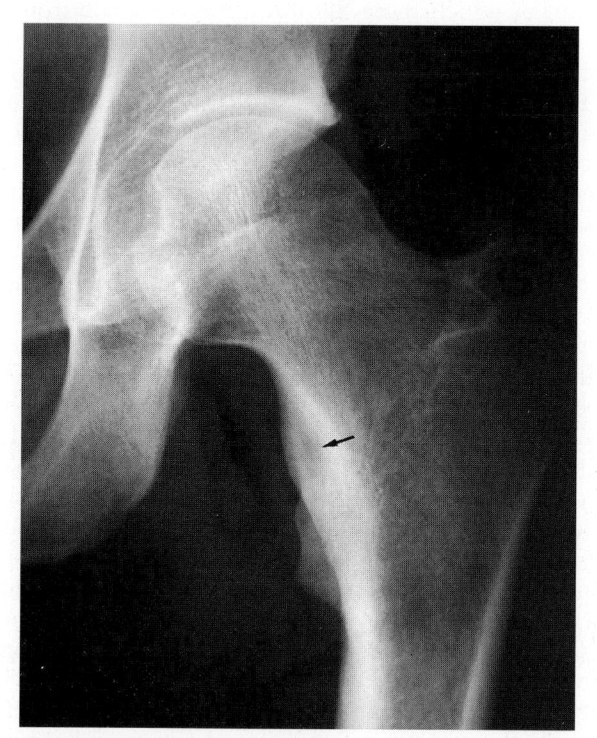

Fig. 13.6 Osteoid osteoma of the medial femoral neck appearing as a small lucent nidus (arrow) surrounded by dense cortical thickening.

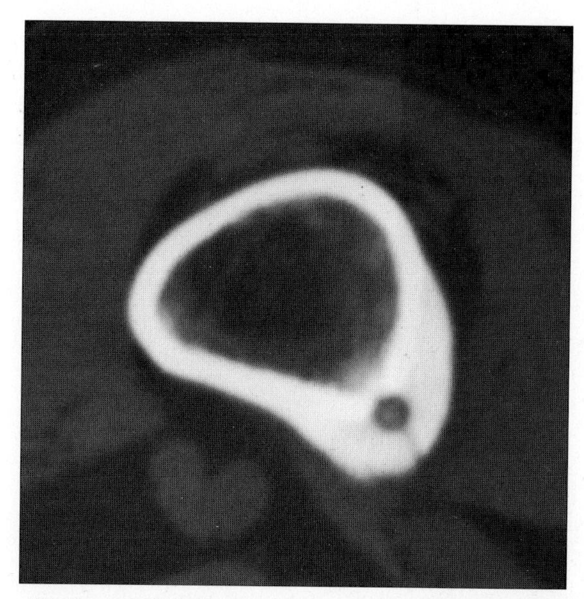

Fig. 13.7 Typical CT features of an osteoid osteoma of the femoral diaphysis. The nidus appears as a round lesion of soft-tissue density containing central calcification. It is surrounded by dense periosteal new bone.

Osteoid osteoma Osteoid osteoma occurs most commonly in the second to third decade, being three times more common in males than females. It accounts for approximately 12% of primary benign bone tumours. Patients classically present with focal bone pain which may be worse at night and relieved by aspirin. The tumour may be cortical, medullary or, rarely, subperiosteal in location. Cortical lesions are commonest and usually occur in long bone diaphyses but have been described in most bones. Intramedullary osteoid osteomas are usually intra-articular, the commonest site being the medial aspect of the femoral neck.

The classic radiological appearance of a long bone osteoid osteoma is of a region of dense, well-defined cortical thickening containing a small (usually < 1 cm), lucent nidus which may be calcified (Fig. 13.6) The nidus represents the actual tumour tissue. Occasionally, the sclerotic response is so marked that the nidus is obscured. In these cases, CT is the best technique for identifying the nidus (Fig. 13.7).

Scintigraphy also shows a characteristic appearance: a focal area of intense activity (the nidus) surrounded by a more diffuse area of less increased uptake due to reactive sclerosis, the 'double-density' sign (Fig. 13.8). A normal radionuclide bone scan virtually excludes the diagnosis.

Tumours in an intra-articular location may produce a periosteal response that is distant from the lesion, and also result in synovitis and joint effusion. Radiographically, such lesions produce diffuse osteopenia and the nidus may not be seen. In these cases, bone scintigraphy will typically show a focal area of intense activity. CT can then be used to demonstrate the nidus.

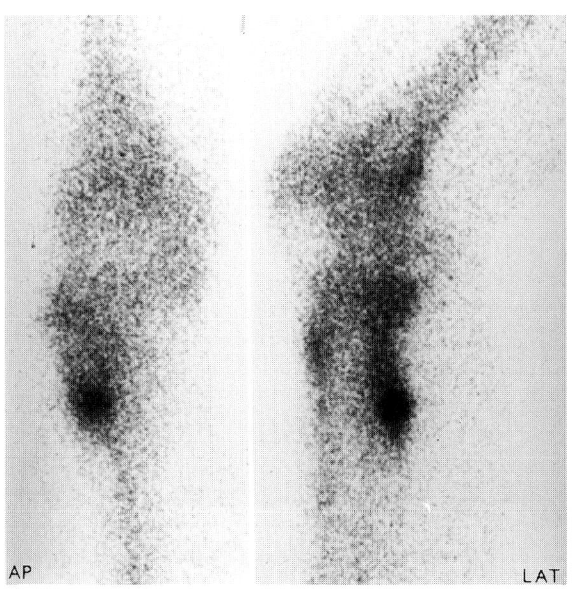

Fig. 13.8 Typical scintigraphic appearance of an osteoid osteoma in the posterolateral tibial cortex demonstrating the 'double density' sign.

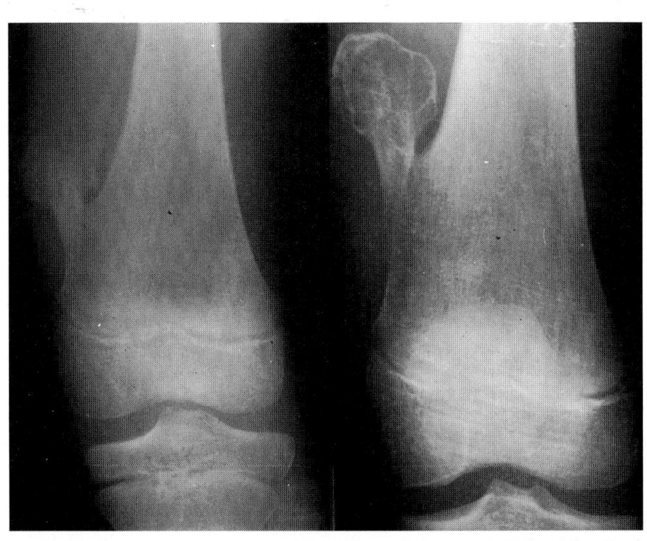

Fig. 13.9 Pedunculated osteochondroma of the medial distal femoral metaphysis. With time, the lesion grows away from the adjacent joint.

CT is also now used to guide percutaneous excision biopsy of this tumour. MRI is less sensitive at identifying the nidus but will identify adjacent marrow and soft-tissue reactive changes.

Osteoblastoma Histologically, osteoblastoma resembles osteoid osteoma but the nidus is larger (usually >1.5 cm). Most lesions occur in the spine (40–50%), flat bones or long bones in young adults (second to third decade).

Radiologically, the lesions are usually lytic and expansile with well-defined sclerotic margins. Variable matrix mineralization occurs. They may occasionally behave in an aggressive manner. The lesions show intense activity on bone scintigraphy due to their osteoblastic nature.

Cartilaginous lesions

Osteochondroma (exostosis) Osteochondroma is a very common benign neoplasm that results from the displacement of a fragment of growth plate cartilage into the metaphyseal region. The underlying bone is normal and the osteochondroma develops as an outgrowth which is continuous with the cortex and marrow cavity at its site of origin. The surface of the lesion consists of a cartilage cap.

Osteochondromas may extend from the host bone on a stalk (pedunculated) or be much more broad-based (sessile). They are usually discovered in the first or second decades; 90% are solitary and 95% are found in the major long bones, especially around the knee. They arise in the metaphysis and, with growth, point away from the adjacent joint (Fig. 13.9). The stalk has the appearance of normal bone and the cap may show chondroid-type calcifications. The lesion ceases to grow at the time of skeletal maturity. Occasionally, a bursa may form over the cartilage cap, which can be demonstrated by ultrasound or MRI.

Complications of osteochondromas include growth abnormalities, mechanical problems and malignant degeneration. Malignant change occurs in less than 1% of solitary lesions and is suggested by the development of pain or further growth after skeletal maturity.

Diaphyseal aclasis is an autosomal dominant condition in which there are multiple osteochondromas. This condition is associated with a relatively high incidence of sarcomatous degeneration (up to 10%).

Enchondroma (chondroma) Enchondromas are usually solitary tumours occurring most commonly in the medulla of tubular bones (40% in hands, 10% in feet, 20% in long bones) or in the flat bones or spine. They are asymptomatic unless complicated by fracture or malignant degeneration.

Multiple lesions occur in multiple enchondromatosis (**Ollier's disease**) or in association with soft-tissue haemangiomas (**Maffucci's syndrome**). The malignant potential is estimated at 1–5%.

Radiologically, they appear as geographic, lytic lesions which may be expansile, especially in the hands and feet. They have thin, sclerotic borders and a calcified matrix (Fig. 13.10). Differentiation from low-grade central chondrosarcoma may be impossible, necessitating biopsy of suspicious lesions. Rarely, chondromas may occur in a juxtacortical location.

Chondroblastoma Chondroblastomas are uncommon tumours typically occurring in children: 65% present in the second decade. The commonest sites include the proximal humerus and femur and around the knee joint.

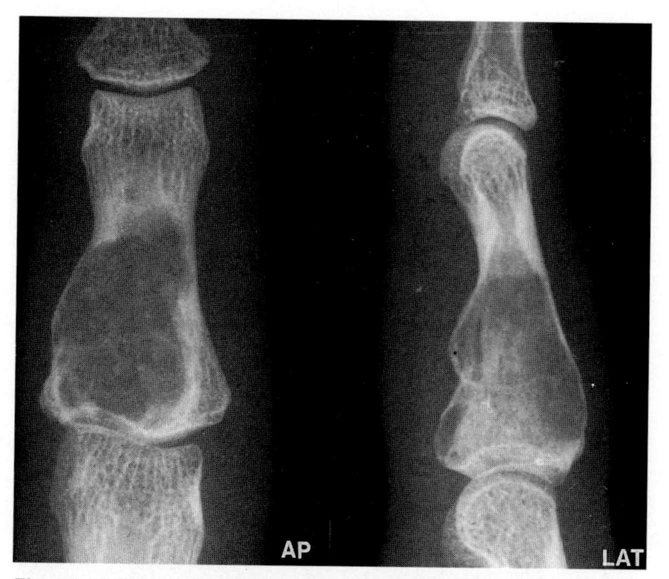

Fig. 13.10 Enchondroma of the middle phalanx appearing as a well-defined, expansile lytic lesion with punctate matrix calcification.

Plain radiographs show a geographic, lytic lesion with thin, marginal sclerosis located in a long bone epiphysis (Fig. 13.11). Matrix calcification and periosteal reaction may be seen. Lesions occurring after closure of the growth plate may extend into the metaphysis. They rarely metastasize.

Chondromyxoid fibroma Chondromyxoid fibromas are very rare tumours classically presenting as a geographic, lobulated lytic lesion in the proximal tibial metaphysis with surrounding sclerosis. Matrix calcification is rare. Other sites include proximal and distal femur, flat bones and tarsals.

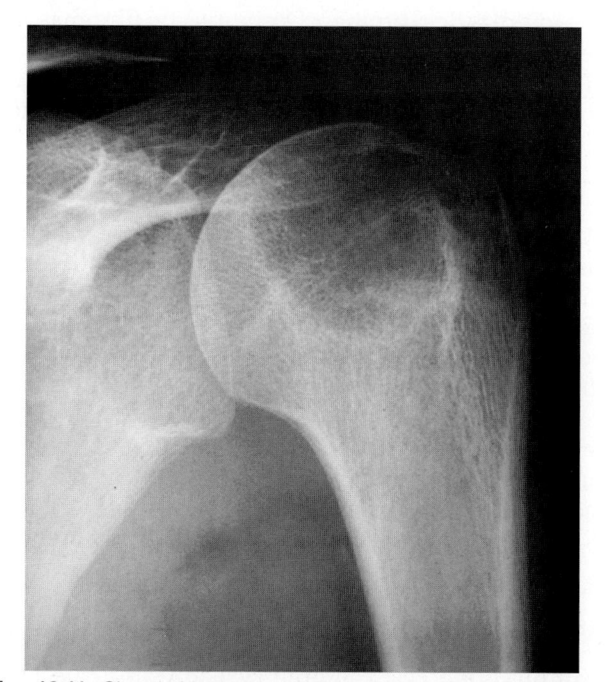

Fig. 13.11 Chondroblastoma of the proximal humeral epiphysis appearing as a well-defined lytic lesion with thin surrounding sclerosis. Multilayered periosteal reaction is present.

Giant cell tumour

Approximately 80% of giant-cell tumours occur in the third to fifth decades. The tumour may behave either in a totally benign fashion, may be locally aggressive or, rarely, may metastasize. The majority of these tumours affect the subarticular regions of long bones, with 50% occurring around the knee. The distal radius is another frequent site. Tumours that arise in an unfused skeleton occur in the metaphysis, adjacent to a growth plate or an apophysis. The flat bones and spine are less commonly affected.

Plain radiographs typically demonstrate a lytic subarticular lesion with an indistinct zone of transition, usually without surrounding sclerosis (Fig. 13.12). Trabeculation is a feature of larger lesions. The lesion is eccentric and thins the cortex, not uncommonly breaking through to form an extraosseous mass. Periosteal reaction is rare.

Fibrous lesions

Fibrous cortical defects and non-ossifying fibroma The appearance, location and histology of these two lesions is identical. They are differentiated only by their size, with larger lesions (>2 cm) being designated non-ossifying fibroma; 95% occur before the age of 20 and 90% involve the lower limbs, especially the tibia and fibula. Most lesions are found incidentally and are of no significance, but larger lesions may present with pathological fracture.

Non-ossifying fibroma is typically metaphyseal, appearing as a geographic, lobulated, intracortical, lytic lesion that may expand into the medulla

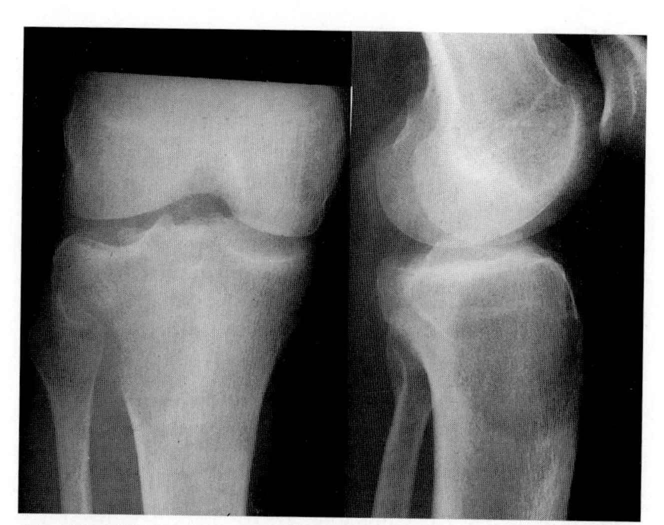

Fig. 13.12 Giant cell tumour of the lateral tibial plateau appearing as a purely lytic lesion with a moderately well-defined margin. Extension to the articular surface is characteristic.

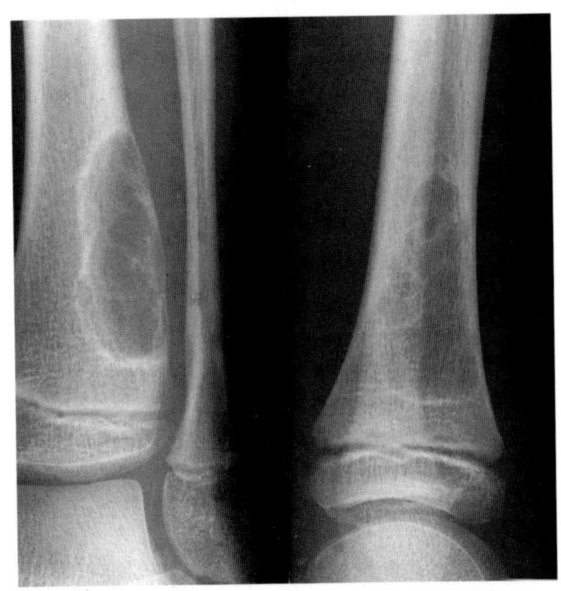

Fig. 13.13 Non-ossifying fibroma of the distal tibia appearing as a lytic cortically based expansile lesion. The appearances are characteristic.

(Fig. 13.13). When multiple, some cases are associated with neurofibromatosis. The plain film findings are usually so characteristic that biopsy is unnecessary.

Fibrous dysplasia and osteofibrous dysplasia Fibrous dysplasia is a relatively common, non-neoplastic condition that may present in a wide age group, but most commonly manifests in the second and third decades; 70% are monostotic, the commonest sites include the metaphyseal regions of the femur and tibia, the ribs (where it represents the commonest benign lesion), the pelvis, skull base and paranasal sinuses. When polyostotic, the condition tends to present in childhood and 90% of lesions are unilateral. Polyostotic fibrous dysplasia may be associated with pigmentation and precocious puberty in young girls (**Albright's syndrome**).

The radiological appearances are very variable. Rib and long bone lesions tend to be expansile with a well-defined, thin, sclerotic rim. The matrix may be predominantly fibrous, giving rise to a 'ground glass' appearance (Fig. 13.14), or show variable mineralization. Deformity is also a feature. Lytic areas within the lesion may represent cystic change, which predisposes to pathological fracture. Pelvic lesions may be very expansile and bubbly. Lesions in the skull and facial bones are often densely sclerotic. Periosteal reaction may accompany pathological fracture. The lesions tend to remain quiescent throughout life, with only a small proportion continuing to enlarge after skeletal maturity.

Osteofibrous dysplasia is a rare lesion similar to fibrous dysplasia, classically occurring in the anterior tibia of young children.

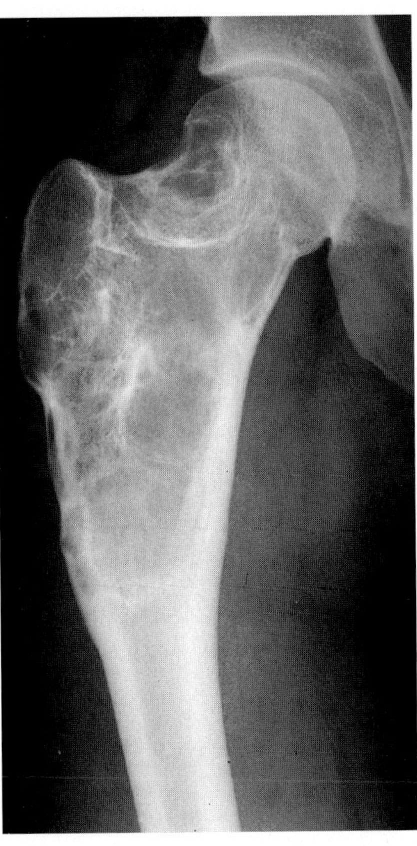

Fig. 13.14 Fibrous dysplasia of the right femoral neck. The lesion is expansile and trabeculated. The 'ground-glass' appearance to the matrix is indicative of a fibrous lesion.

Other connective tissue tumours

Desmoplastic fibroma Desmoplastic fibromas are rare intraosseous lesions, histologically identical to soft-tissue aggressive fibromatosis (extra-abdominal desmoid tumour). The condition may involve various sites, appearing as an expansile lytic lesion.

Cortical desmoid Cortical desmoids are not true neoplasms, but are a post-traumatic fibroblastic response at the insertion of the adductor magnus muscle on the posteromedial cortex of the distal femur. Cortical erosion, soft-tissue mass and periosteal reaction are seen, features that may mimic a surface osteosarcoma.

Intraosseous lipoma Intraosseous lipomas are rare lesions, most commonly occurring in the proximal femur, fibula and calcaneus. Plain radiographs demonstrate a geographic, lytic lesion. A fine sclerotic rim and central calcification may also occur. CT and MRI can be diagnostic because they positively identify fat. The lipoma may also be parosteal.

Miscellaneous lesions

Simple bone cyst Simple cysts are not true neoplasms. They occur most commonly in children; 80% are located either in the proximal humeral or femoral

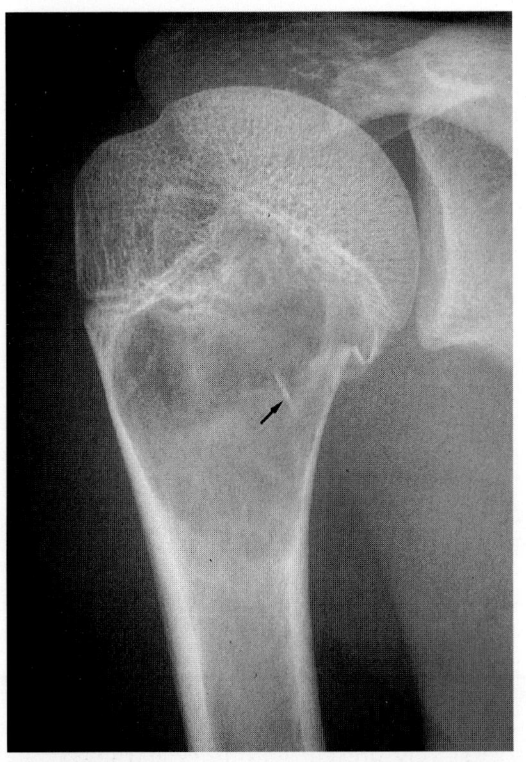

Fig. 13.15 Simple bone cyst of the proximal humerus appearing as a lytic lesion abutting the growth plate. Pathological fracture through the medial cortex has resulted in the 'falling fragment' sign (arrow).

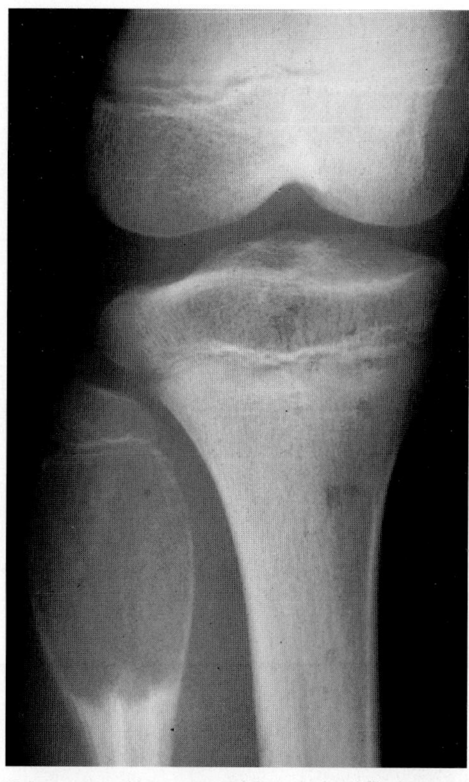

Fig. 13.16 Aneurysmal bone cyst of the proximal fibula appearing as a purely lytic expansile lesion that thins the cortex.

metaphysis. In older patients they may occur in the iliac wing or calcaneus. They usually present with pathological fracture and are otherwise asymptomatic.

Radiologically, simple cysts appear as centrally placed, lytic lesions causing cortical thinning and bony expansion (Fig. 13.15). Initially they are metaphyseal and abut the growth plate. With time they may migrate into the diaphysis and may heal spontaneously by sclerosis. Healing may also be stimulated by fracture or cyst puncture and steroid injection. Fracture may result in the 'falling fragment' sign which is said to be pathognomonic of simple bone cyst.

Aneurysmal bone cyst Aneurysmal bone cysts are also not true neoplasms but probably arise secondarily to a preceding primary tumour; 70% occur between 5–20 years of age and the majority are located in the spine, long bones and pelvis.

Aneurysmal bone cysts in long bones are usually located eccentrically in the metaphysis. However, they may be centrally placed in bones of narrow diameter, such as the fibula and radius. The lesion is purely lytic and expands the bone, resulting in a thin outer layer of cortex over its surface (Fig. 13.16). The cyst may appear trabeculated and rapid growth over a few months is characteristic, resulting in a very aggressive plain film appearance. Aneurysmal bone cysts arising in the diaphysis may be intracortical or subperiosteal.

An interesting, but not pathognomonic, feature on CT and MRI is the presence of fluid–fluid levels within the cysts due to haemorrhage of various ages.

Eosinophilic granuloma Eosinophilic granuloma is the mildest and commonest form of Langerhan's cell histiocytosis (previously referred to as histiocytosis X), accounting for 60–80% of cases. It usually presents in the first to third decade of life with a peak incidence at 5–10 years; 50% are found in the skull, 30% in the spine and pelvis, and 20% in the long bones, most commonly the femur. The disease is usually monostotic at presentation.

The radiographic appearance in the skull is a geographic lytic lesion which may develop marginal sclerosis as it heals. An associated soft-tissue mass is common. In the long bones, eosinophilic granuloma may appear as a solitary lesion of varying aggressiveness, producing relatively well-defined or poorly defined bone destruction with associated periosteal reaction (Fig. 13.17). The proximal femur is the commonest site. The lesion becomes better defined with sclerotic margins as it heals.

Vascular lesions The majority of osseous **haemangiomas** occur in the spine and calvarium. Lesions of tubular bones produce linear striations along the long axis of the bone. In flat bones they may result in geographic, lobulated, lytic lesions. Extension into soft tissues may be identified by the presence of phleboliths. **Lymphangiomas** produce lytic lesions with

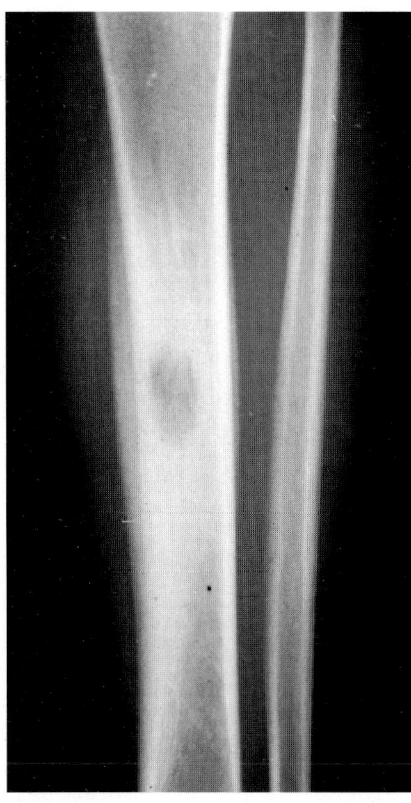

Fig. 13.17 Langerhan's cell histiocytosis (eosinophilic granuloma). Long bone lesions typically appear as moderately well-defined lytic lesions with associated periosteal reaction.

sclerotic margins. Multiple lesions may occur together with lymphoedema and chylous effusions. **Glomus tumours** are painful lesions found in the terminal phalanx, producing a lytic lesion.

Myositis ossificans Myositis ossificans represents post-traumatic soft-tissue bone formation and may be mistaken for osteosarcoma. It is considered in more detail in the section on trauma (p. 306).

Adamantinoma Adamantinomas are rare lesions of unknown origin. Classically, they present in middle age and 90% are found eccentrically in the anterior tibial diaphysis. In children the lesion may arise within an area of osteofibrous dysplasia. The radiological appearance varies from geographic to motheaten. They are locally aggressive and may occasionally metastasize.

PRIMARY MALIGNANT BONE TUMOURS AND METASTATIC DISEASE

Osseous lesions

Osteosarcoma Although rare, osteosarcoma is the commonest primary malignant bone tumour after myeloma. The various forms include classic central osteosarcoma, parosteal, periosteal, high-grade surface osteosarcoma, low-grade intraosseous osteosarcoma and those secondary to Paget's disease and radiotherapy. Rarely, the condition may be intracortical, multicentric or extraskeletal.

Classic central osteosarcoma accounts for 75% of cases. The majority arise between ages 10–25 and there is a 2:1 male to female ratio. The commonest sites are the distal femoral, proximal tibial and proximal humeral metaphyses. However, various sites, including the pelvis and spine, may be affected.

The typical radiographic features in a long bone consist of a permeative area of metaphyseal destruction, poorly defined areas of increased density due to a combination of tumour bone formation and osteoblastic response, and periosteal reaction. At the margin of the tumour this takes the form of a Codman's triangle due to elevation of the periosteum by tumour. A 'sunburst spiculation' pattern may be seen adjacent to the lesion (Fig. 13.18).

Other radiographic appearances include a densely sclerotic lesion or a purely lytic lesion, as may occur with the rare **telangiectatic osteosarcoma**.

Metastases from osteosarcoma are relatively common and occur to other bones, lungs and pleura, where they may present with pneumothorax. Skeletal and soft-tissue metastases may both be detected by scintigraphy.

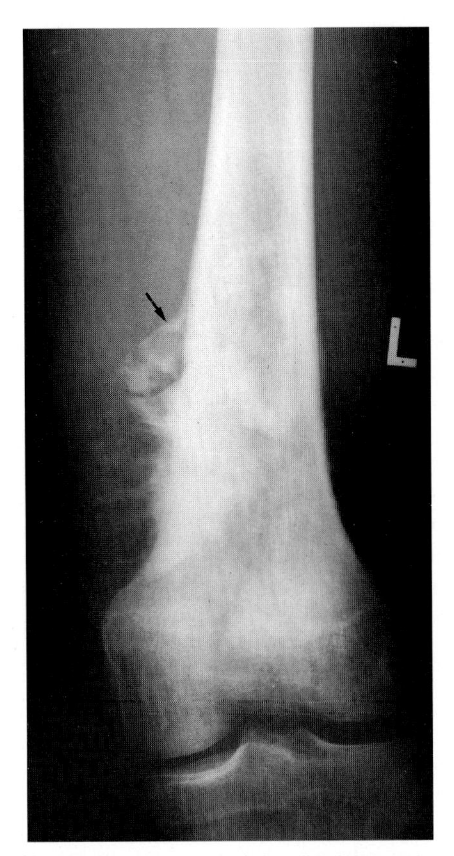

Fig. 13.18 Classic osteosarcoma of the distal femoral metaphysis. Note the Codman's triangle (arrow) and matrix mineralization.

Low-grade intraosseous osteosarcoma accounts for 1% of osteosarcomas. It appears as a mild to moderately aggressive intramedullary destructive lesion in the metadiaphysis, initially without periosteal reaction. It has a better prognosis than conventional osteosarcoma.

Parosteal osteosarcoma is a variant of osteosarcoma generally occurring in the 20–40 age group and has a better prognosis than conventional central osteosarcoma. The majority of lesions affect the distal femur, the tibia or proximal humerus.

Radiographs typically demonstrate a dense mass of mature tumour bone wrapping round the metaphysis of a long bone (Fig. 13.19) with a thin, lucent line separating the tumour bone from the cortex. The bone at the periphery of the tumour is less well formed. Initially, the medulla is not involved but extension through the cortex can occur later. Such extension is best identified by CT or MRI.

Periosteal osteosarcoma is a rare lesion with a prognosis in between that of conventional central osteosarcoma and parosteal osteosarcoma. The distal femoral or proximal tibial diaphyses are most commonly involved. The condition occurs usually in the second to third decades.

The tumour is hemispherical and closely applied to the cortex of the bone. Perpendicular spicules of new bone lie within the tumour and there may be periosteal thickening at its base. The extent of the tumour and status of the medullary cavity, which should not be involved, are best assessed by MRI.

High-grade surface osteosarcoma, which has the same prognosis as conventional central osteosarcoma, has a radiological appearance very similar to periosteal osteosarcoma. The diagnosis is made histologically.

Paget's sarcoma Sarcomatous degeneration occurs in less than 1% of patients with Paget's disease. Of these, 50% are osteosarcomas, 25% fibrosarcomas and 25% anaplastic sarcomas or other cell types.

Paget's sarcomas are usually seen in the femur or pelvis and manifest radiologically as a poorly defined area of bone destruction with a soft-tissue mass. Tumour bone formation may be seen.

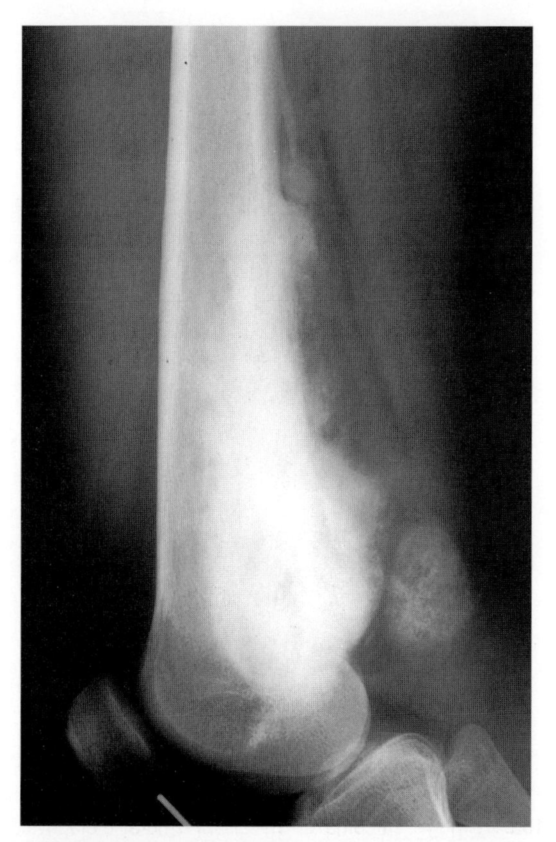

Fig. 13.19 Parosteal osteosarcoma of the femur appearing as a juxtacortical mass of dense tumour bone. The posterior distal femoral metaphysis is a classic site.

Cartilaginous lesions

Chondrosarcoma Chondrosarcoma is the third most frequent primary bone malignancy. It may arise *de novo* within bone or may be secondary to a pre-existing lesion, usually an enchondroma or an osteochondroma, rarely within chondromyxoid fibroma or chondroblastoma. The tumours may therefore be either central, i.e. within the medulla, or peripheral. The mean age at presentation is 50 years with a slight male predominance. The commonest sites include the pelvis, proximal femur and proximal humerus.

The typical radiographic fetaures in long bone lesions include a relatively well-defined, lytic lesion causing endosteal scalloping and mild bony expansion. There may be associated matrix calcification and marked cortical thickening, which is characteristic. Periosteal reaction is variable. In more aggressive tumours, cortical destruction occurs. Pelvic lesions are classically associated with large extraosseous components (Fig. 13.20) which are best delineated with CT or MRI.

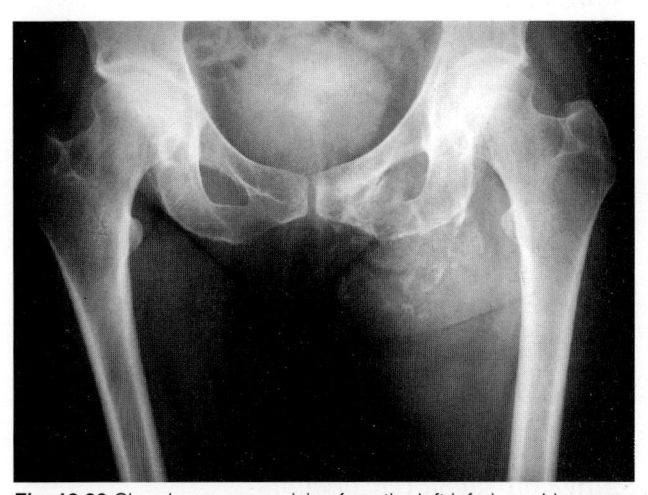

Fig. 13.20 Chondrosarcoma arising from the left inferior pubic ramus. There is a large extraosseous mass containing typical chondroid-type calcification.

Difficulties may arise in the diagnosis of secondary chondrosarcoma. This is suggested clinically when a known benign lesion (osteochondroma or enchondroma) becomes painful and enlarges. Radiological features suggesting malignant change include growth or destruction of part of a calcified cartilage cap or bony stem of an osteochondroma, or enlargement of an enchondroma. The thickness of the cartilage cap can be assessed by ultrasound, CT or, ideally, by MRI. The thicker the cap, the more likely that malignant change has occurred. Occasionally, chondrosarcoma may dedifferentiate, usually into malignant fibrous histiocytoma. This is associated with a poorer prognosis.

Other rare varieties of chondrosarcoma include juxtacortical, mesenchymal and clear-cell types.

Fibrous lesions

Malignant fibrous histiocytoma and fibrosarcoma These are uncommon primary bone sarcomas which usually present in the fourth to fifth decades. Most tumours arise around the knee. Malignant fibrous histiocytomas arise in soft tissues and invade bone secondarily. These tumours may also complicate Paget's disease, chondrosarcoma, bone infarction and sinus tracts in chronic osteomyelitis.

Radiographs typically demonstrate a poorly defined, lytic lesion in a long bone metaphysis, occasionally with associated matrix calcification and little periosteal reaction.

Vascular lesions

Haemangiopericytoma Most haemangiopericytomas are primary soft-tissue neoplasms which may erode the bony cortex. Very rarely, they arise within bone producing a moth-eaten or permeative area of bone destruction. The lesion is monostotic and occurs most commonly in the axial skeleton or in a long bone metaphysis.

Haemangioendotheliomas are rare primary bone tumours occurring in the second to third decade. They are usually polyostotic with lesions tending to involve multiple bones of a single extremity, usually hand or foot. Individual lesions are relatively well-defined and purely lytic. Metastases to the lungs are occasionally seen.

Angiosarcomas are rare primary tumours of bone which usually occur in the fourth and fifth decades. The commonest sites of origin include the major long bones and pelvis. Radiographs demonstrate a permeative lytic lesion with associated soft-tissue mass. The tumour is multifocal in approximately 40% of cases.

Malignant round cell tumours

The term malignant round cell tumour of bone includes Ewing's sarcoma, primitive neuroectodermal tumour, metastatic neuroblastoma and primary lymphoma.

Ewing's sarcoma is a rare, highly malignant tumour which presents most commonly between 5–15 years of age. The common sites include the major long bones, pelvis and ribs. In the long bones, extensive involvement of the diaphysis is typical, although 25% of cases may arise in the metaphysis.

The medullary lesion causes poorly defined, permeative destruction which may be difficult to identify. Periosteal reaction is a common feature and may have a single layer or multilayered ('onion-peel') appearance. A perpendicular type of periosteal reaction may also occur (Fig. 13.21). Characteristically, a very large extraosseous component is present and this is best defined by MRI, as is the extent of medullary involvement. Mineralization of the extraosseous mass is not a feature. Ewing's sarcoma of a flat bone is more commonly densely sclerotic, due to reactive new bone. Once again, a large extraosseous component is characteristic. Bone metastases at presentation occur in up to 10% of patients.

Primitive neuroectodermal tumours occur primarily in soft tissues or bone and produce radiographic changes that may be indistinguishable from Ewing's

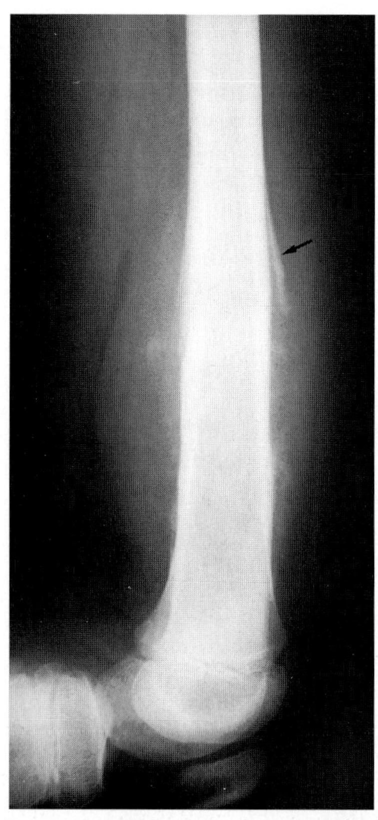

Fig. 13.21 Ewing's sarcoma of the distal femoral metaphysis. The permeative medullary bone destruction, perpendicular periosteal reaction and large extraosseous mass are all characteristic. A Codman's triangle is seen at the margin of the lesion (arrow).

sarcoma. The diagnosis is made by specialized immunohistochemical techniques.

Metastatic neuroblastoma typically occurs in children under 5 years of age who are already known to have a primary abdominal mass. Radiographs may show multiple sites of permeative bone destruction in the metaphyses of the long bones similar to leukaemia or multifocal osteomyelitis. Alternatively, diffuse infiltration of a long bone similar to Ewing's sarcoma may occur. Infiltration of the cranial sutures is relatively common.

Lymphoma of bone

Osseous **Hodgkin's lymphoma** is almost always secondary to primary lymph node disease. Radiographic evidence of bone disease is seen in 20% of patients. The majority of cases (75%) affect the axial skeleton, especially the spine. Two-thirds of cases are multifocal. The radiographic appearances can be either purely lytic with a permeative pattern, sclerotic or mixed. An associated soft-tissue mass is common.

Non-Hodgkin's lymphoma can produce either focal lytic permeative lesions or generalized osteopenia.

Primary lymphoma of bone (reticulum cell sarcoma) The diagnosis of primary lymphoma of bone depends upon involvement of a single site in bone without evidence of extraskeletal lymphoma. The mean age of presentation is in the fifth decade, but the age range is wide. The diaphyses of long bones are most commonly affected but flat bones are also involved.

Radiographs demonstrate an area of permeative bone destruction, commonly with some reactive sclerosis. Rarely, a purely sclerotic tumour is seen. A large associated extraosseous mass is characteristic. Once again, MRI most accurately defines medullary extent.

Leukaemia

Acute leukaemia is the commonest malignancy of childhood and, consequently, radiographic demonstration of bone lesions is not infrequent. In adults, chronic leukaemias predominate and bone lesions are uncommon.

The neoplastic proliferation of white cells initially results in trabecular and endosteal bone destruction which may be followed by extraosseous spread.

The radiographic changes in children are as follows. Metaphyseal lucent bands are a non-specific feature, most commonly seen in the distal femur, proximal tibia and distal radius. The medullary destruction by tumour is of a permeative type similar to Ewing's sarcoma. Endosteal erosion and cortical destruction follow. Focal osteolytic lesions may occur, usually in long bone diaphyses, in over 60% of cases. However, osteosclerotic lesions are rare. These are seen in the metaphysis, either spontaneously or as a consequence of treatment. Periosteal reaction may be due either to subperiosteal tumour or haemorrhage.

As with other malignant marrow tumours, the extent of local involvement is best demonstrated by MRI. The radiographic features described above are not specific to leukaemia, but may also be seen with metastatic neuroblastoma and multifocal osteomyelitis.

Leukaemic bone lesions in adults are rare and have appearances almost identical to a primary malignant tumour or metastasis.

Multiple myeloma and plasmacytoma

Myeloma is a neoplasm of plasma cell origin and is the commonest primary malignancy of bone; 95% of patients are over 40 at presentation with a peak incidence between 60–70 years. Men are affected twice as often as women. The axial skeleton and proximal ends of long bones, the sites of red marrow in adults, are usually affected.

The classic radiological findings are multiple, well-defined, 'punched-out' lytic lesions throughout the skeleton (Fig. 13.22). Marginal sclerosis may be seen with healing. Other findings include diffuse osteopenia (15% of cases) and pathological fractures, especially in the spine. Rarely, myeloma may result in sclerotic or mixed lytic and sclerotic lesions.

Myeloma is the commonest cause of a false-negative ^{99m}Tc bone scan or 'cold' lesion, presumably due to the lack of osteoblastic response to the tumour cells. Scans are positive in 25–40% of myeloma lesions.

The main differential diagnosis is metastatic carcinoma. Features favouring myeloma include presence of an associated soft-tissue mass and involvement of the mandible.

Plasmacytoma, the solitary lesion of myeloma accounting for 30% of cases of myeloma, affects the same sites as multiple myeloma. Radiographs usually demonstrate a well-defined, expansile lesion > 5 cm in diameter with cortical thinning and an associated soft-tissue mass. Plasmacytoma may progress to multiple myeloma.

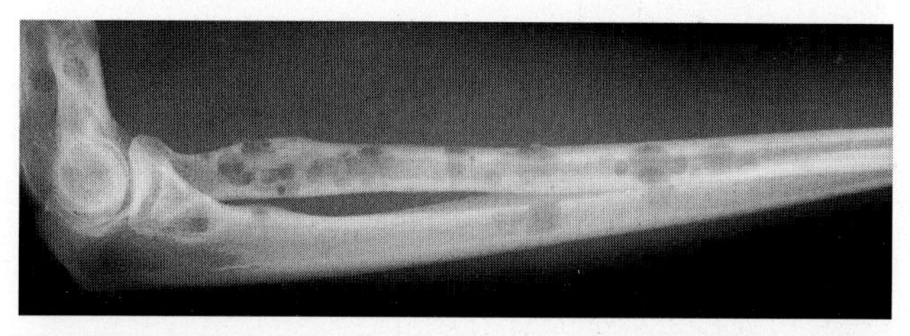

Fig. 13.22 Multiple myeloma affecting the humerus, radius and ulna appearing as well-defined, 'punched-out' lytic lesions without marginal sclerosis.

Metastatic disease

Metastatic deposits from carcinoma are by far the commonest malignant lesions of bone, being 25 times commoner than primary bone tumours. They are solitary in 9% of cases and, therefore, in a middle-aged or elderly patient, a solitary metastasis is more common than a primary bone tumour.

The commonest carcinomas to metastasize to bone are prostate and breast, followed by bronchus (especially small cell tumours). However, primary gastrointestinal and genitourinary carcinomata not uncommonly produce bone metastases.

The most frequent sites involved are those bones containing red marrow. Metastases are, therefore, usually found in the spine, pelvis, ribs, skull and proximal humeri or femora; 50% of peripheral metastases are secondaries from bronchial neoplasms.

Bone metastases have a varied radiographic appearance. Most arise within the medulla, producing multiple lytic lesions without sclerotic borders. They may not be visualized until they reach 2 cm in size or until the adjacent bony cortex has been destroyed (Fig. 13.23). Periosteal reaction and extraosseous extension are occasionally seen. Some carcinomas, particularly prostate, produce predominantly sclerotic metastases due to an osteoblastic response to the tumour (Fig. 13.24). Breast carcinoma may show a lytic, sclerotic or mixed appearance. Expansile lytic lesions are occasionally seen with renal and thyroid metastases.

In a patient with a known carcinoma and bone pain but normal plain radiographs, bone scintigraphy should be performed since it is far more sensitive than plain radiography. If positive, CT or preferably MRI will demonstrate the lesion if there is doubt about the interpretation of the scintigram. Scintigraphy may also demonstrate multiple skeletal lesions and can show a characteristic appearance of multiple areas of increased

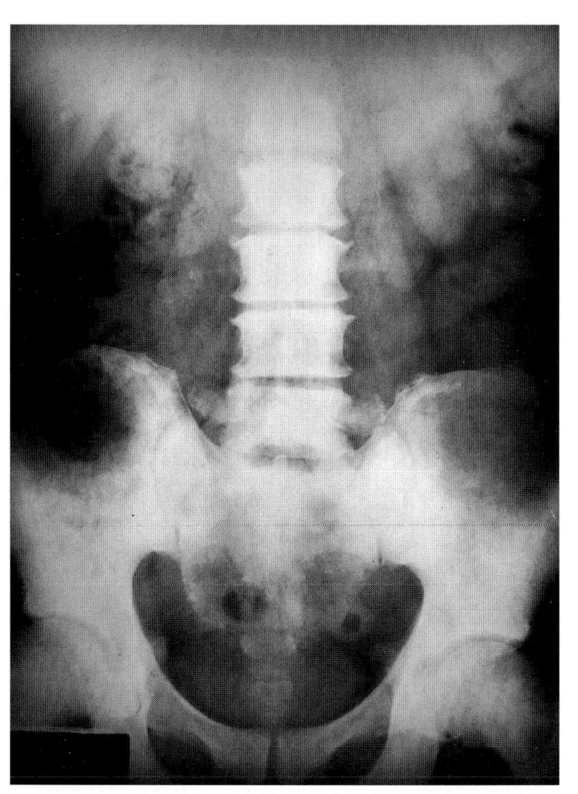

Fig. 13.24 Widespread osteoblastic metastases in the pelvis, proximal femora and spine from a primary prostatic carcinoma.

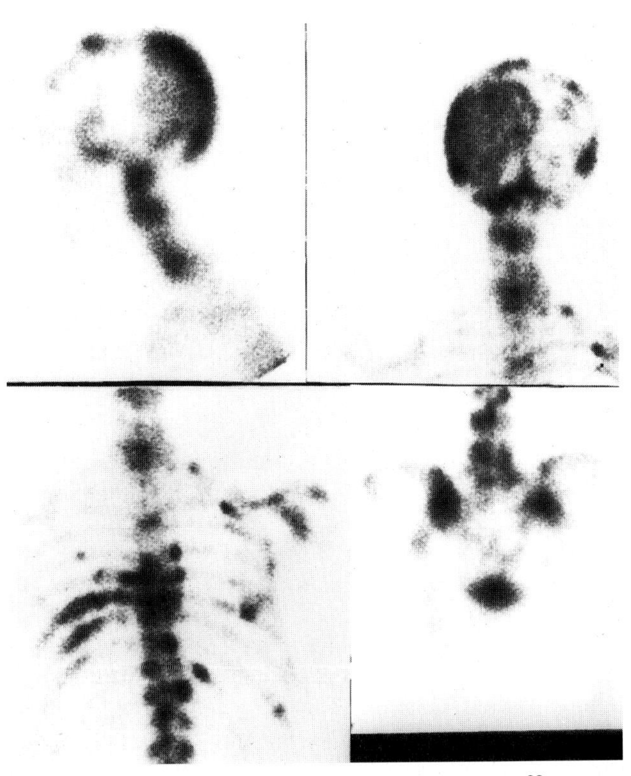

Fig. 13.25 Typical appearances of multiple metastases on ^{99m}Tc-MDP bone scintigraphy. Rib lesions are characteristically linear along the length of the rib, whereas vertebral lesions tend to be focal and related to the pedicles.

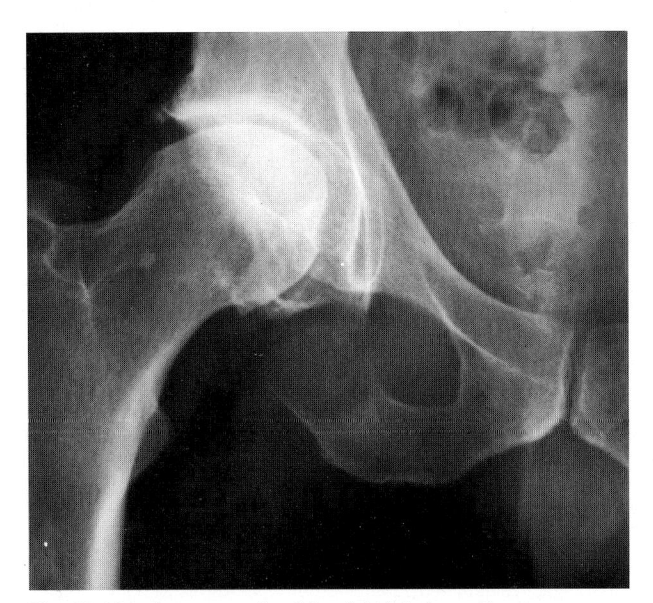

Fig. 13.23 Lytic metastasis of the right inferior pubic ramus.

activity in the spine, ribs and pelvis (Fig. 13.25). In a small proportion of cases the bone scan is normal or shows a focal region of reduced activity. Diffuse metastatic involvement of the skeleton may result in a 'superscan', a term which refers to such uniform increase in skeletal uptake that the scan is incorrectly interpreted as normal. MRI is the most sensitive technique for demonstrating skeletal metastases, but is non-specific, lesions appearing as relatively well demarcated areas of low signal intensity on T1-weighted scans and increased signal intensity on T2-weighted scans, although osteoblastic metastases also show low signal intensity on T2-weighted scans.

METABOLIC BONE DISEASE

OSTEOPOROSIS

Osteoporosis is a condition of unknown aetiology in which there is an abnormal reduction in the quantity of bone. However, the bone that remains is normally mineralized and appears normal histologically. There is no associated abnormality of bone biochemistry.

The commonest cause is senile generalized osteoporosis which typically affects postmenopausal women: 30–50% of women over 60 years of age will show evidence of significant bone loss. The commonest sites affected include the spine, femur (subcapital neck and intertrochanteric region), distal radius and proximal humerus.

Radiographic changes are first seen in the spine but require up to 30–50% of bone loss. There is reduction of bone density due to loss of horizontal trabeculae with accentuation of the vertical trabeculae. There is also thinning of the cortex. In the femoral neck, there may be accentuation of the major stress-bearing trabeculae. Complications include wedge-compression fractures in the spine, and stress fractures as well as complete fractures at other sites, especially the femoral neck and distal radius. Bone mass may be assessed quantitatively either by dual energy X-ray absorptiometry or quantitative computed tomography.

Disorders associated with osteoporosis include excessive endogenous or exogenous corticosteroids, hyperthyroidism, acromegaly, homocystinuria, alcoholism, osteogenesis imperfecta and some drugs. **Idiopathic juvenile osteoporosis** is a rare, specific condition affecting children aged 8–12 years.

Localized forms of osteoporosis include those due to disuse, **reflex sympathetic dystrophy syndrome** (Sudeck's atrophy) and transient regional osteoporosis. In disuse and the reflex sympathetic dystrophy syndrome, the radiographic appearances may be very aggressive with a moth-eaten pattern of bone loss, intracortical tunnelling indicating rapid bone remodelling, and metaphyseal lucent bands. Changes are typically periarticular (Fig. 13.26). The reflex sympathetic dystrophy syndrome is characterized by increased activity in all phases of a triple-phase bone scan.

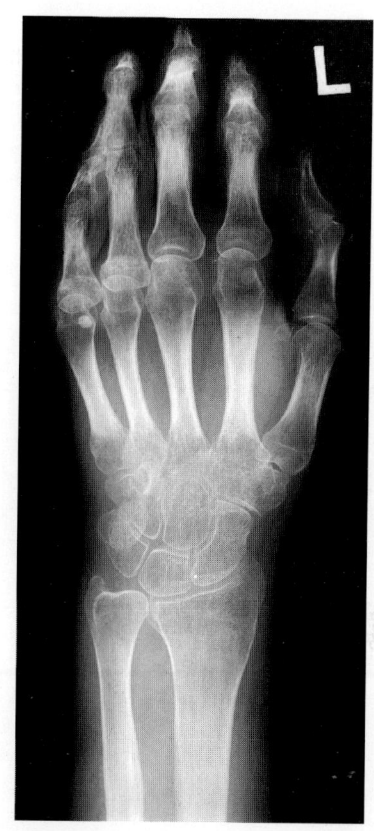

Fig. 13.26 Sudeck's atrophy of the hand. The severe periarticular osteoporosis is a characteristic finding.

Transient regional osteoporosis is a self-limiting condition that takes two forms. The migratory form typically occurs in middle-aged males and usually affects the knee, ankle and foot. It resolves within a year but may recur in another joint. Transient osteoporosis of the hip affects either women in late pregnancy, in which case the left hip is typically involved, or one or other hip in males. MRI is sensitive, but non-specific, showing reduced marrow signal intensity on T1-weighted spin-echo scans. Scintigraphy will demonstrate increased activity but is also non-specific.

RICKETS AND OSTEOMALACIA

Rickets and osteomalacia are characterized by a normal amount of osteoid which, however, shows reduced mineralization. The abnormality of mineralization is related to a deficiency of metabolically active vitamin D. This may be due to dietary causes, malabsorption, liver disease, renal disease, drugs, or, rarely, it may be associated with a variety of tumours.

Both conditions are associated with generalized osteopenia from a decrease in the number of trabeculae, and a coarsening of trabeculae from osteoid deposition without adequate mineralization.

Rickets occurs in childhood with changes predominating at sites of rapid growth, notably the proximal humerus, distal radius, distal femur and both ends of the tibia. Radiographs show widening of the zone of provisional calcification and irregularity and cupping of the metaphyses (Fig. 13.27). Slipping of the epiphysis, bowing of the long bones and vertebral compression fractures may also occur.

Conditions that may mimic rickets include hypophosphatasia and metaphyseal chondrodysplasia (Schmid type).

Osteomalacia is characterized by Looser's zones (pseudofractures) which appear as wide transverse lucent bands, perpendicular to the cortex, that may be incomplete. Characteristic sites include the pubic rami (Fig. 13.28), ribs, axillary borders of the scapulae, medial margin of the proximal femora and posterior border of the proximal ulnae. Bone scintigraphy may show focal lesions representing Looser's zones and/or a generalized increase in bone uptake with reduced or absent renal activity (superscan).

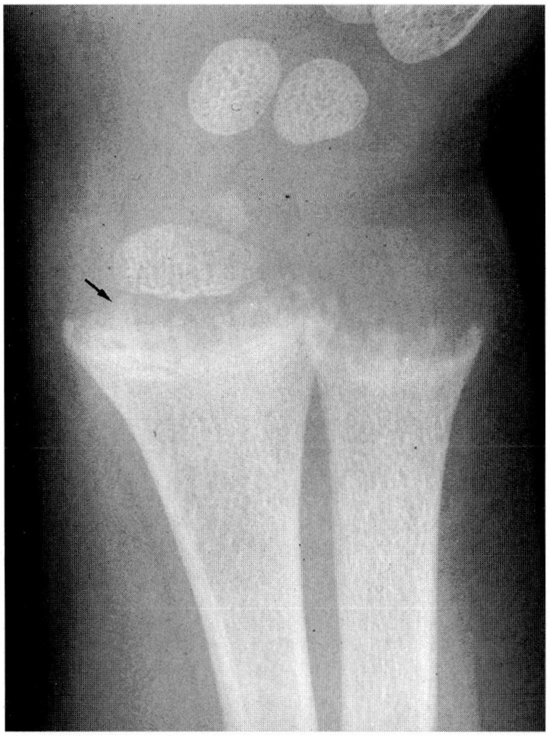

Fig. 13.27 Typical features of rickets in the wrist with widening of the zone of provisional calcification (arrow) and splaying and irregularity of the metaphyses.

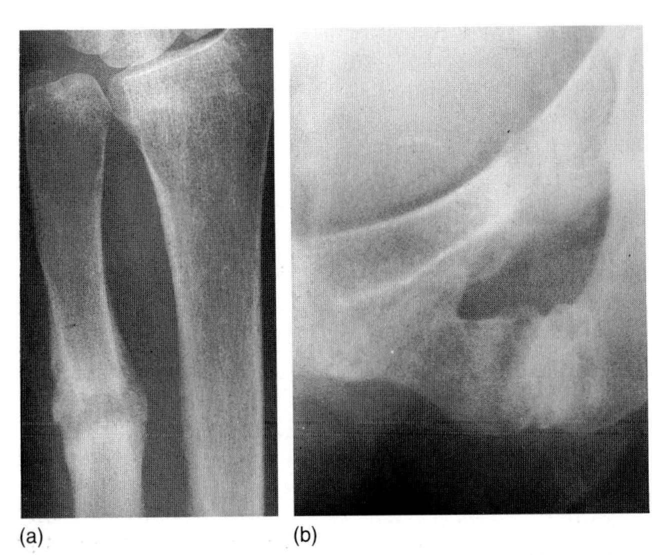

(a) (b)

Fig. 13.28 Radiographs of (a) the wrist and (b) pubic rami in a patient with osteomalacia. Looser's zones appear as lucent bands perpendicular to the cortex. Periosteal reaction occurs as they heal.

HYPERPARATHYROIDISM

Hyperparathyroidism may be either primary, 90% of primary cases are due to adenomas, or secondary due to renal dysfunction. Bone pain and tenderness occur in 10–25% of patients.

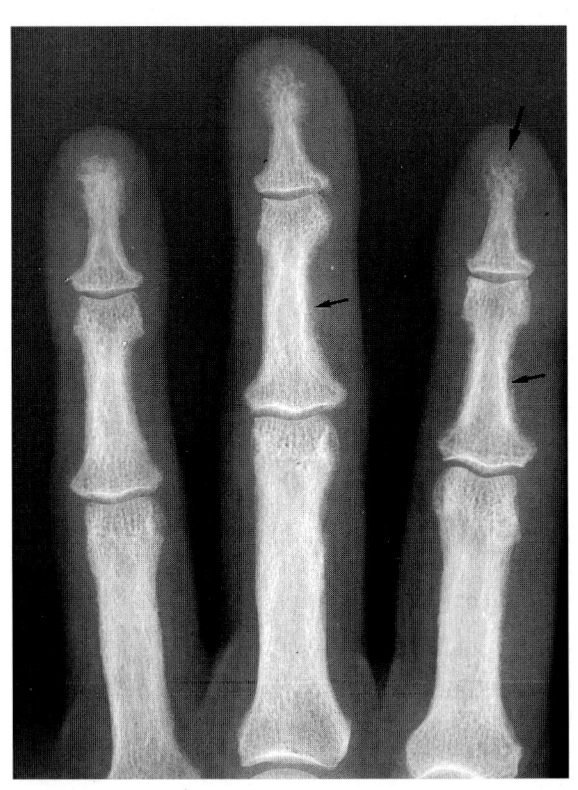

Fig. 13.29 Classic appearances of hyperparathyroidism in the hands, manifest as subperiosteal bone resorption predominantly on the radial side of the digit (fine arrows) and acro-osteolysis of the terminal tufts (arrow).

Radiographically, skeletal abnormalities are seen in 50% of cases. Skeletal manifestations include generalized osteopenia due to excessive bone resorption. Subperiosteal resorption is a classic feature, affecting the radial aspects of the phalanges, especially the middle phalanx of the middle and index fingers, terminal tufts (acro-osteolysis) (Fig. 13.29) and medial cortices of the proximal humerus, femur and tibial shafts. Trabecular resorption is best seen in the diploë of the cranium, resulting in a characteristic 'pepper-pot' skull. Subchondral resorption may result in subchondral collapse and sclerosis with apparent joint space widening. The sacroiliac, temporomandibular, acromioclavicular joints and the symphysis pubis are most commonly affected. Subligamentous resorption is especially seen in the pelvis and calcaneus.

In some patients, bone formation predominates over bone resorption, resulting in patchy or diffuse osteosclerosis. This is much commoner in secondary hyperparathyroidism.

Brown tumours are now an uncommon finding in primary hyperparathyroidism and represent localized accumulation of osteoclasts. Radiographically, they are lytic and expansile, but may become sclerotic after treatment.

Soft-tissue changes include chondrocalcinosis, periarticular, soft-tissue and vascular calcification and 'tumoral calcinosis', most commonly seen in dialysis patients with secondary hyperparathyroidism.

Chronic renal failure results in a combination of bone abnormalities due to rickets/osteomalacia and secondary hyperparathyroidism, known as **renal osteodystrophy**. Also, patients on dialysis may develop bone changes secondary to aluminium poisoning and amyloid.

PAGET'S DISEASE

Paget's disease of bone is a condition of unknown aetiology, typically occurring after 40 years of age with a male predominance. Pathologically, there is simultaneous abnormal osteoclastic and osteoblastic activity, causing abnormal bone remodelling resulting in thickened, disorganized, fragile trabeculae. The condition is often asymptomatic but may cause local bone pain and a variety of other symptoms. Common sites of occurrence include the spine (75% of cases), pelvis (70%), cranium (65%) and tubular bones (35%).

Radiographically, there are three sequential stages, although they may coexist. Initially, there is a predominance of bone destruction. The second stage shows mixed lysis and sclerosis with gradual bony enlargement and deformity. In the third phase, there is further sclerosis with increasing enlargement and deformity.

In the initial phase, radiographs show a geographic area of bone lysis. In the skull, this lytic phase is termed **osteoporosis circumscripta** and usually involves the frontal or occipital areas. In long bones, the lysis typically commences in a subarticular region and extends with a flame-shaped leading margin into the diaphysis (Fig. 13.30). Rarely, in the tibia, the disease may commence in the diaphysis.

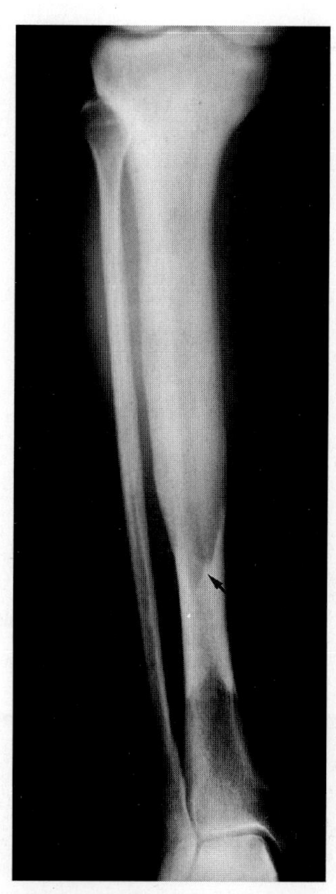

Fig. 13.30 Paget's disease of the proximal tibia. The disease starts at the articular surface and extends into the diaphysis with a 'flame-shaped' leading edge (arrow). Cortical and trabecular thickening are typical features.

Following the lytic phase, areas of sclerosis develop which, in the skull, produce a 'cotton-wool' appearance. In the long bones, sclerosis is due to a combination of cortical and trabecular thickening. In the pelvis, the initial manifestation is thickening of the iliopectineal line. This progresses to patchy or diffuse sclerosis, cortical thickening with loss of corticomedullary differentiation and enlargement of the bone. Deformities occur, since the bone is abnormally soft. This may result in bowing of long bones (Fig. 13.31), basilar invagination and protrusio acetabulae.

Complications of Paget's disease include stress fracture, osteoporosis (if immobilized), arthropathy and sarcomatous degeneration.

The scintigraphic appearances of Paget's disease are also characteristic, with marked increased activity in the involved bone (Fig. 13.32). Scintigraphy is useful in assessing response of the disease to treatment but may be insensitive at identifying stress fractures or sarcomatous change.

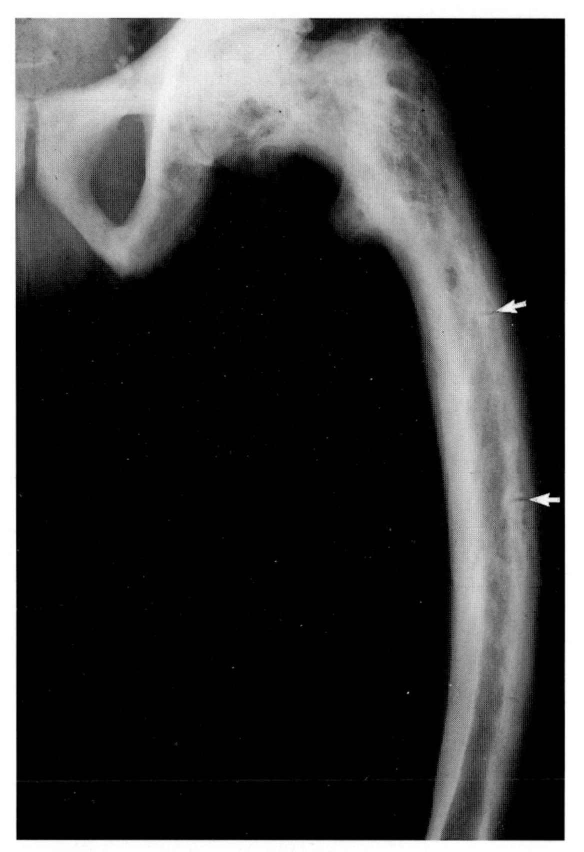

Fig. 13.31 Paget's disease of the left femur and left hemipelvis. There is marked cortical thickening and coarsening of trabeculae. The femur is bowed and multiple stress fractures are seen on the convex aspect of the shaft (arrows).

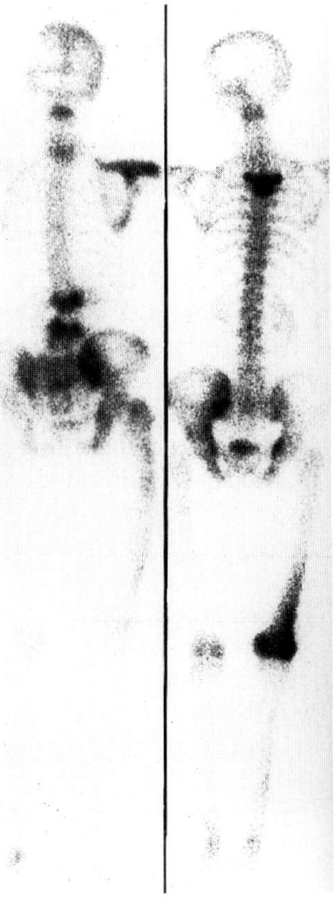

Fig. 13.32 ^{99m}Tc-MDP bone scintigraphy in two patients showing characteristic features of Paget's disease. In the long bones, the disease starts in a subarticular location and spreads into the diaphysis. In the flat bones and spine, the whole of the bone tends to be involved. Enlargement and deformity are also seen.

SCURVY

Scurvy is due to a deficiency of vitamin C, resulting in abnormal collagen formation. There is a tendency toward haemorrhage and abnormal bone formation. It is rarely seen before 6 months of age.

In the infant, subperiosteal haemorrhage raises the periosteum resulting in extensive subperiosteal bone formation. Abnormal bone formation affects particularly the costochondral junctions and ends of long bones. Radiographs demonstrate increased density and widening of the zone of provisional calcification (white line of Frankel), a dense epiphsyeal rim (Wimberger's sign), metaphyseal spurs or corner fractures (Pelkan's sign) and generalized osteopenia.

Radiographic abnormalities in adults are limited to osteopenia and pathological fractures.

MISCELLANEOUS DISORDERS

HAEMOPHILIA

Haemophilic arthropathy is considered in detail in the section on joints. The major non-arthropathic manifestation is the **haemophilic pseudotumour**, which occurs secondary to an intraosseous, subperiosteal or soft-tissue haemorrhage. The commonest sites are the femur, pelvis and tibia.

Radiographs demonstrate an extrinsic and/or intrinsic scalloping and pressure erosion of the affected bone with sharp, sclerotic margins. Other features include a soft-tissue mass and periosteal reaction. As the name implies, this lesion is readily confused radiographically with an aggressive tumour.

SICKLE CELL ANAEMIA AND THALASSAEMIA

Both conditions can result in similar bony abnormalities. Chronic anaemia results in marrow hyperplasia which manifests as osteopenia with coarsened trabeculae, widening of the tubular bones (Fig. 13.33), ribs, mandible and diploic spaces of the skull. Such changes are most spectacular in thalassaemia major. Conversely, osteonecrosis, due to vascular occlusion, is more commonly seen in sickle cell disease (HbSS). Sites of involvement include the small tubular bones of the hands and feet, producing a dactylitis in

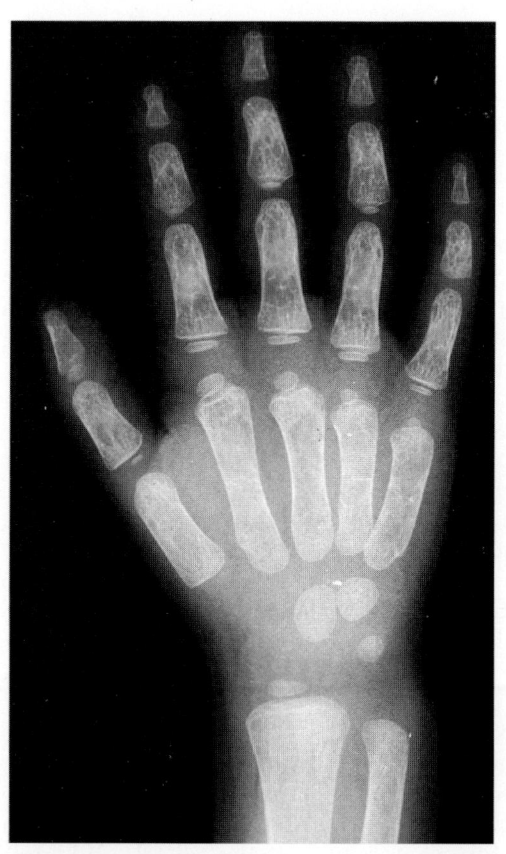

Fig. 13.33 Typical features of thalassaemia in the hands with expansion of the tubular bones, generalized osteopenia and thinning of the cortices.

10–20% of cases, diaphyses of long bones, vertebral end-plates and femoral and humeral heads. There is also a predilection for osteomyelitis, which may be indistinguishable from osteonecrosis. Staphylococcal infection is commonest, but an increased incidence of Salmonella osteomyelitis is recognised. Patients with sickle cell trait (HbAS) have very few musculoskeletal manifestations, but bone infarcts are occasionally seen.

Sickle cell haemoglobin C disease (HbSC) is associated with marrow hyperplasia of the skull and avascular necrosis.

Chronic anaemia due to **hereditary spherocytosis** or **iron deficiency** is rarely associated with radiographic bone changes. Occasionally, widening of the diploic spaces is seen, usually in children or infants.

Bone infarction is also an occasional complication of **polycythaemia rubra vera**, resulting from increased blood viscosity due to the excessive red cell mass.

The marrow hyperplasia or reconversion that occurs in chronic anaemic states is most sensitively demonstrated by MRI as either diffuse or focal areas of medullary low signal on both T1- and T2-weighted spin-echo scans.

MYELOFIBROSIS

Myelofibrosis is a primary disease of marrow resulting in fibrosis of areas of the skeleton normally involved in haematopoiesis. This stimulates reconversion of fatty marrow in long tubular bones to red marrow, which subsequently becomes involved in the fibrotic process. The radiographic features include bone marrow sclerosis, seen in 40% of cases, or patchy increased density with cortical thickening in the involved regions (usually spine, pelvis and ribs). The marrow fibrosis will be manifest on MRI as diffuse or patchy areas of reduced signal on all pulse sequences.

MASTOCYTOSIS

Mastocystosis is a rare proliferative disorder of mast cells. Bone abnormalities include generalized or, rarely, focal osteoporosis due to histamine release, and focal or, rarely, generalized osteosclerosis due to the host response to marrow infiltration.

GAUCHER'S DISEASE

Gaucher's disease is a sphingolipid storage disorder resulting in accumulation of Gaucher cells in the reticuloendothelial system and marrow. The commonest form is seen in children and young adults. Bone abnormalities include expansion of the distal femur, the so-called Erlenmeyer flask deformity, and osteonecrosis, especially of the femoral head. Generalized osteoporosis with vertebral end-plate fractures, marrow infarctions and focal lytic areas are also seen. There is an increased susceptibility to osteomyelitis.

SARCOIDOSIS

Sarcoidosis is a systemic granulomatous disorder of unknown aetiology which affects the bones in 1–15% of cases. Bone involvement in most cases occurs only in the presence of lung and skin lesions. The skeletal manifestations are varied and include generalized osteopenia. Focal lytic lesions with lace-like trabeculae are seen, usually in the middle and distal phalanges, whereas the terminal tufts may show sclerosis. A focal or generalized osteoclerosis is also recognized. The associated clinically apparent arthropathy usually shows no radiographic abnormality.

RADIATION-INDUCED DISORDERS

Radiotherapy is reported to cause a variety of skeletal disorders, including radiation osteitis and osteonecrosis, neoplasia and growth disorders.

In cases of **radiation-induced osteitis** and **osteonecrosis**, the initial radiographic changes may be limited to local osteoporosis. In the later stages of frank osteonecrosis, which usually requires a latent period of several years, local increased bone density containing multiple, small, lytic areas is the characteristic finding. Such bone is brittle and is liable to spontaneous pathological fracture, which is the usual mode of presentation. Calcification in the adjacent soft tissues is common. Typical sites of fracture include the upper humerus and upper ribs following treatment for breast cancer, and the pelvis and proximal femora after treatment for pelvic malignancies.

Large focal osteolytic areas may also occur secondary to radiotherapy and may be confused with osteolytic metastases.

Radiation-induced sarcoma is also a well-recognized, although uncommon, complication. The majority of the early cases were due to radiotherapy as a treatment for various benign bone lesions but now most cases are due to the incidental irradiation of bone during treatment of a primary soft-tissue malignancy. There is usually a latent period of at least 4 years. The commonest radiation-induced sarcoma is osteosarcoma and the tumour has no characteristic radiological features to differentiate it from spontaneous osteosarcoma, although evidence of radiation osteitis may be present.

Growing bone at sites of endochondral ossification is particularly radiosensitive. Radiotherapy may therefore produce various growth disorders due to premature epiphyseal fusion, including limb length inequalities and scoliosis.

DISEASES OF JOINTS

OSTEOARTHRITIS

Osteoarthritis is the commonest joint disease and is characterized pathologically by non-inflammatory cartilage loss accompanied by new bone formation. It may be either primary (where no previous joint pathology is identified) or secondary to a number of predisposing causes, including trauma, inflammatory arthropathy and avascular necrosis.

The radiological manifestations of primary and secondary osteoarthritis, however, are essentially the same. Cartilage loss is always present and tends to be focal, typically in the primary weight-bearing portion of the joint. It is manifest radiographically as reduction in joint space. Erosive changes are not seen, whereas new bone formation, stimulated by abnormal mechanical forces, is common and manifests as osteophyte formation, subchondral sclerosis and cortical buttressing. Osteophytes are small bony protuberances that are in continuity with the underlying medullary cavity and typically occur at the joint margins, though they may be intra-articular. Subchondral sclerosis manifests as focal increased bone density immediately deep to the articular surface. Cortical buttressing is particularly evident along the medial aspect of the neck of femur and appears as thickening of the cortex. Subchondral cyst formation is also common. Cysts usually occur in weight-bearing areas and have thin, sclerotic margins. Intra-articular osteocartilaginous loose bodies are also a relatively common finding. The periarticular bone density is typically preserved.

Soft-tissue abnormalities are not a prominent finding, although chondrocalcinosis can occur. Joint deformities due to osteoarthritis may result in secondary ligamentous abnormalities, such as contractures and laxity, which may produce instability and further degenerative changes.

The common joints involved in primary osteoarthritis are the distal interphalangeal and proximal interphalangeal joints of the hand, the first carpometacarpal and scaphoid–trapezium–trapezoid articulations of the wrist, the hip, knee and first metatarsophalangeal joint. Involvement of the lower cervical spine and lumbar facet joints is also common.

In the hand, **Heberden's** and **Bouchard's nodes** refer to osteophytes at the distal and proximal interphalangeal joints, respectively. The metacarpophalangeal joints are less commonly involved. In the wrist, involvement of the first carpometacarpal joint may result in radial subluxation of the thumb.

In the hip, cartilage loss is usually focal with superior or superolateral migration of the femoral head in 80% of cases. Medial migration with associated protrusio acetabulae is seen in 20% of cases and should suggest the possibility of underlying inflammatory disease, such as rheumatoid arthritis. Typical sites of osteophyte formation are the lateral margin of the acetabulum and in the lateral and medial subcapital region. Subchondral cyst formation is particularly well seen in the weight-bearing portion of the acetabulum. As mentioned previously, cortical buttressing of the medial femoral neck is a classic feature (Fig. 13.34). Superior flattening of the femoral head may occur in advanced disease, simulating avascular necrosis.

In the knee, any of the three joint compartments may be involved, in isolation or in various combinations. Medial compartment disease is commonest and may be associated with a varus deformity and lateral subluxation of the tibia. Patellofemoral osteoarthritis usually involves the lateral facet and may be associated with lateral compartment disease and relative sparing of the medial compartment. Osteophytes may be identified arising from the tibial spines. Osteocartilaginous loose bodies are particularly common in the knee.

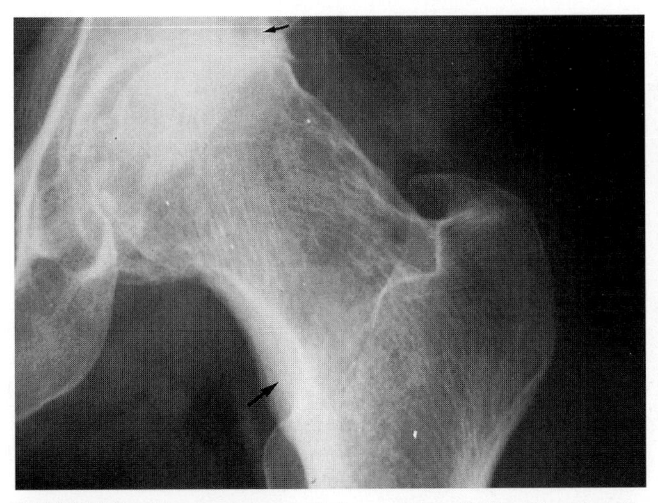

Fig. 13.34 Classic appearances of primary osteoarthritis of the hip with superolateral joint space narrowing, marginal osteophytosis, subarticular sclerosis and cyst formation (short arrow) and cortical buttressing of the medial neck of the femur (long arrow).

Osteoarthritis of the elbow, shoulder and ankle is uncommon and usually secondary to trauma or rheumatoid disease.

Erosive osteoarthritis is an arthropathy seen most commonly in middle-aged women who experience distinct inflammatory episodes, with red, swollen joints similar to rheumatoid arthritis. The distal and proximal interphalangeal joints are involved. Radiographs show loss of joint space, subchondral sclerosis, erosions which tend to be central in the joint, and marginal osteophytes. The appearance may progress to ankylosis. Typical osteoarthritis of the first carpometacarpal and scaphoid–trapezium–trapezoid articulation in the wrist help to differentiate the condition from psoriatic arthropathy.

INFLAMMATORY ARTHROPATHIES

The inflammatory arthropathies comprise a group of disorders that are characterized by synovial inflammation (of unknown aetiology) which results in cartilage destruction and cortical bony erosion. They may be subdivided into seropositive (rheumatoid arthritis, some juvenile chronic arthritides) and seronegative (psoriatic arthritis, Reiter's disease, ankylosing spondylitis, enteropathic arthritis) arthropathies. Since the underlying pathology is similar, the radiographic manifestations at a particular joint are similar, with the pattern of joint involvement being an important factor in differential diagnosis.

The cardinal radiographic signs of inflammatory arthropathies are periarticular soft-tissue swelling, loss of joint space, periarticular osteopenia, marginal erosions and, later, joint deformity and generalized osteopenia (Fig. 13.35).

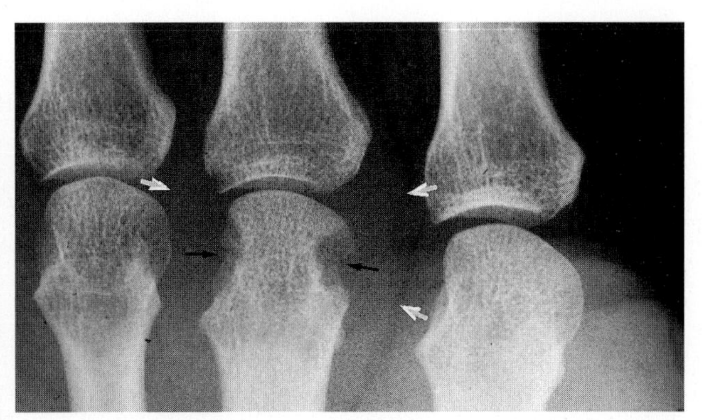

Fig. 13.35 Classic features of inflammatory arthropathy. There is periarticular soft-tissue swelling (white arrows), joint space narrowing and marginal erosions (black arrows).

The initial radiographic abnormality is periarticular soft-tissue swelling which is due to a combination of synovial inflammation, oedema and effusion. Loss of joint space, which tends to be relatively uniform, is due to cartilage destruction by hypertrophied, inflamed synovium (termed 'pannus'). Periarticular osteopenia is a manifestation of the acute stage of the disease and is due to hyperaemia. Erosions are initially manifest as loss of the fine white line of the articular cortex. Larger erosions tend to occur later and are located at joint margins where the bone is not covered by articular cartilage, commonly near capsular or ligamentous attachments. Erosions are due to the direct effect of pannus. Later in the disease, joint deformities occur due to laxity of supporting structures and eventually fibrosis. With chronic disuse, generalized osteopenia is seen; this may be accentuated by steroid therapy.

RHEUMATOID ARTHRITIS

Rheumatoid arthritis is the commonest of the inflammatory arthropathies. Onset is usually in young or middle-aged adults with females affected two to three times more commonly than males. Rheumatoid factor is positive in 90–95% of cases. Extra-articular manifestations include subcutaneous or tendon-sheath nodules, tenosynovitis or bursitis, pleural effusions, rheumatoid pulmonary nodules and diffuse interstitial fibrosis.

The radiographic findings are as described above. In addition, subchondral cysts may be seen, particularly in the hips and knees. These are continuous with the synovium and tend not to have sclerotic borders. Juxta-articular synovial cysts are also a recognized feature and are well imaged with ultrasound or MRI. Bony ankylosis is a rare feature, limited to the carpus and tarsus.

Any synovial joint may be involved by rheumatoid arthritis, although there is a predilection for certain sites. The disease is characteristically a symmetrical polyarthritis.

In the **hand**, the metacarpophalangeal and proximal interphalangeal joints are involved early with relative sparing of the distal interphalangeal joints. Characteristic deformities are ulnar deviation and volar subluxation at the metacarpophalangeal joints (Fig. 13.36), hyperextension at the proximal interphalangeal joints and hyperflexion at the distal interphalangeal joints (**swan-neck deformity**) or, conversely, hyperflexion at the proximal interphalangeal joints and hyperextension at the distal interphalangeal joints (**Boutonnière deformity**). First metacarpophalangeal joint flexion with interphalangeal joint extension (**hitchhiker's thumb**) is also seen. In the wrist, early erosions are seen at the distal radioulnar joint, radial and ulnar styloids, scaphoid waist, triquetrum and pisiform. Intercarpal changes occur later. Wrist deformities include ulnar translocation of the carpus, where more than 50% of the lunate articulates with the ulna, radial deviation of the hand, scapholunate dissociation and other patterns of carpal instability.

In the **shoulder** girdle, early changes include erosions of the distal end of the clavicle, the insertion of the coracoclavicular ligament and marginal erosions at the humeral head. Later signs are those of rotator cuff tear, with elevation of the humeral head and concavity of the undersurface of the acromion.

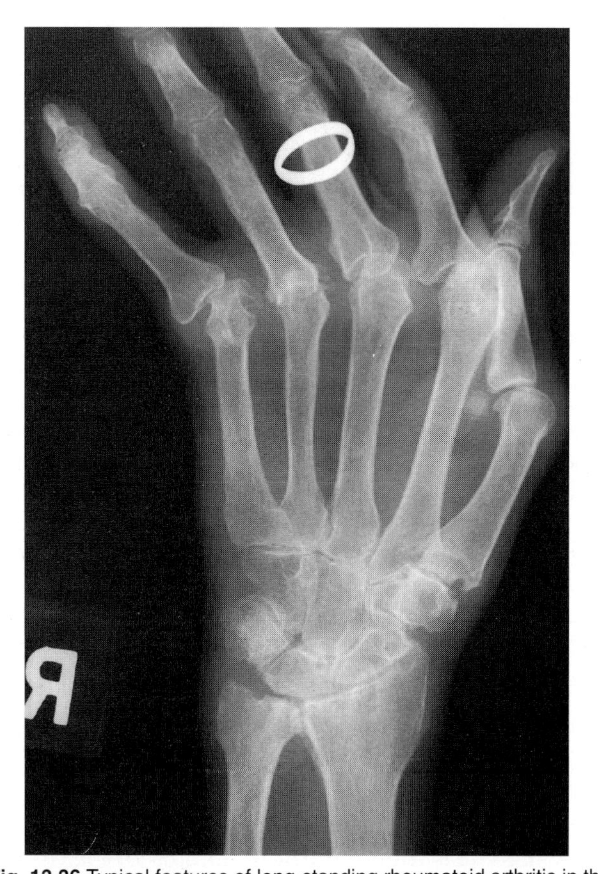

Fig. 13.36 Typical features of long-standing rheumatoid arthritis in the hand with ulnar deviation at the metacarpophalangeal joints, 'hitchhiker's thumb' deformity, ulnar translocation of the carpus and erosion of the ulnar styloid.

In the **foot**, erosive changes typically affect the metatarsophalangeal joints. Associated abnormalities include lateral deviation and/or hyperextension at the metatarsophalangeal joints, and flexion of the proximal or distal interphalangeal joints (**hammer toes**). Intertarsal erosions are a late finding. Calcaneal spurs and retrocalcaneal bursitis are also recognized findings. Involvement of the ankle is relatively uncommon.

In the **knee**, suprapatellar effusions and **popliteal (Baker's) cysts** are characteristic soft-tissue abnormalities. There tends to be symmetrical involvement of all three joint compartments, unlike osteoarthritis. The commonest deformity is a valgus knee.

In the **hip**, again uniform joint space loss helps to distinguish rheumatoid from osteoarthritis. Protrusio acetabulae is also seen.

JUVENILE CHRONIC ARTHRITIS

Juvenile chronic arthritis comprises a group of disorders that includes the various forms of juvenile rheumatoid arthritis and juvenile ankylosing spondylitis. Psoriatic and inflammatory bowel disease associated arthropathies may also be seen in children.

Juvenile rheumatoid arthritis

This disease complex includes Still's disease (~20%), pauciarticular disease (~40%), seronegative polyarticular disease (~25%) and seropositive polyarticular disease (~5%).

Still's disease is an acute systemic illness occurring in children under 5 years of age. The polyarthritis is accompanied by a fever, anaemia, hepatosplenomegaly and lymphadenopathy. In the acute stage, radiographic changes may be minimal, but 25% progress to chronic destructive arthritis. Pauci-articular juvenile rheumatoid arthritis usually occurs in young girls. One to three joints are involved, usually knee, ankle or elbow, and chronic iridocyclitis occurs in 25% of cases. Seronegative polyarticular juvenile rheumatoid arthritis is also commoner in females. Both small and large joints are affected in a symmetrical fashion. **Seropositive polyarticular juvenile rheumatoid arthritis** is generally found in teenage girls. Polyarticular changes typical of adult rheumatoid arthritis are seen.

The radiographic features are similar in all forms of juvenile rheumatoid arthritis. Soft-tissue changes include muscle wasting and fusiform periarticular swelling. Hyperaemia and disuse lead to osteoporosis and metaphyseal lucent lines may be seen during active disease. Periosteal reaction is also an early manifestation. Later findings include loss of joint space due to cartilage destruction, erosive changes and ankylosis, most commonly in the carpus and interphalangeal joints. Joint deformity due to ligamentous rupture are common.

Chronic hyperaemia results in overgrowth of the epiphyses leading to enlargement of the joints involved (Fig. 13.37), and squaring of the carpal and tarsal bones and of the patella. Advanced skeletal maturation results in premature fusion, limb length deformities and overall shortening of limbs. Chronic synovitis also produces distinctive changes, including enlargement of the trochlear notch of the elbow and intercondylar notch of the knee. In the hip, coxa valga and protrusio acetabulae are seen. Hypoplasia of the iliac wings and small size of the femoral shaft may make prosthetic replacement difficult. Spinal disease is also common, as is involvement of the temporomandibular joint, leading to micrognathia.

Juvenile ankylosing spondylitis

This results in bilateral symmetrical sacroiliac joint and lumbar spine changes in adolescent males. However, other joints, particularly the hips, may be involved prior to sacroiliac joint disease, delaying the diagnosis. Also, diagnostic difficulty arises due to the appearance of normal sacroiliac joints in adolescents, which are wide with indistinct cortices.

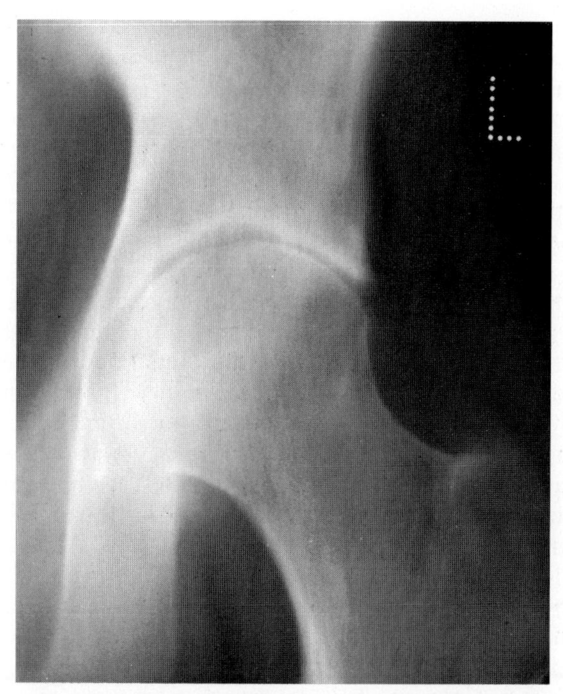

Fig. 13.38 Ankylosing spondylitis involving the left hip. There is concentric loss of joint space, typifying an inflammatory arthropathy, and early osteophyte formation.

ANKYLOSING SPONDYLITIS

Ankylosing spondylitis is the commonest of the seronegative inflammatory spondyloarthropathies, involving primarily the sacroiliac joints, spine and large joints. It is commoner in males (4–10:1/ male:female ratio) and usually presents between ages 15–35 years. More than 90% of patients are HLA-B27 positive. Extra-articular manifestations include iritis, aortic incompetence and upper lobe pulmonary fibrosis.

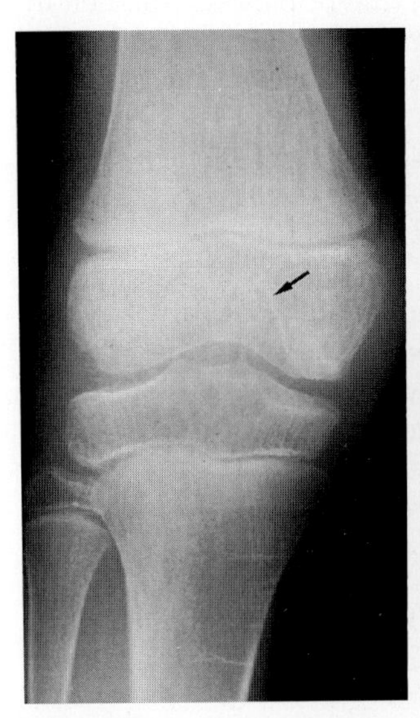

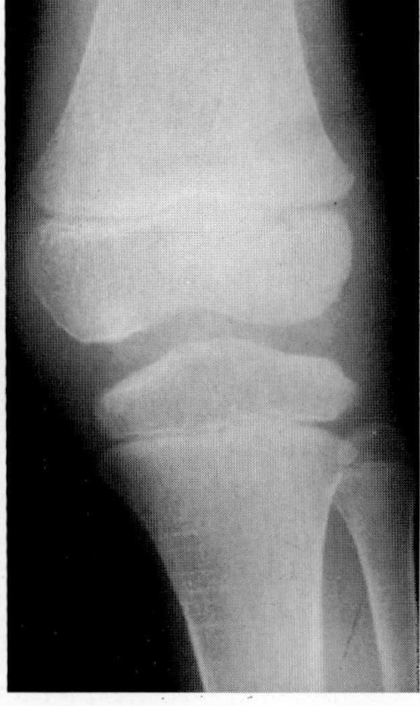

Fig. 13.37 Juvenile rheumatoid arthritis affecting the right knee, manifesting as enlargement of the epiphyses and intercondylar notch (arrow). Similar changes may be seen with haemophilic arthropathy and tuberculous arthritis and are due to chronic hyperaemia and synovitis.

In addition to spinal and sacroiliac joint changes, (see p. 83), involvement of the large joints is relatively common. Up to 50% of patients have hip involvement with concentric loss of joint space due to chondrolysis, mild erosions, protrusio acetabulae and ring osteophytes (Fig. 13.38). Bilateral but asymmetric involvement may be seen. The glenohumeral joint, symphysis pubis, sternomanubrial joint and costovertebral joints are also relatively commonly involved. Joint ankylosis is a late complication. Other radiographic features include enthesopathy, namely the development of bony spurs at sites of ligamentous and tendinous attachments which is particularly common in the pelvis, calcaneum and patella.

PSORIATIC ARTHRITIS

Psoriatic arthritis occurs in 0.5–25% of patients with psoriasis. It generally occurs in young patients with skin disease, but joints may be affected prior to skin changes in 20% of patients. Five distinct forms are described:

- polyarthritis predominantly of distal interphalangeal joints;
- arthritis mutilans (deforming type);
- symmetric polyarthritis resembling rheumatoid arthritis;
- oligoarthritis;
- spondyloarthropathy, occuring in 30–50% of patients with psoriatic arthritis.

The joints commonly involved are the small joints of the hands and feet. In the hands, the interphalangeal joints, together with the intercarpal joints, are involved, commonly in an asymmetrical pattern. Terminal tuft resorption is also a feature. In the foot, the interphalangeal and metatarsophalangeal joints are predominantly involved. Associated retrocalcaneal bursitis and erosions at the insertions of the Achilles tendon and plantar aponeurosis are seen. In 30–50% of cases the sacroiliac joints are involved and spondylitis is also a feature. Involvement of larger joints is much less common.

Characteristic radiographic features include fusiform soft-tissue swelling, leading to a 'sausage' digit if the whole finger is involved. Bone density is generally normal. Early erosions are marginal in location but may progress to the subchondral regions, occasionally producing a 'pencil-in-cup' deformity (Fig. 13.39). Periosteal reaction and, later, joint ankylosis are also features.

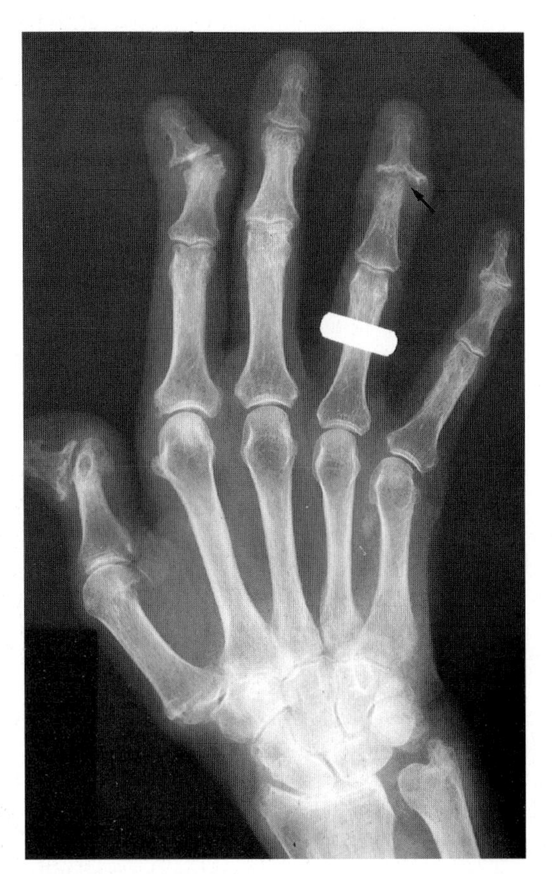

Fig. 13.39 Psoriatic arthritis affecting the hand. Bone density is generally preserved. There is periarticular soft-tissue swelling and central erosion, resulting in a 'pencil-in-cup' deformity (arrow).

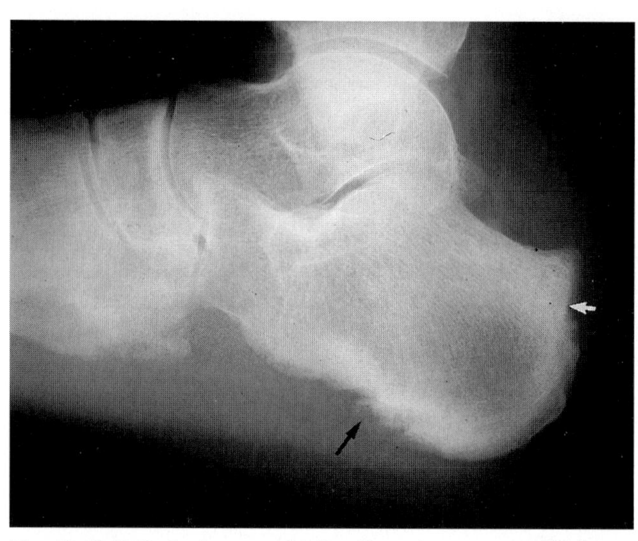

Fig. 13.40 Reiter's disease affecting the calcaneus, manifesting as erosion at the Achilles tendon insertion (white arrow) and plantar aponeurosis (black arrow).

REITER'S DISEASE

Reiter's disease is a syndrome consisting of non-specific urethritis (cervicitis in females) in 85% of cases, conjunctivitis in 60% and arthritis. It typically affects young males, with extra-articular manifestations usually occurring initially. The joint involvement is predominantly distal lower limb (Fig. 13.40). Spondyloarthropathy identical to that of psoriasis is seen in 10–40% of cases. The radiographic abnormalities in the joints are similar to those described for psoriatic arthritis.

ENTEROPATHIC ARTHROPATHY

Sacroiliitis and spondylitis identical to that of ankylosing spondylitis may accompany ulcerative colitis, Crohn's disease and Whipple's disease. Peripheral joint disease is unusual and limited to a mild synovitis with osteopenia, often occurring in conjunction with exacerbation of the bowel disease. Erosive arthritis is rare.

CRYSTAL DEPOSITION DISEASES

GOUT

Gout is a disease caused by the intra-articular and periarticular deposition of monosodium urate crystals secondary to chronic hyperuricaemia. The latter may be idiopathic, secondary to enzyme defects or chronic diseases such as myeloproliferative disorders, renal disease and diuretic therapy.

Acute attacks usually begin in the fourth decade and typically affect the first metatarsophalangeal joint. No radiographic abnormalities may be seen apart from osteopenia and soft-tissue swelling. The classic radiographic findings of chronic tophaceous gout occur after several years, namely the development of deposits of sodium urate crystals within soft tissues (tophi), commonly within the olecranon bursa and adjacent to joints. The tophi typically appear as non-mineralized soft-tissue masses which occasionally calcify. Tophi may also be intraosseous, appearing as subchondral lucent lesions. Bony erosions may be intra-articular, typically eccentrically located at the joint margin, or extra-articular, related to overlying soft-tissue tophi. The erosions have well-defined sclerotic margins and an overhanging edge is characteristic (Fig. 13.41). The bone density is usually preserved and loss of joint space is only a late feature due to the development of secondary osteoarthritis. Chondrocalcinosis is rare but is a recognized finding.

The commonest joints involved are the first metatarsophalangeal joint and, to a lesser extent, the other small joints of the foot. Involvement of the hand, wrist, knee, elbow and, occasionally, sacroiliac joints is also seen.

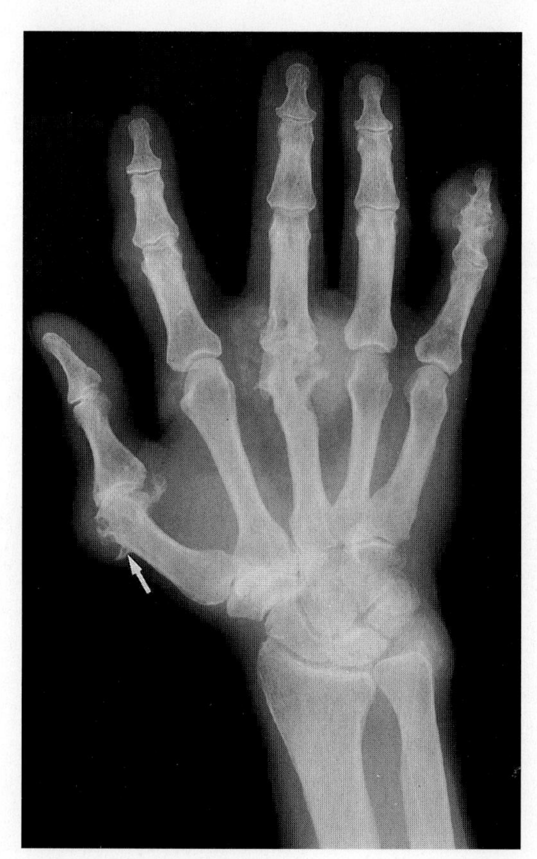

Fig. 13.41 Chronic tophaceous gout of the hand showing multiple calcified tophi and erosions with sclerotic margins and characteristic overhanging edges (arrow).

CALCIUM PYROPHOSPHATE DIHYDRATE (CPPD) CRYSTAL DEPOSITION DISEASE

This condition results from the intra-articular deposition of CPPD crystals. It may manifest as chondrocalcinosis (cartilage calcification) or pyrophosphate arthropathy. The condition is seen in the middle-aged and elderly population and is usually idiopathic.

It presents in several ways, the commonest being as pseudogout (acute self-limiting attacks resembling gout or infection) or a chronic progressive arthropathy with exacerbations. In 10–20% of patients there are no symptoms. Rarely, a rapidly destructive arthritis simulating neuropathic arthropathy may occur. Joint aspiration may yield CPPD crystals.

Radiographic findings include chondrocalcinosis, which occurs in both the articular hyaline cartilage and in the fibrocartilaginous structures, such as the menisci of the knee and triangular fibrocartilage in the wrist. Common sites include the knee, wrist, symphysis pubis and acetabular labrum. CPPD crystals may also be deposited in synovium, capsule, tendons and ligaments. The disease resembles osteoarthritis with loss of joint space, osteophytes, subchondral sclerosis and osteochondral fragments. Subchondral cysts are common and may be very large, simulating neoplasm.

The major differentiating feature from classic osteoarthritis is the specific pattern of joint involvement. In the knee, the patellofemoral joint is typically involved with relative sparing of the femorotibial compartments (Fig. 13.42). In the wrist, the radiocarpal joint is involved and may be associated with scapholunate dissociation and proximal migration of the

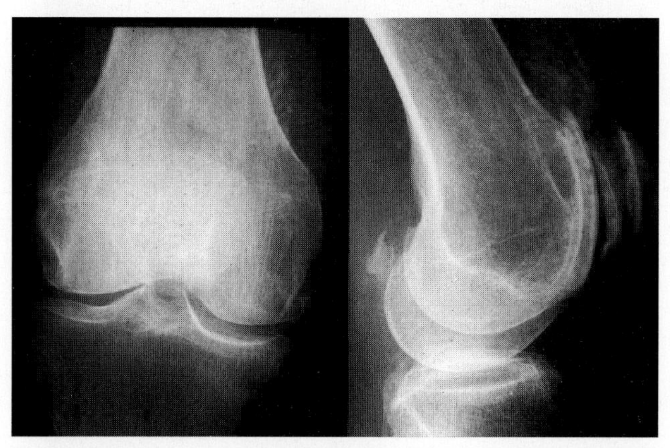

Fig. 13.42 Calcium pyrophosphate dihydrate deposition disease of the knee. Patellofemoral osteoarthritis predominates. There is calcification of the synovium and menisci.

capitate. In the hand, the second and third metacarpophalangeal joints are typically involved. The hip, shoulder and elbow are less common sites of disease. Severe degenerative changes in the spine may also occur.

In patients with **haemochromatosis** 50% develop an arthropathy due to CPPD crystal deposition. The pattern of joint involvement and radiographic features are very similar to those of pyrophosphate arthropathy. Beak-like osteophytes from the second and third metacarpal heads, osteoporosis, extra-articular manifestations and a younger age of onset favour the diagnosis of haemochromatosis.

Other conditions associated with CPPD crystal deposition and chondrocalcinosis include osteoarthritis, trauma, gout, hyperparathyroidism, Wilson's disease and ochronosis.

CALCIUM HYDROXYAPATITE DEPOSITION DISEASE

Calcium hydroxyapatite deposition disease is due to the periarticular deposition of hydroxyapatite crystals. It is usually monoarticular and presents as joint pain in a middle to elderly age group. The commonest joint involved is the shoulder. Other sites include the elbow, wrist and MCP joints.

Radiographs typically demonstrate cloudy or homogeneous periarticular calcification in tendons, ligaments, capsules and bursae, with a normal underlying joint (Fig. 13.43).

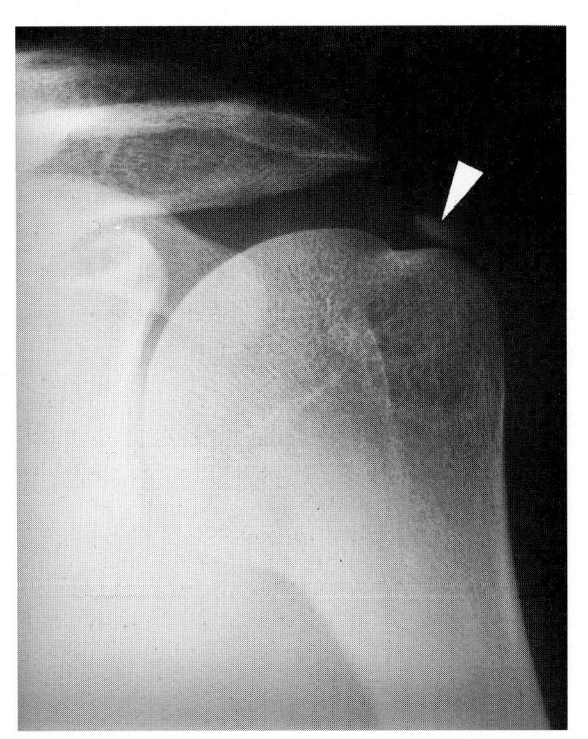

Fig. 13.43 Calcium hydroxyapatite deposition in the supraspinatus tendon (arrow) (calcific tendinitis). The underlying joint is normal.

INFECTIVE ARTHRITIS

ACUTE SEPTIC ARTHRITIS

Joint infection may be due to direct spread of infection from a penetrating wound or compound fracture, from local extension of osteomyelitis or via a haematogenous route. Typically, a single joint is affected. Pathologically, there is joint effusion, synovitis and

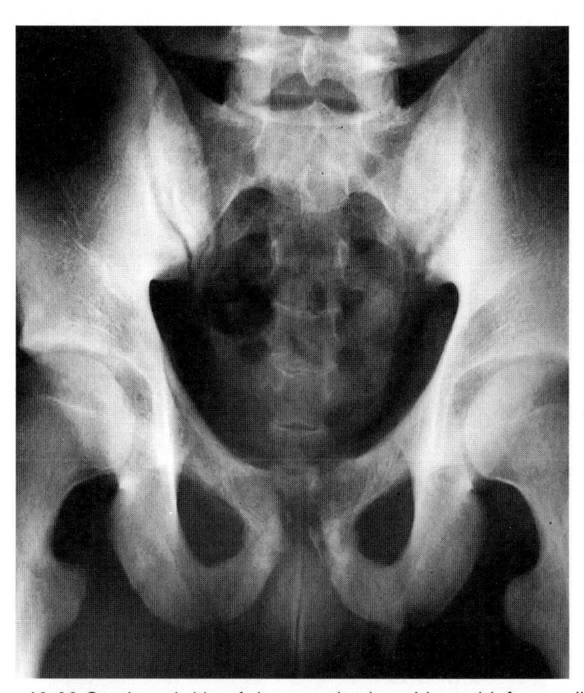

Fig. 13.44 Septic arthritis of the symphysis pubis and left sacroiliac joint. The joints are widened and irregular due to joint destruction.

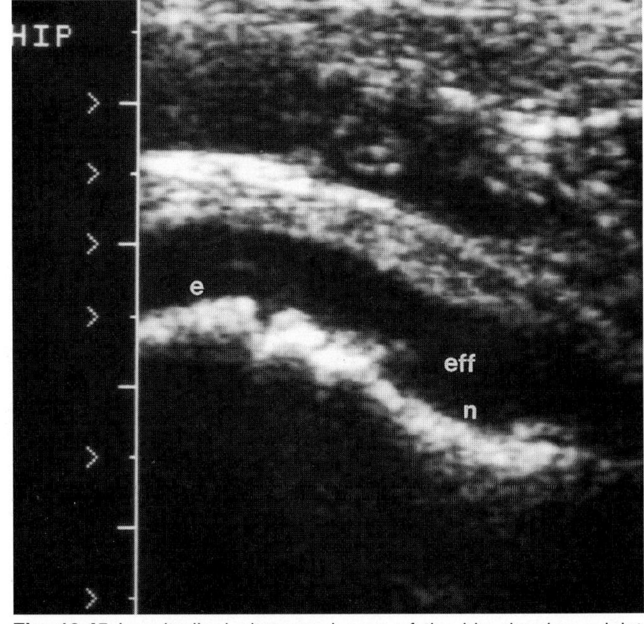

Fig. 13.45 Longitudinal ultrasound scan of the hip showing a joint effusion, manifest as an anechoic space (*eff*) anterior to the femoral neck (*n*) and capital epiphysis (*e*).

cartilage destruction with destruction of cortical bone at the joint margins.

Plain radiographs demonstrate osteopenia, uniform joint space loss and marginal cortical erosions progressing to joint destruction (Fig. 13.44). Joint effusion is the earliest finding and is easily identified radiographically in the elbow, knee and ankle. Ultrasound is much more sensitive for detecting hip effusion (Fig. 13.45) and allows aspiration to be performed. Large hip effusions may result in lateral subluxation of the femoral head on plain radiographs of the pelvis.

Early complications of septic arthritis include avascular necrosis, especially of the femoral head. Late complications include secondary osteomyelitis and ankylosis, either fibrous or bony.

TUBERCULOUS ARTHRITIS

Tuberculosis most commonly involves the hip and the knee, followed by the sacroiliac joints, wrist and elbow. Joint disease is manifest initially as osteopenia and soft-tissue swelling followed by cortical destruction. The bone destruction, which is initially at the edges of the joint, is due to synovitis (Fig. 13.46). In the growing skeleton, chronic hyperaemia may result in accelerated maturation of the epiphyses, resulting in an appearance similar to haemophilic arthropathy or juvenile chronic arthritis. Long-term complications include bony ankylosis.

TUMOURS AND TUMOUR-LIKE CONDITIONS

Primary tumours of the synovium are rare. Benign lesions include *lipoma arborescens* and *synovial haemangioma* which tend to present with pain and swelling, and plain radiographs are either normal or demonstrate evidence of an effusion. Ultrasound, CT or MRI will show either localized or generalized synovial thickening. Areas of fat density/signal in lipoma arborescens may be identified on CT or MRI.

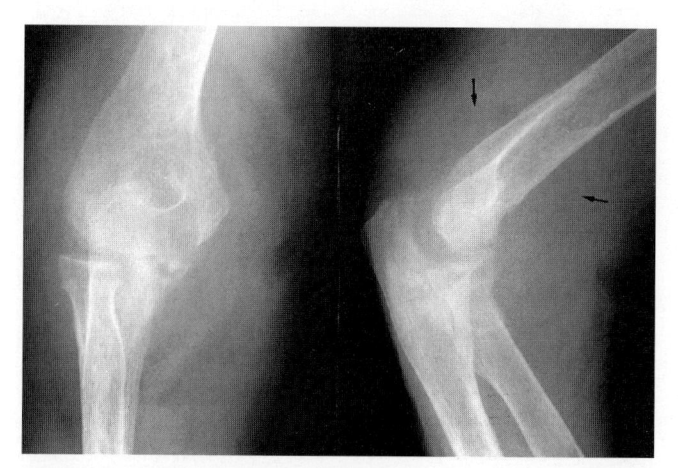

Fig. 13.46 Tuberculosis of the elbow. The anterior and posterior fat pads are elevated (arrows), indicating synovial swelling and/or effusion. The joint is destroyed.

SYNOVIAL SARCOMA (MALIGNANT SYNOVIOMA)

Synovial sarcoma is a rare tumour associated with tendon sheaths, bursae and joint capsules. It occurs predominantly in young adults. Radiographically, a soft-tissue mass is seen which may cause pressure erosion of adjacent bone. Calcification can be identified in approximately 30% of cases. The lesion most commonly arises adjacent to the knee and ankle, or in the foot.

Tumour-like conditions of joints include synovial osteochondromatosis and pigmented villonodular synovitis.

SYNOVIAL OSTEOCHONDROMATOSIS

This rare disorder results from formation of cartilage or bone in relation to the synovium and may be a metaplastic rather than neoplastic condition. Usually a single major joint is involved: 70% of cases affect the knee. Bursae and tendon sheaths may also be affected. It usually occurs in young adults.

Radiographs demonstrate evidence of joint effusion and synovial thickening. If they are calcified, the cartilaginous loose bodies can be seen (Fig. 13.47). Non-calcified loose bodies may be demonstrated by arthrography, ultrasound or MRI. Pressure erosion of adjacent bone and secondary osteoarthritis may occur.

PIGMENTED VILLONODULAR SYNOVITIS

Pigmented villonodular synovitis is a proliferative condition of the synovium of unknown aetiology that usually affects joints but may be extra-articular (giant cell tumour of tendon sheath). It is typically mono-articular, most commonly affecting the knee. It occurs in young and middle-aged adults and may present with a haemorrhagic effusion.

Radiographs show evidence of joint effusion/synovial thickening and articular erosions which progress to large subarticular cysts (Fig. 13.48). The deposition of haemosiderin within the hyperplastic synovium can result in a characteristic appearance at MRI with large areas of synovium showing loss of signal on all sequences.

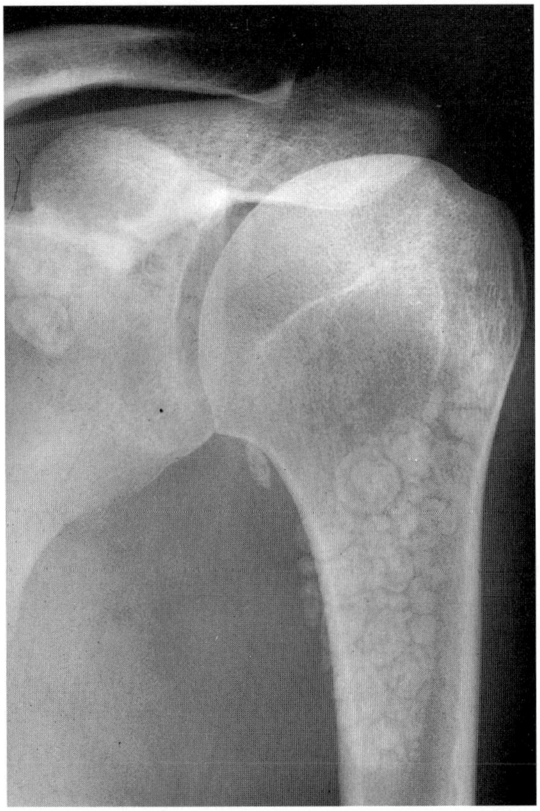

Fig. 13.47 Synovial osteochondromatosis of the left shoulder manifesting as multiple calcified loose bodies in the subscapularis recess and biceps tendon sheath.

MISCELLANEOUS JOINT DISORDERS

NEUROPATHIC ARTHROPATHY

Neuropathic arthropathy (**Charcot joint**) is a severe destructive arthropathy with several aetiologies. The disease is usually monoarticular, the joint affected depending upon the underlying cause. Diabetes, syringomyelia, tabes dorsalis and leprosy are common causes. Clinically, the patient presents with a swollen, unstable but pain-free joint.

The radiographic features depend upon whether the arthropathy is predominantly hypertrophic (20%), atrophic (40%) or mixed (40%). The typical features of the hypertrophic variety are increased bone density, swelling, multiple periarticular bony fragments and a disorganized, dislocated joint (Fig. 13.49). The atrophic variety manifests as relatively well-defined bone resorption adjacent to the joint.

The commonest joints involved include the talonavicular and tarsometatarsal joints in diabetes (usually atrophic or mixed type), the shoulder in syringomyelia (almost always atrophic) and the knee in tabes dorsalis (usually hypertrophic).

An important differential diagnosis of atrophic neuroarthopathy is septic arthritis. The distinction may be particularly difficult in the diabetic foot.

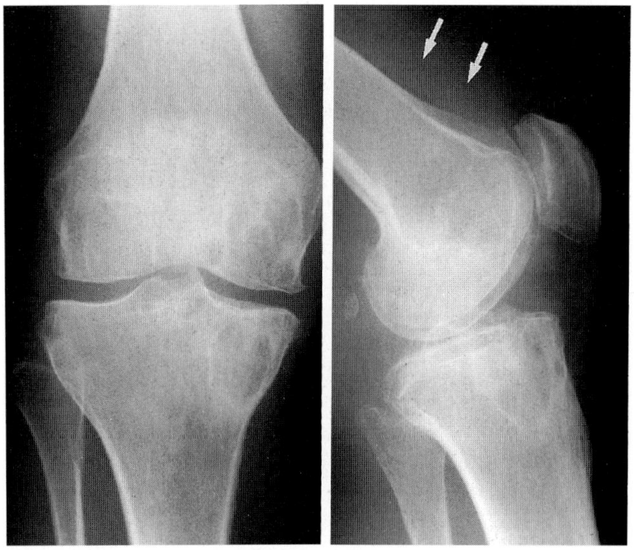

Fig. 13.48 Pigmented villonodular synovitis of the knee. There is synovial thickening in the suprapatellar pouch (arrow); large subchondral cysts are present.

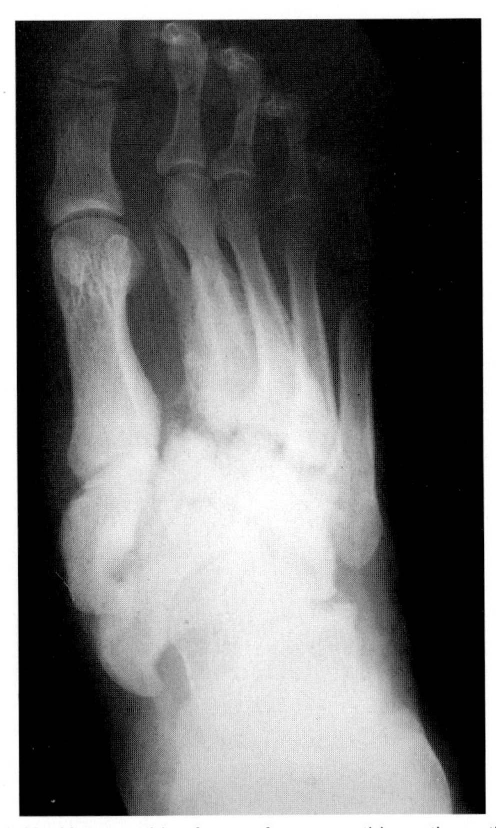

Fig. 13.49 Hypertrophic form of neuropathic arthropathy with increased bone density, periarticular bony fragments and a Lisfranc type tarsometatarsal dislocation.

HAEMOPHILIC ARTHROPATHY

Haemophilia is a bleeding disorder caused by deficiency of Factor VIII (haemophilia A) or Factor IX (haemophilia B). The condition is only found in males since it is an X-linked recessive disorder. Joint changes are a consequence of recurrent haemarthroses which result in synovitis and chronic hyperaemia. The synovitis manifests as soft-tissue swelling which may appear relatively dense due to haemosiderin deposition in the synovium. Hyperaemia in turn results in osteoporosis, epiphyseal overgrowth and early epiphyseal fusion, resulting in short bones.

Cartilage destruction, erosions and subchondral cysts are also seen and secondary osteoarthritis eventually develops. The commonest joints involved are the knee, elbow, ankle, hip and shoulder. The radiographic appearances are similar to those seen in juvenile rheumatoid arthritis.

HYPERTROPHIC OSTEOARTHROPATHY

Hypertrophic osteoarthropathy is a condition of unknown aetiology that presents as an arthropathy but manifests radiologically as symmetrical periosteal reaction along the distal borders of the radius and ulna and tibia and fibula, and occasionally affects the digits (Fig. 13.50). The condition is associated with a variety of intrathoracic and abdominal diseases, the commonest being carcinoma of the bronchus.

EVALUATION OF JOINT PROSTHESES

Causes of a painful hip prosthesis include infection, mechanical loosening and heterotopic ossification. The latter condition manifests as well-developed bone bridging the space between the greater trochanter and lateral margin of the acetabulum.

Difficulties arise in the differentiation between septic and mechanical loosening. Plain radiographic features of loosening include increasing radiolucency at the cement–bone interface and change of position of the components with time (Fig. 13.51), cement fracture and cystic resorption of bone around the femoral component. The presence of periosteal reaction or large amounts of heterotopic ossification are suggestive of infection.

^{99m}Tc-MDP bone scintigraphy has been used extensively to detect loosening and infection. The bone scan

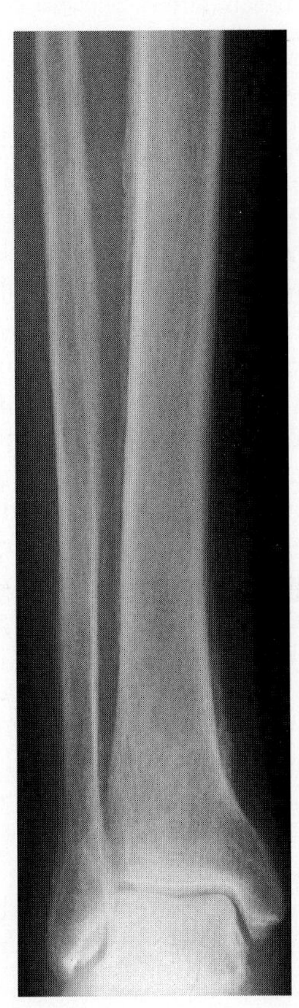

Fig. 13.50 Hypertrophic osteoarthropathy manifesting as fine linear periosteal reaction along the distal tibia and fibula.

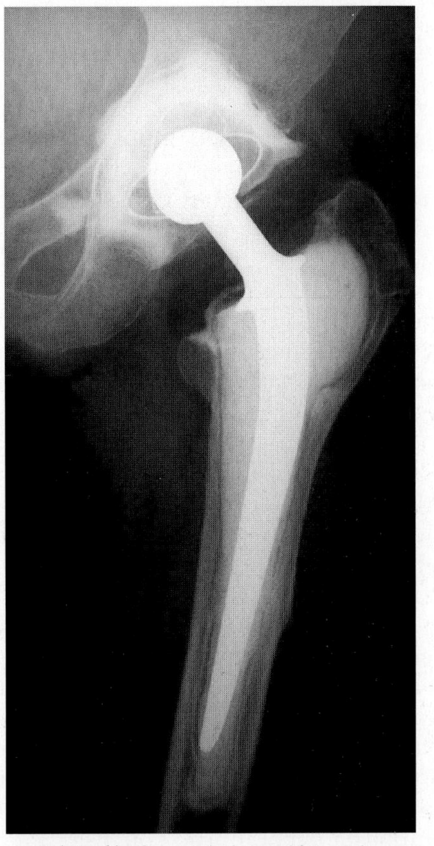

Fig. 13.51 Loosening of both acetabular and femoral components of a left total hip replacement, manifesting as lucency at the cement–bone interface and subsidence of the femoral stem.

remains 'hot' for about 9–12 months postoperatively, then activity gradually subsides. Increased activity at the tip and adjacent to the neck of a femoral prosthesis may be seen with mechanical loosening, whereas infection tends to result in generalized increase in uptake. However, the lack of specificity of these findings reduces the value of routine bone scanning. Increased sensitivity and specificity for infection may be obtained using gallium or labelled white cell scanning.

CT and MRI have no role to play in the assessment of a painful prosthesis due to the artefact caused by the metal implant.

The most specific preoperative technique for diagnosing infection and loosening is the arthrogram, which can confirm loosening by identifying contrast medium within lucent spaces at the cement–bone interface. Aspiration of the joint prior to contrast injection may identify infected prostheses.

OSTEONECROSIS AND THE OSTEOCHONDROSES

Osteonecrosis and the osteochondroses are considered here because they frequently present with pain or abnormality related to joints.

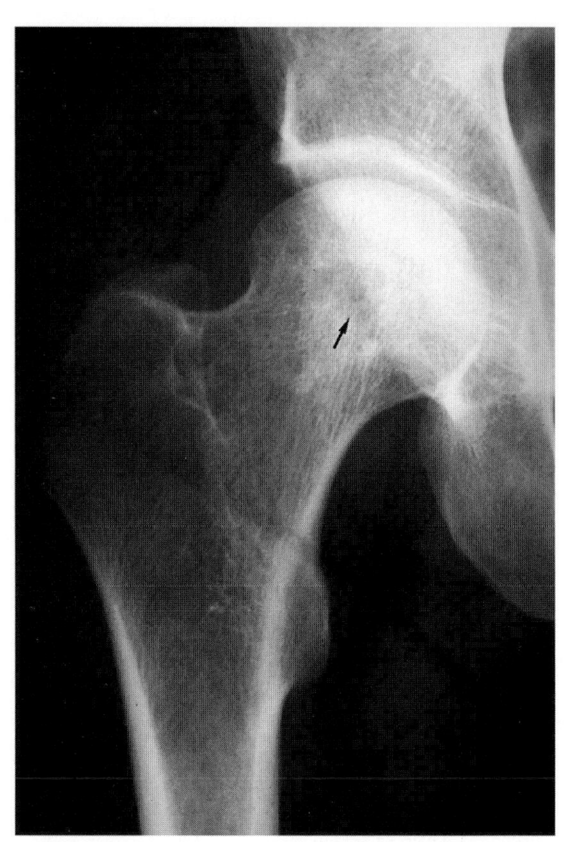

Fig. 13.52 Osteonecrosis of the femoral head. There is subarticular sclerosis and cyst formation (arrow). The joint space is maintained.

OSTEONECROSIS

Osteonecrosis is a term that signifies death of bone due to interruption of blood supply in the absence of infection. When a subarticular site is involved, the term 'avascular necrosis' has been used, whereas the term 'bone infarct' has been used for osteonecrosis involving the metaphysis or diaphysis.

The loss of blood supply may be idiopathic or due to trauma, vascular thrombosis or obstruction, or vascular compression. Other causes include corticosteroid therapy, sickle cell disease, Gaucher's disease, pregnancy, causes of fat embolism (including alcohol and pancreatitis) and caisson disease. The commoner sites of involvement include the femoral and humeral heads, the scaphoid, lunate, talus and shafts of long bones. Idiopathic osteonecrosis is a specific condition usually involving the femoral head or medial femoral condyle.

The plain radiographic features of osteonecrosis are characteristic. In a subarticular site, the findings include an arc-like subchondral lucent line (the crescent sign), which progresses to patchy sclerosis and lysis, cyst formation and eventually collapse of the articular surface (Fig. 13.52). Initially, there is preservation of the joint space but secondary osteoarthritis may complicate femoral head collapse.

Metaphyseal bone infarcts typically appear as poorly defined lucent areas with peripheral sclerosis that do not expand the bone (Fig. 13.53), whereas osteonecrosis affecting smaller bones, such as the scaphoid or lunate, results in mixed sclerosis and lysis with eventual collapse (Fig. 13.54). These changes occur several months after the onset of symptoms and plain radiographs are therefore insensitive for the detection of early disease.

Bone scintigraphy is far more sensitive and will be abnormal in the presence of normal radiographs. Initially, there may be an area of diminished uptake but this is followed within weeks by increased activity. CT is also more sensitive than plain radiographs, but it has now been replaced by MRI which is currently the most sensitive technique for imaging osteonecrosis. Within days there is poorly defined reduced signal intensity on T1-weighted scans and increased signal intensity on T2-weighted scans from oedema associated with acute infarction. This is, however, a nonspecific pattern and must be correlated with clinical findings. The MRI findings in chronic infarction are much more characteristic.

Early detection of osteonecrosis of the femoral head by MRI or scintigraphy, at a time when radiographs are normal, allows treatment with core decompression, which may prevent progression to collapse and secondary osteoarthritis.

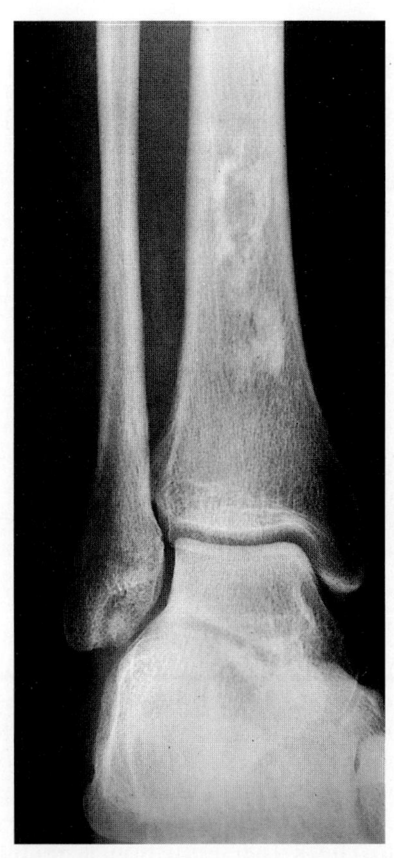

Fig. 13.53 Typical appearances of medullary bone infarct in the distal tibia identified as a region of peripheral serpiginous calcification. Absence of endosteal cortical erosion is a typical feature.

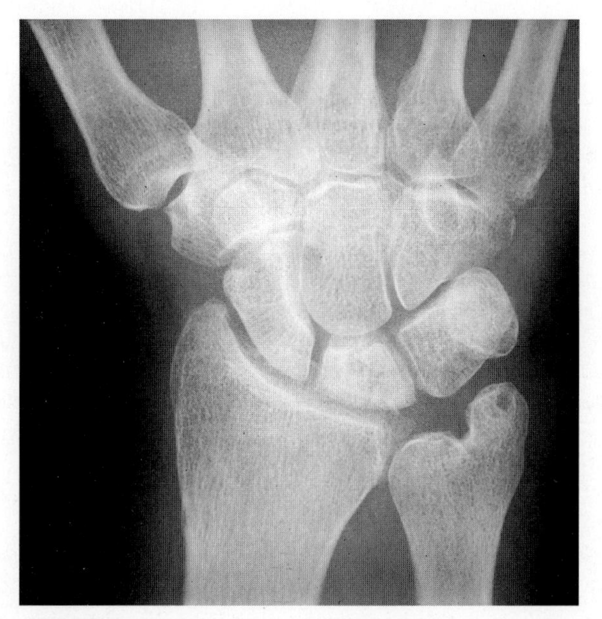

Fig. 13.54 Osteonecrosis of the lunate (Kienböck's disease). There is mixed sclerosis and lysis with early collapse of the distal articular surface.

THE OSTEOCHONDROSES

The osteochondroses comprise a heterogeneous group of conditions that are characterized by involvement, typically in children, of an epiphysis, apophysis or growth plate. The aetiology may be ischaemic, traumatic, either single or repetitive, or due to chronic stress. It is also recognized that some conditions included in this group are normal variants of ossification, e.g. Sever's disease of the calcaneus.

Each of the conditions discussed below appears to be associated with an abnormality of endochondral ossification. Radiologically, they are characterized by fragmentation, collapse, sclerosis and, frequently, gradual re-ossification.

Legg–Calve–Perthes' disease

This condition affects the femoral capital epiphysis. It is a true infarction, usually occurring in the 4–8-year-old age range when the vascular supply to the femoral head is most at risk. It is commoner in boys and bilateral in 10% of cases, although usually there is asymmetrical involvement. The first radiographic sign may be a joint effusion. The initial bony abnormality is the presence of a subchondral lucent line, best seen on a frog-leg lateral view since it involves the superolateral aspect of the femoral head. Progression leads to fragmentation, sclerosis and collapse of the femoral head. Metaphyseal cyst formation and irregularity of the acetabulum are also features.

With healing, there is resorption of dead bone and gradual reossification of the femoral head. Coxa magna and coxa vara may eventally result.

A poorer prognosis is seen in children presenting at an older age and in girls (who are skeletally more mature). Another poor prognostic sign is lateral extrusion of the femoral head ossification centre, when bone fragments are seen lateral to the acetabular rim. This indicates lack of coverage of the femoral head, leading to incongruity between the head and acetabulum (Fig. 13.55). Surgical treatment is aimed at containing the femoral head within the acetabulum to allow optimal development of the head as the child grows. Prior to surgery, hip arthrography is of value in determining the position of maximum congruity and stability. It will also show that the overlying articular cartilage is intact.

The differential diagnosis of Perthes' disease includes other causes of ischaemic necrosis, such as Gaucher's disease and sickle-cell disease, and other causes of fragmented epiphyses, such as hypothyroidism and multiple epiphyseal dysplasia.

Freiberg's disease

This disease is also a true necrosis, usually involving the second or third metatarsal heads (less commonly, the first and fourth). It is usually seen in teenage females.

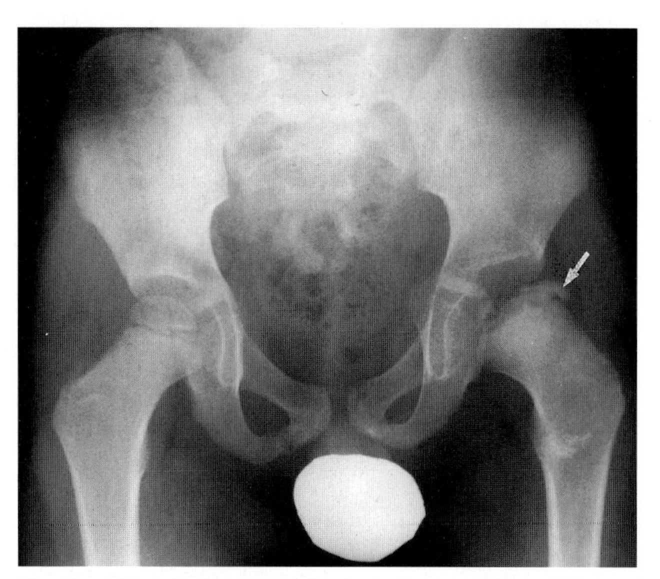

Fig. 13.55 Typical features of Perthes' disease of the left femoral head. The epiphysis is fragmented, flattened and sclerotic. Lateral extrusion is a poor prognostic sign (arrow).

Köhler's disease

A dense, fragmented tarsal navicular may be a normal variant of ossification. Therefore, Köhler's disease should only be suggested when there is fragmentation of a previously normal bone in association with pain.

Osgood–Schlatter's disease

Osgood–Schlatter's disease is thought to be due to traumatic avulsion of the tibial tubercle. The diagnosis is made clinically. Radiographs show soft-tissue swelling and fragmentation of the tibial tubercle.

Sinding–Larsen–Johanssen's disease

This entity is due to traumatic avulsion of the inferior pole of the patella.

Blount's disease

Blount's disease is due to involvement of the medial aspect of the proximal tibial epiphysis growth plate with resulting varus deformity of the knee. The commoner infantile type occurs from a worsening of the normal physiological bowing of the lower extremity with weight-bearing. The increased pressure results in fragmentation of the medial aspect of the metaphysis, which causes epiphyseal deformity. More than 50% of cases are bilateral.

Normal variants of ossification that simulate osteochondroses occur at the lateral femoral condyle posteriorly, calcaneal apophysis, trochlea, lateral epicondyle and ischiopubic synchondrosis.

MISCELLANEOUS PAEDIATRIC CONDITIONS

CONGENITAL DISLOCATION OF THE HIP

Hip instability in the neonatal period is a relatively common clinical finding. However, in 75–95% of cases, the hip will become stable within a few weeks. The incidence of congenital dislocation of the hip after the neonatal period is approximately 1:1000.

Radiography in the neonatal period, before ossification of the femoral capital epiphysis, has now been largely replaced by ultrasound which can demonstrate the dysplasia of the acetabular roof and the degree of coverage of the femoral head. Also, because imaging can be performed in real-time, subluxation or dislocation of the femoral head can be viewed directly. Ultrasound becomes difficult after approximately 6–9 months of age, when ossification begins in the femoral head.

Radiographic signs include slanting of the acetabular roof and acetabular anteversion and, in established dislocation, superior and lateral displacement of the femoral head. The capital epiphysis itself is small compared to the normal side (Fig. 13.56).

Following the initial diagnosis of dislocation and subsequent reduction, follow-up radiographs are obtained to check that reduction is maintained, the acetabulum is developing and ossification of the femoral head is progressing. Avascular necrosis is a recognized complication of treatment for congenital dislocation of the hip and manifests as cessation of epiphyseal growth, sclerosis and fragmentation of the epiphysis.

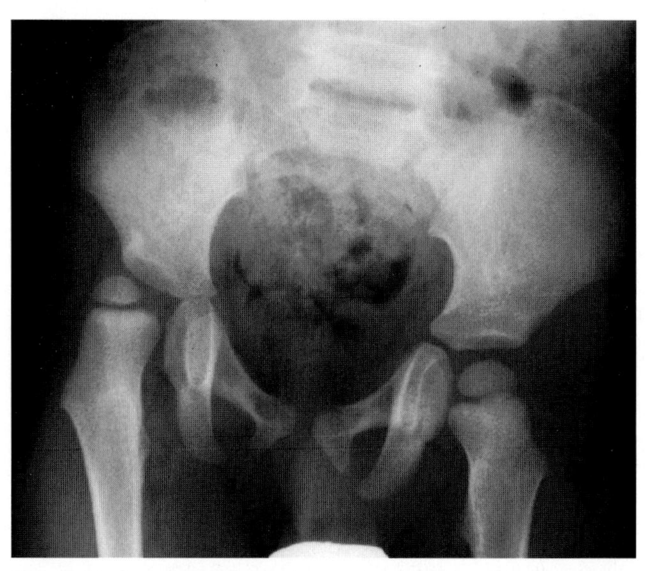

Fig. 13.56 Congenital dislocation of the right hip. There is superolateral subluxation of the femoral head. The capital epiphysis is small and the acetabulum dysplastic.

SOFT TISSUES

SOFT-TISSUE MASSES

The commonest causes of a soft-tissue mass include haematoma, abscess and tumour. It is important to realize that, although plain radiography can demonstrate bone/calcification, air and fat, soft tissue and fluid cannot be distinguished. Ultrasound is the most simple initial technique. Demonstration of a cystic mass by ultrasound can be followed by ultrasound-guided aspiration.

CT and MRI are more sensitive at demonstrating amounts of fat that are too small to see on plain films. However, MRI is relatively poor at identifying gas and calcification compared with CT. MRI is the technique of choice for demonstrating the local relationships of a mass because of its multiplanar imaging capability and also its ability to distinguish solid masses from normal muscle by signal differences on T2-weighted scans. Generally, a solid mass has the same density as muscle on CT.

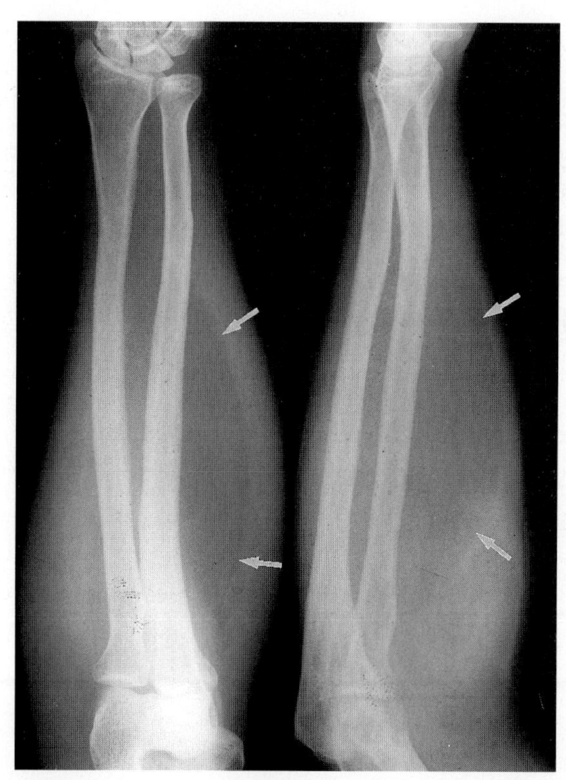

Fig. 13.57 Lipoma of the forearm identified due to the relatively low radiographic density of fat (arrows).

HAEMATOMA

Haematomas may occur secondary to trauma (including iatrogenic) or spontaneously in patients with coagulation deficiencies. CT may be diagnostic in the early stages since fresh blood has a higher density than muscle. As a haematoma resolves, it becomes cystic centrally and therefore must be included in the differential diagnosis of a cystic mass. The MRI appearances of haematoma can also be characteristic and vary with the age of the lesion.

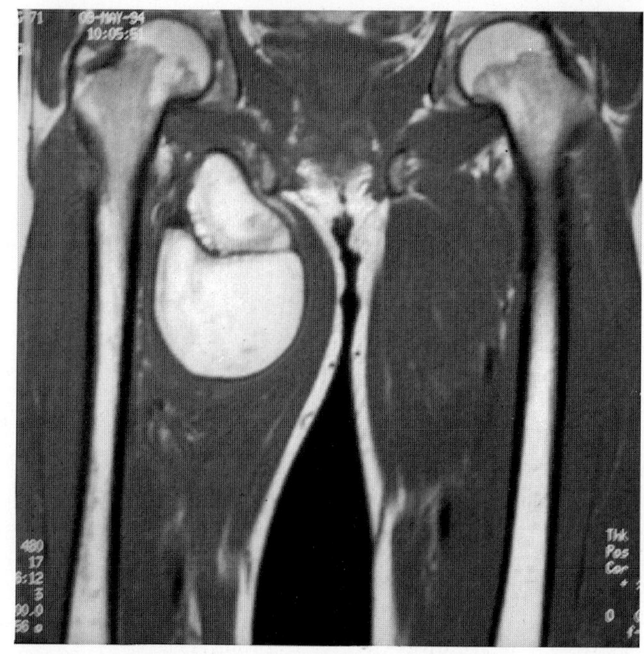

Fig. 13.58 Coronal T1-weighted MRI scan of a liposarcoma of the thigh. The high signal within the mass indicates a high fatty component.

ABSCESS/INFLAMMATORY MASS

The imaging features of an infective inflammatory mass or abscess are also non-specific, although the demonstration of gas in the lesion is suggestive. Initially, the mass may appear solid but, as liquefaction occurs, the central area becomes cystic. This may be identified clearly with ultrasound, CT or MRI. Percutaneous catheter drainage can be performed using ultrasound or CT guidance.

TUMOURS

There are a large variety of both benign and malignant soft-tissue tumours; only a few have specific features that allow a plain film diagnosis. Examples include **lipoma**, with its characteristic low density (Fig. 13.57), and **vascular tumours** which may be identified by the presence of phleboliths.

Plain radiographs can, nevertheless, be useful for assessing the effect of a primary soft-tissue neoplasm on the underlying bone, showing smooth pressure erosion in the case of a slowly growing lesion or frank cortical destruction by an aggressive lesion. Ultrasound is of value in the differentiation of solid from cystic masses. CT is tissue-specific only in tumours with a fatty component (lipoma, liposarcoma). Other soft-tissue tumours tend to be of muscle density. Similarly, MRI has the ability to demonstrate fat as high signal on T1-weighted scans (Fig. 13.58) and may indicate lesions with a predominantly fibrous nature, such as aggressive fibromatosis, because these tend to have low signal on both T1- and T2-weighted sequences. The majority of soft-tissue tumours on MRI are of intermediate signal on T1-weighted sequences and of high signal on T2-weighted sequences.

It is also important to realize that, in the absence of local invasion or distant metastases, the differentiation between benign and malignant neoplasms cannot be confidently made. It is evident, therefore, that a large proportion of soft-tissue tumours will need biopsy for a preoperative diagnosis. This is easily accomplished with either ultrasound or CT guidance. Once a diagnosis of a malignant lesion has been made, further staging includes chest radiography and CT to look for pulmonary metastases, and bone scintigraphy to identify skeletal metastases, although these are rare at presentation.

CHAPTER 14

Breast

A. Robin M. Wilson
and Andrew J. Evans

The investigation and treatment of women with breast problems is best carried out in a coordinated way by a multidisciplinary team. Diagnosis should combine a detailed history, careful clinical examination and, only where clinically indicated, imaging of the breast and fine needle aspiration cytology or needle core biopsy. Ideally, women with breast problems should have all the necessary investigations carried out at a single clinic visit. This is best achieved in a specialist breast clinic with the resources required to provide rapid access to diagnostic procedures with the surgeon able to consult directly with both the radiologist and the pathologist. This type of clinic will usually be part of a specialist breast unit which has the necessary clinical expertise, infrastructure and support from specialist radiology and pathology services and breast care nurses.

This chapter outlines the role of imaging in the assessment of patients with breast problems and in screening asymptomatic women for breast cancer.

GENERAL RULES

- Not all women referred with breast problems require imaging; radiological investigations should only be used in circumstances where they are likely to influence management and according to predetermined diagnostic protocols.
- Wherever possible imaging should be carried out before any needle biopsy is performed; needle biopsy may cause a haematoma in the breast that can cause diagnostic confusion on breast ultrasound and mammography.
- Imaging should be carried out under the supervision of a specialist radiologist.

BREAST IMAGING TECHNIQUES

X-RAY MAMMOGRAPHY

Mammography is the most important and most sensitive of the various methods for imaging the breast. It is carried out using a specially designed X-ray unit (Fig. 14.1). Images are produced on X-ray film or digitally recorded on computer disk. Because the breast is made up of soft tissues the energy of the radiation required to produce an image is considerably less than that required for other X-ray procedures. However, although the radiation dose received by the breast is relatively small, as with all X-ray procedures, mammography should be performed only where it is clinically useful; it should be used judiciously in younger women in whom the breast tissue is potentially more radiosensitive and in whom the sensitivity of mammography for disease is significantly lower.

To obtain a satisfactory mammographic image, the breast must be compressed firmly between the film cassette holder (breast support plate) and a plastic compression paddle (Plate 4, opposite page 354).

Diagnostic and Interventional Radiology in Surgical Practice. Edited by P. Armstrong and M.L. Wastie. Published in 1997 by Chapman & Hall, London. ISBN 0 412 61960 1 (HB), 0 412 61970 9 (PB)

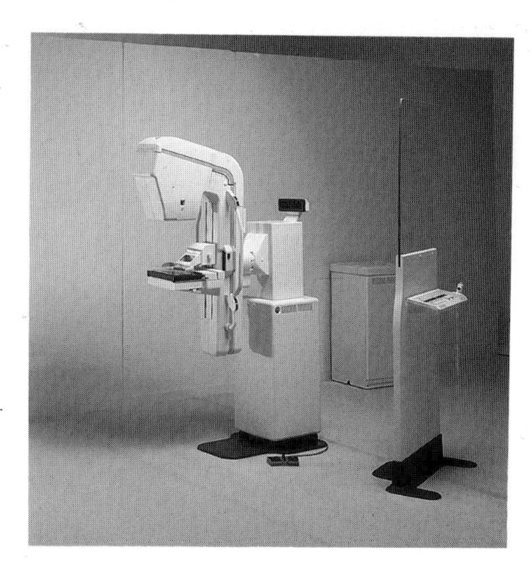

Fig. 14.1 A dedicated mammography X-ray unit.

Compression of the breast achieves uniform breast thickness, reduces the radiation dose required and reduces tissue movement, all of which improve image quality. Because the breast must be compressed many women find the examination uncomfortable and a few find it painful; women referred for mammography should be told that the examination may be uncomfortable. This is particularly so for women who have breast tenderness. When there is no urgency for examination in women with cyclical breast pain, it is better to perform mammography in the first half of the menstrual cycle.

The standard mammographic projection is the medio-lateral oblique view. This single view will image most of the breast tissue and is the view used if only one mammographic view is being obtained. It is performed by placing the film cassette at a 45° angle across the breast. An adequate medio-lateral oblique mammogram will demonstrate the pectoral muscle at an angle across the back of the breast with the nipple in profile, the nipple shown at a level at least up to the margin of the lower pectoral muscle and the infra-mammary angle of the breast clearly demonstrated (Fig. 14.2). Normal anatomical structures can be easily identified on mammograms: fine linear structures represent the normal stroma (ligaments of Astley Cooper); normal ducts are sometimes large enough to be seen immediately behind the nipple; and veins and arteries are often clearly demonstrated. Normal distal ductal and lobular structures are not demonstrated on mammography. There is great variation in the normal background appearances of breast tissue shown on mammography. Some breasts show a predominantly fatty pattern (Fig. 14.3), some a mixed pattern (Fig. 14.4) and others a dense pattern (Fig. 14.5), all of which are normal. Normal anatomy is more difficult to define in the dense breast and background mammographic density is the main determinant of mammographic sensitivity for cancer. Cancers are easier to see in women with a fatty rather than a dense background pattern.

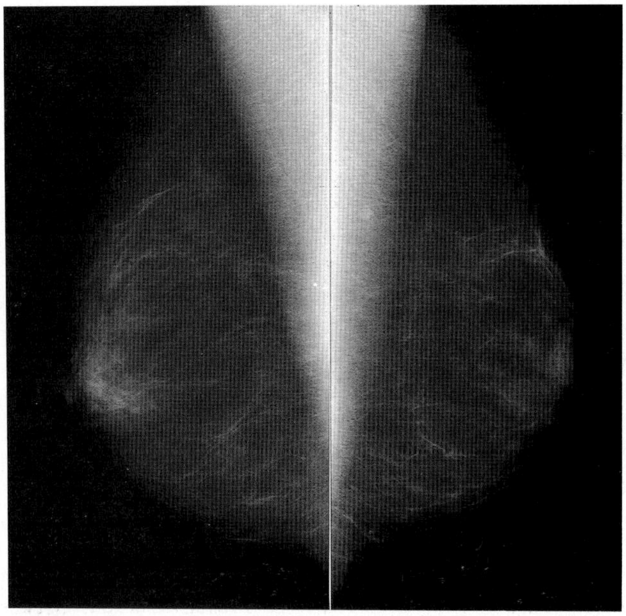

Fig. 14.2 Bilateral, high quality, medio-lateral oblique mammograms.

The companion view to the medio-lateral oblique projection is the cranio-caudal view taken with breast compression applied from above (Plate 5, opposite page 354). In this view a significant proportion of breast tissue is not imaged. As it is the upper inner quadrant of the breast which is often not clearly imaged in the medio-lateral oblique view, the cranio-caudal projection may be rotated to ensure that this area is included.

A standard mammographic examination of the breast should include medio-lateral and cranio-caudal

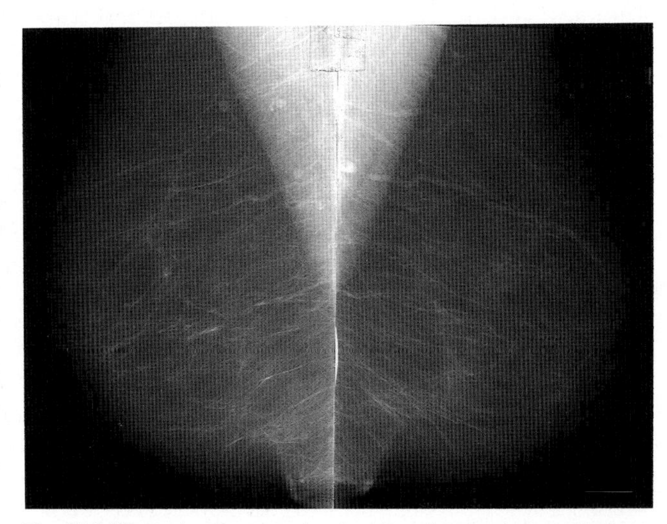

Fig. 14.3 Bilateral mammography showing a fatty background pattern.

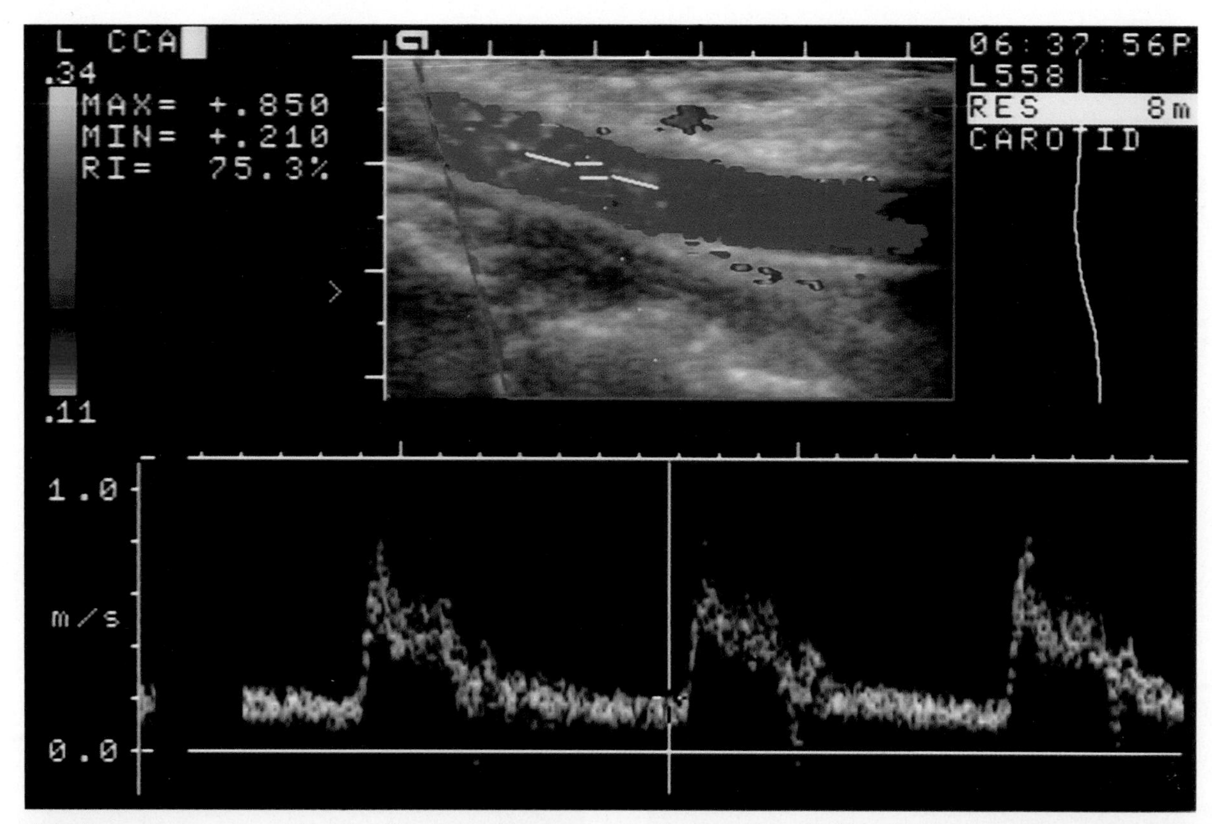

Plate 1 Normal common carotid artery. Top: Colour Doppler showing the gate where the flow velocity waveform has been taken. The dotted line indicates the angle of the beam. Bottom: Flow velocity waveform. The peaks represent systolic blood flow.

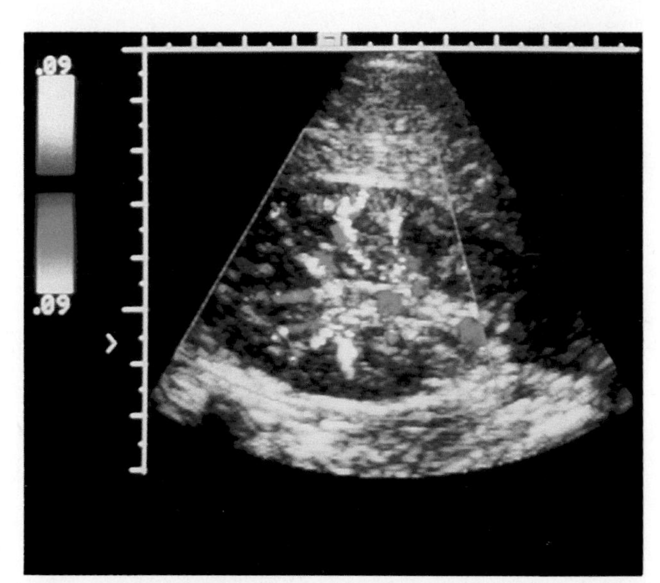

Plate 2a Doppler ultrasound of a normal kidney. Colour Doppler showing flow in the renal vessels as red or blue depending on direction of blood flow. (Courtesy of Acuson Ltd.)

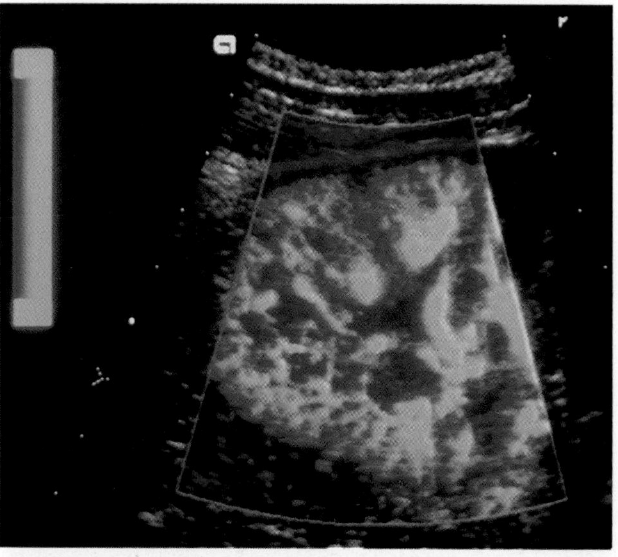

Plate 2b Power Doppler. Perfusion of the kidney is shown to advantage but no information is given on direction of flow. (Courtesy of Acuson Ltd.)

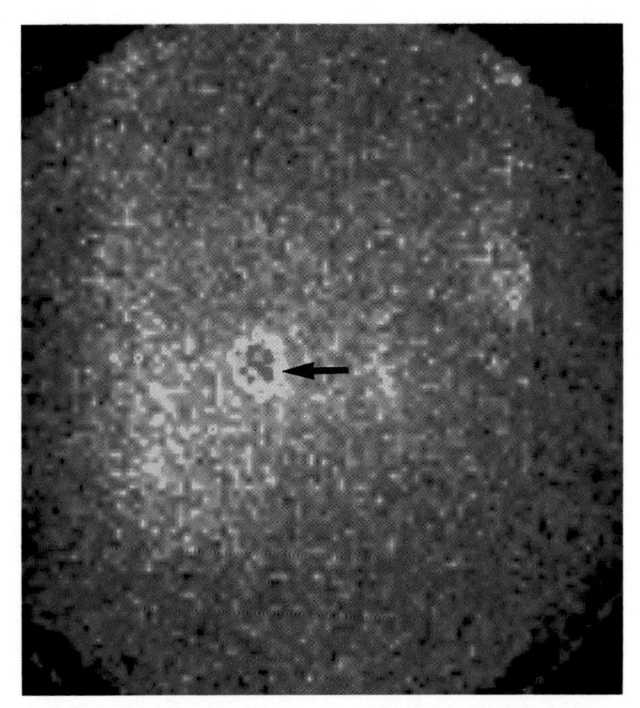

Plate 3 $^{75}Se\text{-}^{6}\beta$-selenomethylnorcholesterol scan showing increased uptake due to small functioning adenoma (arrow).

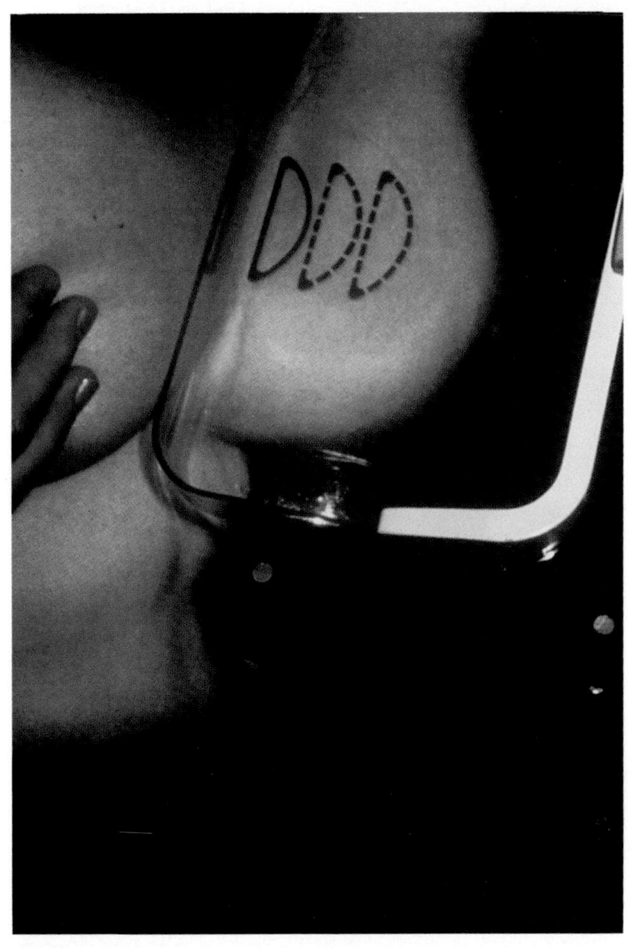

Plate 4 A medio-lateral oblique mammogram being performed. This projection images the whole breast on one film.

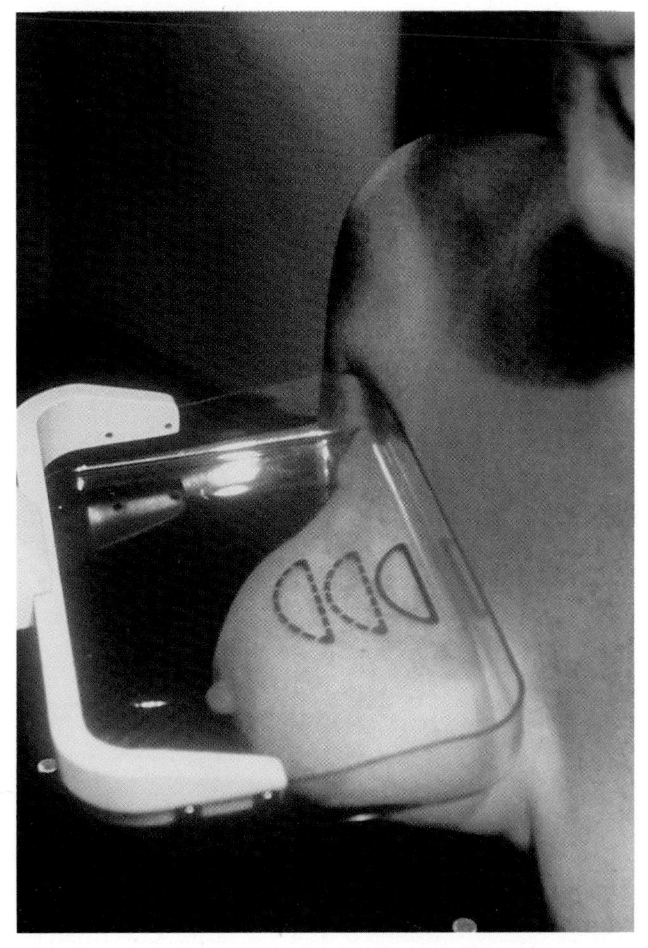

Plate 5 A cranio-caudal view being performed. This is the second standard mammographic view that supplements the oblique view.

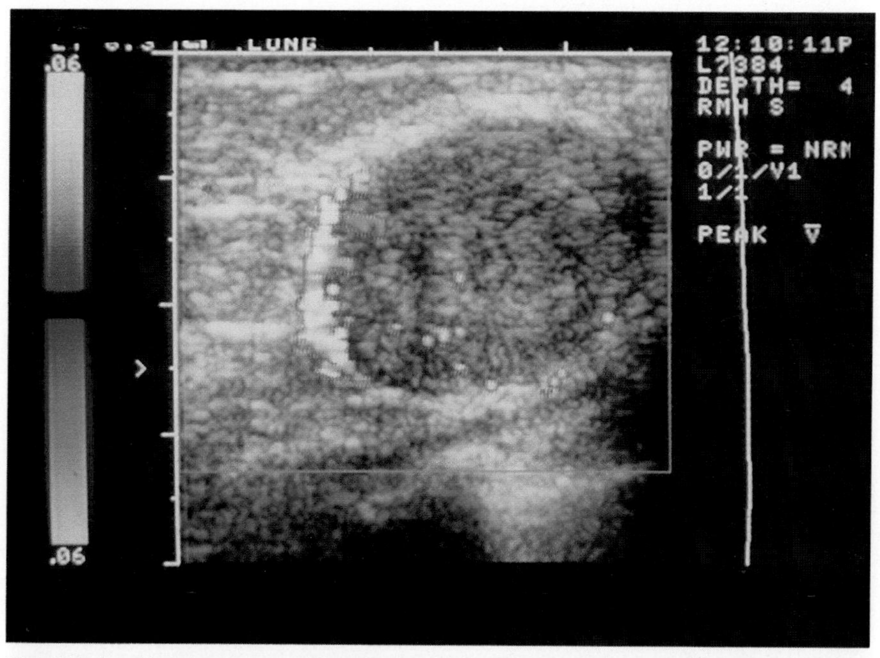

Plate 6 Colour Doppler ultrasound image of a solid breast mass demonstrating some flow signal peripherally. This is typical of a benign lesion, such as a fibroadenoma. (Compare with Plates 7 and 8). (By kind permission of Dr David Cosgrove, Hammersmith Hospital, London.)

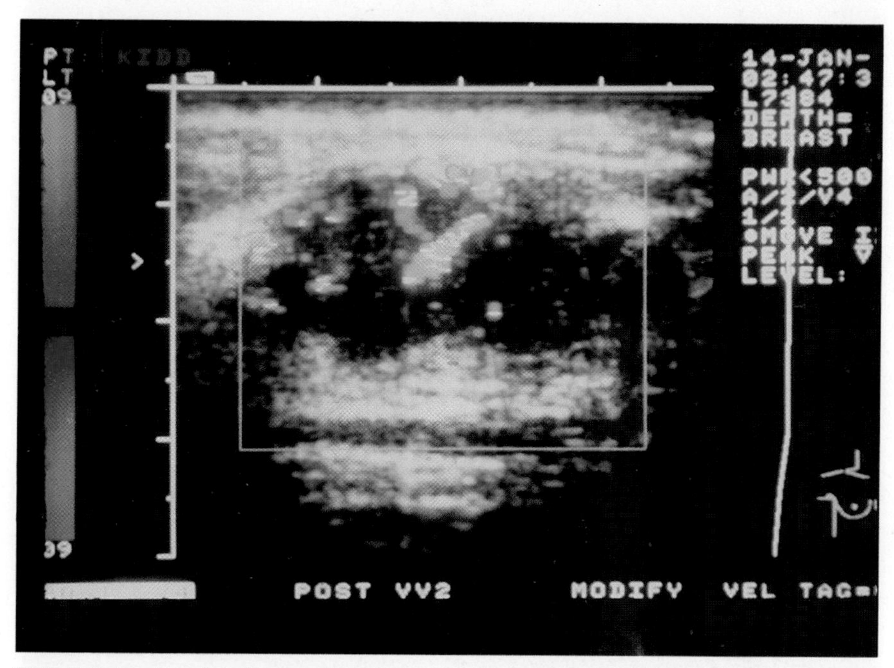

Plate 7 Colour Doppler ultrasound image of a carcinoma of the breast exhibiting abnormal flow signal within and at the periphery of the mass. (By kind permission of Dr David Cosgrove, Hammersmith Hospital, London.)

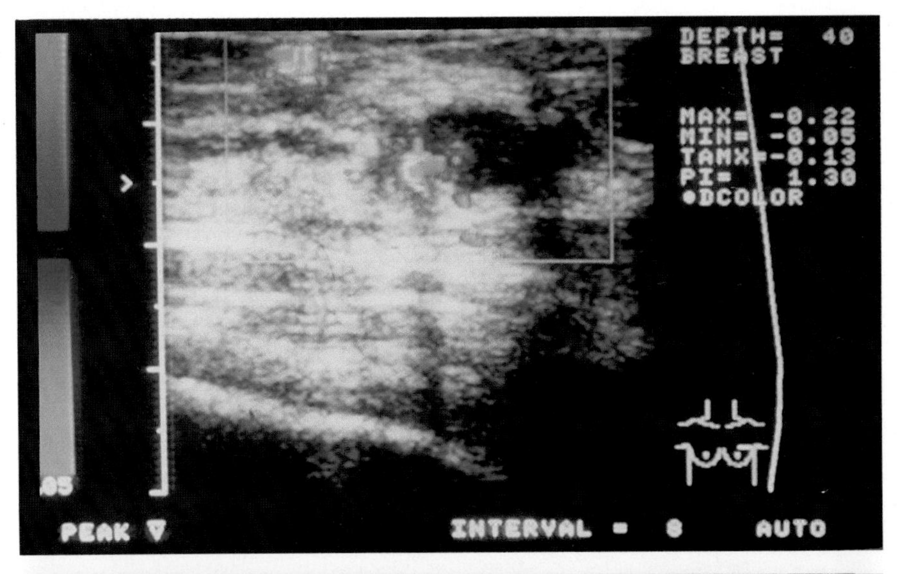

a

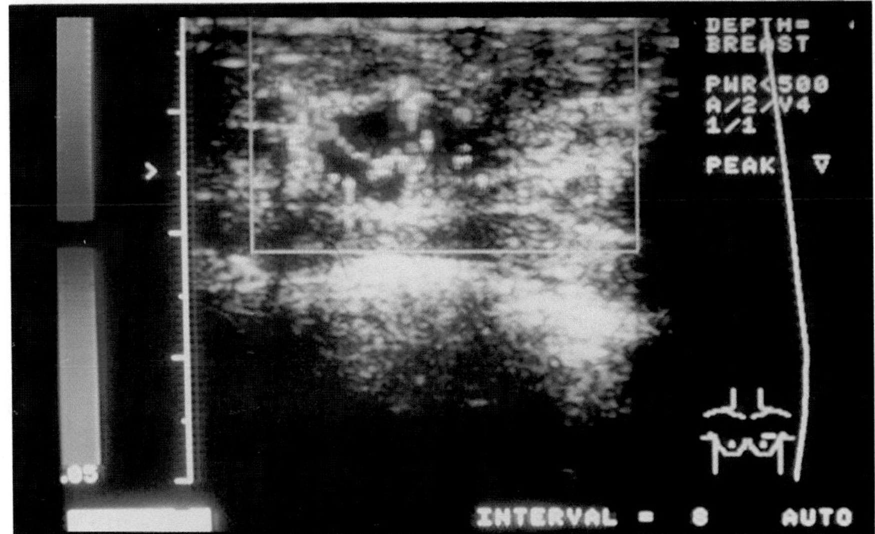

b

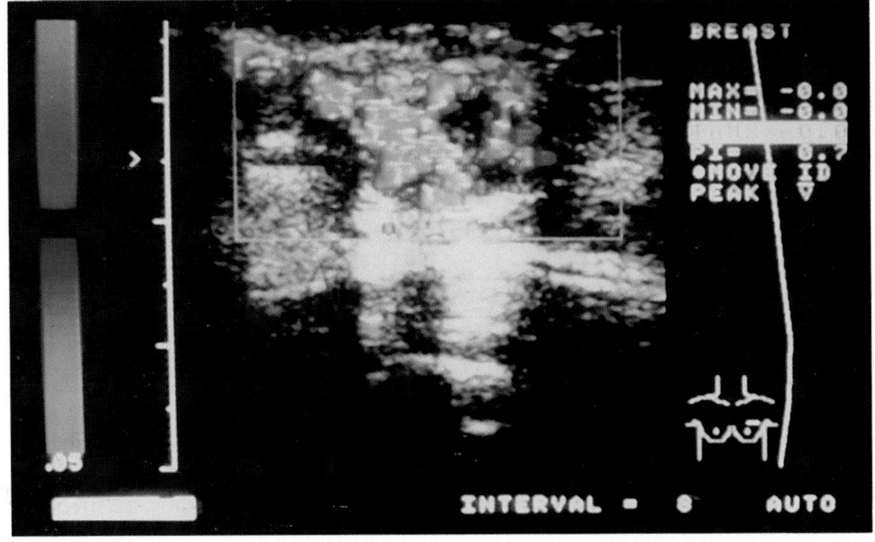

c

Plate 8 A series of three dynamic colour flow Doppler images obtained during injection of an ultrasound contrast agent demonstrating grossly abnormal flow and increasing signal with time in a breast carcinoma. (By kind permission of Dr David Cosgrove, Hammersmith Hospital, London.)

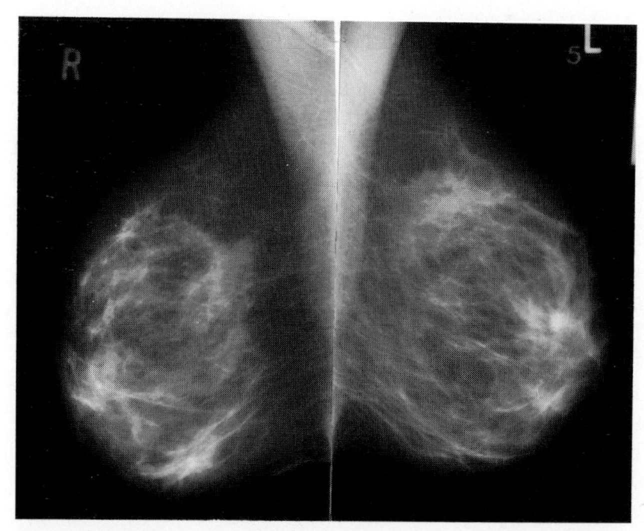

Fig. 14.4 Bilateral mammography showing a mixed fatty dense background pattern.

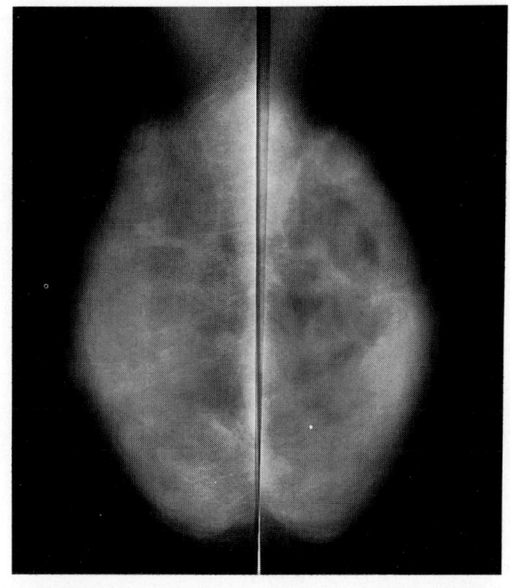

Fig. 14.5 Bilateral mammography showing a homogeneously dense background pattern. This pattern is commoner in younger women and is associated with a decreased sensitivity for malignancy.

views of both breasts and these two views are mandatory for breast screening. Supplementary views, including lateral projections, magnification views and localized paddle compression views, may be performed according to the particular clinical circumstances and as guided by the radiologist.

GALACTOGRAPHY

Galactography is a technique for outlining the duct pattern in the breast by the injection of radiopaque contrast into a duct orifice at the nipple using a small plastic cannula. This procedure is used for further investigation of single duct nipple discharge, which may be a symptom of an underlying carcinoma. However, the cause of single duct nipple discharge is usually benign and galactography is often diagnostically unhelpful. It is now rarely used, as single duct nipple discharge is better managed on the basis of conventional mammographic, clinical and nipple discharge cytological findings.

CYSTOGRAPHY

Cystography is a technique for outlining the inner contours of a breast cyst. After aspiration with a needle a volume of air equal to the fluid aspirated is injected into the cyst lumen. The air acts as an excellent contrast medium and clearly outlines the internal structure of the cyst. The technique is used when cyst aspiration yields frankly blood-stained fluid, the presence of which may indicate that the cyst wall contains a papilloma or carcinoma. With the increasing use and sophistication of breast ultrasound this procedure is now rarely used; ultrasound is able to demonstrate even a small intramural mass in a cyst.

BREAST ULTRASOUND

Ultrasound has been used to image the breast since the early 1970s and is now regarded as a valuable tool in the assessment of both benign and malignant breast problems. Ultrasound differs from X-ray mammography in that it uses high-frequency sound waves to obtain an image. Its advantage over mammography is that it can differentiate solid from cystic lesions (Figs. 14.6, 14.7) and is particularly useful in the mammographically dense breast. Conventional ultrasound

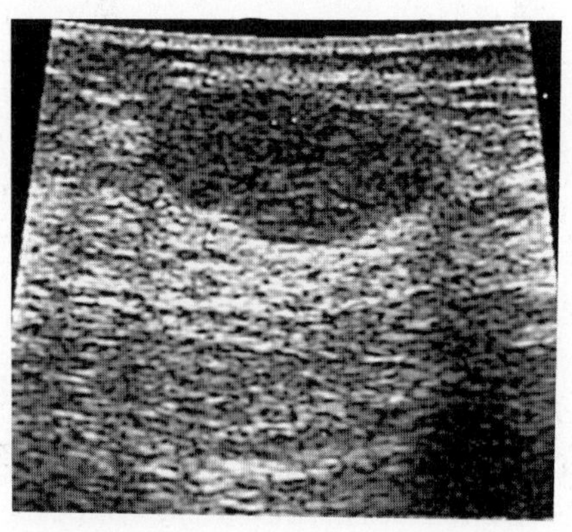

Fig. 14.6 Ultrasound of a fibroadenoma showing a well-defined solid mass with a homogeneous internal echo pattern and distal enhancement of the ultrasound beam.

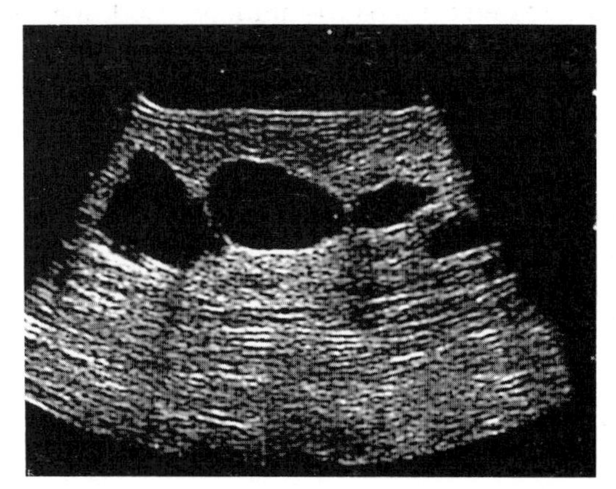

Fig. 14.7 Ultrasound demonstrating three cysts in close proximity. These are very well-defined abnormalities that have no internal echoes and show distal acoustic enhancement. All these features are characteristic of benign cysts.

equipment for breast examination uses higher frequency transducers (7.5–12 MHz) than those used for abdominal ultrasound which allows better spatial resolution. Ultrasound readily demonstrates normal structures in the breast and shows fat, parenchymal tissue and muscle (Fig. 14.8). It also demonstrates distortions of structure in the breast and oedema.

Colour flow Doppler ultrasound is being increasingly used in the evaluation of breast conditions. Generally, malignant lesions show abnormal Doppler patterns indicative of neovascularity whilst benign lesions do not (Plates 6–8, opposite page 354). Unfortunately many benign and malignant masses show significant overlap in their Doppler signal patterns and distinction between the two is not possible with any certainty using this technique. Colour flow Doppler is also useful for diffuse breast problems, such as prominent clinical thickening where the absence of a Doppler signal makes malignancy unlikely. Ultrasound cannot be used to differentiate benign from malignant solid breast lesions.

Ultrasound is significantly less sensitive for malignancy than X-ray mammography. This is, in part, due to the difficulty of demonstrating microcalcifications and architectural distortion on ultrasound. Ultrasound is particularly insensitive for the detection of ductal carcinoma *in situ* which is most commonly manifest as microcalcification on mammography. For this reason mammography is always indicated when there is clinical suspicion of malignancy. It is also inappropriate to use ultrasound as a screening method for breast cancer. The sensitivity of mammography for malignancy increases with age. The normal breast is denser in the younger woman and this largely explains why breast lesions in young women are more difficult to demonstrate on mammography.

MAGNETIC RESONANCE MAMMOGRAPHY

Magnetic resonance mammography is a technique that requires specialized equipment including a dedicated breast surface coil. It is very sensitive for breast pathology but is non-specific. The exact role of magnetic resonance mammography in the evaluation of patients with breast symptoms is yet to be defined but it is of value in the assessment of possible multifocal malignancy, in the exclusion of recurrent disease in patients treated with conservation therapy and in the investigation of patients with breast symptoms who have silicone breast implants (Fig. 14.9). Magnetic resonance mammography should not be regarded as a routine investigation in patients with breast problems.

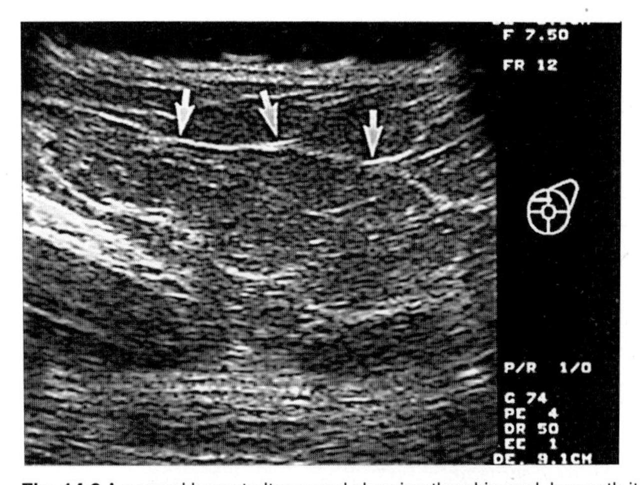

Fig. 14.8 A normal breast ultrasound showing the skin and, beneath it, normal hypoechoic breast tissue with hyperechoic Cooper's ligaments (arrows). Breast ultrasound is particularly useful in differentiating cystic from solid masses.

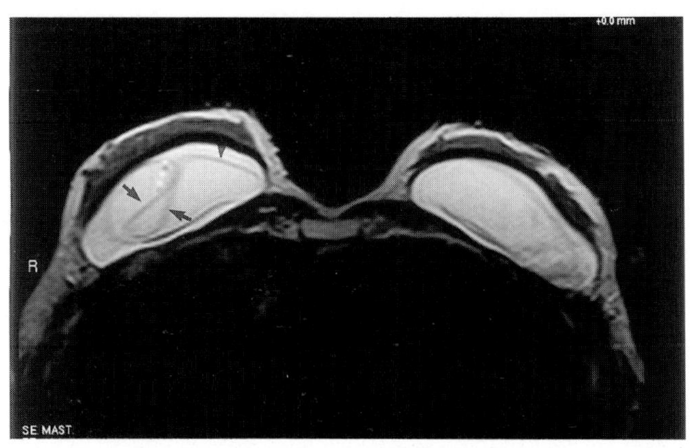

Fig. 14.9 Magnetic resonance mammography showing an intracapsular rupture of both silicone implants. The low signal curvilinear lines (arrows) represent the true implant membrane (Linguini's sign) while the silicone is confined by the fibrous capsule.

COMPUTED TOMOGRAPHY

Computed tomography has no role in the imaging of primary breast disease. However, computed tomography is useful is in the evaluation of metastatic disease, particularly in the axilla, and the assessment of metastatic disease of other parts of the body including the brain, chest and the abdomen. Again, computed tomography should not be regarded as a routine investigation.

IMAGING WOMEN WITH BREAST IMPLANTS

The presence of silicone implants in the breast inevitably compromises the ability of the radiologist to image the breast. Women who have implants placed for augmentation should be informed by the surgeon beforehand that the presence of implants may interfere with subsequent breast imaging and screening.

Mammography of the augmented or reconstructed breast can be carried out safely. Special displacement techniques can be used to ensure that the majority of the breast tissue itself is imaged but the ability to do so depends on the ratio of the size of the implant to the breast tissue.

Patients with breast implants who present with localized breast symptoms should be first assessed clinically. Needling procedures require special care if a prosthesis is not to be punctured and often aspiration of cysts or fine needle aspiration cytology/core biopsy of solid structures are best carried out under imaging control. There is no evidence that silicone implants and silicone leakage are associated with increased risk of malignancy and there is a tenuous link with connective tissue disease. Patients in whom implant rupture is suspected usually request further investigation and, in many cases, removal with or without replacement of the prosthesis. Mammography and ultrasound cannot adequately image breast tissue posterior to the implant and in these circumstances the multiplanar imaging capabilities of magnetic resonance mammography are very useful. Magnetic resonance mammography is an excellent technique for identifying rupture of silicone implants (Fig. 14.9).

CLINICAL APPLICATIONS OF BREAST IMAGING

CLINICAL CONTEXT

Imaging of the breast is best undertaken as part of a multidisciplinary assessment. For women with breast symptoms, using imaging as the sole or initial investigation is not recommended. However, mammography is effective on its own for asymptomatic breast cancer screening.

Problems which most commonly result in a referral to a breast clinic are:

- lump in the breast
- pain and tenderness
- family history of breast cancer
- nipple discharge
- nipple eczema
- skin changes
- other miscellaneous symptoms.

ASSESSMENT OF BREAST LUMPS

Whether imaging of a patient with a lump in the breast is required or not and which imaging technique is appropriate depends upon the age of the patient. The primary role of mammography is the exclusion of malignant disease. Although the radiation dose of mammography is relatively low, any test which involves ionizing radiation should be restricted in its use to circumstances where it is likely to be of clinical benefit. It is, therefore, inappropriate to use mammography where the risk of malignancy is small. Mammography is rarely required in the investigation of women under the age of 35 but should always be performed at any age when there is a strong clinical suspicion of malignancy. Table 14.1 details the criteria, based on triple assessment of clinical examination, imaging and cytology/needle histology, that must be satisfied to make a diagnosis of a benign breast lump, which need not necessarily require surgical excision.

Ultrasound is most useful for further assessment of an abnormality detected on mammography or clinical examination; but should not be regarded as a primary investigative tool. Ultrasound is the imaging technique of first choice in women under the age of 35 with localized breast problems confirmed by clinical assessment.

Patients aged under 25 years

A discrete mobile lump in the breast in a patient under the age of 25 is virtually always benign; the vast majority of lumps in women of this age are fibroadenomas; simple cysts are uncommon. Imaging has little to add to the diagnosis or management of a breast lump at this age, unless there is clinical suspicion of malignancy. The conventional management for a fibroadenoma in a young woman is clinical assessment and fine-needle aspiration cytology to confirm the benign nature of the lesion. A benign lump does not need to be surgically excised unless it is enlarging or the patient requests its removal.

Patients aged 25–35 years

After clinical assessment, ultrasound is the examination of first choice in assessment of a lump in a patient in this age group. Mammography is best avoided

Table 14.1 Benign breast lumps: clinical, imaging and cytological criteria, related to age, required for diagnosis

Technique	*Age*	*Findings*
Clinical examination	All ages	Smooth and mobile
Imaging		
Not required	<25	
Ultrasound	26–35	Well-defined with homogeneous internal echo pattern or not identified
Ultrasound	35 +	Well-defined with homogeneous internal echo pattern or not identified
Mammography		Well-defined mass or not identified
Cytology		
× 1	<25	No abnormal cells
× 2 (4 weeks apart)	26–35	No abnormal cells
× 2 (4 weeks apart)	35 +	Benign epithelial cells seen in both specimens

unless there is suspicion of malignancy. Ultrasound will define the size and nature of the solid lesion in the breast and will also differentiate between a solid and cystic lesion. In this age range, the differential diagnosis of a discrete mobile lump lies between a fibroadenoma and a simple breast cyst. The typical appearance of a fibroadenoma and cyst on ultrasound are shown in Figures 14.6 and 14.7 respectively.

A normal ultrasound examination should not be taken as evidence that no real pathology exists. Some fibroadenomas have appearances very similar to normal breast tissue and are therefore invisible on ultrasound; false-negative ultrasound findings are not uncommon in malignancy particularly with carcinoma *in situ*. If ultrasound examination of a clinically significant abnormality is normal, the patient's management should be based on the clinical and cytological findings.

Patients aged over 35 years

Although breast cancer is rare before the age of 40, its incidence rises significantly after the age of 35 and for this reason mammography is recommended from age 35 as the first imaging investigation where symptoms and clinical signs warrant further investigation. It is helpful to carry out breast ultrasound as well, to define the nature of any mass, except where mammography demonstrates an obvious malignancy. Ultrasound is extremely useful for differentiating solid from cystic lesions and is therefore very helpful in deciding management in the individual case.

Imaging the clinically malignant mass

If a mass is clinically malignant it requires excision irrespective of the imaging and cytological findings. The role of imaging a clinically malignant mass is to define the extent of disease and to screen for malignancy in the contralateral breast. These imaging findings allow the most appropriate treatment to be offered. A clinically small malignant mass may be surrounded by extensive ductal carcinoma *in situ*, which is often impalpable, but which will normally be detected on mammography. In such circumstances it would be inappropriate to offer breast-conserving surgery. Clinical examination has a tendency to overestimate the size of breast carcinomas (Lebourgne's law), while size measured by ultrasound and mammography both show better correlation with the actual size of the excised tumour.

Patients presenting with locally advanced breast carcinoma

Mammography is not clinically useful in these circumstances. Breast-conserving surgery cannot be offered and screening the opposite breast for a second carcinoma is unlikely to alter management because of the poor prognosis of the presenting tumour.

Screening women who attend symptomatic breast clinics

Women over 50 years whose symptoms would not normally warrant imaging assessment should undergo screening mammography, assuming they have not already done so within the previous year. In some centres this protocol applies to all women over the age of 40.

ASSESSMENT OF BREAST PAIN AND TENDERNESS

Breast pain is a very common symptom which on its own does not warrant imaging investigation. Pain as the sole symptom or sign of malignancy is rare. Breast pain is best managed by careful clinical history with appropriate medical treatment.

ASSESSMENT OF WOMEN WITH AN INCREASED RISK OF BREAST CANCER

Some women with a family history of breast cancer or who have certain histological abnormalities detected at a previous breast biopsy are known to be at increased risk of developing breast cancer. The exact role of imaging in their management is controversial as there is no current evidence to suggest that screening reduces mortality in these groups of patients.

Women with family history of breast cancer

There is no conclusive evidence that mammographic screening of women under 50 years with a family history of breast cancer reduces their mortality from breast cancer. It can be argued that it is unethical to inform women of this risk, who may be unaware of the possible increased breast cancer risk, if there is no intervention of proven benefit to offer them. However, if women present with anxiety about their family history, it is reasonable to offer screening once their individual risk has been evaluated. This would normally involve counselling by a specially trained clinician or geneticist. No clear protocols for such screening exist but a combination of counselling followed by clinical and mammographic screening and instruction in breast self-examination is frequently provided. Such screening is best provided by a specialist breast clinic under the supervision of a breast clinician. Usually only a premenopausal first line family history of breast cancer (mother, sister or daughter) is considered significant. Most women over the age of 50 are adequately catered for by routine mammographic screening provided for all women over this age.

Histological risk factors

Certain histological proliferative epithelial abnormalities in the breast are known to be associated with variable increased risk of subsequent breast cancer. In women with a significant histological risk factor the development of breast cancer is highest 10–15 years after the proliferative abnormality has been diagnosed. The increased risk to the individual doubles if there is also a significant family history of breast cancer. Many clinicians recommend regular screening by clinical examination and/or mammography, with professional counselling, for women in this group. Mammography is seldom required more frequently than once a year.

PAGET'S DISEASE OF THE NIPPLE/NIPPLE ECZEMA

Mammography is of limited value in the assessment of patients with Paget's disease of the nipple. The diagnosis can be made by nipple biopsy carried out under local anaesthetic in the clinic. Frequently patients with Paget's disease have no mammographic abnormality and where an abnormality is present, mammography is not useful in defining the extent or nature of the associated malignancy. Because of this difficulty, both clinically and mammographically, patients with Paget's disease of the nipple are not normally offered breast-conserving surgery. Mammography of the opposite breast is recommended to detect synchronous lesions.

NIPPLE DISCHARGE

Imaging is also of little value in the assessment of patients with multiduct nipple discharge. In most circumstances patients with this symptom do not require investigation other than careful clinical assessment. Occasionally, cytological assessment of the discharge may be considered appropriate.

Single duct nipple discharge is a more significant symptom which does require more detailed investigation including imaging. Conventional mammography is helpful in excluding underlying malignancy, and ultrasound will demonstrate duct ectasia. The surgeon can manage this condition conservatively in the absence of mammographic evidence of malignancy. Large duct papillomas are occasionally visible mammographically and are almost always benign and require surgical treatment only if symptoms are troublesome.

IMAGING OF METASTATIC BREAST CANCER

Routine investigation of patients with breast cancer at the time of diagnosis to identify metastatic disease is not indicated as there is a very low yield of true positive results and significant number of false-positive results. Imaging to identify metastatic disease is best reserved for patients who have suggestive symptoms or signs.

SURVEILLANCE AND CHARACTERIZATION OF LOCALLY RECURRENT BREAST CANCER

Follow-up of the treated breast

Where mastectomy has been performed, routine imaging of the mastectomy site or axilla is not helpful; ultrasound is useful in confirming clinical suspicion of recurrence at the mastectomy site. Imaging of suspected axillary recurrence is best performed with either CT or MRI.

In patients treated by lumpectomy (breast conservation), annual routine follow-up mammography is often recommended as part a combined clinical and imaging follow-up strategy. Mammography will identify

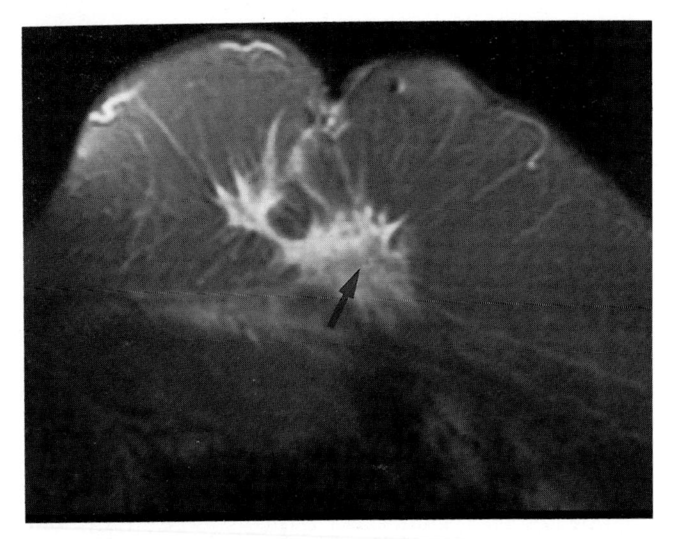

Fig. 14.10 Sagittal magnetic resonance image of the breast after injection of contrast demonstrating enhancing recurrent carcinoma (arrow). (*By kind permission of Dr L Turnbull, Centre for Magnetic Resonance Investigation, Hull Royal Infirmary*)

60–80% of recurrence in the breast and in approximately half of these cases the presence of recurrence will not have been apparent clinically. Mammographic surveillance will thus detect recurrent disease at an earlier stage and, in a significant number of patients, this has prognostic significance. Mammography is particularly effective in detecting recurrent ductal carcinoma *in situ*. The commonest radiological feature of local recurrence is microcalcification, but in the majority of cases microcalcification at the postoperative site is due to fat necrosis or radiotherapy change. If mammographic findings are suspicious of local recurrence, image-guided fine-needle aspiration, core biopsy and magnetic resonance mammography (Fig. 14.10) may be helpful though some cases will require open diagnostic surgical biopsy. Surgical biopsy must be avoided if at all possible after radiotherapy as wound healing may be delayed. Ultrasound is not effective in screening for recurrence. The risk of recurrence in the treated breast is greatest in the first 10 years after treatment and occurs at a rate of approximately 1% per annum.

Surveillance of the opposite breast

Patients who have developed one breast cancer are at significant increased risk of developing a second primary lesion. For this reason, regular mammography of the opposite breast is recommended, especially in those patients whose first tumour had good prognostic features.

IMAGING OF THE MALE BREAST

Enlargement of the breast or breasts is the most common reason for a male patient to be referred to a breast clinician. Simple obesity is a the commonest cause but true gynaecomastia is increasingly common with age. Imaging is rarely necessary as it does not influence clinical management. Breast cancer is rare in men, with < 1% occurring in males; again imaging is rarely contributory as mastectomy is the standard treatment. Mammography can be performed without difficulty in men. It is usually only required when a strong clinical suspicion of malignancy has not been confirmed by other investigations (Fig. 14.11).

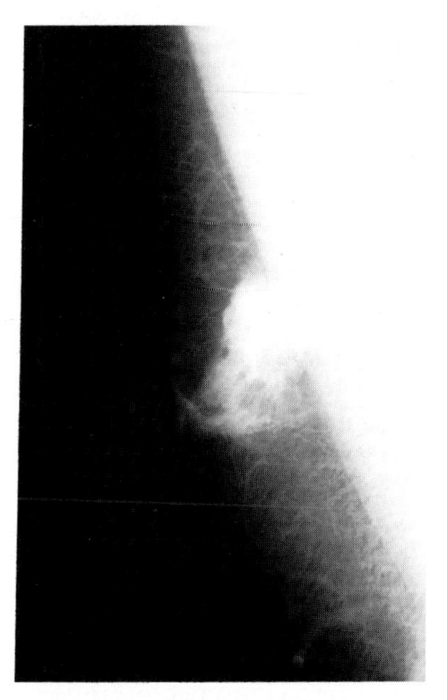

Fig. 14.11 A mammogram of a man with breast cancer showing a spiculate mass in the retroareola region with associated malignant type calcification.

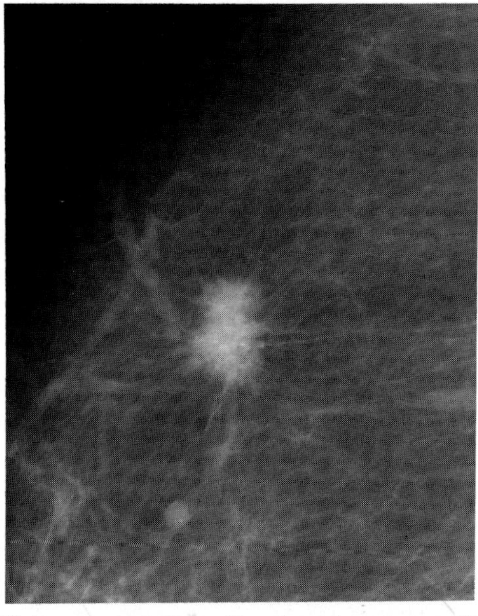

Fig. 14.12 A mammogram showing a breast carcinoma. The appearance is of a spiculate mass with associated calcification. Such an appearance has a greater than 90% chance of being due to breast carcinoma.

IMAGING FEATURES OF THE COMMON PATHOLOGIES

INVASIVE CARCINOMA

The commonest mammographic manifestation of invasive carcinoma is a spiculate mass often associated with calcification (Figs. 14.12, 14.13). Other

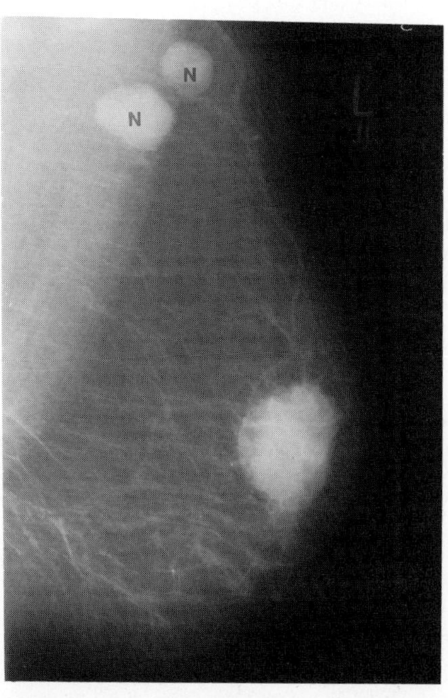

Fig. 14.13 Mammogram demonstrating a clinically obvious large carcinoma behind the left nipple. The mass is lobulated, ill-defined and shows subtle spiculation. Enlarged nodes (N) in the left axilla are seen.

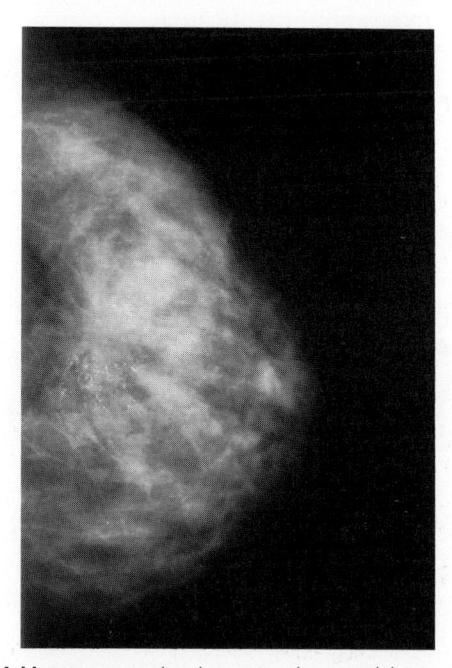

Fig. 14.14 Mammogram showing extensive suspicious calcification and parenchymal distortion due to an invasive carcinoma with associated ductal carcinoma *in situ*.

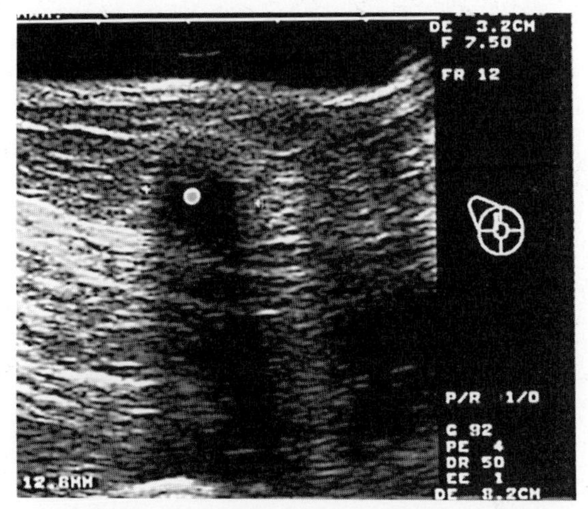

Fig. 14.15 Breast ultrasound showing typical features of a breast carcinoma (circle): an ill-defined hypoechoic mass with an echogenic halo, an ill-defined internal echo pattern and marked distal attenuation of the ultrasound beam.

common appearances of invasive carcinoma are an ill-defined mass, parenchymal distortion and suspicious calcification without a mass (Fig. 14.14). The linear structures seen radiating from spiculate masses and parenchymal distortion represent the inpulling of normal breast structures rather than tumour extending outwards. Up to 10% of clinically apparent carcinomas are not visible on mammography. This is mainly because the tumour is obscured by normal breast tissue which appears dense on mammography in some patients. Normal mammography must never be used to exclude carcinoma in patients with significant clinical findings. Carcinomas are seen on ultrasound as hypoechoic, inhomogeneous, ill-defined masses (Fig. 14.15). Other features often seen are an echogenic halo, distal acoustic shadowing and disturbance of the surrounding architecture.

DUCTAL CARCINOMA IN SITU

Ductal carcinoma *in situ* has become a more common clinical problem with the widespread introduction of mammographic screening; 15–30% of screen-detected cancer is ductal carcinoma *in situ* compared to only 5% of breast cancer presenting with symptoms. Screen-detected ductal carcinoma *in situ* tends to be impalpable and less extensive than symptomatic ductal carcinoma *in situ*. The most common mammographic feature of ductal carcinoma *in situ* is microcalcification, which is found in around 80–90% of those with a mammographic abnormality. The appearance of the

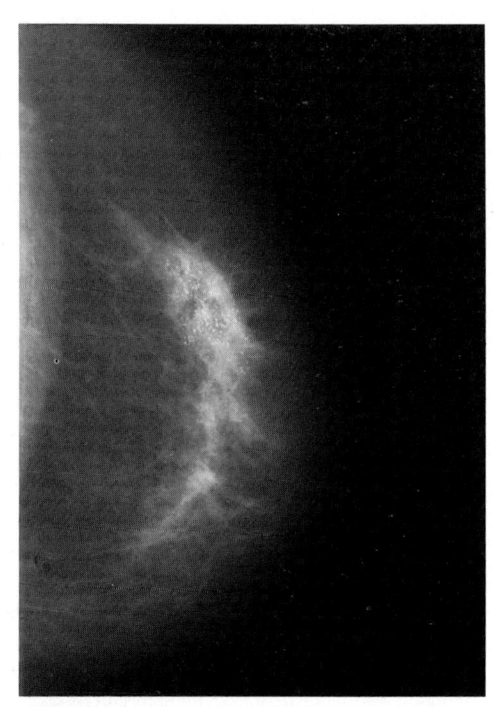

Fig. 14.16 Extensive casting and granular calcifications are demonstrated on mammography in the lateral left breast. The calcifications represent comedo ductal carcinoma *in situ*, the calcification being formed in necrotic intraductal debris.

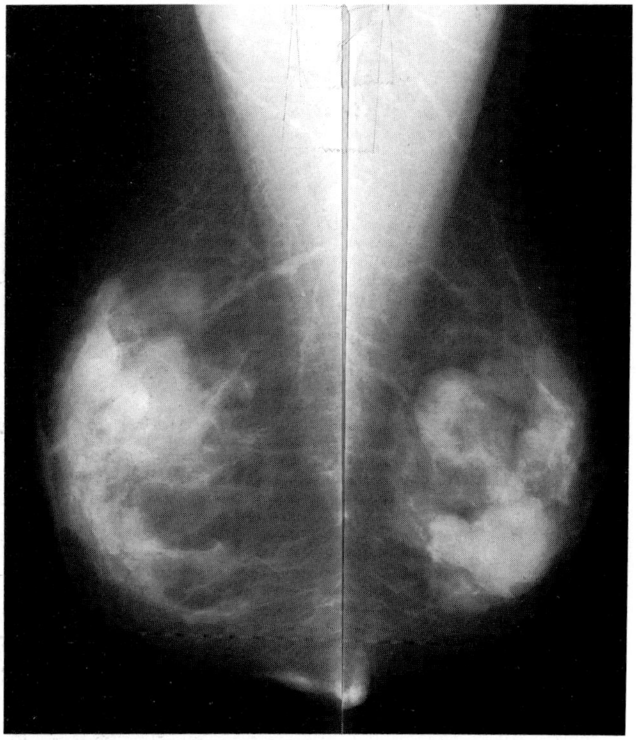

Fig. 14.17 Bilateral mammography showing multiple cysts. These are demonstrated as multiple well-defined masses of varying sizes which do not show calcification.

microcalcifications described as characteristic of ductal carcinoma *in situ* is that of granular particles in a ductal distribution showing a tendency to coalesce to form linear and branching 'casts' with variations in shape, size and density (Fig. 14.16). Such calcifications represent the coalescence of dystrophic calcification formed in necrotic intraluminal debris and are seen in ductal carcinoma *in situ* of high histological grade. Ductal carcinoma *in situ*, normally of low-grade type can also manifest as punctate calcification due to calcification in intercellular spaces.

CYSTS

Cysts are demonstrated on mammography as solitary or multiple well-defined masses (Fig. 14.17). They occur most commonly in the 30–50 age group and frequently subside after the menopause. Cysts do not usually present after the menopause unless the patient is on hormone replacement therapy. Cysts are often multiple and bilateral and may be very large. Ultrasound findings are characteristic with cysts shown as sharply marginated transonic areas with distal acoustic enhancement (Fig. 14.7).

FIBROADENOMA

Fibroadenomas are also demonstrated on mammography as well-defined masses. They most commonly develop in women under the age of 35, but may present for the first time in older women. They are sometimes multiple and bilateral, but are rarely larger than 3 cm. On mammography, calcification is commonly seen within a fibroadenoma and is often coarse and 'popcorn' in character (Fig. 14.18). On ultrasound a

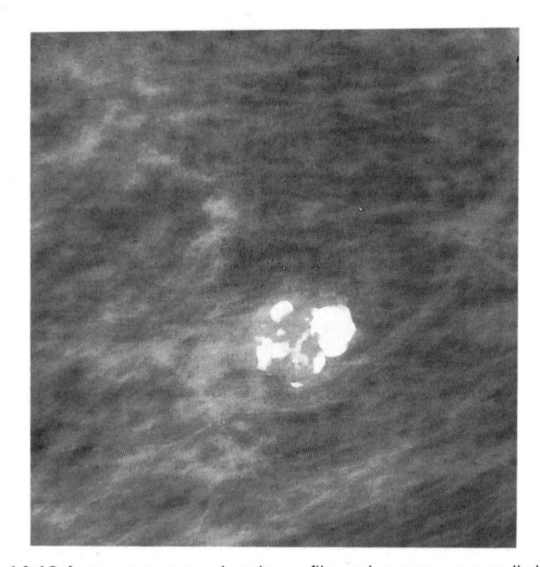

Fig. 14.18 A mammogram showing a fibroadenoma as a well-defined mass containing coarse popcorn shaped calcification.

fibroadenoma is typically a well defined hypoechoic solid mass with a homogeneous internal echo pattern and sharp posterior border, often with distal acoustic enhancement (Fig. 14.6, p. 355).

DUCT ECTASIA

Duct ectasia is seen mammographically most commonly as dense, very well-defined linear 'broken needle' or 'pipe-stem' calcification (Fig. 14.19). Occasionally, dilated ducts can be seen as elongated retroareolar soft-tissue structures without calcification.

BREAST ABSCESS

Breast abscesses are normally seen on mammography as ill-defined or spiculate masses. They are usually found in the retroareolar area in women who are breast feeding but may also occur elsewhere in other patients. The diagnosis is usually suggested by the clinical findings. Ultrasound shows an irregular hypoechoic or transonic mass with distal acoustic enhancement (Fig. 14.20). **Tuberculosis** of the breast is rare and may present as a nodular or ill-defined mass or with diffuse involvement. Abscesses can be successfully treated by aspiration under ultrasound guidance and antibiotic therapy. Repeated aspiration may be necessary but it is usually possible to avoid open surgical drainage.

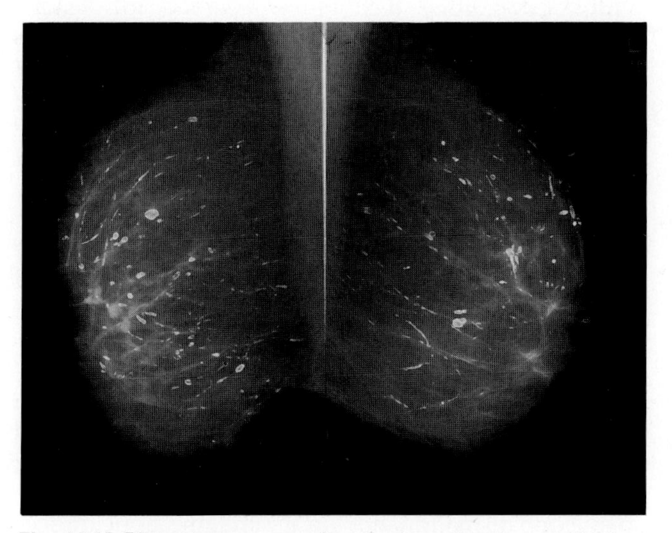

Fig. 14.19 Bilateral mammography showing extensive calcifications diagnostic of duct ectasia.

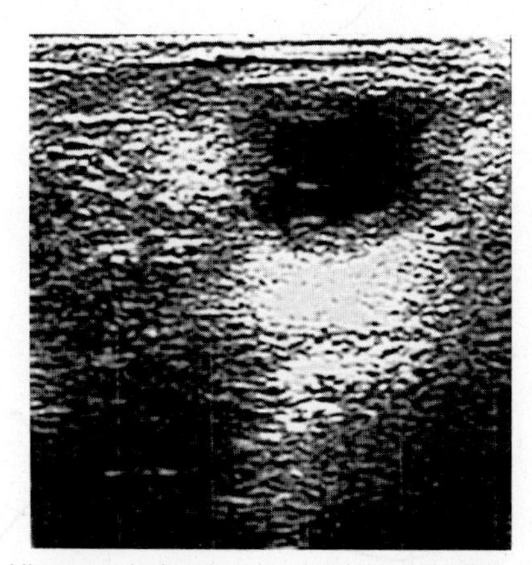

Fig. 14.20 Ultrasound showing a mixed cystic/solid mass due to a breast abscess. There is a peripheral solid component and a central cystic component.

BREAST TRAUMA

On mammography, haematoma in the breast may be shown as an ill-defined mass, spiculate mass or asymmetric density (Fig. 14.21). On ultrasound, haematomas appear as ill-defined cystic/solid masses with distal acoustic enhancement. Fat necrosis can occur following significant or trivial trauma and following surgery (Fig. 14.22). Acute fat necrosis appears as an ill-defined or spiculate mass and ultrasound can show mass lesions suspicous of malignancy. In time, fat necrosis can calcify; such calcification is usually curvilinear and coarse but occasionally calcification due to fat necrosis can mimic malignancy.

FIBROCYSTIC CHANGE

Fibrocystic change (the preferred pathological collective term for combinations of benign breast processes including cyst formation, apocrine metaplasia,

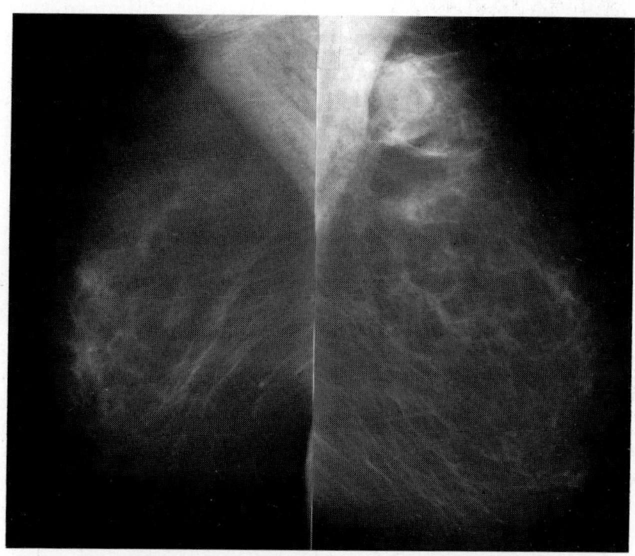

Fig. 14.21 Bilateral mammography showing a large asymmetric density with associated trabecular thickening in the left axillary tail. This was due to haematoma secondary to a seat-belt injury.

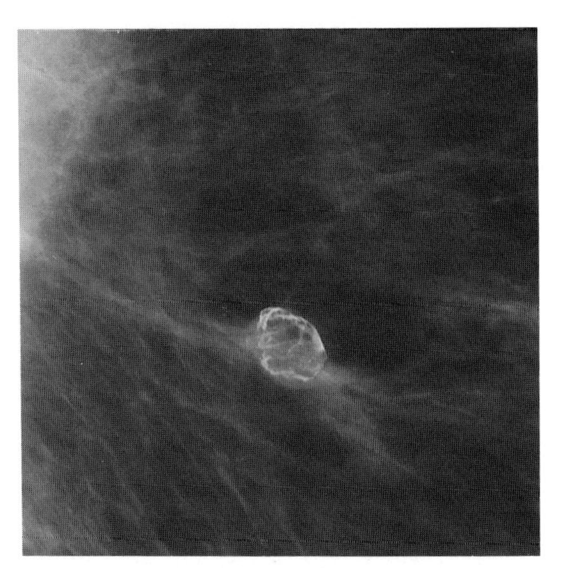

Fig. 14.22 Mammogram demonstrating coarse calcification in an area of architectural distortion. This fat necrosis was secondary to surgery some years before.

blunt duct adenosis, sclerosing adenosis and various benign epithelial hyperplasias) is often shown on mammography as areas of asymmetric density. These asymmetric densities often contain calcification characterized by multiple, often bilateral, round clusters of punctate calcification. The 'teacup' sign, caused by sedimentation of milk of calcium within small cysts, is often seen. On ultrasound, benign breast change shows as diffuse hyperechoic areas. Small cysts are often seen within these areas.

PHYLLODES TUMOUR

Phyllodes tumours are demonstrated mammographically as large, well-defined, often lobulated masses and are often surprisingly large at presentation. On ultrasound, the typical leaf-like echogenic septations may be seen within a homogeneous well-defined mass (Fig. 14.23). Small, round, hyperechoic foci, rather than septations, are more often seen within the mass. About 5% of phyllodes tumours are malignant, but the distinction from benign tumours cannot be reliably made from their imaging features.

ASSESSMENT OF IMPALPABLE LESIONS

IMAGE-GUIDED BREAST BIOPSY AND MARKER LOCALIZATION

The use of mammography for asymptomatic screening and the increasing use of both mammography and ultrasound as part of the assessment of symptomatic breast problems inevitably means that a significant proportion of breast lesions detected are impalpable and require image-guided biopsy. These techniques require special skills on the part of the radiologist and specialist equipment. The technique of first choice for image-guided biopsy is ultrasound, with X-ray-guided techniques reserved for lesions not seen on ultrasound; ultrasound biopsy is quick, relatively cheap and is associated with minimal patient discomfort. Fine-needle aspiration and large-bore needle biopsy under ultrasound guidance are both very accurate techniques and in experienced hands provide a definitive diagnosis in at least 90% of impalpable lesions. Certain lesions cannot be adequately visualized on ultrasound, e.g. areas of architectural distortion and microcalcification, and must be biopsied under X-ray guidance (Fig. 14.24). Stereotactic equipment is more accurate than other X-ray techniques.

Image-guided biopsy should not be considered in isolation and should be part of multidisciplinary triple assessment (clinical examination, imaging and cytology/histology). If a lesion is considered to be suspicious of malignancy on its imaging appearances then open surgical biopsy should proceed even if fine-needle aspiration cytology or core biopsy is benign.

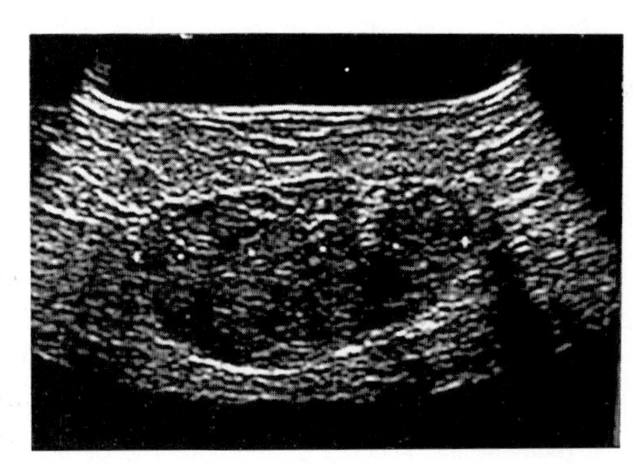

Fig. 14.23 Ultrasound examination of a phyllodes tumour showing a well-defined, hypoechoic solid mass which contains septae.

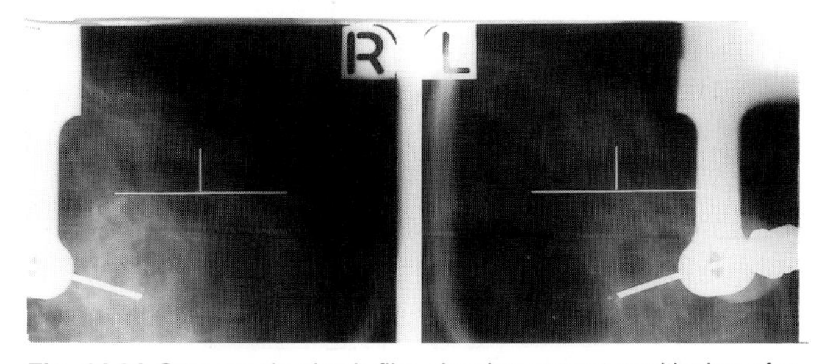

Fig. 14.24 Stereotactic check film showing correct positioning of a needle within a cluster of microcalcifications. Two films are taken at an angle of 30° for an accurate localization.

IMAGE-GUIDED MARKER LOCALIZATION

Impalpable lesions that require surgical biopsy or excision usually require image-guided localization. Some superficial lesions may be localized by marking the overlying skin but most lesions require placement of a marker in the breast. A number of different wire devices are available (Fig. 14.25).

Wire markers have the advantage over other techniques:

- They allow very accurate localization (Fig. 14.26).
- They facilitate excision of small specimens for diagnostic biopsies.
- Accurate wide local excision for malignant lesions is obtained.
- The surgeon can choose the best operative approach to achieve the optimal cosmetic result.

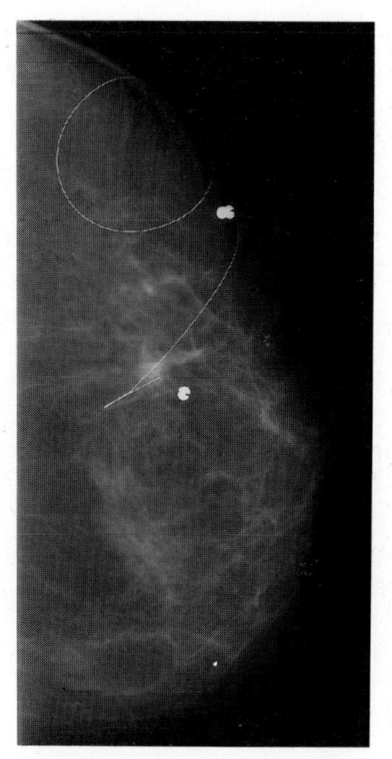

Fig. 14.26 A mammogram performed following insertion of a Nottingham localization wire. The wire is in an ideal position with the lesion transfixed and the 'T' of the wire lying just medially. The radiopaque skin markers represent the site of skin entry of the wire and the position of the lesion closest to the skin.

SPECIMEN RADIOGRAPHY

Specimen radiography is useful to the surgeon for both palpable and impalpable breast lesions. The specimen radiograph will confirm that an impalpable lesion has been successfully excised (Fig. 14.27) and will also allow the surgeon to assess excision margins of palpable abnormalities. When wide local excision for carcinoma is being performed, a specimen radiograph will allow the surgeon to identify a margin that is too close to the lesion and prompt wider excision of this margin. Specimen radiographs are good predictors of inadequate excision but are poor predictors of complete histological excision.

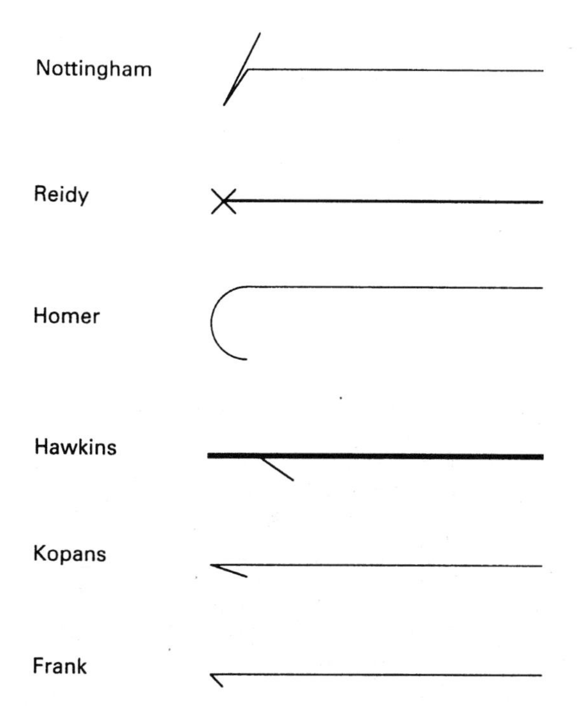

Fig. 14.25 Diagrammatic illustration of some of the various wire markers available for localization of impalpable breast lesions.

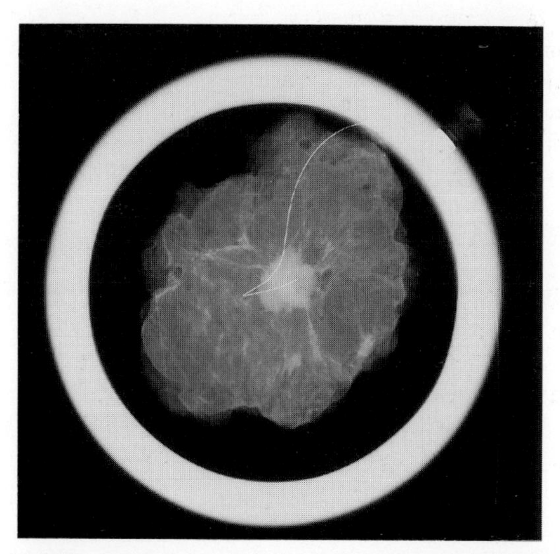

Fig. 14.27 Specimen X-rays showing a spiculate mass in the centre of a therapeutic excision. The lesion appears to be adequately excised with a good clear margin on all sides.

To facilitate re-excision, the specimen must be orientated with respect to the excision bed; this is easily achieved with either radiopaque sutures or surgical staples. Ideally, facilities should be available for carrying out specimen radiographs close to the operating theatre so that the images are available to the surgeon within a reasonable time. This means that further excision or exploration of the excision cavity, if required, can be carried out by the same operative procedure.

BREAST CANCER SCREENING

Screening asymptomatic women for breast cancer with the use of mammography has been shown to reduce breast cancer mortality in women aged 50–70. The mortality reduction may be up to 40% in those who attend for screening. Mammographic screening of women under 50 years and screening for breast cancer by physical examination have not been shown to reduce breast cancer mortality. In the United Kingdom breast screening by mammography is provided for all women over 50 years of age every 3 years.

Hormone replacement therapy (HRT), prescribed in the currently recommended way, may be associated with a small increased risk of breast cancer (relative risk increased by up to 2.5 times). However, it is recognized that the overall benefits of HRT far outweigh the risks. Women about to start HRT do not require baseline mammography and most women receiving HRT do not require screening other than that they would normally be offered according to their age or other risk factors.

From the practical point of view combined oestrogen and progestogen HRT can be associated with increase in mammographic breast density and this may reduce the sensitivity of screening mammography in some women. HRT may also be associated with an increase in the size of pre-existing fibroadenomas and cysts, changes that may cause clinical and imaging concern.

CHAPTER 15

Neck

Brian K. Wignall

IMAGING TECHNIQUES

CONVENTIONAL RADIOGRAPHY

Lateral view of the neck

Excepting suspected vertebral fractures, a lateral view of the neck will suffice for demonstrating most impacted swallowed foreign bodies, and allow initial assessment of laryngeal trauma. Soft-tissue thickening from inflammation or tumour of the larynx, pharynx and thyroid may be demonstrated and any associated airway narrowing identified. A lateral view of the thoracic inlet will indicate intrathoracic extension of a goitre by showing displacement or compression of the trachea.

Chest radiography

A chest radiograph is essential when any primary malignancy is diagnosed to detect metastases in the lungs or mediastinal lymph node enlargement. In addition, malignant lymphadenopathy in the neck can result from a primary bronchial carcinoma. Disease of the larynx and pharynx may cause aspiration pneumonia which will be demonstrated on a chest radiograph.

BARIUM SWALLOW EXAMINATION

This is an initial investigation of patients with dysphagia and is discussed on page 50.

Diagnostic and Interventional Radiology in Surgical Practice. Edited by P. Armstrong and M. L. Wastie. Published in 1997 by Chapman & Hall, London. ISBN 0 412 61960 1 (HB), 0 412 61970 9 (PB)

COMPUTED TOMOGRAPHY

CT provides cross-sectional images in which the contrast between different normal soft tissues, as well as between normal soft tissues and areas of pathology, is much greater than on conventional radiography. This contrast difference can be enhanced by means of intravenous contrast agents. Enhancement of blood vessels allows them to be distinguished from other rounded structures, notably enlarged lymph nodes, and displays the vascular anatomy. CT scanning gives excellent detail of bone and other calcified structures. If a tissue diagnosis has not been established, fine-needle aspiration biopsy may be carried out under CT control. The axial images are also used for mapping radiotherapy fields so that the whole tumour is treated. The information from CT can be transferred by computer disk to a CT integrated therapy planning system.

MAGNETIC RESONANCE IMAGING

With the use of a variety of pulse sequences, images are obtained which, compared with CT scanning, have better contrast between the different soft tissues and between normal soft tissues and tumour. This contrast difference is increased by use of intravenous paramagnetic agents, usually gadolinium DTPA. Additionally, the vascular anatomy can be displayed without recourse to contrast agents. With MRI, there are no artefacts from dental amalgam, a common problem with CT scanning of the neck. Thus, except for assessment of bony structures, MRI is a safer and better scanning technique for the neck than CT.

ULTRASOUND SCANNING

Use of a high frequency (7.5–10 MHz) linear array transducer will give an excellent display of all but the deepest structures in the neck. It is commonly used to examine the thyroid gland and lymph nodes and to act as a guide to fine-needle aspiration biopsy (FNAB) of any mass detected. The scan can be performed in any plane, is rapid and safe and causes no discomfort.

RADIONUCLIDE SCANNING

This involves an intravenous injection of a suitable radiopharmaceutical, after which the patient is scanned by means of a gamma camera in order to produce images which reveal a pattern of uptake of the radionuclide by the various tissues. From this it can be deduced whether these tissues are normal or abnormal.

Investigation of the thyroid and detection of bony metastases are the most common uses of radionuclide scanning in the neck.

CONGENITAL CYSTS OF THE NECK

These arise from duct remnants and often present in adult life due to enlargement as a result of trauma or infection.

BRANCHIAL CLEFT CYST (Fig. 15.1)

This is the most common congenital cyst and usually presents as a smooth fluctuant mass at the angle of the mandible. CT scanning reveals a low-density non-enhancing mass anterior to the sternomastoid muscle and lateral to the carotid sheath. There may be wall thickening or septation, due to infection.

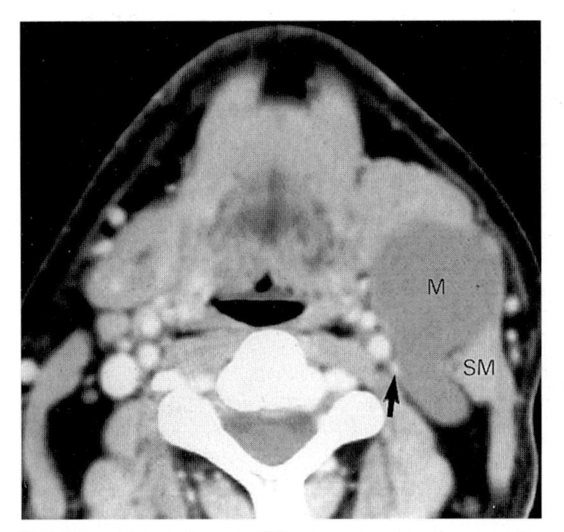

Fig. 15.1 Branchial cleft cyst. CT scan showing the cyst is a low attenuation mass (M) anterior to sternomastoid (SM). The arrow points to a compressed jugular vein.

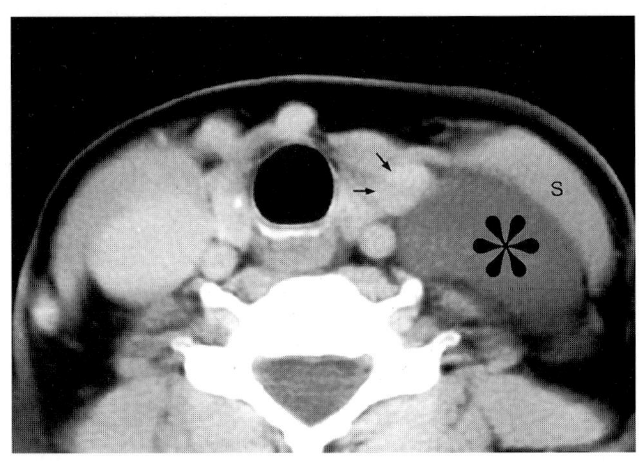

Fig. 15.2 Cystic hygroma. Contrast-enhanced CT scan at C6 level shows low density thin-walled lesion (✻) beneath left sternomastoid muscle (S). Left internal jugular vein (arrows) compressed and displaced medially.

CYSTIC HYGROMA (Fig. 15.2)

This arises from lymphoid tissue and has a similar appearance to a branchial cleft cyst but lies posterior to the sternomastoid muscle, i.e. in the posterior triangle of the neck.

THYROGLOSSAL DUCT CYST

This can arise at any site along the thyroglossal duct but is usually below the hyoid bone. Most thyroglossal cysts present in childhood and are usually midline in position. The cyst is well demonstrated by CT scanning (Fig. 15.3).

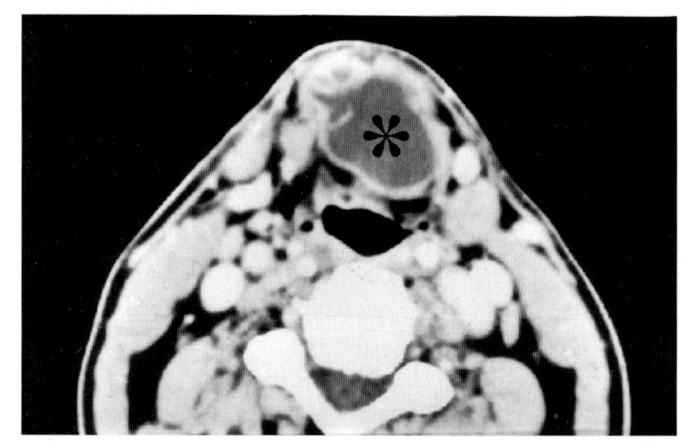

Fig. 15.3 Thyroglossal duct cyst. Contrast-enhanced CT scan just below hyoid bone shows anterior superficial midline low density structure (✻).

BENIGN TUMOURS OF THE NECK

LIPOMAS

Lipomas occur in the neck and are benign encapsulated lesions. Ultrasound scanning (Fig. 15.4a) reveals a very well-demarcated hyperechoic mass which will confirm the clinical impression of a lipoma. CT scanning (Fig. 15.4b) shows the mass to be of very low density with an attenuation value of fat, a finding that is diagnostic for lipoma. CT may be preferred by the surgeon since the anatomy is more clearly demonstrated than with ultrasound.

HAEMANGIOMAS (Fig. 15.5)

This congenital lesion may occur at any site in the face or neck. Rarely it is very extensive and may involve the oropharynx, causing partial obstruction. Radiographs may show multiple opacities representing phleboliths within the tumour and CT scanning reveals a hypervascular infiltrating mass.

PHARYNX

INFLAMMATORY DISEASE

Tonsils and adenoids

Hypertrophy of the pharyngeal lymphoid tissue is usually present in childhood and commonly causes symptoms, i.e. mouth breathing and snoring, and, because of eustachian tube obstruction, may result in deafness. A lateral radiograph of the neck (Fig. 15.6)

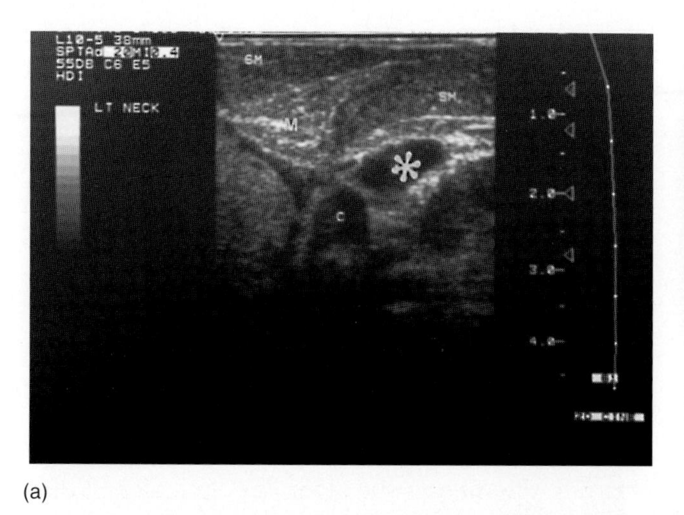

(a)

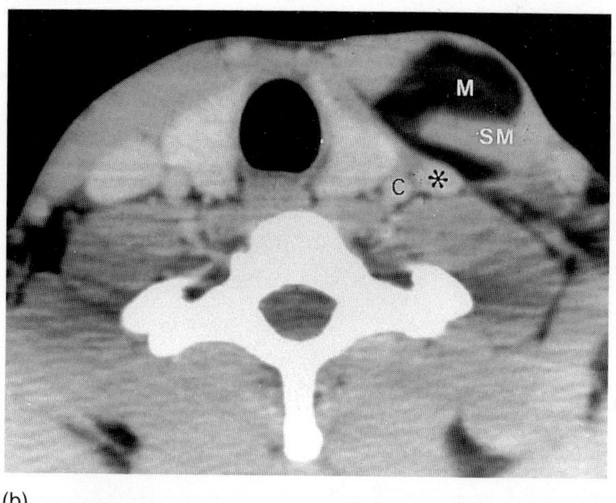

(b)

Fig. 15.4 Lipoma. (a) Ultrasound scan. Echogenic lobulated mass (M) lying between the heads of the sternomastoid muscle (SM). (b) CT scan shows very low density mass (M) indicating fat consistency; C=common carotid artery; ✻ = internal jugular vein.

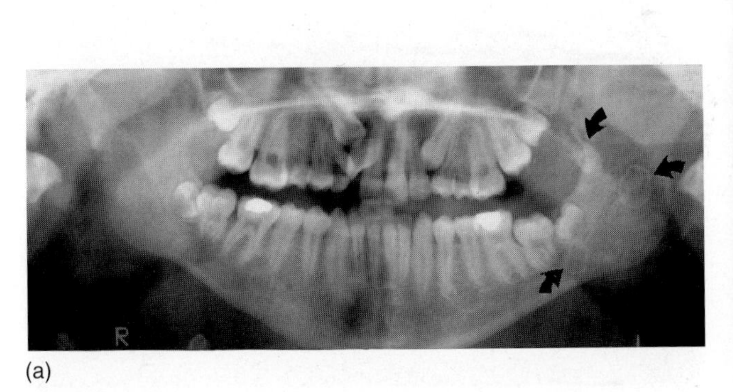

(a)

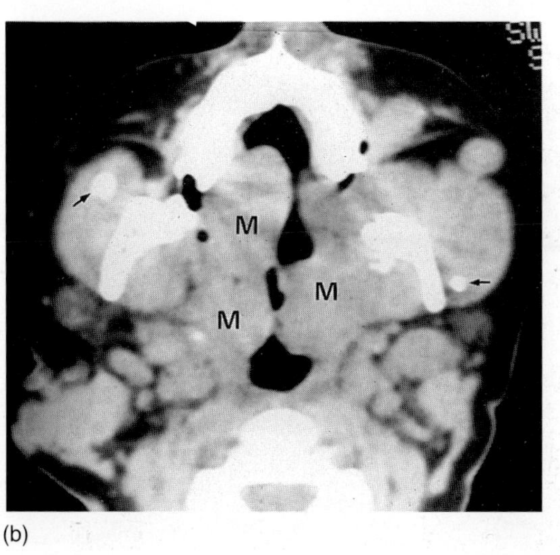

(b)

Fig. 15.5 Cavernous haemangioma in an 11-year-old child. This was present at birth but grew to involve cheeks, oropharynx and right side of neck. (a) Pan-oral view shows multiple ring shadows (arrows) due to phleboliths. (b) CT scan of oropharynx shows widespread soft-tissue masses (M) almost occluding the oropharynx. Phleboliths (arrows) again demonstrated.

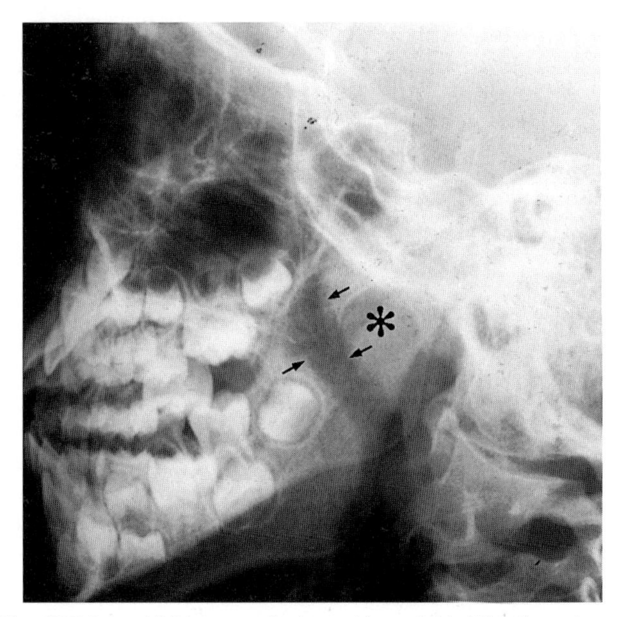

Fig. 15.6 Adenoidal hypertrophy in an 11-year-old child. Note airway narrowing (arrows) by nasopharyngeal mass (✻) posteriorly.

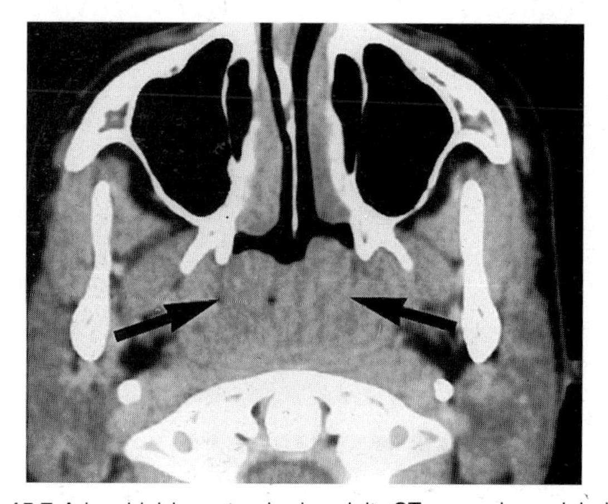

Fig. 15.7 Adenoidal hypertrophy in adult. CT scan shows lobulated soft-tissue mass (arrows) in postnasal space.

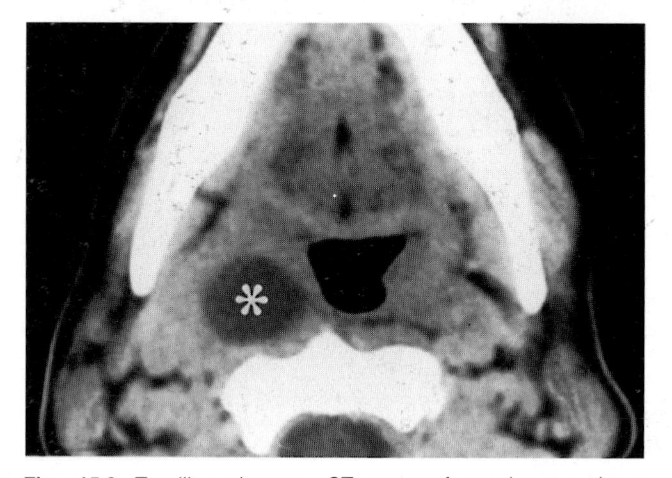

Fig. 15.8 Tonsillar abscess. CT scan of oropharynx shows bilateral tonsillar enlargement with low density abscess (✻) in right tonsil.

will demonstrate the amount of soft-tissue thickening in the postnasal space and indicate the size of the airway. It is unusual for adenoidal hypertrophy to be symptomatic in adult life. Enlargement of the adenoids can be demonstrated on CT scanning (Fig. 15.7) but a biopsy may be required to distinguish hypertrophy from other causes of enlargement such as lymphoma.

Tonsillar enlargement may also be demonstrated but is itself not an indication for radiography. Tonsillar infection, however, may lead to a peritonsillar abscess, the extent of which can be readily assessed by CT scanning (Fig. 15.8). The abscess cavity contains fluid contents which are of low density and its wall is thick, with loss of the adjacent fat planes due to inflammatory oedema.

Retropharyngeal infection

In young children, retropharyngeal infection can lead to abscess formation, the extent of which may be assessed by means of a lateral radiograph of the neck. Infection may spread to the adjacent vertebrae, leading to atlantoaxial subluxation (Fig. 15.9). Conversely, pyogenic or tuberculous infection of the cervical spine may extend to the prevertebral soft tissues, resulting in an abscess (Fig. 15.10).

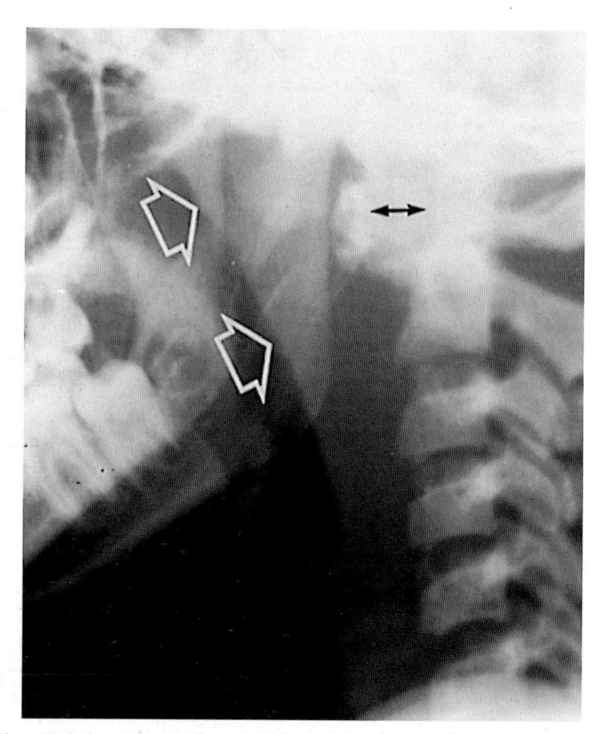

Fig. 15.9 Acute retropharyngeal abscess in a child. Note increased thickness of soft tissues most marked in the nasopharynx (white arrows) and associated atlantoaxial subluxation (arrowheads).

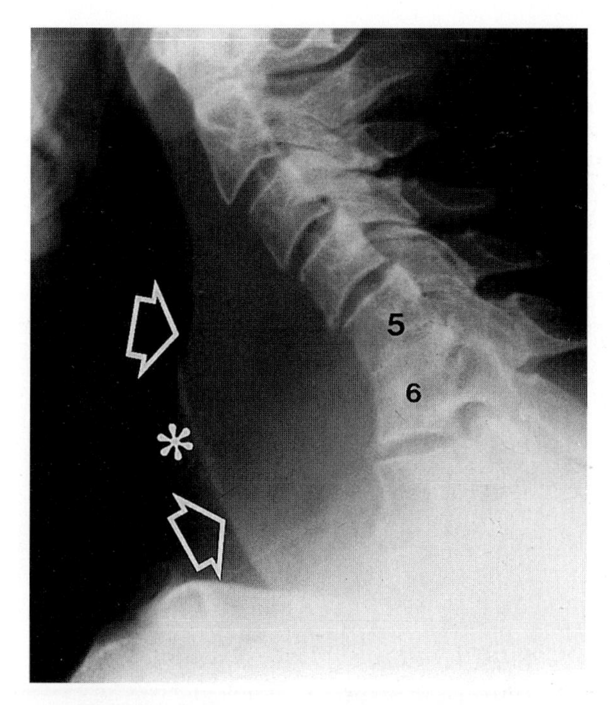

Fig. 15.10 Tuberculous spondylitis causing ankylosis of C5 and C6 vertebral bodies with retropharyngeal abscess (arrows). Note anterior displacement of larynx (*).

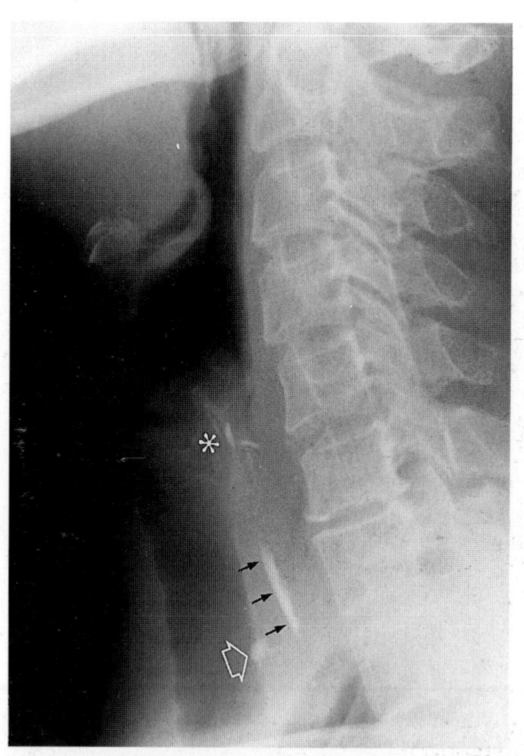

Fig. 15.11 Swallowed chicken bone. Bone fragment (black arrows) impacted at C7 level. Note thyroid cartilage ossification (*) and calcified nodule (white arrow) in thyroid gland.

SWALLOWED FOREIGN BODIES

If there is clinical suspicion of impaction of a foreign body in the pharynx or cervical oesophagus, a lateral radiograph of the neck is indicated. High density material, such as bones (Fig. 15.11) or metallic objects, will be visible. When the impacted foreign body is not radiopaque, e.g. a plastic dental plate (Fig. 15.12), a barium study will demonstrate it as a filling defect within the lumen of the pharynx or oesophagus.

If perforation of the wall of the pharynx or oesophagus has occurred, resulting haemorrhage or oedema causes thickening of the prevertebral soft tissues and may produce surgical emphysema, which may spread into the mediastinum and around the thorax. Abscess formation may develop in the mediastinum. When a perforation is suspected, water-soluble contrast should be used rather than barium because of the risk of barium spreading extraluminally into the soft tissues.

Problems of interpretation of the plain radiograph arise when other opaque structures are present in the neck. These include calcification within lymph nodes and the thyroid gland. Calcification/ossification of the laryngeal cartilages (Fig. 15.13) is commonly incomplete and inhomogeneous. This, as well as the minor laryngeal cartilages, may be mistaken for a swallowed foreign body. It must also be remembered that symptoms may be due to laceration of the mucosa by a foreign body which has not impacted and cannot, therefore, be demonstrated.

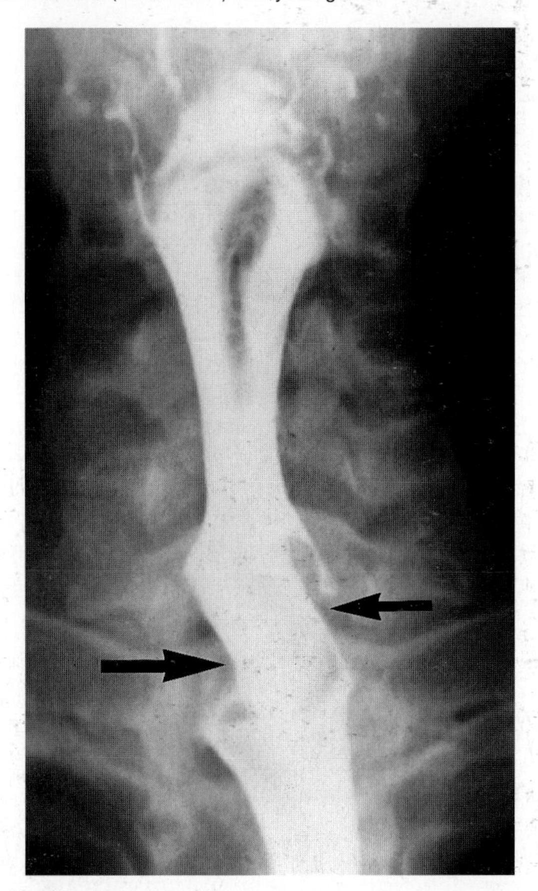

Fig. 15.12 Impacted radiolucent foreign body. Swallowed broken plastic dental plate. Plain radiograph normal. Barium swallow shows plate as irregular filling defect (arrows) at C7/T1 level.

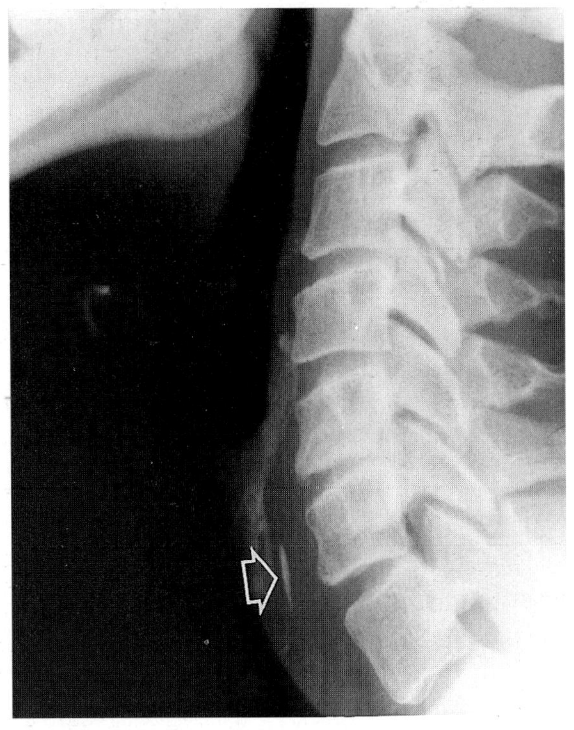

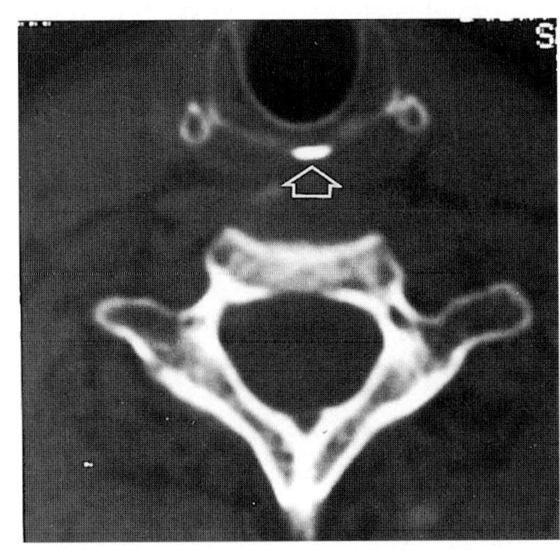

(a) (b)

Fig. 15.13 Cricoid cartilage calcification. Dysphagia after swallowing bone. Endoscopy was normal. (a) Linear density (arrow) at C6 level is due to calcification posteriorly in cricoid cartilage. (b) CT scan confirms this.

PHARYNGEAL DIVERTICULUM (ZENKER'S DIVERTICULUM)

This acquired pulsion diverticulum occurs more commonly in the elderly. A pouch of mucosa protrudes posteriorly through a weakness in the inferior pharyngeal constrictor between its oblique and transverse (cricopharyngeus) portions. Food can accumulate in the pouch, which enlarges, resulting in oesophageal compression causing dysphagia, cough and regurgitation of food eaten hours earlier.

A barium swallow examination (Fig. 15.14) opacifies the diverticulum which, if large, is directed laterally (usually to the left) as well as posteriorly. It may extend downwards into the mediastinum. Resulting oesophageal compression, as well as any aspiration of barium, is also demonstrated.

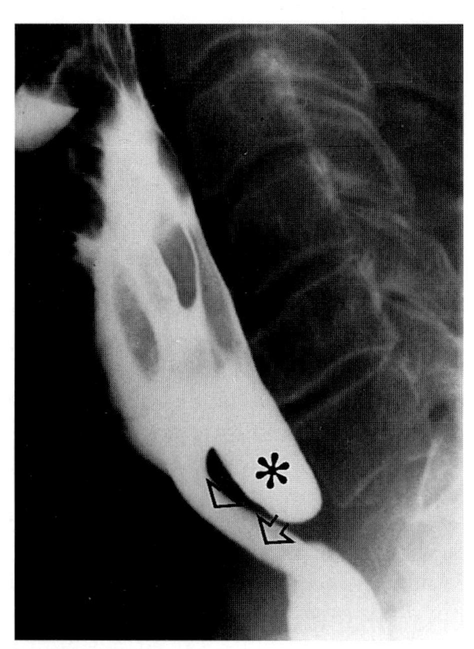

Fig. 15.14 Pharyngeal diverticulum. Barium swallow shows posterior diverticulum (*) at C5 level compressing the pharyngo-oesophageal junction (arrows).

POSTCRICOID WEB

A web is a thin mucosal membrane which projects at right angles from the anterior aspect of the hypopharynx. Webs may be multiple and, when large, are crescentic. A postcricoid web causes dysphagia and, although often an isolated finding, may be associated with iron-deficiency anaemia and an increased incidence of carcinoma. A barium swallow examination shows very clearly on the lateral view even a small web (Fig. 15.15). As with all barium studies of the pharynx and oesophagus, video recording of the examination allows playback in slow motion for closer scrutiny of the abnormal findings.

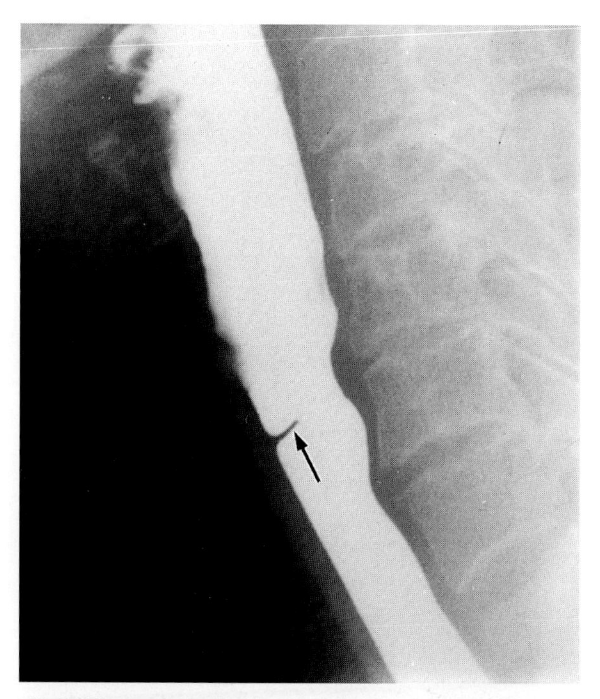

Fig. 15.15 Pharyngeal web. Barium swallow reveals thin shelf-like membrane (arrow) projecting anteriorly into hypopharynx at C5/6 level.

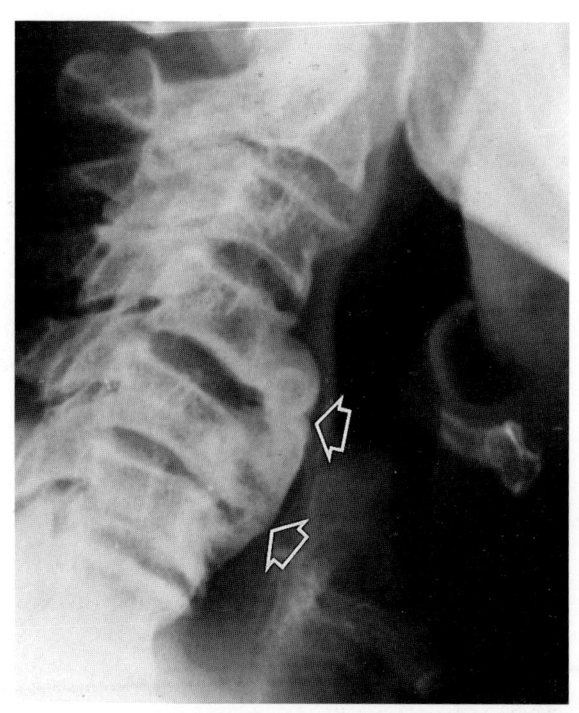

Fig. 15.16 Cervical spondylosis. Large anterior osteophytes (arrows) at C4 to C6 levels causing dysphagia in a patient aged 80 years.

CERVICAL SPONDYLOSIS

In the elderly, osteophytes may impinge on the pharynx (Fig. 15.16) but rarely cause dysphagia.

JUVENILE NASOPHARYNGEAL ANGIOFIBROMA

This uncommon, benign, very vascular tumour of adolescent males, may cause epistaxis and nasal obstruction. Juvenile nasopharyngeal angiofibroma arises in the sphenopalatine foramen and may spread anteriorly into the nasal cavity, or laterally into the pterygopalatine and infratemporal fossae. Superior extension may occur into the sphenoid, ethmoid or cavernous sinuses and through the medial wall of the middle cranial fossa.

Because biopsy of this vascular tumour is contraindicated, diagnosis is made by imaging techniques, which must also show the extent of the tumour as well as its vascular supply since therapeutic embolization may be performed prior to surgery. CT scanning with intravenous contrast enhancement (Fig. 15.17) shows the extent of the tumour which appears hyperdense due to its vascular nature. In addition, CT will demonstrate the characteristic medial pterygoid plate erosion as well as any infiltration of the skull base with intracranial extension. Angiography demonstrates the marked tumour circulation which is derived usually from the internal maxillary branch of the external carotid artery.

PHARYNGEAL TUMOURS

Pharyngeal tumours are discussed on page 375ff.

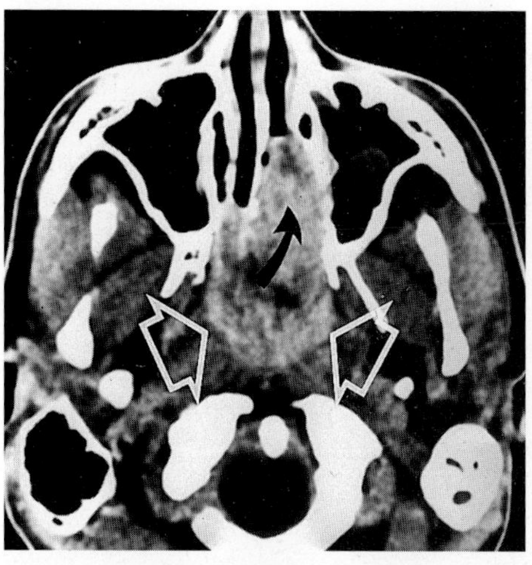

Fig. 15.17 Juvenile nasopharyngeal angiofibroma. Axial CT scan with i.v. contrast. Large enhancing mass (open arrows) obstructs nasopharynx and extends anteriorly into nose mainly on the left side (curved arrow).

LARYNX

LARYNGITIS

Inflammatory oedema of the larynx is a cause of dyspnoea and in children is usually the result of viral or bacterial infections (laryngotracheobronchitis). Swallowed irritant liquids or inhaled toxic gases, as well as allergic reactions, may all result in laryngeal oedema. The soft-tissue swelling of the larynx and any associated airway narrowing is readily appreciated on conventional radiography (Fig. 15.18) or CT scanning.

LARYNGEAL TRAUMA

Laryngeal trauma may occur in road traffic accidents and assault cases and may also occur from knife wounds to the neck. Although a hyoid fracture and any surgical emphysema (Fig. 15.19) are usually detectable on conventional radiographs, fractures of the laryngeal cartilages are unlikely to be diagnosed. However, CT scanning clearly demonstrates fractures or dislocations of these cartilages, together with any resulting narrowing of the airway. Untreated cartilage fractures may lead to laryngeal stenosis.

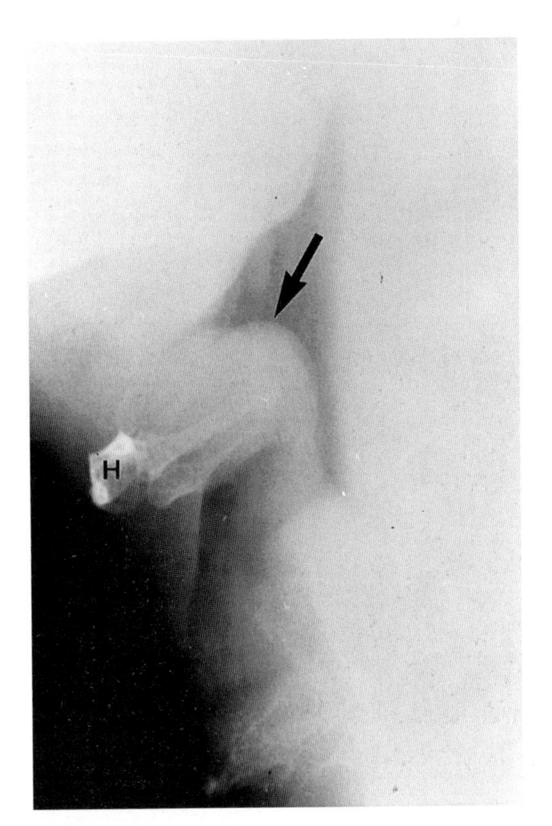

Fig. 15.18 Epiglottitis. Lateral radiograph of neck showing swollen epiglottis (arrow). H=hyoid bone. (Courtesy of Dr Otto Chan, The Royal London Hospital.)

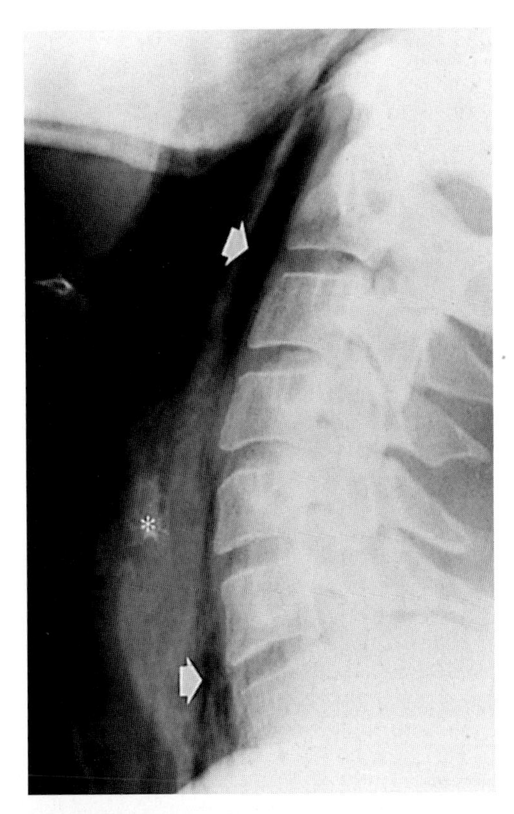

(a)

(b)

Fig. 15.19 Laryngeal trauma. (a) Lateral view of neck with extensive dark streaks (arrows) due to air in soft tissues. Note laryngeal cartilages (✻) but no fracture seen. (b) Chest radiograph indicates spread of emphysema over right supraclavicular region (large arrow) and into mediastinum (small arrows).

LARYNGOCELE

An air- or mucus-filled sac may originate in the laryngeal ventricle, probably as a congenital anomaly. The sac can extend upwards and may cause airway obstruction. An internal laryngocele is one which remains within the thyroid cartilage. If the sac bursts through the thyrohyoid membrane to lie outside the thyroid cartilage it is termed an external laryngocele. Mixed types occur and laryngoceles may be bilateral. CT scanning will allow a precise diagnosis.

MALIGNANT TUMOURS OF PHARYNX AND LARYNX

Squamous cell carcinomas make up 90% or more of the primary tumours in this region. In most cases, the clinician makes the diagnosis by endoscopy and mucosal biopsy. If it is suspected that the tumour extends deeply, or if enlarged lymph nodes are palpable, then imaging with CT or preferably MRI is necessary. Even if no primary tumour is clinically detected, scanning is required if the following signs or symptoms suspicious of malignancy are present:

- nasal obstruction, discharge or bleeding;
- middle ear symptoms (from eustachian tube obstruction);
- cervical lymphadenopathy;
- cranial nerve defects (from skull base infiltration).

CT or MRI scanning is necessary in the following situations:

- As part of the **staging of the tumour**, in accordance with the TNM classification system. Scanning reveals:
  - the size and full extent of the tumour
  - associated destruction of bone or cartilage
  - lymph node involvement;
- **Treatment planning**, i.e. surgery or radiotherapy;
- **Follow-up**, to determine the response to treatment and to detect any tumour recurrence.

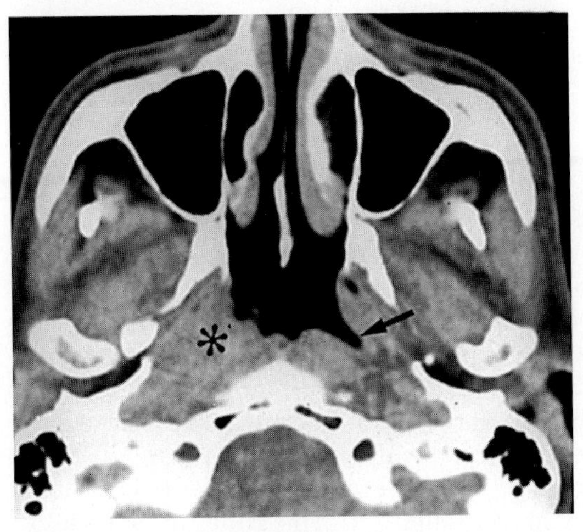

Fig. 15.20 Nasopharyngeal carcinoma. CT scan shows right-sided tumour (*) obliterating lateral pharyngeal recess on that side. Loss of adjacent fat planes indicates infiltration of parapharyngeal space. Note normal left lateral pharyngeal recess (arrow).

NASOPHARYNGEAL CARCINOMA

In 50% of patients, the presenting complaint is a mass in the neck due to lymphadenopathy. Although the nasopharynx extends from the skull base only to the soft palate inferiorly, axial scans are obtained down to the heads of the clavicles whenever a nasopharyngeal carcinoma is identified in order to detect any associated lymphadenopathy. Coronal sections are necessary for proper assessment of the skull base.

The tumour usually arises in the region of the lateral pharyngeal recess and commonly extends to the parapharyngeal space (Fig. 15.20) and may obstruct a eustachian tube orifice, resulting in fluid in the middle

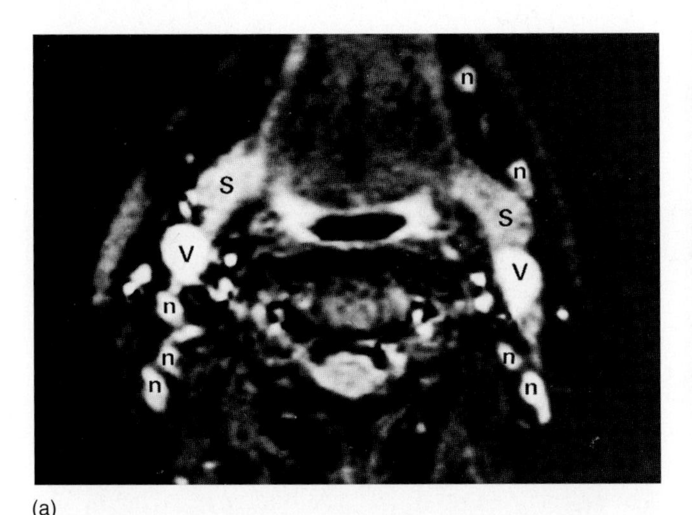

(a)

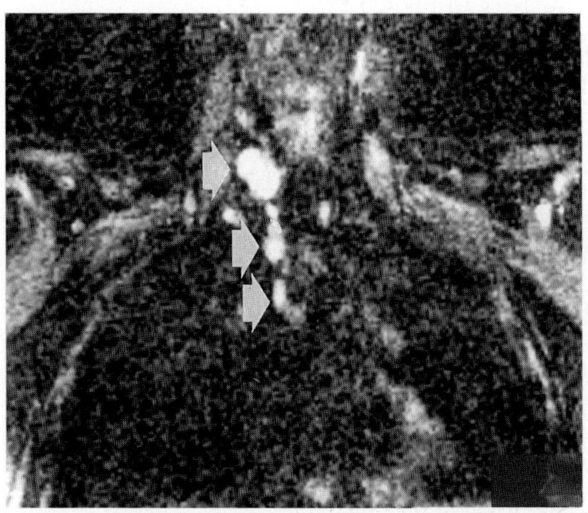

(b)

Fig. 15.21 Lymphadenopathy. MRI using fat-suppression sequence. (a) Reactive: the nodes (n) appear as high signal. V=blood vessels; S=submandibular glands. (b) Malignant: enlarged supraclavicular and mediastinal nodes from breast cancer (arrowed). (Courtesy of Dr Otto Chan, The Royal London Hospital and Dr Wailup Wong, Mount Vernon Hospital, Middlesex.)

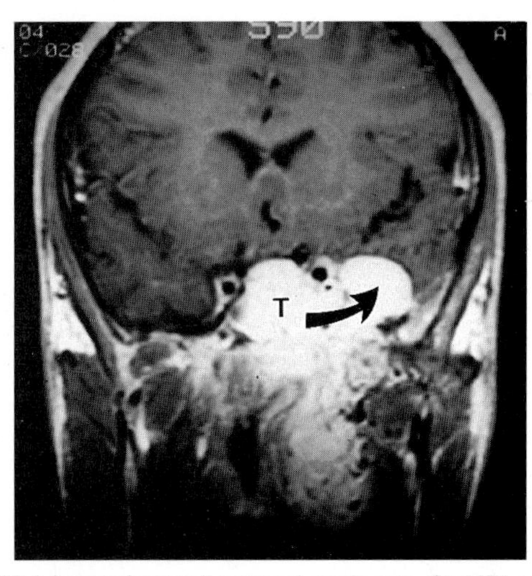

Fig. 15.22 Advanced nasopharyngeal carcinoma. On MRI gadolinium enhanced T1-weighted coronal scan, a large high-signal tumour mass (T) can be seen filling nasopharynx and extending through skull base and cavernous sinus into left middle cranial fossa (arrow). Note excellent definition of tumour margins.

ear or mastoid on that side. The tumour may extend intracranially via the foramen lacerum or foramen ovale and skull base erosion can occur. Lymphadenopathy is detected in approximately 70% of cases, usually in the upper cervical lymph nodes, but, in the minority of cases, extension to the lower cervical nodes occurs.

On T2-weighted MRI images, normal mucosa, tumour and lymph nodes, both reactive or metastatic, are seen as high signal against low signal muscle. Fat also has a high signal and can obscure a tumour or node and, therefore, further imaging is performed using a fat-suppression sequence. Both reactive and malignant lymphadenopathy have a similar appearance on the various sequences (Fig. 15.21).

When a tumour is suspected from these images, a contrast-enhanced MRI scan is required to show the tumour clearly. The tumour margins show a high signal (Fig. 15.22) against the lower signal non-enhancing muscle. Inflammatory oedema does not obscure these margins. In addition, malignant lymph nodes usually show bright outer margins, i.e. peripheral enhancement (Fig. 15.23).

A coronal image is also obtained through the nasopharynx to indicate the extent of the tumour. Coronal images are useful for radiotherapy planning.

CT scanning is an alternative imaging method, although the tumour is less well distinguished from adjacent structures. Contrast enhancement is used in order to increase the density of the tumour tissue and to identify the blood vessels. Malignant lymph nodes are usually > 10 mm in size. The nodes normally show peripheral enhancement but may be seen as low-density masses. Any bone erosion (Fig. 15.24), e.g. of the pterygoid plates, is easily recognized on CT.

OROPHARYNGEAL CARCINOMA

The oropharynx extends from the soft palate inferiorly to the hyoid bone and includes the pharyngeal walls, tonsillar region and base of tongue. The oropharynx is separated from the larynx by the epiglottis and from the hypopharynx by the pharyngo-epiglottic folds.

The patient usually complains of a tonsillar mass, with pain on swallowing, and more than half the patients have nodal metastases in the internal jugular chain at presentation. The tumour is usually more extensive than clinically apparent, i.e. it commonly spreads to other compartments of the pharynx. The tumour often infiltrates the parapharyngeal space, the

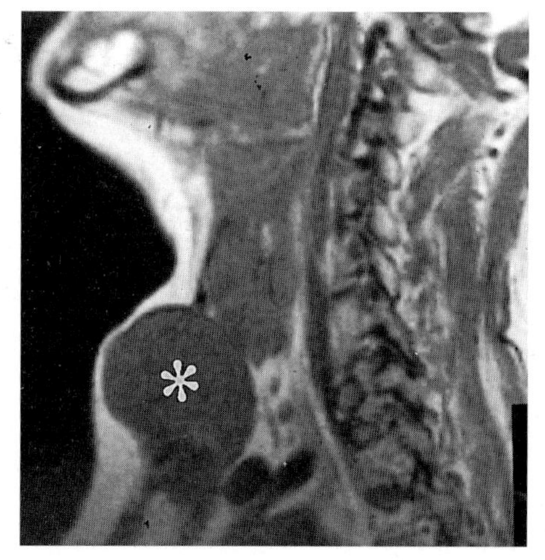

(a)

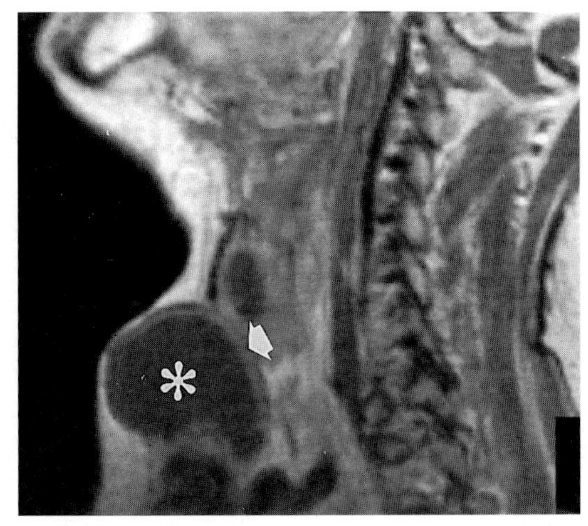

(b)

Fig. 15.23 Malignant lymph node from nasopharyngeal carcinoma (✻). MRI T1-weighted sagittal scans: (a) pre- and (b) post-gadolinium enhanced scans. Note ring enhancement (arrow) of suprasternal node on scan (b). (Courtesy of Dr Wailup Wong, Mount Vernon Hospital, Middlesex.)

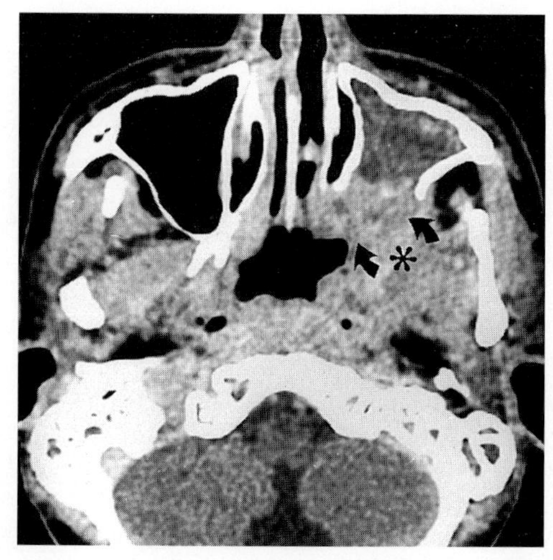
Fig. 15.24 Nasopharyngeal carcinoma stage T3 N1. Axial CT scan indicates large tumour (✻) involving left pterygoid muscles and invading left maxillary sinus, with erosion of left pterygoid plates and posterior wall of left maxillary sinus (arrows).

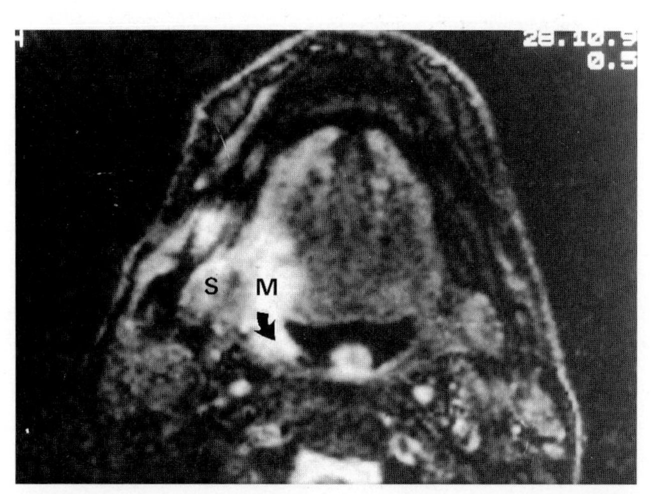

Fig. 15.26 Carcinoma of tongue. Axial MRI with fat-suppression sequence shows high signal tumour mass (M) confined to right side of tongue but involving the adjacent tonsillar fossa (arrow). High signal of right submandibular gland (S) is due to inflammation resulting from duct obstruction by tumour. (Courtesy of Dr Otto Chan, The Royal London Hospital.)

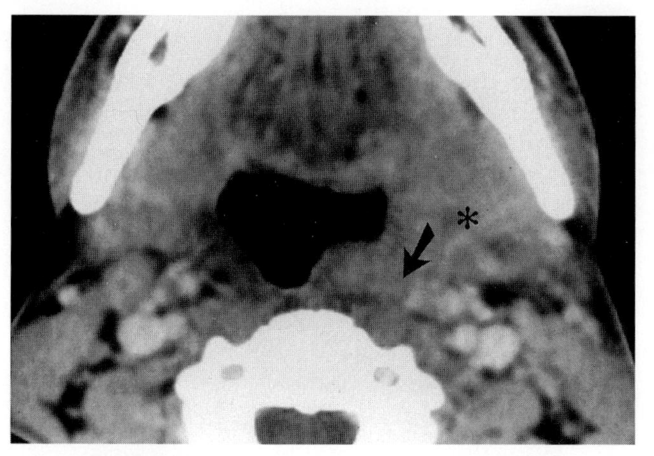
Fig. 15.25 Carcinoma of tonsil. Enhanced CT scan shows poorly enhancing ill-defined mass (✻) extending posteriorly (arrow) to carotid sheath. Note loss of adjacent fat planes.

prevertebral muscles or around the carotid artery (Fig. 15.25) and may extend into the tongue or larynx. Conversely, a primary carcinoma of the tongue not infrequently spreads to the adjacent tonsillar fossa (Fig. 15.26).

CT scanning identifies the tumour and any associated lymphadenopathy as an enhancing mass displacing tissue planes, and the mass may have a low density central region from necrosis. It may, however, be impossible to distinguish between malignant and suppurative lymphadenopathy. CT scan images of the oropharynx are often degraded by streak artefacts from dental amalgam and, because of this and the better demonstration of the soft tissues, MRI is the scanning method of choice for staging oropharyngeal tumours.

HYPOPHARYNGEAL CARCINOMA

The hypopharynx extends from the hyoid bone inferiorly to the cricopharyngeus muscle and includes the piriform sinuses and postcricoid region. The piriform sinuses are situated on either side of the aryepiglottic folds of the larynx and the true vocal cords and are related laterally to the thyroid cartilage. The postcricoid region joins the oesophagus at the lower border of the cricoid.

Symptoms of squamous cell carcinoma of the hypopharynx include sore throat, dysphagia and otalgia, as well as enlarged cervical lymph nodes. Hoarseness indicates laryngeal invasion. On presentation, the tumour is often advanced (T3 or T4 stage).

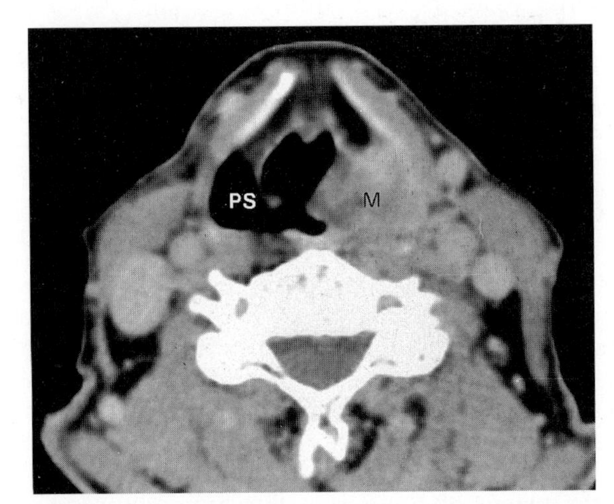

Fig. 15.27 Carcinoma of piriform sinus. CT scan showing large mass (M) obliterating left sinus. Note normal airfilled right pyriform sinus (PS).

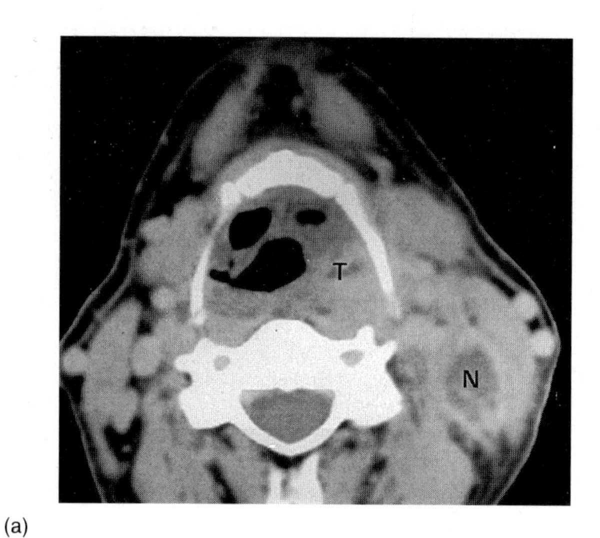

(a)

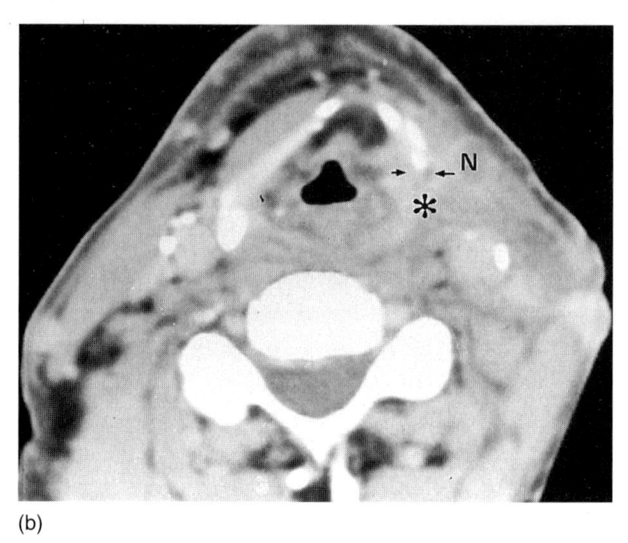

(b)

Fig. 15.28 Carcinoma of piriform sinus. (a) Contrast-enhanced CT scan shows left-sided tumour (T) obliterating left piriform sinus, and also left lymph node metastasis (N) showing ring enhancement and central necrosis. (b) Recurrence 9 months later with tumour extension (✻) in left side of neck and erosion of thyroid cartilage (arrows) on that side. Note malignant lymphadenopathy (N).

The majority of tumours arise in a piriform sinus (Fig. 15.27) and often extend postero-laterally into the soft tissues of the neck and around the carotid artery, and may cause erosion of the thyroid cartilage. Malignant lymphadenopathy is present in 50% of cases, usually at the mandibular angle on the affected side. MRI with contrast enhancement shows well both the extent of the tumour and any lymphadenopathy but CT scanning is better for displaying cartilage erosion (Fig. 15.28).

Postcricoid carcinoma causes dysphagia. The tumour tends to spread early, either upwards, into the oro- and nasopharynx, or inferiorly into the oesophagus. Bilateral internal jugular node involvement is common and the tumour has, therefore, a poor prognosis. MRI or CT scanning will demonstrate the extent of the tumour and nodal involvement, but tumour assessment is difficult in the postcricoid region because of the normal variation of soft-tissue thickness at this site. A barium swallow examination will aid endoscopy in ascertaining the extent of the mucosal spread of tumour (Fig. 15.29).

LARYNGEAL CARCINOMA

As with pharyngeal malignancy, the diagnosis is made and the mucosal extent of the laryngeal carcinoma is assessed by endoscopy and biopsy. If deeper extension of the tumour is suspected, then MRI or CT scanning of the whole neck is required for staging, prior to therapy, in order to reveal:

- the extent of tumour in the supraglottic or subglottic region and any spread to extralaryngeal structures;
- anterior or posterior commissure involvement by glottic tumours;
- cartilage destruction (but assessment is not entirely accurate, due to normal variation in ossification);
- nodal disease.

CT scanning of the larynx is performed during quiet respiration when the vocal cords are abducted. An

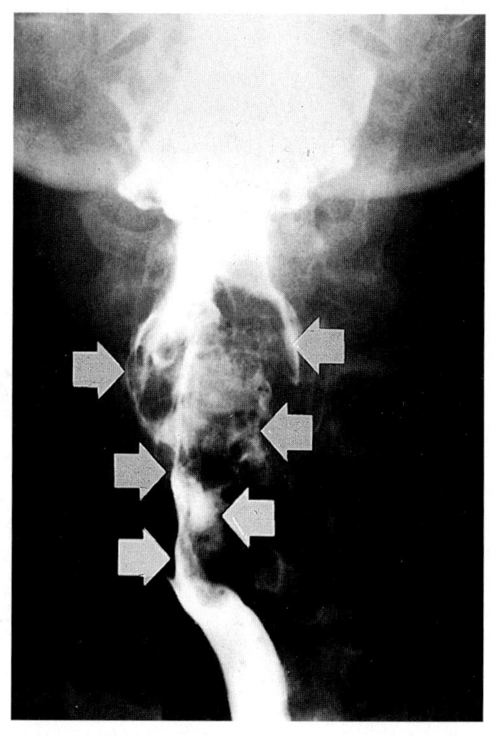

Fig. 15.29 Postcricoid carcinoma. Barium swallow examination showing irregular stricture (arrows) 7 cm long and centred at postcricoid level.

enhanced scan with an intravenous injection of contrast medium is also made to identify blood vessels and detect nodal malignancy. MRI gives better soft-tissue contrast and can differentiate the tumour from muscle and fat. Contrast enhancement aids this differentiation and nodal disease is also better identified on postcontrast images. Coronal images are obtained to verify the origin and extent of glottic and subglottic tumours.

Supraglottic carcinoma

One third of laryngeal tumours arise in the supraglottis, which extends from the epiglottis to the false vocal cords and includes the aryepiglottic folds and laryngeal ventricle. Hoarseness is a late symptom and the tumour is usually advanced at presentation; more than 50% of cases have metastases in the internal jugular nodes. Epiglottic tumours (Fig. 15.30) tend to spread to the pre-epiglottic space and tongue base.

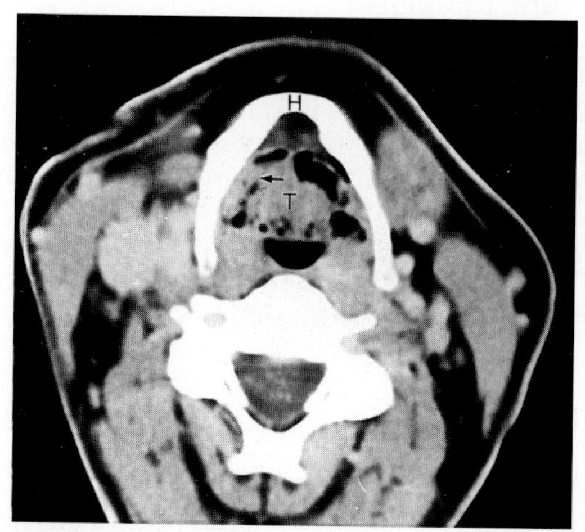

Fig. 15.30 Supraglottic carcinoma of the larynx. CT scan at level of hyoid bone (H) level reveals tumour (T) of epiglottis extending into right pharyngo-epiglottic fold (arrow).

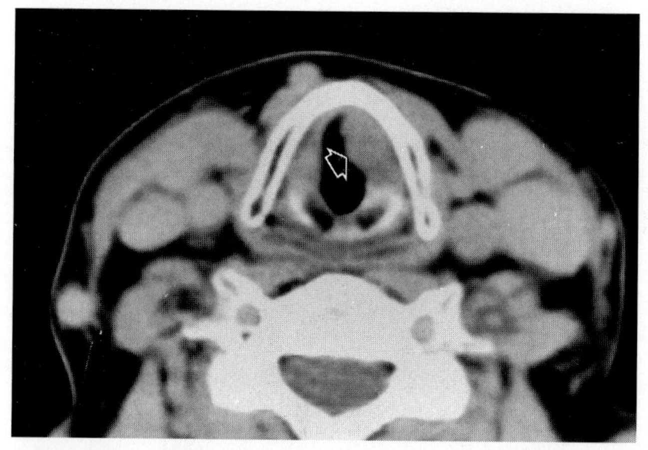

Fig. 15.31 Carcinoma of left vocal cord. Stage T3 N0 tumour. CT scan showing mass (arrow) extending to anterior commissure but no further, i.e. no spread outside larynx and no erosion of thyroid cartilage.

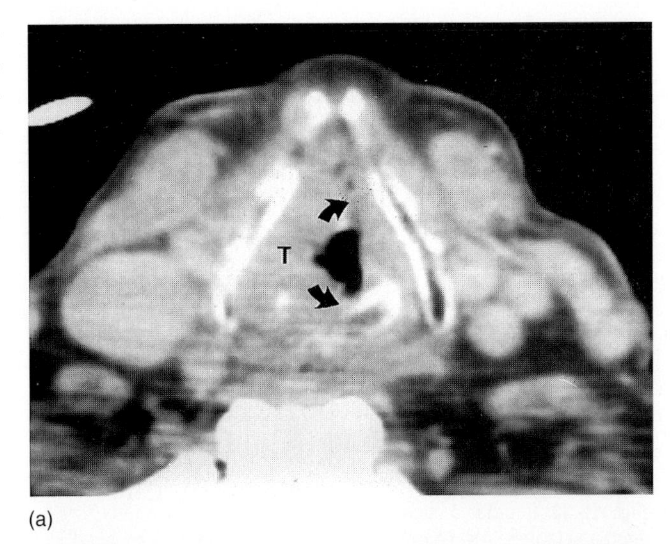

(a)

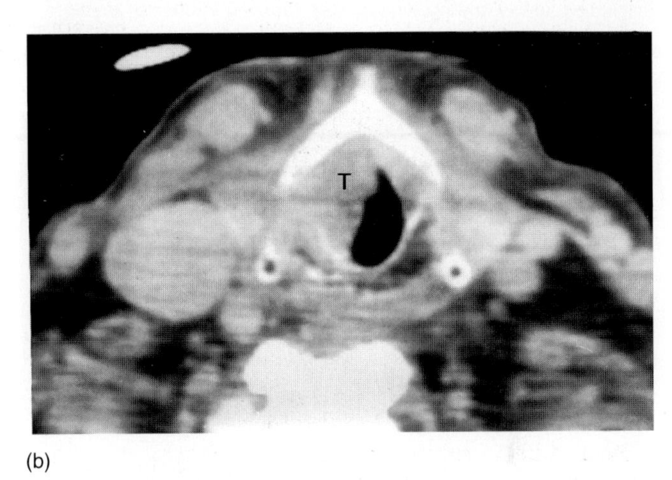

(b)

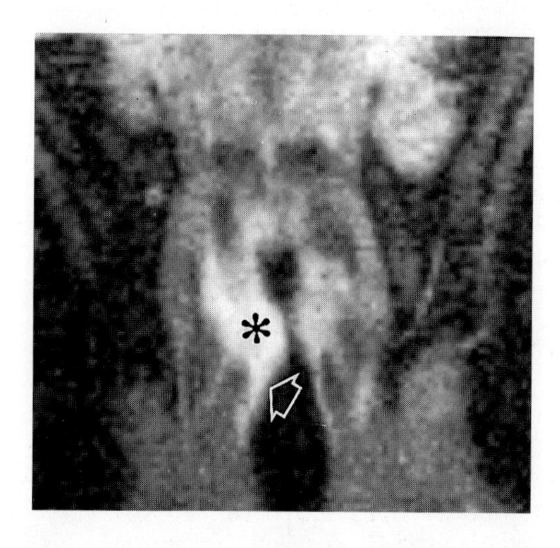

(c)

Fig. 15.32 Carcinoma of right vocal cord with subglottic extension. (a) CT scan at level of true vocal cords shows large tumour (T) of the right cord, extending across midline both anteriorly and posteriorly (arrows). (b) At cricoid level the scan indicates subglottic tumour (T) extension. (c) MRI coronal scan, fat-suppression sequence, shows tumour (*) and subglottic extension (arrow) very well defined. (Courtesy of Dr Wailup Wong, Mount Vernon Hospital, Middlesex.)

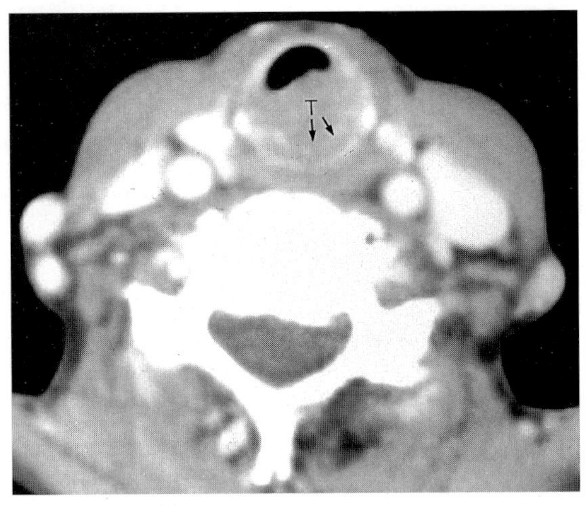

Fig. 15.33 Subglottic laryngeal carcinoma. Contrast-enhanced CT scan just below level of true vocal cord. Note large tumour (T) almost occluding airway and causing erosion (arrows) of cricoid lamina.

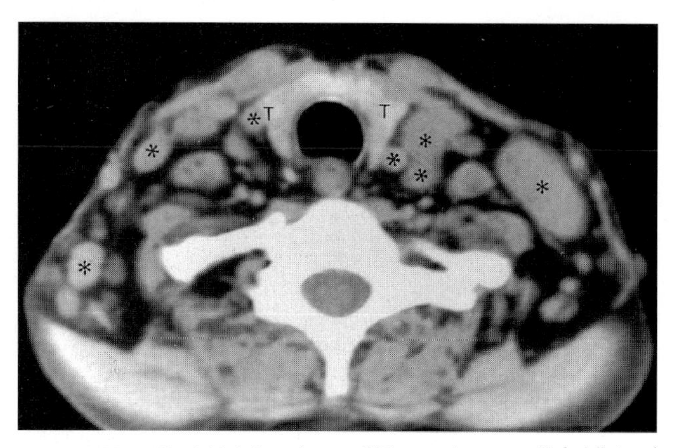

Fig. 15.34 Non-Hodgkin's lymphoma. CT scan shows multiple bilateral homogeneous enlarged lymph nodes (✱) in the neck. Note dense appearance of thyroid gland (T).

Carcinoma of the ventricle and false cords may destroy the thyroid cartilage or extend through the true vocal cords to the subglottis.

Glottic carcinoma

Carcinoma of the vocal cords (Fig. 15.31) is the commonest laryngeal tumour and presents early because of the associated hoarseness. This, together with slow tumour growth and the sparse lymphatic drainage, account for the good prognosis of this malignancy. Thus, most cases are Stage I tumours and do not require radiological imaging. Scanning is reserved for more advanced tumours, which may show spread to the anterior commissure and from the anterior commissure to the opposite cord and supra- or subglottic region (Fig. 15.32), possibly with thyroid cartilage destruction. Some tumours spread to the posterior commissure, with cord fixation and erosion of the arytenoid and cricoid cartilages.

Subglottic carcinoma

The subglottis is the region from the under-surface of the true vocal cords to the lower border of cricoid cartilage. Most tumours in this region are extensions from glottic primary tumours and a true subglottic tumour is rare. A subglottic carcinoma usually presents at an advanced stage and scanning may show spread of the tumour to the vocal cords or extension into the trachea or hypopharynx, with invasion of the cricoid or tracheal cartilages (Fig. 15.33).

LYMPHOMA

Lymphoma usually involves the lymph nodes, tonsils or adenoids but is relatively uncommon elsewhere in the head or neck. The appearances are usually obvious

(a)

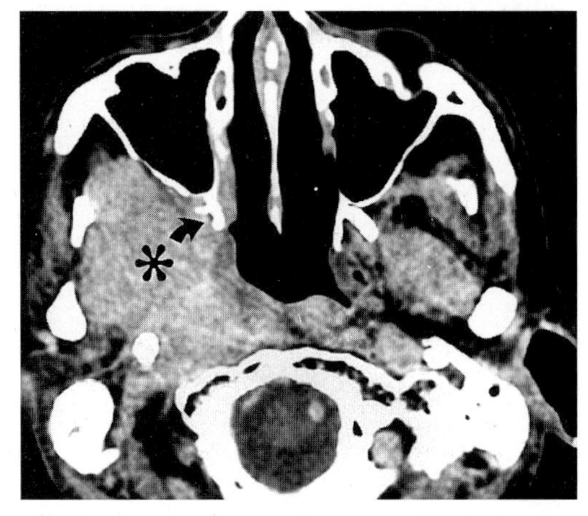

(b)

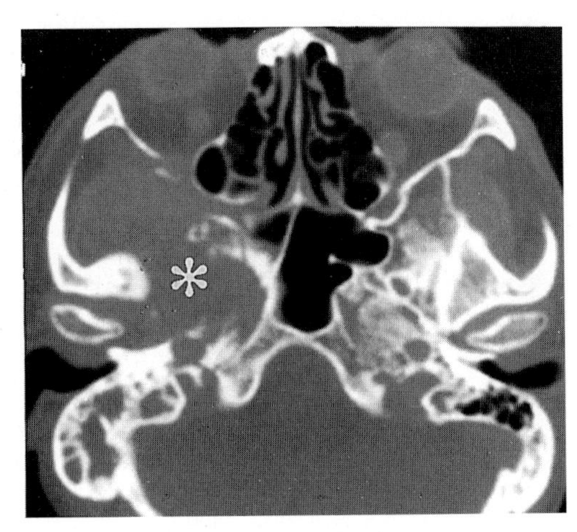

Fig. 15.35 Lymphoma of nasopharynx. (a) CT scan shows large tumour mass (✱) on right side, with obliteration of right lateral pharyngeal recess and parapharyngeal space, and filling infratemporal fossa on that side. Note erosion of right pterygoid plates (arrow). (b) Extensive erosion of skull base (✱) is seen on right side.

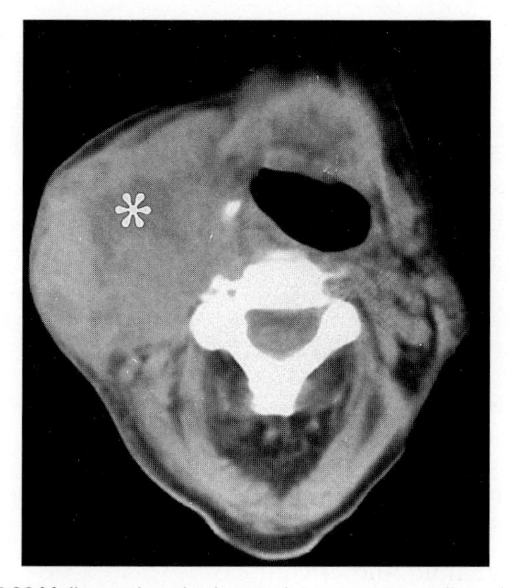

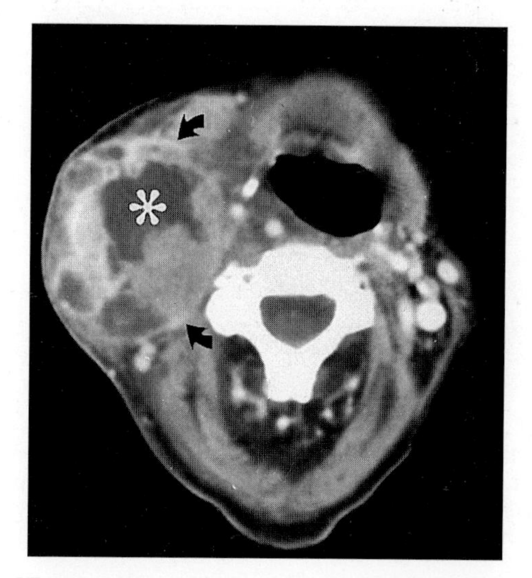

(a) (b)

Fig. 15.36 Malignant lymphadenopathy: squamous cell carcinoma of oropharynx. CT scan at thyrohyoid level shows large lymph node (a) before and (b) after i.v. contrast enhancement. Note ring enhancement (arrows) and necrotic areas (*) in enlarged node. Opacified blood vessels are well shown on the enhanced scan (b).

on MRI or CT scans, which show multiple, often bilateral, enlarged homogeneous lymph nodes (Fig. 15.34). No central necrosis of the nodes is present but, following therapy, necrosis or even calcification can occur. Bone erosion may occur (Fig. 15.35).

Because lymphoma presenting in the neck is, in the majority of patients, part of a more widespread disease, CT scanning of the thorax, abdomen and pelvis may also be required for staging. In the less common instances in which lymphoma occurs as a single extranodal lesion in the neck, CT or MRI scanning will not differentiate lymphoma from any other primary or secondary maligancy.

MALIGNANT LYMPHADENOPATHY

When nodal malignancy is present in the neck, the patient is usually known to have a primary tumour (Fig. 15.36). Sometimes, there is no clinically obvious primary malignancy. If the involved node lies in the upper half of the neck, i.e. above the cricoid, it is likely that the malignancy has spread from the pharynx, larynx or parotid glands. Submandibular node involvement is common in squamous carcinoma of the face or oral cavity.

Malignant lymphadenopathy in the lower half of the neck can be the result of carcinoma of the thyroid, oesophagus or breast. However, bronchial carcinoma is the commonest cause of right supraclavicular lymph node enlargement, whereas left supraclavicular lymphadenopathy is more likely to be due to a subdiaphragmatic primary tumour. Lymphoma or metastatic melanoma may involve lymph nodes at any site in the neck (Fig. 15.37).

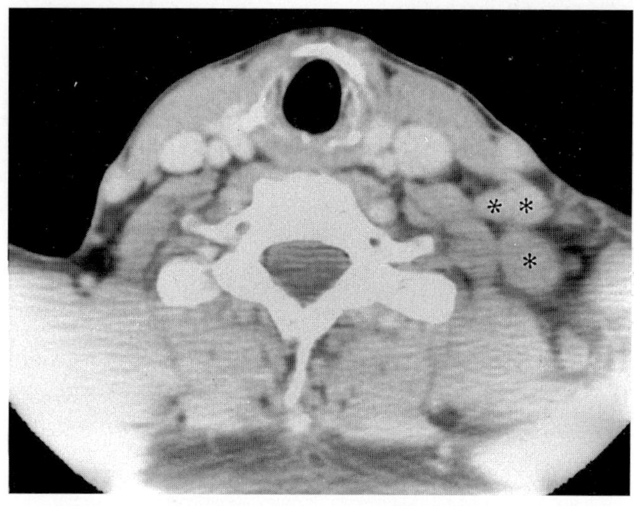

Fig. 15.37 CT scan of malignant lymphadenopathy from melanoma of left forearm. Note several homogeneous enlarged lymph nodes (*) in left lower cervical group.

Although ultrasound can detect nodes as small as 5 mm and can guide a fine-needle aspiration biopsy (Fig. 15.38), contrast-enhanced CT or MRI scanning are better imaging techniques than ultrasound because:

- CT and MRI examine at the same time the likely primary tumour site in the neck. Depending on the clinical presentation, scanning of the thorax and abdomen may also be performed.
- Lymphadenopathy is better demonstrated. Any node with central necrosis, even if <10 mm, is considered malignant.
- CT and MRI assess the deep lymph nodes, e.g. the retropharyngeal group, which are not visualized by ultrasound.

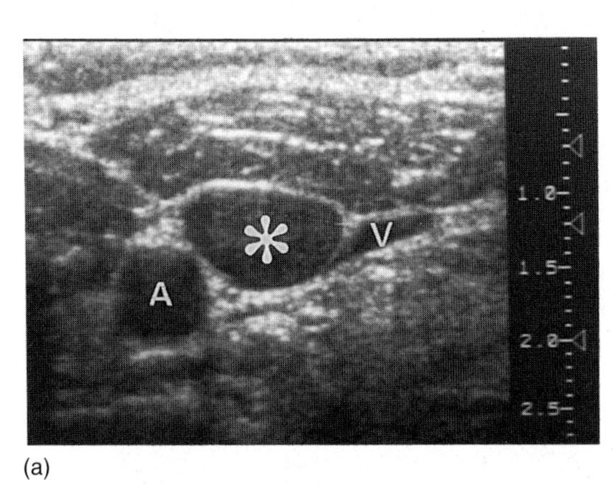

(a)

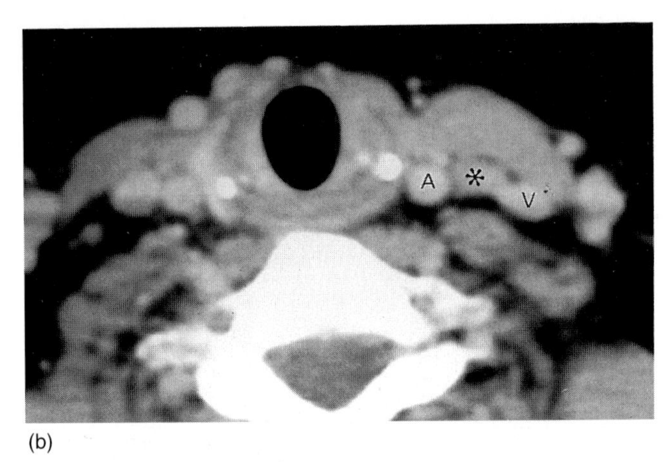

(b)

Fig. 15.38 Enlarged lymph node at cricoid level. (a) Ultrasound and (b) CT transverse scans show node (*) 2.5 cm long, with non-specific appearances. Biopsy indicated squamous cell carcinoma from a nasopharyngeal primary tumour. A=carotid artery; V=internal jugular vein.

Differential diagnosis of lymphadenopathy on CT/MRI

- In reactive lymphadenopathy, i.e. due to adjacent inflammation, the nodes remain homogenous and a nearby inflammatory focus may be demonstrated.
- Suppurative lymphadenopathy, i.e. an intranodal abscess (Fig. 15.39), appears exactly similar to a node with carcinomatous involvement. However, the clinical presentation and demonstration of an inflammatory focus should differentiate between the two.
- Tuberculous lymphadenopathy is usually seen as a mass of nodes matted together and may contain areas of calcification. These appearances are unlike those of malignancy.

Fig. 15.39 Suppurative lymphadenopathy. CT scan with i.v. contrast at hyoid level. Necrotic nodes with ring enhancement and low density centres (N). Note thickening of skin and subcutaneous fat (arrows) due to inflammatory oedema.

Post-treatment scanning

Three months after laryngeal surgery, the patient has a baseline MRI at which time all the postsurgical inflammatory changes should have resolved. Later, if there is recurrence of tumour, this is usually obvious clinically or identified by biopsy. The extent of any submucosal spread of recurrent tumour will require a

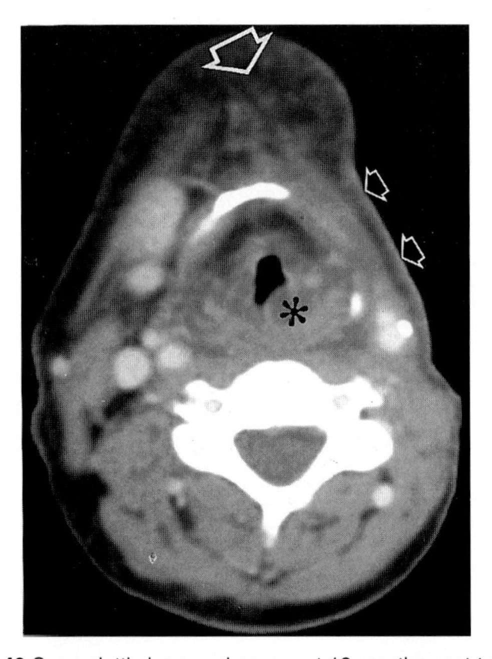

Fig. 15.40 Supraglottic laryngeal cancer at 12 months post-treatment CT scan. Stage T1 N3 tumour treated by left neck dissection and radiotherapy. Scan at thyrohyoid level shows left-sided soft tissue mass (*) in laryngeal vestibule, but endoscopic biopsy showed no tumour recurrence. Note thickening of skin and subcutaneous fat (arrows) due to radiotherapy. Left submandibular gland and sternomastoid muscle have been removed.

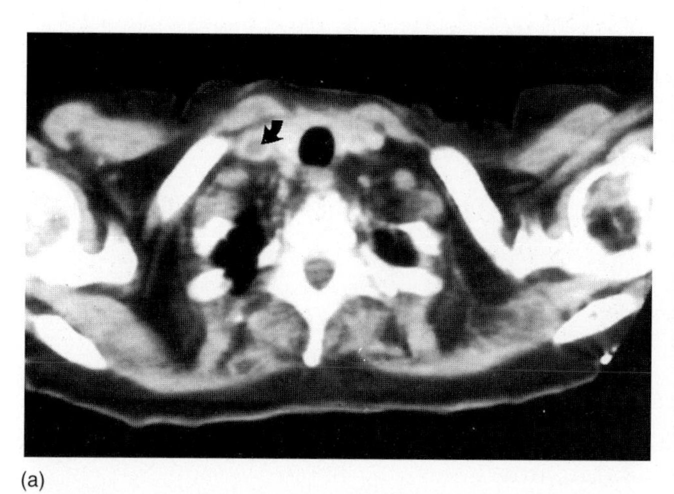

(a)

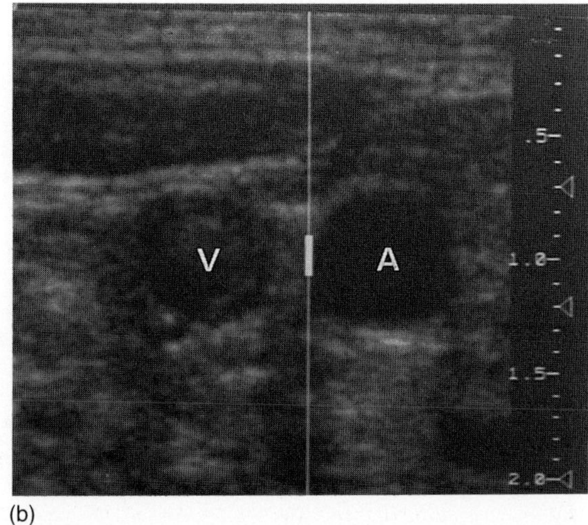

(b)

Fig. 15.41 Thrombosis of right internal jugular vein, complicating supraglottic carcinoma. (a) Contrast-enhanced CT scan. Note distended vein with central low density (arrow) representing thrombus within high density vein wall. (b) Ultrasound scan at same level. Note hyperechoic thrombus totally occluding vein (V). Patent common carotid artery (A) also seen.

repeat MRI scan (T1-weighted with contrast) to compare with the baseline study. Vascular scar tissue has the same appearance as recurrent tumour. Therefore, in doubtful cases, it is often necessary to repeat this scan again in a further 2 months when any tumour recurrence will be obvious.

During a course of radiotherapy, scanning is performed at regular intervals in order to monitor therapy and repeated after the course of radiotherapy has been completed. A major problem is that irradiation causes a generalized thickening of the soft tissues, with loss of fat planes, due to persisting oedema. This can mask or mimic tumour recurrence on MRI or CT images (Fig. 15.40). MRI scanning of the larynx after radiotherapy is only 50% accurate compared with the results of biopsy.

VENOUS THROMBOSIS

Thrombosis of an internal jugular vein is not uncommon and is usually due to compression of the vein by metastatic lymphadenopathy. Other causes of thrombosis of the internal jugular vein include any obstructing mass in the neck or thoracic inlet, an adjacent inflammatory focus and central venous catheterization.

Ultrasound scanning will show clearly the presence and extent of a thrombus and whether it is totally or only partially occluding the vein. A contrast-enhanced CT scan gives less detailed information but will detect a totally occluded vein and will usually better demonstrate the underlying cause of the thrombosis (Fig. 15.41).

CHAPTER 16

Thyroid and parathyroids

Martin L. Wastie

Thyroid disease is common although it is not always diagnosed clinically. The main conditions include hyperthyroidism, hypothyroidism and non-toxic goitre, which are all commoner in females than males. The correct management of thyroid disease depends on an accurate diagnosis.

Hyperthyroidism and hypothyroidism are diagnosed clinically and by the biochemical estimation of the serum levels of tri-iodothyronine (T3), thyroxine (T4) and thyroid stimulating hormone (TSH). Imaging plays no part in the initial diagnosis of hyper- or hypothyroidism. The important role of imaging in thyroid disease is in the investigation of the thyroid nodule, intrathoracic goitre, thyroid eye disease and in the management of thyroid cancer.

THYROID

ANATOMY

The lateral lobes of the thyroid measure 5 cm in length and 2.0–2.5 cm in both thickness and width at their widest diameter. The two lateral lobes are joined by an isthmus of variable thickness that crosses the second and third tracheal rings anteriorly. A third lobe, the pyramidal lobe is sometimes present arising from the isthmus or adjacent portion of either lobe, more commonly the left. There may be asymmetry in the size of the lateral lobes with the right lobe normally being larger than the left. The thin capsule of the gland is connected to the pretracheal fascia outside of which lie the sternothyroid muscles. The gland is fixed to the anterior and lateral aspect of the trachea by connective tissue. The carotid arteries and sternocleidomastoid muscles lie lateral to the gland.

IMAGING TECHNIQUES

PLAIN FILMS

A chest X-ray or views of the thoracic inlet may show a soft-tissue mass due to a goitre in the neck which may be displacing the trachea (Fig. 16.1). An important feature is any compression or narrowing of the trachea. The degree of compression may be judged by assessing the diameter of the trachea on both the frontal and lateral views. The sternoclavicular joints mark the position of the thoracic inlet. Any deviation or compression of the trachea below this level indicates the presence of an intrathoracic or retrosternal goitre. Calcification within a goitre may occur in both benign

Diagnostic and Interventional Radiology in Surgical Practice. Edited by P. Armstrong and M. L. Wastie. Published in 1997 by Chapman & Hall, London. ISBN 0 412 61960 1 (HB), 0 412 61970 9 (PB)

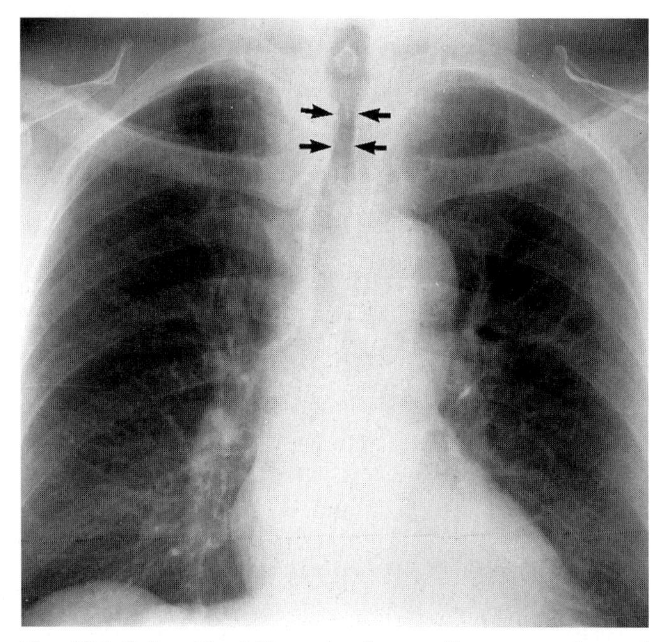

Fig. 16.1 Goitre. Chest X-ray showing a goitre compressing and narrowing the trachea (arrows).

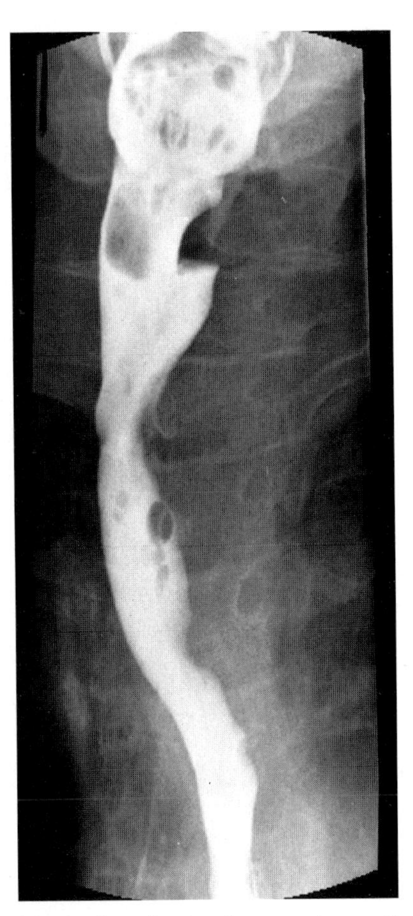

Fig. 16.2 Barium swallow showing the oesophagus displaced to the right by a goitre.

and malignant tumours although any obvious coarse calcification is likely to be benign. Displacement and compression of the oesophagus by a goitre may be demonstrated on a barium swallow (Fig. 16.2).

ULTRASOUND

Ultrasound has now become the most important imaging modality for examining the thyroid. It is easily performed by direct contact scanning with a high frequency (7.5–10 MHz) transducer. The patient lies with the neck extended and the neck is smeared with jelly to ensure acoustic coupling between the transducer and the skin. Ultrasound gives a good demonstration of the isthmus and the lateral lobes lying adjacent to the air-filled trachea with the carotid artery lying lateral to the gland (Fig. 16.3). The gland has a homogeneous pattern due to the numerous follicles and the echo pattern is of higher echogenicity than the adjacent muscles. Images are routinely taken in the axial and sagittal planes. Abnormalities as small as 1 mm in diameter can be detected.

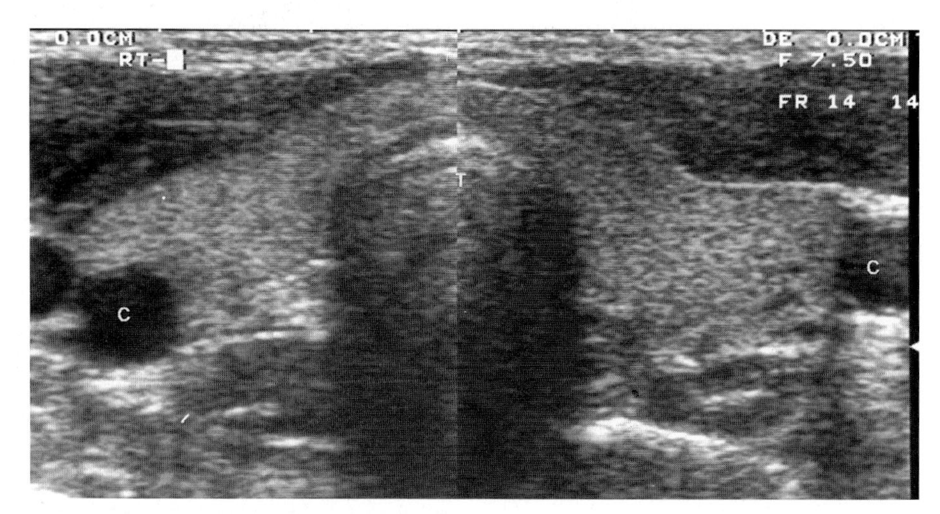

Fig. 16.3 Normal ultrasound. The two lobes of the thyroid lie on either side of the trachea (T). The carotid arteries (C) lie lateral to the gland.

RADIONUCLIDE SCANNING

Scintigraphy has long been the mainstay of thyroid imaging but has to a large extent been replaced by ultrasound scanning, but scintigraphy still has an important role to play. Both ^{99m}Tc pertechnetate and ^{123}I may be used for imaging. The patient is given an intravenous injection of ^{99m}Tc and scans of the neck taken with a gamma camera 20 minutes later. Alternatively scans can be taken 2 hours after an intravenous injection of ^{123}I.

^{123}I is both trapped and organified by the gland whereas ^{99m}Tc is only trapped. ^{123}I gives less background activity and so results in superior pictures of the thyroid compared to ^{99m}Tc but ^{123}I is less readily available and is more expensive. ^{131}I because of its high thyroid and body dose, is used only when investigating patients with known thyroid cancer.

A normal thyroid scan shows homogeneous uptake by the two lobes angled towards each other inferiorly and joined by the isthmus (Fig. 16.4). Any asymmetry of the lobes is easy to recognize.

COMPUTED TOMOGRAPHY

CT is used in selected cases such as determining the spread of malignancy in the neck and demonstrating an intrathoracic goitre. The normal thyroid can be seen as a homogeneous structure with higher attenuation than the adjacent soft tissues, the high attenuation being due to the iodine content of the gland. The thyroid enhances quite markedly after intravenous contrast administration (Fig. 16.5).

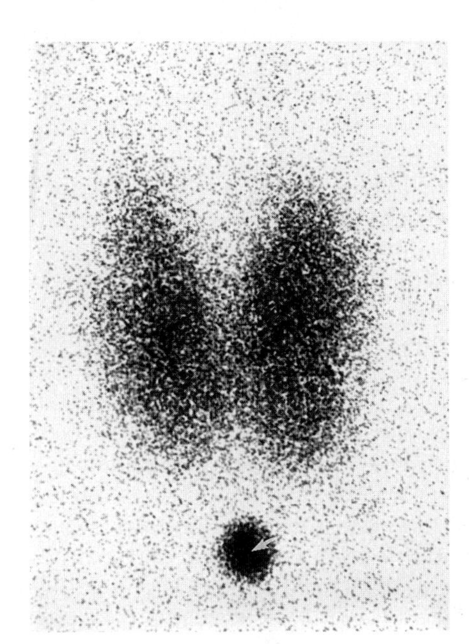

Fig. 16.4 Normal ^{123}I scan. The arrow points to a marker on the suprasternal notch.

MAGNETIC RESONANCE IMAGING

MRI also gives an excellent demonstration of the thyroid (Fig. 16.6), though its role in the management of thyroid disease is not yet clearly defined.

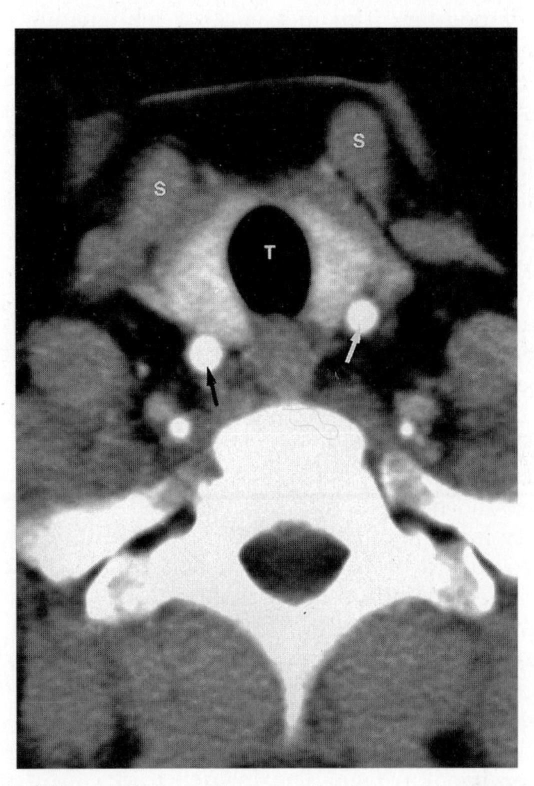

Fig. 16.5 Normal CT scan. The enhancing lobes of the thyroid lie on either side of the trachea (T); the carotid arteries are well opacified (arrows). S = sternocleidomastoid muscle.

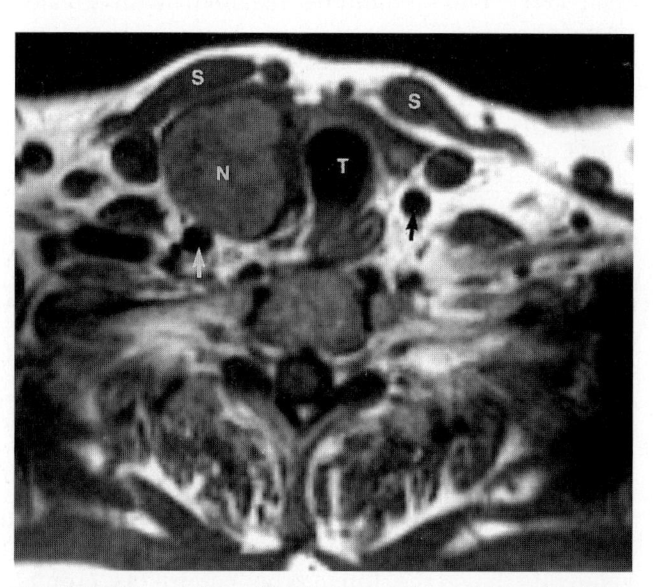

Fig. 16.6 MRI scan. T1-weighted scan showing colloid nodule (N) in the right lobe of the thyroid. T = trachea. S = sternocleidamastoid muscles; arrows = carotid arteries.

THYROID NODULES

The finding of a palpable thyroid nodule is a common clinical problem and is by far the commonest indication for imaging the thyroid. Palpable nodules are found in about 4% of the population with 50% thought to be solitary nodules. The incidence of malignancy in a single nodule is thought to be about 20–30%, so the problem is how to detect this group and avoid unnecessary surgery on the remainder. Different imaging methods have been advocated using both ultrasound and scintigraphy, whilst recently there has been widespread use of fine-needle aspiration cytology which many would regard as the preferred investigation.

The role of imaging is:

- to decide whether a nodule is solitary or multiple;
- to attempt to determine the nature of a solitary nodule;
- to detect a functioning nodule.

Ultrasound is the best initial imaging investigation. Ultrasound may show that a suspected nodule is not solitary but one of several nodules in a multinodular goitre: a third of patients with nodules, thought on clinical examination to be solitary, are shown by imaging to be multiple. The typical nodule has the same echo pattern as the rest of the gland and is recognized by a surrounding lower echogenic zone. There may be a low echogenic cystic component in the nodule due to accumulated colloid, central degeneration or haemorrhage. The incidence of cancer in a multinodular goitre is considerably lower than in a solitary nodule and it has been quoted that ≤ 1% of multinodular goitres are malignant. However, a dominant swelling in a multinodular goitre may indicate malignancy and should be regarded with greater suspicion.

A solitary lesion may be due to an adenoma, colloid nodule, simple cyst, haemorrhagic or degenerating cyst, focus of inflammation or a carcinoma. Ultrasound will go some way to distinguish between these possibilities by showing whether the lesion is solid, cystic or mixed solid and cystic as well as giving information about the edge of the lesion. Simple cysts are rarely malignant. Haemorrhagic cysts may have low level echoes within the cyst. Mixed solid and cystic lesions are mostly benign, due usually to colloid degeneration or degeneration in a follicular adenoma, although cystic degeneration can occur in a carcinoma (Fig. 16.7). Confirmation of the histological nature of the cyst can be obtained by aspiration and cytological examination of the cyst fluid. A problem arises with a solid lesion as ultrasound cannot reliably distinguish between a benign and a malignant mass. Adenomas frequently have the same echo pattern as normal thyroid but may show increased or decreased echogenicity. Carcinomas usually show decreased echogenicity compared to the normal thyroid but the echo pattern alone is not a sufficiently reliable indication to tell whether a nodule is benign or malignant. Even a well-defined edge with a surrounding low echogenic zone around the nodule, the so-called 'halo sign', which was originally thought to indicate a benign lesion, can occur with a carcinoma and is not specific for a benign lesion. An irregular edge suggests a malignant lesion but a definitive diagnosis of malignancy can only be made when there is invasion of adjacent structures and if lymph node metastases are present.

Traditionally **radionuclide scanning** has been used to investigate thyroid nodules although it is now employed much less frequently. The uptake of radioiodine is a reliable index of the rate of secretory activity of the thyroid cells. A cold nodule is one that shows reduced uptake of the radionuclide whilst a hot or functioning nodule shows increased uptake. If the scan shows a solitary cold nodule there is about a 20% probability that the nodule is malignant (Fig. 16.8) but if it is part of a multinodular goitre or if the nodule is hot then the chance of malignancy decreases to a low level (Fig. 16.9). As already mentioned, the probability of malignancy in a multinodular goitre is very much less than for a solitary nodule.

The problem with radionuclide scanning is that although carcinomas normally show as a cold nodule, cysts, adenomas, colloid nodules and foci of thyroiditis also appear as cold nodules. If all cold nodules were excised on the suspicion of malignancy then a large number of unnecessary operations would be performed. Ultrasound is often recommended as the next investigation for characterizing the lesion to see whether it is cystic or solid. If a solitary nodule is hot on a radionuclide scan the likelihood of malignancy is low since functioning nodules are almost all benign; the probability for malignancy is thought to be about 1%.

Some *functioning nodules* appear hot with little or no uptake in the rest of the gland, because the high level of thyroid hormones suppresses the production of thyroid stimulating hormone (TSH) by the pituitary with the result that there is little or no uptake of radionuclide in the normal part of the thyroid gland. A nodule which secretes thyroid hormones independently of TSH control is known as an automonous nodule. There will be no suppression of uptake into the nodule with tri-iodothyromine (T3) on a repeat scan. An injection of TSH stimulates uptake into the suppressed part of the gland. Such a nodule is rarely malignant and is known as a toxic adenoma. If there are multiple nodules the condition is referred to as a toxic multinodular goitre or Plummer's disease.

A hot nodule may rarely be a hypertrophic nodule resulting from thyroiditis. Such a nodule is TSH-dependent and will show suppression with T3.

In the uncommon situation of the patient with hyperthyroidism, who is found to have a thyroid

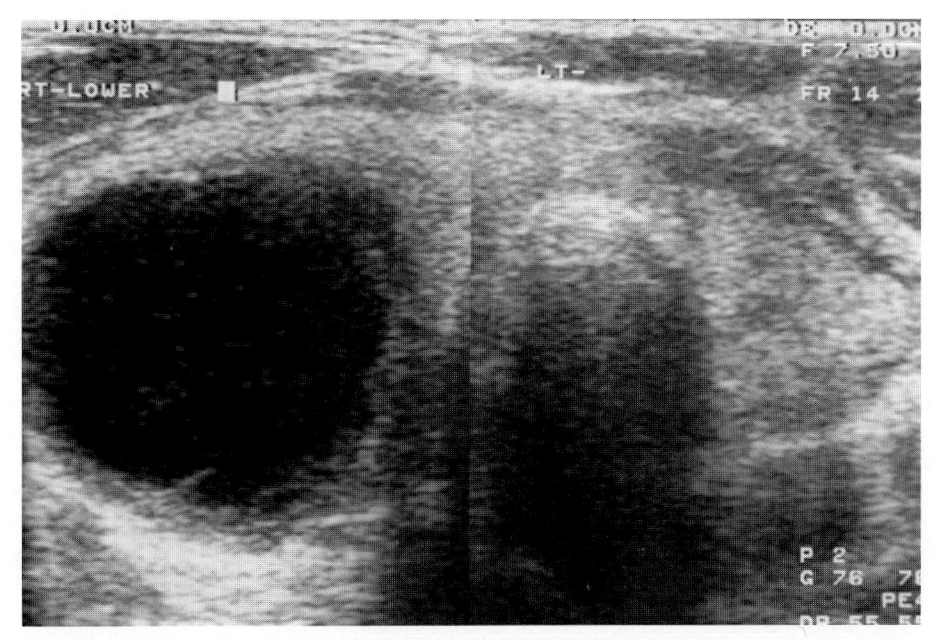

Fig. 16.7a Solitary nodule. Cyst in right lobe of thyroid;

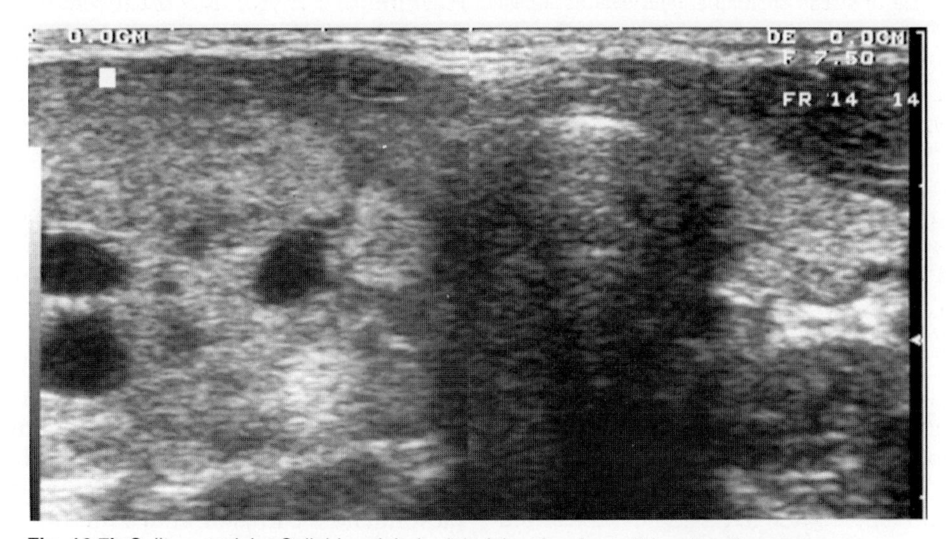

Fig. 16.7b Solitary nodule. Colloid nodule in right lobe showing solid and cystic areas;

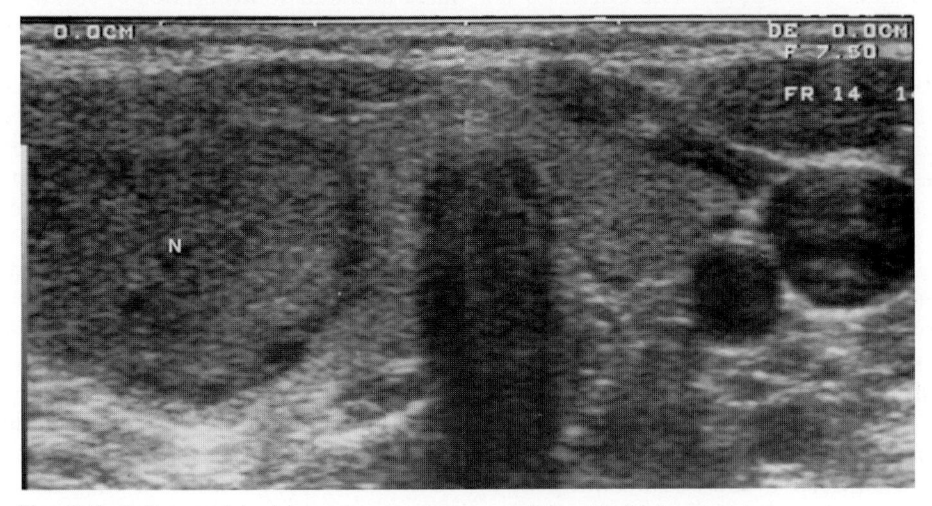

Fig. 16.7c Solitary nodule. Adenoma appearing as a solid nodule (N) in right lobe.

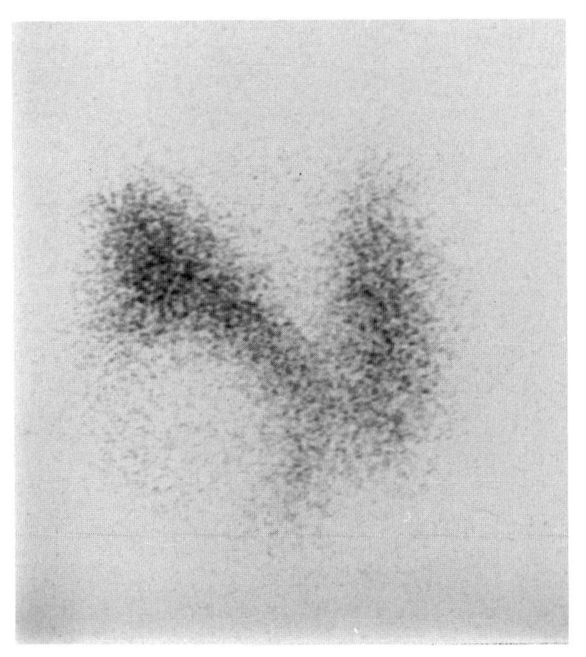

Fig. 16.8 Solitary nodule. ^{123}I scan showing a carcinoma as a cold nodule in the right lobe.

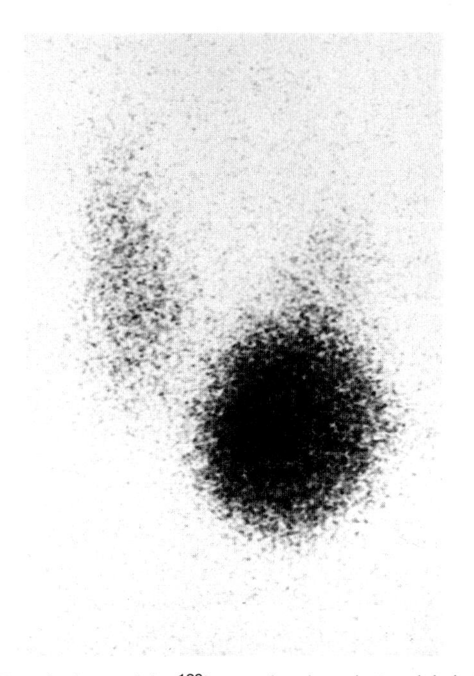

Fig. 16.9 Functioning nodule. ^{123}I scan showing a hot nodule in the left lobe.

nodule, a radionuclide scan will indicate if the nodule is hot and functioning and thus responsible for the hyperthyroidism. If the nodule is non-functioning some other cause such as Graves' disease may be responsible for the hyperthyroidism.

Fine-needle aspiration

Because of the limitations of both ultrasound and radionuclide scanning, the use of fine-needle aspiration for cytological examination has increased considerably over the past few years. The technique is quick, accurate and easy to perform. When fine-needle aspiration yields non-diagnostic results, a not uncommon occurrence, the aspiration is usually repeated. The use of fine-needle aspiration has resulted in a reduction in the number of surgical operations undertaken.

Many centres advocate fine-needle aspiration as the initial investigation of a thyroid nodule because both solid and cystic lesions requires confirmation of the diagnosis.

GOITRE

A goitre is an enlarged thyroid gland which can be due to many causes. Some patients present with hyperthyroidism but many are euthyroid. A clinical history such as iodine deficiency or ingestion of goitrogens may be helpful in making the diagnosis. The age, onset and a family history may suggest Hashimoto's thyroiditis or an enzyme defect. Often the goitre is long-standing but a recent enlargement should raise the suspicion of malignancy.

SIMPLE GOITRE

Simple goitre may be a diffuse hyperplastic (colloid) goitre or a multinodular goitre. Each is thought to represent different stages of the same pathological process and they are the commonest causes of non-toxic goitre.

In a **diffuse hyperplastic (colloid) goitre** there is diffuse uptake of ^{99m}Tc or ^{123}I, whereas in a **multinodular goitre** the uptake is non-homogeneous with discrete areas of reduced uptake. Both types of goitre may show normal or overall reduced uptake of the radionuclide. Ultrasound in a multinodular goitre will show nodules of varying size which may be solid or have a mixed solid/cystic appearance.

X-rays of the thoracic inlet show any tracheal displacement or compression. If there is dysphagia, a barium swallow may demonstrate oesophageal compression. Surgery may be required for a goitre causing tracheal or oesophageal compression. Calcification may be seen in the goitre, particularly in long-standing adenomas, though rarely fine dot-like calcification may be seen within a carcinoma.

Certain complications may arise with a goitre:

- there is a danger of respiratory obstruction due to pressure caused by haemorrhage into a thyroid nodule;
- the possibility of malignancy should be considered in a rapidly enlarging goitre;
- hyperthyroidism may develop in a patient with a long-standing multinodular goitre.

INTRATHORACIC (RETROSTERNAL) GOITRE

A colloid or multinodular goitre may extend downwards into the mediastinum to produce a retrosternal goitre. Invariably, there is a connection between the cervical and mediastinal components of the gland which may sometimes only be a fibrous band or vascular pedicle, but this connection is an important diagnostic feature. Usually an intrathoracic goitre is associated with a palpable enlargement of the thyroid in the neck. Most commonly an intrathoracic goitre is situated in the anterior mediastinum in front of the brachiocephalic vessels but it may occasionally be positioned posteriorly to the trachea. The goitre may be wedged between the oesophagus and trachea or it may extend posterior to the oesophagus. Intrathoracic goitres may cause symptomatic displacement and/or compression of the trachea and oesophagus, but usually they are discovered on a chest X-ray as an asymptomatic mediastinal mass with a well-defined spherical or lobular outline (Fig. 16.10a).

Radionuclide scanning demonstrates that the mass is thyroid tissue and a radioactive marker at the sternal notch confirms the intrathoracic location (Fig. 16.10b). ^{123}I is the agent of choice as the high background activity with ^{99m}Tc prevents satisfactory visualization of an intrathoracic goitre. CT shows the characteristic appearance of thyroid tissue, namely high attenuation values and marked enhancement with intravenous contrast. CT shows the exact position of the thyroid together with any tracheal, oesophageal or vascular compression (Fig. 16.11).

TOXIC GOITRE

Diffuse toxic goitre (**Graves' disease**) is an autoimmune disorder in which an immunoglobulin produced by intrathyroid lymphocytes stimulates the gland to overactivity through TSH receptors on the thyroid cell membranes. Graves' disease is the commonest cause of hyperthyroidism. Usually the diagnosis is made clinically and with the appropriate thyroid function tests without the need for imaging. A ^{99m}Tc or ^{123}I scan will show uniformly increased uptake and this test may be useful in certain cases to distinguish between Graves' disease and the hyperthyroidism occurring in thyroiditis. Ultrasound in Graves' disease shows an enlarged gland with a diffuse hypoechoic pattern (Fig. 16.12).

With a toxic nodular goitre (**Plummer's disease**) one or more hot nodules are seen on the radionuclide scan. On ultrasound these nodules appear as solid or have a mixed solid and cystic appearance.

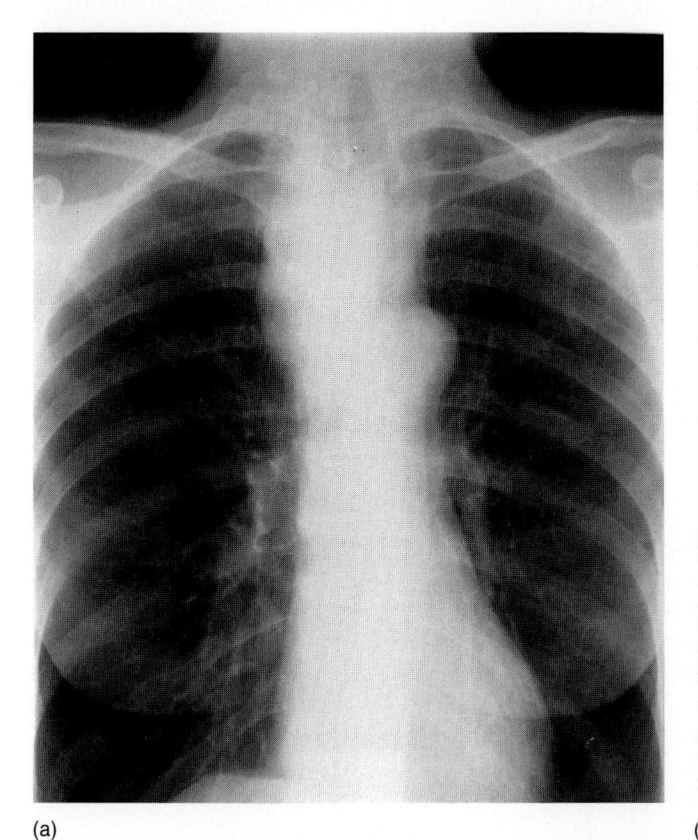

(a)

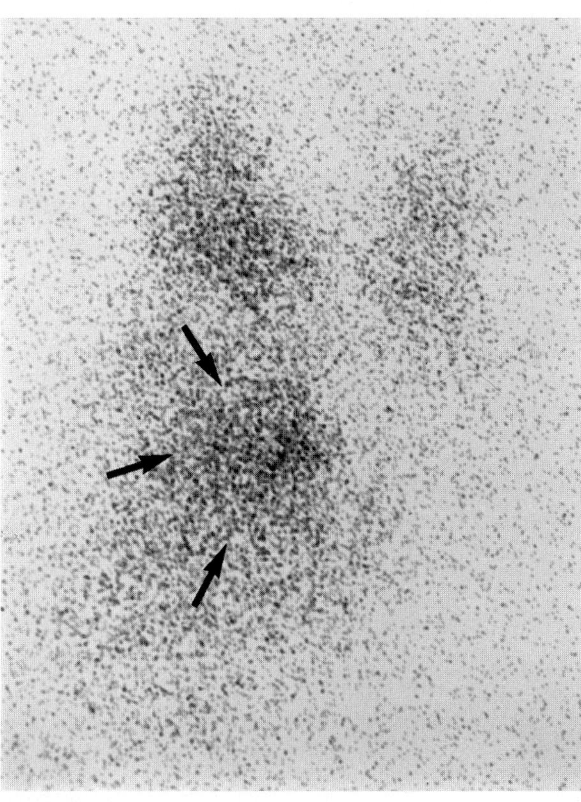

(b)

Fig. 16.10 Intrathoracic goitre. (a) Chest X-ray showing upper right-sided mediastinal mass displacing the trachea to the left. (b) ^{123}I scan showing enlarged thyroid with intrathoracic extension on the right side (arrows).

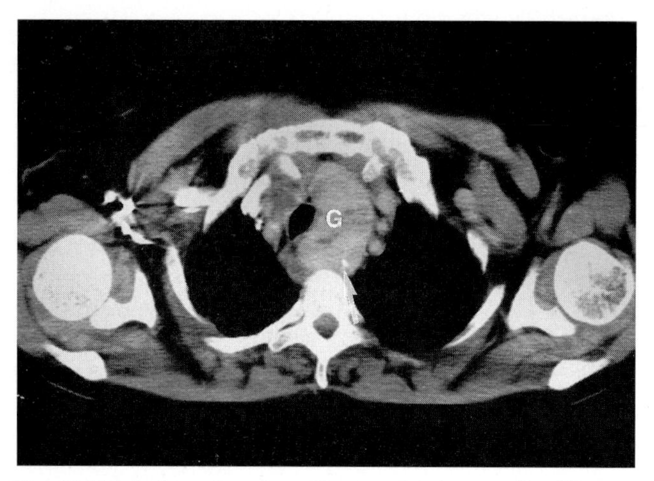

Fig. 16.11 Intrathoracic goitre. CT scan showing a goitre (G) as a mass displacing the trachea to the right. A little calcification is seen within the goitre (arrow).

Thyroid eye disease (ophthalmopathy)

In Graves' disease there may be autoimmune reaction affecting the eye muscles in the orbit which may occur in the absence of clinical or biochemical evidence of thyroid disease. The topic is further discussed on page 430.

THYROIDITIS

Acute thyroiditis is caused by an acute suppurative infection and imaging plays little part except to determine whether an abscess is present.

Subacute thyroiditis, known as **de Quervain's thyroiditis** or granulomatous thyroiditis, is thought to follow a viral infection. Hyperthyroidism may result because of the release of hormones from the damaged gland. A radionuclide scan may show diffusely reduced uptake or focal areas of decreased uptake in the gland.

Hashimoto's thyroiditis (chronic thyroiditis) is an autoimmune destructive disorder causing a goitre and hypothyroidism with positive serum thyroid antibodies. Radionuclide scanning reveals a non-homogeneous pattern and there may be hot or cold nodules present, but scanning alone cannot differentiate Hashimoto's disease from subacute thyroiditis and imaging has little part to play in the diagnosis.

ECTOPIC THYROID

The thyroid is normally situated in the neck but thyroid tissue can be found from the base of the tongue to the mediastinum although mediastinal thyroid tissue almost invariably results from downward extension of a normally situated thyroid. Failure or incomplete descent from its embryological position at the back of the tongue may result in a lingual or sublingual thyroid. This possibility must be considered before a mass at the back of the tongue or upper neck is excised which could result in the necessity of life-long thyroid replacement. The diagnosis of an ectopic thyroid can be readily made with a radionuclide scan with a marker on the suprasternal notch (Fig. 16.13). Any ectopic thyroid tissue and any normal gland will be readily visualized. A thyroglossal cyst, in contradistinction, will show no uptake of the radionuclide as it contains no functioning thyroid tissue.

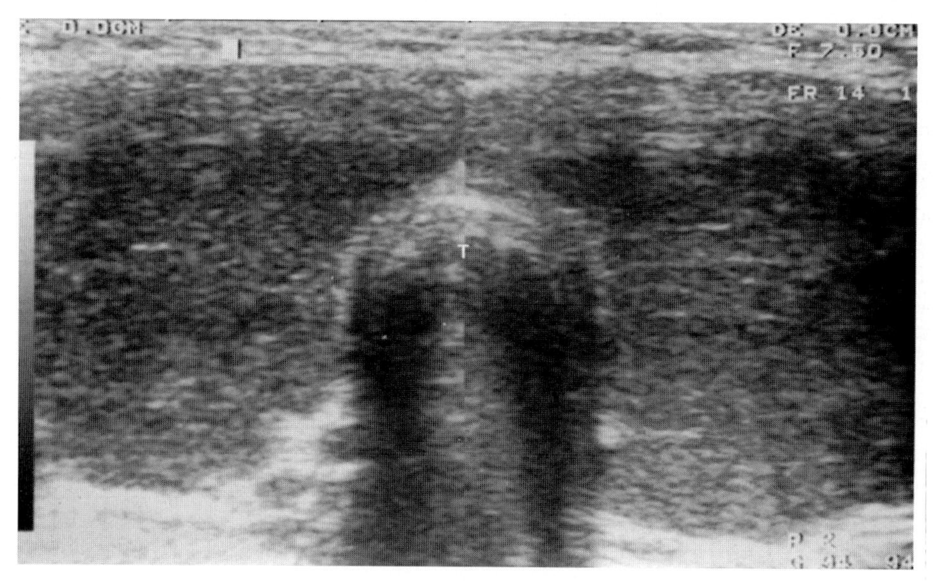

Fig. 16.12 Graves' disease. Ultrasound scan showing a diffusely enlarged gland with a hypoechoic pattern. T = trachea.

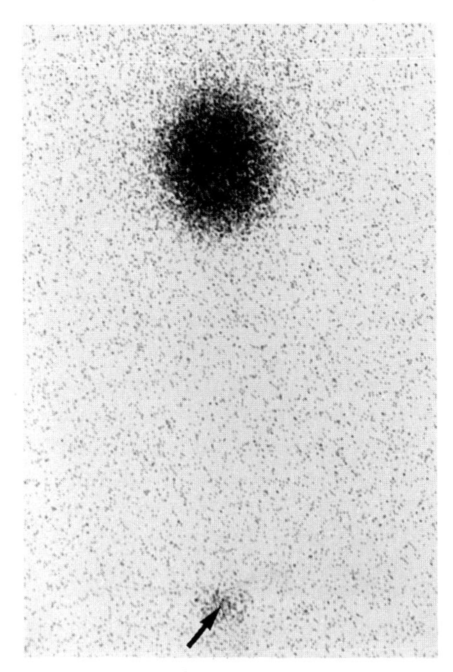

Fig. 16.13 Lingual thyroid. ^{123}I scan showing uptake at the level of the tongue but no uptake in the neck. The arrow indicates a marker on the suprasternal notch.

THYROID CARCINOMA

Thyroid carcinoma may present as a thyroid swelling but at presentation there may be metastases in the lymph nodes, lungs, liver and bone which can be further investigated with conventional X-rays, ultrasound, CT or a radionuclide bone scan.

The management and subsequent imaging depends on the histology of the tumour which is usually classified as papillary, follicular, anaplastic or medullary.

PAPILLARY AND FOLLICULAR CARCINOMA

Papillary and follicular carcinomas are differentiated tumours accounting for 80% of thyroid cancers. As they have some functioning endocrine properties, similar to but less efficient than normal follicles, radionuclide scanning plays a part in their management. The patients often present with a solitary thyroid nodule which characteristically appears as solid on ultrasound and 'cold' on a radionuclide scan. The diagnosis may also be made by fine-needle aspiration cytology or following partial thyroidectomy to remove the nodule. Treatment for a follicular carcinoma is total thyroidectomy but opinions differ as to the treatment for a papillary carcinoma: some surgeons perform a total thyroidectomy while others are content with a partial thyroidectomy. Total thyroidectomy enables the patient to be followed up with ^{131}I scans and further treatment given with a therapeutic dose of ^{131}I if necessary. About 1 month after thyroidectomy a whole body scan using a diagnostic dose of 300 MBq ^{131}I is performed to check for complete ablation of the thyroid and to detect metastases which take up the ^{131}I (Fig. 16.14). Physiological uptake of ^{131}I is normally seen in the salivary glands, stomach, colon or bladder. The uptake in metastases is far less than in the thyroid so metasta-

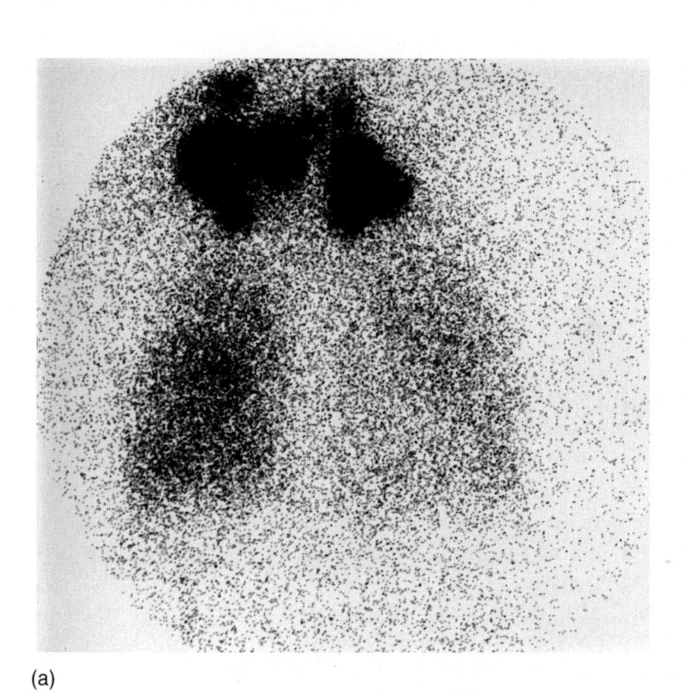

(a)

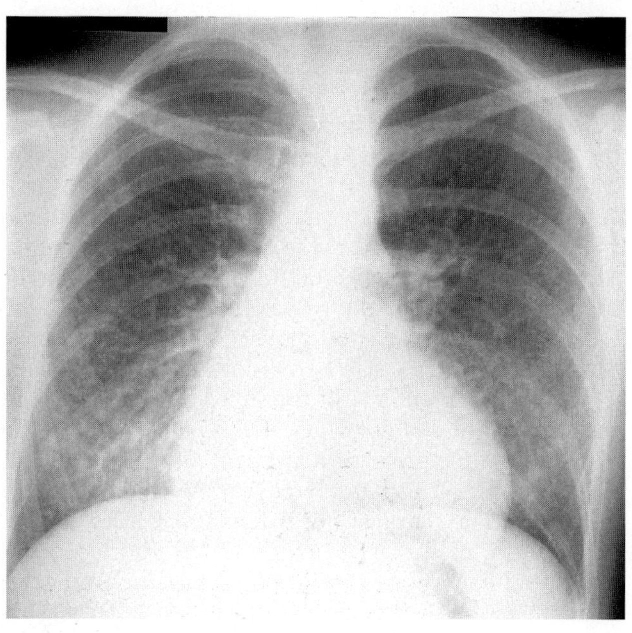

(b)

Fig. 16.14 Carcinoma of thyroid. (a) ^{131}I scan in patient with follicular carcinoma showing uptake in recurrent tumour in the neck and in lung metastases. (b) Chest X-ray showing fine nodular pattern.

ses are detected on a scan only after the thyroid has been ablated either surgically or with a therapeutic dose of ^{131}I. ^{131}I is the radionuclide used for the whole body scan, since its long half-life of 8 days enables sufficient time to elapse between administration and scanning to allow the ^{131}I to accumulate in any metastases.

If residual tumour is present in the neck or if metastases are demonstrated then a therapeutic dose of ^{131}I can be given and the whole body scan repeated every 3–6 months; further therapeutic doses of ^{131}I can be given if necessary. Any pathological uptake may be quantified and if it amounts to > 1% of the administered dose then a further therapeutic dose of ^{131}I is given. When tumour ablation is complete, a follow-up whole body ^{131}I scan may be performed annually. Before any ^{131}I whole body scan is performed, it is essential that the patient stops taking thyroid replacement to allow TSH levels to rise and stimulate ^{131}I uptake into the metastases. T3 should be stopped at least 10 days and thyroxine (T4) 3 weeks before the scan.

ANAPLASTIC CARCINOMA

Anaplastic carcinoma accounts for about 15% of thyroid cancers. It tends to occur in the elderly and has a very poor prognosis. The patients frequently present with lung, liver or bony metastases. This tumour does not concentrate iodine, so radioiodine scanning or treatment with ^{131}I has no part to play in the management.

MEDULLARY CARCINOMA

This tumour arises from the parafollicular or C cells of the thyroid and accounts for about 5% of thyroid cancers. Involvement of the lymph nodes in the neck commonly occurs. The tumour secretes calcitonin which can be measured in the blood. The treatment for medullary carcinoma is total thyroidectomy but as the tumour does not take up iodine, scanning with radioiodine has no part to play in the management of this tumour.

Medullary carcinoma of the thyroid may be part of the **multiple endocrine neoplasm (MEN IIa syndrome [Sipple's syndrome]**) associated with phaeochromocytoma and hyperparathyroidism, either parathyroid hyperplasia or adenoma. Before thyroidectomy for medullary carcinoma is performed, these associated conditions should be excluded by measuring urinary VMA (vanillylmandelic acid) and plasma calcium levels. As the tumour may be inherited as an autosomal dominant condition, screening of the relatives should be carried out.

PARATHYROIDS

Imaging in parathyroid disease is usually performed to detect a surgically amenable abnormality causing primary hyperparathyroidism.

ANATOMY

There are normally four parathyroid glands, two upper and two lower, lying on the posterior aspect of the lateral lobes of the thyroid. Each gland measures 5 mm in length, 3 mm in width and 1 mm in thickness. Some patients have five glands and supernumerary glands are reckoned to occur in 6% of adults, probably arising by division of one or more of the parathyroids during development. The inferior glands develop with the thymus from the third branchial pouch. They migrate caudally and usually settle in the lower poles of the thyroid. Variation in migration results in an ectopic position such as within the thymus, mediastinum or thyroid. The superior glands arise from the fourth branchial pouch; as they migrate little during development they are more constant in position.

HYPERPARATHYROIDISM

Primary hyperparathyroidism occurs when there is elevated serum parathormone, usually caused by a parathyroid adenoma (> 80%) and less commonly by parathyroid hyperplasia (10–15%) or carcinoma (3–4%) or, rarely, from ectopic parathormone produced by a bronchial carcinoma.

Secondary hyperparathyroidism occurs as a response to hypocalcaemia and is most commonly seen in chronic renal failure when the parathyroid glands become hyperplastic. Tertiary hyperparathyroidism occurs when an autonomous adenoma arises following prolonged hypocalcaemia such as untreated malabsorption or chronic renal failure.

IMAGING TECHNIQUES

Once hyperparathyroidism has been diagnosed it is generally agreed that surgical removal of the abnormal gland or glands should be performed in symptomatic patients, in asymptomatic patients with high calcium levels, and in younger patients. There is no consensus as to the precise role of localizing tests prior to neck exploration. An experienced surgeon will localize up to 95% of adenomas at the initial operation by identifying and if necessary biopsying all four parathyroid glands; 90% of cases of primary hyperthyroidism are due to a single adenoma. It has been shown that preoperative localization does shorten the operating time. Preoperative localization is, however, important in those patients undergoing reoperation which is invariably technically much more difficult. Initial surgery may be unsuccessful if there is an ectopic gland in the neck or mediastinum, if hyperplasia has not been recognised or if a fifth gland has not been discovered.

Rarely a parathyroid tumour may cause a palpable mass in the neck and may even indent the oesophagus on a barium swallow but usually parathyroid adenomas are small and impalpable.

RADIONUCLIDE IMAGING

The ^{201}Tl and ^{99m}Tc subtraction technique is frequently used and probably should be the initial test to localize a parathyroid abnormality. Thallium given intravenously will be taken up both by the thyroid and by any hyperactive parathyroid tissue which may be present. The thyroid is visualized with ^{99m}Tc and this image is subtracted from the combined thallium image (Fig. 16.15). Normal parathyroid glands are not visualized so any residual uptake will be in a parathyroid abnormality. The thallium and technetium images are acquired consecutively with a gamma camera and the subsequent subtraction is computer generated. It is important that the patient stays still during the examination so that an accurate subtraction can be performed.

This technique gives good results in localizing adenomas both in normal and ectopic positions (Fig. 16.16) but the results are inferior for the detection of parathyroid hyperplasia in both primary and secondary hyperparathyroidism. False positive results

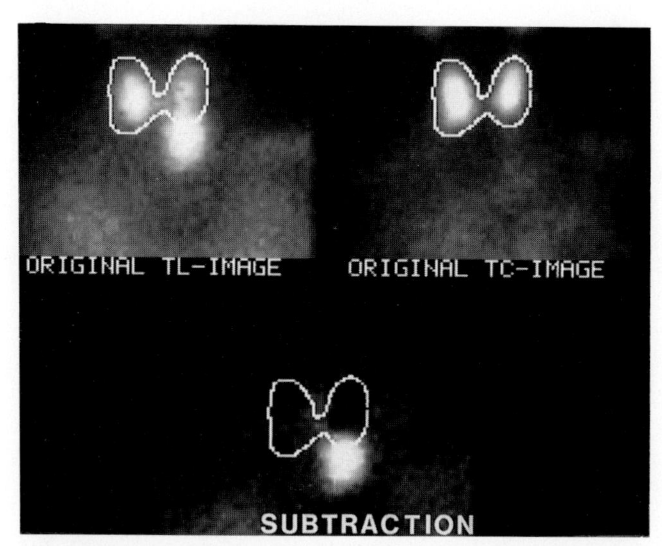

Fig. 16.15 Parathyroid adenoma. Thallium/technetium subtraction scan showing an adenoma of the left inferior parathyroid gland.

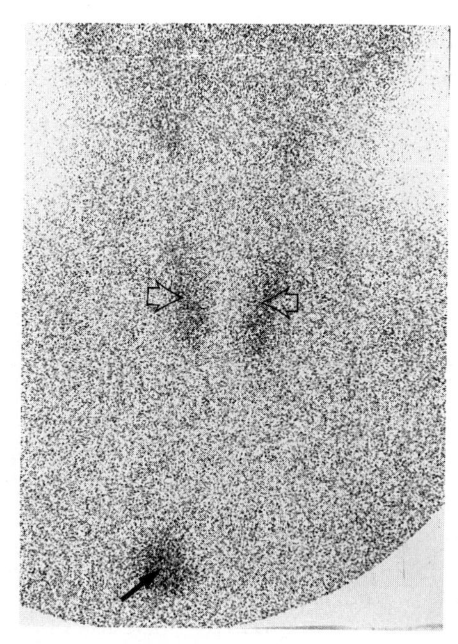

Fig. 16.16 Ectopic parathyroid. Thallium scan showing uptake in a parathyroid adenoma in the mediastinum (arrow). The open arrows point to the lobes of the thyroid.

may occur with coexisting thyroid disease as a thyroid adenoma will trap ^{201}Tl and show reduced uptake with ^{99m}Tc.

A similar subtraction technique can be employed using ^{99m}Tc-sestamibi and ^{123}I to visualize the thyroid.

ULTRASOUND

The neck is scanned using a high frequency 7.5–10 MHz transducer. Normal parathyroid glands cannot usually be identified but an adenoma can be identified as a mass of low echogenicity frequently measuring as much as 1 cm in length and usually lying behind the thyroid in the angle between the trachea and oesophagus. (Fig. 16.17) Hyperplasia can be recognized when all four glands are enlarged in contradistinction to an adenoma which involves one or possibly two glands. Ultrasound has difficulty in demonstrating glands in an ectopic position and cannot show a parathyroid gland in the mediastinum.

Neither ultrasound nor radionuclide scanning can reliably demonstrate small adenomas less than 0.3 g in weight.

OTHER TECHNIQUES

CT can localize a parathyroid tumour and its accuracy is largely dependent on the size of the tumour. CT has the advantage that it can locate tumours in the mediastinum. **MRI** gives excellent soft-tissue contrast and can be used to image the neck, thoracic inlet and mediastinum. It appears to be a technique with great

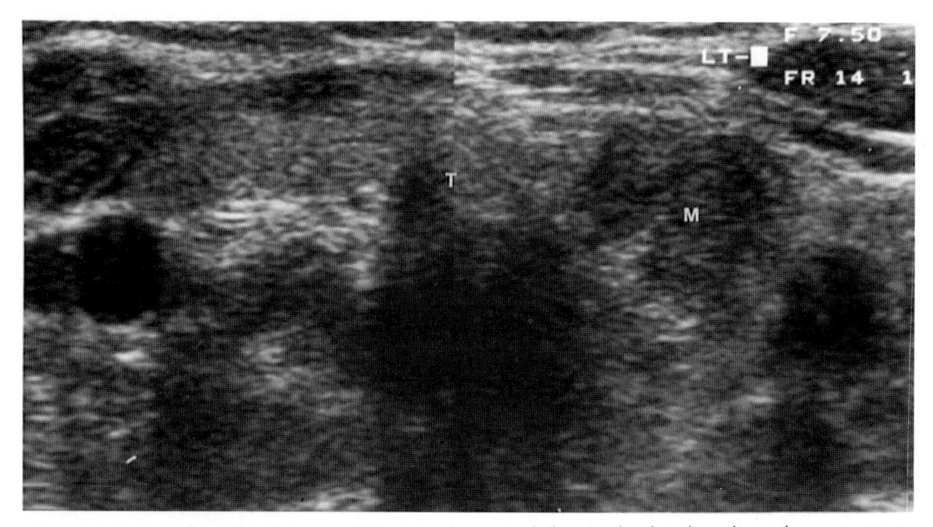

Fig. 16.17 Parathyroid adenoma. Ultrasound scan of the neck showing the adenoma as a hypoechoic mass (M) at the lower pole of the thyroid on the left in the same patient as illustrated in Fig. 16.15. T = trachea.

promise for demonstrating parathyroid abnormalities.

Venous sampling involves introducing a catheter into the neck or upper mediastinal veins via the internal jugular vein or from a femoral vein puncture. Parathormone levels in the blood are measured at various sites in an attempt to localize a hyperactive parathyroid gland. **Arteriography** entails injecting contrast into the carotid or subclavian arteries or their branches to try to demonstrate a parathyroid tumour which may show a vascular blush. Both venous sampling and arteriography are invasive techniques that are only used when other non-invasive methods have failed to demonstrate any parathyroid abnormality.

MULTIPLE ENDOCRINE NEOPLASIA (MEN)

Hyperparathyroidism may coexist with disorders of other endocrine glands. The commonest combination occurs with abnormalities of the pituitary and pancreas known as the MEN I syndrome in which there may be parathyroid adenomas or hyperplasia, a prolactin-secreting or other adenoma of the pituitary and a pancreatic tumour which may secrete gastrin (Zollinger–Ellison syndrome), insulin, glucagon, somatostatin or vasoactive intestinal peptide.

In the MEN IIa syndrome, parathyroid hyperplasia or adenoma may be associated with medullary carcinoma of the thyroid and a phaeochromocytoma.

CHAPTER 17

Maxillofacial region, jaws and salivary glands

James McIvor

Plain films still have an important role in the initial imaging of the maxillofacial region and jaws and are still the best technique for demonstrating pathological conditions limited to the teeth and adjacent bone. Intraoral dental films provide very detailed images of a small area and panoramic radiographic techniques such as orthopantomography will show the whole dentition on a single film. However, CT and MRI are playing an increasingly important role in this region and are of particular value in diagnosing complex fractures and defining the extent and nature of soft tissue lesions.

FRACTURES OF THE MAXILLA

LE FORT FRACTURES

Maxillary fractures are still classified according to the system of Le Fort (Fig. 17.1) who defined three principal patterns of fracture after applying blunt trauma to the faces of cadavers at the beginning of the twentieth century.

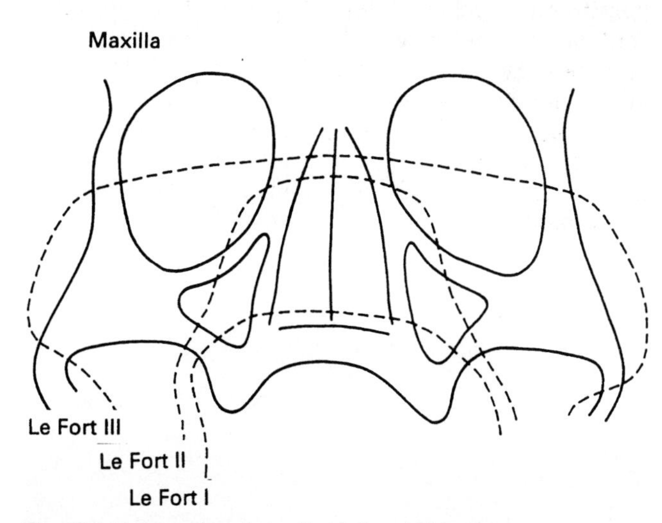

Fig. 17.1 Fracture lines in Le Fort I, II and III fractures

In a Le Fort I fracture the tooth-bearing part of the maxilla becomes separated from the rest of the maxilla by fractures through the medial and lateral walls of the maxillary sinuses, and by a fracture through the lower part of the nasal septum.

The Le Fort II fracture (Figs 17.2, 17.3) is more extensive and the separated fragment is pyramidal. The apex of the pyramid is the lower part of the nasal bones and the fracture lines run inferiorly and

Diagnostic and Interventional Radiology in Surgical Practice. Edited by P. Armstrong and M.L. Wastie. Published in 1997 by Chapman & Hall, London. ISBN 0 412 61960 1 (HB), 0 412 61970 9 (PB)

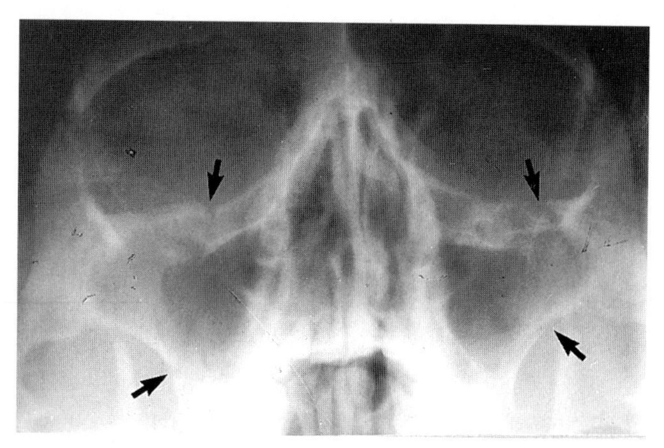

Fig. 17.2 Le Fort II fracture. The fractures of the inferior margins of the orbits and of the lateral walls of the maxillary sinuses can be seen (arrows) but the fracture of the nasal bones is not visible on this projection.

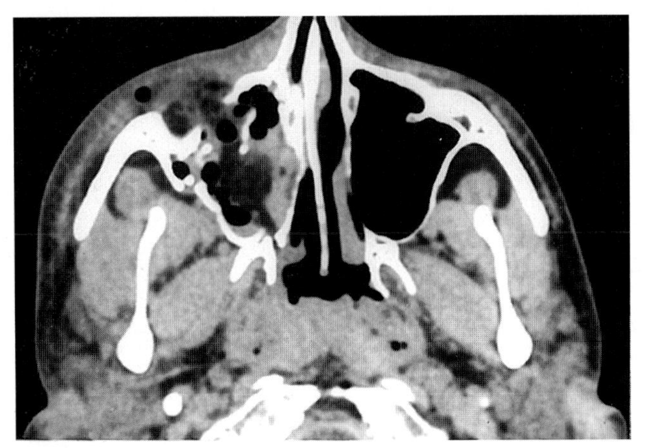

Fig. 17.3 Axial CT of a Le Fort II fracture of the right maxilla. There are fractures of the anterior and postero-lateral walls of the right maxillary sinus.

laterally through the medial and inferior walls of the orbits.

In the Le Fort III fracture (Fig. 17.4a) there is complete craniofacial disjunction. The fracture line runs through the nasal bones as in the Le Fort II fracture, and then posteriorly and laterally through the medial and lateral walls of the orbits, and through the zygomatic arches.

In practice, many fractures do not fit these descriptions exactly. Fractures caused by sharp-edged objects can produce comminuted fractures. Some fractures are unilateral (Fig. 17.3), and a Le Fort I or II fracture may coexist with a Le Fort III. However, the Le Fort classification is still in general use, as it allows these complicated fractures to be described in a few words, and has the additional advantage of grouping the fractures according to the pattern of subsequent surgical management. In Le Fort I and II fractures the detached maxillary fragment is usually wired or plated to the zygomatic arches, but if the arches are fractured, as in a Le Fort III fracture, it may be necessary to resort to a more complicated type of pin and rod fixation to the skull vault (Fig. 17.4b).

FRACTURES OF THE ZYGOMA (Fig. 17.5)

The zygomatic bone contributes to the lateral and inferior margins of the orbit, the lateral wall of the maxillary sinus and the anterior end of the zygomatic arch A fracture of zygomatic bone results in fractures of these regions (Fig. 17.6). It is usually impossible to

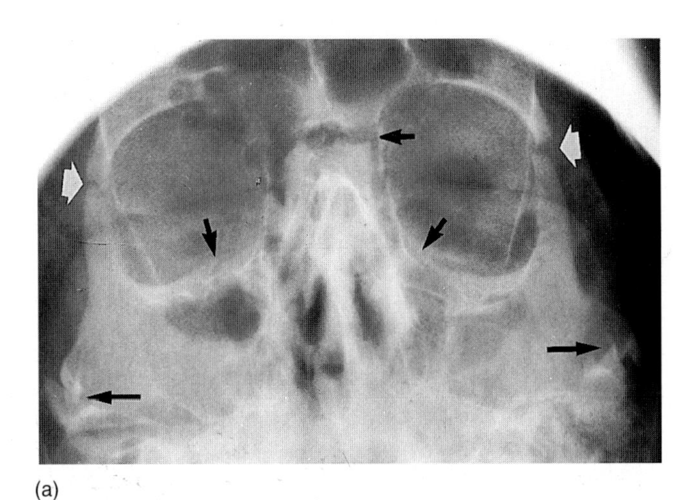

(a)

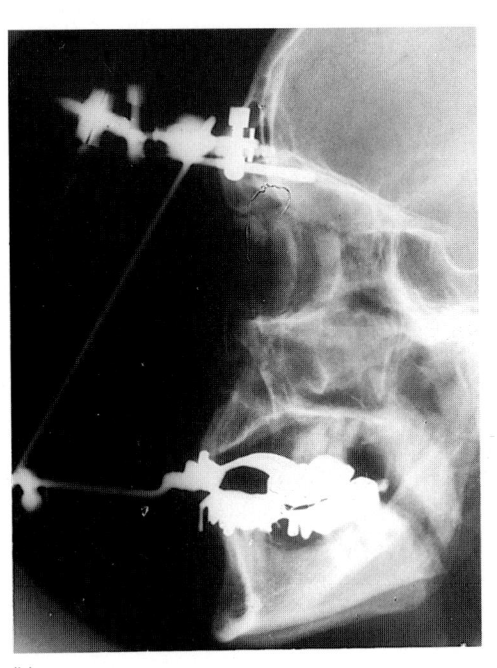

(b)

Fig. 17.4 Combined Le Fort II and Le Fort III fractures. (a) There are fractures of the nasal bones, lateral orbital margins, inferior orbital margins and zygomatic arches (arrows). There is a fluid level in the right maxillary sinus and opacification of the left maxillary sinus. (b) The fracture is reduced using metallic dental splints and interosseos pins in the skull base.

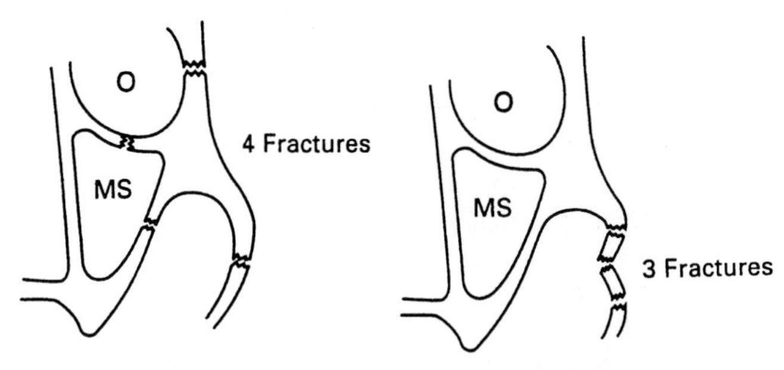

Fig. 17.5 Usual sites of fracture of the zygoma and of the zygomatic arch. 0 = orbit; MS = maxillary sinus.

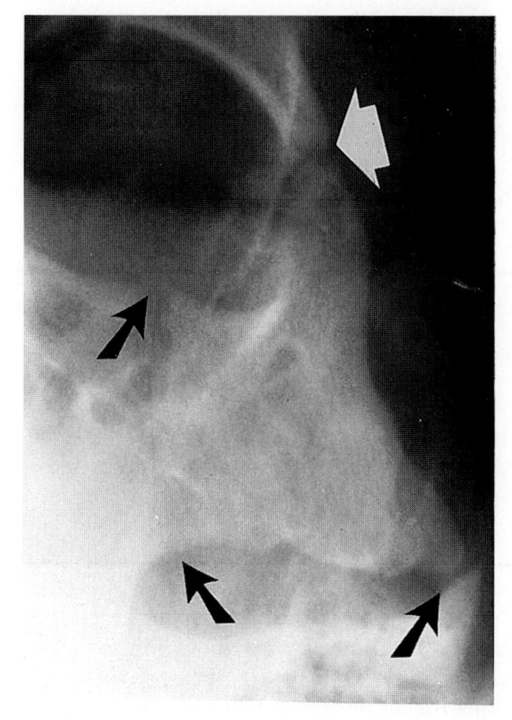

Fig. 17.6 Displaced fracture of the zygoma (black and white arrows).

see all four fractures on a single film but the presence of even one fracture should raise the suspicion that other fractures are present and is an indication for further imaging.

The zygomatic arch may be fractured in association with a fracture of the zygoma as described above, or it may be fractured as a result of direct trauma, when it fractures in three places (Figs. 17.7).

Fractures of the zygoma also occur in Le Fort II and III fractures.

BLOW-OUT FRACTURES OF THE ORBITAL FLOOR

A 'blow-out' fracture of the orbital floor is an uncommon sequel to blunt trauma applied to the front of the orbit. The orbital rim remains intact, but the temporary increase in pressure within the orbit causes the thin floor to fracture and the soft tissues of the orbit to herniate through the defect into the maxillary sinus.

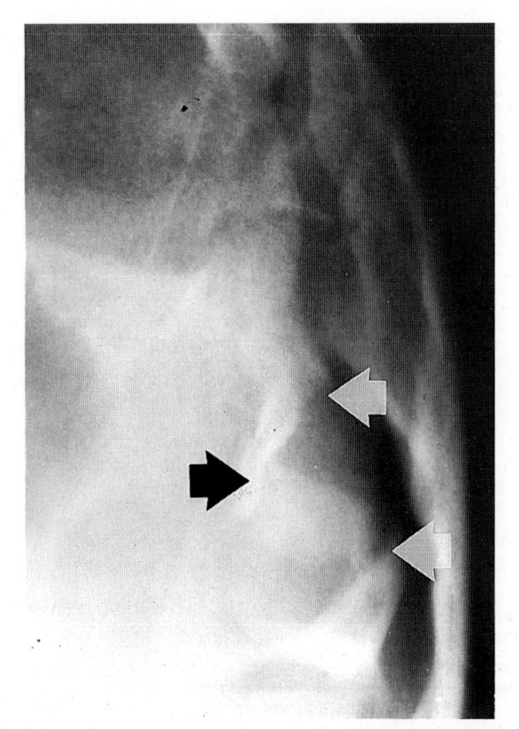

Fig. 17.7 Fracture of the zygomatic arch (arrows).

The herniated orbital contents may show as a soft-tissue shadow in the upper part of the maxillary sinus on a plain radiography, but the fractured bony floor rarely shows. If a blow-out fracture is suspected, coronal CT of the orbital floor is indicated as it will demonstrate soft-tissue herniation and the fractured orbital floor (Fig. 17.8).

The clinical importance of a blow-out fracture is that the inferior rectus and oblique muscles become attached to the orbital floor by fibrous tissue, resulting in permanent limitation of upward rotation of the

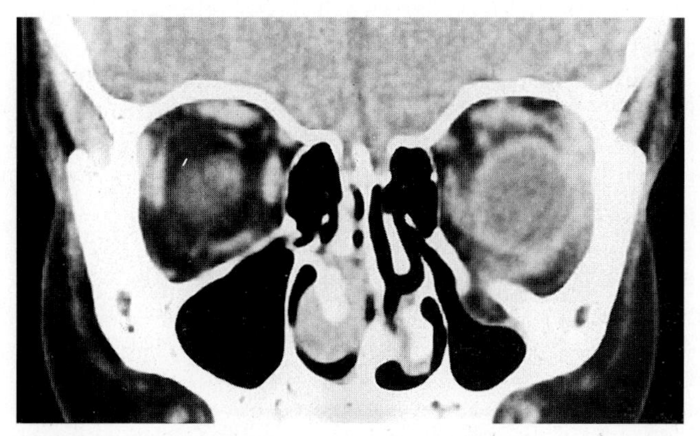

Fig. 17.8 Coronal CT scan showing a blow-out fracture of the floor of the left orbit with posterior displacement of the globe of the eye.

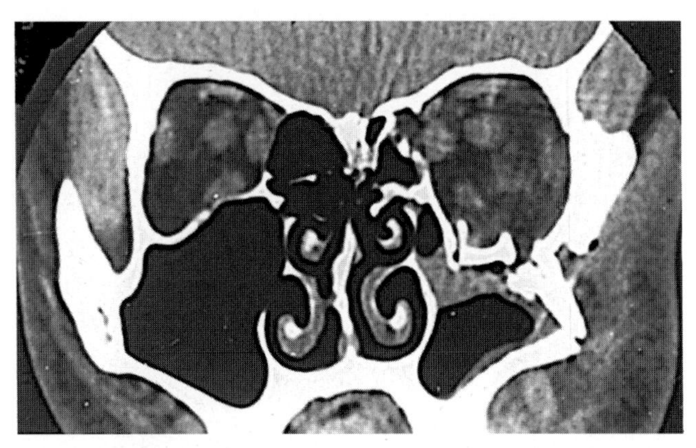

Fig. 17.9 Coronal CT of a comminuted fracture of the left zygoma showing a fracture of the orbital floor and herniation of the orbital contents into the maxillary sinus.

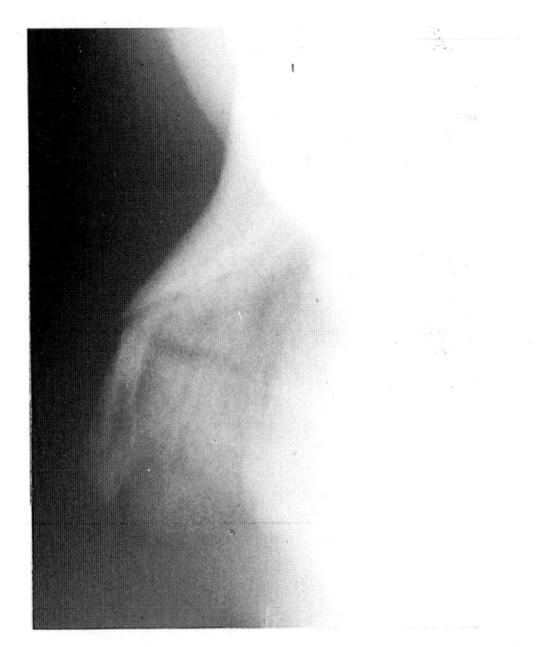

Fig. 17.10 Fracture of the nasal bones on a lateral radiograph.

eyeball and permanent diplopia on looking upwards. The changes are best shown by coronal MRI imaging.

Fractures of the orbital floor can occur in association with Le Fort II and III fractures and with zygomatic fractures (Fig. 17.9).

RADIOLOGICAL INVESTIGATION OF MAXILLARY FRACTURES

The initial radiographic investigation of a patient with a suspected fracture of the maxilla should be limited to three films: a standard occipito-mental, a 30° occipito-mental and a lateral film centred on the maxilla. These films may provide the diagnosis but further imaging is often necessary.

Recent undisplaced or 'crack' fractures may be difficult or impossible to demonstrate even on plain films of the highest quality and one should be very cautious about 'excluding' a recent, undisplaced fracture on the basis of a normal plain film examination.

Fractures of the nasal bones which occur in Le Fort II and III fractures are best shown on standard lateral films of the nasal bones (Fig. 17.10).

Fractures of the teeth and alveolar bone show most clearly on non-screen intraoral dental films.

Computed tomography (CT) is indicated if the fractures cannot be satisfactorily demonstrated on plain radiographs or if there is a discrepancy between the clinical findings and the fractures shown on the plain films.

Axial slices parallel to the occlusal plane of the teeth are convenient for detecting maxillary fractures as slices in this plane can be repeated at a later date and artefacts produced by metallic dental restorations will be limited to a few slices. Thin slices of 2 mm at 5 mm intervals are adequate in most cases.

Direct coronal slices at right angles to the occlusal plain demonstrate fractures of the orbital floor more clearly than axial slices but coronal views suffer from the disadvantage that the neck has to be fully extended and this may not be possible in elderly, uncooperative or recently injured patients.

Three-dimensional CT reconstruction is a very elegant technique demonstrating fractures of the facial skeleton and can provide an excellent overview of a complex fracture (Fig. 17.11). The main disadvantages are that a high quality reconstruction requires the patient to remain completely immobile for 10–20 slices and the radiation dose is about twice as high as a standard CT examination of the same region.

INDIRECT SIGNS OF MAXILLARY FRACTURES ON PLAIN RADIOGRAPHS

Soft-tissue swelling and opacification of the maxillary sinus are two radiological abnormalities which are often due to maxillary fractures, but which may occur in other conditions. Thus, their presence in patients with a history of facial trauma should increase the suspicion that a fracture is present, and should be an indication for furtner films.

Soft tissue swelling is a common and non-specific sign which is almost invariably present if there is a recent fracture.

Opacification of the maxillary sinus is usual in fractures which involve its wall (Le Fort I, II and III fractures, zygomatic fractures) and a fluid level is occasionally seen (Fig. 17.4a). Both these abnormalities should suggest haemorrhage into the sinus.

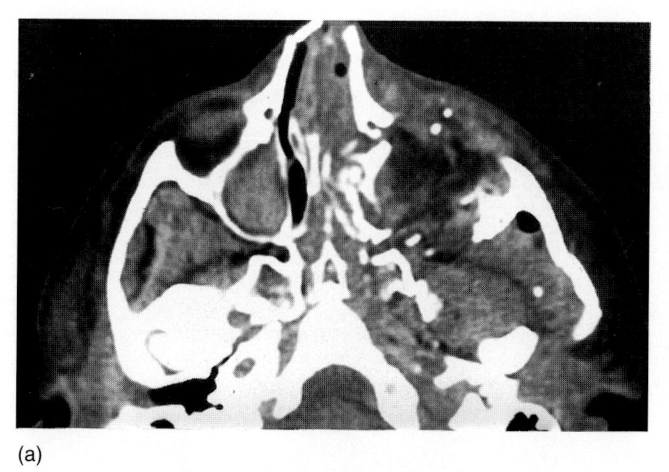

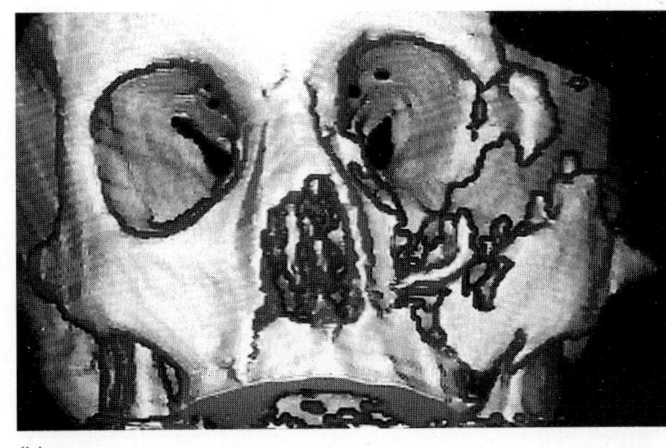

(a) (b)

Fig. 17.11 (a) Comminuted fracture of the left zygoma on axial CT. There are multiple fractures of the anterior, postero-lateral and medial walls of the maxillary sinus. (b) Three-dimensional CT reconstruction of the left zygoma.

FRACTURES OF THE MANDIBLE

CLASSIFICATION

Fractures of the mandible are classified according to the site of fracture. The most common sites are the condylar neck (Fig. 17.12), the ramus (Fig. 17.13), the angle (Fig. 17.14) and the body (Fig. 17.15), but fractures can occur elsewhere. Pathological fractures secondary to tumours (Fig. 17.15), osteomyelitis (Fig. 17.31, p. 408) and large cysts are uncommon but do occur.

Undisplaced fractures of the body and angle are classified as being 'vertically favourable' if the fracture line runs inferiorly and anteriorly, as the muscles

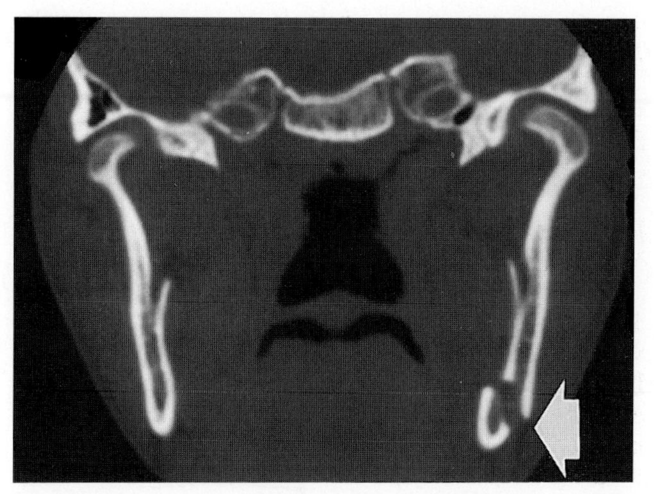

Fig. 17.13 Fracture of the ramus of the mandible on coronal CT (arrow).

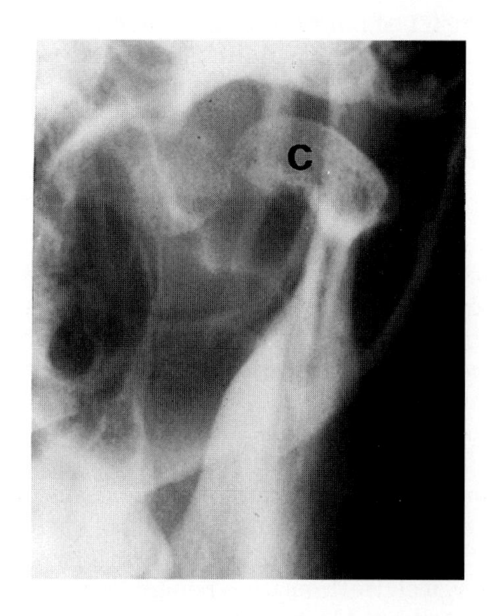

Fig. 17.12 Fracture of the condylar neck of the mandible on an AP radiograph showing displacement of the condyle (C) of the mandible out of the glenoid fossa.

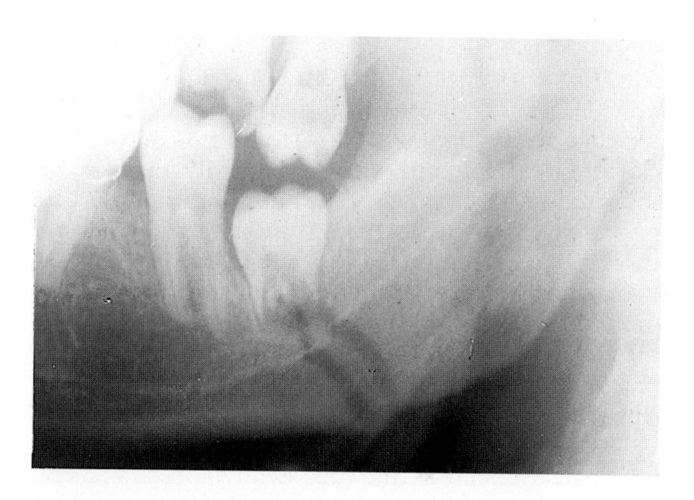

Fig. 17.14 Vertically unfavourable fracture through the angle of the mandible. The two radiolucent lines represent fractures through the inner and outer plates.

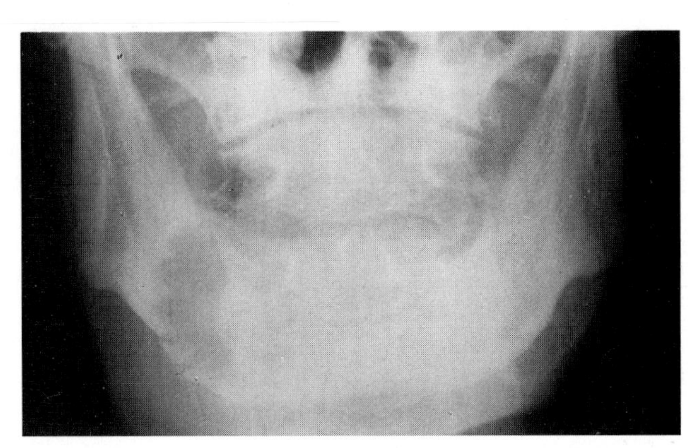

Fig. 17.15 Pathological fracture of the right side of the mandible secondary to carcinoma of the oral mucosa that has extended into the mandible.

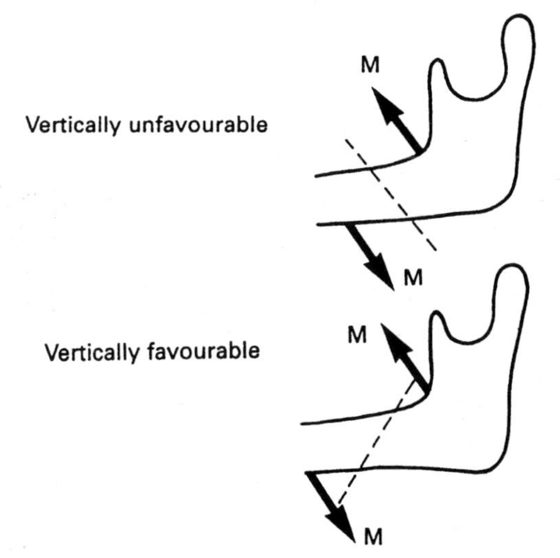

Fig. 17.16 Fracture lines in vertically favourable and unfavourable fractures of the body of the mandible (M). Arrows indicate the direction of muscle pull on the anterior and posterior fragments.

attached to the fragments tend to pull them together. Conversely, a fracture running inferiorly and posteriorly is described as vertically 'unfavourable', as the fragments tend to be pulled apart by the muscles inserted into them (Fig. 17.16).

Fractures through the tooth-bearing part of the mandible are almost invariably compound into the mouth but, despite this, osteomyelitis is very rare unless the patient is immunologically compromised (Fig. 17.17).

The mandible is commonly fractured at two sites, as the bone is U-shaped and held firmly at both ends by the capsules of the temporomandibular joints. A fracture of the body on one side is often accompanied by a fracture of the condylar neck on the other.

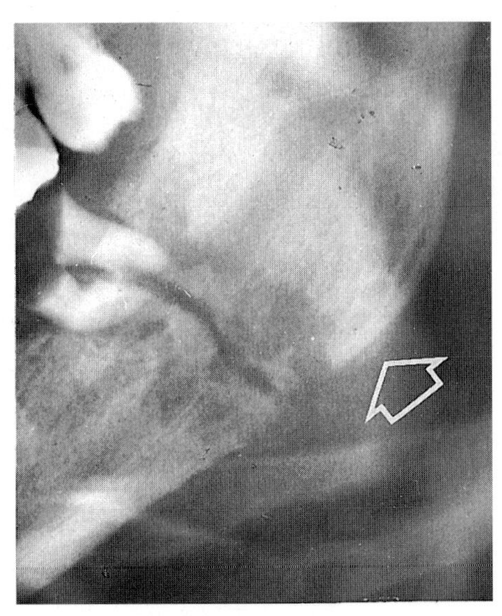

Fig. 17.17 Osteomyelitis following a vertically unfavourable fracture of the angle of the mandible. There is bone rarefaction around the fracture lines and subperiosteal new bone formation (arrowed). The patient was HIV positive.

RADIOLOGICAL INVESTIGATION OF MANDIBULAR FRACTURES

Recent, undisplaced fractures of the mandible can be difficult to demonstrate and may not show on plain films until some days after the injury, when there will be some resorption at the fracture site. The initial films should consist of a postero-anterior view of the facial bones, plus oblique views of the injured side of the mandible. If the patient is able to cooperate, a panoramic radiograph of the mandible should also be taken.

Coronal CT should be used to demonstrate undisplaced fractures of the mandibular ramus and condyle that may be impossible to demonstrate on plain films (Fig. 17.13).

BENIGN CYSTS

Benign cysts of the jaws differ pathologically from benign cysts in other bones as they are usually of dental origin. Cysts are common lesions which usually present when they rupture into the oral cavity and become infected.

In general, benign cysts and tumours displace the roots of adjacent teeth without resorbing them, but malignant tumours often resorb the roots of teeth. Benign cysts can become very large before they present clinically.

The surgical treatment of benign cysts is usually curettage, followed by primary closure, but large cysts are occasionally marsupialized into the oral cavity. As in other bone lesions, the final diagnosis depends on a

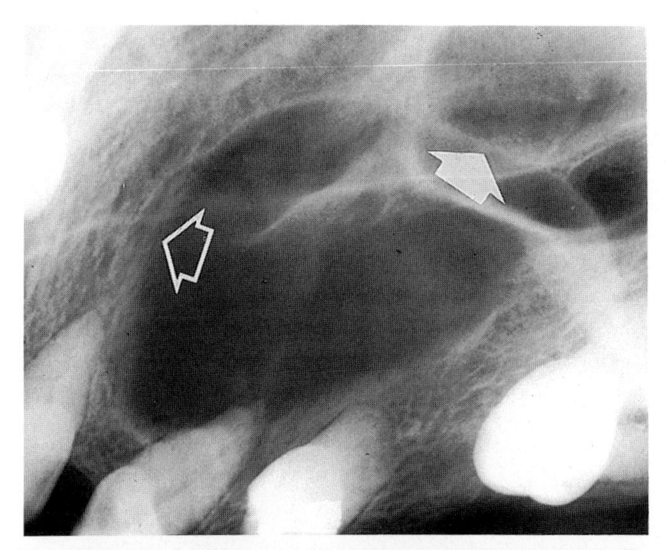

Fig. 17.18 Apical dental cyst arising from an upper canine tooth. The cortical margin of the cyst has been partially destroyed anteriorly (open arrow) by infection but is intact posteriorly (solid arrow).

combination of the clinical, radiological and histological features.

A dental cyst (periodontal cyst) is the most common cyst of the jaws, and accounts for almost half of all radiolucent jaw lesions. It develops at the root apex of a non-vital permanent tooth, and can present at almost any age above 18 years (Fig. 17.18). Large cysts expand the cortical outline of the maxilla or mandible, and maxillary cysts may expand into the maxillary sinus (Fig. 17.19). Some cysts appear multilocular radiologically, but they are always unilocular at operation.

A **residual dental cyst** (residual periodontal cyst) is an apical or lateral dental cyst that was left behind when the tooth from which it developed was extracted. It is, therefore, more common in the older age groups (Fig. 17.19).

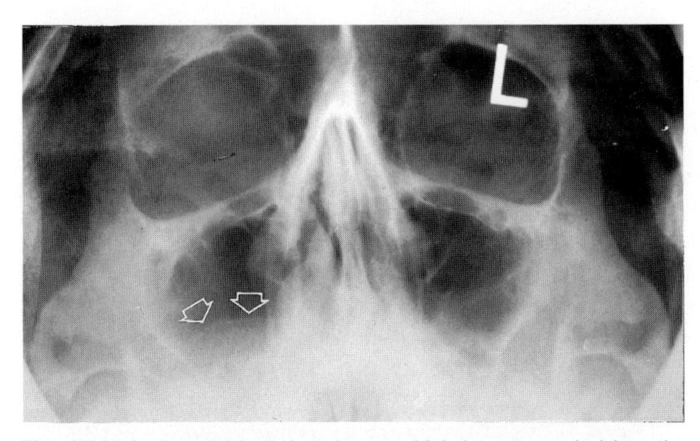

Fig. 17.19 Large residual dental cyst which has expanded into the right maxillary sinus. The radiopaque line at the upper margin of the soft-tissue shadow (arrows) indicates that the lesion has originated outside the maxillary sinus and expanded into it.

A **dentigerous cyst** develops from the enamel-forming tissue (enamel organ) of a developing permanent tooth. These cysts usually present during the second decade and commonly develop around the crowns of lower third molars (Fig. 17.20). The cortical outline is continuous in the absence of infection. Adjacent teeth are often displaced, but their roots are rarely resorbed. Dentigerous cysts can become very large and may develop a multilocular appearance on plain radiographs. However, they are always unilocular at operation.

An **incisive canal cyst** (nasopalatine cyst) arises within the incisive canal of the maxilla. The diagnosis can be made with some confidence if the diameter of the incisive canal measures > 20 mm and should be suggested if the diameter is > 15 mm. These cysts usually present as painless, palatal swellings.

A **globulomaxillary cyst** is an uncommon fissural cyst which develops at the junction between the premaxilla and maxilla, where it appears as a radiolucent area between the roots of the lateral incisor and the canine teeth.

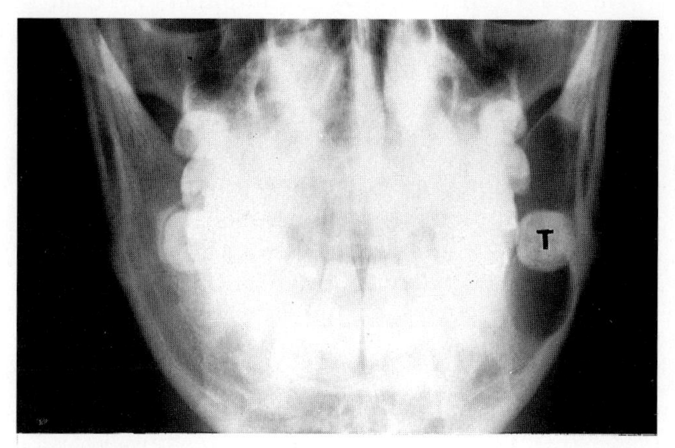

Fig. 17.20 Dentigerous cyst around the crown of an unerupted lower third molar tooth (T).

Odontogenic keratocysts (primordial cysts) occur most commonly in the ramus of the mandible, and are often associated with a missing lower third molar. However, keratocysts can arise from any tooth-bearing part of the jaws. The diagnosis depends entirely upon the histological appearance of the lining, which consists of a thin layer of keratinized, stratified, squamous epithelium. Microscopic daughter cysts are occasionally seen beyond the bony margin of the main cyst, and this may account for the high rate of recurrence about 10–20% after simple curettage. Multiple odontogenic keratocysts are a feature of Gorlin's syndrome.

The **non-epithelial bone cyst** (solitary bone cyst, haemorrhagic bone cyst, traumatic bone cyst, unicameral bone cyst) is always located in the body of the mandible below the premolar and molar teeth. They are rare lesions which are usually discovered incidentally in young adults. These lesions should not really be classified as cysts, as they have no epithelial lining. The pathology is uncertain and it has been suggested that they are bone infarcts. There are a few reports of untreated 'cysts' resolving completely on follow-up radiographs.

BENIGN TUMOURS

Benign tumours of the jaws are rarer than benign cysts. The radiological abnormalities produced by benign tumours are similar to cysts, but tumours are more likely to be multilocular and are more likely to resorb teeth.

The **giant cell tumour** (osteoclastoma) is an uncommon tumour of the jaws, and like giant cell tumours elsewhere, usually occurs in adults between 20 and 40 years. Radiologically it appears as an expanding multilocular lesion with a scalloped margin. Recurrence after excision is common.

The **giant cell reparative granuloma** is peculiar to the jaws and has the same radiological features as a giant cell tumour (Fig. 17.21). However, it occurs in a younger age group (10–25 years) and, although it grows more rapidly than a giant cell tumour, it rarely recurs after removal.

Ivory osteomas and **osteochondromas** occasionally arise from the maxilla and mandible, and have the same features as in other bones (Fig. 17.22). Multiple ivory osteomas are a feature of Gardner's syndrome.

The **chondroma** is a rare tumour of the maxilla, that usually develops after the age of 40 years. It appears as an area of bone destruction and often erodes the roots of teeth without displacing them. Complete excision is difficult, and recurrence is common.

The **fibromyxoma** is a rare tumour of children and young adults, and appears radiologically as a multilocular expanding lesion.

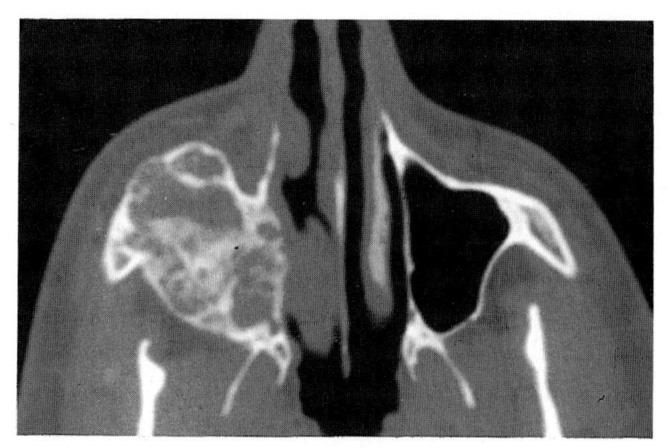

Fig. 17.21 Giant cell reparative granuloma of the right maxilla on axial CT showing the typical multilocular appearance.

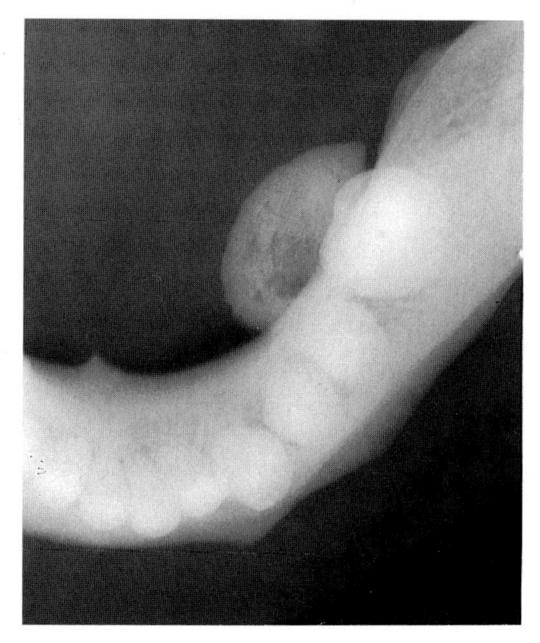

Fig. 17.22 Benign 'ivory' osteoma arising from the lingual plate of the mandible.

Haemangioma of the mandible is an extremely rare tumour that appears radiologically as a multilocular radiolucency (Fig. 17.23), with occasional ring opacities in the soft tissues due to calcified phleboliths. It is important to diagnose haemangiomas as they can result in torrential haemorrhage if teeth are extracted from the affected bone, and the diagnosis should always be considered for any multilocular radiolucent lesion in the mandible.

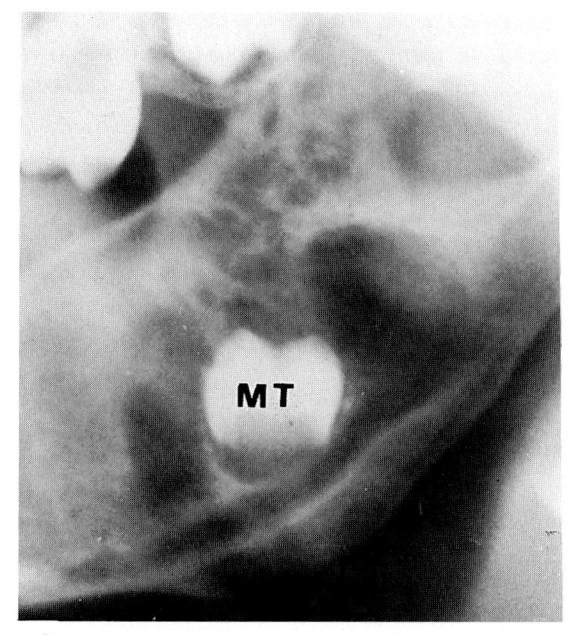

Fig. 17.23 Haemangioma of the body and ramus of the mandible in a child aged 6 years. The developing second molar tooth (MT) has been displaced posteriorly.

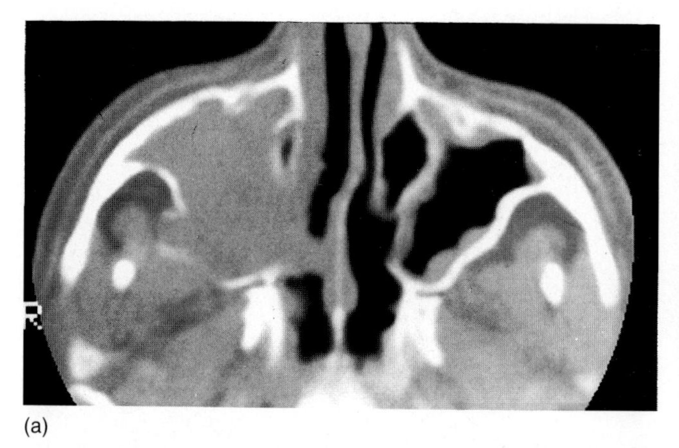

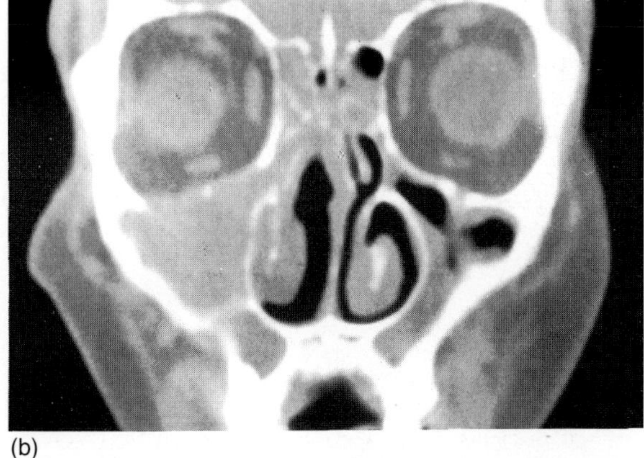

(a) (b)

Fig. 17.24 Ameloblastoma of the right maxilla. (a) Axial CT shows the tumour has extended through the postero-lateral wall of the sinus into the infratemporal fossa and through the medial wall of the sinus into the nasal cavity. (b) Coronal CT shows tumour extension into the maxillary sinus and the ethmoid sinuses on both sides, and destruction of the bony floor of the right orbit. (Courtesy of Dr Otto Chan, The Royal London Hospital, London.)

A **neurilemmoma** or **neurofibroma** occasionally arises from the inferior dental nerve, and may cause widening of the inferior dental canal.

Fibromas, lipomas and **ganglioneuromas** may rarely develop in the maxillofacial region.

AMELOBLASTOMA

Ameloblastoma (adamantinoma) is a remarkably well-known tumour despite the fact that it accounts for only 1–2% of tumours in the maxillofacial region. Radiologically it appears as an expanding multilocular radiolucent lesion, that may erode the roots of adjacent teeth.

Recurrence is common after simple curettage, so the tumour should be removed along with a margin of apparently normal bone. These tumours are slow growing and can reach an enormous size. Ameloblastoma is a locally invasive tumour and its behaviour has been compared to basal cell carcinoma. Pulmonary metastases have been reported in a few cases. Large tumours are best shown by CT (Fig. 17.24).

Ameloblastomas usually present in early adult life, but can occur at any time after the age of 12 years.

NON-NEOPLASTIC BONE LESIONS

An **odontome** is an abnormal growth of calcified dental tissue, which behaves like a hamartoma rather than a neoplasm and stops growing when the individual stops growing.

A complex composite odontome is a mass of enamel, dentine and cementum which shows as a dense radiopacity with an irregular but clearly defined margin (Fig. 17.25). Sometimes there are small radiolucencies within this radiopaque mass due to small cysts.

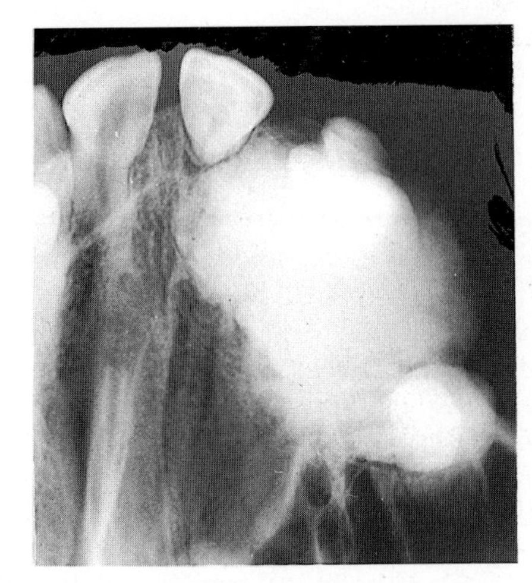

Fig. 17.25 Complex composite odontome in the upper premolar and molar regions which appears as a very dense radiopacity with a well-defined lobulated margin.

A compound composite odontome is a mass of small 'denticles', most of which contain enamel, dentine and cementum (Fig. 17.26). It is more commonly situated anteriorly than posteriorly. Multiple compound composite odontomes have been described in association with Gardner's syndrome.

Dilated composite odontomes and germinated composite odontomes are abnormally formed teeth.

Fibrous dysplasia in the maxillofacial region is usually monostotic but can be a feature of polyostotic fibrous dysplasia or of Albright's syndrome. Fibrous dysplasia is more common in the maxilla than the mandible, and presents as painless bony swelling, usually in adolescence.

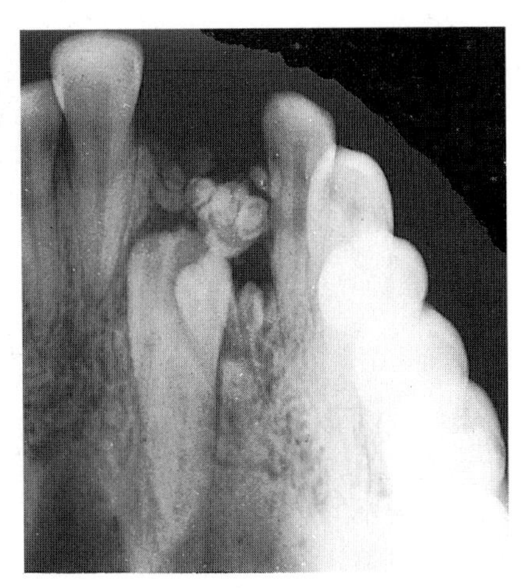

Fig. 17.26 Compound composite odontome in the incisor region. It appears as a mass of 'denticles' or small deformed teeth and has delayed the eruption of an upper first incisor tooth.

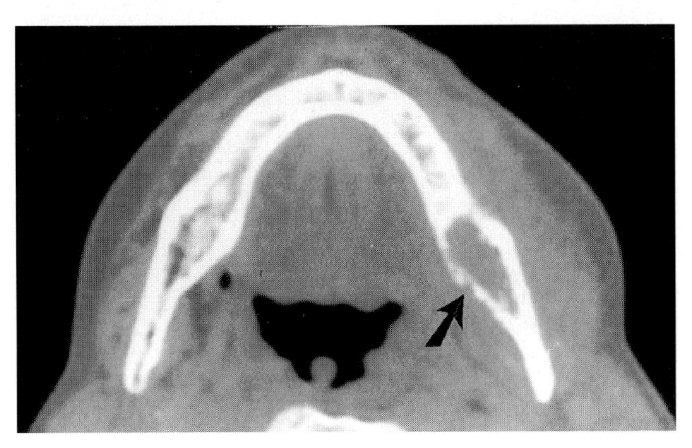

Fig. 17.27 Carcinoma of the left mandibular ramus on axial CT showing irregular destruction of the medial cortex (arrow), destruction of trabecular bone and marked soft-tissue swelling laterally.

Fibrous dysplasia begins as an expanding radiolucent lesion. Sclerotic areas soon develop within the radiolucency and gradually enlarge and coalesce until there is dense, homogeneous opacification of the expanded bone, sometimes described as a 'ground-glass' appearance.

CT shows generalized expansion of the affected bone with thickened irregular trabeculae plus sclerotic and radiolucent areas.

The teeth in the affected bone are often displaced. The eruption of developing teeth is usually delayed or prevented.

Paget's disease can affect the maxilla and the mandible and is usually bilateral. In most cases it is preceded by Paget's disease of the skull vault. As in other bones, the radiological features are bone expansion with a coarse trabecular pattern. Areas of dense bone sclerosis may develop, and masses of radiopaque cementum may develop adjacent to the roots of teeth (**hypercementosis**).

MALIGNANT TUMOURS

Carcinoma is the most common malignancy of the maxillofacial region and usually presents in the middle-aged and elderly, with pain, anaesthesia and loosening of teeth. Most tumours are squamous cell carcinomas or adenocarcinomas. The carcinoma usually arises from the oral mucosa, but occasionally develops within the mandible or maxilla.

Radiologically, carcinomas are purely destructive and there is little evidence of bone expansion or of subperiosteal new bone formation. The margin of the lesion is irregular (Fig. 17.27) and erosion of the roots of teeth is common.

Osteogenic sarcoma is the most common malignant tumour of the jaws in young adults, and usually presents between the ages of 15 and 30 years, with pain, local anaesthesia and loosening of the teeth. Radiologically it appears as an ill-defined area of bone destruction, often associated with resorption of the roots of adjacent teeth and with thickening of their periodontal membranes. In a few cases, sclerosis is more marked than bone destruction, and these tumours are said to have a slightly better prognosis. However, the most striking bone abnormality is the presence of subperiosteal new bone, which may have a lamellar (onion-skin) or spiculated (sun-ray) appearance (Fig. 17.28a). Histologically the tumour is always much more widespread than the bone abnormalities suggest and MRI is currently the best technique for demonstrating extension into the soft tissues (Fig. 17.28b, c).

Metastatic carcinoma rarely affects the maxillofacial region, but when it does the primary tumour is usually situated in the breast, bronchus, colon or kidney. Radiologically there may be a single ill-defined area of bone destruction, or multiple coalescing radiolucent areas scattered throughout the maxillofacial bones. Occasionally a single metastasis lodges in the inferior dental canal and widens it.

Multiple myeloma may produce multiple radiolucencies in the mandible in the absence of similar radiolucent areas of the skull vault.

Burkitt's lymphoma of the maxilla and mandible is very common in some parts of Africa, where it affects children of all ages. Radiologically it is a highly destructive lesion, usually accompained by massive soft tissue swelling, with patchy radiolucencies, destruction of the cortex, resorption of the lamina dura and destruction of the developing teeth.

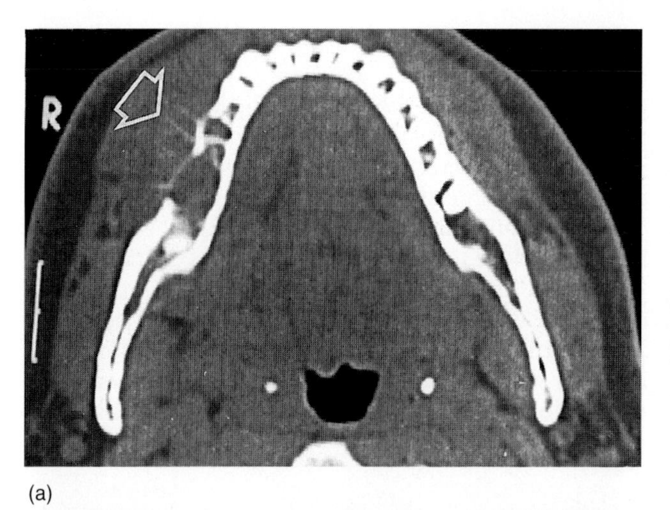

(a)

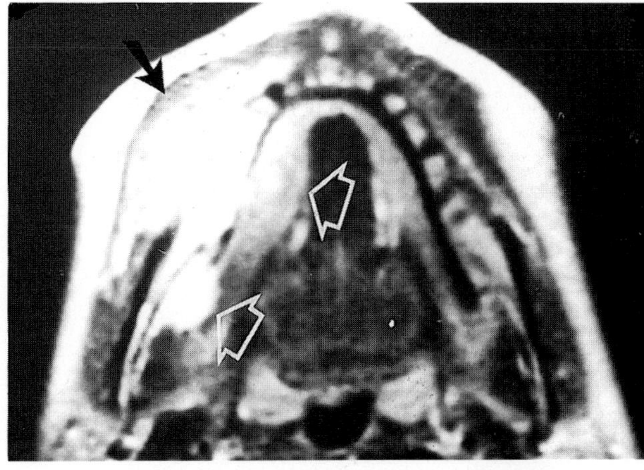

(b)

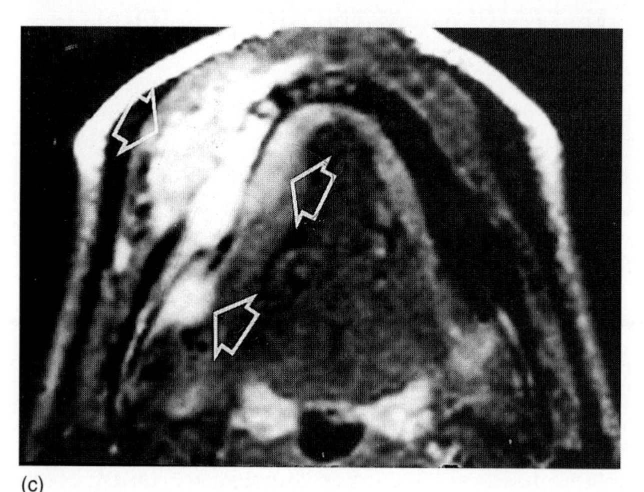

(c)

Fig. 17.28 Osteogenic sarcoma of the right mandible. (a) Axial CT shows bone destruction in the molar region and new bone formation ('sun-ray' spiculation) in the soft tissues laterally (open arrow). (b) On T2-weighted axial MRI, the high signal areas medially and laterally indicate soft-tissue extension (open and closed arrows) but a high signal is also produced by fat. (c) On fat-suppressing STIR sequence axial MRI the high signal areas medially and laterally (open arrows) indicate soft-tissue tumour extension. (Courtesy of Dr Otto Chan, The Royal London Hospital.)

INFECTION

A **dental alveolar abscess** results from bacterial infection spreading from the pulp of a tooth through the root apex into the periapical bone. The earliest radiological change is widening of the radiolucent periodontal membrane around the tooth root and this is followed in a few days by localized rarefaction of the periapical bone and bone destruction (Fig. 17.29).

Pyogenic osteomyelitis of the mandible is usually precipitated by local conditions, such as a dental abscess or a fracture. Considering the frequency of dental alveolar abscess, osteomyelitis is surprisingly rare. The infecting organism is usually a staphylococcus.

Acute osteomyelitis in children may complicate severe infections such as measles and typhoid, and is presumably a blood-borne infection. Acute osteomyelitis may also be a complication of local pyogenic infections such as tonsillitis. The incidence of infection is higher after radiotherapy (osteoradionecrosis, see below) and in HIV-positive patients (Fig. 17.17).

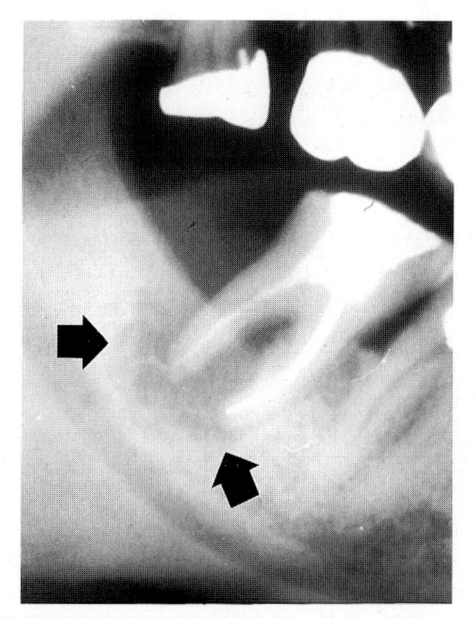

Fig. 17.29 Dental alveolar abscess (arrows) around the root apices of a root-treated lower molar tooth.

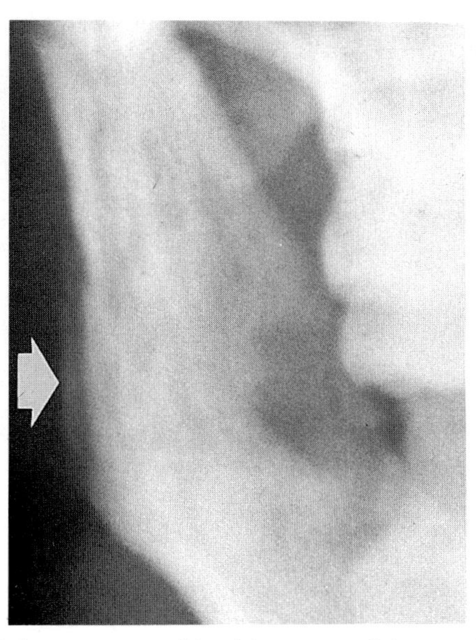

Fig. 17.30 Acute osteomyelitis of the ramus of the mandible with a periosteal reaction laterally (arrow).

As in other bones, the radiological features do not appear until the clinical symptoms of pain, tenderness and soft-tissue swelling have been present for some days. The earliest change is an ill-defined area of bone rarefaction which rapidly progresses to more extensive bone destruction. Subperiosteal new bone formation develops in most cases (Fig. 17.30). Sequestra are inevitable, unless the appropriate antibiotic is given early, and appear as opacities lying in cavities. A pathological fracture may occur if the mandible is seriously weakened (Fig. 17.31).

Chronic osteomyelitis may follow acute osteomyelitis and has similar radiological features, with patchy osteoporosis, patchy sclerosis and sequestra lying in cavities. Subperiosteal new bone is a relatively uncommon feature.

Garré's osteomyelitis (subperiosteal sclerosing osteomyelitis) presents as a tender bony swelling and often responds to antibiotics and conservative surgery.

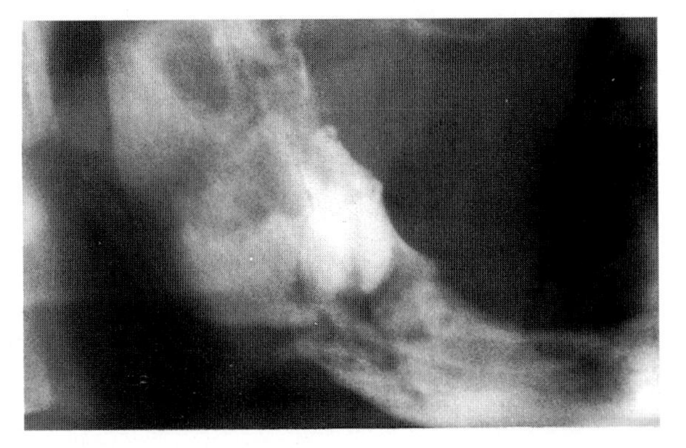

Fig. 17.31 Chronic osteomyelitis around an infected unerupted tooth with a pathological fracture through the angle of the mandible.

The dominant radiological feature is the formation of dense subperiosteal new bone. There is sometimes patchy sclerosis in the underlying bone and, rarely, patchy rarefaction and sequestrum formation.

Osteoradionecrosis is the name given to a particularly intractable form of chronic osteomyelitis, that can occur following radiotherapy. Radiotherapy itself rarely produces any radiological change in the bone pattern of the maxilla or mandible, but very high doses occasionally result in rarefaction or sclerosis. The radiological abnormalities produced by this infection are widespread patchy sclerosis, with areas of rarefaction and multiple sequestra.

THE TEMPOROMANDIBULAR JOINT

The temporomandibular joint is a synovial joint, divided into upper and lower compartments by a fibrocartilaginous disc. These compartments may communicate through acquired disc perforations.

INTERNAL DERANGEMENT

The fibrocartilaginous disc may become displaced and is then often associated with pain, tenderness, limited opening and 'clicking'.

Magnetic resonance imaging is the best technique for demonstrating the disc and its relationship to the glenoid fossa. T1-weighted images are taken in an oblique parasagittal plane with the mouth closed and open. Techniques have been described for obtaining images of the joint in intermediate positions to give a dynamic picture of movements of the disc and mandibular condyle. Coronal images can also be obtained. T2-weighted images will demonstrate soft-tissue inflammation around the joint as a high-signal area.

In **disc displacement without reduction**, the disc is fixed against the anterior wall of the glenoid fossa with the posterior margin of the disc anterior to the superior convexity of the articular surface of the mandibular condyle. Anterior movement of the condyle on opening is considerably reduced (Fig. 17.32).

In **disc displacement with reduction**, the disc is also fixed against the anterior wall of the glenoid fossa anterior to the superior convexity of the articular surface of the condyle when the mouth is closed, but the condyle moves anterior to the displaced disc on opening (Fig. 17.33).

The **pain-dysfunction syndrome** is the clinical diagnosis most frequently applied to patients with temporomandibular joint pain. The aetiology is uncertain, but most cases are probably due to internal derangement of the joint. The joint is usually normal on plain radiographs.

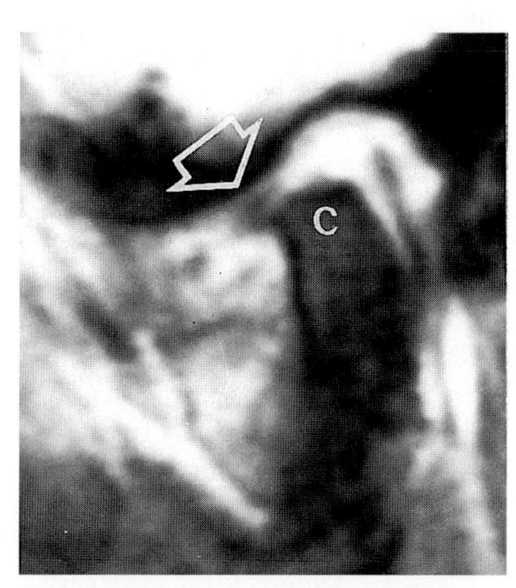

Fig. 17.32 Disc displacement without reduction. Parasagittal T1-weighted image with the mouth open showing anterior displacement of the disc (arrow), against the anterior wall of the glenoid fossa. There is limited forward movement of the condyle (C) on opening. (Courtesy of Dr Richard Nakielny, Royal Hallamshire Hospital, Sheffield.)

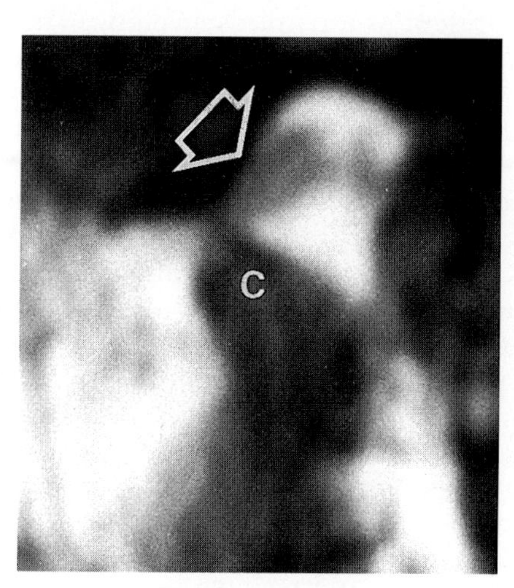

Fig. 17.33 Disc displacement with reduction. T1-weighted parasagittal MRI taken with the mouth open. There is anterior displacement of the disc against the anterior wall of the glenoid fossa (arrow) and the condyle (C) has moved anterior to the displaced disc, on opening. (Courtesy of Dr Richard Nakielny, Royal Hallamshire Hospital, Sheffield.)

ARTHRITIS

Inflammatory arthritis due to systemic disease is uncommon, but can be a feature of connective tissue diseases such as rheumatoid arthritis and psoriasis. Erosions develop in the articular surface of the condyle and they can be very extensive. The glenoid fossa remains radiologically normal.

Degenerative arthritis (osteoarthritis) (Fig. 17.34) can occur in the elderly and eventually results in the same abnormalities as osteoarthritis in other synovial joints, namely joint space narrowing, sclerosis and osteophyte formation. The sclerosis is confined to the

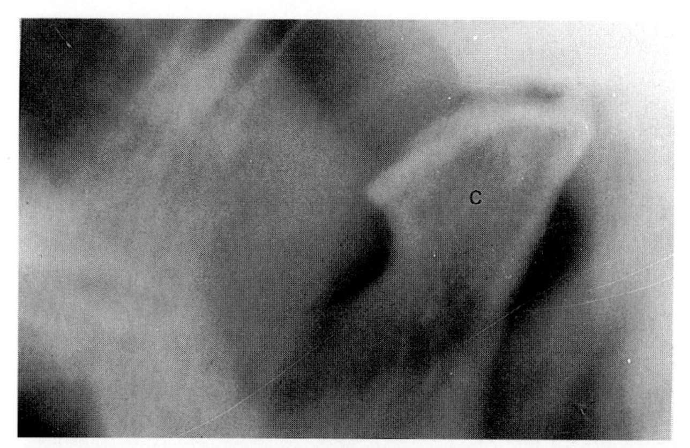

Fig. 17.34 Degenerative arthritis (osteoarthritis). There is flattening and sclerosis of the mandibular condyle (C).

mandibular condyle and osteophytes arise only from the anterior margin of the condyle. The articular surface of the glenoid fossa remains normal.

Ankylosis of the temporomandibular joint may follow infective arthritis or traumatic haemarthrosis. As these disorders usually occur in childhood, most cases are complicated by hypoplasia of the mandibular condyle due to the epiphyseal cartilage of the condylar neck having been damaged at the same time. CT is usually required to demonstrate bony ankylosis between the temporal bone and the mandibular condyle.

DISLOCATION

The diagnosis of dislocation is made clinically rather than radiologically as the mandibular condyle may move anterior to the maximum convexity of the articular eminence in normal individuals. The role of imaging in dislocation is to exclude a fracture or some other pathology such as a bone tumour. Recurrent dislocation may be a feature of Marfan's syndrome and of the Ehlers–Danlos syndrome.

SALIVARY GLANDS

IMAGING THE SALIVARY GLANDS

Lesions of the gland parenchyma such as tumours and abscesses are best shown by CT, MRI or ultrasound which can usually distinguish between lesions situated in the salivary glands and those situated in adjacent structures.

Imaging is particularly useful in lesions of the parotid glands as the retromandibular vein (posterior facial vein) can often be identified on axial CT images (Fig. 17.35) and T1-weighted MRI images. This vein is a useful anatomical landmark for the facial nerve (VIIth cranial nerve) which supplies the facial muscles

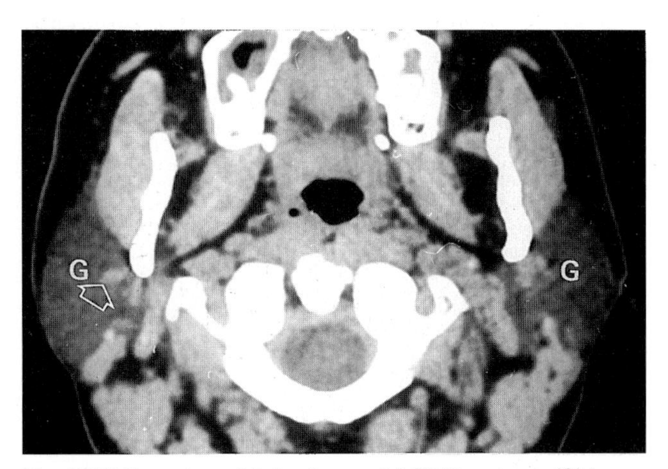

Fig. 17.35 Normal parotid glands on axial CT. The glands (G) have a lower attenuation than the surrounding muscles owing to the presence of fat. The retromandibular vein on the right has been arrowed.

and runs immediately lateral to the vein. The facial nerve divides the parotid gland into a large superficial lobe and a much smaller deep lobe. The clinical importance of this distinction is that tumours in the superficial lobe can be surgically removed with little risk of damaging the nerve, but tumours in the deep lobe have to be dissected from the nerve and its branches and there is always a risk of temporary or even permanent nerve damage.

Coronal MRI is particularly useful for showing the submandibular glands and adjacent structures (Fig. 17.36).

Disorders of the duct systems, such as calculus, stricture and sialectasis of the parotid and submandibular glands, are best demonstrated by sialography. The examination should be preceded by plain radiographs to show any radiopaque calculi. Cannulation of the parotid ducts is usually straightforward, but the orifices of the submandibular ducts can be extremely difficult to identify and cannulate. Water-soluble low-osmolar media should always be used as any extravasation into the soft tissues is relatively painless and has no complications.

Delayed radiographs should be taken 10 minutes after the cannula has been removed, as the presence of contrast medium remaining within the duct system indicates duct obstruction or reduced function.

Disorders of function and some inflammatory conditions are best shown by radionuclide scanning. ^{99m}Tc pertechnetate will outline normally functioning parotid, submandibular and sublingual glands, as the isotope is excreted in the saliva. Most tumours produce a localized area of reduced uptake.

Gallium scanning with ^{67}Ga citrate is an effective technique for diagnosing infectious and inflammatory processes such as sialadenitis, sarcoid and benign lymphoepithelial infiltration.

TUMOURS

Salivary gland tumours can develop at any age, and usually present as a painless swelling. They are more common in the parotid than in the submandibular glands. The overall incidence of malignancy is 10–20%, being higher in the submandibular gland than in the parotid. The pathological classification is complex.

Benign pleomorphic adenoma is the commonest tumour of the salivary glands and accounts for over 50% of all tumours. CT usually shows a well-defined homogeneous lesion with a higher attenuation than in normal parotid gland parenchyma (Fig. 17.37) Malignant change occurs rarely and usually results in an area of low attenuation within the tumour and blurring of the tumour margin. Sialography of benign lesions shows displacement of the intraglandular ducts but malignant lesions may occlude ducts. Myxoid tissue or fluid in the stroma of benign and malignant pleomorphic adenomas will produce a

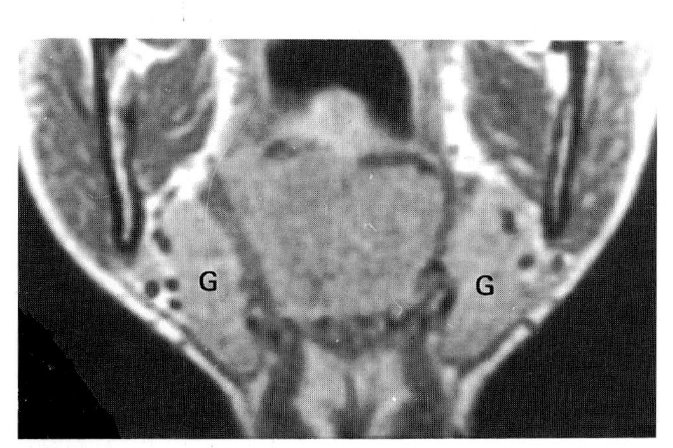

Fig. 17.36 Normal submandibular glands (G) on a coronal T1-weighted MRI.

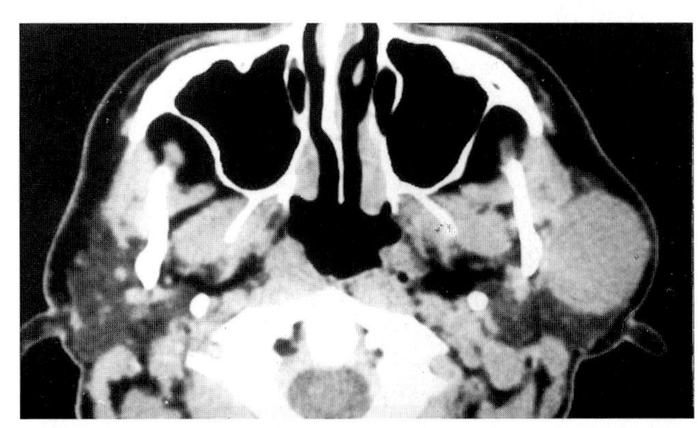

Fig. 17.37 Benign pleomorphic adenoma of the superficial lobe of the left parotid gland on axial CT. The lesion is homogeneous and has a higher attenuation than normal gland parenchyma. The border is well defined.

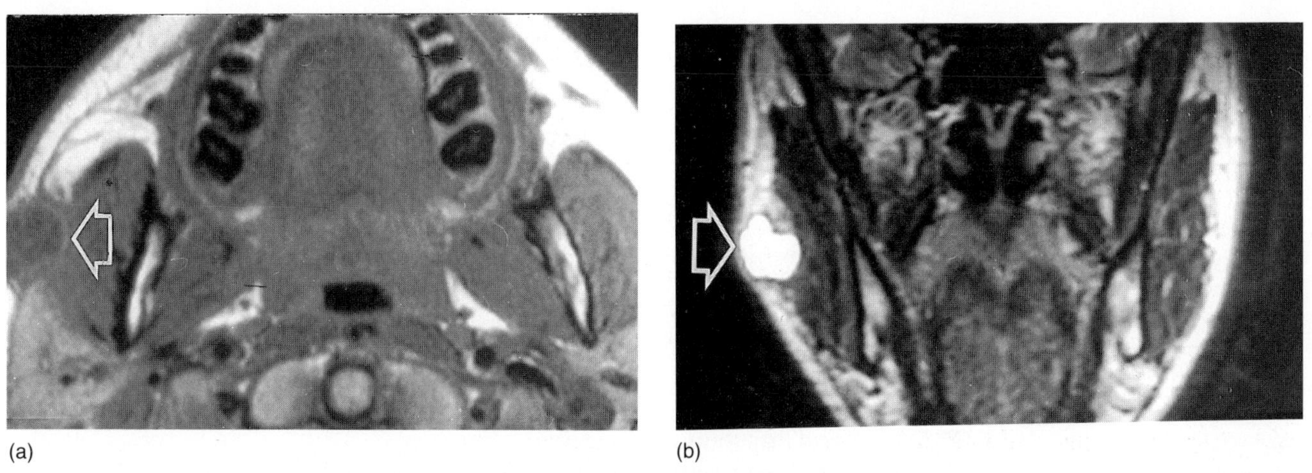

(a) (b)

Fig. 17.38 Benign cystic pleomorphic adenoma (arrow). (a) Axial T1-weighted MRI, shows the adenoma as a low signal area. (b) Coronal T2-weighted MRI shows the adenoma as a high-signal area (arrowed) due to fluid in the cyst. (Courtesy of Dr R. Phillips, St. Bartholomews Hospital, London.)

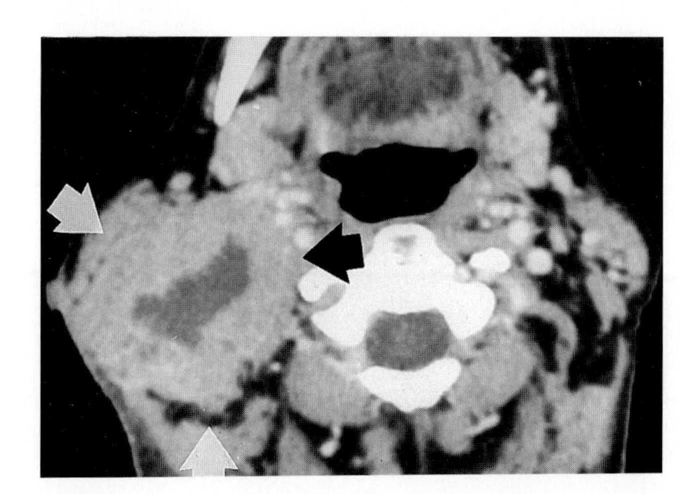

Fig. 17.39 Huge mucoepidemoid carcinoma (arrows) of the right parotid gland on enhanced axial CT. The lesion contains an area of low attenuation and has a poorly defined margin which merges with adjacent structures.

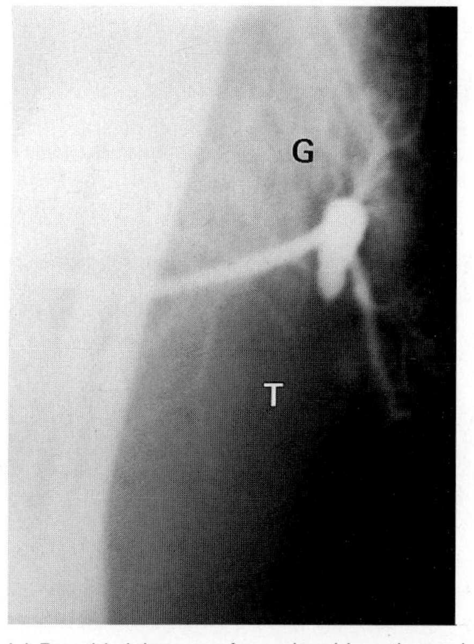

(a)

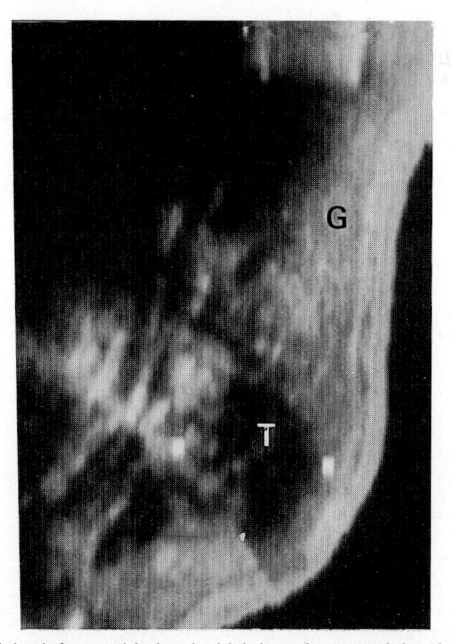

(b)

Fig. 17.40 (a) Parotid sialogram of an adenoid cystic carcinoma of the lower pole of the left parotid gland which has destroyed the duct system G = upper pole; T = tumour. (b) The ultrasound examination (slice in the coronal plane) shows an area of reduced and mixed echogenicity (T) in the lower part of the gland. The lesion has poorly defined margins which is typical of a malignant tumour.

characteristically high signal on T2-weighted MR images (Figs 17.38a,b).

Adenocarcinomas are rarely true adenocarcinomas and usually have a distinctive histological appearance. The commonest histological types are adenoid cystic carcinoma and mucoepidermoid carcinoma. These tumours grow slowly but are difficult to eradicate and the 10-year survival rate is $< 50\%$. The larger tumours often contain areas of low attenuation on CT and have an irregular border which merges with adjacent structures (Fig. 17.39). Sialography usually shows obstruction of the intraglandular ducts and there may be complete absence of a normal duct system in the affected part of the gland (Fig. 17.40a). Ultrasound usually shows an ill-defined area of reduced and mixed echogenicity. (Fig. 17.40b).

Rare tumours include the benign adenolymphoma (**Warthin's tumour**) which has a high uptake on radionuclide scanning and malignant lymphoma which is characteristically hypoechoic on ultrasound.

CALCULI AND DUCT STRICTURES

Calculi are more common in the submandibular region than in the parotid region, and are usually a sequel to infection or stasis. Most calculi are radiopaque on plain films but show as relatively radiolucent lesions on sialography (Fig. 17.41).

Strictures of the main ducts and of the intraglandular ducts are usually due to infection or calculi, and predispose to sialectasis and calculus formation. Strictures at the orifices of the parotid ducts may be caused by cheek biting, and strictures at the anterior ends of the submandibular ducts may be caused by trauma from an ill-fitting denture.

Sialography will demonstrate strictures quite clearly (Fig. 17.42) and may show dilation of the duct system behind the stricture.

SIALECTASIS

Sialectasis is usually associated with recurrent infection and describes a radiological appearance. The terms 'punctate' or 'globular' are sometimes used to

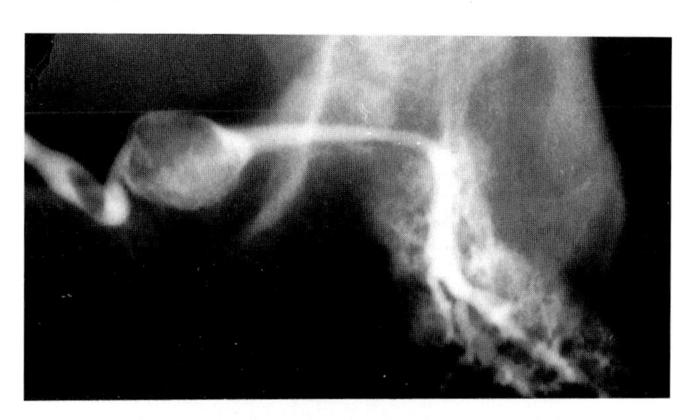

Fig. 17.41 Submandibular sialogram showing two calculi in the main duct (Wharton's duct). The calculi appeared radiopaque on the preliminary films taken before injecting contrast medium.

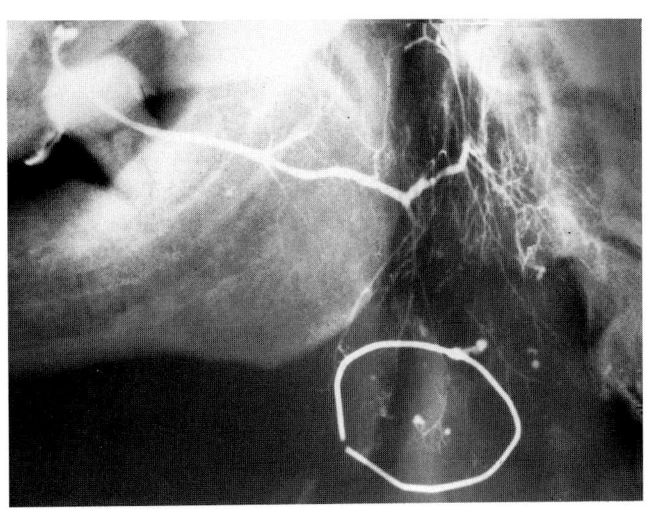

Fig. 17.43 Parotid sialogram showing punctate sialectasis localized to the inferior pole of the gland. The area of clinical swelling has been outlined with a radiopaque wire.

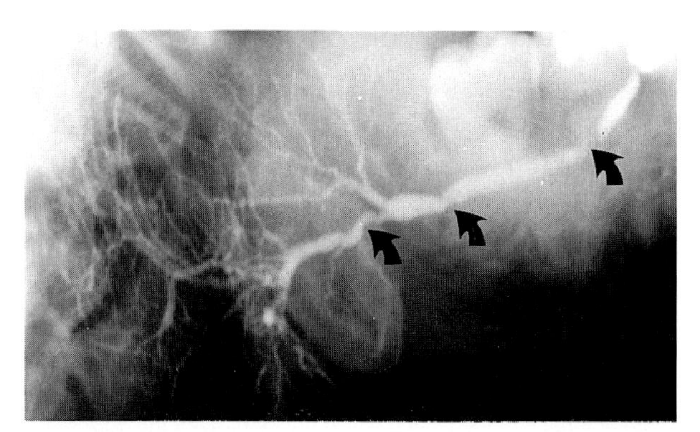

Fig. 17.42 Multiple strictures of the main parotid duct (Stensen's duct) on sialography (arrows).

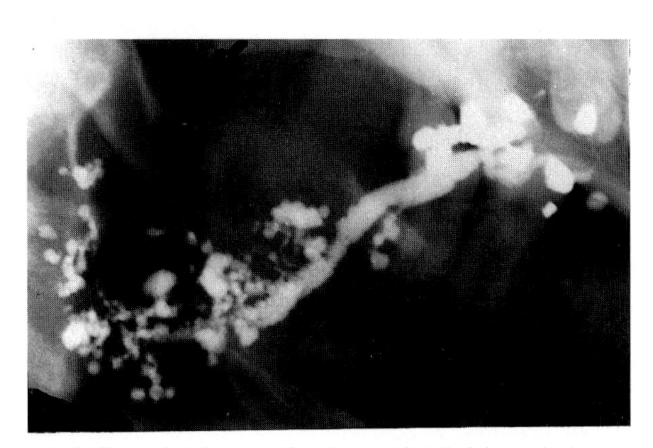

Fig. 17.44 Parotid sialogram showing 'cavitary' sialectasis throughout the gland.

describe small regular cavities measuring < 2 mm in diameter (Fig. 17.43), and the term 'cavitary' to describe larger cavities with irregular walls (Fig. 17.44). A cavity which is > 5 mm in diameter is likely to be an abscess. Infective sialectasis can produce any of these abnormalities, and may be accompanied by calculus formation in the main duct or in the sialectatic cavities within the gland.

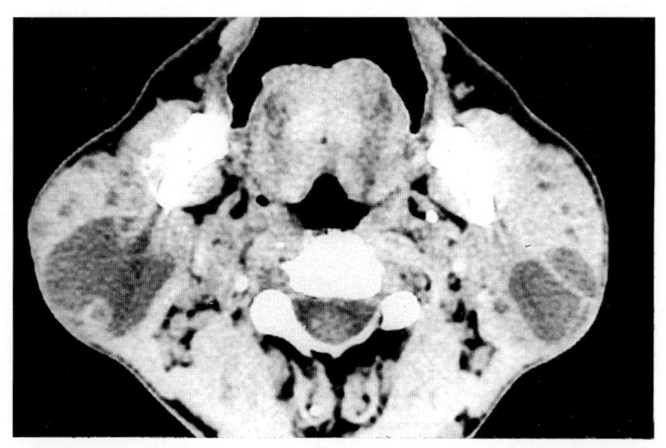

Fig. 17.45 Benign lymphoepithelial infiltration of the parotids on axial CT. The glands are grossly enlarged and contain multiple round areas of low attenuation.

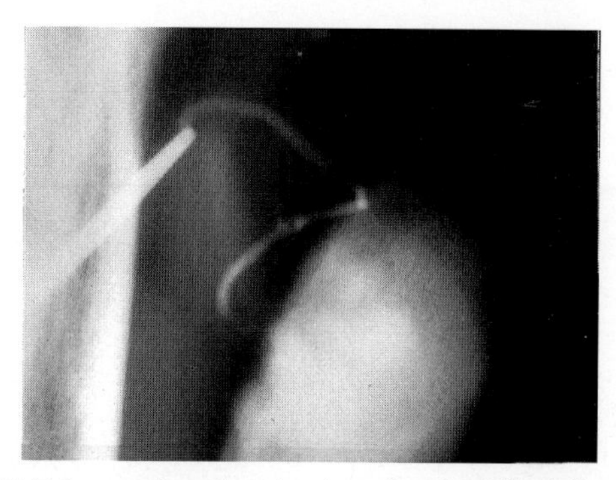

Fig. 17.46 Extravasation of contrast medium from the left parotid duct into the soft tissues. The duct had been damaged at surgery 2 weeks earlier.

Sjögren's syndrome and other connective tissue diseases are also associated with sialectasis. Most patients with Sjögren's syndrome have sialectasis and there is often dilation of the main duct.

MISCELLANEOUS CONDITIONS

Infective sialadenitis of viral or bacterial origin causes generalized glandular enlargement and there is usually increased attenuation on CT. Abscess formation will produce an area of low attenuation on CT and an area of low echogenicity on ultrasound. Sialography in cases of recurrent infection may show calculus, duct stricture or sialectasis.

Benign lymphoepithelial infiltration can occur as an isolated abnormality (Mikulicz' disease) but is more commonly a feature of Sjögren's syndrome or HIV disease. The CT appearance in advanced disease is quite characteristic. The glands are grossly enlarged and contain multiple well-defined areas of low attenuation (Fig. 17.45). The condition is not as benign as the name implies; it is complicated by malignant lymphoma in 5% and anaplastic carcinoma in about 1% of patients.

Trauma to the main parotid duct, or to one of its larger intraglandular branches, occasionally results from penetrating facial injury and is a very rare complication of surgery. Sialography will show extravasation of contrast medium from the duct system into the soft tissues (Fig. 17.46).

CHAPTER 18

Sinuses

Iain R. Colquhoun

ANATOMY
INFLAMMATORY DISEASE
BENIGN TUMOURS
MALIGNANT TUMOURS

Conventional X-ray examinations have a limited role for investigation of sinus pathology. A single occipitomental (OM) view is recommended for assessment of inflammatory disease. This film is taken with the patient erect with a horizontal X-ray beam to demonstrate fluid levels. More detailed assessment of the sinuses requires CT or MR imaging.

ANATOMY

The sinuses develop as pouches from the nasal cavity, lined by ciliated columnar epithelium. The maxillary and ethmoid sinuses are present at birth, but fluid-filled. The ethmoid sinuses reach near adult size by 12 years of age. The maxillary sinuses have two major growth periods at 0–3 and 7–12 years. The frontal sinuses, usually derived from the anterior ethmoid sinuses, are visible by the age of 2 and well pneumatized by the age of 12. The sphenoid sinuses pneumatize from the age of 3.

The maxillary sinuses drain via a single ostium into the middle meatus, lateral to the middle turbinate. Accessory ostia within the medial maxillary wall occur in 15–40% of patients. In general the frontal, anterior and middle ethmoid sinuses also drain via the middle meatus. Each sphenoid sinus drains via a single ostium, which is located 10–15 mm above the floor of the sinus, into the sphenoethmoidal recess in the superior meatus, where the posterior ethmoid sinuses also drain.

Sinus anatomy is ideally demonstrated with coronal CT, developed as a 'road map' to facilitate functional endoscopic sinus surgery. One key structure for endoscopic sinus surgery is the 'osteomeatal complex' within the middle meatus, where the frontal, ethmoid (anterior and middle) and maxillary sinuses drain (Fig. 18.1). Obstruction to the osteomeatal complex typically results in opacification of this group of sinuses (Fig. 18.2).

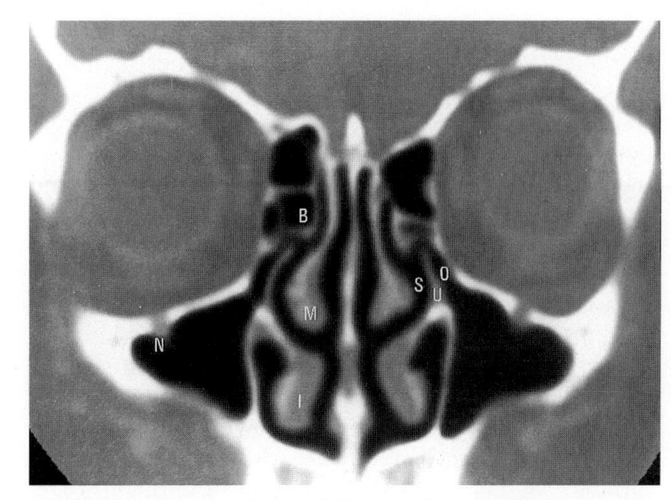

Fig. 18.1 Normal coronal sinus CT through the osteomeatal complex. N = infraorbital nerve; M and I = middle and inferior turbinates; O = ostium in osteomeatal complex; U = uncinate process; S = middle meatus; B = ethmoidal bulla.

INFLAMMATORY DISEASE

Sinusitis can be related to acute or chronic infection, allergy, altered immunity or a combination of these factors. In the absence of trauma, fluid levels usually denote acute infection. The degree and extent of mucosal thickening is very variable. Involvement of a

Diagnostic and Interventional Radiology in Surgical Practice. Edited by P. Armstrong and M. L. Wastie. Published in 1997 by Chapman & Hall, London. ISBN 0 412 61960 1 (HB), 0 412 61970 9 (PB)

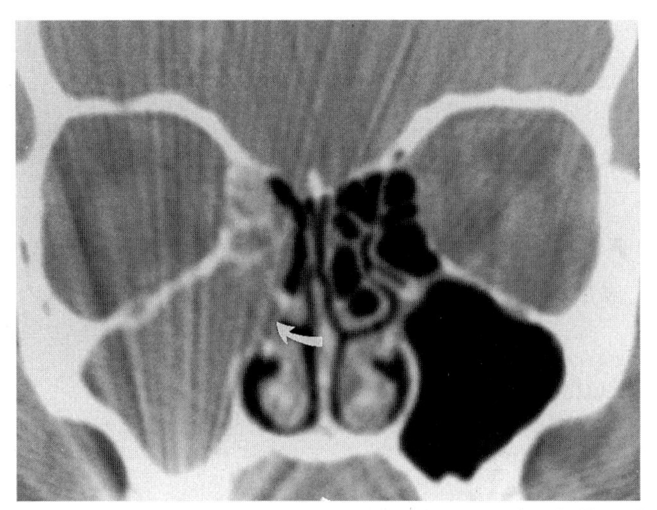

Fig. 18.2 Coronal CT in acute sinusitis demonstrating unilateral osteomeatal complex disease (curved arrow) and consequent opacification of the maxillary and middle ethmoid sinuses. Anterior ethmoid and frontal sinus opacification was also present.

single sinus usually denotes infection, whereas multiple sinus and nasal mucosal involvement, often with polypoidal mucosal thickening, suggests an allergic aetiology. Chronic sinusitis usually produces thickening and sclerosis of the bones surrounding the involved sinus. Infective, as opposed to allergic, mucosal thickening will exhibit enhancement with intravenous contrast on both CT and MRI. This enhancement is typically peripheral as opposed to the solid or uniform enhancement of tumours. Inflammatory mucosal thickening is markedly hyperintense on T2-weighted MRI sequences, whereas tumours are of more intermediate intensity. However, in chronic sinus disease, resorption of water will result in variable signal intensities, making exclusion of a tumour difficult on MRI. The major complication of sinus infection is spread of infection to the orbit, brain or cavernous sinus.

Because of the excellent contrast between bone, soft tissue and air, CT is the most suitable technique for assessment of inflammatory sinus disease. The major disadvantage of MRI is that neither cortical bone nor air produces a signal, thereby reducing anatomical detail. MRI is, however, better than CT for assessing cavernous sinus and early intracranial involvement.

ASPERGILLOSIS

Aspergillosis is the commonest fungal infection. The invasive form frequently originates in one maxillary sinus, producing extensive bone destruction resembling carcinoma; intracranial extension can also occur. Fungal infections typically contain hyperdense foci on CT and corresponding hypointense areas with a T2-weighted MRI sequence.

POLYPS

Polyps are associated with infection, allergy, aspirin sensitivity, asthma and cystic fibrosis. Polyps are frequently multiple and expansile, involving the nasal cavities and sinuses and can produce complete opacification of these structures. In such severe cases CT demonstrates opacification with soft-tissue density material in the nasal cavities and sinuses and often marked thinning, or even absence, of the intervening bony septa (Fig. 18.3). The degree of bone loss can occasionally mimic a malignant process. Typical MRI characteristics of polyps are similar to acute infectious mucosal thickening with low to intermediate T1-weighted intensity and T2-weighted hyperintensity. Chronic polyposis produces heterogeneous

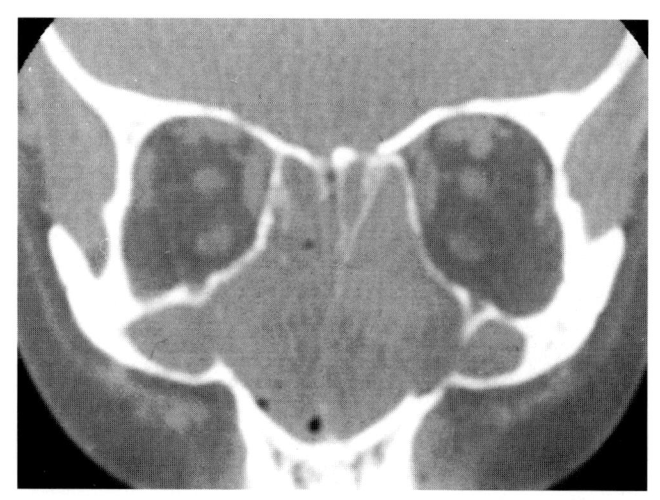

Fig. 18.3 Coronal CT in gross polyposis with opacification of all the sinuses, resulting in marked loss of definition of the bony septa.

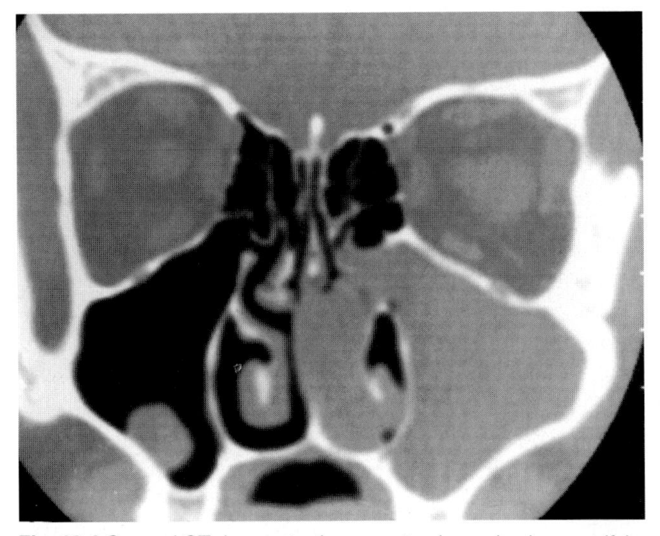

Fig. 18.4 Coronal CT demonstrating an antrochoanal polyp opacifying the maxillary sinus and extending through an expanded ostium into the nasal cavity and bowing the nasal septum. A small polyp is present at the base of the opposite maxillary sinus.

intensity of the nasal cavities and sinuses even exhibiting areas of signal void which can be mistaken for air.

Antrochoanal polyps are benign polyps that grow within and usually fill the maxillary sinus before expanding the ostium and extending posteriorly into the nasal cavity towards the nasopharynx (Fig. 18.4). Similar sphenochoanal polyps occasionally occur.

MUCOCELE

Mucoceles are expansile lesions of the sinuses, caused by obstruction of the ostium, usually secondary to infection or, rarely, by tumour or trauma. The ostial obstruction causes an accumulation of secretions within the sinus with absorption of trapped air, thereby creating an opaque sinus. The slow increase in pressure within the sinus produces expansion with bowing and thinning of the bony margins. Mucoceles occur most frequently in the frontal sinuses and with decreasing frequency in the ethmoid, maxillary and sphenoid sinuses. Acute infection produces a **pyocele**, with bone destruction and an associated soft-tissue abscess. Chronic infection leads to thickening and sclerosis of the expanded bony margins of the sinuses.

A mucocele is shown on CT as an opaque expanded sinus with bony thinning of its walls (Fig. 18.5). MRI demonstrates an opaque, expanded sinus, the contents of which are typically homogeneous and of low to intermediate intensity on T1-weighted and hyperintense on T2-weighted sequences. However, the intensity varies with the relative composition of the contents and the intensity is frequently either hypo- or hyperintense on both the T1- and T2-weighted sequences.

GRANULOMATA

Wegener's and midline granuloma both produce destructive soft-tissue masses involving the nasal cavities and sinuses. **Sarcoidosis** produces irregular mucosal thickening usually confined to the nasal cavities.

BENIGN TUMOURS

Osteomas are benign tumours, usually formed from dense compact bone (ivory osteoma), which commonly occur in the frontal sinus. They are generally an incidental finding unless ostial occlusion produces a mucocele.

Inverted papilloma frequently occurs on the lateral nasal wall and can be expansile and locally invasive, tending to involve the adjacent maxillary and ethmoid sinuses (Fig. 18.6). Local recurrence following excision is not uncommon.

MALIGNANT TUMOURS

Squamous cell carcinoma is the commonest malignant tumour to affect the sinuses and most frequently arises in the maxillary sinuses and nasal cavities. Early tumours are radiologically indistinguishable from, and frequently coexist with, inflammatory mucosal thickening. Consequently, on diagnosis there is often a large tumour mass, the radiological characteristics of which are bone destruction and infiltration into adjacent structures, particularly the orbit and infratemporal fossa. Coronal and axial CT are required to

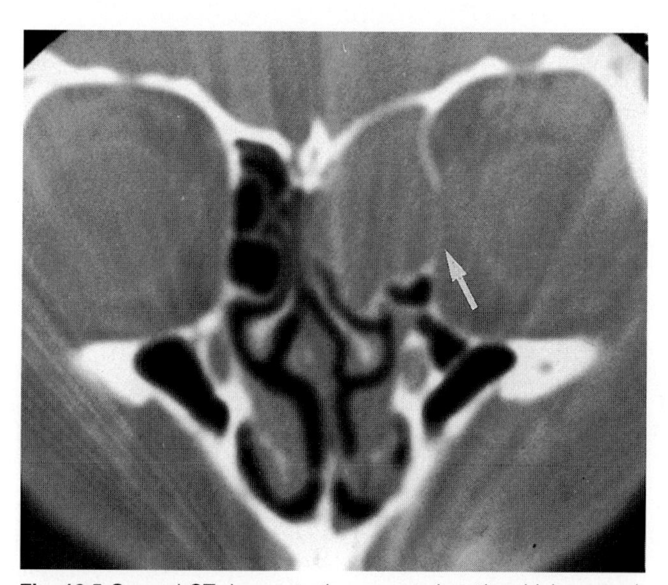

Fig. 18.5 Coronal CT demonstrating an anterior ethmoidal mucocele producing marked bony expansion with thinning but preservation of the lamina papyracea (arrow).

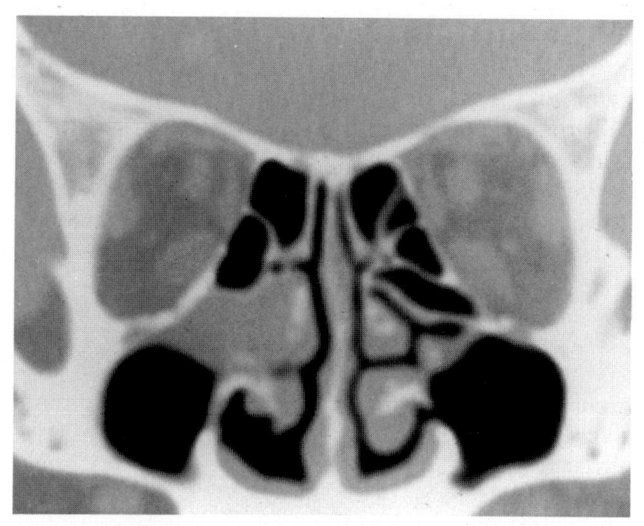

Fig. 18.6 Coronal CT demonstrating an inverted papilloma originating from the middle turbinate and extending into the maxillary sinus with erosion of the medial wall.

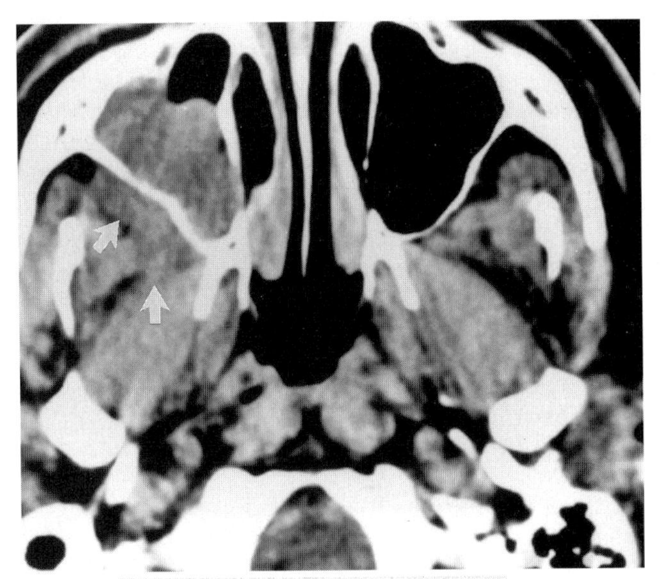

Fig. 18.7 Axial CT of a squamous cell carcinoma originating within the maxillary sinus but demonstrating early extension into the infratemporal fossa (arrows) with an intact posterior wall.

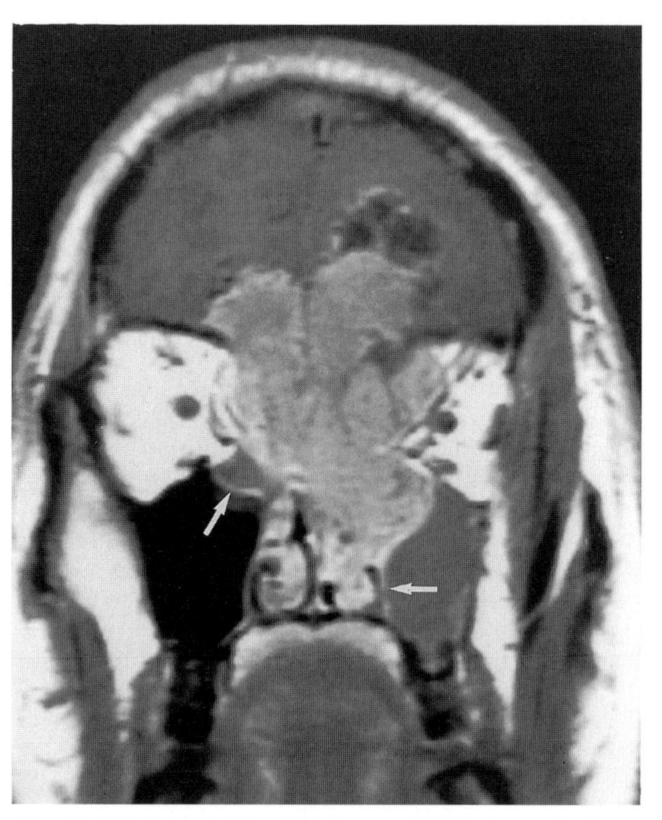

Fig. 18.8 Enhanced T1-weighted coronal MRI demonstrating an olfactory neuroblastoma involving the nasal cavity, frontal lobes (with capping cysts), orbits, ethmoid and maxillary sinuses. Note the intermediate signal intensity material in both maxillary sinuses which exhibits peripheral enhancement (arrows) consistent with secondary acute and chronic inflammatory reaction from ostial obstruction.

assess fully the extent of bone destruction and tumour infiltration. Early infratemporal spread, which can occur without demonstrable bone destruction, is more easily appreciated on axial images (Fig. 18.7). Squamous cell carcinoma often occurs against a background of chronic inflammation and the tumour frequently produces acute inflammatory change secondary to ostial occlusion. The soft-tissue opacification seen with CT is a combination of tumour and inflammation and therefore the actual tumour bulk is overestimated. MRI is frequently able to distinguish tumour from inflammatory change as the inflammation generally appears more hyperintense than tumour on T2-weighted sequences. However, areas of haemorrhage and necrosis can produce heterogeneous foci within the tumour on both T1- and T2-weighted sequences. Tumours usually exhibit diffuse enhancement with intravenous contrast on both CT and MRI as opposed to the peripheral enhancement of acute inflammation.

Adenocarcinoma also appears as a destructive soft-tissue mass with similar MRI characteristics to squamous cell carcinoma, except that adenocarcinoma usually exhibits less marked enhancement. An adenocarcinoma commonly originates within the ethmoid sinuses and frequently extends intracranially.

Non-Hodgkin's lymphoma is the commonest variety of lymphoma to involve the sinuses. Lymphoma generally appears as a more infiltrative rather than destructive mass and is of intermediate intensity on all MRI sequences.

Olfactory neuroblastoma (or aesthesioneuroblastoma) arises from the olfactory mucosa superiorly within the nasal cavities. The tumour is locally

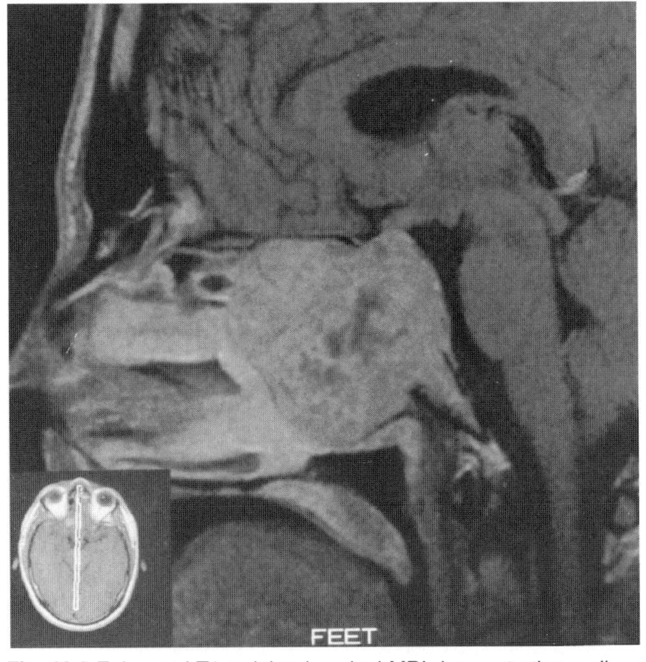

Fig. 18.9 Enhanced T1-weighted sagittal MRI demonstrating a clivus chordoma presenting as a nasopharyngeal mass.

invasive, extending into the adjacent ethmoid sinuses, orbits and anterior cranial fossa and is ideally imaged with MRI (Fig. 18.8).

Other malignancies involving the sinuses and nasal cavities include **primary sarcomas** and **melanoma, metastases** and **myeloma**. Infiltration from adjacent salivary gland and dental tumours occurs and some tumours arising from nearby structures may present as nasal masses, including **clivus chordomas** (Fig. 18.9) and **juvenile nasopharyngeal angiofibromas**.

CHAPTER 19

Eye and orbit

Ivan Moseley

With the development of modern imaging techniques, a range of methods is available to image the orbits:

- plain radiographs
- ultrasonography
- arteriography
- dacryocystography
- computed tomography
- magnetic resonance imaging.

IMAGING TECHNIQUES

Since so many techniques are available, an informed choice is essential.

PLAIN FILMS

Plain films now have very limited applications. They are mainly used in the management of suspected foreign bodies within the orbit, fractures and a few cases where bone disease such as fibrous dysplasia is suspected. There are virtually no indications for 'optic foramen' views. Plain films, however, do offer a simple means of confirming the presence of paranasal sinusitis.

Diagnostic and Interventional Radiology in Surgical Practice. Edited by P. Armstrong and M.L. Wastie. Published in 1997 by Chapman & Hall, London. ISBN 0 412 61960 1 (HB), 0 412 61970 9 (PB)

SONOGRAPHY

The role of sonography is essentially in the investigation of ocular disease. Although it is quick and simple, its use as a 'screening' test in patients with suspected orbital masses does not obviate more definitive studies.

INTRAVASCULAR PROCEDURES

Intravascular procedures have become much less common in recent years. There is now no place for **orbital phlebography** except as part of an interventional procedure. With the very rapid and striking improvements in magnetic resonance angiography, diagnostic **carotid arteriography** is performed less frequently, but it is the examination of choice for interventional procedures, including embolization of vascular malformations and tumours in and around the orbits and cavernous sinus region. Both diagnostic and therapeutic angiograms should be performed and interpreted only by experts. **Dacryocystography** has specific indications which are discussed below.

COMPUTED TOMOGRAPHY

CT is especially suited to examination of the orbit, because the orbital walls and soft-tissue structures have high natural radiographic contrast. It does, however, have the disadvantage that the lens is particularly sensitive to ionizing radiation, so that the examination should not be undertaken lightly, especially in children or when repeated studies seem probable. The ophthalmologist should insist on high-quality, high-resolution studies with sections no more than 2 mm thick. Resolution can be increased by 'coning down' on the orbits, but for many orbital problems, particularly unilateral visual loss, it is highly desirable that the pituitary fossa be included in the field of view. The adjacent paranasal sinuses should also be covered, as an apparently intraorbital mass may arise from one of the sinuses. In many institutions it is a general rule that CT is carried out first without intravenous contrast medium and repeated after injection, should that prove necessary. Because of constraints on radiation dose, orbital CT is best performed with contrast medium *ab initio*; the injection rarely assists in diagnosis of orbital lesions, but extension of pathological processes beyond the orbits may be much more accurately assessed. When imaging CT examinations of the orbits it is often helpful to have both bone and soft-tissue 'windows'.

MAGNETIC RESONANCE IMAGING

MRI does not use ionizing radiations and is therefore theoretically preferable to CT for examination of the orbit. However, the spatial resolution of many current imagers is rather unsatisfactory, and the long data acquisition times sometimes necessary for MRI mean that movement of the eyes can occur. Special considerations arise because of the presence of the orbital fat. The high signal from the orbital fat and the major differences in MRI characteristics of the orbital tissues may give rise to chemical shift artefact, so that structures such as the optic nerve have a dense white line along one side and a black one along the other. Special sequences can be employed to reduce these effects. Furthermore, pathological enhancement with intravenous gadolinium is manifest on T1-weighted images as high signal, which paradoxically has the effect of making a mass outlined by high-signal orbital fat less conspicuous. Contrast-enhanced images of the orbit should therefore be obtained using fat-suppression sequences. Mascara contains iron and degrades the images of the anterior orbit; it should be removed before the examination.

TRAUMA TO THE ORBIT

A blow to the orbit can involve the eye, the other soft tissues (including the lids and extraocular muscles) and the surrounding bones. The eye may be subject to blunt trauma or a penetrating injury.

FOREIGN BODIES

One of the commonest indications for imaging is the suspicion of an intraocular foreign body. If it lies within the globe, it should be removed because of the risks of premature cataract and sympathetic ophthalmitis, but small extraocular foreign bodies are usually left *in situ*. Imaging of any kind should follow expert clinical examination, as the detection rate for intraocular foreign bodies is very low when an ophthalmologist believes that none is present.

The basic technique is plain film radiography. With advances in vitreoretinal surgery, very precise localization of intraocular particles is less critical than previously, and a simple technique usually suffices. A single lateral film, which shows the corneal surface clearly, is all that is usually required for screening. This must be obtained with the eye open, in the primary position, the side being investigated next to the film. All metallic foreign bodies of sufficient size should be visible, as will the large majority of glass fragments and some other foreign bodies composed of, for example, stone. If no foreign body is visible, the plain film examination is over. When a radiopaque foreign body is identified as a white blob or streak on the film, a postero-anterior film (with the face against the film) is required for localization. A second lateral exposure, with the patient looking up or down may be helpful if the preceding films do not make it clear that the foreign body is intra- or extraocular (Fig. 19.1). If the fragment moves with the eye, it is within it although, rarely, a foreign body in one of the extraocular muscles can cause confusion. Simple measurements on the postero-anterior and lateral views, suitably corrected for magnification, can be transferred to a chart for presurgical localization.

When the plain film shows no foreign body in the face of strong clinical suspicion, ultrasonography may reveal a fragment which is not radiopaque. If the long axis of a shard of foreign material lies in the plane of the ultrasound beam, however, it can be overlooked.

If the foregoing studies are inconclusive as to the presence and/or intraocular location of a foreign body, or if multiple fragments preclude localization from two films in two planes, CT can be employed. Fine (1.5–2.0 mm) axial or coronal sections, with reformats in appropriate planes, are required. Wooden foreign bodies may appear of less than soft-tissue density.

Not only is MRI not indicated in a suspected intraocular foreign body, any patient who might have a metallic foreign body in the orbit (metal workers, for example) must not undergo MRI of any part of the body, as the movement of the fragment in the magnetic field can cause serious damage. Plain films of the orbits should be obtained before carrying out MRI for other indications in patients at risk. Most, but importantly not all, metal-containing surgical

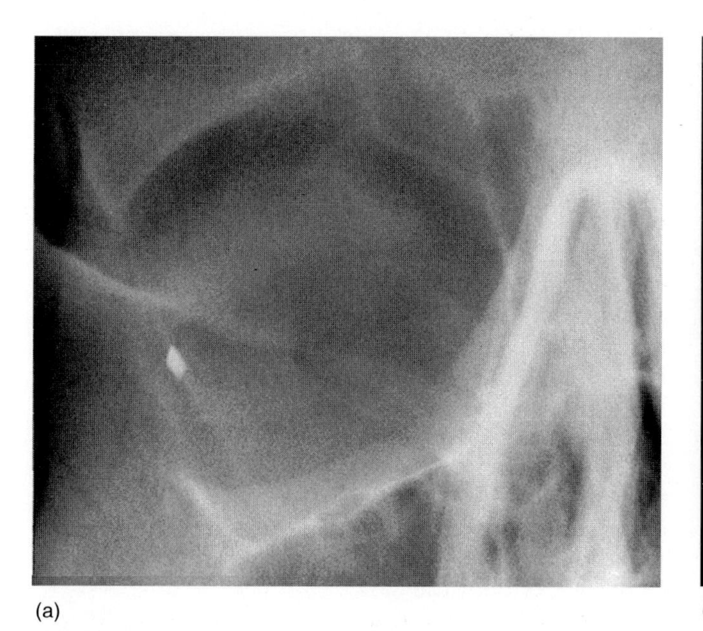

(a)

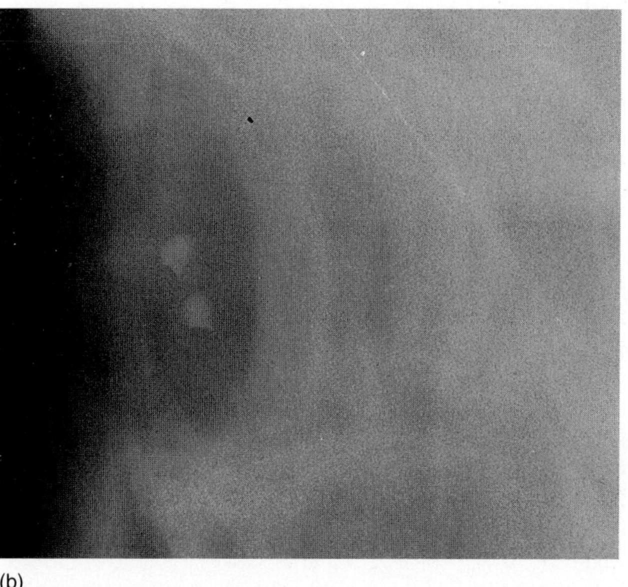

(b)

Fig. 19.1 Plain film localization of a metallic foreign body. (a) Postero-anterior and (b) double-exposed 'eye-mover' lateral plain films. A metallic fragment is seen laterally in the right orbit; although it might be thought too laterally placed to be intraocular, it does move with eye movement.

materials placed within the orbits, such as intraocular lenses, wire sutures, retinal tacks, do not contraindicate MRI as the material is not ferromagnetic. However, ocular implants containing magnets are an absolute contraindication to MRI. If there is any doubt about safety, the radiologist should be consulted **before** the patient is referred for imaging.

OTHER OCULAR INJURIES

Ultrasonography is the method of choice for the detection of other traumatic injuries such as dislocation or rupture of the lens (Fig. 19.2), intraocular haemorrhage or retinal detachment. CT or MRI may sometimes be necessary for demonstration of rupture of the globe, particularly if the media are opaque. The long-term result of severe ocular trauma is a shrunken globe, with calcification in the coats. On CT or MRI the characteristics of the media are different from those of the opposite eye.

Injuries to other soft-tissue structures in the orbit

Imaging usually plays little part in the assessment of orbital soft-tissue injuries, but CT or MRI can be used to demonstrate division of the extraocular muscles.

Orbital fractures

Other than in major, widespread facial injuries, fractures usually involve the thin floor and medial wall of the orbit. The mechanism of injury is most commonly a direct blow to the eye by a fist or an object of similar size. The major indications for imaging are enophthalmos and/or diplopia, particularly if these features are persistent.

Radiographic examination is not an emergency and may be delayed until some of the overlying soft-tissue swelling has subsided. In the acute phase, plain radiographs may show direct evidence of downward displacement of the floor of the orbit (a 'blow-out' fracture), frequently centered on the infraorbital canal. Medial displacement of the lamina papyracea, which separates the orbit from the ethmoid air cells, is more difficult to recognize because of normal bone anterior

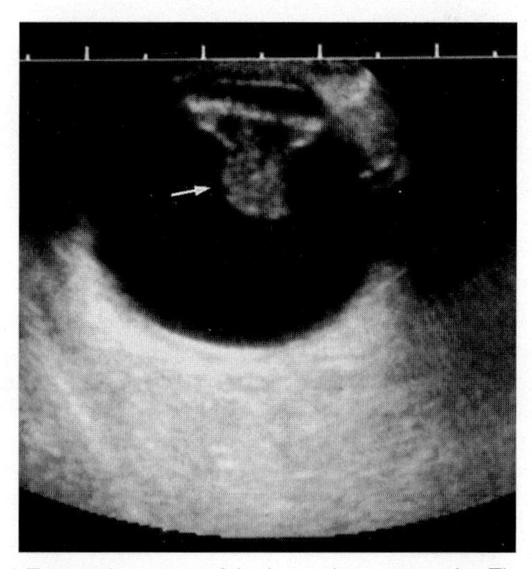

Fig. 19.2 Traumatic rupture of the lens: ultrasonography. The probe is positioned at the top of the image. The aqueous and vitreous are very hypoechoic, whereas the retrobulbar fat appears very bright. The nucleus of the lens (arrow) has been extruded through a defect in the posterior capsule.

and/or posterior to the displaced fragment. Indirect signs of fractures include:

- non-specific soft-tissue swelling, evident as increased density of the affected side;
- air within the orbital cavity 'orbital emphysema' (Fig. 19.3) which, in the absence of a penetrating injury, indicates a fracture involving one of the paranasal sinuses;
- protrusion of orbital soft tissues (the 'hanging drop') through the fracture in the orbital floor;
- a fluid level in the maxillary antrum.

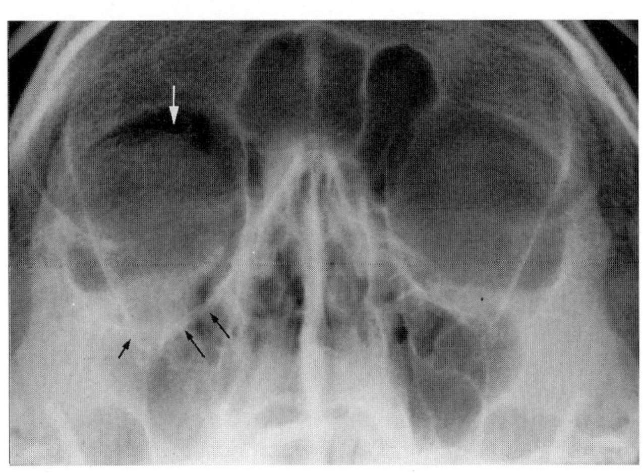

Fig. 19.3 Blow-out fracture; anteroposterior plain film. Orbital emphysema is evident as low-density bubbles within the superior (white arrow) and medial parts of the right orbit. There is a blow-out fracture of its floor, centred on the infraorbital canal, with downward angulation of the fragments medial (two black arrows) and lateral (single black arrow) to it.

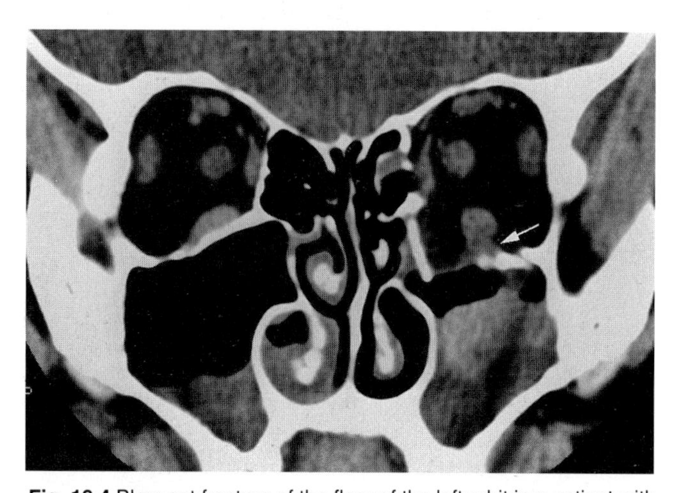

Fig. 19.4 Blow-out fracture of the floor of the left orbit in a patient with persistent restriction of elevation: direct coronal CT. The fracture has occurred in the centre of the floor, with downward displacement of medial and lateral fragments. Orbital fat has herniated into the fracture site, and there is abnormal soft tissue, probably representing scar tissue (arrow), between the inferior rectus muscle and the lateral fragment. There could well be disruption of the medial wall of the orbit, adjacent to the medial rectus muscle. High-density blood is seen in the upper part of the left maxillary antrum, above presumably pre-existing mucosal thickening.

In many cases diplopia resolves quite rapidly after injury, but when double vision or enophthalmos persists, CT is the investigation of choice. Thin sections in the direct coronal plane are most useful in order to show not only the details of fractures (particularly those fractures involving the floor of the orbit) but also the position of the extraocular muscles and retrobulbar fat, either of which may become trapped in the fracture (Fig. 19.4).

Investigation and treatment of acute traumatic optic neuropathy is the subject of intense debate. The case for active decompressive treatment is as yet unproven, and there is thus no indication to search for orbital fractures and/or haematomas. It may, however, be wise to examine the orbital apices, where compression or trapping of the optic nerve is most likely to occur, in a patient with normal vision who is to undergo surgical fixation of extensive facial fractures; CT is the technique of choice.

OCULAR LESIONS

The position of a mass relative to the cone formed by the extraocular muscles and eye may give a clue to its nature. Thus, ocular and optic nerve tumours are, by definition, **intraconal**. Some tumours, such as cavernous haemangiomas, most commonly arise within the muscle cone, while others, including those arising from the lacrimal gland, are primarily **extraconal**. Yet others, such as lymphoma and metastases can arise in either site.

TUMOURS

Primary diagnosis of ocular tumours is by fundoscopy, but imaging may be required if the media are opaque, when a retinal detachment is thought to be secondary to an underlying neoplasm (Fig. 19.5), or when a retrobulbar extension of a tumour is suspected.

In children, **retinoblastoma** is the principal ocular tumour; it may be bilateral. Sonography, CT or MRI can be used to confirm the presence of a fundal mass and to assess any retrobulbar extension, although CT and MRI may necessitate sedation or even general anaesthesia in a young child. Small tumours can be rendered more conspicuous with intravenous contrast medium enhancement on both CT and MRI. Calcification of the tumour, visible on CT and occasionally dense enough to be seen on plain films, is highly suggestive of the diagnosis. Distinction from Coats' disease, which is an exudative retinopathy, may be problematical; retinoblastoma, however, tends to give lower signal than subretinal fluid on T2-weighting.

In adults the common ocular tumour is **malignant melanoma of the choroid**. In the early stages this is

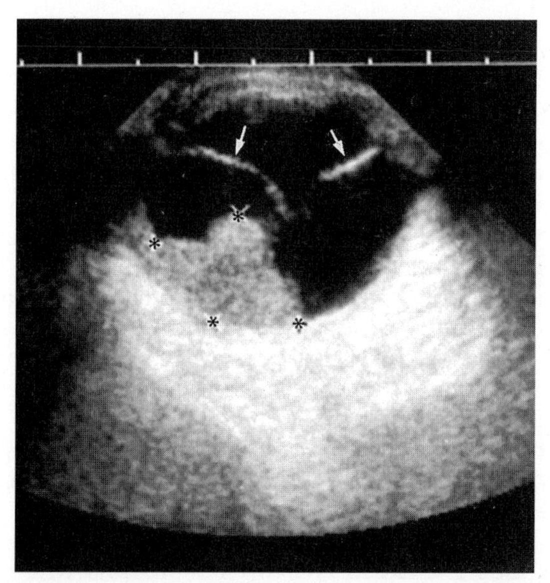

Fig. 19.5 Ocular tumour causing retinal detachment: ultrasonography. Image configuration as in Fig. 19.2. The leaves of the detached retina (arrows) are clearly seen, and were shown to change position with eye movement. A solid mass underlying the detachment (indicated by asterisks) arises from the posterior surface of the eye.

best imaged by ultrasonography or MRI; these show a localized area of thickening of the choroid. Ultrasound is much simpler and although MRI may be specific, showing high signal on T1-weighted images due to the T1 shortening effect of melanin, MRI is less reliable in cases where the clinical diagnosis is in doubt. Similar high signal has been described not only in uveal naevus, for example, but also in choroidal haemangioma, metastases, osteoma and retinal gliosis. Fat-suppressed, contrast-enhanced T1-weighted images may show trans-scleral spread of the tumour, which is a bad prognostic sign (Fig. 19.6). If treatment is to consist of topical radiotherapy, a chest radiograph is essential to exclude dissemination. When the patient with advanced disease presents with a shrunken phthisical eye, the observation on CT or MRI of a retrobulbar mass that also involves the eye itself is highly suggestive of melanoma; invasion of the globe by orbital tumours is very uncommon.

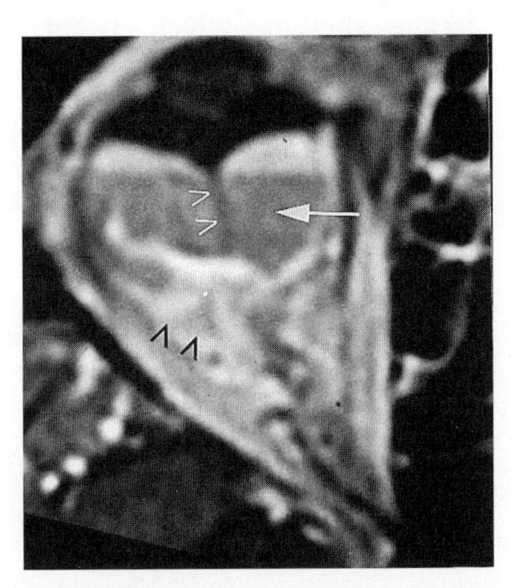

Fig. 19.6 Ocular malignant melanoma with subretinal haemorrhage: axial T1-weighted MRI after intravenous gadolinium. The remaining vitreous overlies subretinal fluid which has divided into high-signal anterior and intermediate-signal posterior (arrow) layers; the high signal of the former is due to methaemoglobin. The retina is still attached in the region of the optic disc (white arrowheads). A contrast-enhancing mass (black arrowheads) is seen in the macular area and behind the posterior pole, indicating trans-scleral extension.

OTHER OCULAR DISEASES

Imaging may be required in **malformations of the globe**. When there is apparent anophthalmos, sonography, CT or MRI may reveal a buried globe, for which surgery may potentially be beneficial. Some malformations, such as colobomas, can be associated with more complex anomalies, such as basal encephaloceles; CT or MRI can be of great importance in showing that an external soft-tissue mass in such cases is not an associated soft-tissue tumour that might be thought suitable for excision, but consists of brain herniating through a bone defect. Some children have a developmentally large (buphthalmic) eye, probably because of congenital glaucoma; differentiation from proptosis may require imaging.

Retinal and choroidal detachments can be documented rapidly and simply by sonography. The classic retinal detachment shows as a fine, V-shaped line whose base is at the optic disc. If the patient is instructed to move the eye during the examination, the mobility of the detached retina, of significance as regards surgical repair, can be assessed. The ultrasonographer can also examine the fundus of the eye to detect a tumour as the cause of the detachment. MRI may be useful for distinguishing a simple detachment from a subretinal haemorrhage. After intraocular tamponade, some investigations such as ultrasound or MRI may be hindered by artefact.

Uveitis can be clinically isolated or found as part of a large spectrum of systemic diseases. Imaging is directed at the latter and can include a plain film of the chest (for sarcoidosis or tuberculosis); sacroiliac joints (for ankylosing spondylitis) and heels (for calcaneal spurs in Behçet's disease). Brain imaging may be required if systemic lymphoma or multiple sclerosis are suspected.

When **scleritis** involves the anterior portion of the globe, the diagnosis can often be made clinically, but imaging techniques can aid in the assessment of posterior scleritis, showing soft-tissue thickening, often centered around the most anterior portion of the optic nerve.

LACRIMAL SYSTEM

In patients who present with epiphora or masses at the medial canthus, dacryocystography can be informative. It should be performed only after probing and syringing of the canaliculi by an ophthalmologist. Two major methods are employed, involving either plain radiographs with introduction of positive contrast medium into the lacrimal system, or a gamma camera following instillation of a radioactive material into the conjunctival sac. The former method gives much more precise anatomical detail, but the latter is perhaps more physiological.

With the patient prone and after topical anaesthesia of the conjunctival sac, a soft plastic cannula is introduced into the inferior canaliculus, and an oil-based or water-soluble iodinated contrast medium is injected. A general anaesthetic may be required in children. Films are exposed just before and during injection; digital subtraction equipment can be used. It is customary to inject both sides, for comparison and because asymptomatic contralateral disease is not rare. If obstruction is shown, a further film may be obtained in the erect position. If the inferior punctum cannot be cannulated, the superior one may be employed. The system may be obstructed at any point; the proximal common canaliculus, the lower border of the lacrimal sac (with the formation of a mucocele) (Fig. 19.7) and the inferior ostium of the nasolacrimal duct are common sites. For planning surgery, precise localization of proximal obstructions is required, as the exact site determines the surgical procedure. Filling defects within the system may represent dacryoliths, and are relatively common with fungal infections; however, air bubbles must be considered. Dacryocystography may be particularly informative as regards the patency of the surgical tract when an operation for lacrimal pathway obstruction has been unsuccessful, in order to show re-stenosis, occlusion or formation of a 'sump' in which the tears collect.

CT may be employed to show involvement of the bony portion of the nasolacrimal duct by disease in adjacent structures.

Transnasal balloon dilatation of the lacrimal pathways can be employed as an alternative to surgery.

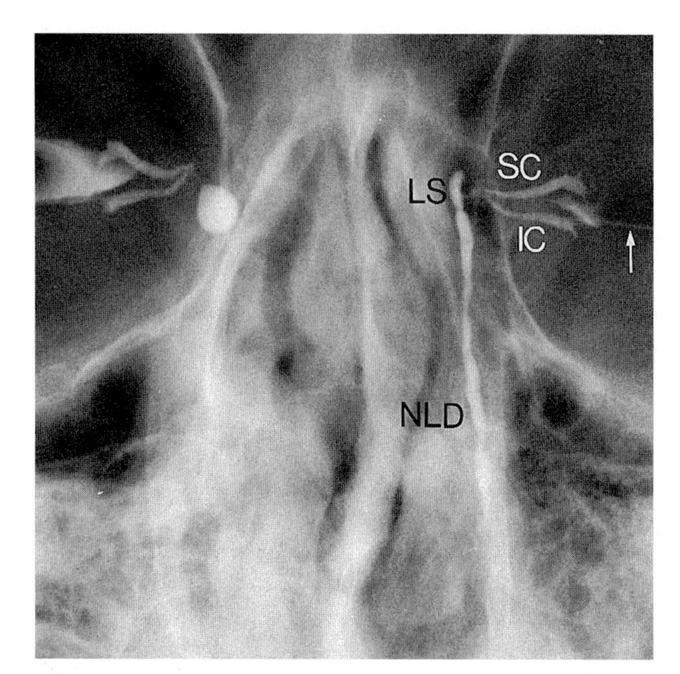

Fig. 19.7 Mucocele of the right lacrimal sac on dacryocystogram: anteroposterior projection during injection. Both inferior canaliculi have been cannulated; note the fine polyethylene catheter (arrow). On the left the lacrimal system is patent, but on the right no contrast medium passes further distally than the dilated lacrimal sac. There is considerable reflux of contrast medium, mainly via the superior canaliculus, into the conjunctival sac. IC, SC = inferior and superior canaliculi; LS = lacrimal sac; NLD = nasolacrimal duct.

MASSES IN THE LACRIMAL GLAND REGION

The superolateral angle of the orbit is a relatively common site for a number of masses, only some of which are associated with the lacrimal gland. The masses include developmental lesions (dermoid cyst), primary tumours (carcinoma, pleomorphic adenoma, lymphoma), inflammatory swellings (acute and chronic dacryoadenitis, orbital pseudotumour, sarcoidosis – often bilateral, primary amyloidosis) and post-traumatic lesions (cholesterol granuloma).

Dermoid cysts may arise anywhere around the orbital margin, or within the orbit, but the lateral canthus is the most common site. If a clinically typical dermoid cyst is freely mobile in all directions on clinical examination surgery can be carried out without imaging, especially in children, but relatively immobile lesions, or those which appear to extend posteriorly, require radiological investigation. Plain radiographs are inadequate; CT is probably the optimal technique, although high-quality MRI may be satisfactory. A dermoid cyst is seen on CT as a mass of water or lower density (depending on the fatty

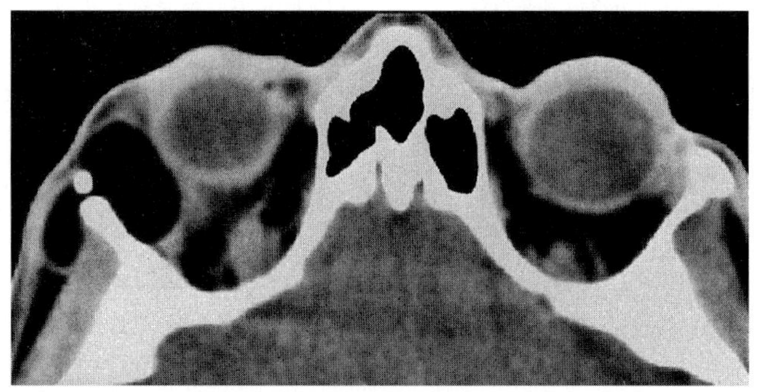

Fig. 19.8 Lateral canthus dermoid cyst on axial CT. A large cyst, whose contents are similar in density to the orbital fat, has displaced the right globe anteriorly and inferiorly. It is clearly seen to communicate with a loculus in the temporal fossa via a cleft in the lateral wall of the orbit.

content), with a fine soft-tissue density rim, but larger lesions are frequently more complex. The orbital walls should be carefully examined for evidence of the cyst extending into a canal in the bone; 'collar-stud' cysts extending from the orbit to the temporal fossa, or vice versa, are not rare (Fig. 19.8).

Carcinomas of the lacrimal gland are most commonly of adenoid-cystic type, but adenocarcinomas occur. On CT or MRI they are manifest as a soft-tissue lesion, often moulded to the eye. Curiously, calcification within the tumour is more common than with benign lacrimal gland lesions. Infiltrative bone destruction is highly suggestive of the diagnosis of carcinoma. Evidence of deep, often perineural extension towards the orbit, cranial cavity or infratemporal fossa may be present. Follow-up frequently shows spread of this type.

Pleomorphic adenomas ('benign mixed tumours') of the lacrimal gland are characteristically hard. They therefore tend to indent the adjacent globe (Fig. 19.9) and, as they enlarge slowly, have often also caused smooth pressure erosion of the lacrimal fossa by the time of presentation. *En bloc* removal, without biopsy, is the treatment of choice for these tumours, so preoperative diagnosis is important.

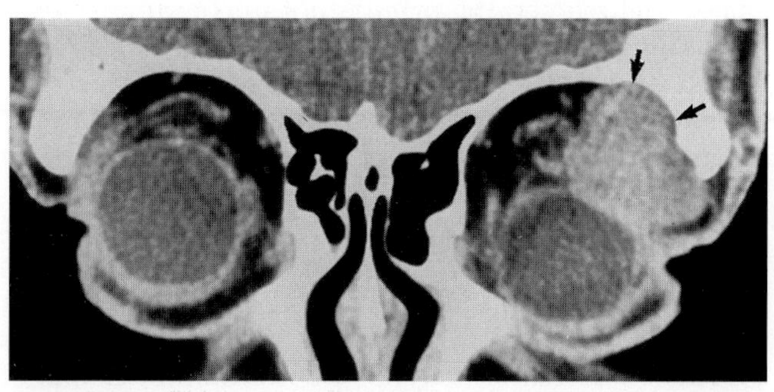

Fig. 19.9 Pleomorphic adenoma of the lacrimal gland on direct coronal CT. A rather dense soft-tissue mass occupies the position of the left lacrimal gland. It displaces the globe downwards, flattening its superolateral aspect, and has caused smooth erosion of the adjacent bone (arrows).

Primary orbital lymphoma not uncommonly involves the lacrimal gland region, although it can arise anywhere within the orbit. On CT the tumour appears of soft-tissue density; it may appear infiltrative, but is often rather well-defined (Fig. 19.10). Signal characteristics on MRI are variable, but nonspecific. The only factor which reliably differentiates lymphoma from benign idiopathic inflammatory disease is that lymphoma may cause bone destruction, but it does so only in a small minority of cases. Either condition may be bilateral, and biopsy is necessary to make the diagnosis.

In **acute inflammatory dacryoadenitis** the diagnosis is usually obvious, but pain is relatively mild in some patients. A chronically inflamed gland may simply be swollen, but if the inflammatory process spreads to the surrounding tissues, the margins of the gland may become blurred on CT or MRI. In such cases, differentiation from carcinoma or lymphoma will require a biopsy.

When **sarcoidosis** involves the lacrimal glands, the swelling is frequently bilateral and imaging simply shows expansion of the glands. However, this appearance can also be seen in lymphoma. The chest radiograph, showing the classic bilateral hilar adenopathy, may clinch the diagnosis, but the chest X-ray is sometimes normal.

Cholesterol granuloma is thought to be the result of haemorrhage into bone, with formation of a granulomatous reaction around blood products, and progressive bone erosion. The superolateral angle of the orbit is, for unknown reasons, a prime site. Plain films show ragged bone destruction, more suggestive of a malignant tumour. CT reveals that the soft-tissue mass associated with the granuloma projects inferomedially

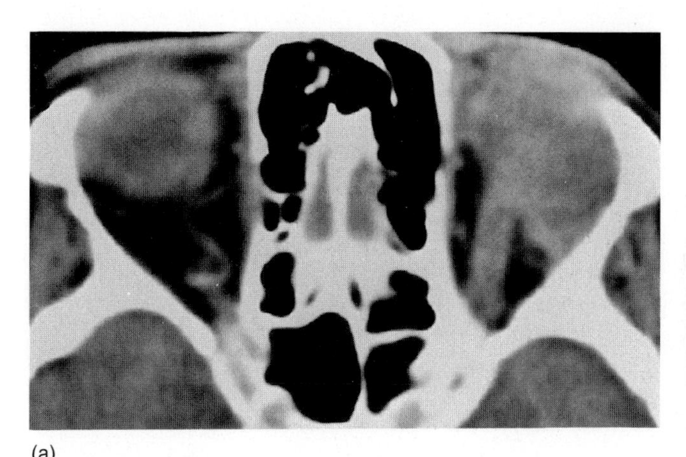

(a)

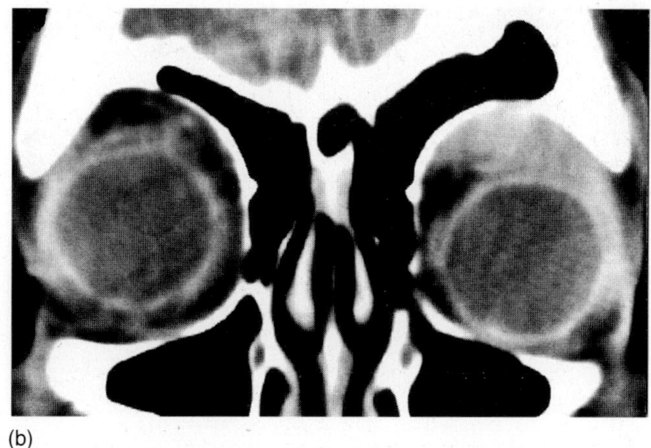

(b)

Fig. 19.10 Primary orbital lymphoma. (a) Axial and (b) direct coronal contrast-enhanced CT showing an amorphous, but well-defined, soft-tissue density mass extending across the roof of the anterior half of the left orbit, moulded to the globe, which it has displaced anteriorly and downwards. There are no bone changes. Biopsy would be necessary to distinguish this lymphoma from other infiltrative lesions such as a metastasis or even a benign inflammatory orbital pseudotumour.

into the orbit and is characteristically of lower density than brain; this is a valuable observation which allows distinction from a carcinoma. MRI shows high signal on both T1- and T2-weighted images. After curettage, imaging procedures may show remarkable resolution of the bone destruction.

PRIMARY ORBITAL NEOPLASMS

Benign orbital neoplasms are relatively uncommon in young children; the most frequent tumour is **rhabdomyosarcoma**. Often presenting with an inflammatory clinical picture, a rhabdomyosarcoma is manifest on imaging as a non-specific and often moderately well-defined orbital mass. Since the tumour arises from primitive rests within the orbit, it characteristically does not simulate an expanded extraocular muscle. Contrast enhancement on CT or MRI is typically marked. Bone destruction is not characteristic.

The commonest benign retrobulbar tumour is the **cavernous haemangioma** which presents, usually in adult life, with proptosis and occasionally also with visual impairment, particularly if the tumour arises at the apex of the orbit. CT or MRI show a discrete, rounded retrobulbar tumour, typically lying within the cone formed by the extrocular muscles lateral to the optic nerve. Contrast enhancement is characteristically intense and homogeneous, although rapid imaging may show enhancement spreading through the tumour from a 'hilum' (Fig. 19.11).

Neurofibromas or **neurilemmomas** can arise from the intraorbital branches of the cranial nerves. Imaging procedures show them as solid masses, commonly in the upper half of the orbit. The tumours tend to be more elongated in the anteroposterior plane than haemangiomas and may extend posteriorly through the superior orbital fissure towards the cavernous sinus. Fibrous histiocytoma and haemangiopericytoma also form rounded masses, but are more common in the anterior half of the orbit. Angiography may be indicated, if a mass looks hypervascular or appears pulsatile, to confirm the vascular nature of the tumour and show the origin of feeding vessels; in some cases, preoperative embolization may be possible. Several of these solid tumours also have malignant forms, and primary sarcomas also arise within the orbit. Liposarcoma may be particularly difficult to recognize if its imaging characteristics are similar to those of the adjacent orbital fat.

The orbit is a common site for **metastases**. Their imaging features are very varied, but a poorly defined soft-tissue mass, which fails to respect normal tissue planes, is most common. Some fibrotic tumours, such as scirrhous carcinoma of the breast, cause volume loss, resulting in enophthalmos.

Meningiomas arising within the orbit, other than from the sheath of the optic nerve, are extremely rare, although it is a common error to include meningioma in the differential diagnosis of discrete intraorbital masses. However, the orbit is not uncommonly invaded by meningiomas of the sphenoid bone, and proptosis and/or visual disturbance may cause the patient to consult the ophthalmologist rather than the neurologist. The cardinal abnormality on imaging is thickening (hyperostosis) and increased density (sclerosis) of the greater wing of the sphenoid; the soft-tissue component may be relatively small, and may be visible on CT only following intravenous contrast medium. The lateral rectus muscle often appears swollen. Differential diagnosis is from other causes of focal bone thickening, such as fibrous dysplasia (in which there is no soft-tissue lesion) (Fig. 19.12) or osteoblastic metastasis.

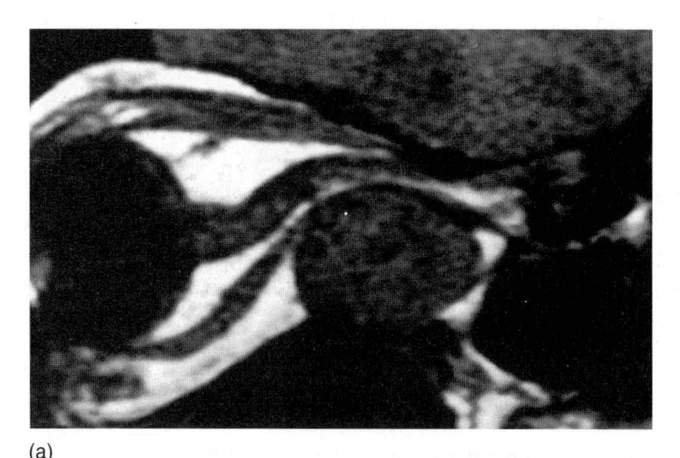

(a)

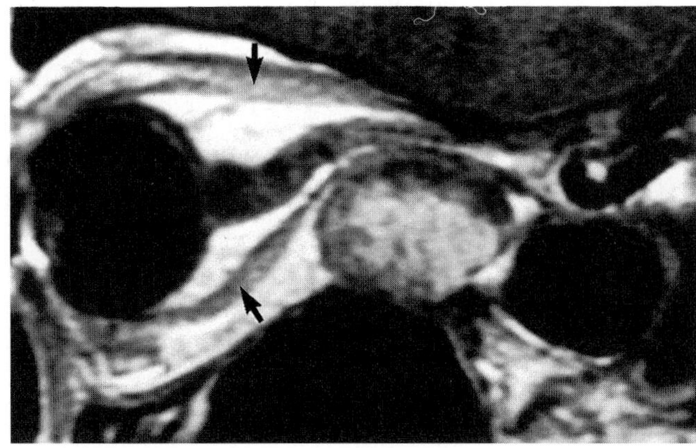

(b)

Fig. 19.11 Retrobulbar cavernous haemangioma on parasagittal MRI (a) before and (b) after intravenous gadolinium. A strikingly smooth, elliptical mass lies beneath the inferior rectus muscle, with the optic nerve draped over it. The mass shows inhomogeneous contrast enhancement, spreading out from its centre, because of the very slow blood flow within it; for the same reason, these lesions do not 'blush' on angiography. Note the normal contrast enhancement of the extraocular muscles (arrows).

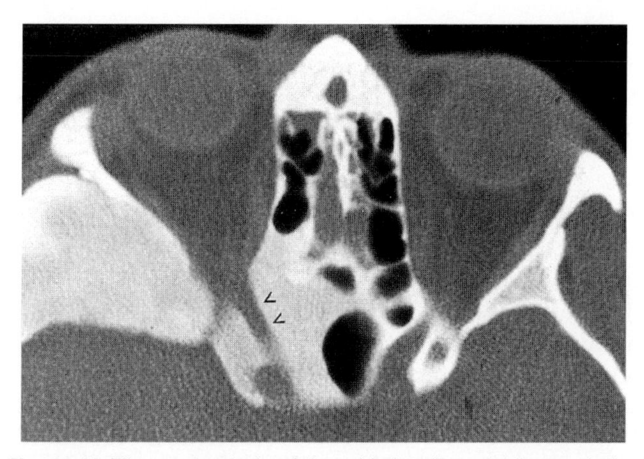

Fig. 19.12 Fibrous dysplasia of the orbital walls: axial 'bone-window' algorithm CT. Gross thickening of its lateral wall is encroaching on the right orbit, displacing the globe anteriorly. Note the very characteristic, featureless, 'ground-glass' texture of the abnormal bone. Although the bone surrounding it is involved, the optic canal (arrowheads) is not significantly narrowed. The granular texture of the soft tissues is an imaging artefact typical of high-resolution 'bone-window' imaging.

Mucoceles or tumours of the paranasal sinuses can present as orbit masses, so that adequate imaging for an orbital mass should always include the adjacent sinuses.

OPTIC NERVE AND MENINGEAL COVERINGS

TUMOURS

Glioma

The optic nerve itself effectively gives rise to only one tumour: the optic nerve glioma, which occurs almost invariably in children, and is usually a relatively benign lesion. This uncommon tumour is manifest on CT as a swelling of the optic nerve, often rather bulky by the time of presentation, with a waist between the mass of the tumour and the posterior pole of the globe. Contrast enhancement is variable. Coronal sections sometimes reveal a 'target' appearance, the central portion of the nerve appearing denser than the periphery. Posterior extension to the intracranial optic pathways is an important prognostic observation. It may not be obvious whether a mass, particularly one which is rather elongated in the anteroposterior plane, arises from the optic nerve or lies alongside it; MRI may be particularly helpful in such cases.

Meningioma

The meninges surrounding the optic nerve can give rise to meningiomas. Unlike optic nerve gliomas, meningiomas occur almost exclusively in adults. On CT the optic nerve appears thickened, in a more fusiform manner than in cases of glioma (Fig. 19.13) and plaques of calcification are diagnostic. Abnormally intense contrast enhancement may be seen. MRI is insensitive to calcification of the meningeal sheath of the nerve, but shows intracranial extension of the tumour to better advantage than CT. Since in most patients vision is at least moderately impaired by the time of presentation, surgery on the nerve itself is unlikely to be beneficial, but imaging is particularly important for detection of intracranial tumour, which may compromise not only the chiasm, but also the contralateral optic nerve. Bilateral optic nerve sheath meningiomas are frequently associated with intracranial meningiomas.

Swelling of the optic nerve/sheath complex can also be seen in raised intracranial pressure since the

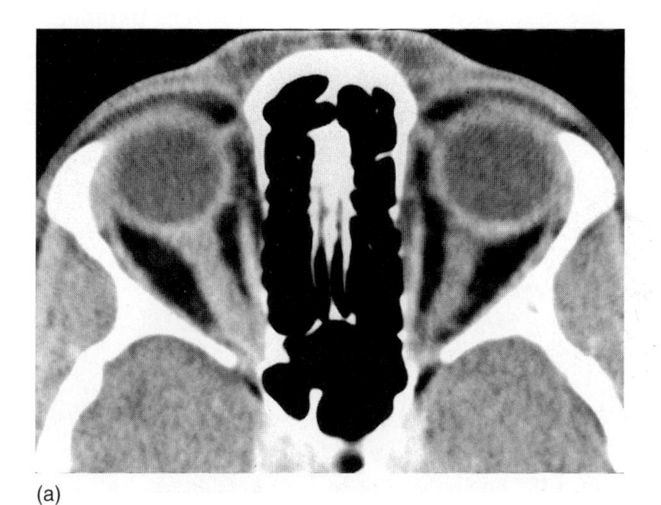

(a)

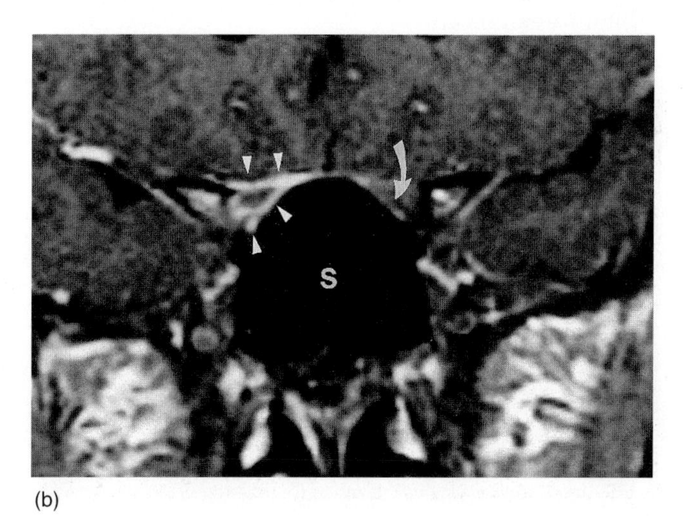

(b)

Fig. 19.13 Meningioma of the sheath of the optic nerve. (a) Axial CT section in the plane of the optic nerves shows the right nerve/sheath complex to be wider, denser and more irregular in outline than its fellow. Other images showed no evidence of intracranial extension. (b) Coronal contrast-enhanced T1-weighted MRI section through the cranial end of the optic canals in the same patient shows a thin layer of pathologically enhancing tissue (arrowheads) surrounding the optic nerve as it enters the head; it almost reaches the midline, and threatens eventually to involve the contralateral optic nerve (arrow). S = sphenoid sinus.

subarachnoid space surrounding the nerve is in continuity with the intracranial cerebrospinal fluid spaces and inflammatory conditions (retrobulbar neuritis, sarcoidosis).

Chronic fungal infections may produce large soft-tissue masses in the orbit, which have non-specific appearances on CT, but characteristically give low signal on MRI.

OTHER INTRINSIC DISEASES OF THE OPTIC NERVE

A number of inflammatory and idiopathic diseases can affect the optic nerve without causing morphological changes. These conditions are not generally of surgical significance, but may be revealed by imaging. In **retrobulbar neuritis**, typified by multiple sclerosis, inflammation in the acute stage, gliosis in the chronic stage and plaques of demyelination can be demonstrated on MRI as areas of altered signal, without mass effect. Contrast enhancement is shown in the acute phase. Similar signal changes can be seen in some cases of acute disseminated encephalomyelitis or sarcoidosis, with optic nerve involvement, or conditions such as Leber's hereditary optic neuropathy.

INFLAMMATORY DISEASE

PYOGENIC INFECTION OF THE ORBITS

Orbital cellulitis is a condition requiring urgent treatment. Imaging with CT or MRI can be employed to determine whether the disease extends posterior to the orbital septum and, more rarely, whether there is an orbital abscess, although differentiation of confluent cellulitis and abscess may be difficult. Plain films are a simple way of diagnosing associated paranasal sinusitis and may also show an unsuspected orbital foreign body.

THYROID OPHTHALMOPATHY

Graves' disease characteristically causes swelling of the rectus muscles; the superior oblique may also be involved. Although this is a systemic disease, imaging often shows the muscle involvement to be asymmetrical, or even unilateral (Fig. 19.14); the medial rectus and inferior rectus muscles are most commonly affected. In a relatively small proportion of patients the muscles appear normal, but the retrobulbar fat appears increased in volume. In some patients the expanded muscles show fatty replacement. There is typically marked proptosis with forward herniation of orbital fat. The orbits may be enlarged with medial bowing of the lamina papyracea on one or both sides. The optic nerve often appears stretched in advanced cases, but optic neuropathy is probably due to compression of the nerve by the expanded muscle bellies near the orbital apex. The superior ophthalmic vein may also be engorged. CT may be useful for determining the anatomical efficacy of surgical decompression.

OTHER IDIOPATHIC INFLAMMATORY CONDITIONS

Idiopathic inflammation of the orbit ('orbital granuloma' or 'pseudotumour') is one of the commonest causes of pain and/or proptosis in adults. By definition, no infective organism is found, although some cases are associated with systemic illness or paranasal

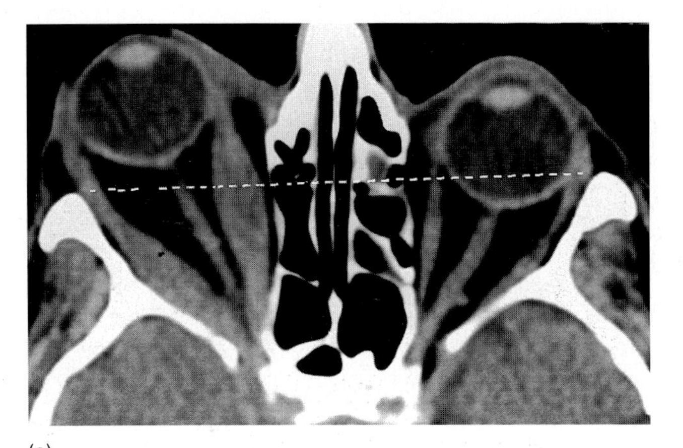

(a)

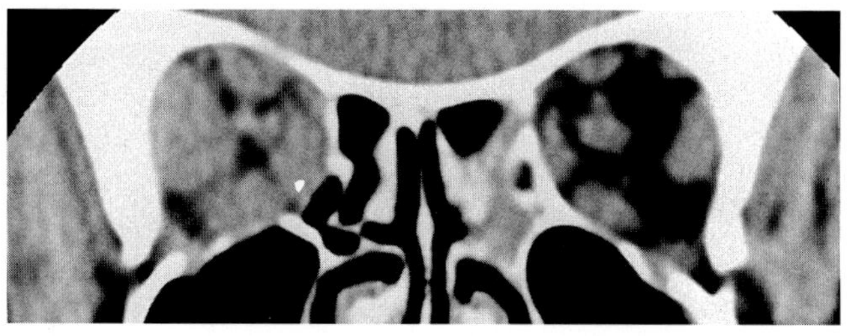

(b)

Fig. 19.14 Unilateral thyroid ophthalmopathy. (a) Axial and (b) reformatted coronal CT show marked swelling of all the rectus muscles on the right, with exophthalmos and expansion of the orbit. The optic nerve appears stretched and the coronal image shows the potential for compression of the nerve at the apex. Note that on the healthy side only about three-quarters of the globe is anterior to an imaginary line joining the anterolateral bony margins of the two orbits.

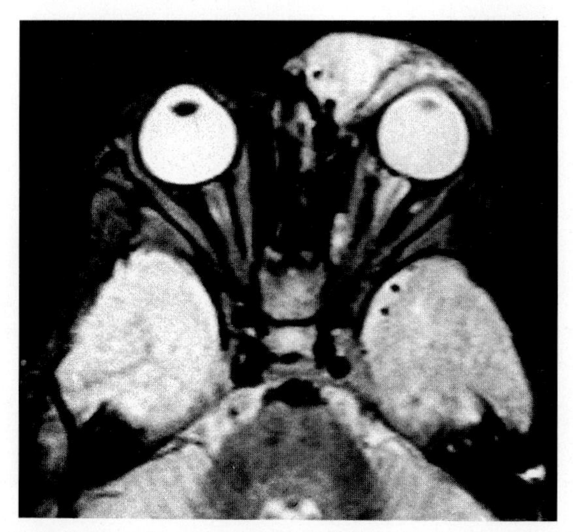

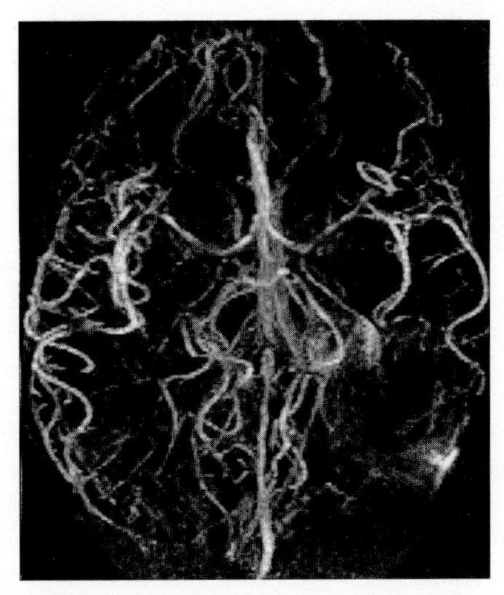

(a) (b)

Fig. 19.15 Capillary haemangioma in a 15-month-old child. (a) Axial T2-weighted MRI shows a heterogeneous high-signal mass anterior to the left eye, which is displaced laterally. (b) Magnetic resonance angiography shows high-flow intracranial arteries, but no abnormal vasculature related to the slow-flow haemangioma.

sinus disease. Imaging procedures show proptosis, usually unilateral, with a soft-tissue mass which can involve the orbital fat, extraocular muscles, lacrimal gland and optic nerve. The tissue planes around these structures are frequently obliterated and vessels may be prominent in the fat. In some patients, enlargement of a single muscle ('orbital myositis') may be seen. The 'pseudotumour' may show marked contrast enhancement. Extension intracranially via the superior orbital fissure is infrequent but well documented; the cavernous sinus can appear expanded. The process may also extend out of the orbit onto the facial soft tissues and, via the inferior orbital fissure, down to the infratemporal fossa and pterygoid region. Bone erosion is uncommon but in chronic disease the adjacent orbital walls may become thickened. There is considerable overlap between the imaging features of orbital pseudotumour, lymphoma and metastases. Moreover, differentiation on clinical and histological grounds may be problematic. As management of each condition is different, biopsy is essential; localization of the lesion for biopsy is a major contribution of imaging.

Other inflammatory processes can involve the orbit. Quasimalignant diseases such as Wegener's granuloma and lethal midline granuloma frequently involve the paranasal sinuses, and can cause widespread bone destruction affecting the orbits.

VASCULAR LESIONS OF THE ORBIT

In young children, **capillary haemangioma** is the commonest developmental vascular lesion. Although congenital, the bluish periorbital mass develops after birth and may enlarge until about the age of 18 months. The nature of the lesion is usually evident clinically; ultrasonography, CT or MRI (Fig. 19.15) usually demonstrate a rather homogeneous soft-tissue mass that shows marked contrast enhancement. Closure of the palpebral fissure in early life threatens to produce amblyopia. Angiography may be helpful prior to surgery and intravascular therapy may be possible.

Venous malformations ('orbital varices') are also relatively common. Plain films may show enlargement of the orbit. CT shows serpinginous or multinodular masses within the orbit, which on MRI characteristically show mixed signal intensity, due to both fast and slowly flowing blood or thrombus. Phleboliths, evident as small, punctate areas of increased density seen on CT within the mass, are more readily seen on CT than on plain films and are diagnostic (Fig. 19.16).

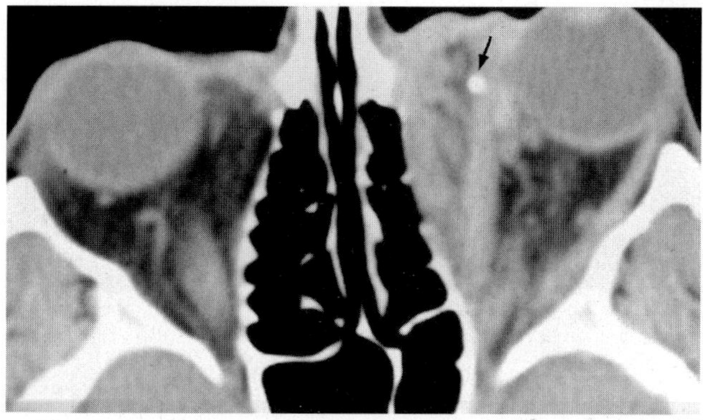

Fig. 19.16 Orbital varices on axial CT. The left globe is displaced forwards and laterally by a mass composed of multiple serpiginous structures, containing a phlebolith (arrow). The left orbit is enlarged.

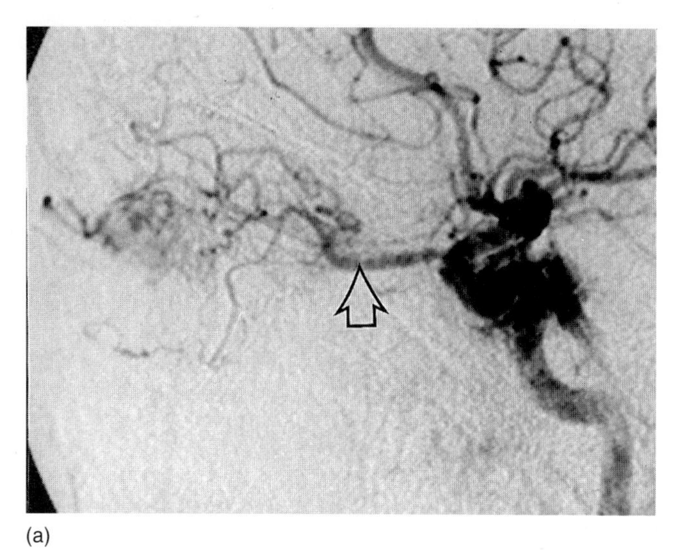

(a)

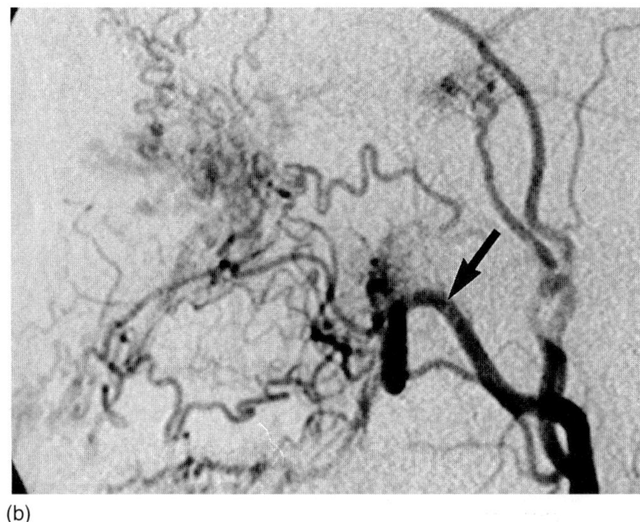

(b)

Fig. 19.17 Orbital arteriovenous malformation on digital subtraction angiography, with arterial phase (a) internal and (b) external carotid artery injections. Extensive pathological vessels within the orbit fill from both the ophthalmic artery (open arrow) and from several branches of the external carotid artery, mainly the internal maxillary artery (arrow).

Paradoxically, arteriography and phlebography are unrewarding investigations. The nosology of 'orbital lymphangioma' is contested; some workers suggest that these lesions are simply chronic venous malformations with lymphocytic infiltration.

The imaging manifestations of **arteriovenous malformations** within the orbit depend on their size and flow characteristics. High-quality superselective arteriography is required for planning treatment (Fig. 19.17). With the development of fine catheters that may be introduced into the branches of not only the external carotid, but also the ophthalmic artery, occlusion by embolization is a serious therapeutic option.

The orbit may also be secondarily involved in patients with arteriovenous fistulae or malformations in the region of the cavernous sinus, in which abnormal drainage occurs via the veins of the orbit. Imaging may show the superior ophthalmic veins to be dilated; there is commonly proptosis and swelling of the orbital soft tissues, notably the extraocular muscles, because of the increased venous pressure within the orbit.

Orbital haemorrhage usually has typical clinical features, particularly a very acute onset. Although bleeding may be secondary to an underlying lesion such as varices or an arteriovenous malformation, in many cases no source is found. Management is conservative so extensive investigation is not required. In children particularly, the clot tends not to spread through the orbit; the septa within the fat limit the haemorrhage, giving rise to a rounded 'haematic cyst', which can be documented on CT or MRI. The density on CT or signal characteristics on MRI may make its nature unmistakable, especially if a fluid level between solid and liquid components is shown. A follow-up examination usually demonstrates resolution. In the elderly, the laxer soft tissues do not confine the bleeding, which is often manifest clinically as subconjunctival extension.

CHAPTER 20

Ear

Iain R. Colquhoun

ANATOMY
CONGENITAL ABNORMALITIES
OTOSCLEROSIS
TRAUMA
INFLAMMATORY DISORDERS
CHOLESTEATOMA
CHOLESTEROL CYSTS AND GRANULOMAS
NEOPLASMS

Computed tomography and magnetic resonance imaging are the principal radiological investigations for assessing petrous bone pathology. The fine structural detail requires high resolution CT techniques (HRCT), comprising 1–2 mm thick contiguous sections, ideally in both the axial and coronal planes. MRI has improved soft-tissue resolution, and the development of fast imaging sequences with thinner sections and greater spatial resolution has significantly increased the use of MRI.

ANATOMY

The petrous bone is pyramidal, lying horizontally, the apex directed medially and anteriorly towards the clivus. The upper surface forms the posterior floor of the middle cranial fossa, the posterior surface of the petrous bone forming the anterior border of the posterior cranial fossa with the clivus (Figs 20.1, 20.2).

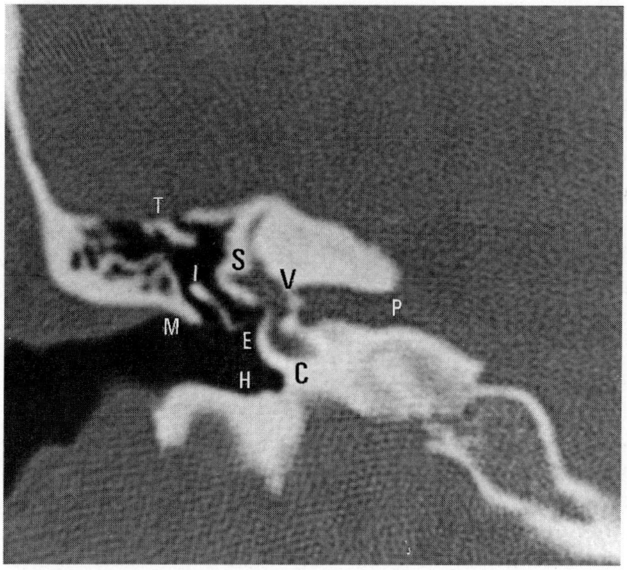

Fig. 20.1 Coronal HRCT of normal anatomy. C = basal turn of cochlea; E = stapes articulating in oval window above the promontory; H = hypotympanum; I = incus in epitympanum; M = scutum; P = porus of internal auditory canal; S = semicircular canals; T = tegmen tympani; V = vestibule.

MIDDLE EAR

The middle ear cavity is divided into three sections. Superiorly is the epitympanum containing the head of the malleus and body and short process of the incus. Inferiorly is the hypotympanum, the smallest of the three divisions and empty. Between these is the mesotympanum containing the handle of the malleus, long process of the incus and the stapes. The lateral wall is formed by the tympanic membrane and above this by a pointed bony projection, the scutum. The anterior wall is shortened by approximation of the floor and roof and contains the opening for the bony portion of the eustachian tube. The floor is a thin plate of bone separating the middle ear from the jugular foramen posteriorly and the carotid canal anteriorly.

Diagnostic and Interventional Radiology in Surgical Practice. Edited by P. Armstrong and M.L. Wastie. Published in 1997 by Chapman & Hall, London. ISBN 0 412 61960 1 (HB), 0 412 61970 9 (PB)

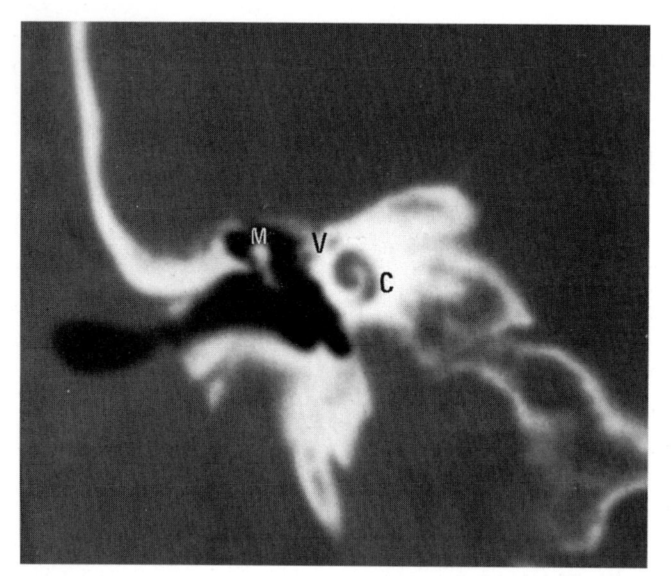

Fig. 20.2 Coronal HRCT of normal anatomy (2 mm anterior to Fig. 20.1). C = cochlea; M = malleus; V = hairpin turn of facial nerve canal.

The roof is another thin plate of bone, the tegmen tympani, separating the middle ear from the middle cranial fossa dura and extending posteriorly to cover the antrum. The posterior wall is perforated superiorly by an opening into the mastoid antrum – the 'aditus ad antrum' – and blends into the medial wall, the main feature of which is 'the promontory' for the basal turn of the cochlea. Behind and above this is the oval window, closed by the stapes footplate. Above the promontory and oval window is a ridge containing the horizontal portion of the facial nerve canal.

INNER EAR

Deep to the middle ear cavity is the otic capsule formed of dense compact bone. Within this is the labyrinth consisting of the cochlea, vestibule and semicircular canals. The cochlea has two and three-quarter turns, the basal turn being the largest and easily visualized, the middle and apical turns being difficult to separate. The vestibular system consists of the three semicircular canals and the vestibule, the membranous components of which (the saccule and utricle) cannot be separately visualized. The lateral semicircular canal lies near the axial plane, its apex directed laterally; the posterior lies along, and the superior lies across the long axis of the petrous bone, their apices directed cranially.

INTERNAL AUDITORY CANAL

The medial end of the internal auditory canal, the porus, is divided into quadrants. Through the anterior two quadrants pass the facial nerve superiorly and the cochlear branch of VIII inferiorly. The two divisions of the vestibular branch of VIII pass through the posterior quadrants.

FACIAL NERVE

The facial nerve leaves the pons at the pontomedullary junction and traverses the cerebellopontine angle cistern to the porus. In the internal auditory canal it passes laterally and anteriorly to a point above and lateral to the cochlea where it is expanded by the geniculate ganglion and takes a hairpin turn to run posteriorly through the medial wall of the middle ear cavity, immediately below the lateral semicircular canals before turning vertically downwards to exit via the stylomastoid foramen.

IMAGING STRATEGIES

HRCT is the method of choice for demonstrating the bony anatomy but the fluid-containing structures of the inner ear, the cochlea, vestibule and semicircular canals are well shown on T2-weighted MRI sequences, appearing hyperintense against the surrounding hypointense bone.

CONGENITAL ABNORMALITIES

Atresia of the external auditory canal is relatively common and may involve the cartilaginous or bony sections. HRCT is essential for assessment of the

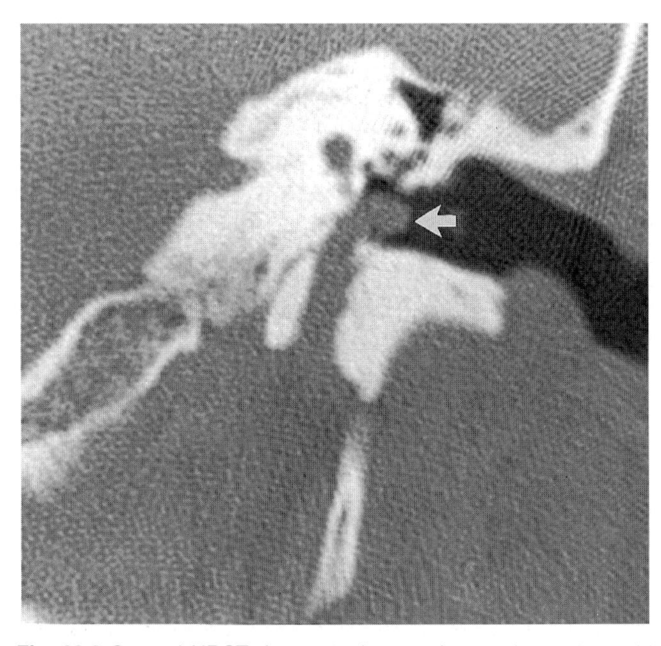

Fig. 20.3 Coronal HRCT demonstrating an aberrant internal carotid artery within the middle ear cavity (arrow).

extent of the atresia, associated anomalies and for excluding a concomitant primary cholesteatoma of the middle ear. The cochlea may be hypoplastic as in the Mondini deformity, with an intact basal turn and a common cavity for the middle and apical turns. Anomalies of the semicircular canals most frequently involve the lateral semicircular canal, which is dilated, often in conjunction with the vestibule.

The major congenital vascular anomalies relate to variations in position of the internal carotid artery and jugular bulb. An aberrant internal carotid artery passes through the middle ear cavity anterior to the cochlear promontory (Fig. 20.3). Variations in size and position of the jugular bulb can result in it protruding into the middle ear cavity. Vascular variations are readily evaluated by HRCT or MRI with flow-sensitive sequences.

OTOSCLEROSIS

Otosclerosis is an idiopathic disease of the labyrinthine capsule with replacement of the normal lamellar bone by initially spongy and later denser bone, and is best assessed by HRCT. Active disease (**otospongiosis**) appears as focal or diffuse areas of reduced density, whereas areas of calcification or sclerosis denote mature disease.

The process most frequently involves the oval window (fenestral), where in the active stage there is apparent widening due to the surrounding bone resorption. Cochlear otosclerosis may involve the basal turn or be more diffuse, appearing as a zone of reduced density around the labyrinth (Fig. 20.4).

TRAUMA

Temporal bone fractures may be longitudinal (80%), transverse (15%) or mixed (5%). Longitudinal fractures pass through the long axis of the temporal bone,

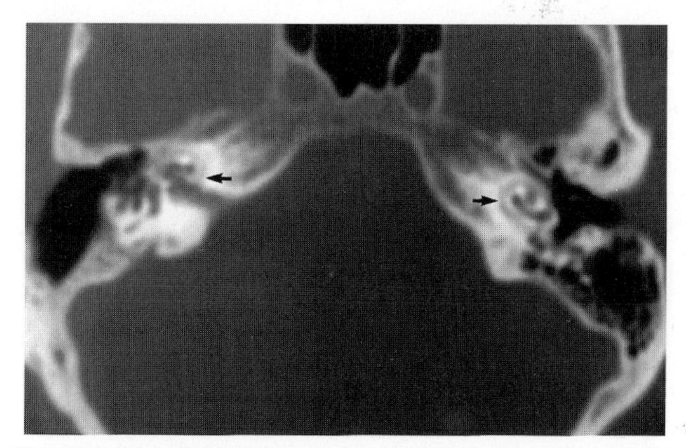

Fig. 20.4 Axial HRCT demonstrating bilateral cochlear otosclerosis (arrows).

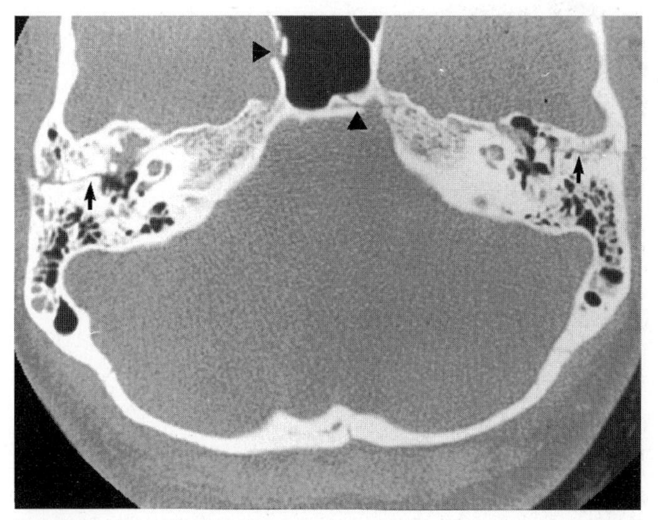

Fig. 20.5 Axial HRCT demonstrating bilateral longitudinal petrous bone fractures (arrows). Note extension of the fractures through the sphenoid sinus (arrowheads).

along the external auditory canal and roof of the middle ear to the inner ear (Fig. 20.5), whereas transverse fractures are perpendicular to the long axis. Complications include facial nerve injury (particularly with transverse fractures), CSF fistula, post-traumatic meningoencephalocoeles and rarely internal carotid artery aneurysm. Ossicular disruption can occur in conjunction with petrous fractures or in isolation, the incus being most frequently involved. HRCT is ideally suited for assessment of petrous fractures and associated complications.

INFLAMMATORY DISORDERS

Acute otitis media and **acute mastoiditis** are common infections, clinically evident and responsive to antibiotic therapy. Imaging is only required if complications are suspected. Occasionally the infection can extend medially into the petrous apex, **apical petrositis**.

Chronic otitis media and **mastoiditis** are usually the result of eustachian tube dysfunction or secondary to the presence of a cholesteatoma. Evaluation of the extent of disease and degree of bony erosion is best performed with HRCT. The limitation of this technique is the inability to differentiate fluid, inflammatory or fibrous tissue and cholesteatoma, all appearing as non-specific soft tissue density material.

Malignant otitis externa is an aggressive infection, usually caused by *Pseudomonas aeruginosa*, and frequently seen in elderly diabetics. Infection originates in the external auditory canal and, if untreated, rapidly spreads inferiorly and medially to involve the bone and soft tissues of the skull base; direct spread into the middle ear cavity is rare. Initial radiological assessment is principally by axial HRCT (Figs. 20.6, 20.7).

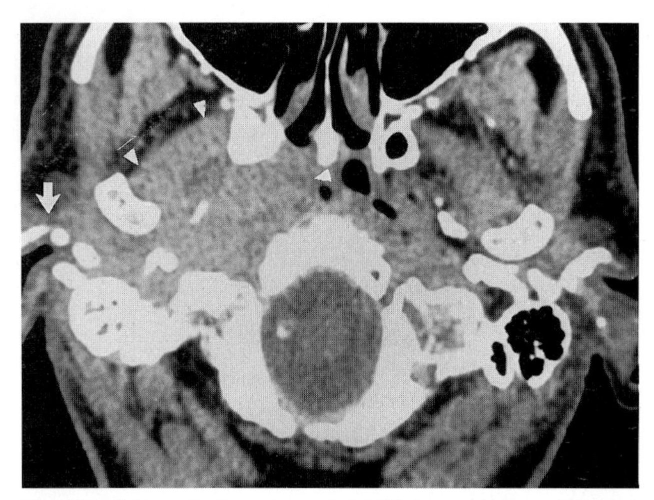

Fig. 20.6 Malignant otitis externa. Axial CT demonstrating a large soft-tissue mass below the skull base (arrowheads), extending medially from the external auditory canal (arrow).

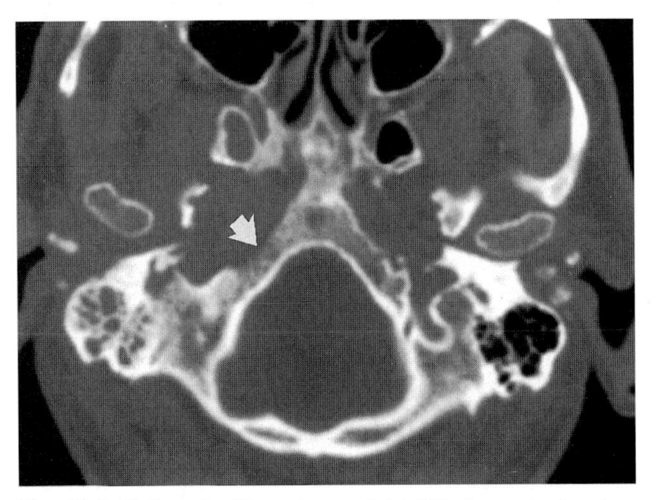

Fig. 20.7 Malignant otitis externa. Axial CT demonstrating bone erosion of the skull base with loss of cortex (arrow). Note the ipsilateral mastoid air cell opacification.

Bell's palsy is the commonest cause of lower motor neurone facial paralysis. Thin section T1-weighted MRI can demonstrate the facial nerve, diffuse linear enhancement of the nerve occurring with Bell's, herpes zoster, postoperative and post-traumatic facial nerve palsies.

CHOLESTEATOMA

Cholesteatomas are epidermoids of the petrous bone, composed of keratinizing stratified squamous epithelium which constantly desquamates keratin.

Congenital cholesteatomas, though rare, occur most frequently at the petrous apex or within the middle ear. Lesions at the petrous apex are discussed with cholesterol granulomas. Congenital cholesteatomas of the middle ear are rare, occurring behind an intact ear drum without a history of otitis media, and are difficult to distinguish from acquired lesions.

Acquired cholesteatomas are associated with prior otitis media. They can occur anywhere within the middle ear, but typically originate laterally in the epitympanum, between the scutum and malleus (Prussak's space). Radiological diagnosis is primarily by direct coronal HRCT with visualization of a soft-tissue mass in the appropriate location and erosion of the scutum and ossicles (Fig. 20.8). With a larger mass occupying the middle ear cavity and extending into the mastoid antrum, differentiation from fluid or granulation tissue is not possible with CT. MRI may be of use, cholesteatomas being low to medium intensity on T1-weighted, and relatively hyperintense on T2-weighted sequences, whereas granulation tissue is less intense on T2-weighted and may enhance with gadolinium. Fluid is more intense on T2-weighted sequences. However, extensive cholesteatomas are usually associated with fluid, granulation tissue and often cholesterol crystals (hyperintense on both T1 and T2-weighted sequences) resulting in a non-specific lesion of heterogeneous intensity. Coronal HRCT will demonstrate local complications including destruction of the medial wall of the middle ear cavity, usually involving the lateral semicircular canal (leading to a labyrinthine fistula) and horizontal segment of the facial nerve, and superior extension into the mastoid antrum with destruction of the tegmen. Contrast-enhanced CT or MRI is essential to exclude the intracranial complications associated with perforation of the tegmen tympani, or more rarely of the posterior mastoid cortex, namely epidural empyema, or temporal or cerebellar abscess.

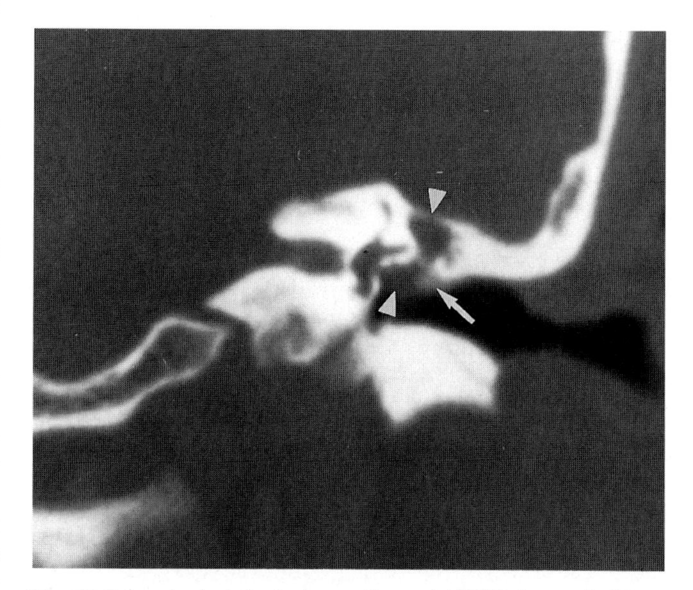

Fig. 20.8 Acquired cholesteatoma. Coronal HRCT demonstrating a soft-tissue mass in the epitympanum and mastoid antrum (arrowheads) with early erosion of the scutum (arrow)

CHOLESTEROL CYSTS AND GRANULOMAS

Small cholesterol cysts are frequently seen within the normal petrous apex on MRI. When larger, they are termed giant cholesterol cysts or cholesterol granulomas and produce a well-defined expansile and usually destructive mass. The appearances are very similar to those of congenital cholesteatomas of the petrous apex. Differentiation is facilitated by MRI, cholesterol granulomas being hyperintense on both T1 and T2-weighted sequences, whereas congenital cholesteatomas are low to medium intensity on T1-weighted and relatively hyperintense on T2-weighted sequences.

NEOPLASMS

ACOUSTIC NEUROMA

Acoustic neuromas are the commonest tumours involving the temporal bone and cerebellopontine angle. Approximately 90% arise from the superior division of the vestibular nerve close to the porus. Bilateral acoustic neuromas are found in neurofibromatosis type II. Occasionally vestibular neuromas can arise at the fundus of the internal auditory canal or within the vestibule. Cochlear neuromas are rare, usually arising near the porus, or rarely within the labyrinth.

On both MRI and CT acoustic neuromas usually appear as well-defined masses of homogeneous texture and exhibit marked contrast enhancement. They can contain cystic areas from either necrosis or previous haemorrhage. MRI is the radiological screening test of choice, with the use of thin section axial and coronal T2-weighted images through the internal auditory canal, acoustic neuromas appearing as hypointense masses compared to CSF (Fig. 20.9). If detail is obscured by artefact, usually from CSF flow, post-gadolinium T1-weighted axial and coronal images are necessary.

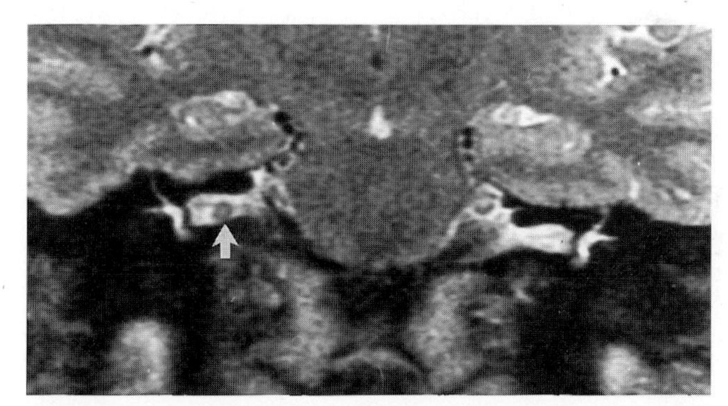

Fig. 20.9 Coronal fast spin-echo T2-weighted image through the internal auditory canal clearly demonstrating a small intracanalicular acoustic neuroma (arrow).

FACIAL NERVE NEUROMA

Facial nerve neuromas have the same CT and MRI characteristics as acoustic neuromas and mimic them when they occur within the internal auditory canal or cerebellopontine angle cistern. The commonest site is at the geniculate ganglion where the neuroma produces local erosion of the petrous bone.

PARAGANGLIOMA

Paragangliomas or glomus tumours are highly vascular tumours, usually benign in nature but locally invasive. Glomus tumours of the temporal bone are divided into two groups, tympanicum or jugulare. The tumours originate from glomus cells within the adventitia of the jugular bulb or along the course of the tympanic branch of the glossopharyngeal nerve (Jacobson's nerve) or the auricular branch of the vagus (nerve of Arnold).

Glomus tympanicum tumours arise within the mucosa overlying the cochlear promontory on the medial wall of the middle ear cavity and frequently present with pulsatile tinnitus, due to tumour vascularity, or conductive hearing loss from mass effect on the ossicular chain. The tumour is usually visible otoscopically as a reddish-blue pulsatile mass behind an intact tympanic membrane. Radiological examination with coronal and axial HRCT, supplemented by MRI aims to demonstrate that the tumour is confined to the middle ear cavity, in which case surgical removal is generally straightforward. If the tumour breaches the middle ear cavity it usually extends through the floor into the jugular foramen.

Glomus jugulare tumours originate within the jugular foramen. Presentation depends upon tumour size and pattern of extension. Growth within the jugular foramen leads to palsies of the IXth, Xth and XIth cranial nerves. Upward extension into the middle ear cavity commonly occurs (Fig. 20.10), producing symptoms similar to those of a glomus tympanicum tumour but there is usually more extensive bone destruction with involvement of the VIIth cranial nerve. These tumours also frequently grow superiorly into the posterior cranial fossa and inferiorly into the neck.

HRCT in the axial and coronal planes will show a mass centred on the jugular foramen with varying degrees of erosion and expansion of the foramen. Initially the bone erosion is subtle with slight irregularity and loss of definition of the cortex (Fig. 20.11). Attention to detail is important when assessing the

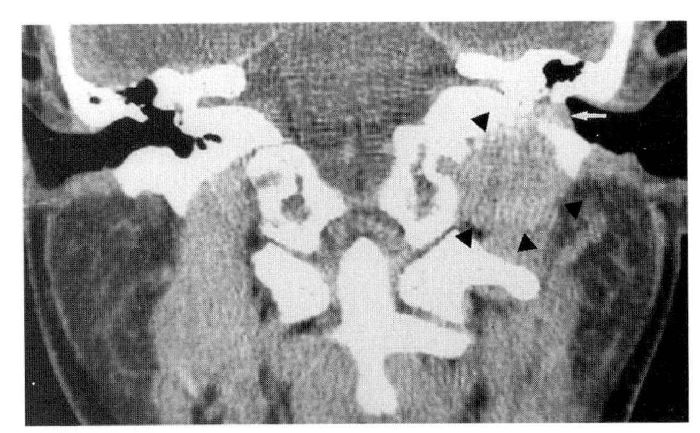

Fig. 20.10 Coronal CT demonstrating a large glomus jugulare tumour (arrowheads), extending into the middle ear (arrow).

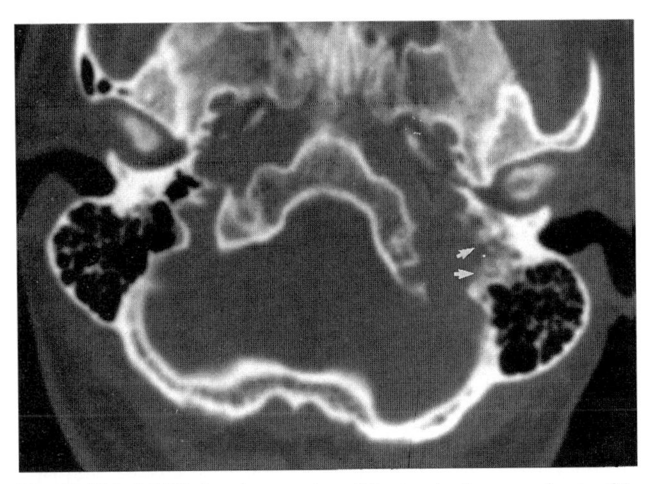

Fig. 20.11 Axial CT showing erosion of the jugular foramen (arrows) by a glomus jugulare tumour. Compare with the normally corticated contralateral jugular foramen.

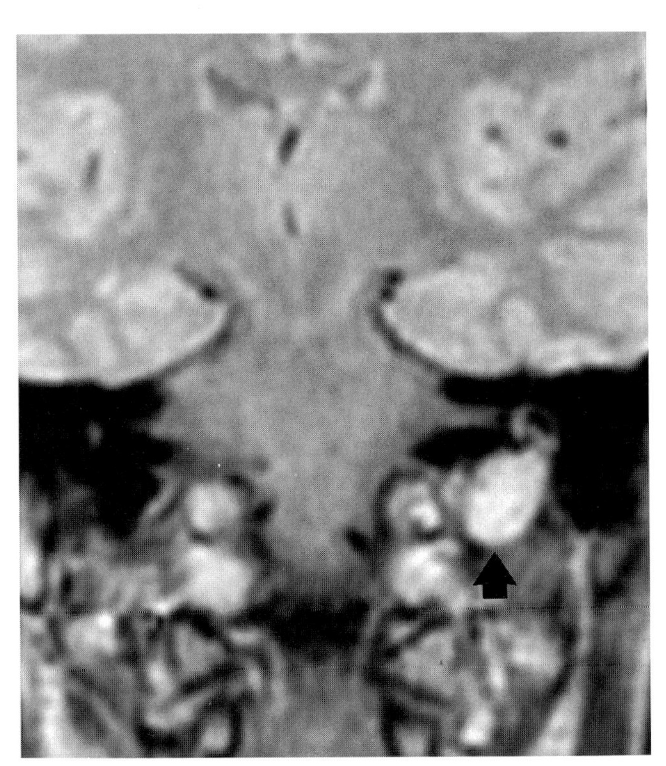

Fig. 20.12 Coronal MRI clearly demonstrating a small hyperintense glomus jugulare tumour (arrow).

jugular foramina as there is marked developmental variation in size and shape, the right foramen being generally the larger.

The full extent of the extraosseous spread is most easily appreciated with MRI. The tumours are hypointense on T1-weighted and hyperintense on T2-weighted sequences (Fig. 20.12) and exhibit marked enhancement. Serpiginous hypointensities present within the tumour represent flow-voids from tumour vessels. Where possible, treatment is by surgical excision, the safety and completeness of which is facilitated by preoperative endovascular embolization of the tumour.

CHORDOMA

Chordomas are rare tumours arising from remnants of notochord. Between 35–40% occur intracranially, typically within the clivus, but unilateral petrous bone tumours do occur. Chordomas appear as well-defined extra-axial soft-tissue masses of heterogeneous density, associated with bone destruction, and characteristically contain areas of calcification. On MRI they are heterogeneously hypointense on T1-weighted and markedly hyperintense on T2-weighted images, the heterogeneity probably representing calcification and areas of haemorrhage as these are very vascular tumours. Marked contrast enhancement with gadolinium usually occurs. Chordomas are predominantly locally invasive, usually presenting with local cranial nerve palsies. Metastases are uncommon.

CARCINOMA

Squamous cell carcinoma of the ear although rare, is the commonest primary malignant tumour of the ear. It usually originates from the external auditory canal or middle ear, but localization of the site of origin is rarely possible due to the marked bony destruction frequently present at diagnosis. Extensive local spread occurs but metastases are rare.

The degree of bone destruction is best assessed with HRCT, as is bony sclerosis of the adjacent middle cranial fossa that is frequently associated with this tumour, possibly reflecting previous chronic infection.

MRI is more sensitive for demonstrating soft-tissue extension.

PRIMARY BONE TUMOURS

Osteomas can occur within the external auditory canal. Giant cell tumours occur at the petrous apex, producing irregular expansion. Osteosarcomas and chondrosarcomas both produce soft-tissue masses with extensive bone destruction.

METASTASES

The petrous bone can be the site of metastatic deposits, commonly from carcinoma of the breast. The petrous bone may also be involved by myeloma, usually as part of widespread disease, but occasionally as the site of a solitary plasmacytoma. Direct extension of adjacent advanced malignant tumours, particularly nasopharyngeal and parotid carcinomas can involve the petrous bone.

CHAPTER 21

Skull and brain

Donald M. Hadley

IMAGING TECHNIQUES
SCALP AND SKULL
CONGENITAL STRUCTURAL ABNORMALITIES OF BRAIN
INTRACRANIAL NEOPLASMS
HEAD INJURY
INFECTION
VASCULAR ABNORMALITIES
HYDROCEPHALUS

In no other area of the body are so many of the available imaging modalities used to provide complementary information. The information may be structural, functional or a mixture of both. Unfortunately the increasing sensitivity of the more recently introduced examinations has not been matched by improved specificity. Fundamental radiological criteria based on a thorough knowledge of the common sites of the possible lesions, their structure and growth patterns are still essential to narrow the differential diagnosis. In many patients a final diagnosis will only be obtained when the radiological findings are matched with the microscopic examination of tissues obtained by image-directed biopsy or surgical resection.

Technical developments in therapeutic radiological intervention have already revolutionized the treatment of many intracranial and intraspinal vascular lesions and promise to change the role of the clinical neuroradiologist in the care of patients presenting with CNS symptoms.

IMAGING TECHNIQUES

Since the development of computed tomography and magnetic resonance imaging, plain skull radiographs now seldom give additional information in the evaluation of CNS disease and have lost their pivotal role as the initial examination of the brain and skull. Plain radiography may be justified:

- to assess conditions that affect the density of the skull (Fig. 21.1);
- to assess conditions that cause remodelling of the skull either secondary to local destruction or increased intracranial pressure;
- to assess cases of gross facial and skull fractures;
- to exclude radiopaque foreign bodies, e.g. before MRI.

Intravenous contrast agents are used with CT and MRI to assess the vascularity of lesions and their effect on the blood–brain barrier, a functional barrier formed by the tight junctions in the capillary endothelial cells of the brain and spine. This barrier, which prevents hydrophilic molecules from entering the interstitial compartment by passive diffusion from the vascular space (as happens in the rest of the body), is disrupted by most neoplasms, infections, inflammation, infarction and certain stages of maturation of haemorrhage. With CT, iodinated agents show patterns of increased attenuation in areas of blood–brain barrier breakdown, whilst with MRI, paramagnetic agents, such as those based on gadolinium, result in an increased signal on T1-weighted images. These enhancement characteristics help to narrow the differential diagnosis, provide information about the 'activity' of a lesion and can show abnormalities invisible on unenhanced images.

Diagnostic and Interventional Radiology in Surgical Practice. Edited by P. Armstrong and M.L. Wastie. Published in 1997 by Chapman & Hall, London. ISBN 0 412 61960 1 (HB), 0 412 61970 9 (PB)

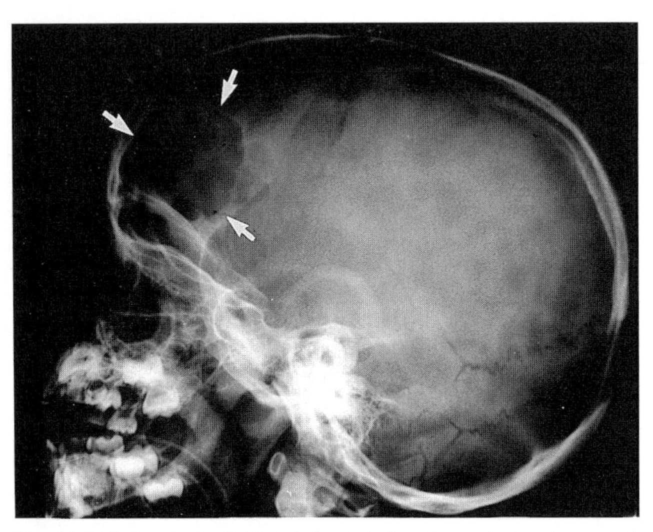

Fig. 21.1 Histiocytosis-X. Plain lateral skull radiograph showing a well-defined punched out lytic lesion with a bevelled appearance of the inner margins (arrows). The extent of the skull lesion is more apparent on a plain film than on CT but even with a typical pattern there are still several differential diagnoses.

Tissue contrast in the brain on CT is inferior in comparison to MRI and iodinated intravenous contrast is frequently required. However CT has advantages:

- it is widely available and well understood;
- it can be performed quickly and is relatively inexpensive;
- it is excellent in the examination of patients with:
  - suspected acute subarachnoid haemorrhage;
  - acute trauma;
  - subtle bony abnormalities, such as those in the temporal and facial regions;
  - calcified intracranial lesions;
  - contraindications to MRI, e.g. patients with a cardiac pacemaker.

MRI is now an alternative to CT for the investigation of nearly all cranial disorders and competes with angiography and ultrasound for the non-invasive assessment of the larger extra-and intracerebral arteries and veins. The increased tissue contrast and spatial resolution produced by MRI together with the multiplanar imaging capability allows earlier detection of many intracranial lesions. This is especially so in regions enclosed by dense bone such as the middle and posterior fossae which degrades the CT image. However MRI has disadvantages:

- it is relatively insensitive to calcification;
- it is more expensive and tends to be less readily available than CT;
- it requires more patient preparation;
- it is contraindicated in those patients with electronic implants such as cardiac pacemakers, most aneurysm clips and any metallic foreign bodies in the orbits.

SCALP AND SKULL

Imaging can play a role in defining the origin and extent of lesions presenting in the scalp. The skin, subcutaneous tissue, galea (epicranial aponeurosis) and subaponeurotic areolar layer overlying the skull are all shown on CT when soft-tissue windows are used but are better seen on MRI (Fig. 21.2). Haematomas and infection usually result from trauma and can involve any of these layers or the underlying bone. Imaging is not usually required to define the commonly found sebaceous cyst or lipoma but, if there is any clinical doubt or the lesion is unusually large, its morphology can be shown on CT or MRI. Differentiation from dermoids, which usually occur at the outer upper angle of the orbit and may have an intracranial component, is important. A full imaging evaluation is mandatory for midline abnormalities as they may represent the superficial portion of an intracranial lesion such as a cephalocele or meningomyelocele.

Focal involvement of the inner and outer tables of skull may be shown on plain radiography. If the lesion lies posteriorly a Towne's view will best show the occipital bone. Tangential views of the lesion may be required to assess bone erosion or calcification but these features are better shown on CT, which will also show any additional involvement of the intracranial contents. Plain films often give a better geographical overview of the site and extent of the lesion but plain films are now being superseded by the use of the digital 'scout' view obtained routinely with CT.

Normal variants producing focal areas of **decreased bone density** include venous lakes, parietal foramina,

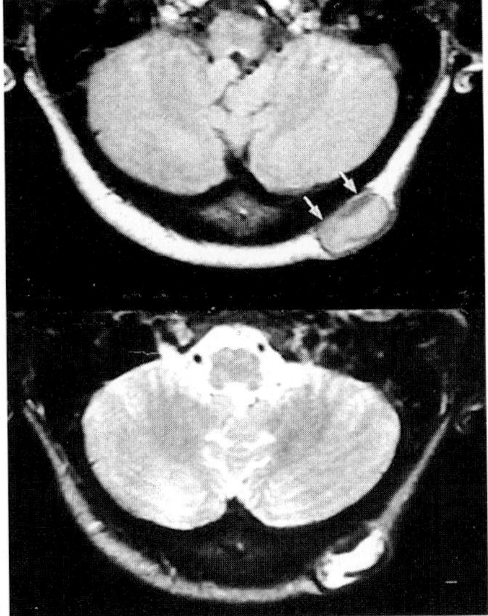

(a) and (b)

Fig. 21.2 Subcutaneous occipital scalp lump on (a) proton density and (b) T2-weighted axial sections. The lump is a cyst which contains fatty components. Note intact outer skull table (arrows) under the lesion.

pacchionian granulations and parietal thinning. These normal findings have to be differentiated from epidermoids, haemangiomas, eosinophilic granulomas and multiple myeloma. Slowly growing lesions, or those producing a long-standing pressure erosion, tend to be well demarcated with some reactive sclerosis in their margins. The lesions of untreated multiple myeloma appear 'punched out' and sharply delineated without sclerosis. Metastatic lesions in the skull are nearly all lytic, although the same primary may produce sclerotic lesions elsewhere. Metastases are poorly marginated, irregular in size and shape, may be single or multiple and produce varying destruction of the inner or outer table of the skull with infiltration of the diploë. Common primary tumours that metastasize to the skull are carcinomas of the breast, thyroid and prostate.

Hyperostosis frontalis interna is a common normal variant seen most frequently in middle-aged women which results in sclerosis and thickening of the inner table and diploë of the frontal bone with relative sparing of the midline. This density change must be differentiated from fibrous dysplasia which produces sclerotic, lytic or mixed lesions involving mainly the outer table. Fibrous dysplasia usually shows 'ground-glass' appearance on plain film; it causes expansion of the bone which may encroach on the paranasal sinuses or skull base foramina. Meningiomas may induce secondary effects which result in hyperostosis and increased density with eventual obliteration of the diploë of the adjacent involved bone. Enlarged vascular grooves on the inner table of the skull may be noted running to the lesion. These are formed by hypertrophied external carotid artery branches supplying this dural based tumour. Occasionally, destructive changes are found and a meningioma may be indistinguishable from a solitary metastasis (Fig. 21.3). Osteomas and exostoses show typical densities on imaging and can arise from the inner or outer tables of the skull.

Lesions producing **mixed density** include the various stages of Paget's disease. Its lytic phase involves the frontal or occipital bones and spreads to the vertex affecting the outer table of the skull. The sclerotic phase shows recalcification and dense skull thickening that often produces compression of the skull base foramina. The new bone is soft, and basilar invagination causes compression at the cervical medullary junction. Infection of the skull may be the result of direct extension from surrounding soft tissues, from the paranasal sinues or mastoids, or from blood-borne infection. Infection causes resorption of bone and a

(a)

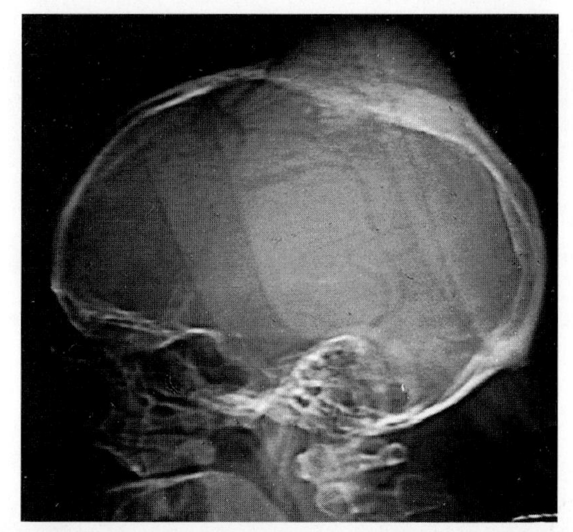

(c)

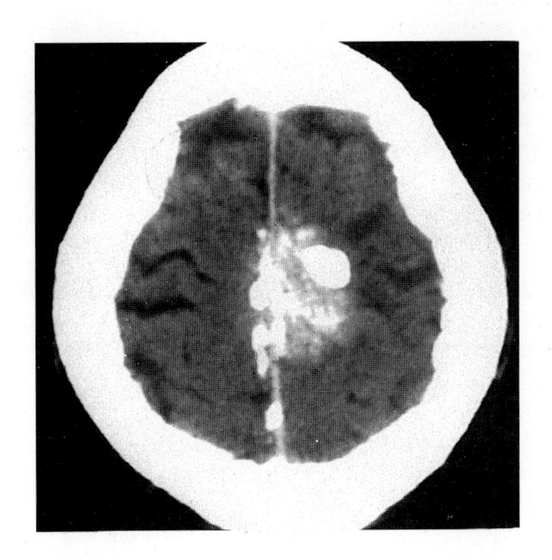

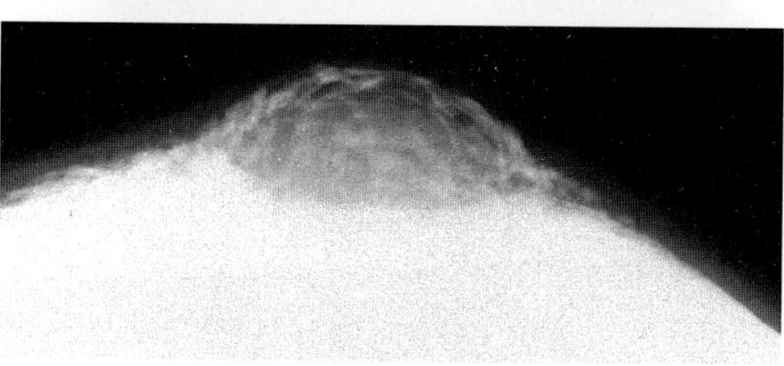

(b)

Fig. 21.3 Meningioma presenting as skull lump in a 60-year-old. (a) Digital lateral CT 'scanogram' shows a calcified mass expanding through the skull. (b) Soft-tissue tangential plain radiograph shows 'eggshell' thinning and expansion of the outer skull table. (c) Axial CT through the lesion shows craggy calcification associated with the dural-based mass expanding through the skull provoking only minimal oedema in the adjacent brain.

lytic lesion may be shown associated with periosteal reaction and a soft-tissue mass. The main reason for cross-sectional imaging in bony osteomyelitis is to define any intracranial spread so that adequate decompression and appropriate antibiotic therapy is instituted. Occasionally a 'button' sequestrum will form with an island of bone in the lytic area. This is unusual as the skull has such a good blood supply; sequestrum formation occurs most often with tuberculous osteitis and staphylococcal infections. Sclerotic lesions occur when the infection is chronic, as may happen with an inadequately treated acute osteomyelitis or with infections due to organisms which have a low virulence, such as fungi, spirochetes and tuberculosis.

Trauma is now the commonest cause of a skull lesion. Fractures and their effects will be discussed in the section on craniocerebral injuries.

Calcification in the pineal, choroid plexus and habenula, if sufficiently dense, is seen on plain films and must not be mistaken for a lesion. Occasionally, displacement of these normal calcifications reveal the presence of an intracranial mass lesion although this is more readily demonstrated by CT or MRI.

In young children **increased intracranial pressure** may cause widening of sutures. After suture fusion the effects of chronic increased intracranial pressure may be shown on plain lateral and anterior skull views as thinning of the cortex of the dorsum sellae extending to the floor of the sella turcica. Eventually enlargement of the whole sella may be seen. Although thinning of the calvarium may occur and prominent convolutional markings may develop, these findings may also be seen in normal people. These signs of raised intracranial pressure are only found after a considerable period of raised pressure but are often seen at first presentation. CT or MRI is required to assess the cause of the increased pressure and the size of the ventricles. If fontanelles are not closed they can be used as a window for ultrasound to assess ventricular size.

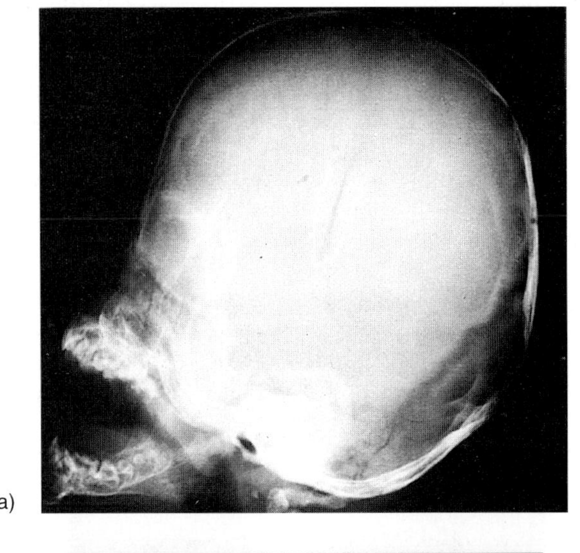
(a)

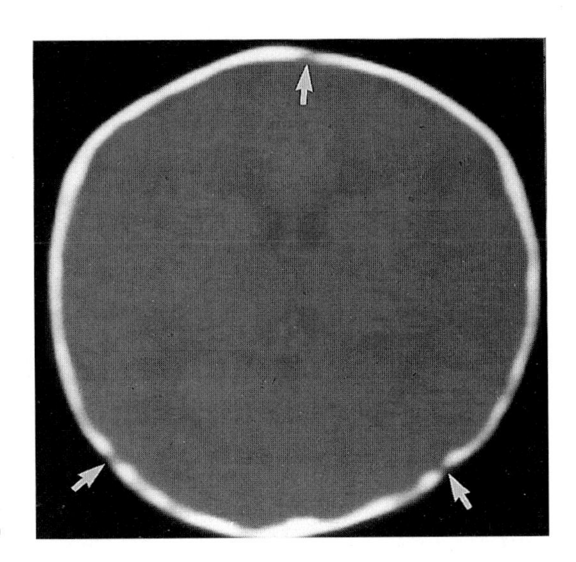
(b)

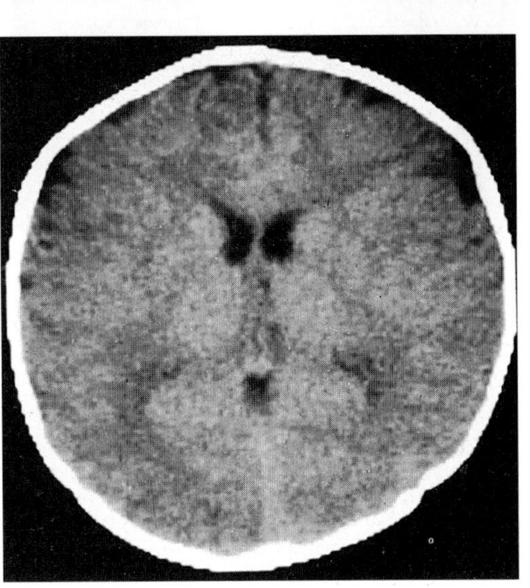
(c)

Fig. 21.4 Bilateral coronal synostosis producing turricephaly in a 9-month-old infant. (a) Plain lateral radiograph shows the typical skull shape while CT with (b) bone and (c) soft-tissue windows shows that the coronal sutures are fused while the lambdoid and sagittal sutures are normal (arrows); the brain has formed normally and there is no hydrocephalus.

Cranial synostosis, the premature fusion of one or more of the sutures, results in deformity of the skull. An overview of the skull shape and assessment of the sutures is usually made on plain films. CT is used to document the effect on the brain and ventricles. The bone adjacent to the fused suture becomes thickened with a band of increased density parallel to the suture. Involvement of the sagittal suture, the commonest fusion, results in compensatory overgrowth of the sutures perpendicular to it, namely the lambdoid and coronal, producing an elongated narrow skull (dolichocephaly or scaphocephaly). Unilateral coronal synostosis, which is the most common fusion to be treated, results in elongation of the orbit and greater wing of sphenoid producing an oblique-shaped or plagiocephalic skull. With bilateral coronal synostosis there is general shortening of the skull with compensatory upward growth, resulting in turricephaly (Fig. 21.4). Lambdoid synostosis similarly can be bilateral or unilateral and result in turricephaly or plagiocephaly. Follow-up examinations, plain films or CT may be required after surgical treatment. Changes in ventricular size are noted particularly.

CONGENITAL STRUCTURAL ABNORMALITIES OF BRAIN

Normal mature brain structure depends on incredibly complicated repeated cycles of development and remodelling. Disturbance at a particular stage occurs in up to 1% of live births although in less than half can an identifiable genetic, vascular or infectious cause be found. A wide range of congenital malformations may be recognized by using ultrasound in the fetus and infant.

MRI is the optimal imaging modality once the fontanelles close because of the propensity for lesions to lie in the sagittal plane and because of the excellent soft-tissue definition and multiplanar sections possible with MRI.

The abnormalities may be classified according to the timing of the insult with disturbances of dorsal induction (3rd and 4th week of gestation), ventral induction (5th to 10th week), neuronal proliferation, differentiation and histogenesis (8th to 16th week) and neuronal migration disorders (2nd to 5th month) producing distinct groups of lesions. Over 2000 malformations have been described but only those of 'surgical interest' will be discussed here.

DORSAL INDUCTION

Failure of dorsal induction causes the neural tube defects which include cephaloceles, the Chiari malformations and spinal dysraphic abnormalities (p. 291). These abnormalities are best shown on midline sagittal T1-weighted MRI but suspicious features on a routine axial CT such as an abnormal fourth ventricle, a 'full' foramen magnum and absent cisterna magna must be recognized and followed-up with MRI.

Chiari I Malformation

Chiari I is the mildest of the hindbrain malformations and is characterized by displacement > 5 mm downwards of deformed cerebellar tonsils through the foramen magnum. The brain stem and fourth ventricle retain their normal position although the ventricle may be small and slightly distorted. A Chiari I malformation is not usually associated with other cerebral abnormalities but a syrinx may be found in the spinal cord in up to 25% of cases.

Chiari II Malformation

A Chiari II malformation is a more extensive and complex abnormality than the Chiari I malformation with infratentorial and supratentorial abnormalities. The cerebellar tonsils, inferior vermis, fourth ventricle and brain stem are herniated from a shallow posterior fossa through a wide foramen magnum (Fig. 21.5). There is nearly always a meningocele or meningomyelocele with some associated hydrocephalus. Partial or complete agenesis of the corpus callosum is found in many patients. A degree of spinal dysraphism is usually present together with a tethered cord and filum lipoma.

Chiari III Malformation

A Chiari III malformation is very rare. There is herniation of the posterior fossa contents into an associated occipital or high cervical cephalocele together with the other features of a Chiari II malformation.

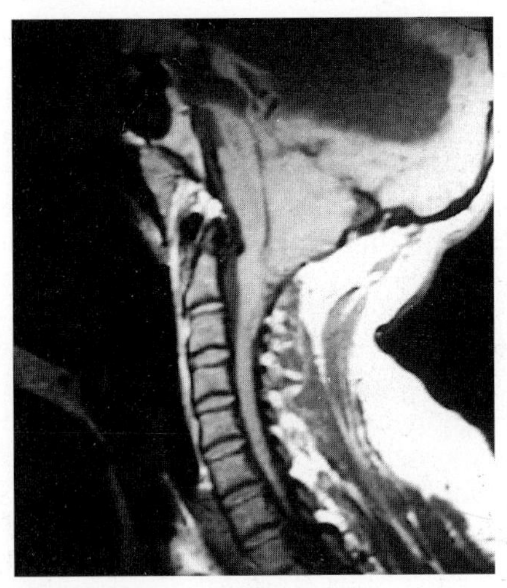

Fig. 21.5 Midline sagittal T1-weighted section showing a Chiari II malformation associated with hydrocephalus.

Cephalocele

The term cephalocele refers to an abnormal protrusion of an intracranial structure through a skull defect. It can include brain, ventricles, cerebrospinal fluid (CSF) and meninges either alone or in combination. A cephalocele is commonest in the occipital region in the Caucasian population, but may also occur through the frontal, basal and parietal bones. Although large occipital, parietal and frontal cephaloceles are usually diagnosed on clinical examination, small cephaloceles may be misdiagnosed as a skull lump and should therefore, be imaged before biopsy or excision. They usually lie in the midline and T1-weighted MRI is the best way to identify their contents and any connection with intracranial structures. Cephaloceles involving the nasofrontal or sphenoethmoidal bones may present to the otorhinolaryngologists as masses with a wide clinical differential diagnosis. Imaging is essential to prevent possible biopsy of the frontal lobe protruding through a defect. Axial or reformatted sagittal CT sections show the bony defect but T1-weighted coronal and sagittal MRI shows the whole lesion more clearly.

VENTRAL INDUCTION

Ventral induction results in the formation of the brain and face. Disorders of ventral induction result in holoprosencephaly, septo-optic dysplasia and the Dandy–Walker syndrome. The Dandy–Walker syndrome is the commonest and the most important surgically.

Dandy–Walker syndrome and variant

The Dandy–Walker syndrome comprises partial or complete cerebellar vermis aplasia so that the cerebellum is displaced and the fourth ventricle replaced by a cyst which does not communicate with the subarachnoid CSF. The condition is thought to be due to obstruction of CSF flow at the foramina of Luschka and Magendie. More than 50% of patients have other congenital anomalies including agenesis of the corpus callosum, holoprosencephaly, schizencephaly, polymicrogyria, cephaloceles and grey matter heterotopia. The clinical signs and symptoms usually relate more to these associated conditions than to the main defect.

The Dandy–Walker variant is a less severe form of the complex in which the vermis and fourth ventricle are better developed. Communication between the fourth ventricle and the posterior fossa cyst is variable. Hydrocephalus, heterotopias and callosal dysgenesis occur much less commonly in the variant. CT axial sections show the CSF space and the cerebellar dysplasia but these are all best shown with MRI using sagittal and axial sections of the posterior fossa and foramen magnum. The many associated anomalies are readily shown on MRI.

The Dandy–Walker syndrome and variant must be differentiated from a giant cisterna magna which is a normal variant and a posterior fossa arachnoid cyst which does not communicate with the fourth ventricle and is not associated with other anomalies.

NEURONAL PROLIFERATION, DIFFERENTIATION AND HISTOGENESIS

Disorders of these stages of development result in neoplastic and vascular malformations often with cutaneous manifestations, hence they are also called neurocutaneous disorders or phakomatoses.

Neurofibromatosis I

Neurofibromatosis I is the commonest type of neurofibromatosis accounting for 90% of cases. The defect is known to lie on the long arm of chromosome 17 and in half the patients the disorder is transmitted as an autosomal dominant; it is sporadic in the remainder. In this type of neurofibromatosis there are prominent skin manifestations associated with tumours of neurones and astrocytes often with distinctive osseous and dural lesions such as sphenoid dysplasia or vertebral scalloping and lateral meningoceles. Spinal neurofibromas, which are often small and single, may develop.

Neurofibromatosis II

Neurofibromatosis II is much less common than neurofibromatosis I and the cutaneous manifestations are less marked. Neurofibromatosis II is also an autosomal dominant disorder but the defect is on chromosome 22. There are associated tumours of the meninges and Schwann cells, the hallmark of the condition being bilateral acoustic schwannomas. Ependymomas and astrocytomas of the spinal cord may develop.

Von Hippel–Lindau disease

Von Hippel–Lindau disease is an autosomal dominant multisystem disorder in which the short arm of chromosome 3 has been implicated. Screening has been implemented for at-risk families. Patients usually develop posterior fossa or spinal haemangioblastomas associated with retinal angiomas, renal cell carcinomas, phaeochromocytomas, and cysts of the kidney, pancreas and liver. Multiple haemangioblastomas which develop in the third or fourth decades are pathognonomic.

The cerebellar tumours are seen with CT and MRI either as a strongly enhancing mass (20%) or a cystic lesion with an enhancing mural nodule (80%). They are usually located in the vermis, the brain stem being a less common site; cerebral hemisphere lesions are rare. The cystic component usually gives a higher signal than CSF on T1-weighted MRI due to its raised protein content. Vertebral angiography may define a vascular blush in the nodule. Angiography can assist in differentiating a haemangioblastoma from a cystic astrocytoma or metastasis.

Spinal cord lesions are seen with MRI in 8–35% of patients. These are similar to the intracranial haemangioblastomas but may be associated with larger, more syrinx-like cysts. Angiography may be required to define the vascular supply.

Sturge–Weber syndrome

The Sturge–Weber syndrome is characterized by a vascular naevus of the face, the so called 'port-wine stain', which occurs in one or more divisions of the fifth cranial nerve. The accompanying intracranial lesion is an ipsilateral angioma of the meninges which results in hemiparesis, seizures and mental retardation. Typically, unilateral curvilinear calcification in the gyri in the occipitoparietal regions may be seen on plain films and CT, which also demonstrates cerebral atrophy.

Tuberous sclerosis

Tuberous scelerosis is characterized by multisystem hamartomatous tumours. Cranial involvement results in mental retardation, seizures, adenoma sebaceum of the face with calcified retinal hamartomas. Intracranial hamartomas are seen most typically as subependymal lesions which usually undergo calcification, best detected by CT. In 10–15% of patients malignant transformation into a subependymal giant cell astrocytoma occurs within a hamartoma located at the formen of Monro. Cortical tubers are best appreciated on MRI, appearing as iso- or hypointense areas on T1-weighted images and hyperintense foci on a T2-weighted sequence (Fig. 21.6). Lesions may also be seen in the kidneys, heart, lung, liver, spleen and bones.

MIGRATION DISORDER

Migration disorder occurs between 2 and 5 months of intrauterine life when there is a disorder of the systematic migration of the proliferating neurones from the periventricular region to the cortex and deep nuclei, resulting in schizencephaly, agyria, pachygyria, heterotopia and dysgenesis of the corpus callosum. Although MRI can now clearly define the abnormal brain structure, functional imaging with positron emission tomography or single photon emission computed tomography (SPECT) may be required for assessment of associated abnormal function such as epilepsy. Corpus callosum abnormality is associated with many of the other lesions already mentioned and is discussed in more detail below.

DYSGENESIS OF THE CORPUS CALLOSUM

During months 3 and 4 of fetal life the corpus callosum develops from the front to the back beginning with the genu. An interruption of growth affects the body, splenium or rostrum. Agenesis results from an insult before 12 weeks of gestation and is associated with many anomalies including Dandy–Walker, Chiari malformations and midline lipoma (Fig. 21.7). CT and MRI show absence or underdevelopment of

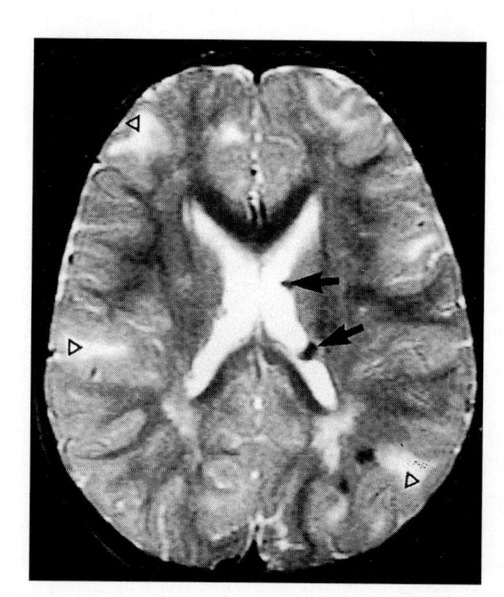

Fig. 21.6 Tuberous sclerosis. T2-weighted axial section in a 2-year-old showing hypointense subependymal calcified tubers (arrows) and hyperintense cortical hamartomas (arrow heads).

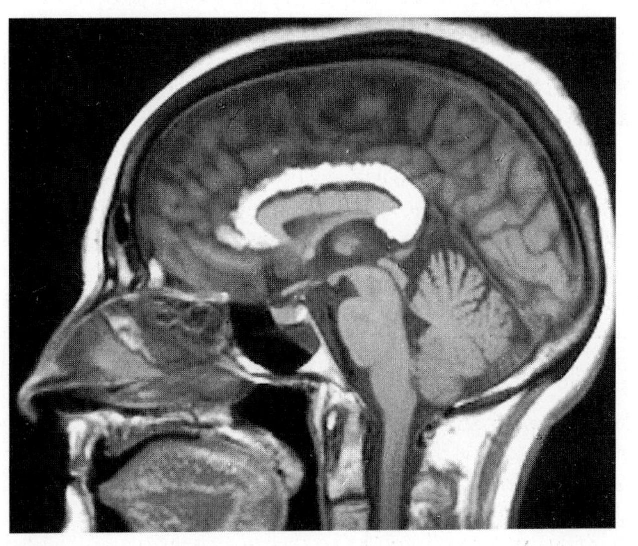

Fig. 21.7 T1-weighted midline sagittal section showing hyperintense lipoma of the corpus callosum.

the corpus callosum with separation of the lateral ventricles and elevation of the third ventricle between them.

INTRACRANIAL NEOPLASMS

Primary tumours can arise from any intracranial cell line other than mature neurones which do not divide, except for ethesioneuroblastoma which is derived from still dividing neural tissue in the olfactory mucosa. Metastatic disease is commonest from lung, breast, kidney, melanoma and colon tumours while prostatic secondaries and myeloma are found in the dura and calvarium.

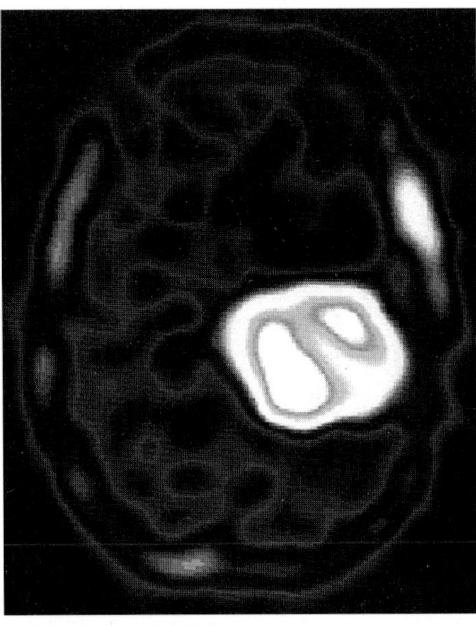

Fig. 21.8 Intense ^{201}Tl uptake in a deep left temporoparietal glioma; baseline assessment before resection.

CT is still the first modality for the investigation of most patients presenting with signs or symptoms of a tumour but the advantages of MRI in terms of increased contrast sensitivity, direct multiplanar capability and lack of bone artefact are now being realized. MRI is especially useful for detecting and managing tumours in the brain stem, middle and posterior cranial fossae. Angiography is still used to assess the vascularity of selected tumours such as meningiomas and may be combined with presurgical embolization. SPECT with ^{201}Tl shows selective uptake in malignant tumours (Fig. 21.8) as well as meningiomas, and thallium scanning is useful both for measuring the functional volume of the tumour before and after treatment and in the differential diagnosis between radiation necrosis and recurrent tumour, both of which may present as enhancing masses on CT or MRI.

Tumours are characterized on CT and MRI by showing a central mass causing variable displacement (or mass effect) on adjacent normal structures which can lead to obstructive hydrocephalus. Tumours are frequently surrounded by oedema, the most severe oedema being seen with fast-growing and aggressive tumours. In general, the density of the mass on CT is reduced compared to normal brain, and after intravenous contrast, if there is blood–brain barrier breakdown due to 'leaky' immature neovascularity, various patterns (homogeneous, ring, patchy) of enhancement are identified. On MRI the T1- and T2-relaxation times

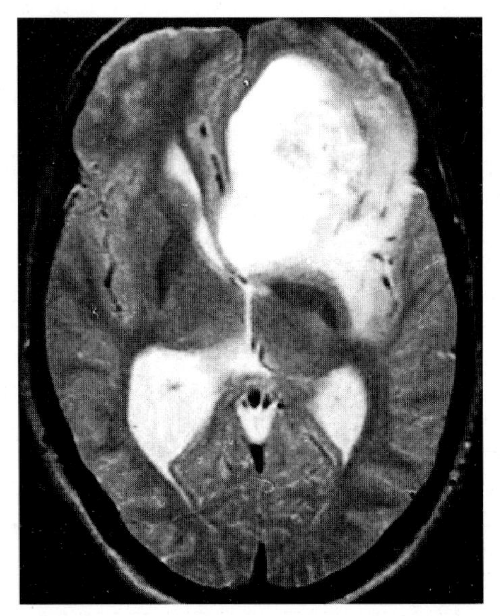

(a)

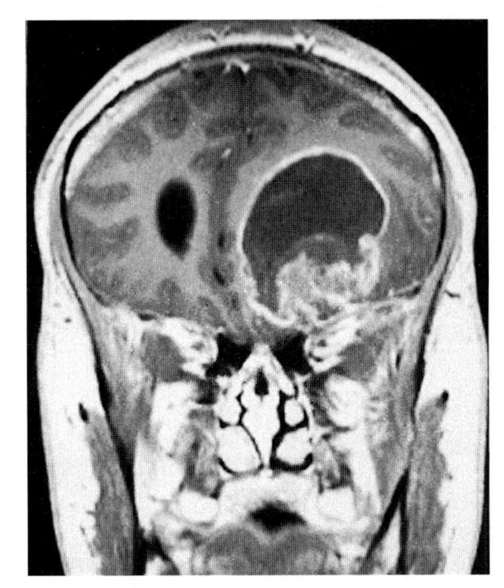

(b)

Fig. 21.9 Intermediate grade glioma in a 29-year-old with personality change, headaches and papilloedema. (a) T2-weighted axial and (b) T1-weighted coronal post-gadolinium enhancement sections show a left frontal cystic mass surrounded by oedema with an enhancing irregular solid nodule and cyst wall, together with marked ventricular compression and displacement.

of tumour are increased, so it appears hypointense on T1-weighted and hyperintense on T2-weighted images. Any surrounding oedema follows a similar but more pronounced set of signal patterns which can sometimes make it difficult to separate tumour mass from oedema. Blood–brain barrier breakdown can be highlighted in a similar way to that with CT, with intravenous gadolinium-based contrast agents; these cause a shortening of T1-relaxation time resulting in increased signal on T1-weighted images (Fig. 21.9). It is important to avoid equating the extent of a tumour shown radiologically with the limits of its growth because CT and MRI stereotactic biopsy studies have shown that malignant cells often extend into the peritumoural oedema beyond the enhancing margins of the mass.

Neoplasms are generally classified according to their site and original cell type:

- **Intra-axial:** *glial tumours*
  - astrocytoma
    - low-grade astrocytoma
    - anaplastic astrocytoma
    - glioblastoma
  - oligodendroglioma
  - ependymoma
  - choroid plexus tumour
- **Intra-axial:** *non-glial tumours*
  - haemangioblastomas
  - primitive neuroectodermal tumour (PNET)
  - lymphoma
  - metastasis
  - hamartoma
- **Intraventricular**
  - colloid cyst
  - choroid plexus tumour
  - ependymoma
  - astrocytoma
  - meningioma
  - subependymal giant cell astrocytoma
- **Extra-axial**
  - meningioma
  - nerve sheath tumours
    - schwannoma
    - plexiform neurofibroma
  - glomus tumour
  - chordoma
  - chondroma, chondrosarcoma
  - epidermoid
  - dermoid
  - teratoma
  - arachnoid cyst
  - pituitary tumours
  - metastatic tumours

Unfortunately the cell type is only known with certainty after histological examination and often requires specialist immunological stains directed at individual cellular components. It is sometimes possible to identify a particular tumour type with a high degree of confidence on both CT and MRI but since many tumours contain calcification, haemorrhage, cysts or necrotic areas it is not surprising that there is a huge overlap in the appearance of the different types of tumour.

Once a tumour is imaged the first critical decision, which will narrow the differential diagnosis, is whether it is an intra-axial lesion arising from brain substance or an extra-axial lesion arising in the dura, meninges, extradural or intraventricular space. On CT or MRI extra-axial lesions buckle the cortex and white matter, displace the subarachnoid veins inwards, expand the ipsilateral subarachnoid space and sometimes cause reactive bone changes. Axial lesions lie within the brain and expand the cortex with no separation by the underlying leptomeninges. They spread across parenchymal boundaries and the dura is seen to lie peripherally. If a lesion is aggressively invasive the distinction between an intra- or extra-axial lesion may be blurred and, rarely, a dural meningioma invades the brain while a parenchymal metastasis may invade the meninges.

INTRA-AXIAL TUMOURS

Intra-axial tumours include metastases, glial and non-glial neoplasms. Glial tumours, which cause up to 45% of primary brain tumours, arise from astrocytes, oligodendrocytes, ependymal cells and the choroid plexus. The non-glial tumours include those arising from primitive bipotential precursors (primitive neuroectodermal tumour or PNET), mesenchymal cells (haemangioblastoma), the lymphoreticular system (lymphoma) and those associated with the phakomatoses.

Developmental tumours (dermoid/epidermoid tumours) although strictly extra-axial are frequently seen within the brain substance and are considered in this section.

Metastases

Metastases are usually multiple, well-defined enhancing masses that characteristically grow from the grey-white matter junction (Fig. 21.10). They are typically low density on non-contrast CT unless haemorrhagic or hypercellular. On T1-weighted MRI they are either hypointense or isointense, while on T2-weighted sections they have variable intensity depending on cellularity, haemorrhage, necrosis and cyst formation. Nearly all metastases enhance to some degree on CT and MRI in either a homogeneous ring, or patchy manner, MRI being more sensitive to tiny lesions. The surrounding oedema is often out of proportion to the size of the metastases.

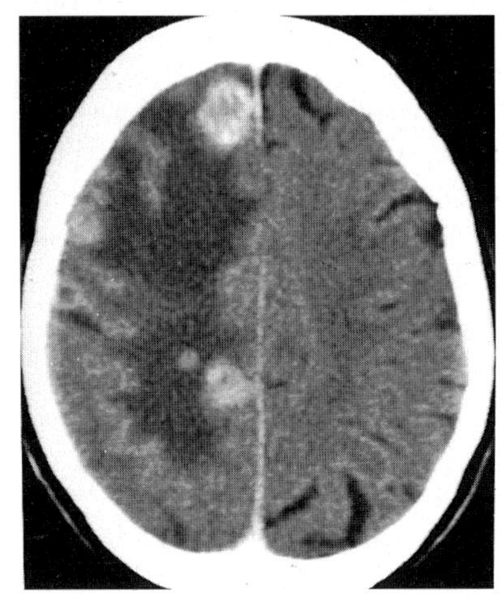

Fig. 21.10 Metastases in a 67-year-old with a previous resection of a colonic carcinoma presenting with ataxia, left-sided sensory symptoms and headache. CT with contrast shows multiple small ring enhancing masses surrounded by extensive disproportionate oedema.

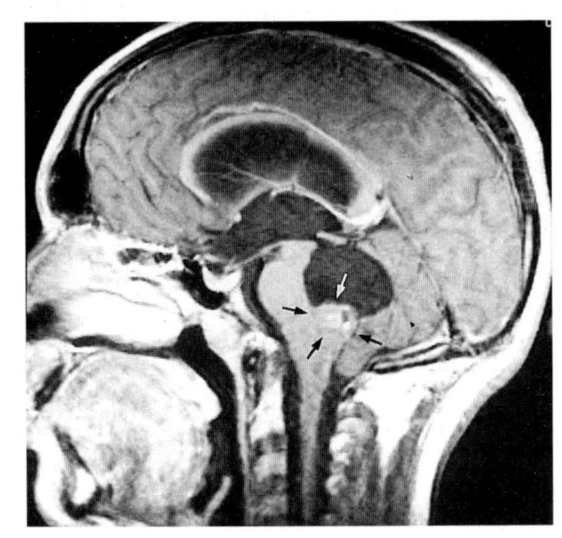

Fig. 21.11 T1-weighted contrast enhanced sagittal section showing an ependymoma (arrows) involving the exits of the fourth ventricle causing an obstructive hydrocephalus.

Glial tumours

Astrocytomas are graded from I to IV depending on their malignant potential with the grade IV type being considered as **glioblastomas**. The lowest grade tumours have variable CT appearances with mixed attenuation and poorly defined margins in which tumour and oedema merge. Calcification may be present. MRI shows these low-grade tumours as areas of hyperintensity on T2-weighted and hypointensity on T1-weighted scans with mild enhancement following intravenous contrast. Calcification, if dense, will produce signal voids. MRI is usually no better at showing tumour margins than CT. Cystic astrocytomas are low grade and are most often seen in children, frequently in the cerebellum. Occasionally cyst wall or nodular enhancement will be seen on CT or MRI. **Oligodendrogliomas** are slow growing, tend to be large and are mainly found in adults. Calcification is an important diagnostic feature being seen in 80% on CT. They may undergo malignant astrocytic behaviour.

With the most malignant grades such as anaplastic astrocytomas (III) and glioblastomas (IV), CT shows areas of mixed attenuation with central low attenuation often representing necrosis. After intravenous contrast there is marked irregular enhancement. These aggressive tumours invade grey and white matter producing extensive surrounding oedema. MRI demonstrates heterogeneous intensity which is increased on T2-weighted and decreased on T1-weighted images. Contrast enhancement is even more marked than on CT. Haemorrhage in various states of maturation is often seen on MRI.

Ependymomas most often arise in the posterior fossa in children although there is a second smaller incidence in the third decade. An ependymoma presents on CT as a midline mass which shows variable enhancement (Fig. 21.11); 50% show calcification. The tumour is often cystic and may extend into the cerebellopontine angles and the foramina of the fourth ventricle and spread in the subarachnoid space.

Choroid plexus tumours are intraventricular and should really be considered as extra-axial. They are unusual in adults and are most commonly found in the atria of the lateral ventricles in children <5 years old. On CT they appear as well marginated, lobulated isodense intraventricular masses that show strong uniform contrast enhancement. There is calcification in up to 80% of the tumours. On MRI both T1- and T2-weighted images may show intermediate intensities with foci of dense calcification showing as signal voids. The mass enhances strongly. Old haemorrhage seen on T2-weighted images as hypointensity is common. Malignant change should be syspected if the tumour extends into brain parenchyma. Hydrocephalus can be caused by haemorrhage obstructing the flow of CSF or possibly by overproduction of CSF by the tumour. Both the benign and malignant forms can seed through the CSF pathways.

Non-glial tumours

Primitive neuroectodermal tumours now include tumours that pathologists previously classified as medulloblastomas and pineoblastomas in addition to other undifferentiated small cell tumours. Most medulloblastomas are seen on CT as well defined, hyperdense midline posterior fossa masses which nearly all show uniform strong enhancement. A few tumours calcify but haemorrhage is rare. Most patients present because of the accompanying obstructive hydrocephalus. On MRI the features are variable with the mass iso- to hypointense on T1-weighted and iso- to hyperintense on T2-weighted images. Strong contrast enhancement is common. The extent of the mass and its relation to the fourth ventricle is shown best on sagittal sections. Metastases which have seeded via the CSF can be shown on enhanced T1-weighted images in over 25% of patients. These metastases can involve the cerebral subarachnoid space in addition to the spinal cord, causa equina and thecal sac.

Pineal region tumours are a heterogeneous group of neoplasms which includes the primitive neuroectodermal tumours described above in addition to germinomas, teratomas, pineocytomas and tumours arising from other cell types such as gliomas, meningiomas, melanomas and metastases. All are best imaged with MRI using a combination of axial and sagittal plane T1- and T2-weighted sections. MRI also demonstrates the site of the obstruction responsible for hydrocephalus, which is frequently the presenting complaint.

Haemangioblastomas have already been described earlier as part of von Hippel–Lindau disease (p. 446). Most occur sporadically in young or middle-aged adults and although a benign tumour some 25% recur after surgery.

Lymphomas are uncommon but the incidence is rising with the increasing population of immunocompromised patients with AIDS and from transplant programmes. Lymphoma usually forms a solitary mass but multiple lesions clustered around the ventricles may be seen. On CT there is slightly increased attenuation with marked homogeneous contrast enhancement and surrounding oedema. MRI demonstrates the expected hyperintensity on T2- and hypointensity on T1-weighted images. The mass frequently abuts a CSF surface such as the pia or ependyma of the ventricles. After steroid treatment the mass may temporarily disappear. In patients with possible concurrent infections, such as AIDS-associated toxoplasmosis, a thallium radionuclide scan will show uptake in tumour but not abscess.

Epidermoids arise from the inclusion of epidermal tissue. They most commonly involve the cerebellopontine angles but are also found in the Sylvian fissures or basal cisterns. CT shows a lobulated mass of low attenuation without enhancement unless there have been reactive changes in the surrounding brain. Occasionally flecks of marginal calcification may be seen. It can be difficult to differentiate these tumours from arachnoid cysts but an epidermoid mass is extra-axial and invaginates into the brain substance.

Dermoids arise from the inclusion of ectoderm, mesoderm and endoderm and are generally midline tumours frequently involving the posterior fossa. Dermoids contain varying amounts of fat and calcification. The fat is seen as low attenuation on CT associated with high attenuation due to calcification. Occasionally the fat leaks into the surrounding CSF space to cause a ventriculitis or meningitis. On MRI the fat is seen as a high signal on T1-weighted images. As with epidermoids, dermoids are really extra-axial but are generally seen within brain parenchyma and so are considered here.

Tumours associated with the phakomatoses have been discussed under the neurocutaneous syndromes (p. 446).

EXTRA-AXIAL TUMOURS

Extra-axial tumours include neoplasms of mesenchymal cell origin (meningiomas), nerve sheath tumours, schwannomas, tumours related to maldevelopment with inclusions and metastatic neoplasms. Pituitary tumours are also discussed in this section.

Meningiomas

Meningioma is the most common extra-axial tumour. In order of frequency it is found in the parasagittal regions, convexities of the skull vault, sphenoid wing, cerebellopontine angle, olfactory groove and planum sphenoidale. On unenhanced CT more than 50% of these tumours have a higher attenuation than brain with calcification in 20%. The lesions commonly invaginate into and buckle the brain parenchyma but because they grow slowly they have less mass effect than would be expected for their size (Fig. 21.12). Some tumours grow *en plaque* along the dura, especially in the posterior fossa and the parasellar regions. Hyperostosis of adjacent bone which may be appreciated on plain films of the skull is common. After intravenous contrast there is marked enhancement of the tumour seen on CT, although areas of necrosis or fatty degeneration remain unenhanced. Surrounding oedema is variable with most large tumours invoking oedema, but small tumours may have no oedema, although occasionally they show considerable oedema, especially if adjacent to the skull base. On MRI the signal from the tumour is usually similar to grey matter on both T1- and T2-weighted images, making it difficult to identify small tumours without contrast. Avid enhancement after contrast is seen in meningiomas of all sizes. An adjacent tail of dural enhancement may be seen which is due either to dural reactive changes or frank invasion but this appearance is also occasionally seen with other tumours such as metastases and gliomas. Signal voids due to flow in enlarged vessels and dense calcification are often seen. As meningiomas grow extra-axially they often have a large external carotid arterial supply with a typical vascular pattern which can be shown with angiography. Preoperative embolization by the neuroradiologist can be used to make subsequent resection easier (Fig. 21.12).

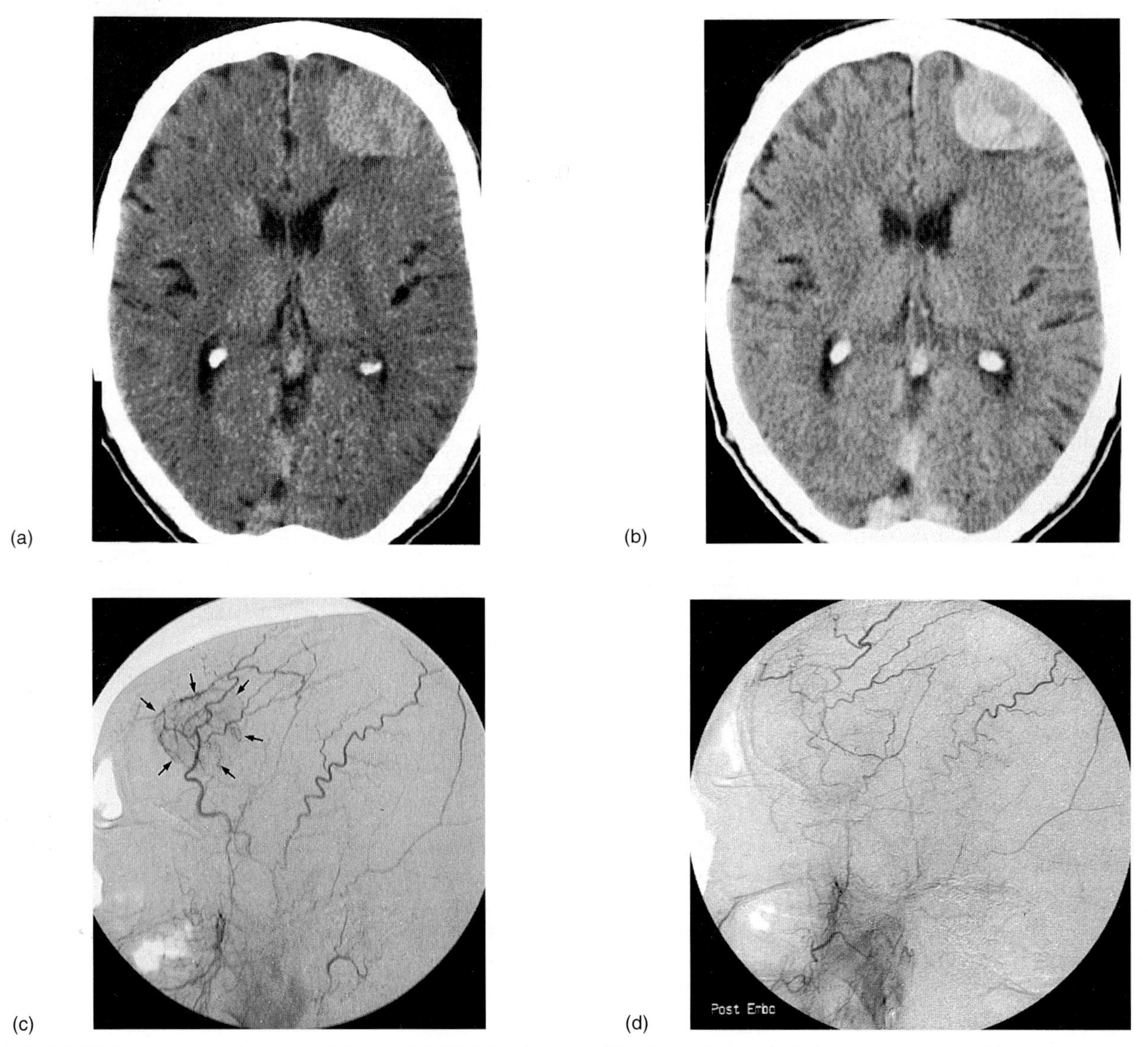

Fig. 21.12 Frontal meningioma in a 54-year-old. CT (a) before and (b) after enhancement shows a dense dural-based mass lesion which enhances strongly after contrast. Selective digital subtraction angiography of the external carotid artery (c) before and (d) after flow-directed particulate embolization shows obliteration of the arteriolar blush (arrows) of the tumour prior to resection.

Schwannomas

Schwannomas are the usual cranial nerve sheath tumours, whereas most cutaneous and peripheral nerve sheath tumours are neurofibromas. Schwannomas are associated with neurofibromatosis II. Schwannomas affect the cranial nerves III–XII, most commonly the vestibular division of the eighth nerve known as an **acoustic neuroma**. These tumours are well defined iso- or hypodense masses which enhance strongly on CT and occasionally calcification is present. On MRI the tumours are hypo- or isointense on T1-weighted and hyperintense on T2-weighted images and show marked enhancement after contrast (Fig. 21.13). An enlarged internal auditory meatus and canal may accompany the VIIIth nerve lesion. When screening for tumours very high definition T2-weighted axial sections are made. Small tumours may be obscured by the high signal from the CSF but the presence of a tumour may be suspected by blurring of the normal outline of the individual nerves; a tumour can be confirmed by contrast enhanced T1-weighted sections which will show marked enhancement in tumours as small as 1–2 mm (Fig. 21.14).

Colloid cysts

Colloid cysts though not neoplastic are important intraventricular mass lesions which arise in the anterior portion of the third ventricle close to the foramen of Monro. Even small colloid cysts can cause an acute obstructive hydrocephalus of the lateral ventricles

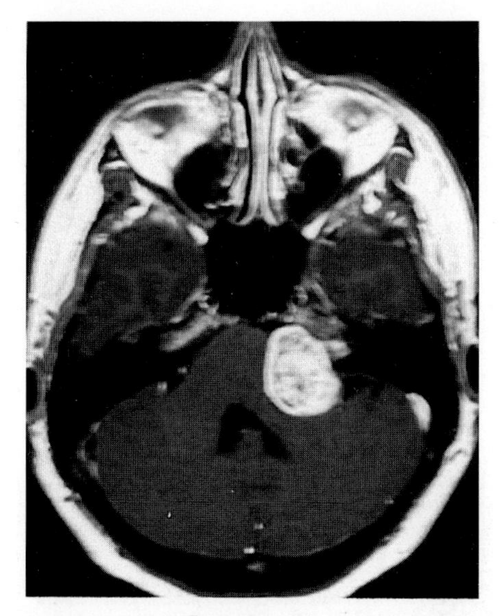

Fig. 21.13 Large acoustic schwannoma in a 49-year-old with left-sided sensorineural deafness. T1-weighted contrast enhanced axial section shows a 28 mm diameter extra-axial cerebellopontine angle enhancing mass compressing the brain stem and fourth ventricle extending from the internal auditory canal.

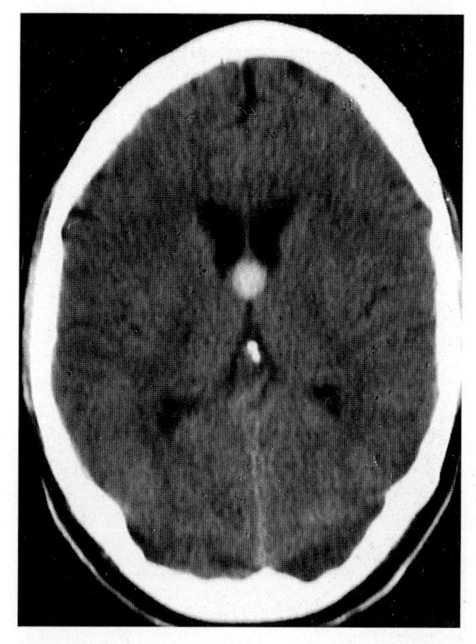

Fig. 21.15 Unenhanced axial CT showing a high attenuation colloid cyst in a typical position at the foramen of Monro.

which may initially be intermittent. Colloid cysts are well defined, often pedunculated round lesions, with increased attenuation on CT due to their high protein content (Fig. 21.15). On MRI they are usually hyperintense on both T1- and T2-weighted sections. Sagittal and coronal sections are best for defining the lesions which do not usually enhance after contrast.

Metastases

Metastases involving the dura occur most commonly with tumours of the lung, breast, prostate and melanoma. Dural metastases tend to spread as plaque lesions and there may be associated parenchymal lesions. On CT, metastases appear as isodense thickening of the meninges which enhances after contrast. Increased signal is seen on T2-weighted and decreased signal on T1-weighted MRI and, again, marked enhancement is a feature. With subarachnoid seeding small plaques or minute foci of tumour may be found with enhanced T1-weighted MRI. CT is considerably less sensitive for the detection of metastases than MRI. Subarachnoid metastases are found typically in the

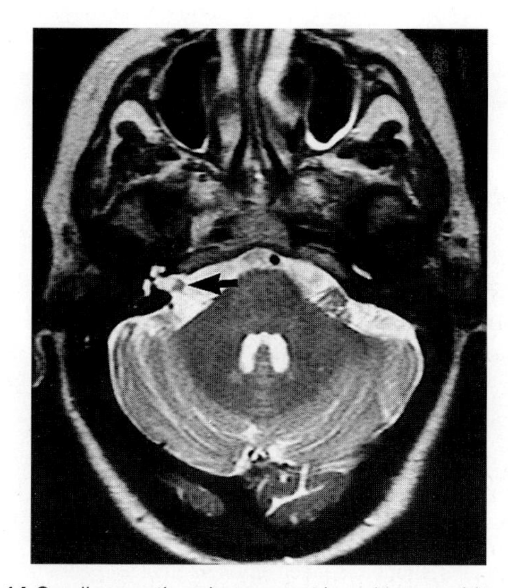

(a)

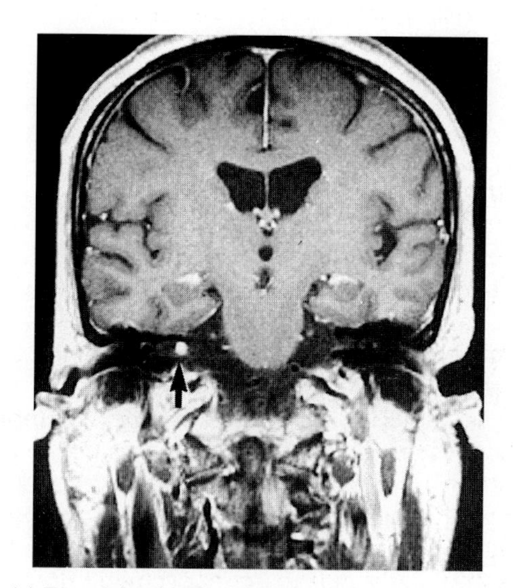

(b)

Fig. 21.14 Small acoustic schwannoma in a 41-year-old complaining of tinnitus. (a) T2-weighted high definition axial section shows 3 × 3 × 2 mm diameter filling defect in the right internal auditory meatus (arrow) displacing the VIIth and VIIIth cranial nerves. (b) T1-weighted contrast enhanced coronal section confirms the tiny enhancing hyperintense tumour (arrow).

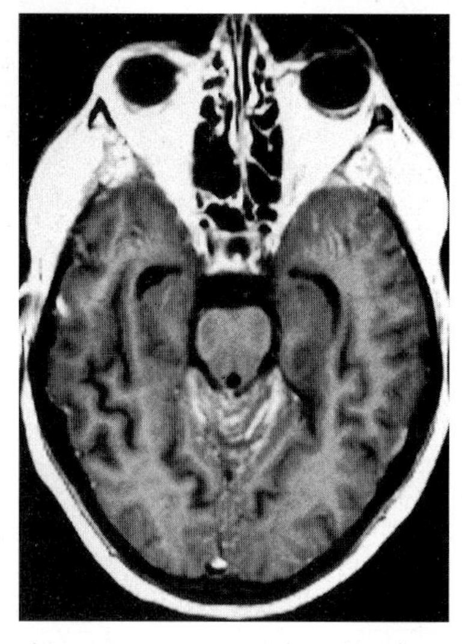

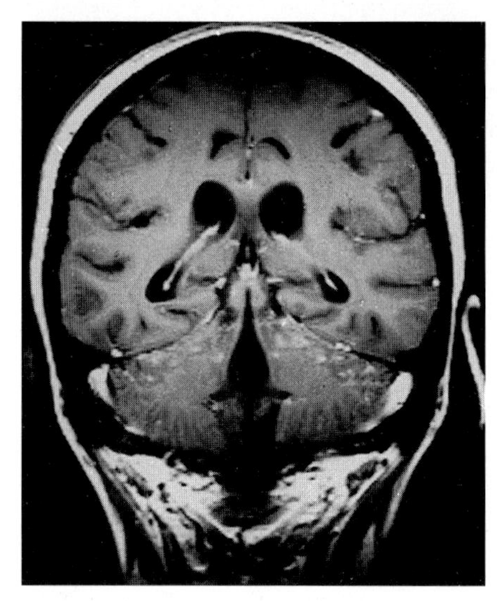

(a) (b)

Fig. 21.16 Subarachnoid and pial metastases shown as focal and coalescing hyperintensities over the superior cerebellum and vermis on (a) axial and (b) coronal enhanced T1-weighted MRI.

cerebellopontine angles and the basal cisterns but there is a broad differential diagnosis including infection and granulomas (Fig. 21.16).

Chordomas

Chordomas arise from notochord remnants and are most frequently seen in the clivus and sacrum. Chordomas produce focal bone destruction eroding into the adjacent structures, compressing cranial nerves and eventually vessels. CT shows the extent of bone erosion and a mass of inhomogeneous density with focal calcification and patchy enhancement with intravenous contrast. Chordomas are best demonstrated with T1-weighted MRI when they appear as a mass replacing the normal high intensity marrow signal (Fig. 21.17a). On MRI, chordomas have an inhomogeneous intensity which is generally hypointense on T1-weighted and hyperintense on T2-weighted images and show patchy contrast-enhancement. Metastatic lesions and bone tumours such as sarcomas and chondrosarcomas may initially appear very similar to a chordoma.

Pituitary tumours

Pituitary tumours are arbitrarily divided into macroadenomas (>1 cm) and microadenomas (<1 cm).

Macroadenomas usually enlarge and expand out of the pituitary fossa to produce symptoms eventually

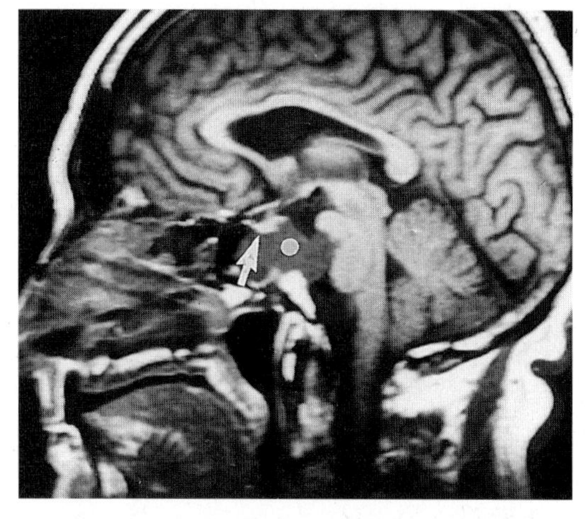

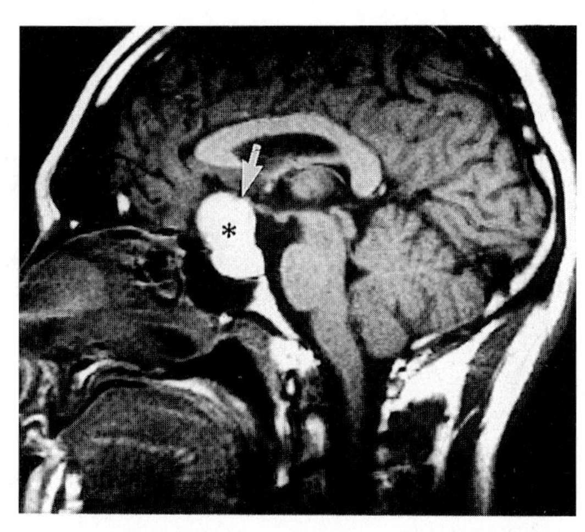

(a) (b)

Fig. 21.17 Differentiation of sellar and parasellar tumours is made easier by identifying the structures involved on sagittal and coronal MRI. (a) Chordoma. T1-weighted sagittal section showing a hypointense mass (circle) replacing the normally hyperintense marrow of the clivus while the pituitary (arrow) remains intact. (b) Pituitary macroadenoma. T1-weighted contrast enhanced sagittal section showing an enhancing mass (asterisk) expanding out of the sella to impinge on the optic chiasm (arrow) and floor of the third ventricle.

by impinging on the optic nerves and optic chiasm. Endocrine abnormalities are a less prominent feature. Macroadenomas should be recognized on routine axial CT but are better outlined by direct coronal dynamic enhanced CT. Sagittal and coronal MRI T1-weighted sections will define the limits of the mass and its relation to adjacent structures such as the chiasm, floor of third ventricle, pituitary stalk, cavernous sinuses, intracranial carotid arteries and sphenoid sinus. The tumours are usually homogeneous appearing iso-hypointense on T1-weighted images with hyperintensity on T2-weighted images and show moderate enhancement with intravenous contrast (Fig. 21.17b). The occasional presence of haemorrhage, cysts or necrosis influences the MRI appearances.

Microadenomas are more common than macroadenomas and present with hormone imbalance rather than mass effects. Prolactin-secreting tumours are the most common tumours but adrenocorticotrophic and growth hormone secreting lesions are also found. Again high definition, dynamic enhanced direct coronal CT will identify lesions >5 mm in diameter which are silhouetted as a low density against the normally enhancing pituitary gland. The pituitary stalk may be displaced away from the lesion and there may be localized erosion of the floor of the pituitary fossa. MRI is more sensitive than CT for the detection of microadenomas. With dynamic enhanced coronal and sagittal T1-weighted thin sections a microadenoma appears as a non-enhanced focus against a background of enhancing normal pituitary gland (Fig. 21.18). The displaced stalk can be assessed while the relation of the adenoma to the cavernous sinus and adjacent carotid arteries is clearly displayed. These are important features to note prior to trans-sphenoidal surgery.

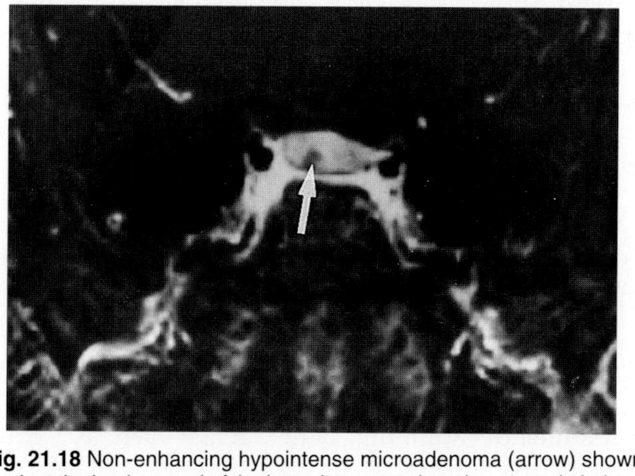

Fig. 21.18 Non-enhancing hypointense microadenoma (arrow) shown against the background of the hyperintense enhancing normal pituitary on a dynamic T1-weighted contrast-enhanced thin-section MRI in a patient with Cushing's disease.

HEAD INJURY

Head injuries now represent a major cause of death and disability especially in young otherwise healthy people. The main cause of head injury is still road traffic accidents in spite of seat belt, alcohol and crash helmet legislation reducing hospital admissions by 25%. Falls, assaults and sports injuries form an increasing proportion of the workload in neurosurgical units.

CLASSIFICATION OF INJURIES

With a combination of clinical and imaging information, injuries may be classified into primary lesions, secondary consequences and late sequelae (Table 21.1). Primary lesions are due to damage at the moment of impact and immediate complications. Primary lesions include skull fractures, diffuse axonal injury, contusions, lacerations and intracranial haemorrhage which may be found both intra- and extracerebrally. Secondary consequences occur later and include brain swelling, raised intracranial pressure, ischaemic damage and infarction due to brain herniation or vascular injury. Late sequelae include cerebromalacia, cerebral atrophy, hydrocephalus, CSF fistula, infection and vascular lesions.

CT is still the examination of choice in the immediate assessment of a patient with a head injury. While CT is adequate for making acute surgical management decisions, it has become increasingly clear that MRI is more sensitive to minute alterations in cerebral water content and blood products and MRI can show injuries invisible to CT. MRI is particularly useful in the subacute and chronic phases. Radionuclide scanning can show the functionally disrupted metabolism

Table 21.1 Clinical and Imaging Classification of Head Injury

Primary lesions	*Secondary consequences*	*Late sequelae*
Skull fracture	Raised intracranial pressure	Cerebromalacia
Diffuse axonal injury	Ischaemic damage	Cerebral atrophy
Contusions	Brain herniation	Hydrocephalus
Lacerations	Vascular injury	CSF fistula
Haemorrhage	Infarction	Infection
intracerebral		Vascular lesions
intraventricular		
subarachnoid		
subdural		
extradural		

and ischaemia prevalent in most types of brain injury. The cerebral protection therapies currently under development are directed at potentially reversible damage and confirm the increasing complementary role for functional and structural imaging.

PLAIN SKULL FILMS FOLLOWING HEAD INJURY

Skull radiographs remain important in the triage of minor injuries but if neurosurgical referral is already deemed necessary or if CT is indicated on clinical grounds, performing a skull X-ray will just delay the patient's transfer or the definitive CT examination and give no additional management information. A skull X-ray should now be performed in those patients with a minor head injury to identify a skull fracture so that they may be scanned electively within the following 24 hours.

If a skull X-ray is required, at least two views at right angles should be taken. The lateral view should be taken with the patient supine and a horizontal X-ray beam to ensure that a fluid level may be seen in the paranasal sinuses and that any intracranial air can be detected. Moreover the cervical spine is not moved and the upper cervical region is included on the radiograph. A fluid level caused by blood within the sphenoid sinus is a common indirect sign of a skull base fracture but CT is usually required to show the fracture line. Fractures are shown on plain films as sharply demarcated black lines without corticated margins. Fractures do not branch, tend to run in straight lines and stop at sutures which may themselves be diastased. A depressed fracture may be suspected if there is an area of reduced density with an associated area of increased density corresponding to displaced bone superimposed upon adjacent normal skull. A tangential view will confirm the degree of displacement.

Plain films and direct coronal CT are used to assess complex facial fractures but can be delayed until the patient has been stabilized, is fit enough to cooperate or reparative surgery is imminent. Three-dimensional surface reconstruction of a stack of CT sections can give the surgeon a dynamic interpretation of the image, highlighting bony displacements or distortions. However, the algorithms used in the formation of the 3D-image can obscure or falsify fracture lines and the value of 3D-reconstruction in patient management is therefore limited.

CERVICAL SPINE INJURY

It may be impossible to exclude a cervical spine injury without radiology in the head-injured patient with a severely impaired conscious level. Lateral and frontal films, which include the craniocervical junction and the first thoracic vertebra, are first obtained. As the cervicothoracic region is frequently not satisfactorily imaged on the plain films, axial thin-section CT from C6 to T2 should be carried out and midline and oblique sagittal re-formations obtained to show any fractures or subluxation. MRI may be required to demonstrate or exclude soft-tissue injury involving the cord, ligaments, discs or paraspinal tissues.

CT IN HEAD INJURY

When blood clots, its large protein molecules become compacted, water is excluded and a high electron density develops. This attenuates X-rays more than in normal brain and the clot is displayed as a bright area. Conversely, oedema or ischaemia produce an increase in water content and hence a reduction in electron density. This reduced attenuation is displayed as a dark area. Normal grey and white matter lie between these two extremes.

Patients are usually scanned supine but if restless a decubitus position may settle them long enough to enable a diagnostic scan to be carried out without sedation or anaesthetic. The scan should extend from the foramen magnum to the vertex. Both soft-tissue and bone-window images can be obtained from the same data set.

MRI IN HEAD INJURY

Now that MRI-compatible cardiorespiratory monitoring and support equipment are available, critically ill patients can be imaged safely at any stage after a head injury. However, if the patient is not unconscious or paralysed and ventilated, a higher degree of patient cooperation is required than for CT. These patients may have sustained multiple injuries and screening is required to exclude ferrometallic foreign bodies or electronic implants which would preclude MRI.

With appropriate choice of sequence the contrast between normal and pathological tissues can be many times that shown by CT. Certain sequences are very sensitive to acute and chronic haemorrhage. Rapid sequences have been developed recently and the increased speed of acquisition can be used to carry out a quicker study in children or severely injured patients. Alternatively more acquisitions can be acquired in the same time as a conventional scan to improve anatomical detail markedly.

RADIONUCLIDE SCANNING IN HEAD INJURY

Radionuclide scanning with agents such as ^{99m}Tc-hexamethyl propylene amine oxime (^{99m}Tc-HMPAO) are used to map regional cerebral blood flow. Because HMPAO is lipophilic, it crosses the blood–brain

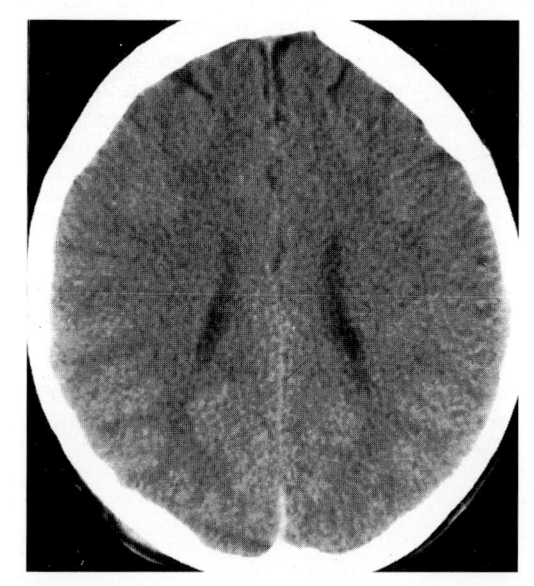
(a)

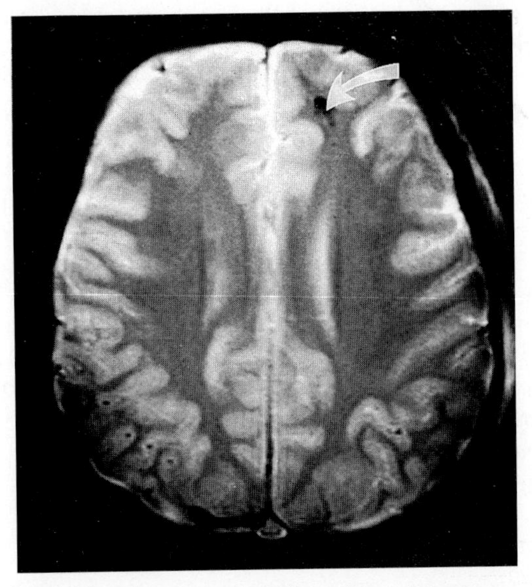
(b)

Fig. 21.19 Diffuse axonal injury in a patent unconscious 8 h after an acute head injury from a road traffic accident. (a) CT normal. (b) T2*-weighted MRI section shows the hypointensity of deoxyhaemoglobin in acute haemorrhage in the parasagittal frontal white matter (arrow), one of the hallmarks of diffuse axonal injury.

barrier where it is rapidly converted into a hydrophilic compound and is trapped for several hours while the distribution is recorded.

PRIMARY INJURY OF THE BRAIN

Diffuse axonal injury

Axonal injury is due to the stresses in the brain caused by severe acceleration and/or deceleration of the head at the moment of injury. Varying degrees of white matter tract disruption may occur often with involvement of adjacent capillaries. It has recently been shown that the lesion may progress and so treatment to limit its progression is being sought. Sometimes the damage due to diffuse axonal injury may only be apparent when diffuse atrophy is found on follow-up examination.

Axonal damage occurs in a 'top down' pattern. With a mild concussive injury small lesions with increased water content are seen paramedially at the junction of the cortical grey/white matter on MRI, while on CT these lesions are usually invisible (Fig. 21.19). These lesions are thought to represent the 'gliding contusions' described neuropathologically, although direct correlation is unavailable. With increasing severity other lesions become apparent in the corpus callosum and extend downward into the brain stem. MRI is very sensitive to these lesions even in the absence of macroscopic haemorrhage, a feature which has to be present before the diagnosis can be made on CT. The full classic triad of haemorrhage in the brain stem, the corpus callosum and the cortical grey/white matter junction on CT or MRI is rarely found. Small haemorrhages in the basal ganglia region and intraventricular haemorrhage may also be seen (Fig. 21.20). As the injury ages the blood becomes isodense on CT and if the CT scan is delayed beyond a few days from the injury the scan may be falsely interpreted as normal. If the scan is delayed still further low attenuation mass lesions may be seen at the site of the resolving haemorrhage. MRI is the best method of detecting haemorrhage and diagnosing the extent of injury.

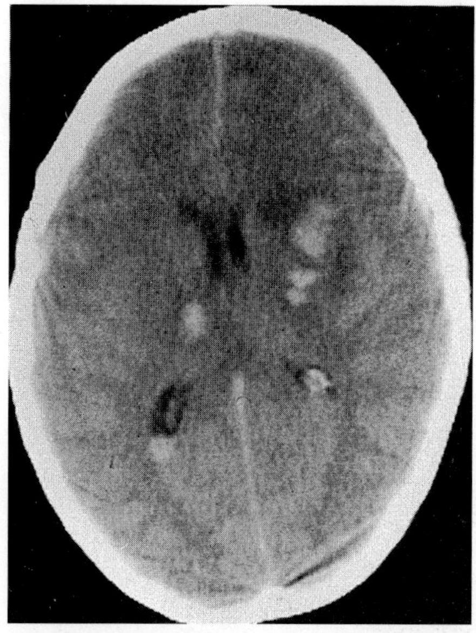

Fig. 21.20 Thalamic, basal ganglia and grey/white matter interface haemorrhages with intraventicular haemorrhage on acute CT following a 20 m fall. These features are associated with diffuse axonal injury.

Contusions and lacerations

Contusions are bruises of the brain formed by coalescing petechial haemorrhages caused by direct contact of the brain with the inner table of the skull. Contusions are seen most frequently on the under surfaces of the frontal and temporal lobes and are the most common complication of head injury. Lacerations are due to direct tearing of the brain by penetrating sharp objects such as bone spicules, bullets or stabbing. A variable amount of ischaemic brain, which further enlarges the area of swelling, surrounds the contusion or laceration. Although blood–brain barrier breakdown occurs in the surrounding ischaemic area, contrast enhancement on CT or MRI adds nothing to the diagnosis and may be toxic to the damaged brain.

Contusions are recognized on CT as areas of low attenuation. Haemorrhage is always present pathologically but may be microscopic and undetectable on CT. However, the amount of blood present varies from a small quantity on the brain surface to substantial collections extending deeply into the subcortical white matter (Fig. 21.21).

INTRACEREBRAL HAEMATOMA FOLLOWING HEAD INJURY

Most intracerebral haematomas develop as a complication of a contusion. On CT, acute haemorrhage is seen as a hyperdense area with a rim of surrounding oedema which is darker than normal brain. As the haematoma ages it becomes isodense with the brain

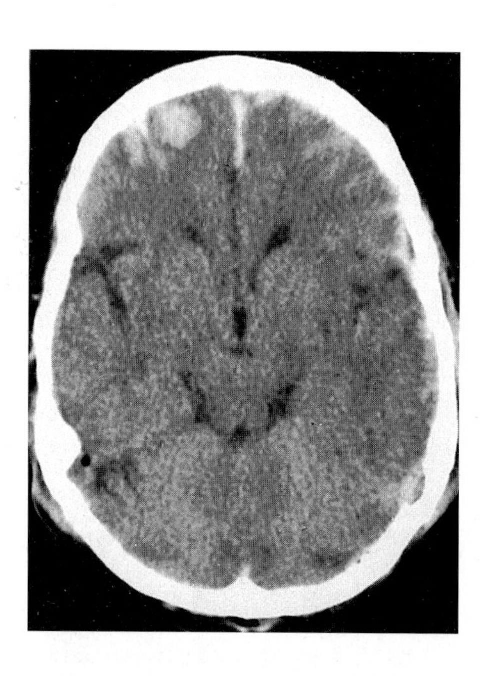

(a)

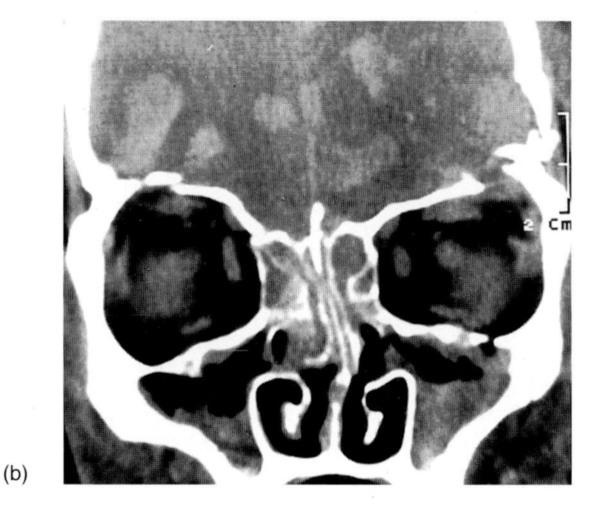

(b)

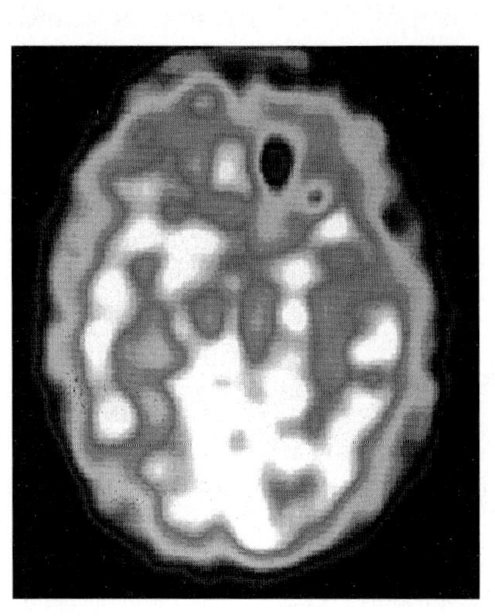

(c)

Fig. 21.21 Bilateral frontal contusions following a fall down steps shown on (a) axial and (b) coronal CT (note the bilateral orbital rim fractures). (c) ^{99m}Tc HMPAO-SPECT section showing bilateral frontal hypoperfusion worse on the left than the right.

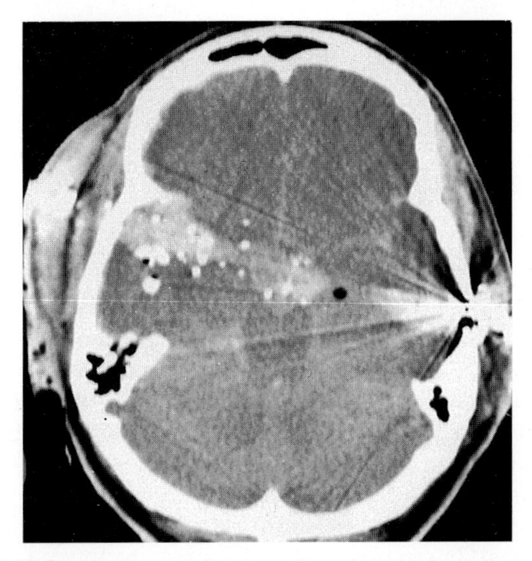
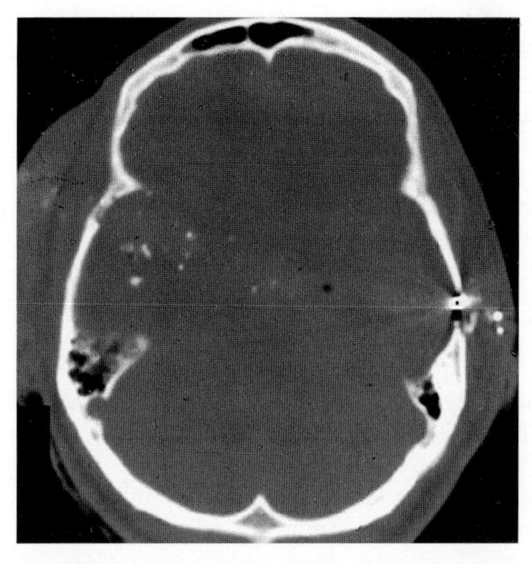

(a) (b)

Fig. 21.22 Gunshot wound showing a linear haemorrhagic laceration across the brain with intracranial air, bony and metallic debris seen on CT on (a) soft tissue and (b) bony windows.

over the course of the next 1–4 weeks. Occasionally angiography is required to exclude aneurysmal rupture as the cause of an unexplained haematoma.

A penetrating injury should be suspected if a laceration is demonstrated and haemorrhage is seen in a peripheral-to-deep linear orientation or if a foreign body is present (Fig. 21.22).

Delayed haematomas are now being seen more frequently. Patients tend to be scanned soon after their head injury before the haematoma has time to develop and then subsequently have a repeat scan. Delayed haematomas usually occur at the site of a contusion but may develop in the extradural or more rarely the subdural space. These haematomas are also seen more frequently if surgery has been performed, or after resuscitation in patients with major injury when there may have been cerebral hypoperfusion.

Brain-stem haematomas occur in three circumstances:

- in the rostral brain stem lateral or anterolateral to the fourth ventricle when associated with diffuse axonal injury (Fig. 21.23);
- centrally in the pons and mesencephalon when secondary to tentorial herniation (Duret haematoma);
- in a similar central location after severe primary trauma.

Trauma is thought to cause an acute transient descent of the brain stem at the time of the impact resulting in stretching and rupturing the perforating vessels.

MRI is more sensitive to haemorrhage than CT but the appearance of haemorrhage on MRI is complex and depends on multiple factors including the paramagnetic form of haemoglobin present, clot matrix formation, changes in erythrocyte hydration and changes in the degree of red blood cell packing. There is a characteristic sequence of intensity patterns as the haematoma forms, serum is absorbed, haemoglobin matures, becomes denatured to methaemoglobin and is engulfed by macrophages. The methaemoglobin is metabolized and eventually a haemosiderin-lined cleft remains. At this stage the blood–brain barrier is intact and the degradation products are trapped. The pattern on MRI of haemorrhage and haematoma formation is summarized in Table 21.2.

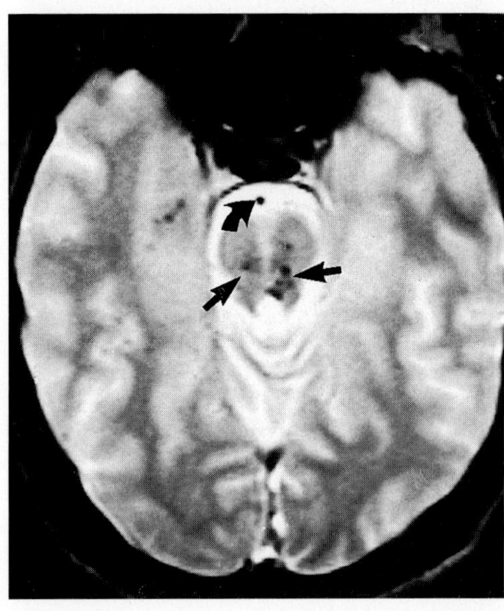

Fig. 21.23 Hypointense acute brainstem haemorrhage (arrows) associated with diffuse axonal injury shown only on T2*-weighted MRI (CT normal). Note basilar artery (curved arrow).

Table 21.2 Maturation of Haemorrhage on MRI

Stage	*Biochemistry*	*T1*	*T2*
1. Hyperacute (up to 2–3 hours)	Oxyhaemoglobin	Dark	Bright
2. Acute (3 hours–4 days)	Deoxyhaemoglobin	Isointense	Dark
3. Subacute (early) (4–7 days)	Methaemoglobin (intracellular)	Bright	Dark
4. Subacute (late) (6 days–8 weeks)	Methaemoglobin	Bright	Bright
5. Chronic (8 weeks onwards)	Ferritin/Haemosiderin	Isointense	Dark

INTRAVENTRICULAR HAEMORRHAGE FOLLOWING HEAD INJURY

Intraventricular haemorrhage is unusual even in severe head injury occuring in only 3% of all head injuries. It occurs most commonly when an intracerebral haemorrhagic contusion or haematoma breaks into the ventricle. In this situation the prognosis is poor, especially if there is a large amount of clot in the ventricle. Intraventricular haemorrhage is commonly associated with a callosal tear and so in the correct clinical setting intraventricular haemorrhage can act as one of the markers for diffuse axonal injury. In elderly patients intraventricular haemorrhage can sometimes occur as an isolated finding, where it is likely to be due to rupture of a subependymal vein. In this situation the prognosis is usually less dire.

SUBARACHNOID HAEMORRHAGE FOLLOWING HEAD INJURY

Up to a third of severely head injured patients have associated subarachnoid haemorrhage lying between the arachnoid membrane and the pia covering the brain. Subarachnoid haemorrhage may coexist with any type of traumatic lesion but is usually found isolated in the basal cisterns after a skull base fracture while a subarachnoid haemorrhage over the hemispheres may be related to a vault fracture, local haemorrhage or cerebral contusion. A traumatic subarachnoid haemorrhage is not associated with vasospasm, as may occur with rupture of an aneurysm.

Subarachnoid haemorrhage can only be shown by MRI in the acute stage if special sequences are used. If there is sufficient clot left in the subacute stage it will be seen as hyperintense on T1-weighted images.

SUBDURAL HAEMORRHAGE

Subdural collections lie between the arachnoid membrane and the inner meningeal layer of the dura, most commonly over the convexity of the brain but can also arise along the falx and the tentorium. A subdural haemorrhage is usually caused by tearing of the relatively unsupported veins which cross the subdural space but can also form directly from adjacent severe contusions and subarachnoid lacerations. When severe contusions are associated with an adjacent subdural haematoma the lesion is termed a 'burst lobe'.

On CT it is important to look at soft-tissue and bone windows to distinguish hyperdense clot from bone. Occasionally a thin subdural haematoma may be suspected only from the compressive pattern it causes. MRI has shown that small subdural haematomas are almost universally present with moderate to severe contusions but a surgically significant subdural haematoma will not be missed on CT.

Within the first week the haematoma appears hyperdense (Fig. 21.24) but a week or more after the trauma a more mature clot will be shown. The haematoma then becomes isodense with brain at

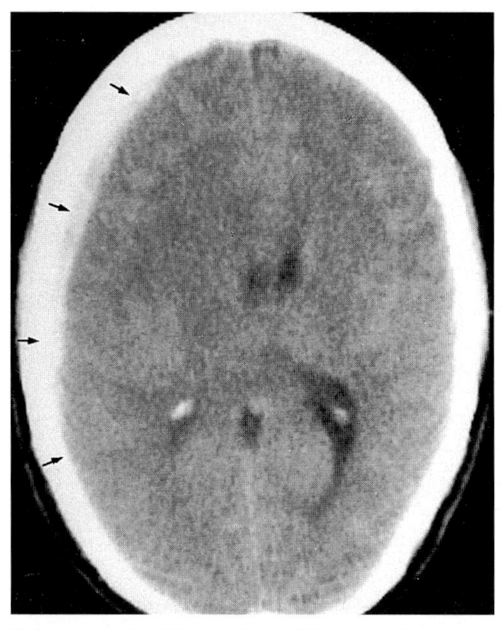

Fig. 21.24 Acute subdural haematoma. CT shows the haematoma as a thin dense rim (arrows) overlying the surface of the brain.

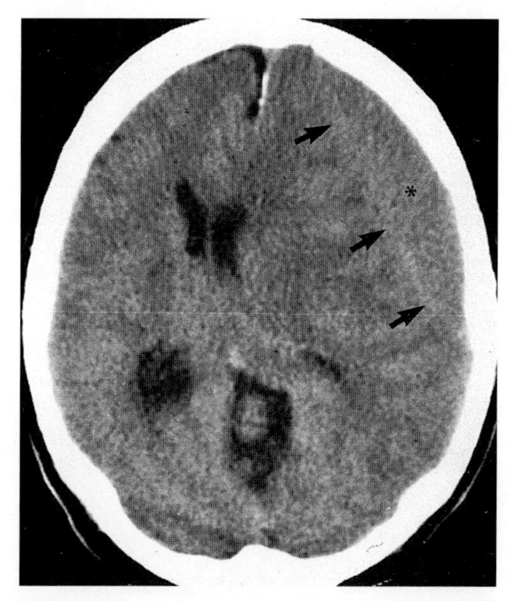

Fig. 21.25 Extensive isodense left subdural haematoma (*) causing severe brain compression with 2 cm of midline shift, compression of the ipsilateral lateral ventricle and dilatation of the contralateral lateral ventricle following a fall 10 days earlier. The arrows mark the inner border of the haematoma.

approximately 7–10 days (Fig. 21.25) and hypodense by 21–30 days. Fresh haemorrhage can also occur within a subacute subdural haematoma to produce a mixed or layered pattern of high- and low-attenuation clot.

It is important to realize that occasionally an isodense bilateral subdural haematoma without midline shift can occur, in which case the CT diagnosis of subdural haematoma can be overlooked. An increase in apparent cortical thickness, symmetrical posterior displacement of the anterior horns of the lateral ventricles and compression or absence of the third ventricle will suggest the correct diagnosis.

MRI always shows a subdural haematoma separate from the underlying brain. The full extent of the haematoma can be assessed ideally by coronal MRI. Collections lying along the falx, the peritentorial space and along the floor of the middle cranial fossa are clearly demarcated while the volumetric perception of those collections lying over the convexity can be accurately assessed by coronal scans (Fig. 21.26).

EXTRADURAL HAEMORRHAGE

Haemorrhage occurs in the potential space between the inner table of the skull and the dura when the dura is stripped off in association with a fracture. The blood comes from the marrow in the skull, from torn meningeal arteries or veins or from a laceration of the dural sinuses. The clot is usually limited by the adjacent skull sutures where the dura is tethered. Classically, CT shows a uniformly high attenuation biconvex lesion based against the skull vault (Fig. 21.27). As more patients are being scanned immediately after injury many extradural clots are now seen as mixed or even mainly low attenuation lesions because the blood is still liquid and the clot is still forming and does not yet have the same appearance on CT as a mature haematoma. An extradural haematoma is usually very obvious, although clots in the floor of the middle fossa can be mistaken for an

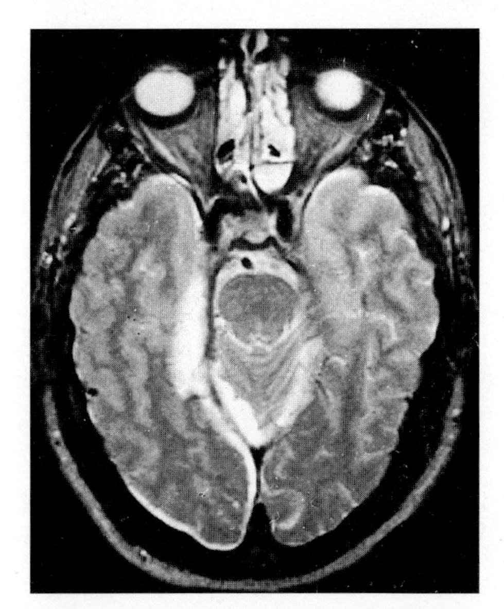

(a)

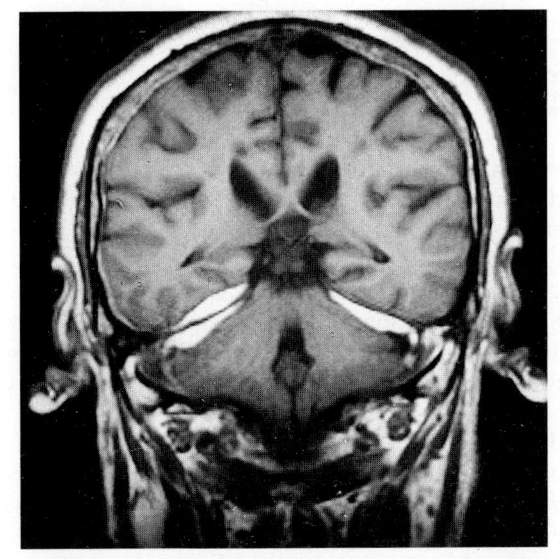

(b)

Fig. 21.26 Subacute subdural haematomas appearing as high signal around the occipital and right temporal lobes seen on (a) T2-weighted axial and (b) T1-weighted coronal scans. They demonstrate high signal subdural collections on either side of the tentorium.

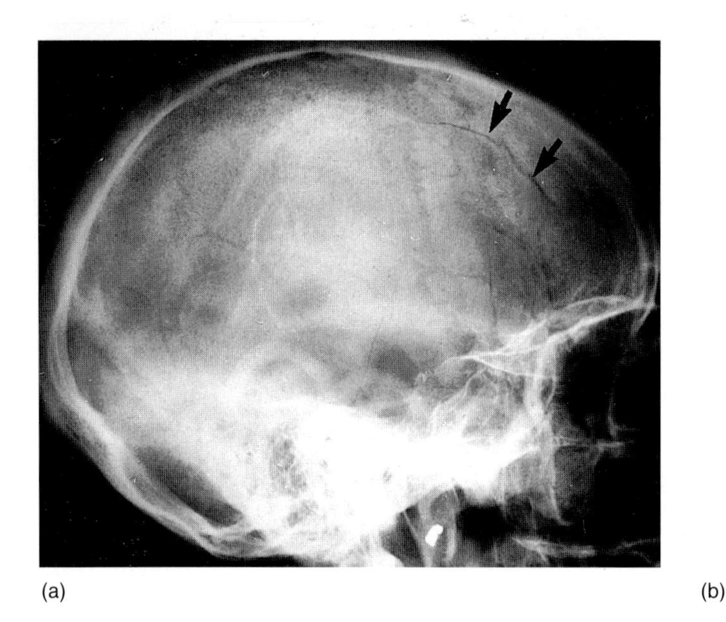

(a)

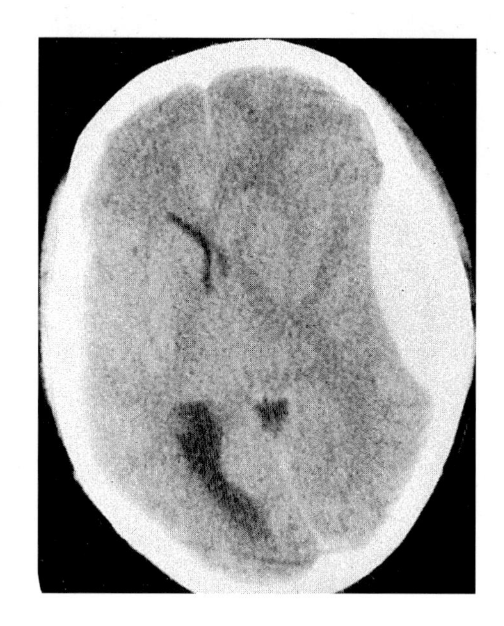

(b)

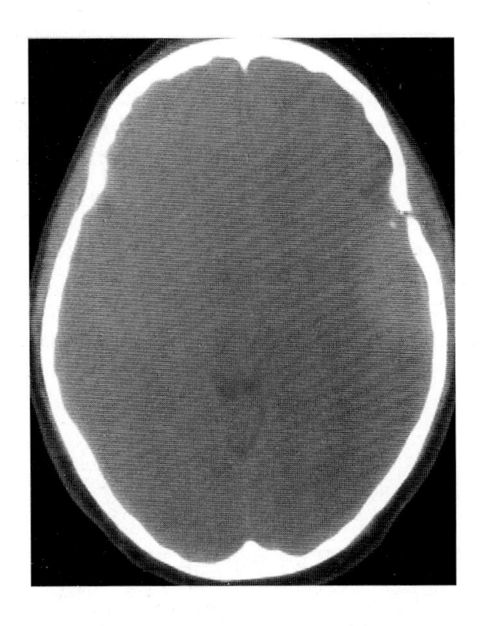

(c)

Fig. 21.27 Extradural haematoma following an assault. (a) Plain radiograph shows a frontal fracture (arrows). CT shows (b) biconvex dense haematoma on soft tissue windows and (c) the relation of the haemorrhage to the fracture on bone-windows settings.

intratemporal lesion and those on the vertex of the skull missed altogether if the scan is not continued to the top of the head.

On MRI, subdural and extradural haematomas age in a similar way to intracerebral haemorrhage, but in the acute and subacute stages there is less reabsorption of serum and varying degrees of liquefaction so extracerebral haematomas mature more quickly than their intracerebral counterparts. If air enters the collection through a compound fracture, attempted aspiration or surgery, the formation of methaemoglobin from deoxyhaemoglobin is accelerated giving an early hyperintense signal on T1-weighted images.

Unlike haemorrhage into the subdural space a chronic extradural haematoma is rare (Fig. 21.28).

PNEUMOCEPHALUS FOLLOWING HEAD INJURY

Pneumocephalus usually follows a fracture involving the paranasal sinuses, most often the frontal, the mastoid air cells or the middle ear, and occasionally air will enter either the subdural, subarachnoid space or the brain. A CSF leak commonly develops.

RAISED INTRACRANIAL PRESSURE AND HERNIATION FOLLOWING HEAD INJURY

Raised intracranial pressure > 20 mmHg is a frequent and serious complication of head injury. Focal mass lesions such as haemorrhage and generalized cerebral

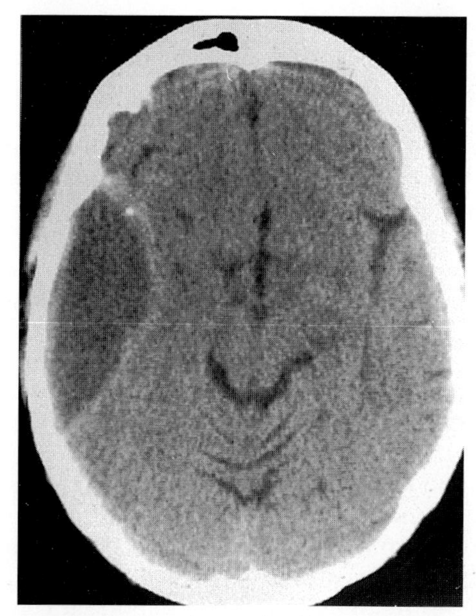

Fig. 21.28 Low-density chronic extradural haematoma with thickened dense dural membrane containing calcification on CT.

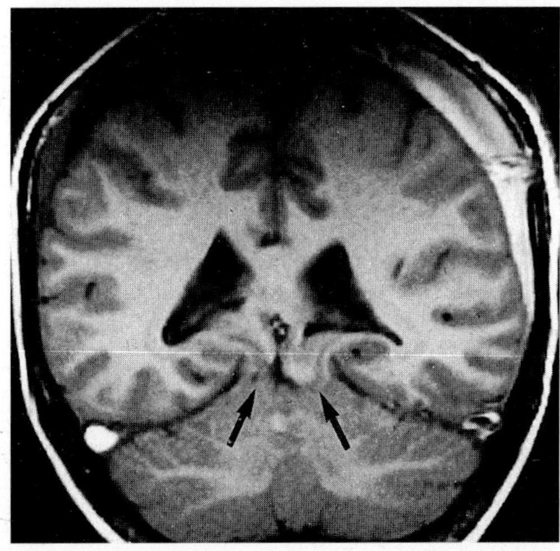

Fig. 21.29 T1-weighted coronal MRI with a left subdural haematoma causing uncal herniation (arrows) through the tentorial notch.

swelling are responsible for the elevation of pressure. General swelling or multiple diffuse contusions cause effacement of the cerebral sulci of the involved lobes. Shift of the adjacent ventricle will be localized if the mass lesion is small. The fourth ventricle should always be visible, lying centrally in a reasonably well-positioned axial scan. If the fourth ventricle is displaced or compressed, a local cause should be sought and a thin extracerebral collection excluded by viewing the CT scan at different window levels or carrying out MRI.

Large supratentorial masses produce lateral and downward herniation of the brain. There is compression of the ipsilateral ventricle, shift of the midline structures below the falx and dilatation of the contralateral trigone and temporal horn of the lateral ventricle once the foramen of Monro is occluded. This ventricular dilatation is often associated with periventricular oedema and the third ventricle is occluded. At this stage there is usually transtentorial herniation. Transtentorial herniation is well shown on coronal MRI on which subcallosal and uncal herniation can be appreciated (Fig. 21.29). Such downward shift of the brain is associated with raised intracranial pressure and is a life-threatening condition. On the other hand even severe lateral shift can be tolerated if the third ventricle and the basal cisterns remain patent.

Tonsillar herniation cannot be shown directly by CT although it is clearly demonstrated by sagittal sections on MRI. Isolated masses within the posterior fossa can cause an acute obstructive hydrocephalus of the third and lateral ventricles by compressing the fourth ventricle. The earliest sign of hydrocephalus is dilation of the temporal horns that, in normal young people, are seen only as narrow curved slits. Upward tentorial herniation is unusual because isolated infratentorial traumatic lesions are uncommon.

The midline may remain undisplaced when there are bilateral masses of similar size or if there is general swelling of the hemispheres, but significant downward herniation and raised intracranial pressure can still be present. Normally it should always be possible to identify the third ventricle and basal cisterns as low attenuation CSF-containing spaces. If either the third ventricle or the basal cisterns are obliterated with <5 mm of midline shift, the intracranial pressure lies between 25 and 30 mmHg (Fig. 21.30). If both the third

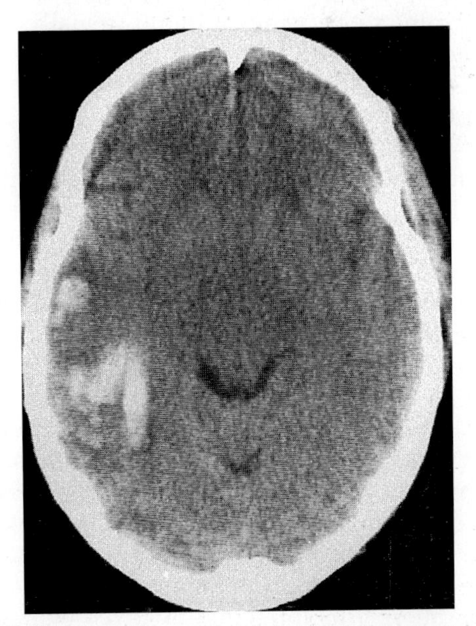

Fig. 21.30 Brain swelling and right temporal contusion following severe trauma. Although the basal cisterns contain CSF, the third ventricle is not visible confirming raised intracranial pressure between 25 and 30 mmHg.

ventricle and basal cisterns are obliterated the intracranial pressure is > 35 mmHg.

It is not clear whether the generalized hemisphere swelling occurring after head injury is due to hyperaemia or ischaemia. This hemisphere swelling is most commonly seen in children and young adults.

ISCHAEMIC DAMAGE, VASCULAR INJURY AND INFARCTION FOLLOWING HEAD INJURY

On CT, ischaemia which may be reversible and infarction are both shown as areas of reduced attenuation. Cerebral ischaemia is universal in fatal head injuries but it is rarely demonstrated by CT in life as it is almost impossible to separate necrotic brain from the coexistent cytotoxic oedema of ischaemia. The diffuse multifocal ischaemia seen commonly by the pathologist cannot be shown by CT although it has been demonstrated with radionuclide studies.

Arterial vascular territory ischaemia is the most commonly recognized ischaemic complication. It frequently involves the posterior cerebral artery ipsilateral to a mass lesion causing severe midline shift. Pericallosal artery ischaemia can be produced in a similar way.

Visible middle cerebral territory ischaemia suggests damage to the carotid artery in the neck or skull base, local dissection or embolic thrombosis from more proximal dissection. Early angiography will identify lesions which can be treated surgically although treatment for traumatic small vessel dissection or thrombosis remains controversial. Ischaemia in the basilar territory causes diffuse low attenuation on CT in the brain stem and midbrain usually on CT contrasted against the preserved normal density pattern of the cerebellum. Vertebral dissection may show only as infarction in the territory of the ipsilateral posterior inferior cerebellar artery.

All ischaemia is much better visualized with MRI than with CT, especially ischaemia in the posterior fossa and medial aspects of the temporal lobes. Ischaemia appears on MRI as well-defined focal regions of hyperintensity on T2-weighted sequences with corresponding less prominent areas of hypointensity on T1-weighted sections.

Cortical venous infarction can be caused by a fracture involving a major venous sinus or secondary infection which results in dural venous sinus thrombosis. On CT, venous infarction shows as peripheral high attenuation areas owing to haemorrhage, surrounded by low attenuation areas from oedema. These changes do not conform to an arterial territory distribution. Venous infarction involves white matter more than grey matter and can occasionally mimic gliding contusions. Both venous occlusion and consequent infarction are better defined by MRI than CT. MRI shows thrombosis of the occluded sinus on routine sequences but can be most convincingly demonstrated on a magnetic resonance venogram. Venous infarcts give similar signal characteristics on MRI to arterial infarcts but are less well defined.

Ischaemia in watershed territories can develop after a period of global hypotension. On CT, areas of reduced attenuation will be seen whilst MRI shows hyperintensity on T2-weighted images with hypointensity on T1-weighted images. These changes are seen in the watershed area between the anterior and middle cerebral artery territories, in the frontal and parafalcine regions, and in the area between the middle and the posterior cerebral artery territories in the parietal region.

Profound persistent hypotension, ischaemia or generally elevated intracranial pressure usually results in loss of the normal grey/white matter differentiation in both hemispheres and is associated with an apparent increase in the attenuation of the normal cerebellum and tentorium on CT. These appearances are limited to children and young adults and are pathognomonic of a non-perfused cerebrum.

Radionuclide scanning is more sensitive to perfusion changes than CT or MRI and often shows regions of both abnormally high and abnormally low cortical blood flow. All focal traumatic mass lesions such as contusions and intracerebral haemorrhage show zones of severely reduced cerebral blood flow which can persist for days to months particularly in the surrounding oedematous areas. Occasionally the abnormal perfusion pattern persists over several months even though the structural appearance on CT or MRI returns to normal. This abnormal perfusion may correlate with some of the late neuropsychological sequelae found after head injury.

CEREBROMALACIA FOLLOWING HEAD INJURY

As contusions heal by progressive degradation and maturation of haemorrhage with eventual gliosis they shrink to leave a low-attenuation area on CT with loss of cortex and adjacent white matter. This lesion, known as cerebromalacia, is commonly found in a subfrontal and/or temporal location. After the acute space-occupying effects of haemorrhagic contusion have resolved, an *ex vacuo* effect supervenes resulting in enlargement of adjacent sulci and ventricles.

CEREBROSPINAL FLUID FISTULA

An overt CSF leak is present in about 25% of patients with pneumocephalus demonstrated on CT but in the majority the leak ceases spontaneously within 7 to 10 days. If it persists or if there is evidence of meningitis

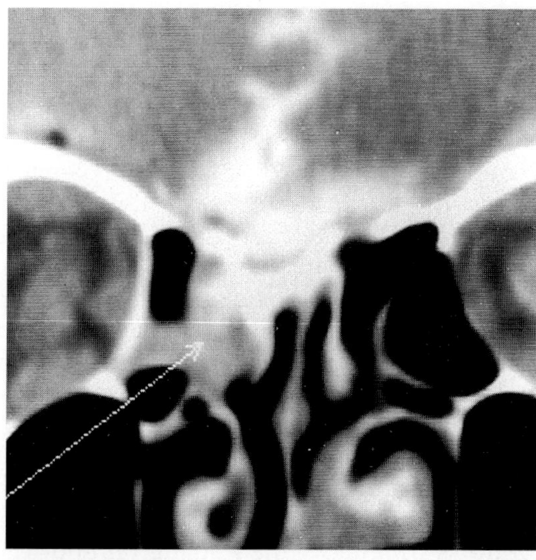

Fig. 21.31 CSF fistula shown by leakage of intrathecal contrast (arrow) into the posterior ethmoid air cells on coronal CT.

then the fracture site should be sought. Direct coronal high resolution CT of the anterior fossa is used to investigate CSF rhinorrhoea and axial and coronal high resolution sections of the petrous bones are used in patients with CSF otorrhoea. If CT fails to demonstrate an opaque sinus adjacent to a bone defect the examination should be repeated following contrast opacification of the cisternal CSF by instillating 5 ml of non-ionic contrast medium via a lumbar puncture. The contrast is then run up to the basal cisterns and positioned over the appropriate portion of the skull base and the CT repeated to detect any leak (Fig. 21.31).

VASCULAR LESIONS FOLLOWING HEAD INJURY

Penetrating injuries must be recognized in the acute stage and any associated vascular lesion demonstrated by urgent angiography. Arteriovenous fistula or a pseudoaneurysm can form secondary to a skull fracture and tear of the meningeal vessels. Delayed or recurrent intracranial haematomas can follow penetrating injuries. When the intracavernous segment of the carotid artery is damaged, with or without a skull-base fracture, a caroticocavernous fistula may form with unilateral or bilateral pulsing exophthalmos or, much less commonly, a pseudoaneurysm may form. Although either can be present at the time of injury both are more frequent after several weeks have elapsed. Angiography is required for the full definition of the vascular components but the abnormal vessels will be shown on enhanced CT and MRI. Either an endovascular approach with embolization or a combined neuroradiological–neurosurgical treatment plan is now used to occlude the fistula, aneurysm or parent vessel preserving as much of the normal vasculature as possible.

HYDROCEPHALUS FOLLOWING HEAD INJURY

Localized dilatation of the ventricles may be seen adjacent to a large area of cerebromalacia following head injury but generalized hydrocephalus is unusual and most often follows intraventricular or subarachnoid haemorrhage. In hydrocephalus there is disproportionate ventricular enlargement compared to the cortical sulci and cisterns. Although the temporal horns should be involved, care has to be taken as their enlargement can also be a local complication of cerebromalacia. With severe hydrocephalus, CT or MRI may show periventricular white matter oedema. Progressive ventricular dilation associated with enlarged cortical sulci and cisterns owing to cerebral atrophy that may be seen four to six months after an injury, may be the only sign of diffuse axonal injury.

INFECTION FOLLOWING HEAD INJURY

Infection is still a serious problem but nowadays is usually pre-empted by prophylactical treatment.

Meningitis is a common complication of compound skull fractures. It is diagnosed clinically and a CT or plain film usually simply confirms the fracture site. CT and MRI with intravenous contrast enhancement shows generalized meningeal enhancement although in the acute phase the examination may be normal.

Cerebral abscess may present as an intracranial mass, most often associated with a penetrating injury or a foreign body even though the primary breach in the dura may not have been suspected.

Bone infection is unusual and is seen most frequently in association with a craniotomy bone flap or an infected scalp wound. Plain films or CT show the abnormalities once the infection is established.

CEREBRAL ATROPHY, EPILEPSY AND POSTCONCUSSION SYNDROME FOLLOWING HEAD INJURY

Cerebral atrophy usually starts to show around four months after a head injury. It may be progressive with ventricular dilatation and enlarged sulci and cisterns. The presence of the enlarged sulci and cisterns differentiates atrophy from the obstructive forms of hydrocephalus.

Epilepsy is commonest in patients who had seizures in the acute phase of a head injury, in patients who had a depressed fracture or who underwent a craniotomy. Other than defining that an injury has occurred, imaging does not have a role to play in these patients with epilepsy.

Postconcussion syndrome is being increasingly recognized and comprises symptoms such as headache, dizziness, lack of concentration and poor memory. Although the syndrome may relate to minor diffuse cerebral injury, CT and MRI show similar abnormalities in patients with postconcussive syndrome as in patients with no complaints following head injury.

INFECTION

Intracranial infections include abscess, encephalitis and meningitis. Imaging plays a central role in the management of abscesses and encephalitis but has a lesser role in meningitis. The brain reacts to an insult such as an infection in a limited way by becoming hyperaemic, swollen and oedematous; consequently many infections have a similar appearance. The blood–brain barrier is breached and shows leakage of contrast following intravenous contrast injection. If there is focal brain damage the tissue shrinks leaving an area of gliosis and malacia in the healing phase.

ABSCESS

Abscesses can be caused by pyogenic, tuberculous, fungal or parasitic organisms. They may lie within brain parenchyma, the subdural or epidural (extradural) spaces or may involve each compartment. Radiological localization is essential prior to biopsy, drainage or definitive resection. Localization can be carried out with a few MRI or CT sections through the lesion with a suitable skull marker in position. Formal stereotactic localization can be performed with CT or MRI now that special frames are available.

An established abscess is a focal parenchymal infection with a central zone of liquefaction and necrosis surrounded by a fibrocollagenous capsule which localizes the infection. An abscess may be surrounded by oedema. The imaging appearances depend on the maturity of the abscess at the time of scanning. Initially there is a cerebritis with minimal or no CT change. At this stage MRI is more sensitive than CT and shows hyperintensity on T2-weighted sections with irregular enhancement on T1-weighted images. Later the abscess increases in size, becomes rounded and a central necrotic zone develops with a thick wall which shows irregular enhancement on both CT and MRI. With more maturity the abscess wall becomes thinner and less irregular while the centre undergoes liquefaction (Fig. 21.32).

Abscesses within the brain substance often occur by spread from the epidural and subdural spaces. Epidural infection is most often the result of spread of infection from the mastoids, paranasal sinuses or cranium. CT shows a focal low attenuation epidural mass but MRI is more sensitive with hypointensity on T1- and hyperintensity on T2-weighted images. Dural thickening or a ring configuration is seen after contrast enhancement. Epidural infection may cross the midline so differentiating it from a subdural empyema.

Subdural abscesses occur as acute or chronic lesions appearing as extracerebral collections over the convexities and within the interhemispheric fissure. On CT, a subdural abscess shows as a low or isodense extra-axial mass. MRI demonstrates an isointense signal on T1-weighted and hyperintense signal on

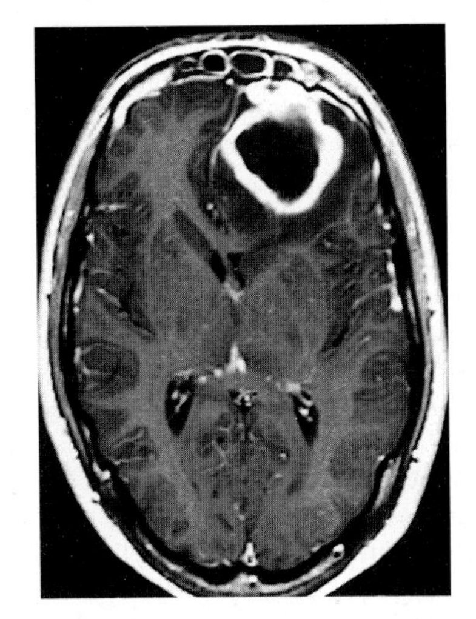
(a)

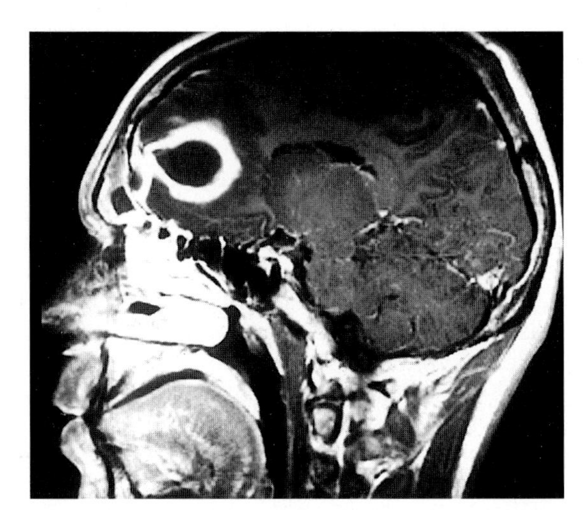
(b)

Fig. 21.32 T1-weighted post contrast on (a) axial and (b) sagittal sections of left frontal brain abscess associated with frontal sinus infection and adjacent epidural abscess in a 19-year-old with headache, lethargy and progressive reduction in conscious level.

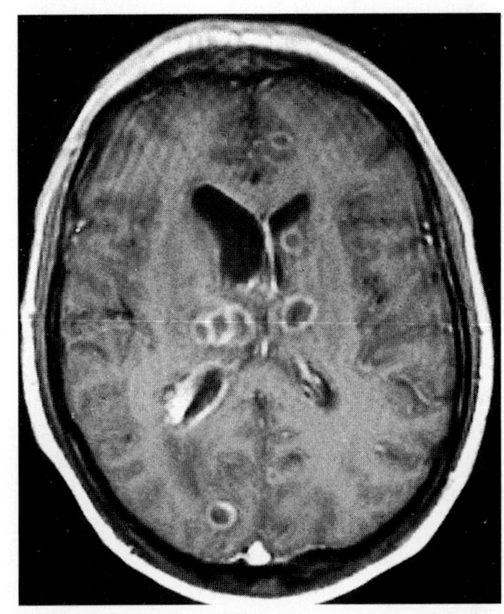

Fig. 21.33 Toxoplasmosis. Multiple small ring enhancing abscesses shown on a T1-weighted section in a 43-year-old HIV-positive patient.

T2-weighted sections. Depending on the amount of granulation tissue the mass shows contrast enhancement on CT and MRI. The underlying brain may be affected and there may be enhancement of the cortical gyri.

Many parasitic infections can invade the brain. **Cysticercosis** from the pork tapeworm is one of the commonest worldwide demonstrated by multiple small rounded ring enhancing lesions on CT and MRI. **Toxoplasmosis** is a ubiquitous protozoan infection and in immunocompromised hosts, such as in AIDS, may reactivate. In toxoplasmosis, abscesses form most commonly in the basal ganglia, corticomedullary junction, white matter or periventricular regions. Ring or nodular enhancement is seen on CT and MRI (Fig. 21.33). **Paragonimiasis** from the lung fluke produces clusters of abscess-like ring-enhancing masses with surrounding oedema. **Hydatid cysts** from the dog tapeworm can produce large cysts of CSF density on CT and MRI without enhancement in cysts that are not secondarily infected.

ENCEPHALITIS

Encephalitis can be caused by a wide variety of organisms (most commonly viruses) or immune-mediated reactions to actual infections (acute disseminated encephalomyelitis). CT shows asymmetrical unilateral or bilateral focal areas of reduced attenuation causing a mass effect especially with herpes encephalitis. The typical distribution involves the temporal lobe, orbitofrontal region and insula. The changes are much better defined with MRI which shows hyperintensity on T2-weighted and hypointensity on T1-weighted sections. The infection mainly affects the cortical grey matter and later spreads to the subcortical white matter. The basal ganglia are spared. Haemorrhage is not uncommon. Enhancement with intravenous contrast on CT and MRI varies with the stage and severity of disease. If imaging is delayed or if the patient does not respond to antiviral therapy, blood–brain barrier breakdown occurs and linear, subarachnoid or gyriform enhancement is seen.

Acute disseminated encephalomyelitis produces a reactive multifocal acute inflammatory demyelination in the white matter of the brain or spinal cord which may be indistinguishable from an acute episode of multiple sclerosis. MRI is the most sensitive method for assessment. Contrast enhancement distinguishes acute enhancing plaques of demyelination from established non-enhancing more chronic lesions.

MENINGITIS AND VENTRICULITIS

Meningitis and ventriculitis present with inflammation of the meninges or ependyma following haematogenous dissemination of organisms or following direct inoculation after a compound fracture, or, more rarely, following surgery particularly mastoid/paranasal sinus surgery or shunt insertion. The diagnosis of meningitis or ventriculitis is made clinically with bacteriological examination of the CSF and imaging is used only to evaluate complications.

In acute meningitis, CT and MRI are usually normal. In severe cases there may be some brain swelling with obliteration of the basal cisterns and sulcal CSF spaces. Leptomeningeal inflammation, showing enhancement extending to the depths of the sulci, develops, and is most clearly seen on T1-weighted coronal post contrast MRI. The inflammation may cause ischaemia producing further generalized brain swelling, focal infarction or communicating hydrocephalus.

Granulomatous meningitis, such as tuberculosis, produces more prominent meningeal reaction with obliteration of the cisterns and involvement of the branches of the circle of Willis with ischaemia which often results in haemorrhagic infarction of the basal ganglia.

Ventriculitis is seen on CT or MRI as enhancement of the ependyma. Ventriculitis is often associated with retrograde spread of infection from the meninges, the presence of foreign bodies such as shunts, or rupture of an abscess into the ventricle. Occasionally with severe ventriculitis a pus – CSF level may be seen in the occipital horns of the lateral ventricles which are the most dependent parts of the ventricular system when the patient is scanned in the supine position. Ventriculitis can result in an obstructive hydrocephalus.

VASCULAR ABNORMALITIES

INTRACRANIAL ANEURYSMS AND SUBARACHNOID HAEMORRHAGE

Berry aneurysms are the most important intracranial aneurysms from the surgical point of view. They occur at the arterial bifurcations in or near the circle of Willis and are due to acquired conditions such as atherosclerosis superimposed on a congenital propensity to a deficient internal elastic lamina and collagen disorder. These aneurysms show a familial tendency and are associated with inherited conditions such as Ehlers–Danlos syndrome, Marfan's syndrome, neurofibromatosis and polycystic kidney disease. Approximately 33% of intracranial aneurysms occur on the anterior communicating arteries, 33% at the origin of the posterior communicating arteries, 20% in the middle cerebral artery, 5% each at the basilar bifurcation and rest of the posterior fossa, with 1–3% in sites distal to the circle of Willis; 15–20% of patients have multiple aneurysms.

Aneurysms can rupture to cause subarachnoid haemorrhage but may cause symptoms because of mass effect even when only 6 mm in diameter. Posterior communicating aneurysms can present with a third nerve palsy due to direct pressure on the nerve. The aneurysm in this case is usually of sufficient size to be demonstrated by dynamic bolus contrast high-definition CT. Giant middle cerebral and basilar tip aneurysms impinge on adjacent structures and can cause pressure effects.

CT is the best way to demonstrate acute subarachnoid haemorrhage but if CT is delayed it is progressively less sensitive as the blood is washed away in the CSF. If subarachnoid haemorrhage is diagnosed on CT (Fig. 21.34), a lumbar puncture and CSF examination is not required. Lumbar puncture could be hazardous if there were an intracerebral mass and raised intracranial pressure. Unfortunately in a patient with clinically suspected subarachnoid haemorrhage, a normal CT examination does not exclude the diagnosis.

CT also shows associated intracerebral haemorrhage and any direct or retrograde spread of haemorrhage into the ventricles that is best appreciated in the dependent trigones and occipital horns. The site of maximal haemorrhage often gives a clue to the site of the aneurysm. MRI can show subarachnoid haemorrhage but special sequences are required that depend on the increased protein content of bloody CSF. MRI is sometimes useful to identify small associated intracranial haemorrhages which indicate which aneurysm has ruptured when multiple aneurysms have been found at angiography.

Once the patient is stable, angiography is required to identify the cause of the haemorrhage, which is most commonly due to an aneurysm and less commonly to an arteriovenous malformation or other anomaly. Preshaped catheters are used to catheterize the carotid and vertebral arteries selectively via the transfemoral route. The entire intracranial vascular tree can be visualized in arterial, capillary and venous phases. Aneurysms as small as 1–2 mm may be defined, whilst most are around 5–10 mm. Aneurysms > 10 mm may well contain clot and only the lumen will fill with contrast on the angiogram, thus underestimating its size. A contrast-enhanced CT may well

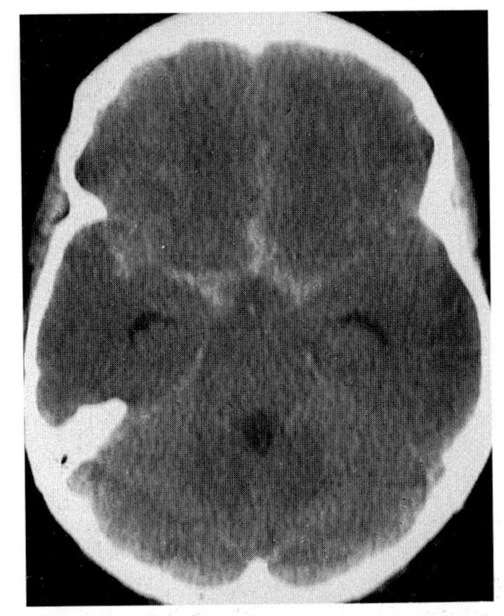
(a)

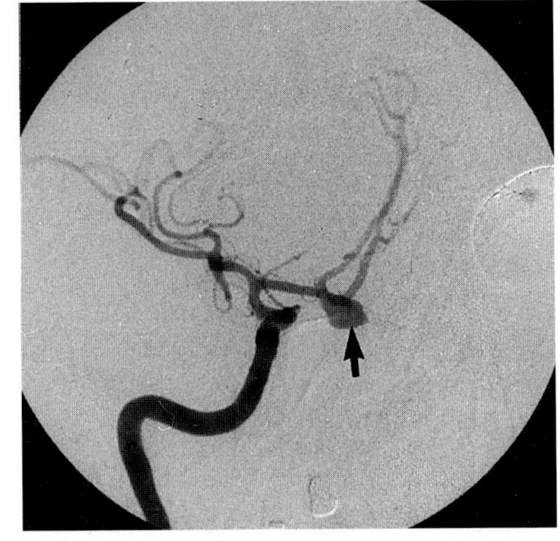
(b)

Fig. 21.34 Anterior communicating artery aneurysm in a 60-year-old with sudden severe headache, meningism and photophobia. (a) CT shows extensive basal cistern and interhemispheric subarachnoid haemorrhage. (b) Oblique view from a selective internal carotid artery angiogram shows the aneurysm (arrow); its rupture had caused the haemorrhage.

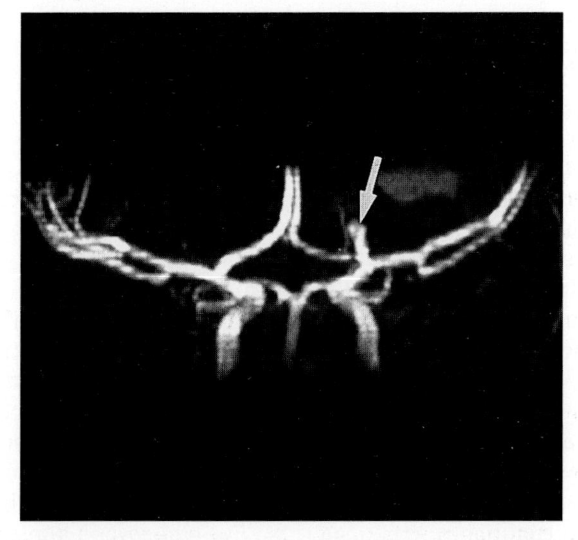

(a)

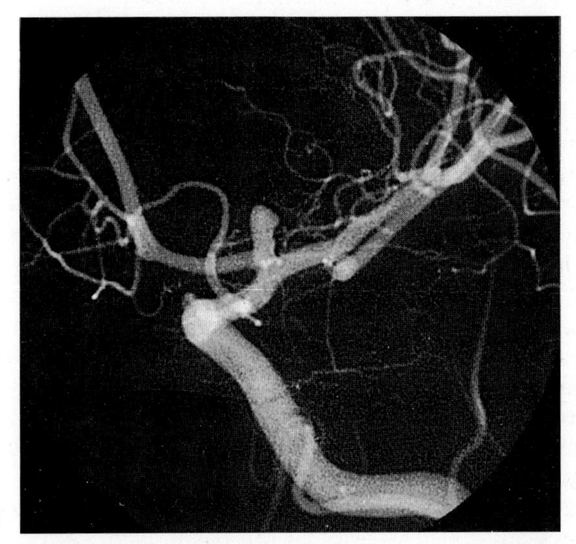

(b)

Fig. 21.35 Terminal internal carotid artery aneurysm (arrow) demonstrated on (a) magnetic resonance angiography with (b) conventional common carotid angiogram for comparison.

show the organized clot and the enhancing lumen if the aneurysm is sufficiently large.

MR angiography can also be used to demonstrate aneurysms and the vascular tree non-invasively, using the magnetic properties of flowing blood (Fig. 21.35). At present aneurysms as small as 5 mm can be shown reliably but at the present stage of development of MR angiography, the gold standard remains conventional angiography.

Most aneurysms are treated by isolating them from the circulation with an aneurysm clip at open craniotomy with the use of an operating microscope. Percutaneous transarterial interventional radiological catheter techniques are now being used to treat increasing numbers of selected aneurysms: platinum microcoils are threaded through the catheter and released in the aneurysm to form a small 'nest' (Fig. 21.36). This invokes thrombosis in the aneurysm and over time the thrombus becomes endothelialized and the aneurysm is excluded from the circulation preventing further haemorrhage.

Subarachnoid haemorrhage is often accompanied by arterial spasm induced by vasoactive substances released in response to the haemorrhage. Spasm can be severe enough to cause ischaemia, infarction and even death. The angiogram will show irregular narrowing of the intracranial vessel usually close to the ruptured aneurysm but spasm can be extensive

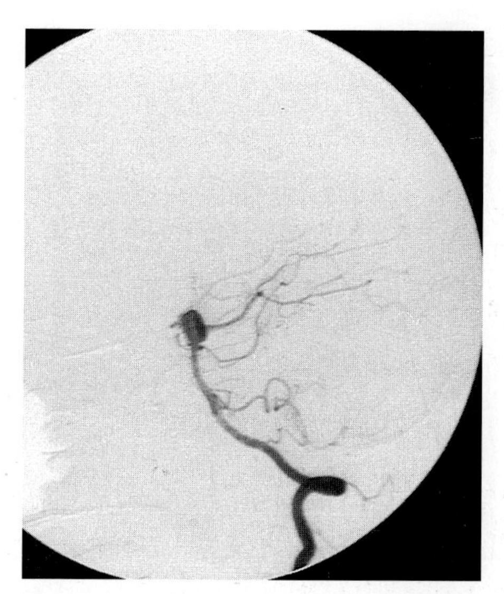

(a)

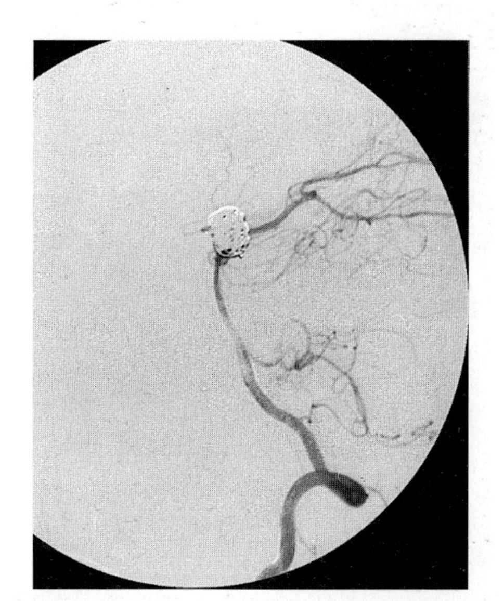

(b)

Fig. 21.36 Treatment of a terminal basilar artery aneurysm with microcoils. (a) Lateral view of aneurysm before endovascular introduction of coils and (b) exclusion of the aneurysm from the circulation by the tight coil nest preserving the parent and distal vessels.

involving many vessels. Transcranial Doppler ultrasound can be used to monitor the blood flow in the circle of Willis and can indicate the presence of spasm.

Other causes of subarachnoid haemorrhage include arteriovenous malformation, intracerebral haemorrhage, trauma, dural fistula and, rarely, haemorrhagic infarcts and tumours. CT shows the abnormality, and angiography is required in many of these patients to show the vascular aspects of the lesion.

ARTERIOVENOUS ANOMALIES

Arteriovenous anomalies are divided into:

- arteriovenous malformations;
- venous angiomas which are composed entirely of veins;
- cavernous angiomas which show large sinusoidal vascular spaces;
- telangiectases which are tiny capillary angiomas.

Arteriovenous malformations, the commonest vascular anomaly, are congenital lesions consisting of a coiled mass of arteries and veins. Arteriovenous malformations generally involve the cerebral hemispheres but may occur anywhere in the brain and can have single or more usually multiple arterial supply. Aneurysms are sometimes found on the feeding arteries. Venous drainage can be by single or multiple veins running to the deep or superficial venous systems. CT shows serpiginous densities that enhance markedly after contrast, representing the draining veins. There may be associated calcification in the lesion but little or no mass effect if the lesion has not bled. Intracerebral and intraventricular haemorrhage and, less often, subarachnoid haemorrhage result if the arteriovenous malformation bleeds (Fig. 21.37). MRI is particularly useful in defining the relationship of the arteriovenous malformation to other midline and posterior fossa structures by observing the flow voids produced by the arteries and veins. MRI is better than CT in defining any subacute and chronic parenchymal haemorrhage which may have occurred. Treatment is by endovascular occlusion, surgical excision, 'gamma knife' stereotactic radiotherapy or a mixture of each with the aim of obliterating the maximum amount of the arteriovenous malformation whilst doing least damage to the normal surrounding brain. Angiography enables the normal and abnormal vascular tree to be outlined and the feeding and draining vessels to be identified. In selected patients microcatheters can be guided into the malformation and cyanoacrylate glues or coils introduced to occlude the lesion.

Cavernous angiomas are usually high attenuation-enhancing lesions on CT and usually produce no mass effect. They are often occult and do not show on angiography. Calcification may occasionally be seen within the lesion. On MRI, cavernous angiomas show a typical pattern consisting of a hypointense ring owing to haemosiderin around an inhomogeneous hyperintense lesion on T2-weighted scans. Cavernous angiomas rarely bleed and are usually only removed if they cause symptoms such as focal epilepsy.

ARTERIAL OCCLUSIVE DISEASE

Atherosclerosis affects the extracranial carotid or vertebral arteries and is the commonest cause of intracranial artery stenosis. However, the intra- and extracranial vessels may be affected by a variety of

(a)
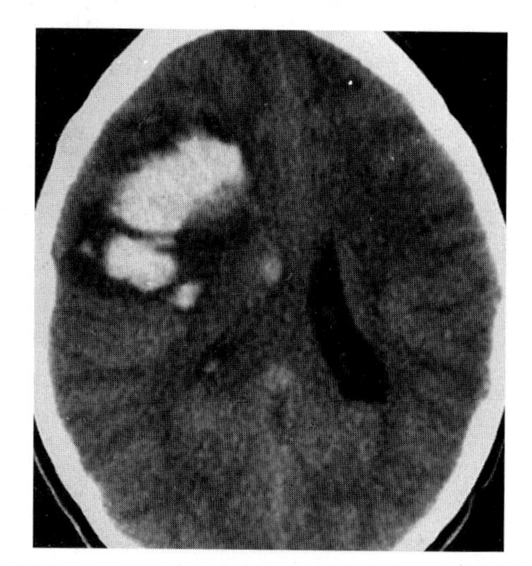

(b)
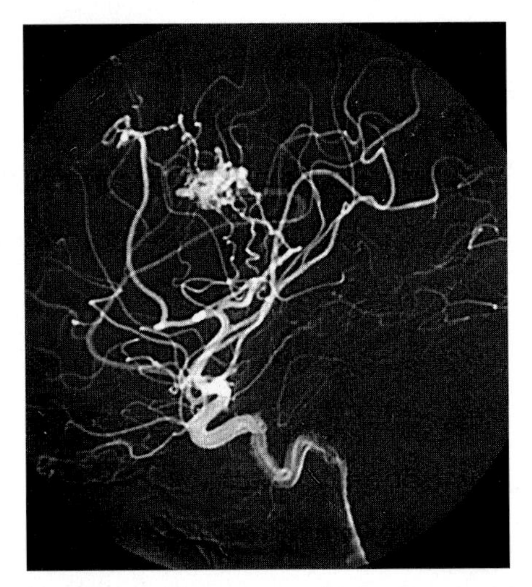

Fig. 21.37 Arteriovenous malformation in a 14-year-old. (a) CT shows a right frontal intracerebral haematoma. (b) Internal carotid arteriogram shows the malformation is supplied by abnormal branches of the anterior and middle cerebral arteries.

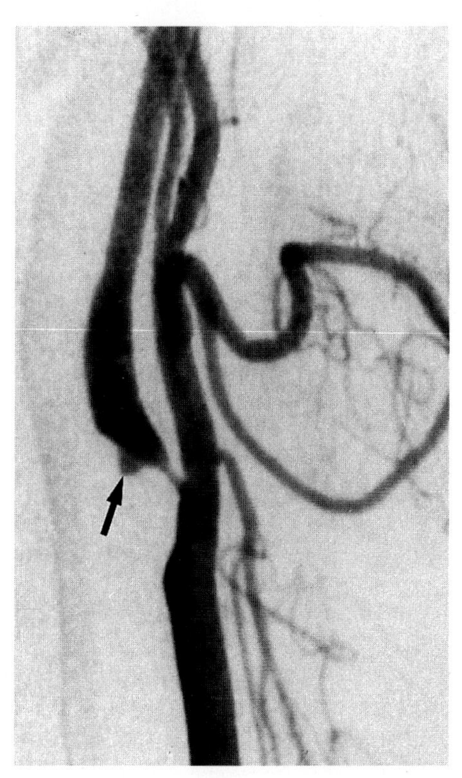

Fig. 21.38 Internal carotid artery stenosis in a 57-year-old with transient ischaemic attacks. Carotid angiography shows > 70% stenosis of the internal carotid artery with an atheromatous ulcer (arrow) distal to the stenosis, the source of emboli.

conditions including arteritis, sickle cell disease, neurofibromatosis, and many rare congenital diseases. Stenosis can lead to territorial or watershed infarction due to emboli or ischaemia. The origin of the internal carotid artery is the commonest site for cranial vessel arterial stenosis and endarterectomy may be indicated if a stenosis > 70% is present. Stenosis can be shown by conventional angiography, but non-invasive MR angiography and Doppler ultrasound compete very favourably with angiography (Fig. 21.38).

ARTERIAL DISSECTION

Arterial dissection is being demonstrated more commonly as a cause of stroke in young people. Dissection usually involves the extracranial internal carotid and vertebral arteries. Angiography or MRI will show the typical tapering of the lumen of the affected vessel.

SINOVENOUS OCCLUSIVE DISEASE

Although facial and mastoid infection used to be the commonest cause, thrombosis is now most frequently associated with dehydration, often after gastrointestinal infections on long aeroplane flights, hormone treatment, trauma or tumours directly affecting the sinus. Occlusion of the dural venous sinuses and intracerebral veins with subsequent venous infarction or brain swelling and increased intracranial pressure is much less common than arterial infarction. The imaging appearances are less predictable and a high index of suspicion is required to make an early diagnosis. Dynamic contrast CT will usually show non-enhancement of a whole segment of sinus or may show filling defects in the sinus. On MRI the absence of normal flow phenomenon in the sinus will be seen. MR venography is excellent in the superior sagittal sinus, straight sinus and parts of the transverse sinuses but around the torcula and the sigmoid sinuses the normal turbulent flow patterns can easily be confused with partial occlusions. Late views in the venous phase of conventional angiography remain the definitive diagnostic method.

HYDROCEPHALUS

CSF is formed from a mixture of plasma ultrafiltrate produced by the choroid plexus and of cerebral extracellular fluid permeating through the ependyma into the ventricles. It functions as a homeostatic medium and provides a protective hydrostatic cushion for the brain. CSF is dynamic, pulsing with the arterial pressure wave but also circulates from its production site in the ventricles, into the subarachnoid spaces, around the brain and spinal cord with reabsorption back into the vascular system, through the arachnoid villi that project into lacunae along the superior sagittal sinus.

Strictly defined, hydrocephalus just means an increased amount of CSF in the cranial cavity. It is usually associated with enlarged ventricles but not all patients with enlarged ventricles have clinical hydrocephalus as the enlargement may be an *ex vacuo* effect due to loss of brain substance as in the physiological atrophy of ageing or following head injury, infection or dementia. Hydrocephalus is now usually defined as an imbalance between CSF production, circulation and reabsorption and radiology plays a key role in defining its presence and cause.

Excessive production of CSF associated with hydrocephalus has been attributed to intraventricular choroid plexus papillomas but there is increasing evidence that there is obstruction of the foramina of Luschka and Magendie by tumoral haemorrhage, high protein levels or intraventricular debris rather than just overproduction of CSF.

Headaches, nausea and vomiting are the cardinal symptoms of hydrocephalus once it causes increased intracranial pressure in the older child or adult. In the infant, accelerated head growth with widening of the sutures is often the first sign. Gradual increases in intracranial pressure may be accommodated for a short time and the onset of symptoms may be delayed.

Radiology is used to confirm the presence of abnormal CSF circulation and make an estimate of ventricular size. Comparison with previous imaging is essential for progression to be assessed. CT is most frequently used because of its wide availability but MRI with axial and sagittal sections will give a more complete impression of the disruption to CSF flow. Multiple measurements of ventricular size and shape have been defined but in routine clinical practice they are seldom used.

With increasing CSF pressure the lateral ventricles first show subtle enlargement of the normally slit-like temporal horns. Their size provides a sensitive indication of increased pressure. There is then symmetrical rounding of the anterior horns leading to an increase in the angle between the frontal horn and the median sagittal plane and finally, if there is no obstruction at the foramen of Monro, the ventricles dilate. The third ventricle is surrounded by relatively compact brain and so dilates later in the presence of increasing intracranial pressure and tends to be the first region to resume normal size after the pressure is relieved. Sagittal MRI now makes the assessment of the aqueduct easier and dilatation or focal stenosis can be seen directly. The fourth ventricle may also dilate later with increased CSF pressure. It assumes a more rounded shape on axial section while on sagittal sections an enlarged triangular shape is maintained (Fig. 21.39). The caudal foramina must be assessed and those that are seen to be wide and dilated differentiated from those appearing stenotic or closed by a membrane.

Periventricular oedema, seen on CT as a rim of decreased attenuation or on T1- and T2-weighted MRI imaging as hypo- and hyperintense signal, may occur with increased intraventricular pressure, especially if there has been an acute pressure rise. Periventricular

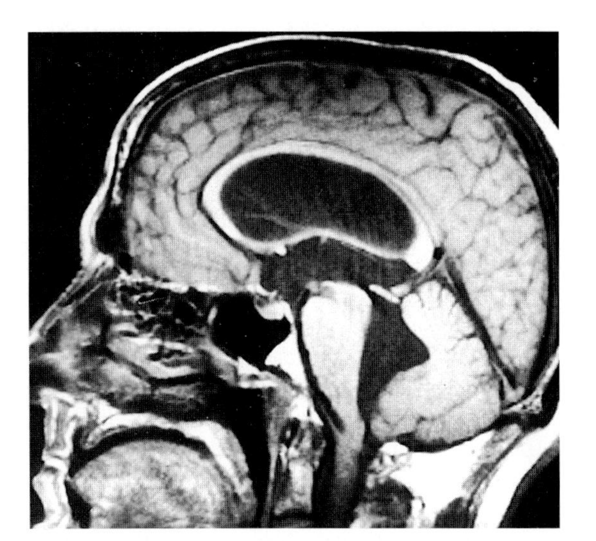

Fig. 21.39 Hydrocephalus in a 55-year-old following meningitis. The lateral, third and fourth ventricles are all dilated due to obstruction around the basal cisterns.

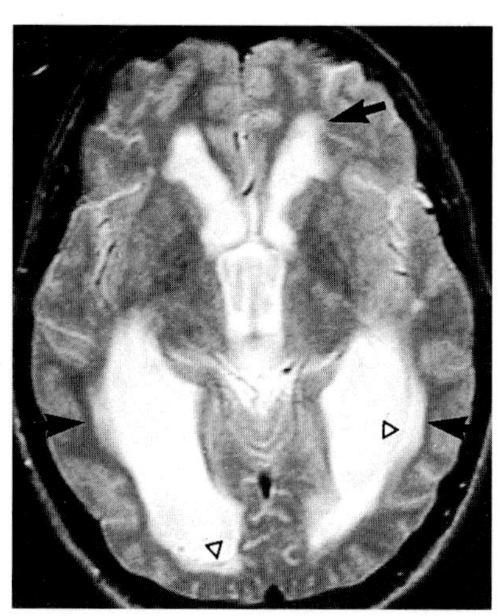

Fig. 21.40 Acute hydrocephalus of the lateral and third ventricles with periventricular oedema (arrows) on T2-weighted axial sections. Arrow heads mark lateral border of the ventricle.

oedema initially represents the 'damming back' of the transependymal flow of extracellular fluid towards the ventricles, and then with increasing pressure flow reverses with leakage from the ventricles through the damaged, stretched ependyma into the periventricular white matter (Fig. 21.40). When chronic, a degree of demyelination can occur. Hydrocephalus rarely becomes compensated but a new equilibrium may be established at a higher intracranial pressure owing to the opening of other pathways of absorption through the arachnoid membrane, the stroma of the choroid plexus and with reversed transependymal flow through the cortical mantle.

The ventricular dilatation compresses the brain against the skull vault and displaces CSF from the sulci and cisterns. This differentiates hydrocephalus from atrophy where the increase in ventricular size is proportionate to the increase in sulcal and cisternal CSF volumes. Another feature of cortical atrophy is that atrophy causes less dilation of the third ventricle compared to the lateral ventricles.

The flow pattern and absorption of CSF can be followed directly with radionuclide studies by injecting ^{111}In-DTPA into the lumbar or cisternal theca and following the activity period over 48 hours. This technique has been largely superseded by the indirect visualization of CSF flow by MRI.

CONGENITAL HYDROCEPHALUS

Congenital hydrocephalus is usually caused by insults during the 3rd and 4th week after conception. It most frequently results from aqueduct stenosis (43%) followed in frequency by forms of communicating hydrocephalus (38%), Dandy–Walker syndrome (13%) and other anatomical lesions (6%). Hydrocephalus is usually recognized on ultrasound but MRI is required for a full anatomical assessment of the site of CSF flow blockage and for detecting any of the frequently associated congenital abnormalities, such as cephaloceles, absent corpus callosum, Chiari malformation and neural tube closure defects.

INTRAVENTRICULAR OBSTRUCTIVE (NON-COMMUNICATING) HYDROCEPHALUS

When the ventricular CSF is unable to communicate with the subarachnoid space, the ventricles proximal to the obstruction dilate. The cause of the obstruction may arise within the ventricular system such as an ependymoma, glioma or a colloid cyst of the third ventricle and cause an obstruction at the foramen of Monro; more commonly the abnormality arises outside the ventricular system such as a craniopharyngioma, pituitary macroadenoma or primitive neuroectodermal tumour. A third possibility is a congenital lesion such as an aqueduct stenosis.

EXTRAVENTRICULAR OBSTRUCTIVE (COMMUNICATING) HYDROCEPHALUS

This term is used when the obstruction is distal to the outlets of the fourth ventricle and is due either to impeded flow around the convexities or to impeded reabsorption by the arachnoid villi. The condition most commonly follows subarachnoid haemorrhage when absorption through the arachnoid villi is blocked. Similar blockage may also occur with widespread subarachnoid neoplasm (primitive neuroectodermal tumour, lymphoma, adenocarcinoma) and infections such as purulent or tuberculous meningitis. In some cases the obstruction to free flow will be at the level of the tentorial hiatus or basal cisterns.

For normal absorption to occur there must be a pressure difference across the arachnoid villi of about 3–6 cm of water. If there is venous hypertension or venous sinus thrombosis absorption is impaired and hydrocephalus supervenes. This can be shown on dynamic contrast enhanced CT or MR venography.

CONCLUSION

Imaging has a key role:

- in deciding whether hydrocephalus is present;
- in categorizing the type;
- in assisting in the choice of treatment;
- in assessing the effect of treatment with shunting or internal diversions;
- in monitoring the side effects of treatment.

CT is usually adequate but MRI will give a more complete understanding of the CSF pathways.

CHAPTER 22

Thorax

Peter Armstrong

A wide range of intrathoracic diseases can be diagnosed with modern imaging techniques. The first imaging examination is almost invariably a plain chest radiograph and more complex tests may follow. Computed tomography is an increasingly used modality having almost entirely replaced conventional tomography. Techniques such as ultrasound, magnetic resonance imaging, radionuclide examinations and angiography all have specific indications, which are discussed in the appropriate sections of this chapter.

TECHNIQUES

PLAIN CHEST RADIOGRAPHY

The frontal view is the routine plain radiographic projection taken either as a postero-anterior (PA) or antero-posterior (AP) view; the PA view is preferable but may not be practicable in sick patients. A lateral view may be needed as a supplementary view. Routine examinations are exposed on full inspiration with the patient in the upright position (Fig. 22.1). Portable examinations are technically inferior to films taken with fixed equipment and should, therefore, be restricted to patients who are too ill to be moved to the radiology department. Technical evaluation of a film is necessary, since incorrect exposure, poor centring or faulty projection may hide or mimic disease. The correctly exposed routine PA chest film is one in which the ribs and spine behind the heart can be identified. Unless one can see through the heart, lower-lobe lesions and cardiac calcifications may be completely overlooked. A straight film is one where the medial ends of the clavicles are equidistant from the edges of the thoracic vertebrae. Unless the film is exposed on full inspiration, the heart may appear enlarged and the lung bases may be hazy or show ill-defined densities (Fig. 22.2). Such an appearance may mimic pulmonary oedema, pneumonia or pulmonary infarction. The degree of inspiration is adequate when the dome of the right hemidiaphragm is in the sixth anterior interspace.

Additional plain films of the chest may provide details of lesions seen on routine films or may even enable a previously invisible abnormality to be detected:

- **Oblique views** (films taken with the patient turned to one or other side) are useful for demonstrating the chest wall and ribs, particularly fractures, and, occasionally, for showing intrathoracic shadows to better advantage.

Diagnostic and Interventional Radiology in Surgical Practice. Edited by P. Armstrong and M. L. Wastie. Published in 1997 by Chapman & Hall, London. ISBN 0 412 61960 1 (HB), 0 412 61970 9 (PB)

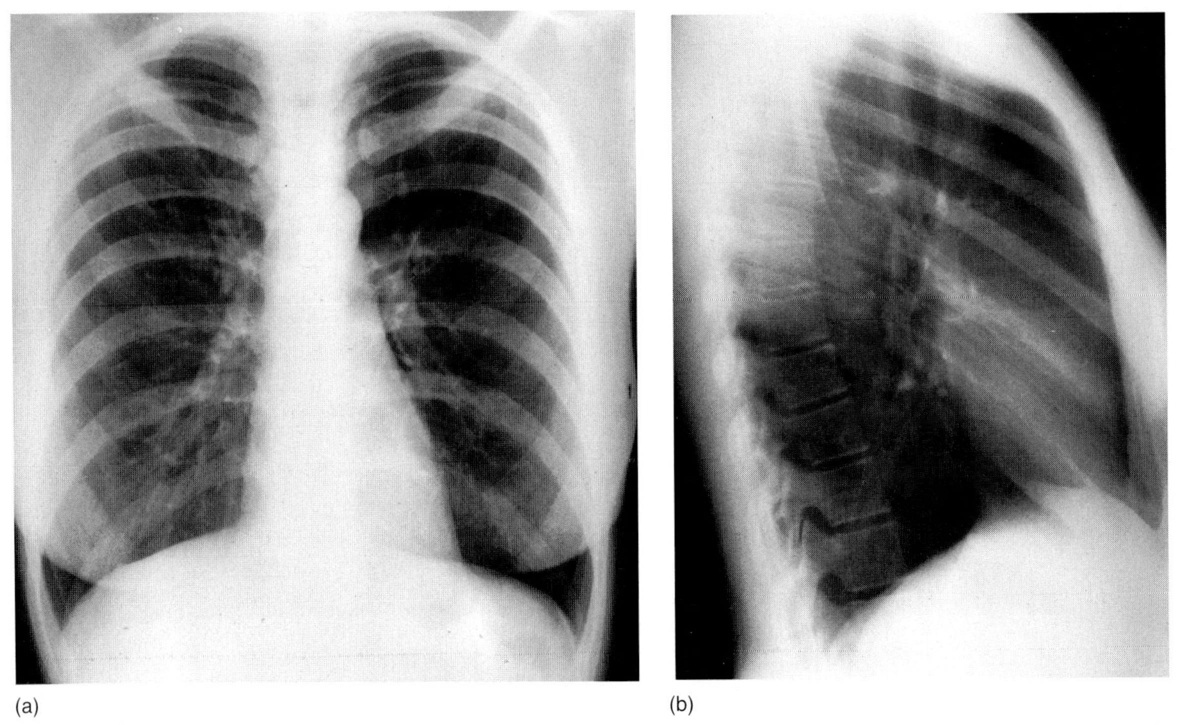

Fig. 22.1 Routine normal postero-anterior (PA) and lateral views of chest. Note that the patient is straight and the films have been exposed on deep inspiration. (a) The heart and mediastinal borders are clearly seen as are the left and right upper surfaces of both hemidiaphragms, except where the aorta passes through the diaphragm. Lung behind the heart can be seen; (b) on the lateral view, the vertebrae appear darker as the eye travels down the spine.

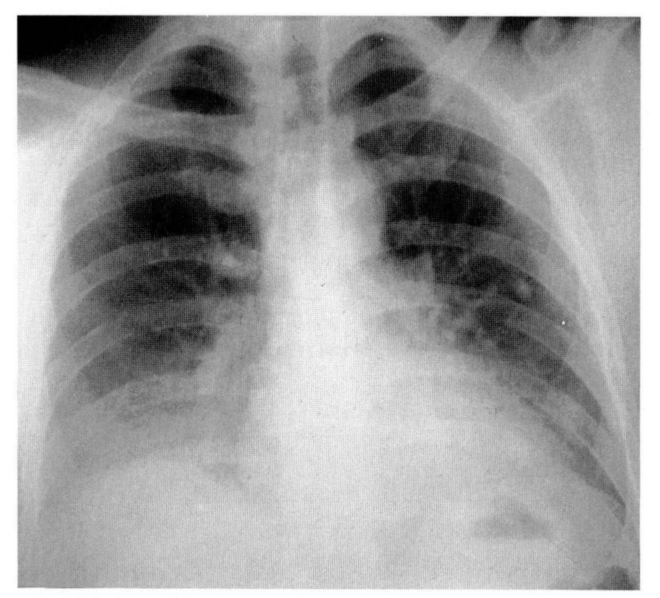

Fig. 22.2 Chest film in normal patient exposed on expiration. The heart appears enlarged and the lung bases are hazy due to poor inflation of the lungs. The appearance mimics congestive heart failure or bilateral basal pneumonia.

- **Lateral decubitus views** are not, as the name suggests, lateral views: they are frontal projections taken with the patient lying on one or other side. Their principal use is to demonstrate mobile fluid in the pleural cavities.
- **Expiration films** are frontal films deliberately exposed on expiration in order both to demonstrate diaphragmatic movement or the ability of the lung to deflate and to detect a pneumothorax which may be more obvious on an expiration than an inspiration film.

COMPUTED TOMOGRAPHY

CT is now widely used to examine the chest:

- to demonstrate enlarged hilar and mediastinal lymph nodes or mediastinal invasion when patients with neoplastic disease, notably lung cancer and lymphoma, are being staged;

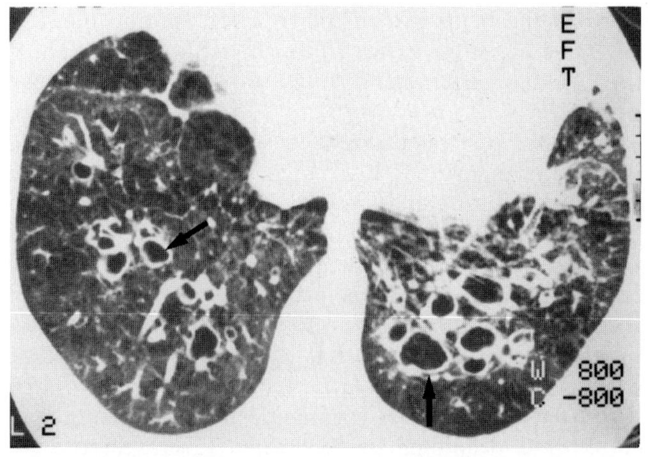

Fig. 22.3 HRCT of lungs showing bilateral lower lobe bronchiectasis. There are numerous greatly dilated bronchi (arrows), many of which have thick walls.

- to show the presence and extent of mediastinal masses (sometimes it is possible to diagnose the nature of the mass based on shape, precise location and density characteristics);
- to show the precise shape of a focal intrapulmonary or pleural lesion and to detect any calcification in the lesion, features which may help to decide whether an abnormality is malignant or benign;
- to localize a mass prior to biopsy;
- to demonstrate the presence of disease when the plain chest radiograph is normal in those cases where the possibility of intrathoracic abnormality is suspected on other grounds, e.g. detecting pulmonary metastases; finding a primary carcinoma in patients whose sputum cytology shows neoplastic cells; and demonstrating thymic tumours in patients with myasthenia gravis;
- to diagnose chest wall disease;
- to diagnose the presence, extent and severity of bronchiectasis and certain pulmonary parenchymal processes, such as fibrosing alveolitis, when a high resolution technique is employed.

Routine chest CT examinations consist of adjacent 8–10 mm sections through the area of interest. Intravenous contrast medium may be injected when the primary purpose of the examination is to show the mediastinal or hilar structures. The images are usually viewed at two distinct window settings: lung and mediastinal windows (p. 10). If the CT scan has been performed for bone lesions then bone settings are used.

High-resolution CT (HRCT) utilizes very thin sections 1–2 mm thick. HRCT of the lungs (Fig. 22.3) is a specialized application designed primarily to diagnose bronchiectasis and other airway disorders or to determine the presence, extent and, if possible, the diagnosis in patients with diffuse lung disease, of which fibrosing alveolitis is the commonest.

OTHER TECHNIQUES

Magnetic resonance imaging

MRI of the chest provides similar information to chest CT with respect to pleural, mediastinal or chest wall disorders, but has advantages in certain specific circumstances. The multiplanar imaging capability allows images to be obtained in any desired plane. Coronal, sagittal and oblique planes may provide superior information to images taken in an axial plane, the usual plane for CT. This is particularly true for showing the extent of tumours or lymphadenopathy in the aortopulmonary window, the subcarinal region or the lung apices. Because it is possible to obtain cardiac-gated MR images, the pericardium, myocardium and cardiac chambers can be shown with less degradation from cardiac movement. Also, using surface coils it is possible to obtain very high-resolution MR images of the chest wall.

With spin-echo sequences, fast flowing blood produces a signal void. This allows structures such as the aorta, central pulmonary vessels, great veins and cardiac chambers to be imaged without the need for contrast agents. It also allows small masses to be distinguished from blood vessels in areas of complex vascular anatomy such as the hilar regions.

There is no such examination as a routine chest MRI: all chest MRI is tailored to answer specific questions. The most frequently used sequences are T1-weighted, cardiac-gated images and a variety of magnetic resonance angiography techniques.

Radionuclide imaging

The use of radionuclide imaging in diagnosing pulmonary embolic disease is discussed on page 492.

Pulmonary angiography

The pulmonary arteries and veins can be demonstrated by taking serial films following the rapid injection of angiographic contrast media into the pulmonary arterial circulation through a catheter introduced from the groin or antecubital fossa. The catheterization is carried out under fluoroscopic control with continuous electrocardiographic and pressure monitoring by an operator skilled in cardiac catheterization. Pulmonary angiography carries a small but definite risk to the patient. Its major use is to diagnose pulmonary emboli. Occasionally, it is needed to demonstrate congenital vascular anomalies.

Bronchography

Bronchography involves introducing an iodinated contrast material into the bronchial tree. The only remaining indication is for the assessment of selected cases of bronchiectasis.

Fluoroscopy

The image at fluoroscopy is poor compared to that which can be achieved with X-ray film. Fluoroscopy is limited to observing the movement of the diaphragm and shift of the mediastinum caused by air trapping in cases of suspected inhalation of a foreign body.

BASIC PRINCIPLES OF INTERPRETING PLAIN CHEST RADIOGRAPHS

THE ABNORMAL CHEST RADIOGRAPH

There are many ways of looking at chest films. The trained radiologist often uses a problem-oriented approach: the search pattern is varied according to features present on the films, with constant integration of the clinical information. For example, if a nodule representing a possible lung carcinoma is seen, the shape of the nodule itself, other lung lesions and evidence for spread of disease are sought. Those observers with less radiological experience should follow a routine to avoid overlooking important information. One approach is presented here.

NORMAL CHEST RADIOGRAPH (Fig. 22.1)

The upper surface of the diaphragm extending from one costophrenic angle to the other should be clearly outlined by aerated lung, except where the mediastinal structures including the heart are in contact with the diaphragm. The costophrenic angles are usually sharp, but if the hemidiaphragms are flattened, the angles may become meniscus-shaped, simulating pleural fluid. Failure to see the diaphragm outline clearly suggests either pleural or pulmonary disease.

The normal right hemidiaphragm is usually 1–3 cm higher, but may be level with, or even slightly lower, than the left; the midpoint of the right hemidiaphragm is usually level with the anterior end of the sixth rib.

The lateral borders of the heart and mediastinum should be clearly defined between the clavicles and the diaphragm. Any lack of clarity indicates pulmonary or, less often, pleural disease. Above the clavicles the normal mediastinal border may be indistinct. Aortic unfolding often modifies the appearance of the superior mediastinum and may hide pathology or simulate disease.

On the PA view the centre of the trachea lies midway or slightly to the right of the midpoint between the medial ends of the clavicles. The trachea courses vertically or slightly to the right as it descends into the chest. The position of the heart is variable, making it difficult to diagnose all but the most severe degrees of cardiac displacement. On average, one third of the heart lies to the right of the midline, but the normal range varies from one fifth to one half of the cardiac diameter lying to the right of the midline.

The cardiothoracic ratio is a widely used but crude method of measuring heart size. In normal people the transverse diameter of the heart is usually less than half the internal diameter of the chest. Knowing whether or not the heart has increased in size compared with previous films is often more useful than the cardiothoracic ratio in isolation. It should, however, be realized that the transverse cardiac diameter varies with the phase of respiration and, to a lesser extent, with the cardiac cycle. Thus changes in transverse diameter of less than 1.5 cm should be interpreted with caution.

In children under the age of seven, the thymus may be visible as an anterior mediastinal mass. In babies the thymus is usually a prominent structure. Its shape is variable, a 'sail' configuration being characteristic, but rounded outlines are frequent and may be mistaken for true mediastinal masses or pulmonary shadowing. As the thymus is soft it does not deform adjacent structures, such as the trachea.

The hilar shadows are produced by the pulmonary arteries and veins. The lower lobe arteries are 9–16 mm in diameter, with parallel walls except where they branch. The hilar lymph nodes cannot be identified as separate shadows, and the walls of the bronchi are thin and contribute little to the image seen on the radiograph. The left hilum is usually slightly higher than the right. Any lobulation of the hilar shadows, any local expansion or increase in density compared with the opposite side, indicates a mass.

The only structures that can be identified within normal lungs are blood vessels, interlobar fissures and the walls of certain larger bronchi seen end-on. The blood vessels show an orderly decrease in diameter as they progress from the hila outward. In the upright patient, equivalent vessels in the upper zones are smaller than in the lower zones, although this difference is not seen if the patient is examined supine. The fissures can be seen only if they lie tangential to the X-ray beam. Usually, the minor fissure is the only visible fissure in the frontal projection; it can be identified in over half the population, running from the right hilum to the sixth rib in the axilla. In about 1% of the population an extra fissure, the so-called azygos fissure, is visible in the frontal view. On the lateral view each main fissure runs obliquely across the chest from the T4 or T5 vertebral body to reach a point on the hemidiaphragm close to the anterior chest wall.

Care should be taken not to confuse chest wall structures such as pectoral muscles, breasts, or costal cartilages with intrathoracic diseases. In particular, the nipples or any skin lumps may mimic pulmonary nodules, and hair braids or clothing may cause shadows that resemble pulmonary densities. The nipples are usually in the fifth anterior rib space and in general, if one nipple is visible, the other will also be seen.

Finding abnormal pulmonary shadows in the frontal film is usually fairly easy, since it is possible to compare one lung with the other. Detecting shadows on the lateral view may be difficult. A useful rule is that as the eye travels down the vertebrae towards the diaphragm each vertebral body should appear more lucent than the one above. Also, but less reliably, the density of the retrocardiac space in most patients is similar to that of the retrosternal space, and the density over the heart shows no abrupt change.

The ribs, sternum, clavicles, scapulae and spine need to be examined for fractures and areas of lysis and sclerosis. The upper cortical line of the ribs is continuous and easy to assess. The inferior cortical line, however, is normally indistinct in the posterior portions of the ribs and its absence should be not interpreted as a lytic lesion. Each scapula casts two linear shadows on the lateral view which can be mistaken for disease or misplaced fissures.

Rib disease may be accompanied by soft tissue swelling and, not infrequently, the swelling is more obvious than the bone abnormality. Therefore, the outer lung edge should always be scanned for extrapleural soft tissue swelling, and the frontal film should be reviewed for ill-defined densities that may lead to the discovery of a rib lesion which may be clearer with detailed rib views.

RADIOLOGICAL SIGNS IN LUNG DISORDERS

Before the radiological signs of intrathoracic diseases are considered, it is worth discussing a sign with widespread application, namely the **silhouette sign** (Figs 22.4, 5). The information on a chest film is largely dependent on the transradiancy of air in the lung compared with the heart, blood vessels, mediastinum and diaphragm, all of which have a similar density, known as 'soft tissue density'. An intrathoracic lesion in contact with the heart, mediastinum or diaphragm will cause normal borders to become ill-defined or invisible. This sign, known as the silhouette sign, may be very helpful both in recognizing and localizing chest disease. The silhouette sign makes it possible to localize a shadow by observing which borders are lost (e.g. loss of the heart border must mean that the shadow lies in the anterior half of the chest). Alternatively, loss of part of the diaphragm outline indicates disease of the pleura or lower lobes.

The silhouette sign also makes it possible, on occasion, to diagnose disorders such as pulmonary

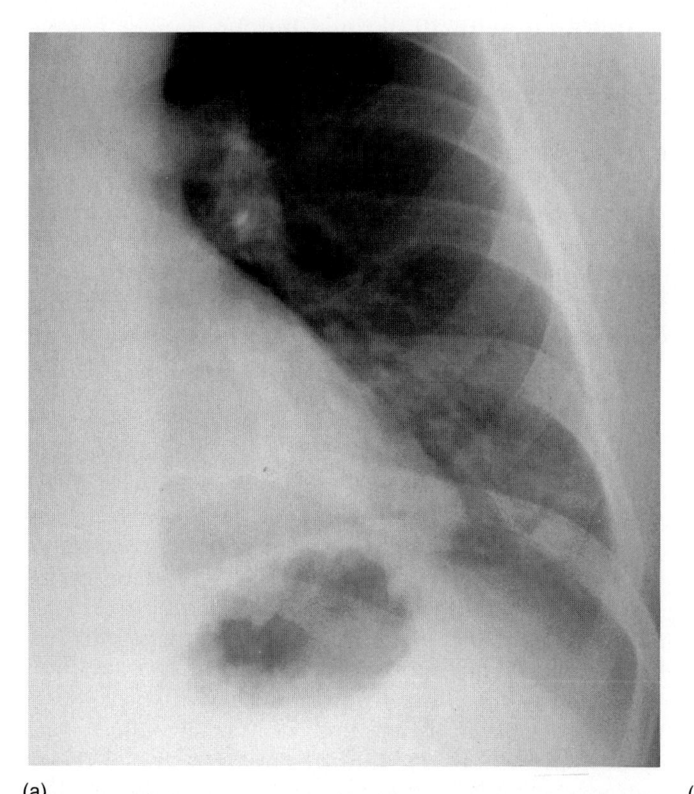

(a)

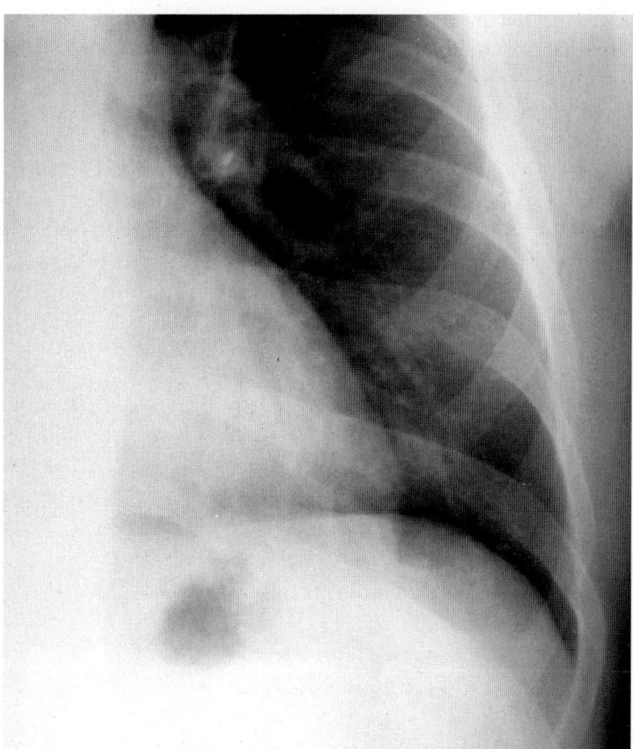

(b)

Fig. 22.4 Silhouette sign. (a) An area of pneumonia in the anterior segment of the left lower lobe has rendered the diaphragm outline lateral to the heart invisible. (b) The same patient after the pneumonia has resolved. The left hemidiaphragm is now clearly visible.

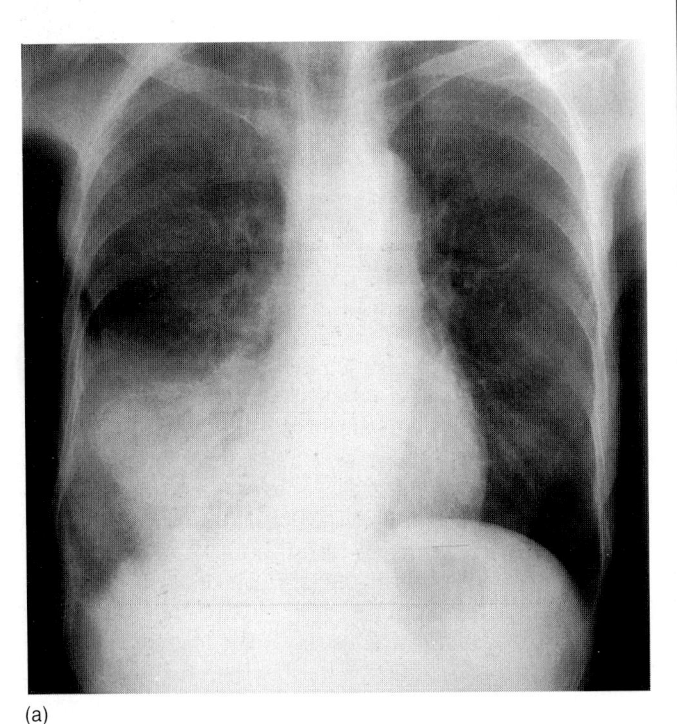

(a)

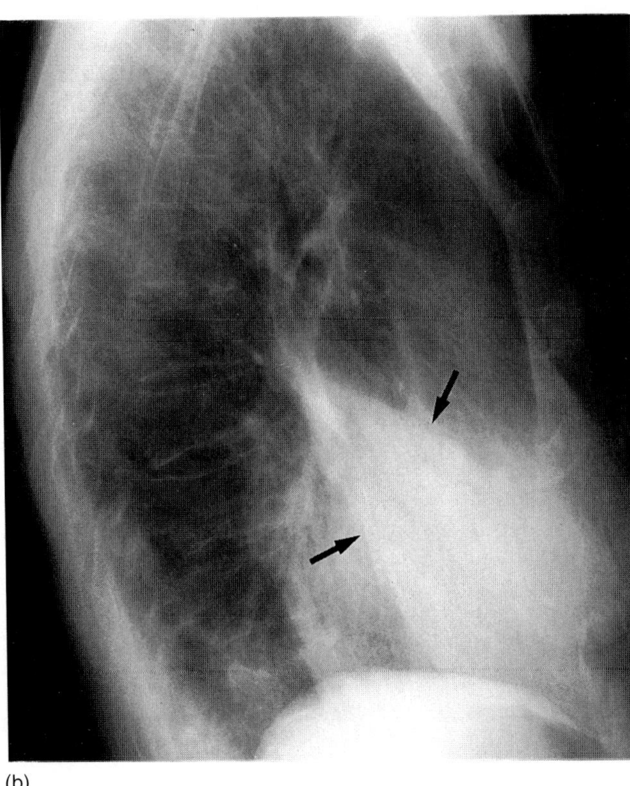

(b)

Fig. 22.5 Silhouette sign. (a) PA view. In the lateral view (b), the consolidation of the right middle lobe (arrows) has rendered the adjacent right heart border invisible. (The lobe has also lost volume).

consolidation, even when one is uncertain whether an opacity is present. It is a surprising fact that a wedge- or lens-shaped opacity may be very difficult to see because of the way the shadow fades out at its margin, but if such a lesion is in contact with the mediastinum or diaphragm, the normal sharp boundary of these structures is lost.

When the lungs are being viewed, it is helpful to try to categorize the abnormalities into one or more basic patterns in order to limit the differential diagnostic possibilities for lung disease:

- pulmonary consolidation or collapse (or a mixture of the two);
- pulmonary oedema;
- spherical shadows;
- line shadows;
- widespread small shadows.

PULMONARY CONSOLIDATION

Consolidation and collapse (atelectasis) often coexist. It is, however, convenient to consider these two phenomena separately. The signs of pulmonary consolidation (Fig. 22.5; see also Fig. 22.20, p. 490) are:

- a **shadow with ill-defined borders** except where the disease process contacts a fissure, in which case the shadow has a well-defined edge corresponding to the fissure;
- an **air bronchogram**. Normally, it is not possibly to identify air in bronchi within the lung substance because the bronchial walls are too thin and are surrounded by air in the alveoli, but if the alveoli are filled with fluid or inflammatory exudate, then air in the bronchi stands out against the background of fluid or exudate in the lung. An opacity containing an air bronchogram is almost always due to either pneumonia or pulmonary oedema.

Consolidation of a whole lobe or the great majority of a lobe (Figs 22.5 and 22.6; see also Fig. 22.20) is virtually diagnostic of pneumonia.

Patchy consolidation, i.e. one or more patches of ill-defined shadowing up to the size of one or more segments, is usually due to infection, but may occasionally be due to infarction, or, even less commonly, to eosinophilic pneumonia or vasculitis. There is no reliable way of telling from the films which of these possibilities is the cause but, in most instances, the clinical and laboratory findings point to one of these options. Another major diagnostic difficulty is distinguishing widespread patchy consolidation, e.g. due to pneumonia, or from pulmonary oedema.

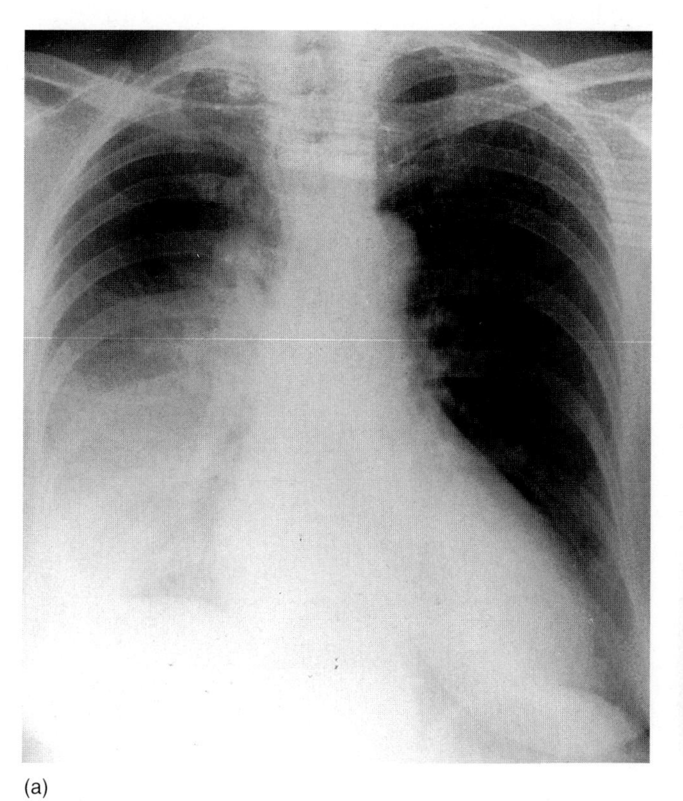

(a)

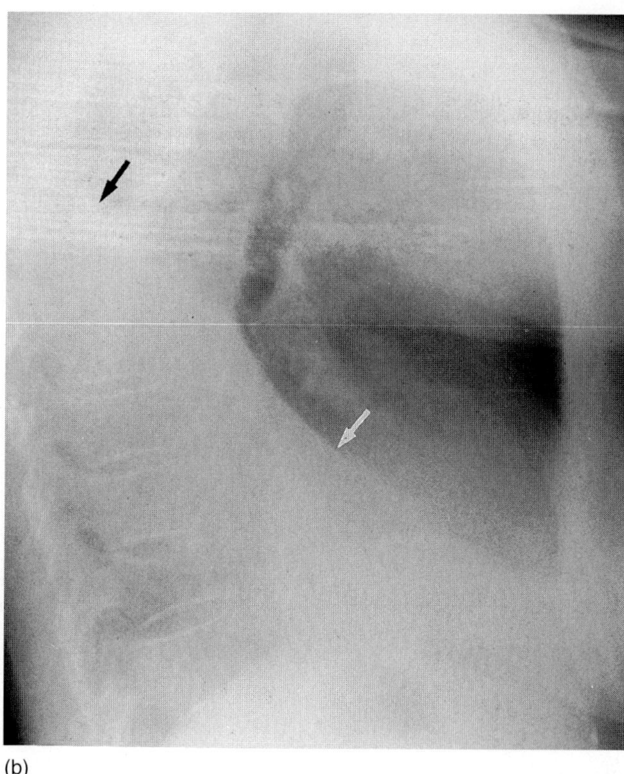

(b)

Fig. 22.6 Lobar pneumonia. The whole of the right lower lobe is consolidated. The lobar shape is best seen in the lateral view (b) where the opacity is sharply demarcated by the oblique fissure (arrows).

Cavitation within consolidation The diagnosis of cavitation depends on recognizing an air space or an air-fluid level within the consolidation. Patchy consolidation with intervening normal or emphysematous areas of lung can easily be mistaken for cavities and CT may be helpful to make the distinction. Infectious agents particularly liable to produce cavitation are *Staphylococcus aureus,* klebsiella spp., *Mycobacterium tuberculosis* (Fig. 22.7), anaerobic bacteria and various fungi. Cavitation is occasionally seen in other forms of pulmonary consolidation, e.g. infarction and Wegener's granulomatosis.

Fig. 22.7 Cavitation (arrow) within consolidation of the right upper lobe in active tuberculosis. The right upper lobe shows extensive consolidation and some loss of volume. Further foci of tuberculous infection are seen in the adjacent lower lobe.

CAVITATION

Cavitation without consolidation is seen as a spherical shadow containing a central lucency due to air within the cavity. This air may be difficult to appreciate without tomography. The air is often accompanied by fluid, in which case an air-fluid level will be visible on erect films.

A cavity may be due to:

- **infective lung abscess** – the most frequent cause of an infective lung abscess is aspiration of food or secretions; such abscesses are usually in the apical (superior) segments of the lower lobes or in the posterior segments of the upper lobes; lung abscesses may also be due to infection beyond an obstructing lesion in the bronchus or infected emboli, particularly in drug addicts;
- **lung neoplasm** (Fig. 22.8);
- **Wegener's granulomatosis**.

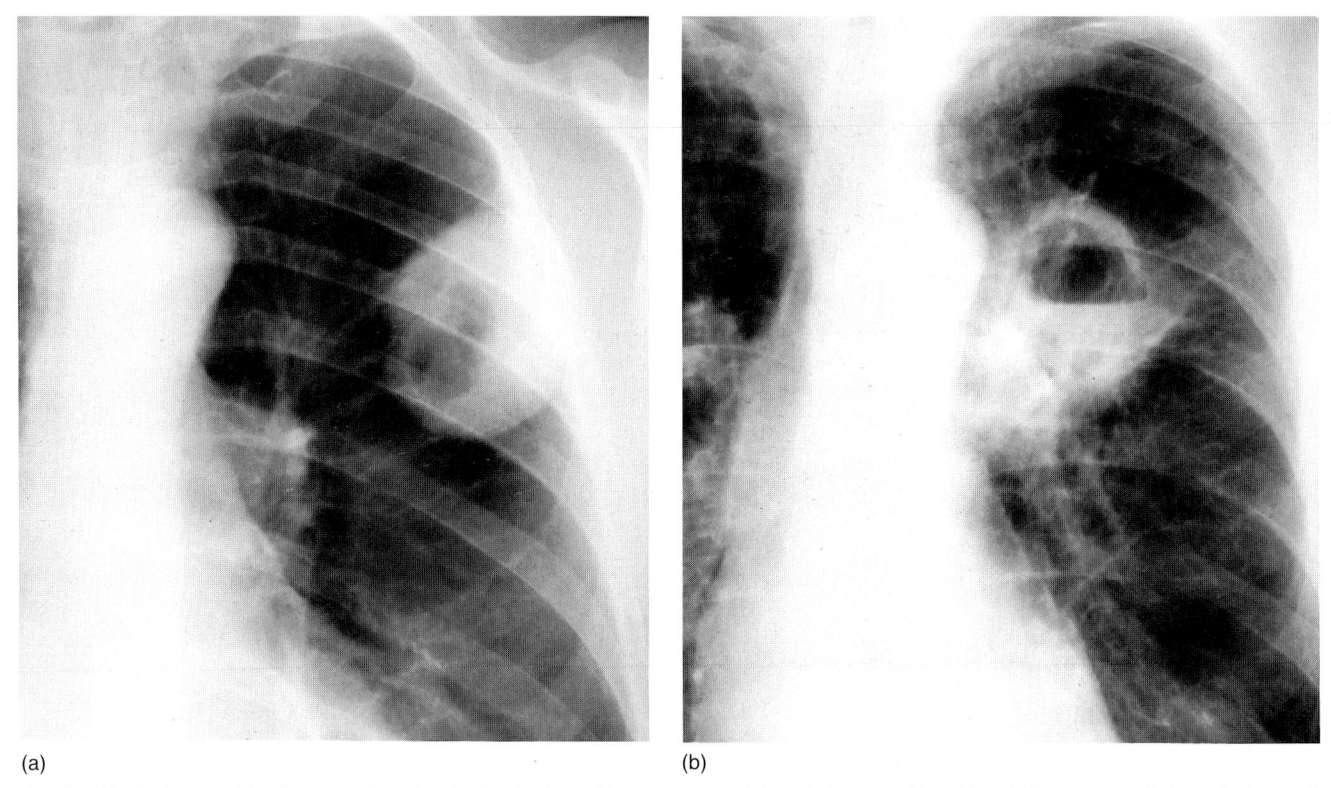

(a) (b)

Fig. 22.8 Spherical cavities in two different patients with bronchial carcinoma. (a) Note the variable width of the cavity wall; in parts the wall thickness is 2–3 cm; (b) thin-walled cavitating squamous cell lung carcinoma showing an air–fluid level within the cavity.

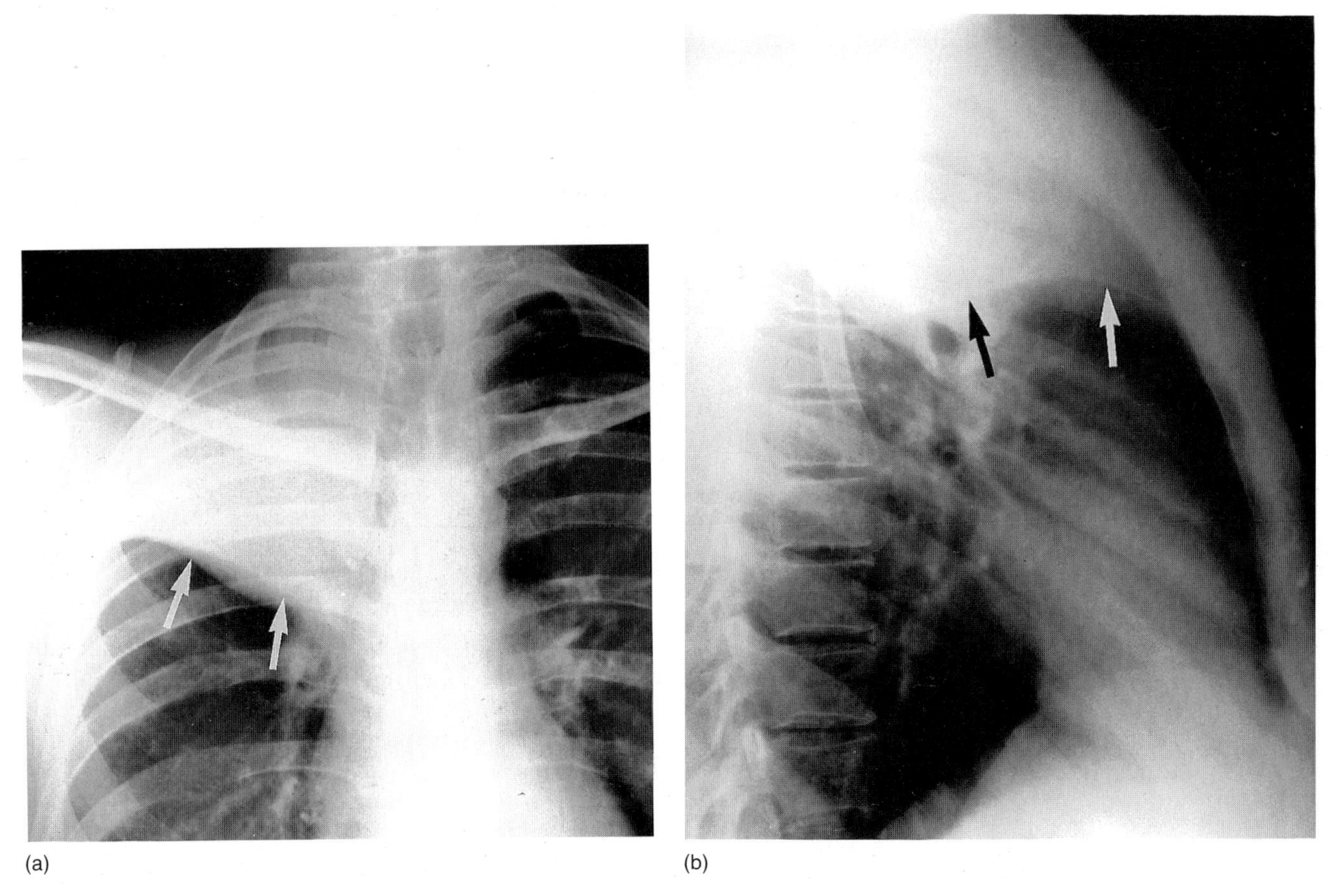

(a) (b)

Fig. 22.9 Right upper lobe (RUL) collapse with complete consolidation. Note the opaque RUL with elevation of the horizontal fissure (arrows). The trachea is deviated towards the collapsed lobe. The lobar shape is well shown in both (a) PA and (b) lateral views.

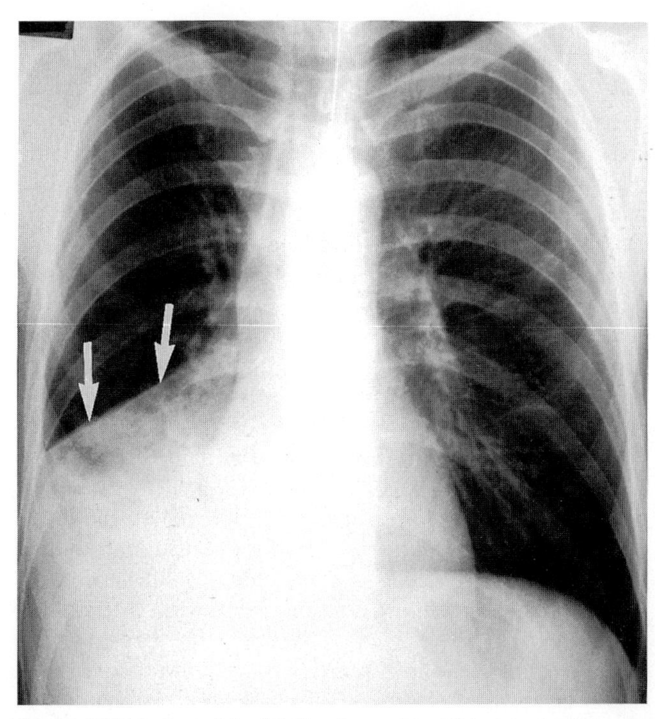

Fig. 22.10 Right lower lobe (RLL) collapse. The RLL shows substantial opacity and the oblique fissure (arrows) is pulled downward and angled so it can be seen in the frontal view. The trachea is deviated towards the side of the collapse.

It can be difficult or impossible to distinguish an infective lung abscess from a cavitating lung neoplasm or cavitation due to Wegener's granulomatosis on the basis of imaging, but if either the inner or outer walls are irregular the diagnosis of carcinoma is highly likely. Clinically it is usually straightforward to distinguish between cavitating neoplasms and infective lung abscesses.

PULMONARY COLLAPSE (ATELECTASIS)

Collapse (loss of volume of a lung or lobe) may be due to:

- bronchial obstruction
- fibrosis of a lobe, usually following tuberculosis
- bronchiectasis
- pulmonary embolus
- pneumothorax
- pleural effusion.

Collapse due to bronchial obstruction and to pleural effusion warrant further discussion.

Collapse due to bronchial obstruction

Collapse due to bronchial obstruction occurs because no air passes into the lung to replace the air absorbed from the alveoli. Consolidation almost invariably accompanies lobar collapse, so the resulting shadow is usually obvious. The likely causes are:

- **Bronchial wall lesions**
  - usually primary carcinoma
  - rarely, other bronchial tumours such as carcinoid
  - rarely, endobronchial tuberculosis

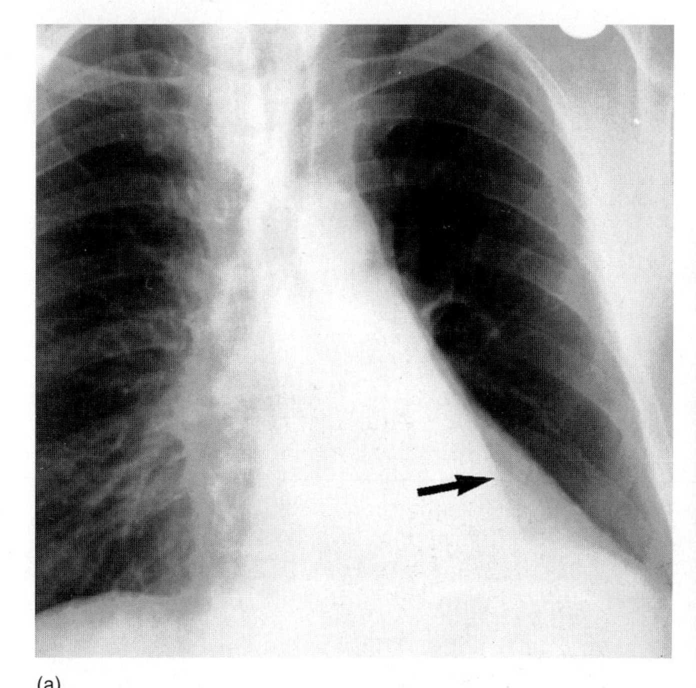

(a)

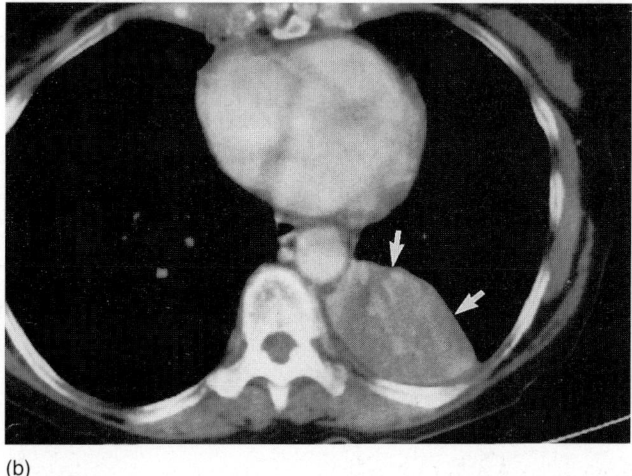

(b)

Fig. 22.11 Left lower lobe (LLL) collapse. (a) LLL collapse can be much more difficult to diagnose than other collapsed lobes on plain chest radiographs because, as in this case, the collapsed lobe lies entirely behind the heart. The triangular density of the collapsed lobe has a straight linear border (arrow). Note the lack of visibility of the descending aorta and left hemidiaphragm outlines. (b) On CT scanning the collapsed lobe is easy to identify. Note the clear-cut curvilinear anterior margin formed by the backwardly displaced oblique fissure (arrows).

- **Intraluminal occlusion**
  - mucus plugging, particularly in postoperative, asthmatic or unconscious patients, or in patients on artificial ventilation
  - inhaled foreign body
- **Invasion or compression by an adjacent mass**
  - malignant tumour
  - enlarged lymph nodes.

The signs of lobar collapse on plain chest radiography (Fig. 22.9–12) are the shadow of the collapsed lobe, the silhouette sign, and displacement of structures to take up the space normally occupied by the collapsed lobe. The diagnosis of lobar collapse is easy at CT when the opaque lobe of reduced volume is readily identified (Fig. 22.11b).

Occasionally, the lobe becomes so shrunken that, unless the lobe is precisely tangential to the X-ray beam, it may be difficult to see on a plain chest radiograph in one or other projection (Fig. 22.12). The silhouette sign can be very useful in this situation, since the mediastinal and diaphragmatic borders are ill-defined adjacent to the collapsed lobe. The silhouette sign also helps in deciding which lobe is collapsed. Collapse of the anteriorly located lobes (the upper and middle) obliterates portions of the mediastinal and heart outlines, whereas collapse of the lower lobes obscures the outline of the adjacent diaphragm and descending aorta.

When a lobe collapses, the ipsilateral unobstructed lung expands so that the hilum and fissure move toward the collapsed lobe. The hemidiaphragm may become elevated. With collapse of the whole of one lung, the entire hemithorax is opaque and there is substantial mediastinal and tracheal shift (Fig. 22.13).

When atelectasis is due to lobar fibrosis or bronchiectasis, the lobe usually remains aerated. The signs are, therefore, displacement of structures.

Collapse in association with pleural abnormality

The presence of air or fluid in the pleural cavity allows the lung to collapse. In pneumothorax, the diagnosis is obvious but if there is a large pleural effusion with underlying pulmonary collapse it may be difficult on a chest radiograph to diagnose the presence of collapsed lung. Even if the collapsed lobe is identified it can be difficult to tell whether the collapse is due to pleural fluid or whether both the collapse and the effusion are due to the same process, e.g. carcinoma of

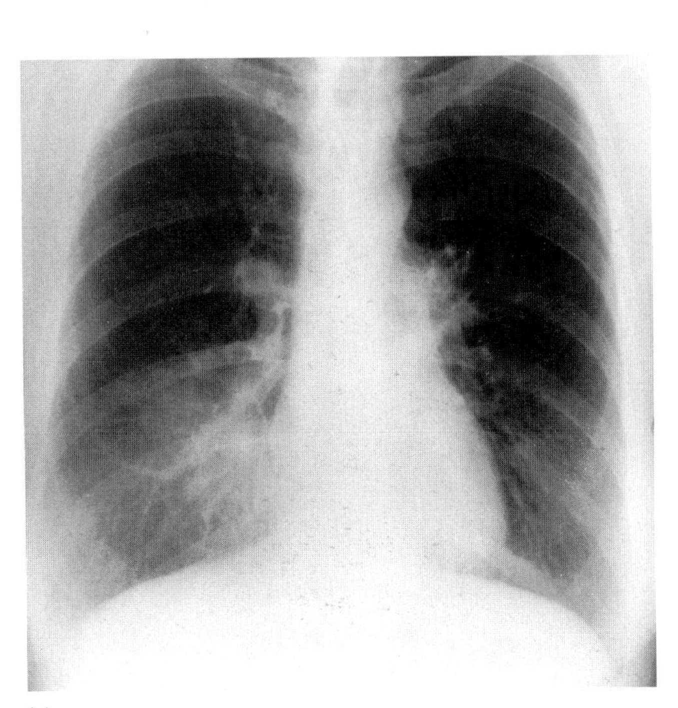

(a)

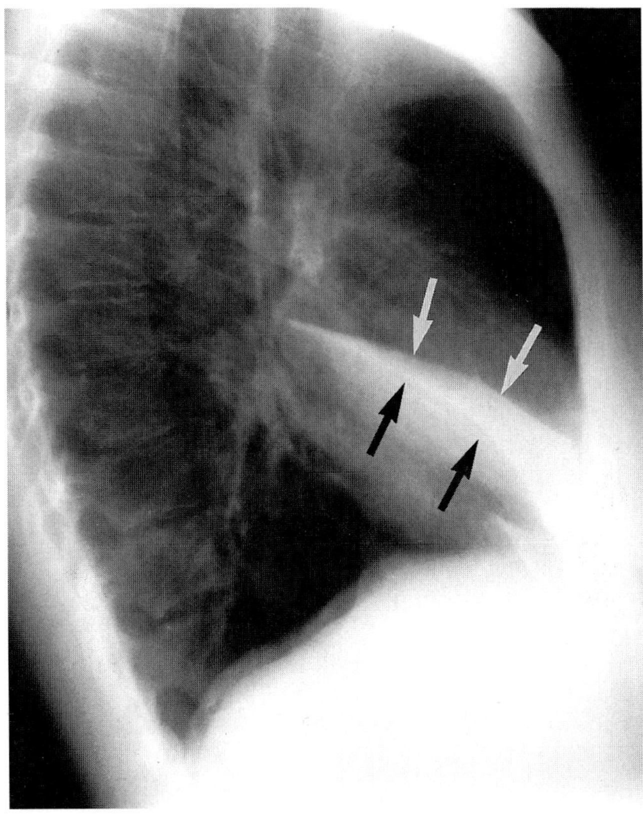

(b)

Fig. 22.12 Severe collapse of the right middle lobe. (a) On the frontal view the opacity of the collapsed lobe is ill-defined and quite difficult to see. Note the lack of clarity of the lower right border due to the silhouette sign. (b) The lateral view shows a wedge-shaped density with a clear-cut upper margin due to the downwardly displaced horizontal fissure (white arrows) and a well-defined lower margin due to the upwardly displaced right oblique fissure (black arrows).

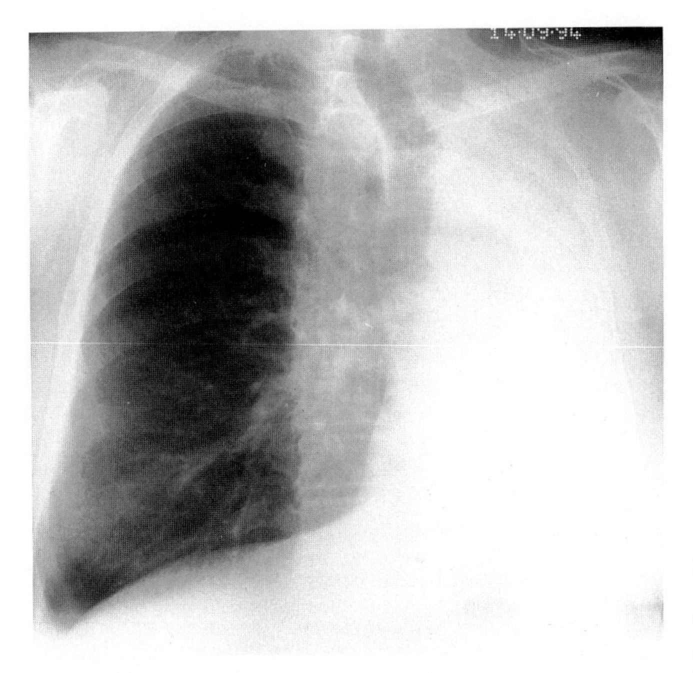

Fig. 22.13 Collapse of left lung. Both the left upper and left lower lobes are airless and severely collapsed. The whole left hemithorax is opaque with no visible left heart border or left hemidiaphragm. The trachea is greatly displaced towards the side of the opacity.

the bronchus. At CT it is usually easy to recognize pulmonary collapse despite the presence of a pleural effusion.

PULMONARY OEDEMA

When pulmonary oedema floods the alveoli it gives rise to widespread pulmonary opacification which is usually bilateral and is most severe in the central and dependent portions of the lungs. This form of pulmonary oedema, known as alveolar oedema, can be difficult to distinguish from widespread pneumonia. Pulmonary oedema has a number of causes and a variety of patterns, including basal shadowing and **septal lines** (see p. 518).

SOLITARY PULMONARY NODULE (MASS)

The diagnosis of a solitary spherical shadow (solitary pulmonary nodule) in the lung is a common problem (Fig. 22.14). The usual causes are:

- **bronchial carcinoma** or bronchial carcinoid;
- **benign tumour of the lung**, hamartoma being the most common;
- **infective granuloma**, tuberculoma being the most common in the UK, fungal granuloma the most frequent in the USA;
- **metastasis**;
- **lung abscess**.

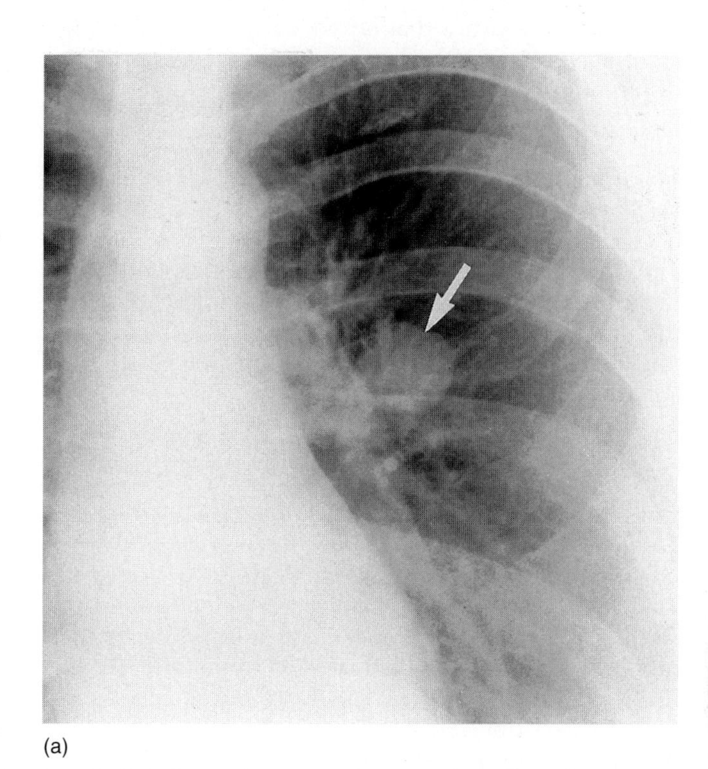

(a)

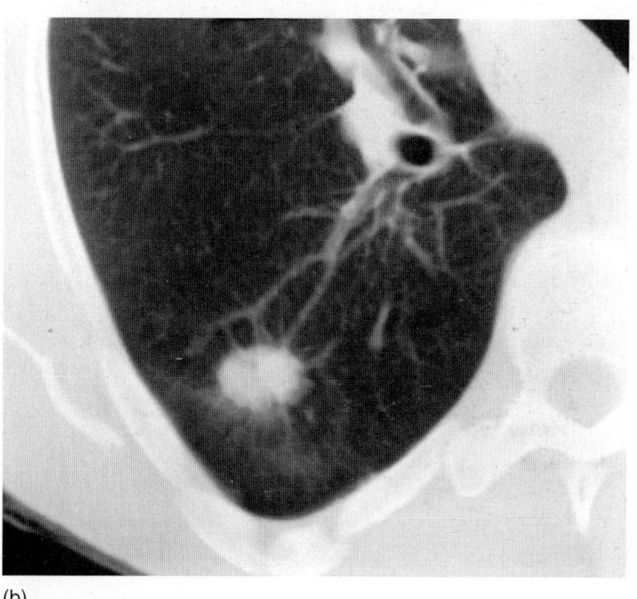

(b)

Fig. 22.14 Solitary pulmonary nodule (arrow). (a) The differential diagnosis for this 2 cm rounded, well-defined nodule with no calcification or cavitation and no previous examination with which to compare would be wide (see text). (b) CT scan in a different patient showing a 2 cm nodule with an irregular margin with infiltrating edges. The appearances are highly suggestive of bronchial carcinoma; this proved to be the diagnosis in this particular case.

With the exception of lung abscess, the nodule itself is often asymptomatic, the lesion being first noted on a routine chest film. When a nodule is discovered in a patient who is over 40 and a smoker, bronchial carcinoma becomes the major consideration.

The various possible lesions require totally different forms of management. Hamartomas and granulomas are best left alone, whereas bronchial carcinoma or carcinoid, active tuberculosis and lung abscess require treatment. Curative resection is possible for bronchial carcinoma/carcinoid. Careful observation of the following features may help in making the diagnosis.

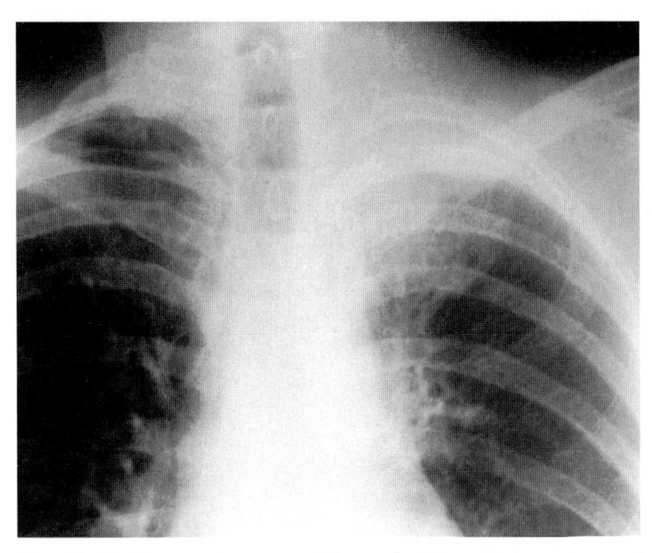

Fig. 22.16 Pancoast's tumour. The apical bronchial carcinoma is causing opacity of the uppermost portion of the left lung. The left first rib is almost totally destroyed by the tumour. This destruction is difficult to appreciate at first glance, but when the right and left first and second ribs are compared it is obvious that apart from a tiny residue of the head of the left first rib, the posterior portion of the rib in question is totally destroyed.

Comparison with previous films

Assessing the rate of growth of a spherical lesion by comparing previous examinations is one of the most important observations, because lack of change over a period of 18 months is a strong indication of a benign tumour or inactive granuloma. Almost all primary lung cancers double their volume between one month and 18 months (a 26% increase in diameter corresponds to a doubling in volume).

Calcification

The presence of calcification is the other vital observation, because substantial calcification virtually rules out the diagnosis of a malignant lesion; bronchial carcinoids may, however, show extensive calcification. Calcification is a common finding in hamartomas, tuberculomas and fungal granulomas. In hamartomas the calcification is often of the 'popcorn' type (Fig. 22.15). CT is of great value in detecting calcification and confirming that the calcification is within the lesion, not just projected over it. Uniform calcification can be difficult to recognize on plain chest radiography but is readily diagnosed with CT, and in such cases carcinoma of the lung can be excluded from the differential diagnosis.

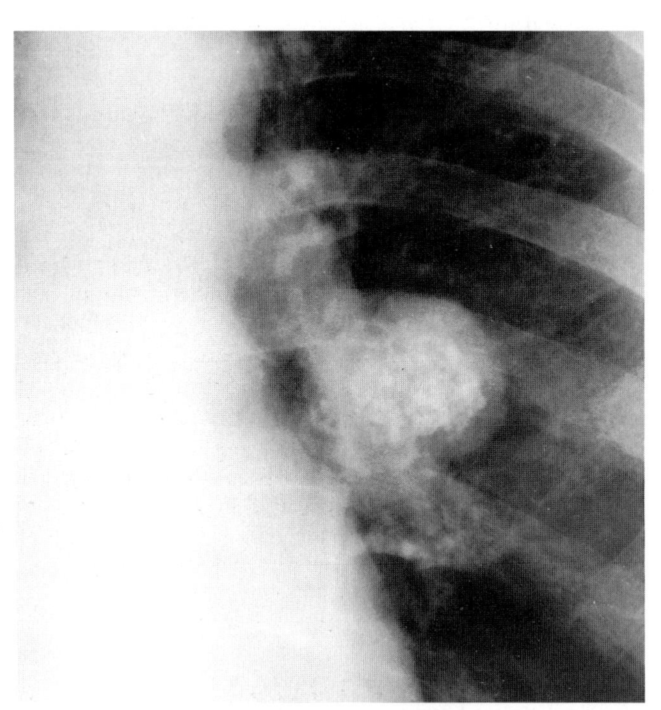

Fig. 22.15 Hamartoma of the lung. The central 'popcorn' calcification typical of cartilage calcification is diagnostic of hamartoma in this case.

Involvement of the adjacent chest wall

Destruction of the ribs adjacent to a pulmonary mass is virtually diagnostic of invasion by carcinoma. Tumours of the lung apex are particularly liable to invade adjacent bones, the chest wall and the root of the neck (Pancoast's tumour) (Fig. 22.16). CT, MRI or radionuclide bone scan may be indicated to demonstrate this invasion.

The shape of the shadow

Primary carcinoma nearly always shows a lobulated, notched or infiltrating outline. Even if only a small portion of the lesion has an ill-defined edge, the diagnosis of primary lung carcinoma should be seriously considered. A markedly infiltrating edge is highly suggestive of bronchial carcinoma (Fig. 22.14b). If the shadow is perfectly spherical and the edge very well defined the lesion is likely to be a hamartoma, a tuberculoma or a metastasis.

The shape may be obvious from plain films but CT can be used to show the edge of a pulmonary nodule to advantage.

Cavitation

If the centre of the tumour undergoes necrosis and is coughed up, air is seen within the mass. Such air is often accompanied by fluid, in which case an air–fluid level will be visible on erect films. The air, which may be difficult to appreciate, is seen as a translucency within the mass. This feature is particularly well seen at CT.

Size

A solitary lesion over 4 cm in diameter which does not contain calcium is nearly always either a primary carcinoma or a lung abscess; rarer causes include hydatid cyst and Wegener's granulomatosis. Lung abscesses and Wegener lesions of this size virtually always show cavitation, whereas carcinoma may or may not undergo recognizable cavitation.

Other lesions

The rest of the film should be checked carefully after a solitary lung mass has been found. Finding a small pleural effusion or a rib metastasis alters the management of the patient. Alternatively the nodule may not be solitary; multiple pulmonary nodules are likely to be due to metastases.

The role of CT for evaluating solitary pulmonary nodules

CT is performed in a patient with a solitary pulmonary nodule in order to:

- diagnose the nature of the nodule – the role here is limited since the plain film signs and knowledge of the rate of growth provide adequate information in most cases; CT is better able to detect calcification in a nodule than conventional films; as mentioned above, extensive calcification of a nodule effectively excludes primary carcinoma of the lung;
- stage the extent of disease in those cases where the nodule is likely to be a primary carcinoma;
- localize accurately the nodule prior to bronchoscopic or percutaneous needle biopsy in cases where localization is difficult from conventional films;
- establish whether or not the nodule is solitary or multiple when the lesion in question is likely to be a metastasis and when surgical resection of metastases is being considered.

MULTIPLE PULMONARY NODULES

Multiple well-defined spherical shadows in the lungs are virtually diagnostic of metastases (Fig. 22.17). Occasionally, such a pattern is seen with abscesses or with granulomatous disorders such as collagen vascular disease, sarcoidosis and tuberculous or fungal infections.

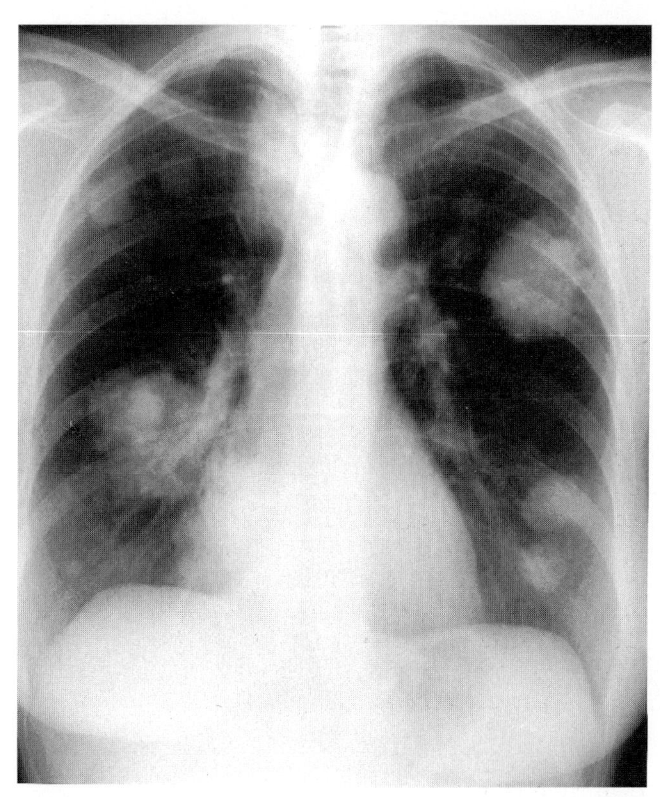

Fig. 22.17 Pulmonary metastases presenting as multiple pulmonary nodules.

LINE SHADOWS

Long line shadows, other than normal fissures and the pleural edge of a pneumothorax, are usually due to pleuropulmonary scars from previous infection or infarction. Mostly, these scars reach the pleura and are often associated with visible pleural thickening. They are of no significance to the patient. Emphysematous bullae are often bounded and traversed by thin line shadows.

An important cause of line shadows are **septal lines** (Fig. 22.18). They are usually due to pulmonary oedema or lymphangitis carcinomatosa. The pulmonary septa are interlobular connective tissue planes which are only visible radiologically when thickened. The most readily seen are the so-called **Kerley B lines**: small horizontal lines, never more than 2 cm in length, which are best seen at the periphery of the lung bases. In contrast to the blood vessels, they often reach the edge of the lung. So-called Kerley A lines are longer and situated more centrally. They radiate outward from the hila.

WIDESPREAD SMALL SHADOWS

Nodular and reticular shadows

Plain chest radiographs with widespread small (2–5 mm) pulmonary shadows often present a

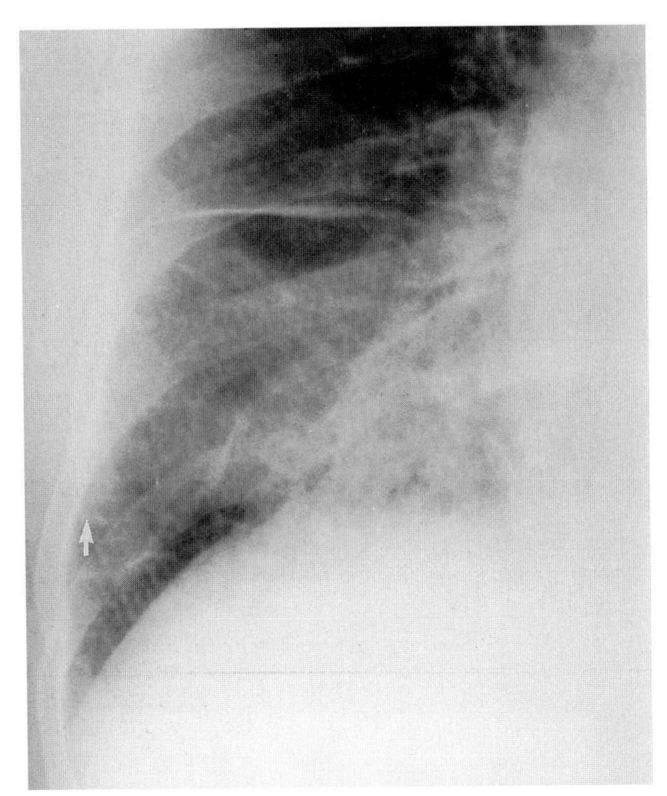

Fig. 22.18 Septal lines (Kerley B lines) due to pulmonary oedema. The short horizontal lines (one of which is arrowed) are parallel to one another and reach the pleura. Note also the thickening of the horizontal fissure which is also due to interstitial oedema.

diagnostic problem. With few exceptions it is only possible to give a differential diagnosis when faced with such a film. A final diagnosis can rarely be made without an intimate knowledge of the patient's symptoms and signs. High-resolution computed tomography (often abbreviated to HRCT) may enable a more confident diagnosis in many cases (Fig. 22.19).

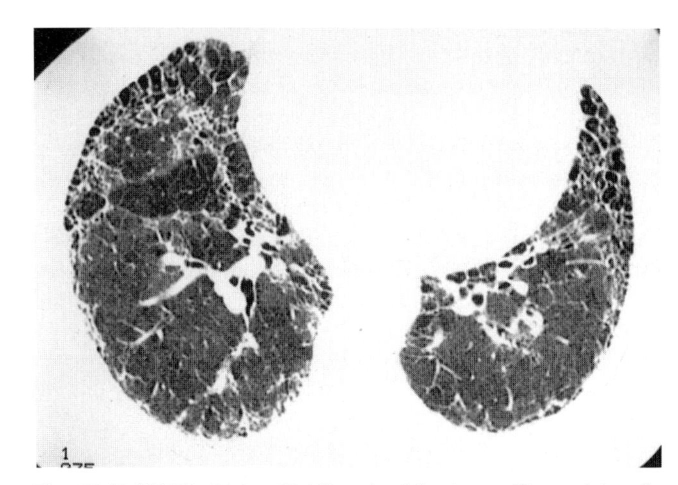

Fig. 22.19 HRCT of interstitial fibrosis of the lungs. The peripherally predominant reticular shadowing is typical of end-stage fibrosing alveolitis, in this case cryptogenic fibrosing alveolitis.

Many descriptive terms have been applied to widespread small pulmonary shadows, notably 'nodular', to signify discrete small round shadows and 'reticular' to describe a net-like pattern of small lines. Often there are both nodular and reticular elements and this is called 'reticulonodular'.

These patterns are due to very small lesions in the lung, no more than 1 or 2 mm in size. Individual lesions of this size are invisible on a chest film. That these very small lesions are seen at all is explained by the phenomenon of superimposition: when myriads of tiny lesions are present in the lungs it is inevitable that several are superimposed.

How to decide whether or not multiple small pulmonary shadows are present

Often, the greatest problem is to decide whether widespread abnormal shadowing is present at all, since normal blood vessels can also appear as nodules and interconnecting lines. To be confident involves looking carefully at many hundreds of normal films to establish a normal pattern in one's mind. The normal vessel pattern shows a branching system which connects in an orderly way: the vessels are larger centrally and they become smaller as they travel to the periphery. Vessels seen end-on appear as small nodules, but these nodules are no bigger than vessels seen in the immediate vicinity and their number corresponds to the expected number of vessels in that area.

When abnormal shadowing is found and its pattern determined, the next step is to construct a differential diagnostic list. The features of diagnostic importance are the pattern of shadowing, the distribution of abnormal shadows and other features such as mediastinal or hilar lymph node, or associated pleural effusion (Table 22.1). HRCT may be helpful in selected cases.

INCREASED TRANSRADIANCY OF THE LUNGS

Localized increase in transradiancy

When one hemithorax appears more transradiant than normal the following causes should be considered:

- **true or compensatory emphysema** (compensatory emphysema occurs when a lobe or a lung is collapsed or has been excised and the remaining lung expands to fill the space);
- **pneumothorax** – the diagnosis of a pneumothorax depends on visualizing the lung edge with air peripheral to it, and checking that the space believed to be a pneumothorax does not contain any vessels;
- **reduction in the chest wall soft tissues**, e.g. mastectomy;

Table 22.1 Commoner causes of nodular and reticular shadowing

Diagnosis	*Radiographic pattern*	*Distribution of shadows*	*Other features which may be seen*	*High-resolution CT (HRCT)*
Miliary tuberculosis	Small nodules of uniform size	Uniform	± Mediastinal/hilar lymph nodes One or more patches of consolidation	Not necessary
Sarcoidosis	(a) Fine nodular	Uniform	Hilar and paratracheal lymph nodes	Shows disease well but adds little of diagnostic value
	(b) Reticulonodular	Often predominant in mid and upper zones	Hilar and paratracheal lymph nodes	
Coal miners' pneumoconiosis	Nodular	Predominant in upper zones	Progressive massive fibrosis in the complicated form of the disease Emphysema	Adds little of diagnostic value
Asbestosis	Fine reticulonodular	Predominant in lower zones	Pleural thickening and/ or calcification	Useful for documenting the severity of fibrosis, and for showing pleural plaques where the diagnosis is in doubt
Fibrosing alveolitis	Reticulonodular	Often predominant in lower zones, but may show a variety of patterns	Diaphragm often high and indistinct	Characteristically shows peripherally predominant reticulonodular shadowing
Lymphangitis carcinomatosa	Reticulonodular	No predominant pattern	Septal lines Bronchial wall thickening Hilar adenopathy Other signs of carcinoma	The combination of septal lines and small nodules produces a characteristic pattern
Pulmonary oedema	Ill-defined nodules	Often central predominance with clear zone at periphery of lobes	Cardiac enlargement Left atrial enlargement Septal lines	Not indicated

- **air-trapping due to central obstruction** – most obstructing lesions in a major bronchus lead to lobar collapse; occasionally, particularly with an inhaled foreign body, a check valve mechanism occurs leading to air-trapping;
- **rarely massive pulmonary embolus** and **McLeod's syndrome** (Swyer–James syndrome), a condition that follows severe pneumonia in childhood.

Generalized increase in transradiancy

Generalized increased transradiancy of the lungs is one of the signs of emphysema. The other signs include reduction of vessel size and increased lung volume.

LUNG DISEASE WITH A NORMAL CHEST RADIOGRAPH

Serious respiratory disease may exist in patients with a normal chest radiograph:

- **Pulmonary emboli without infarction**. The chest radiograph may be normal in patients with pulmonary emboli, even those with life-threatening emboli;
- **Obstructive airways disease**. Asthma and acute bronchiolitis may produce overinflation of the lungs, but in many cases the chest film is normal. Emphysema, when severe, gives rise to the signs

described above, but when moderate, the chest radiograph may be normal or very nearly so. Uncomplicated acute or chronic bronchitis in adults does not produce any radiological signs and a considerable proportion of patients with productive cough due to bronchiectasis shows no plain film abnormality;

- **Infections**. Most patients with acute bacterial pneumonia present with recognizable consolidation, but in other infections, notably *Pneumocystis carinii* pneumonia, the recognizable pulmonary consolidation may only develop after the onset of symptoms. Patients with miliary tuberculosis may initially have a normal chest film;
- **Small lesions**. It is rarely possible to see solitary lung masses or consolidations of less than 1 cm in diameter. Even 2–3 cm lung cancers may be difficult to identify on routine films if they are partially or wholly hidden behind rib or clavicle shadows, of if they lie behind the heart or diaphragm. Endobronchial lesions, such as carcinoma, cannot usually be diagnosed on routine films unless they cause collapse/consolidation;
- **Diffuse pulmonary disease** may be responsible for breathlessness with substantial alteration in lung function tests before clear-cut abnormalities are evident on plain chest radiography.

SPECIFIC PULMONARY DISEASES

PNEUMONIA

The primary purpose of the chest radiograph in patients with suspected chest infection is to establish whether or not pneumonia is present. Clearly, the chest radiograph cannot replace bacteriological and laboratory information for diagnosing the infective agent. The principal radiographic features of pneumonia are one or more areas of pulmonary consolidation, which may show cavitation and may be accompanied by pleural effusion. The appearance of individual consolidations within the lung varies from a small, ill-defined density to large shadows involving the whole or most of one or more lobes (Fig. 22.20), the pattern depending on the infecting organism and the integrity of the host defences. Where pneumonia lies against a pleural fissure, it has a well-defined edge, but otherwise the margin is hazy. Occasionally, well-defined, rounded consolidation is seen.

Postobstructive pneumonia

Bacterial pneumonia may be secondary to obstruction of the bronchus. In a patient over 35 years of age, the obstruction is likely to be neoplastic, usually carcinoma. Occasionally, the central mass is so large

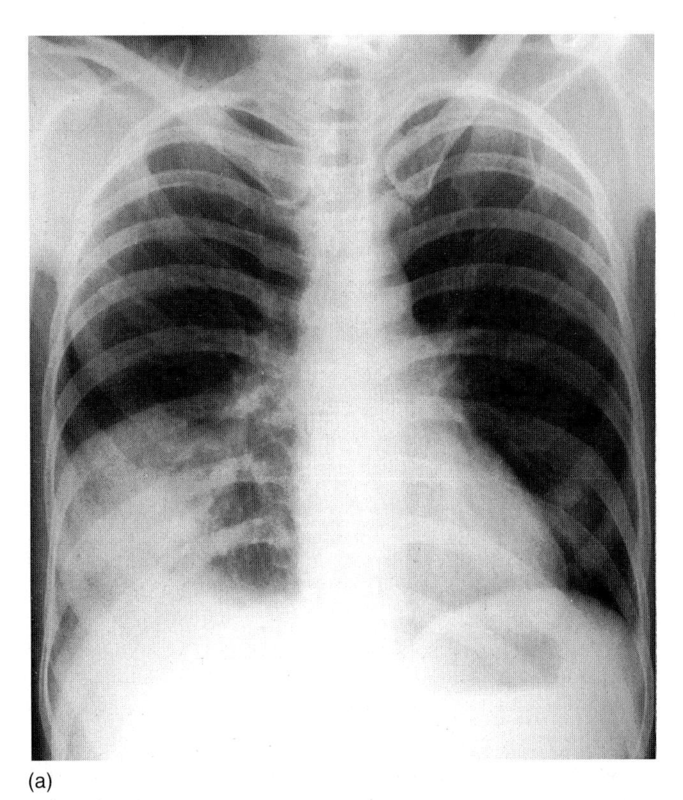

(a)

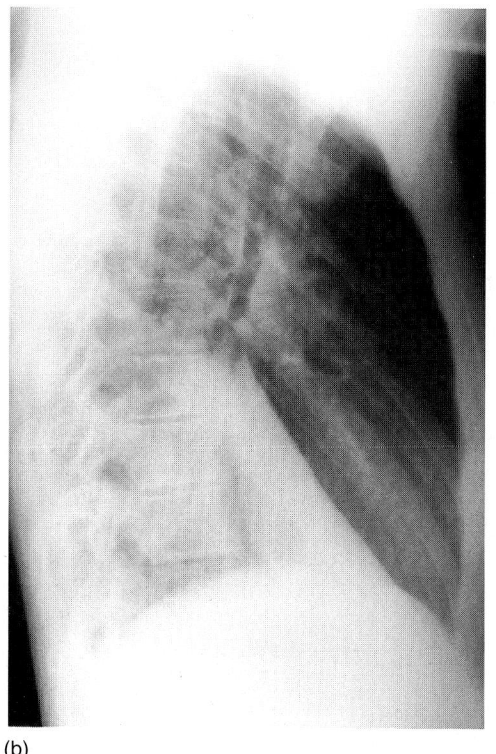

(b)

Fig. 22.20 Pneumonia causing consolidation of the basal segments of the right lower lobe. The superior segment is spared and, therefore the upper border of the consolidation is ill-defined in both (a) the PA and (b) the lateral views. The 'lobar' shape of the consolidation is particularly well seen in the lateral view. Note that in the lateral view the lower vertebrae are much whiter than the upper vertebrae.

that it deforms the outline of the affected lobe. In children, the common causes of obstruction in a major bronchus are an inhaled foreign body or a mucus plug.

Postobstructive pneumonia is usually confined to one lobe, but if more than one lobe is involved the two lobes usually share a common bronchus; for example, the right lower and middle lobes can be involved due to a lesion in the bronchus intermedius. The lobe almost invariably shows some loss of volume: air bronchograms are rarely visible within the area of consolidation. Typically, the pneumonia does not resolve radiologically on antibiotic therapy, although partial improvement of the radiological appearances is frequently seen.

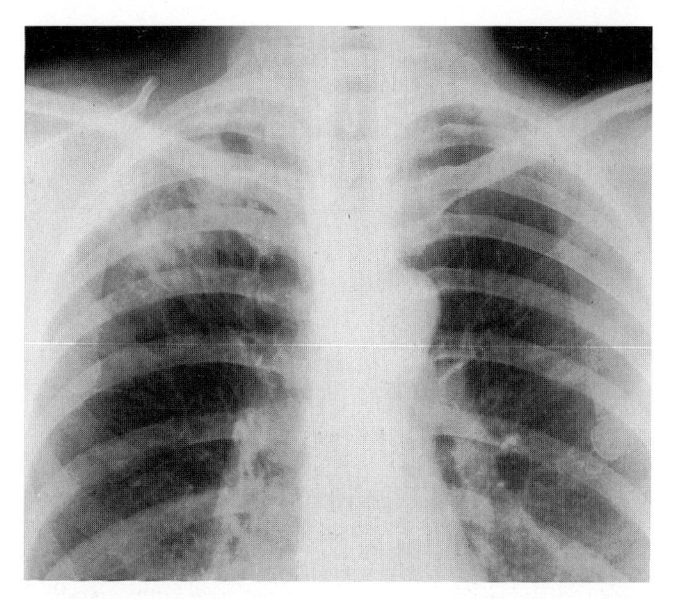

Fig. 22.22 Active postprimary pulmonary tuberculosis. There is patchy, moderately well-defined, consolidation in the right upper lobe. In this case the left upper lobe appears normal.

PULMONARY TUBERCULOSIS

Pulmonary tuberculosis is often divided into primary and postprimary forms, even though these divisions are not clear-cut. Primary tuberculosis follows the initial infection with *Mycobacterium tuberculosis* and usually occurs in childhood. Postprimary tuberculosis is the usual form seen in adults. It is believed to be a reinfection in a patient who has developed relative immunity.

Primary tuberculosis appears radiographically as an area of consolidation in the lung (Ghon focus) usually in the middle and upper zones, together with enlarged hilar or mediastinal nodes; a combination known as the primary complex. The disease may progress, giving rise to tuberculous bronchopneumonia, which often cavitates, or miliary tuberculosis, which produces innumerable small pulmonary nodules on chest X-ray (Fig. 22.21). The nodules are all much the same size, usually well-defined and fairly evenly distributed. Early in the clinical course the chest radiograph may be normal.

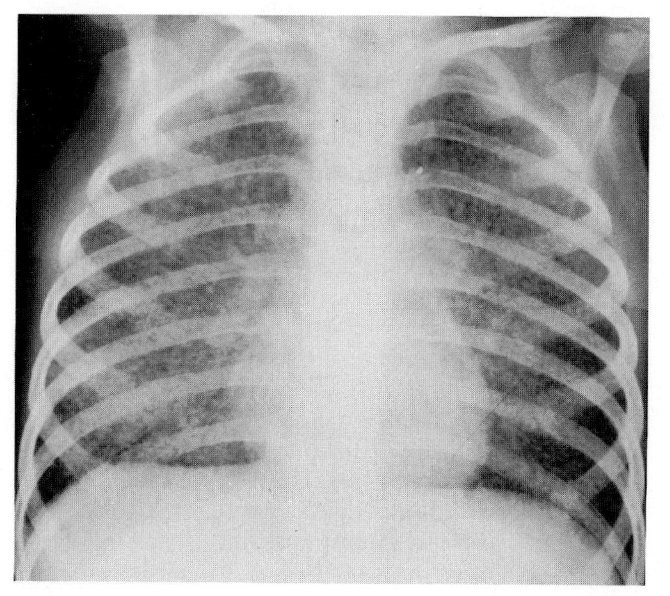

Fig. 22.21 Miliary tuberculosis in a child. Note the innumerable, uniformly distributed, small nodular shadows.

Pulmonary involvement in postprimary tuberculosis is usually greatest in the upper portions of the lungs, the apical and posterior segments of the upper lobes (Fig. 22.22), and the superior segments of the lower lobes. Multiple small areas of consolidation are seen initially. As the infection progresses, the consolidations enlarge and frequently cavitate. Extensive bronchial spread may occur, giving rise to multilobar bronchopneumonia, usually including one or both upper lobes, with cavitation being a frequent phenomenon. Healing occurs with fibrosis and calcification, but signs of healing may be seen despite continuing activity. Occasionally, tuberculosis takes the form of lower or middle-lobe bronchopneumonia and may even resemble lobar pneumonia. As with the primary form, the infection may spread via the bloodstream to give rise to miliary tuberculosis.

Pleural effusions are frequent in both primary and postprimary tuberculosis and may be the only manifestation of the disease.

Tuberculoma refers to a tuberculous granuloma in the form of a spherical mass, usually less than 3 cm in diameter (Fig. 22.23). The edge is usually sharply defined and these lesions are often partly calcified. Computed tomography may be needed to demonstrate the calcification. Most tuberculomas are inactive but viable tubercle bacilli may be present even in the calcified lesions.

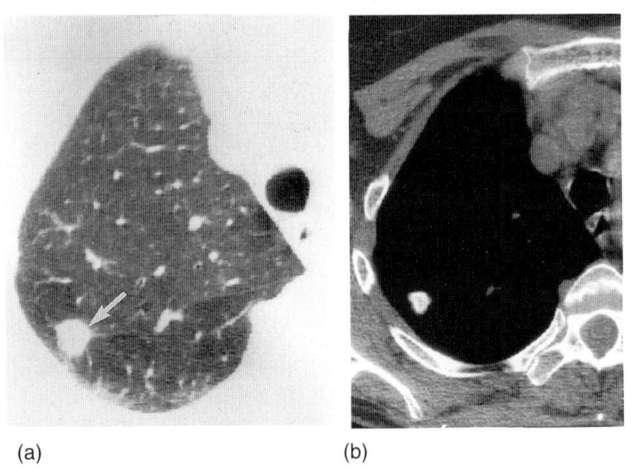

(a) (b)

Fig. 22.23 Tuberculoma in posterior segment of right upper lobe. (a) CT scan displayed at lung windows shows a 1 cm diameter round nodule (arrow) with irregular edges (closely resembling a primary lung carcinoma). (b) Same CT image, but displayed at soft-tissue windows showing extensive calcification of the nodule. Note that the nodule is the same 'whiteness' as the calcified bone.

MYCETOMA

The fungus *Aspergillus fumigatus* may colonize old tuberculous or other cavities to produce a ball of fungus (mycetoma) lying free within the cavity. Since the fungus ball usually occupies only a portion of the available space, air is seen between the mycetoma and the wall of the cavity (Fig. 22.24). The shape and position of this rim varies with the position of the patient. Cavities containing mycetomas are usually surrounded by evidence of old tuberculous infection, particularly fibrosis and calcification of the adjacent lung.

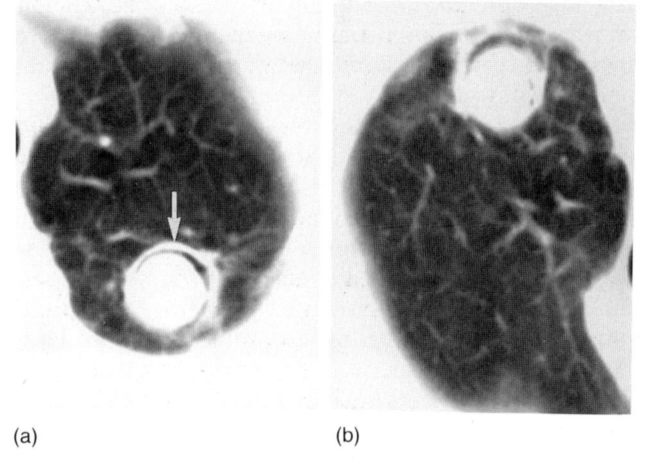

(a) (b)

Fig. 22.24 Mycetoma. CT scans taken in (a) usual supine position and (b) in prone position. The mass of the mycetoma is seen lying within an old thin-walled tuberculous cavity (arrow). Note that the mass moves to lie respectively on the posterior wall of the cavity when the patient is supine and on the anterior wall when the patient lies prone. In other words the mycetoma lies in the most dependent portion of the cavity in both positions.

PULMONARY EMBOLISM AND INFARCTION

Although many plain chest radiographic signs are described in pulmonary embolism and infarction, they are all non-specific. It is, therefore, impossible to decide from plain chest radiographs alone whether a patient has or has not had a pulmonary embolus. However, significant, even life-threatening, pulmonary embolism may occur in patients with normal chest radiographs. One of the principal values of the chest radiograph is to exclude clinically similar diseases that may show radiographic abnormalities, e.g. pneumothorax or dissecting aneurysm.

A simple way to consider pulmonary embolism is to regard it as either embolism without infarction or embolism with infarction. Pulmonary embolism without infarction usually produces no recognizable abnormality. Enlargement of a major arterial trunk at the hilum is a well-known, but very rarely seen, sign. Discoid (linear) atelectasis may be seen, but this phenomenon occurs with numerous disorders and is a reflection of poor diaphragmatic excursion rather than vascular occlusion. Elevation of one hemidiaphragm, a common finding in pulmonary embolism, is non-specific and can be normal.

Pulmonary embolism causing infarction gives rise to consolidation which tends to be wedge-shaped and based on the pleura, but many patterns are seen. The consolidation may have a round medial edge (Hampton's hump). This shape is uncommon and, although very suggestive of pulmonary infarction, is also seen with pneumonia. Small ipsilateral pleural effusions are often present in patients with pulmonary infarction.

Radionuclide lung scanning for pulmonary embolism

Since plain film radiology is so non-specific for diagnosing pulmonary embolism, further investigation with radionuclide imaging is often needed. There are two major types of lung scan, namely perfusion and ventilation scans.

For **perfusion scans**, often called Q scans, particulate material such as technetium-99m labelled macroaggregates of albumin, with an average particle size of 30 μm, are injected intravenously. These particles become trapped in the pulmonary capillaries and the distribution of radioactivity, when imaged by a gamma camera, accurately reflects blood flow.

For **ventilation scans**, often called V scans, the patient inhales a radioactive gas such as xenon-133 or krypton-81m and the distribution of radioactive gas is imaged using a gamma camera. Aerosols labelled with technetium-99m may be used instead of gases.

Interpretation of radionuclide lung scanning The cardinal sign of pulmonary embolism on radionuclide lung scanning is a perfusion defect. Perfusion defects are usually segmental in shape and extend to the pleural surface. A normal perfusion scan excludes the diagnosis of pulmonary embolism, but the presence of a perfusion defect is non-specific, because many other disease processes can cause focal reduction in blood flow. These include obstructive airways disease (either acute or chronic), pneumonia, atelectasis, pulmonary oedema and vasculitis. Increased specificity for pulmonary embolism can be obtained by adding a ventilation scan to the procedure. The major patterns are:

- **Mismatched ventilation/perfusion defects** (V/Q mismatches)
  - perfusion defects in an area with normal ventilation strongly suggest pulmonary embolism without infarction (Fig. 22.25).
  - perfusion defects which are larger than the corresponding ventilation defects suggest pulmonary infarction. Such cases often show consolidation on plain chest radiograph.
  - There are, however, a number of conditions that can cause perfusion defects without disturbing ventilation and without recognizable abnormality on the chest radiograph, including previous pulmonary emboli, obstruction to pulmonary arteries by vasculitis, neoplasm or inflammation, primary pulmonary arterial hypertension and systemic arterial blood flow to a portion of the lung. This long and varied list highlights the lack of specificity even of mismatched defects.
- **Matched ventilation/perfusion defects** may be seen with pulmonary infarction, pneumonia, pulmonary oedema, or airway disease.

Abnormal ventilation–perfusion scan results are expressed in terms which indicate the probability that the diagnosis of pulmonary embolism is correct but the radionuclide scan findings alone cannot provide a reliable estimate of likelihood without factoring in the clinical probability of pulmonary embolism. Unfortunately, this important concept is often overlooked.

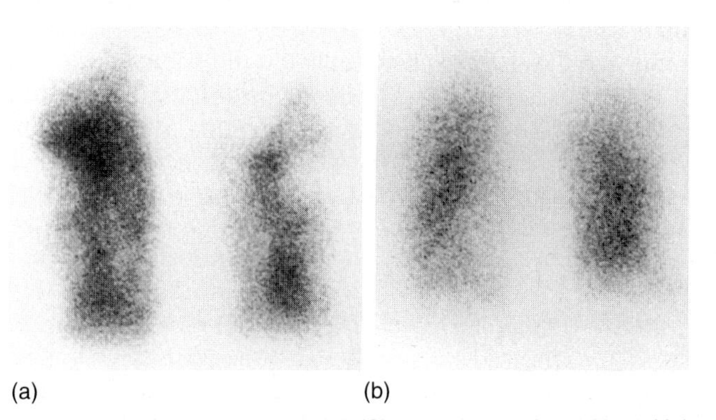

Fig. 22.25 Ventilation–perfusion (V/Q) scans in a patient with multiple large pulmonary emboli. (a) The perfusion scan shows multiple large segmental-shaped perfusion defects (the distribution of radioactivity should closely resemble the distribution of radioactivity in the ventilation scan). (b) The ventilation scan shows normal distribution of the inhaled radionuclide.

A ventilation–perfusion scan interpreted as low probability, typically a scan with matched ventilation perfusion defects, is associated with a 10% incidence of pulmonary embolism. The term 'high probability' in general means a likelihood greater than 85%. It is worth noting that when the diagnosis is clinically likely and there are multiple segmental or larger defects in the presence of a normal ventilation scan, the probability of pulmonary embolism exceeds 90%.

Pulmonary angiography for pulmonary embolism

Pulmonary angiography is the most sensitive and specific available test for pulmonary embolism, but because it is an invasive test the procedure is reserved for those patients who require a precise diagnosis of pulmonary embolism. The diagnostic feature is an intraluminal filling defect within the opacified arterial tree on two or more films. Occlusion of an artery is less specific and may be seen in a variety of conditions, including previous embolus or occlusion due to direct involvement by neoplasm or inflammatory disease.

ADULT RESPIRATORY DISTRESS SYNDROME (NON-CARDIOGENIC PULMONARY OEDEMA)

Adult respiratory distress syndrome is characterized by unexpected or severe respiratory distress in patients whose lungs were previously normal. There are many precipitating disorders, including hypotension, septic shock, aspiration of gastric contents, haemorrhagic pancreatitis, near drowning, ingestion of drugs, fat embolism, inhalation of toxic fumes and severe trauma. The common feature appears to be damage to the pulmonary capillaries which leads to increased permeability.

Radiologically, the oedema of adult respiratory distress syndrome is initially identical to cardiogenic alveolar oedema, namely ill-defined pulmonary shadowing in both lungs, maximal close to the hila fading out towards the periphery of the lobes. Cardiac enlargement and pleural effusions are not features. The pulmonary oedema seen on the chest radiograph may sometimes be identified only a few hours after the onset of hypoxaemia, in contrast to cardiogenic pulmonary oedema, which is visible coincident with the development of hypoxaemia. With time, the patient develops increased lung density involving the whole of both lungs (Fig. 22.26). Such patients invariably require artificial ventilation and are therefore liable to complications of ventilation such as interstitial emphysema, pneumothorax and pneumomediastinum.

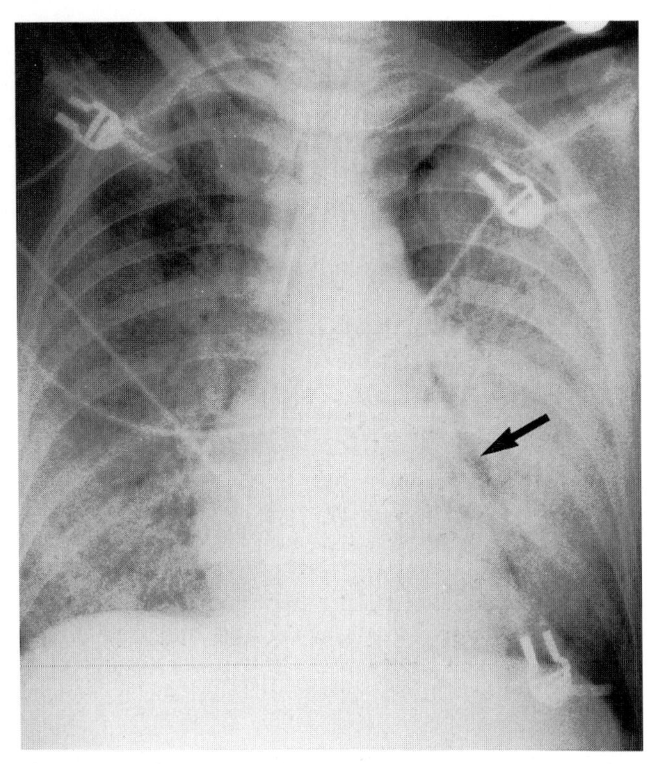

Fig. 22.26 Adult respiratory distress syndrome. Note the widespread opacity of the lungs. Air bronchograms are visible. The patient is on positive pressure ventilation via an endotracheal tube and a left-sided pneumomediastinum (arrow) has developed.

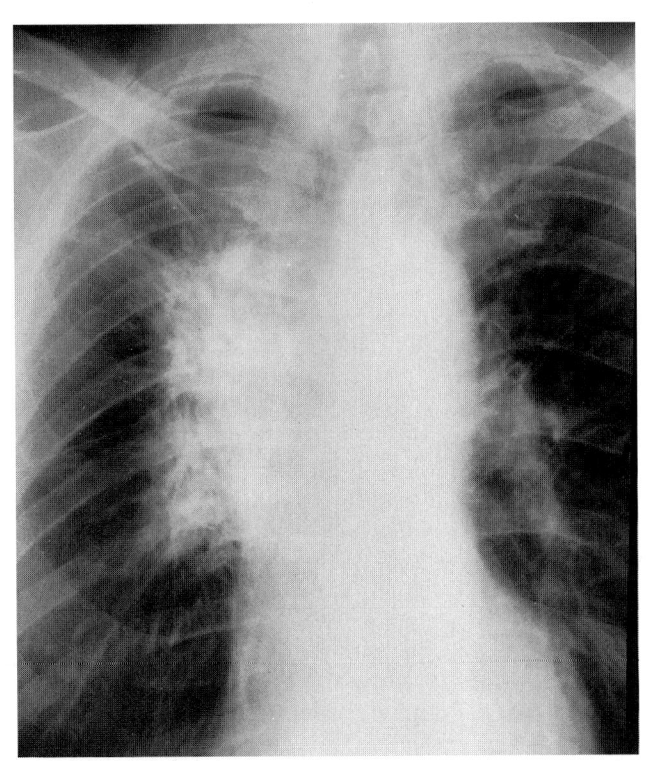

Fig. 22.27 Radiation fibrosis. The dense opacity within the lung adjacent to the right hilum and upper mediastinum has a geometric shape in this case conforming to the rectangular radiation field. Note the fibrotic contraction which has caused the trachea to shift towards the fibrotic area.

RADIATION PNEUMONITIS AND FIBROSIS

The response of normal lung to radiation varies from patient to patient. Initially, there is no radiological change, but within a few weeks ill-defined small shadows, indistinguishable from infective consolidation, are seen in the radiation field. If the inflammatory change progresses to fibrosis, there is dense coarse shadowing which may be sharply demarcated from the normal lung in a geometric fashion, conforming to the field of radiation rather than the lobar boundaries of the lung (Fig. 22.27). There is loss of volume of the fibrosed areas and extensive pleural thickening is often seen.

BRONCHIAL FOREIGN BODIES

Metallic foreign bodies in the bronchial tree are usually readily visualized and localized radiographically. Teeth fragments, however, may be difficult to recognize. Most foreign bodies, e.g. nuts, sweets and small plastic objects, are not radiopaque. The radiographic signs are, therefore, those of the effects of the foreign body on the lungs, namely the signs of major airway obstruction. In children, the obstruction is usually of the ball-valve type, and evidence of air trapping is the commonest sign. A minority show atelectasis or postobstructive pneumonia. A significant proportion of children with a proven foreign body in the trachea or bronchi have normal plain chest radiographs.

Air trapping is rarely severe enough to be appreciated on standard films taken on full inspiration. The sign is always more obvious on expiration. Indeed, the inspiratory film may be completely normal in cases when the diagnosis is obvious on expiration. The signs of air trapping are increased radiolucency of the affected lung with a decrease in the size of the vessels within that lung, together with the signs of increased or fixed volume, flat hemidiaphragm and mediastinal shift to the opposite side.

CARCINOMA OF THE BRONCHUS

The majority of bronchial carcinomas arise in larger bronchi at, or close to, the hilum. These tumours are usually confirmed or excluded by bronchoscopy and transbronchial biopsy. The remainder arise peripherally and their investigation can be more problematic.

Signs of a central tumour

The tumour itself may present as a hilar mass and the effects of obstruction by the tumour may be seen: usually a combination of collapse and consolidation (Fig. 22.28).

Signs of a peripheral tumour

A peripheral primary carcinoma usually presents as a rounded shadow with an irregular border showing lobulated, notched or infiltrating edges (Fig. 22.29). Cavitation may be seen within the mass. Peripheral squamous cell carcinomas show a particular tendency for cavitation (Fig. 22.30). The walls of the cavity are classically thick and irregular, but thin-walled smooth cavities due to carcinoma do occur. On very rare occasions primary lung carcinomas may show calcification on computed tomography.

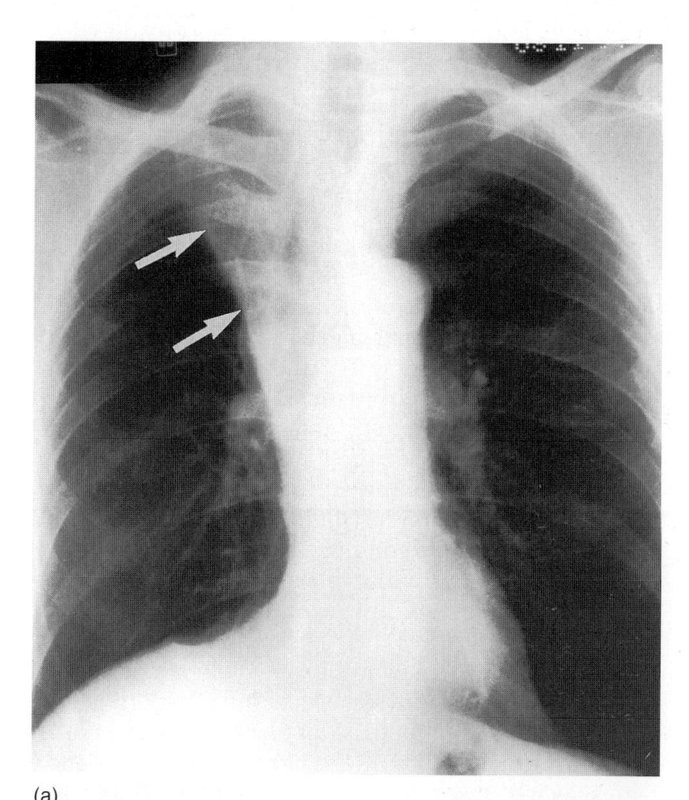

(a)

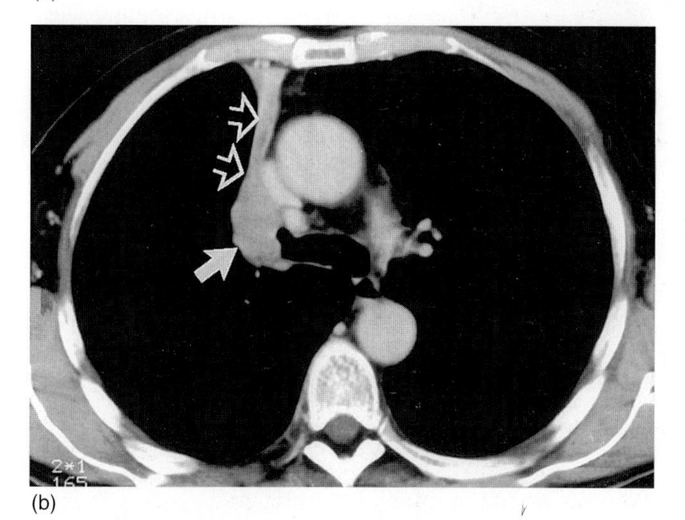

(b)

Fig. 22.28 Bronchial carcinoma causing right upper lobe collapse and a right hilar mass. (a) The chest radiograph shows right upper lobe collapse. (The arrows point to the greatly elevated horizontal fissure). (b) The mass of tumour at the right hilum is best seen at CT (solid arrow). The greatly collapsed right upper lobe is seen as a sliver of tissue plastered against the mediastinum anteriorly (open arrows).

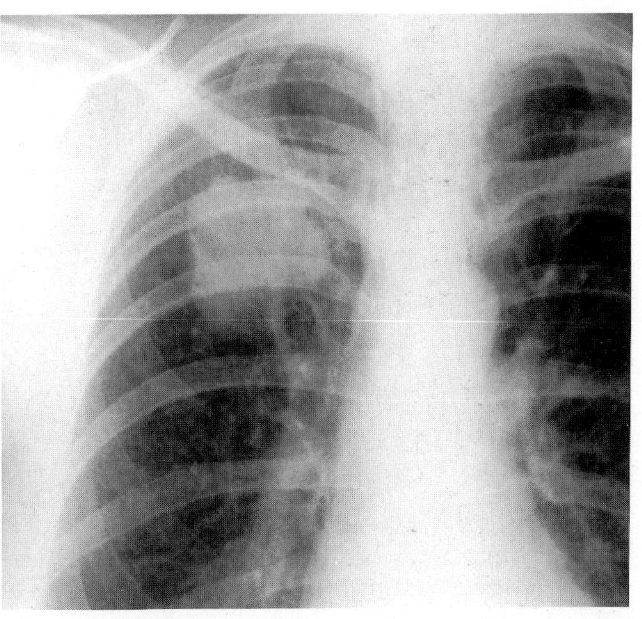

Fig. 22.29 Peripheral bronchial carcinoma presenting as a 4 cm diameter lobulated mass in the right upper lobe.

Signs of spread of bronchial carcinoma

The signs of spread of bronchial carcinoma may be visible on plain chest radiography. Computed tomography has made a major contribution to the staging of lung cancer, because CT may show mediastinal lymph

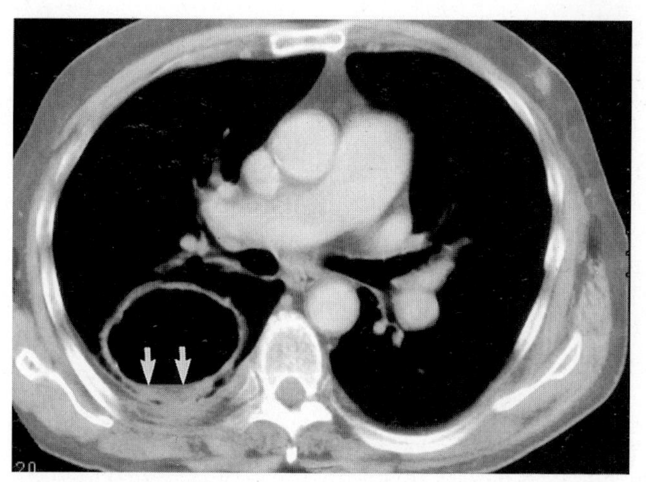

Fig. 22.30 Squamous cell carcinoma of the lung. CT scan showing a strikingly thin-walled cavitating tumour. A little fluid is seen lying in the dependent portion of the cavity (arrows).

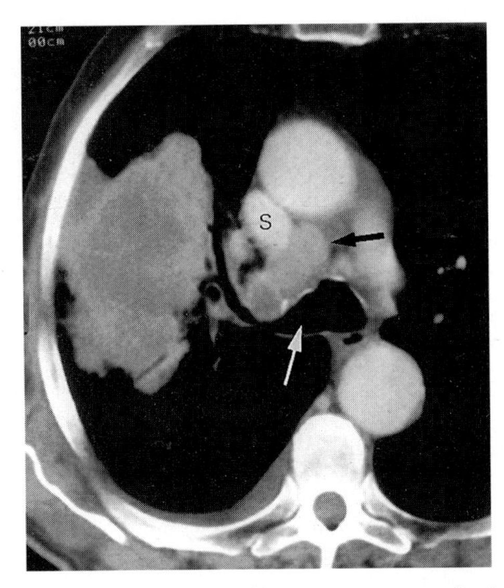

Fig. 22.31 Bronchial carcinoma with metastases to mediastinal lymph nodes. The large primary bronchial carcinoma in the right upper lobe has metastasized to mediastinal lymph nodes lying between the superior vena cava (S) and the right main bronchus (white arrow). The black arrow points to the largest of the enlarged nodes.

node enlargement or direct invasion of the mediastinum that is invisible or questionable on the plain chest film – information that may save the patient an unnecessary thoracotomy. MRI is used only to solve specific problems following CT.

- **Hilar and mediastinal lymph node enlargement** due to lymphatic spread of tumour. Only greatly enlarged lymph nodes can be recognized on the plain chest radiograph. The sites in which nodes are most readily identified are at the hilum and in the right paratracheal area. Computed tomography (Fig. 22.31), on the other hand, has the ability to show even mildly enlarged nodes in any site in the mediastinum and hila. However, enlargement of lymph nodes does not necessarily mean metastatic involvement, since reactive hyperplasia to the tumour or associated infection can be responsible for nodal enlargement as can pre-existing disease such as granulomatous infection, sarcoidosis or pneumoconiosis. In practice, the role of CT is to decide which patients are unsuitable for surgery, which patients need mediastinoscopy or mediastinotomy prior to thoracotomy, and to show the surgeon which nodes to biopsy preoperatively. Nodes below 1 cm in diameter can be considered as normal in size and need not be biopsied prior to thoracotomy. Nodes above 1 cm in diameter should be biopsied prior to surgical resection of the primary tumour, though it should be borne in mind that nodes of 2 cm or greater in the lymphatic drainage of a bronchial carcinoma almost invariably contain metastatic neoplasm. MRI, in general, has no advantages over CT for demonstrating mediastinal lymph node enlargement.
- **Pleural effusion**, particularly if bloody, in a patient with lung cancer is usually due to malignant involvement of the pleura. If so, the tumour is classified as a T4 tumour and is considered unsuitable for surgical resection. Pleural effusion may also be secondary to associated infection of the lung or coincidental, as in heart failure. Pleural aspiration and biopsy is, therefore, indicated.
- **Invasion of the mediastinum**. On plain films the signs of mediastinal invasion are widening of the mediastinal shadow; elevation of one or other hemidiaphragm may indicate involvement of the phrenic nerve by tumour. Mediastinal widening can be difficult to evaluate, particularly in older people with aortic unfolding. Computed tomography and, in selected cases MRI, are accurate methods for assessing mediastinal invasion by tumour because the neoplasm and the mediastinal structures can be directly visualized (Figs. 22.32, 22.33).

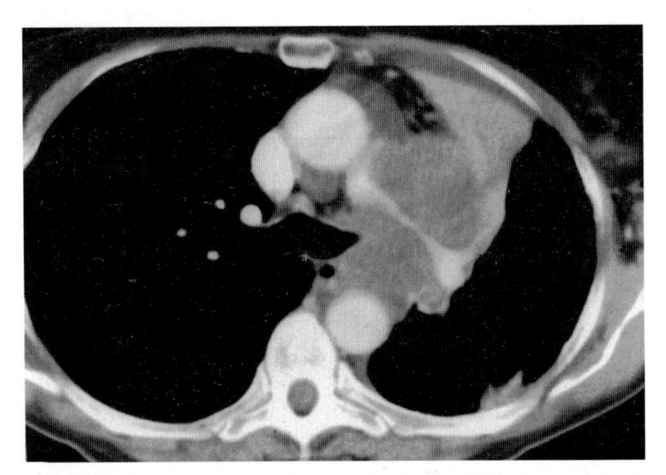

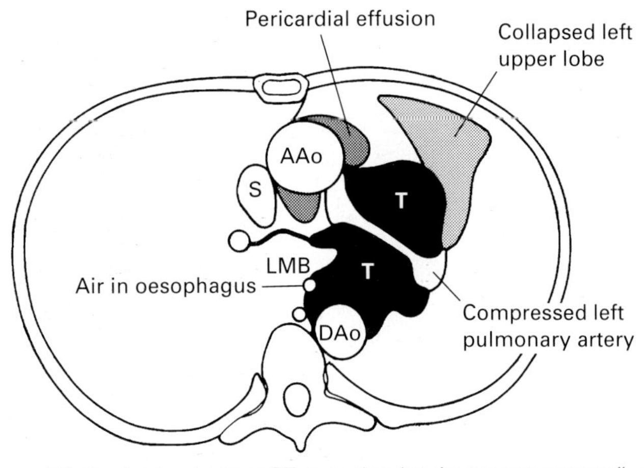

Fig. 22.32 Extensive mediastinal invasion by a left hilar bronchial carcinoma (T). Contrast-enhanced CT scan showing the tumour surrounding, invading and narrowing the main and left pulmonary arteries and the descending aorta. The tumour obstructing the left upper lobe bronchus has caused left upper lobe collapse. AAo = ascending aorta; DAo = descending aorta; LMB = left main bronchus; S = Superior vena cava.

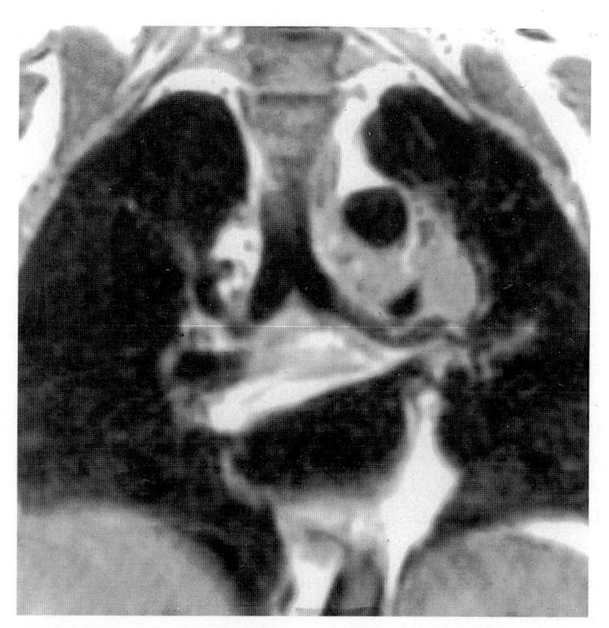

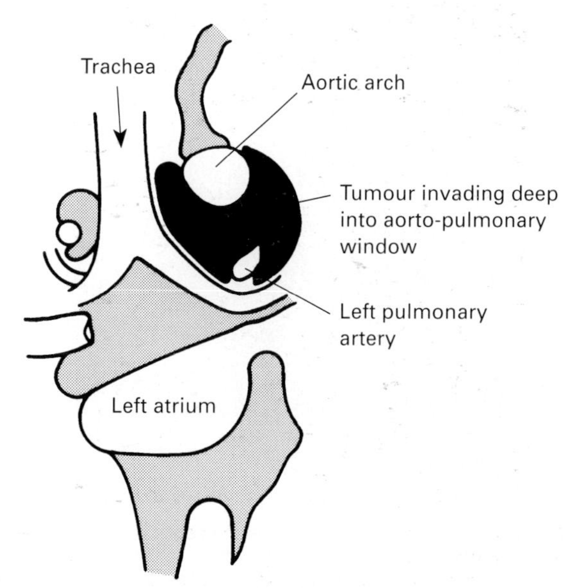

Fig. 22.33 Extensive mediastinal invasion by a left hilar bronchial carcinoma shown by coronal MRI scan. Note the tumour extending into the aortopulmonary window and lying medial to the aortic arch. The mediastinal fat is bright white (tinted areas in the diagram).

- **Invasion of the chest wall**. Destruction of a rib immediately adjacent to a pulmonary shadow indicates chest wall invasion. Recognizing rib destruction can be difficult unless a conscious effort is made to look at the ribs directly. Oblique views may be helpful in detecting bone destruction. CT can demonstrate chest wall invasion to advantage (Fig. 22.34) and may show soft tissue invasion even when the bone is not visibly eroded. Imaging techniques, even CT and MRI, may not always be reliable for diagnosing chest wall invasion and local chest wall pain remains the most important feature indicating that the tumour has crossed the pleura.

  Invasion of the root of the neck by so-called Pancoast's tumours (superior sulcus tumours) may be difficult to diagnose by CT. MRI, because of its multiplanar imaging capability, is particularly useful for showing the full extent of such tumours.

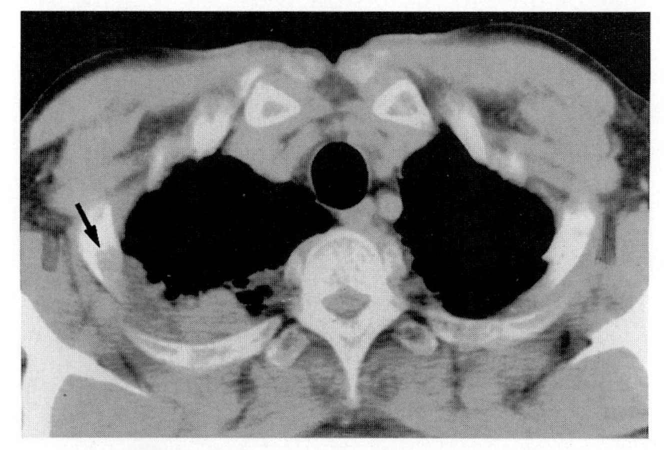

Fig. 22.34 Chest wall invasion by a peripheral bronchial carcinoma. The tumour has invaded the adjacent rib (arrow).

- **Lymphangitis carcinomatosa**. Lymphangitis carcinomatosa can be due to spread from abdominal, breast and other extrathoracic cancers as well as from carcinoma of the lung. The lymphatic vessels become grossly distended and the lungs become oedematous. When bilateral, the signs on plain film radiography can be identical to those seen in interstitial pulmonary oedema (septal lines, loss of vessel clarity and peribronchial thickening), but if the heart is normal in size and there is hilar adenopathy and/or lobar consolidation, or if the changes are unilateral, the diagnosis of lymphangitis carcinomatosa deserves serious consideration (Fig. 22.43b, p. 504). The clinical story is very helpful, since if the changes are due to pulmonary oedema, the patient usually complains of sudden onset of breathlessness, whereas a patient with lymphangitis carcinomatosa gives a story of slowly increasing dyspnoea over the preceding weeks or months. Computed tomography, particularly high resolution CT (HRCT) has proved very valuable in demonstrating lymphangitis carcinomatosa, because the appearances, in the correct clinical circumstances, are highly specific (Fig. 22.35). The cardinal HRCT signs are non-uniform thickening of the interlobular septa with thickening of the broncovascular bundles in the centre of the pulmonary lobules.
- **Haematogenous metastases**. Distant metastases may be seen in the lung, bones, liver and adrenals.

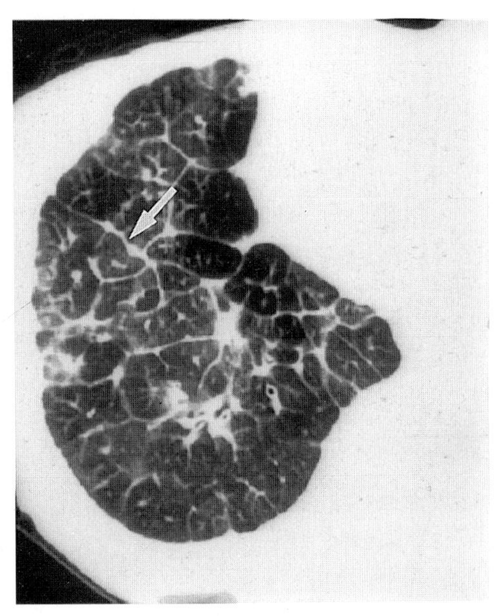

Fig. 22.35 Lymphangitis carcinomatosa. HRCT showing thickening and nodularity of the interlobular septa of the lung. The arrow points to one septum which shows the abnormality particularly well.

PULMONARY METASTASES

The hallmark of blood-borne metastases to the lungs on imaging studies is one or more discrete pulmonary nodules, maximal in the outer portions of the lungs. Metastases vary in size from microscopic to many centimetres in diameter, are usually multiple, and have well or moderately well defined outlines. On occasion, particularly when due to metastatic adenocarcinoma or if the metastases have bled into the surrounding lung, they show irregular or ill-defined edges. Cavitation is seen from time to time, particularly with metastatic squamous cell carcinoma.

Detectable calcification in metastases is very unusual indeed, except in metastases from sarcomas, notably osteosarcoma and chondrosarcoma, in which the calcification is then part of the tumour matrix just as it is in the primary tumour.

Miliary nodulation, a pattern of innumerable tiny nodules resembling miliary tuberculosis, is occasionally encountered but is decidedly rare. Miliary metastases are most likely to be due to thyroid or renal carcinoma.

The standard initial test for the detection of pulmonary metastases is the plain chest radiograph. As with primary lung tumours, metastases have to be almost a centimetre in diameter or larger to be visible on plain chest radiographs or conventional tomograms. CT, particularly spiral (helical) CT, is currently the most sensitive technique available for the detection of pulmonary metastases and can detect metastases as small as 3 mm in diameter. There is, however, a disadvantage attached to the excellent sensitivity of CT. Some small nodules are benign processes such as tuberculomas or fungal granulomas. This is a major diagnostic problem in those parts of the world where tuberculosis and fungal infections are common. Currently, MRI plays no part in diagnosing pulmonary metastases.

CT is only used in selected cases, because it is rarely necessary to demonstrate further metastases once the presence of definite pulmonary metastatic disease has been established. CT can be used in:

- patients with a normal chest radiograph in whom the presence of pulmonary metastases is likely and would significantly alter patient management, e.g. osteo-sarcoma;
- patients who are being considered for surgical resection of known pulmonary metastases;
- distinguishing solitary from multiple pulmonary nodules where the diagnostic dilemma is metastasis versus new primary bronchial carcinoma.

THE PLEURA

PLEURAL EFFUSION

Fluid in the pleural cavity has the same appearance on plain chest radiographs regardless of whether the fluid is a transudate, an exudate, pus or blood. With rare exceptions this is also true even for CT and MRI, though ultrasound may show numerous echoes within the fluid when it is due to pus. Fluid that is free to move collects in the most dependent portions of the pleural cavities which clearly will vary with the position of the patient.

CT and MRI examinations are routinely conducted with the patient in the supine position, whereas ultrasound examination is carried out with the patient in any position that seems desirable to the operator. Position becomes a very important issue when deciding where to place a thoracentesis needle or chest tube as the fluid may well be in a different position at the time of the procedure than when the imaging was performed.

On plain chest radiographs, free pleural effusions assume a variety of shapes, the commonest of which is similar to the shape that would be seen if a large balloon were pressed down into a container of water. The water would be forced around the outer surface of the balloon up the sides of the container. Similarly, in most pleural effusions some fluid is seen running up the sides of the lungs (Fig. 22.36) and into the fissures. With large effusions, fluid may be seen extending over the lung apex. The smooth edge between lung and pleural fluid can often be recognized on an adequately penetrated film, provided the underlying lung is aerated. The fluid itself casts a homogeneous shadow whereas pulmonary consolidations often show patchy air shadows or air bronchograms. In the upright

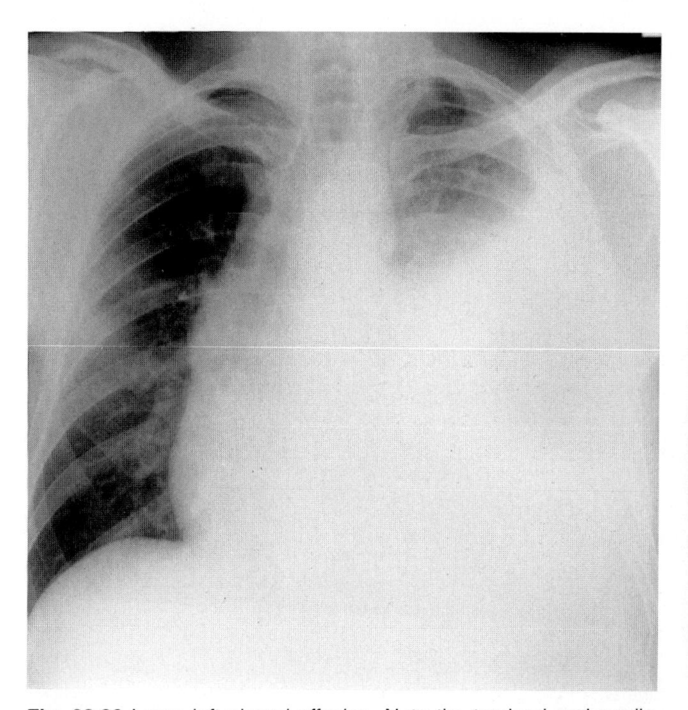

Fig. 22.36 Large left pleural effusion. Note the tracheal and mediastinal shift to the opposite side and the homogeneous opacity of the pleural fluid. The opacity can be seen running up the side of the chest wall to extend over the lung apex, a feature typical of large pleural effusions.

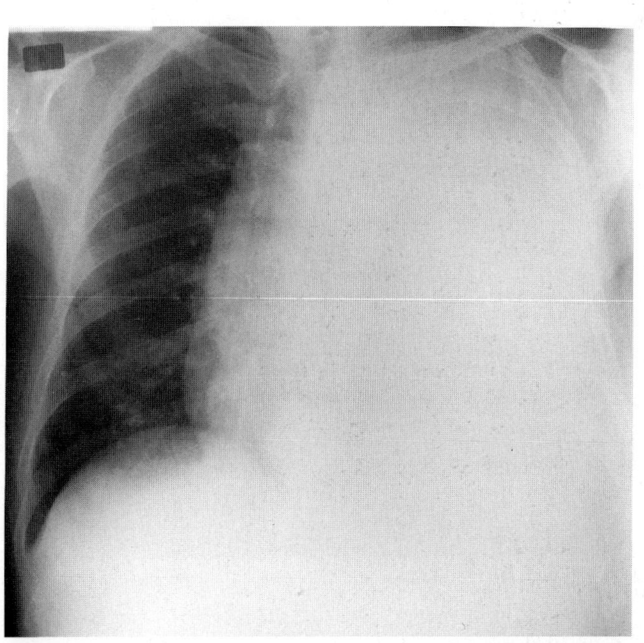

Fig. 22.37 Massive left pleural effusion leading to total opacity of the left hemithorax. The distinction from left lung consolidation or left lung collapse is made by noting the displacement of the trachea away from the side of the opacity. (See Fig. 22.13 for illustration of complete left lung collapse.)

position, all the fluid may lie in a subpulmonary location and the upper border of the fluid may assume a shape similar to the normal hemidiaphragm.

Free pleural effusions have a different appearance on supine compared to upright examinations. In the supine position, the posteriorly layered fluid causes an ill-defined increase in density of the hemithorax and the hemidiaphragm outline is often indistinct. Fluid may be seen over the lung apex, forming a well-demarcated band of density. With large effusions this band of density extends around the outer edge of the whole lung and the entire hemithorax is clearly denser than normal.

Up to 300 ml of pleural fluid may be difficult or impossible to see on standard PA and lateral chest films. If there is doubt about the presence or the amount of fluid, a lateral decubitus view can be of great help. The fluid, if free to move, settles along the dependent lateral chest wall where it can be recognized.

Very large effusions with little underlying pulmonary collapse displace the mediastinum and trachea to the opposite side (Fig. 22.37). Pulmonary collapse is seen in association with larger pleural effusions: the pleural effusion and the pulmonary collapse can both be due to the same basic process, e.g. pneumonia or carcinoma of the lung, or the effusion may have caused compression and collapse of the underlying lung. If the trachea is displaced to the side of the effusion, there must be substantial collapse of the lung, more than could be accounted for by compression collapse alone.

Loculated pleural effusions occur whenever the movement of pleural fluid within the pleural cavity is prevented by pleural adhesions. Loculation occurs in many types of effusions, but it is a particular feature of empyema. The loculations may be anywhere in the pleural cavity, including the fissures. Loculated fluid collections cause oval, lens-shaped or rounded expansions of the pleura and may be confused with pulmonary consolidation or lung abscess, but these misdiagnoses can be avoided by recognizing the clearly defined curved border of a pleural-based density (Fig. 22.38). Often, one or more interfaces with the lung are not tangential to the X-ray beam, and the density, therefore, fades off with an imperceptible border. On a lateral view, a loculated effusion within the oblique or horizontal fissure is clearly lens-shaped and lies within the known position of one of the fissures.

It may be difficult to tell from plain chest radiographs whether an opacity at a lung base is due to pleural effusion or whether it is due to pulmonary consolidation or collapse. The shadow of pleural fluid is usually higher laterally than medially, is homogeneous in density and lies outside the lung, being bounded by a sharp concave interface with the lung. Where the effusion runs into a fissure, both sides of the fissure are visible. The trachea and mediastinum are either central or are pushed to the opposite side.

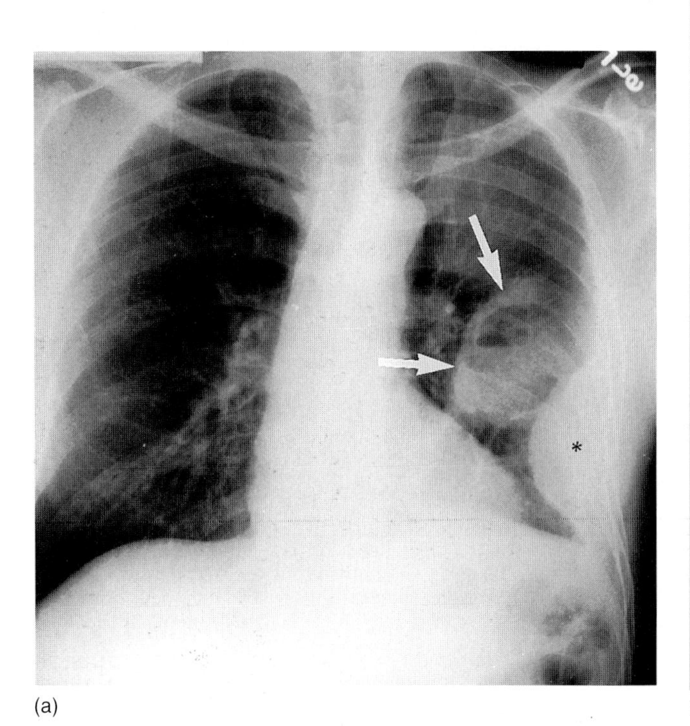

(a)

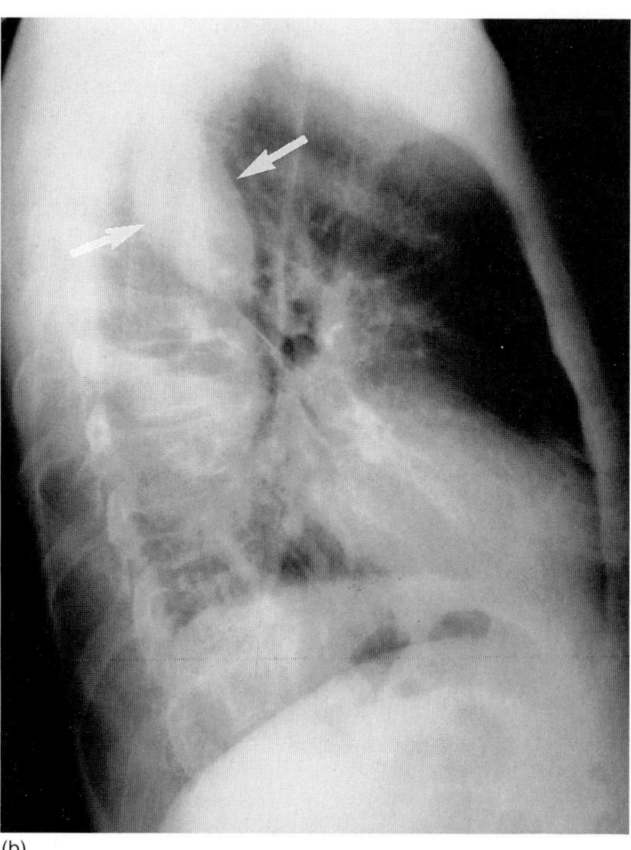

(b)

Fig. 22.38 Comparison of loculated pleural fluid and an intrapulmonary lung abscess. (a) The asterisk is in the centre of a loculated pleural fluid collection lying against the left chest wall. Note the flat base on the parietal pleura and the smoothly curved edge gently fusing with the chest wall pleura. The arrows point to a lung abscess in the left lower lobe. The abscess is round and has a less well-defined interface with surrounding lung. (b) Another loculated fluid collection is present in the upper portion of the left oblique fissure. This collection is best seen in the lateral projection as a lens-shaped opacity, sometimes called an interlobar effusion (arrows).

Conversely, with consolidation or collapse, the shape of the shadow conforms to that of a lobe or segment, an air bronchogram may be present and, where the consolidation abuts a fissure, the fissure is seen as an edge with only one side being visible. With consolidation or collapse, the trachea and mediastinum are either central or pulled toward the side of the shadow.

Computed tomography of pleural effusion

The basic signs of pleural effusion on CT are similar to those on plain film, with the additional information that the density of pleural fluid is homogeneous and, characteristically, pleural fluid is of lower density than most soft tissues (Fig. 22.39), being in the range expected for water, namely –10 to +10 Hounsfield units (HU). Distinguishing between pleural effusion and lobar collapse is very easy with CT, but CT is only occasionally needed because the lateral decubitus view is a simpler method. At CT, the density of the collapsed lobe is usually appreciably greater than that of the pleural effusion, even more so if intravenous

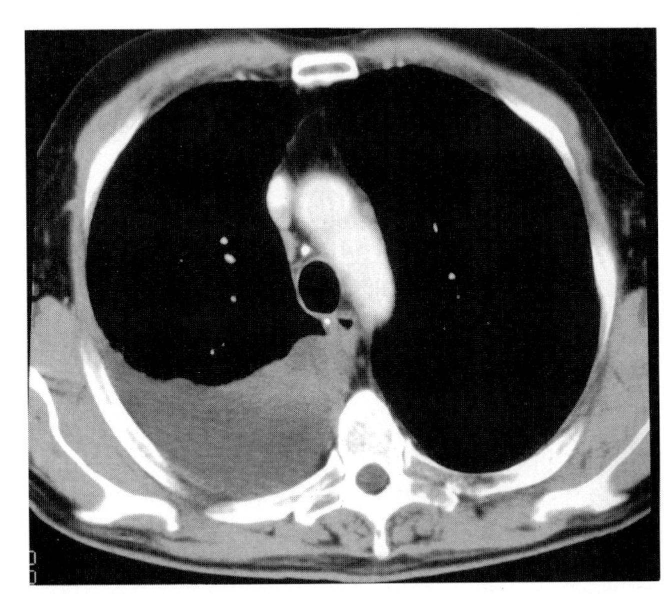

Fig. 22.39 Pleural effusion on CT scan. Note the shape of the opacity, conforming to the shape of the pleural cavity, the smooth interface with lung and a CT density lower than muscle. (The measured density was in the range expected for water.)

contrast enhancement is used. Also, air within the bronchi can often be traced into the compressed lung. The MRI features are essentially the same as for CT.

Surprisingly, it is sometimes difficult to say at CT whether fluid is pleural effusion or ascites. The distinction is made by noting the relationship of the fluid to the diaphragm. Pleural fluid collects outside the diaphragmatic dome and can be seen posterior to the portion of diaphragm that covers the bare area of the liver.

Ultrasound of pleural effusion

Ultrasound examination can be very useful for investigating pleural effusion. At ultrasound, pleural fluid can be recognized as a transonic area between the lung and diaphragm. Since the diaphragm is so well seen there is no confusion with ascites. When pleural fluid loculates against the chest wall, it is possible to place the ultrasound probe directly over the fluid collection, show its size and extent, and determine the best site for needle or chest tube placement.

The main causes for pleural effusion are:

- **Infection**. Pleural effusions due to pneumonia are on the whole small, and the pneumonia is usually the dominant feature on the chest film. Large loculated effusions in association with pneumonia often indicate empyema formation. In some cases of tuberculosis the effusion is the only visible abnormality and the effusion may be large. Subphrenic abscess nearly always produces a pleural effusion.
- **Malignancy**. Effusions are seen with pleural metastases, but it is unusual to see the pleural deposits themselves on plain chest radiographs. Malignant effusions are frequently large. If the effusion is due to bronchogenic carcinoma, other signs of tumour are usually evident.
- **Cardiac failure**. Small bilateral pleural effusions are frequently seen in acute left ventricular failure. Larger pleural effusions may be present in long-standing congestive cardiac failure. The effusions are usually bilateral, often larger on the right than the left. Other evidence of cardiac failure, such as alteration in the size or shape of the heart, pulmonary oedema or the signs of pulmonary venous hypertension, are usually present.
- **Pulmonary infarction**. Effusions in pulmonary infarction are usually small and accompanied by a lung shadow due to the pulmonary infarct itself.

PARAPNEUMONIC PLEURAL EFFUSIONS AND EMPYEMA

There is no generally accepted definition that distinguishes an uncomplicated parapneumonic pleural effusion from an empyema. The factors used to make the distinction centre on the protein levels and white blood cell count of the pleural fluid.

The diagnosis of parapneumonic effusion and empyema depends on recognizing fluid in the pleural cavity and performing thoracentesis to analyse the fluid. Because empyemas are so protein-rich, there is a strong tendency for the pleural fluid to loculate and, therefore, ultrasound or CT may be required to appreciate the full size of the pleural fluid collection.

The distinction between pulmonary consolidation/abscess and loculated pleural fluid has important therapeutic consequences. Empyema requires early tube drainage, whereas adequate antibiotic therapy obviates the need for drainage in most cases of lung abscess. The distinction on conventional radiographs can be difficult. The inner margin of the empyema, like all loculated fluid collections is sharply defined with a curved smooth interface with the adjacent lung when tangential to the X-ray beam.

Computed tomography can be very valuable in deciding between empyema (Fig. 22.40) and a peripherally positioned lung abscess in those cases when the plain chest radiographic features are ambiguous. The distinguishing features at CT are:

- **Shape**. Empyemas, unless very large, are basically lenticular in shape. The angle formed at the interface with the chest wall is obtuse or tapering. Lung abscesses, on the other hand, tend to be spherical and show acute angles at their margins with the chest wall.
- The **walls** of an empyema are formed by thickened visceral and parietal pleura. This thickened pleura is of uniform thickness, enhances following intravenous contrast injection and has a smooth inner

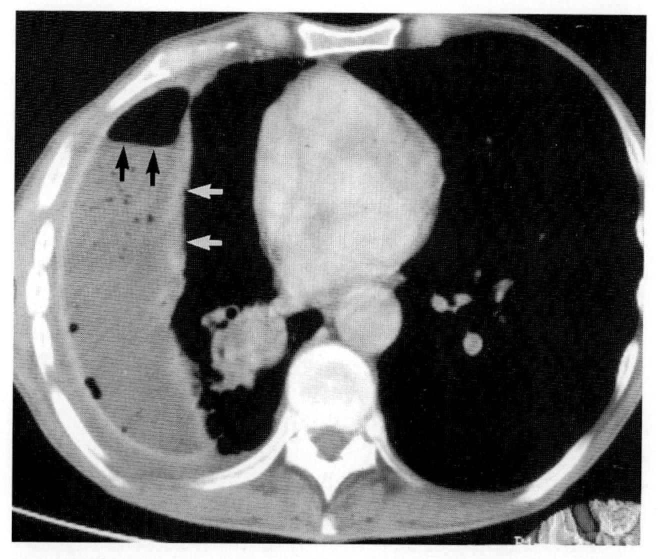

Fig. 22.40 Empyema. CT scan shows a lens-shaped, loculated fluid collection in the right pleural cavity. Note the thickened pleura (horizontal arrows) and the air–fluid level (vertical arrows). There are multiple bubbles of gas trapped in the empyema. Enlarged right hilar nodes are also present.

and outer wall, enclosing the empyema fluid. The wall of a lung abscess is irregular in thickness and has an irregular inner and outer margin. An abscess may contain multiple dots of air and, on occasion, may even show distorted air broncho-grams.

PRIMARY PLEURAL TUMOURS

Primary pleural tumours, namely localized fibrous tumour of the pleura and diffuse malignant mesothelioma, are relatively uncommon.

Localized fibrous tumour of the pleura

Localized fibrous tumour of the pleura has been given a variety of names, including pleural fibroma and benign mesothelioma. These tumours are mostly benign though some may be locally invasive. Unlike diffuse mesothelioma, the localized tumour is not related to asbestos exposure.

On plain chest radiography, the usual finding is a slow-growing, rounded or oval, often lobulated, homogeneous mass in contact with a pleural surface. The lesions vary in size from less than 1 cm to 30 cm diameter, but are usually 7 cm or more at initial presentation.

On CT and MRI, the lesions are well marginated, based on a pleural surface, and show acute angles at their margins. In other words they grow outwards from a relatively narrow base or pedicle. Smaller lesions show uniform soft tissue density, and enhance after intravenous contrast injection, whereas a substantial proportion of the larger lesions show the CT or MRI features of central necrosis.

Diffuse malignant mesothelioma

Malignant mesothelioma is a rare tumour except in patients exposed to asbestos. The imaging features are similar on plain chest radiographs, CT and MRI, but the extent of the tumour and any accompanying pleural fluid is shown with greater accuracy by CT and MRI than by plain radiography.

The imaging findings typically consist of extensive nodular thickening of the pleura (Fig. 22.41), which may conglomerate to form a circumferential lobular sheet of soft tissue density encasing the lung. The tumour often runs into the fissures, accompanied by varying amounts of pleural fluid. Sometimes the accompanying pleural effusion is very large, and if it obscures the pleural masses, the chest radiographic appearances may be indistinguishable from other causes of pleural effusion. At CT (and MRI scanning), the soft tissue density of the tumour tissue can be readily distinguished from the adjacent pleural effusion, but the nodules may on occasion be so tiny that they are unrecognizable and the only imaging feature in these cases is a pleural effusion.

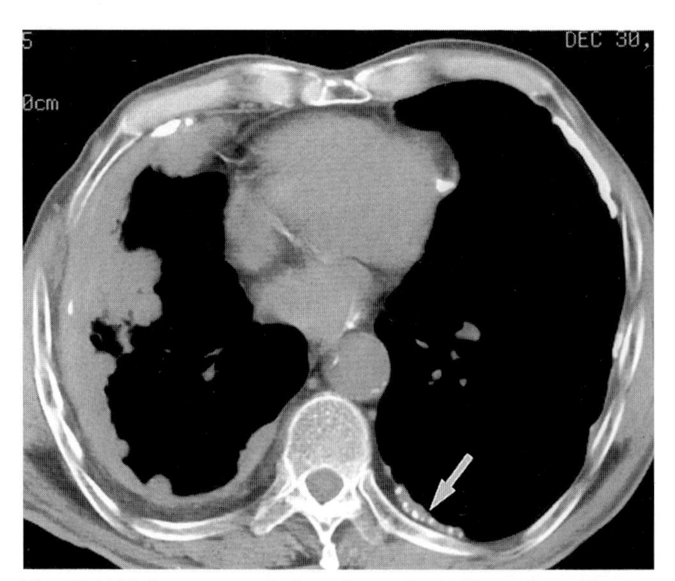

Fig. 22.41 Malignant mesothelioma in a patient with previous asbestos exposure. The sheet of tumour masses in the pleura surrounding the right lung is well demonstrated. Note the calcified pleural plaques in both the right and left pleural cavities (the arrow points to one of the partially calcified asbestos-related pleural plaques in the left pleural cavity).

Chest wall invasion, bone destruction and direct extension to the pericardium and other mediastinal structures, involvement of mediastinal lymph nodes and invasion through the diaphragm into the upper abdomen are all best seen on CT (or MRI). Since many malignant mesotheliomas are secondary to asbestos exposure, asbestos-related pleural plaques may be seen in either pleural cavity.

Very occasionally malignant mesothelioma may take the form of a focal mass similar to localized fibrous tumour of the pleura.

PLEURAL THICKENING

Pleural thickening can be due to fibrosis following previous pleural effusion or haemorrhage, pleural plaque formation in asbestosis or, on occasion, pleural neoplasm. It may be impossible to distinguish pleural fluid from pleural fibrosis on conventional radiographic projections. Comparison with previous films may be necessary to show that the pleural shadow is not changing and is, therefore, likely to be fibrosis. Alternatively, the problem can be tackled by taking a lateral decubitus view, in which free fluid changes its appearance as it falls to lie along the lateral chest wall, whereas pleural thickening or loculated fluid is unaltered in appearance.

The distinction between pleural fluid and soft tissue thickening such as fibrosis or neoplasm is readily made at CT because most pleural fluid shows a CT density of –10 to +10 HU whereas fibrosis/neoplasm shows a density similar to muscle (30–50 HU). The distinction is particularly easy with ultrasound because fluid and solid have such different ultrasonic characteristics. Pleural fibrosis usually produces a smooth edge to the pleural echoes, whereas pleural tumours produce lobulated pleural masses typical of neoplasm. Asbestos-related pleural plaques are flat, sharply demarcated and usually show minimal, if any, lobulation.

PLEURAL CALCIFICATION

Irregular plaques of calcium may be seen with or without accompanying pleural thickening. When unilateral and focal they are likely to be due to either an old empyema, usually tuberculous, or an old haemothorax. Bilateral, patchy pleural calcification is often related to asbestos exposure. Sometimes no cause for pleural calcification can be found.

PLEURAL METASTASES AND MALIGNANT PLEURAL EFFUSION

Metastases to the pleura can originate from carcinoma of almost any organ, but the lung appears to be the most frequent primary site, followed by breast, pancreas, stomach and ovary.

Usually the findings on plain chest radiograph, CT, MRI and ultrasound are those of free or loculated pleural effusion without any specific features to the effusion itself. There may be recognizable tumour nodules in the pleura on CT, ultrasound, or even, occasionally, on chest radiographs.

PNEUMOTHORAX

The diagnosis of pneumothorax depends on recognizing the line of the pleura separated by air from the chest wall, mediastinum or diaphragm with no vessels beyond this line (Fig. 22.42). Lack of vessel shadows alone is insufficient evidence on which to make the diagnosis, since there may be few or no visible vessels in emphysematous bullae. There is often no appreciable increase in the density of the collapsed lung beneath the pneumothorax unless the pneumothorax is very large.

The detection of a small pneumothorax can be very difficult. It is easy to confuse the pleural edge with the cortex of normal ribs and a skin fold can, on occasion, be confused with a pneumothorax. Sometimes a pneumothorax is more obvious on a film taken in expiration.

With tension pneumothorax, there is mediastinal shift, and the hemidiaphragm is often flattened. It is worth noting that tension pneumothoraces are almost invariably large because the underlying lung collapses due to increased pressure in the pleural space.

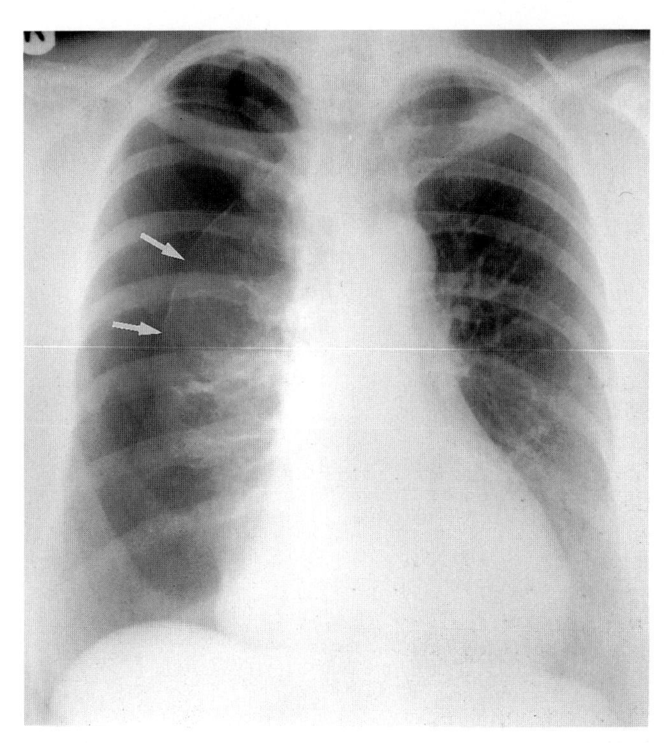

Fig. 22.42 Pneumothorax. The lung edge can be identified (arrows) with a large air collection between the partially collapsed right lung and the right chest wall.

Causes of pneumothorax

Pneumothorax is associated with many underlying disorders of the lung including emphysema, trauma, certain forms of pulmonary fibrosis, tuberculosis and rarely metastases.

The majority, however, occur in young people who have no recognizable lung disease but who have small blebs or bullae at the periphery of their lungs which burst.

Hydropneumothorax, haemopneumothorax and pyopneumothorax

In most cases of pneumothorax, whatever the cause, some fluid is present in the pleural cavity. In spontaneous pneumothorax the fluid is often bloody but the amount is small.

Fluid in the pleural cavity, whether it be a pleural effusion, blood or pus, assumes a different shape in the presence of pneumothorax. The diagnostic feature is the air–fluid level which extends across the hemithorax.

PULMONARY HILA

Hilar enlargement presents two main diagnostic questions. Firstly, is the enlarged hilum due entirely to large blood vessels or to a mass? Secondly, if a hilar

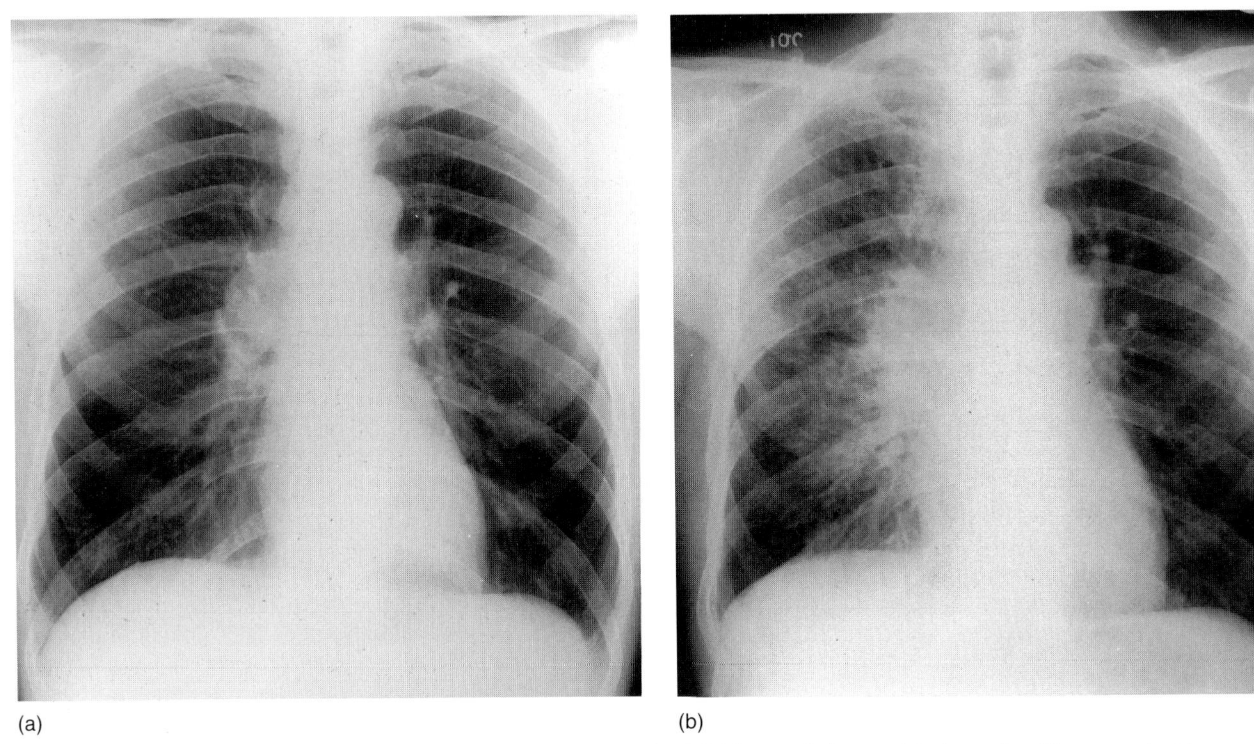

(a) (b)

Fig. 22.43 Hilar mass. (a) The right hilum is substantially larger than the left hilum and shows a lobular outline. The cause in this case was a bronchial carcinoma at the right hilum together with enlargement of the adjacent lymph nodes. (b) Two years later the patient developed right-sided lymphangitis carcinomatosa.

mass is present, what is its nature? The chief possibilities for a hilar mass are enlarged nodes, a bronchial carcinoma or a combination of the two (Fig. 22.43).

It is usually possible to decide on plain chest radiographs whether hilar enlargement is due to large pulmonary arteries by appreciating the branching nature of the shadows and the fact that vascular enlargement is usually bilateral and accompanied by enlargement of the main pulmonary artery and heart. On occasion, it is necessary to perform contrast-enhanced CT which will differentiate between enlarged pulmonary arteries and adenopathy.

MRI is the single best technique for elucidating hilar enlargement. It is, however, rarely required because plain films and CT usually give the necessary information. The advantage of MRI is that there is very little signal from the hilar structures in normal individuals using the usual spin-echo sequences, because there is no signal from fast-flowing blood in the major hilar vessels and no signal from the air within the bronchi. Thus, any hilar mass stands out clearly against the low signal background.

HILAR LYMPH NODE ENLARGEMENT

Usually more than one lymph node is enlarged, so the hilum appears lobulated in outline on plain films.

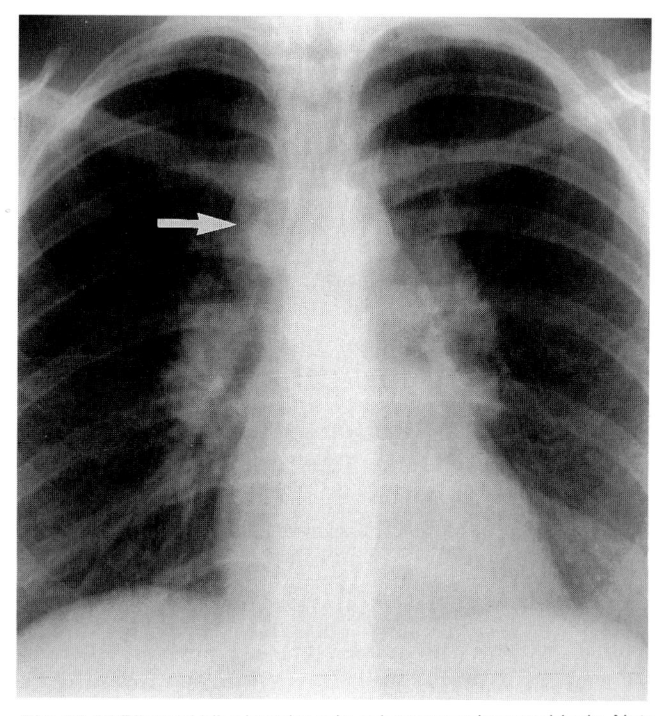

Fig. 22.44 Bilateral hilar lymph node enlargement in sarcoidosis. Note the symmetrical enlargement, the lobular outline of the hila and the enlargement of nodes in the right paratracheal area (arrow).

- **Unilateral enlargement** of hilar lymph nodes may be due to:
  - metastases from carcinoma of the bronchus, in which case the primary tumour is often visible. Metastases from other sites are rare;
  - malignant lymphoma;
  - infections, particularly tuberculosis and histoplasmosis in endemic areas. Hilar adenopathy is occasionally seen accompanying acute bacterial infection. Tuberculosis is the commonest cause of unilateral hilar adenopathy in children.
- **Bilateral enlargement** of hilar nodes occurs in:
  - sarcoidosis (Fig. 22.44), which is far and away the commonest cause. The diagnosis is almost certain if the hilar enlargement is symmetrical and if the patient is asymptomatic, or has either erythema nodosum or iridocyclitis; simultaneous enlargement of the right paratracheal nodes is common and lung changes are sometimes visible;
  - malignant lymphoma;
  - tuberculosis; the African and Asian races show this form of the disease but it is rare in Caucasians;
  - fungus disease, which is a rare cause of hilar enlargement.

THE MEDIASTINUM

CT AND MRI OF THE NORMAL MEDIASTINUM

The appearances at four levels of the thorax are illustrated in Fig. 22.45. The mediastinal structures are surrounded by fat. Important features to note are:

- The bulk of the mediastinum is due to the heart and blood vessels. Blood vessels are easy to recognize as tubular structures retaining a near constant diameter on several adjacent sections. For CT they can be opacified by intravenous contrast medium (in some centres such opacification is used almost routinely). On standard MRI spin-echo sequences, the larger mediastinal blood vessels are seen as signal void due to fast-flowing blood.
- The only other normal structures of appreciable size are the thymus, oesophagus, trachea and bronchi. The thymus is the most difficult to assess because it is so variable in size.
- Normal lymph nodes are small, usually less than 6 mm in short-axis diameter (maximum 10 mm), and most are too small to recognize.

MEDIASTINAL MASSES

Mediastinal masses are usually classified according to their position in the mediastinum; so the first step in diagnosis is to establish the likely anatomical origin using frontal and lateral radiographs supplemented, when necessary, by CT scans.

Plain chest films in mediastinal masses

The presence of a mediastinal mass is often first observed on plain chest radiography. The following general points are helpful when deciding the next steps in management.

- Intrathoracic thyroid masses (**goitres**) are the most frequent cause of a mediastinal mass. The characteristic feature is that the mass extends from the superior mediastinum into the neck and almost invariably compresses or displaces the trachea.
- **Lymphadenopathy** is the next most frequent cause of a mediastinal swelling. Lymphadenopathy may occur in any of the mediastinal compartments. It is often possible to diagnose enlarged lymph nodes from their multiplicity and their lobulated outlines.
- **Neurogenic tumours** are by far the commonest posterior mediastinal lesions. They frequently cause pressure deformity of the adjacent ribs and thoracic spine.
- Certain tumours, such as **dermoid cysts** and **thymomas**, are, for practical purposes, confined to the anterior mediastinum.
- **Calcification** occurs in many conditions but almost never in malignant lymphadenopathy. Occasionally, the calcification is characteristic in appearance, e.g. in aneurysms of the aorta.
- A mediastinal mass due to a **hiatus hernia** is usually easy to diagnose on plain films because it often contains air and may have an air-fluid level, best seen on the lateral view. A film taken after a mouthful of barium has been swallowed will confirm the diagnosis of hiatus hernia.
- Most masses in the **right cardiophrenic angle** anteriorly are benign, e.g. large fat pads, benign pericardial cysts or hernias through the foramen of Morgagni. However, neoplastic involvement of lymph nodes should be considered in patients with known lymphoma or breast carcinoma.

Computed tomography of mediastinal masses

Computed tomography is usually the best method of assessing mediastinal abnormalities when problems remain unanswered from the plain chest radiographs.

- Abnormalities can be accurately localized. Knowledge of the precise shape, position, size and multiplicity of masses frequently narrows the differential diagnosis. For instance, contiguity of the mass with the thyroid in the neck suggests a goitre and multiple oval-shaped masses suggest lymphadenopathy.

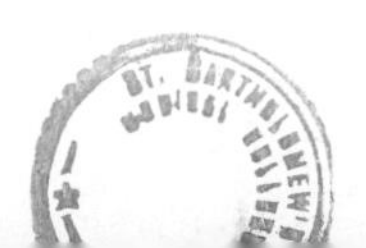

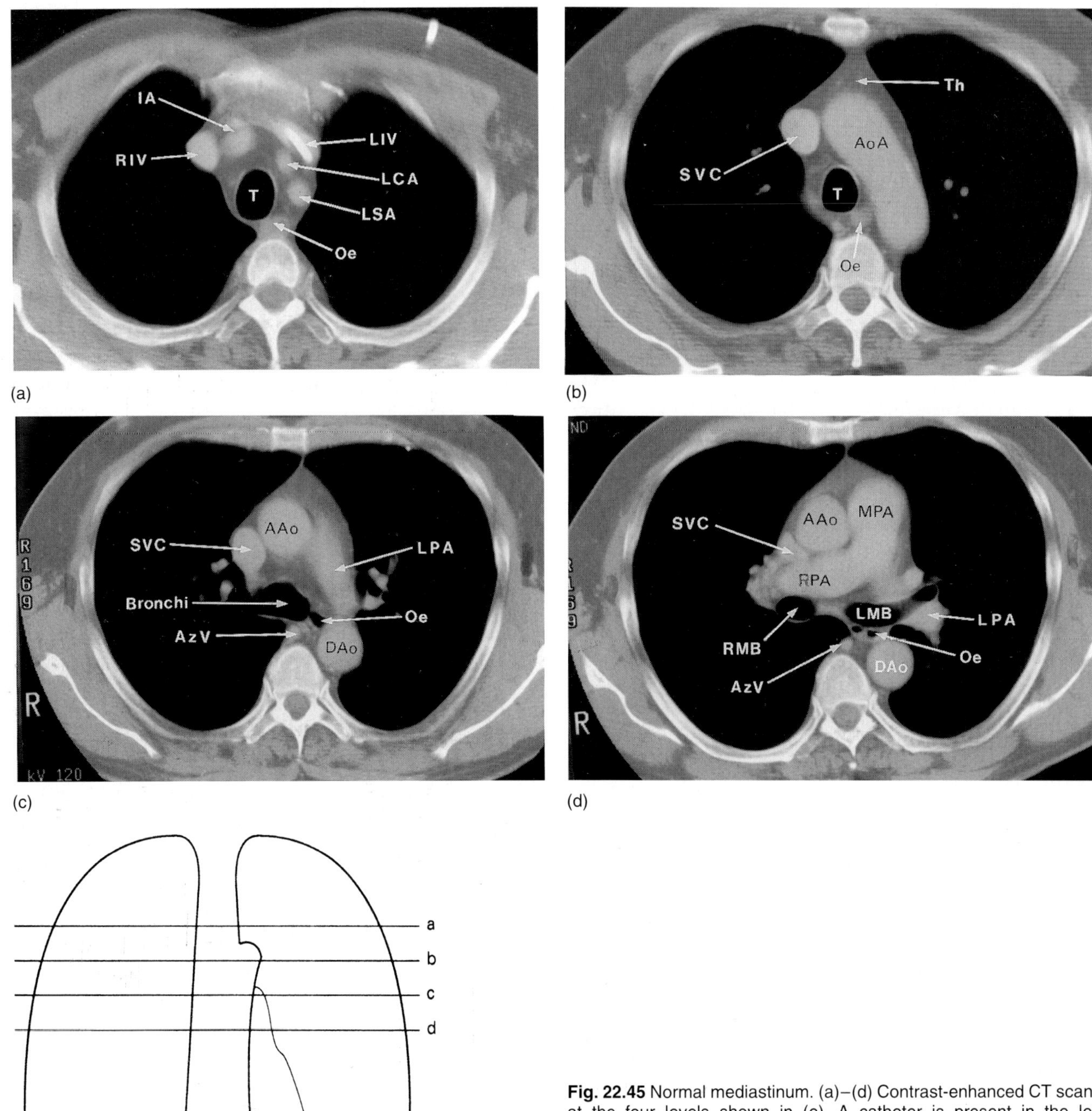

Fig. 22.45 Normal mediastinum. (a)–(d) Contrast-enhanced CT scans at the four levels shown in (e). A catheter is present in the left innominate vein. AoA = aortic arch; AAo = ascending aorta; AzV = azygos vein; DAo = descending aorta; IA = innominate artery; LIV = left innominate vein; LCA = left carotid artery; LPA = left pulmonary artery; LSA = left subclavian artery; MPA = main pulmonary artery; Oe = oesophagus; RIV = right innominate vein; RPA = right pulmonary artery; SVC = superior vena cava; T = trachea; Th = thymus.

- Occasionally, the density of the abnormality reveals its nature.
  - Fat can be recognized as such. This is useful in distinguishing tumours from large cardiophrenic angle fat pads or unusual fat collections. Cystic teratomas (dermoid cysts) may contain recognizable fat.
  - Thyroid tissue has a characteristic higher density than muscle both before and after contrast enhancement.
  - Intravenous contrast enhancement permits ready differentiation of aneurysms and anomalous blood vessels from other masses.
  - Calcification is more readily seen at CT than on plain radiographs. The presence of calcification in a mass excludes untreated malignant neoplastic adenopathy.
  - Cysts containing clear fluid, e.g. pericardial cysts and some bronchogenic cysts, can be diagnosed based on a CT number close to water (0 HU) provided the mass has smooth thin walls and a smooth outline.

Magnetic resonance imaging of mediastinal masses
MRI gives similar information to CT regarding most mediastinal masses, but, because it is a more complex and more expensive examination, it is rarely indicated. MRI does, however, have certain specific advantages. For example, aneurysms and vascular anomalies are readily demonstrable without the need for contrast medium. Also, in some instances, the ability to image in coronal, sagittal or oblique planes may show anatomical relationships that are difficult to demonstrate with CT. This information may help with surgical planning and, on rare occasions, may be of diagnostic value.

INTRATHORACIC THYROID MASSES

Intrathoracic thyroid masses are usually benign multinodular colloid goitres or adenomas, but may occasionally be carcinomas. They are almost invariably downward extensions of thyroid masses that originate in the neck and descend into the mediastinum; the continuity between the mediastinal mass and the thyroid gland in the neck is, therefore, an important diagnostic feature both on conventional films and at CT or MRI (Fig. 22.46).

On plain films, intrathoracic thyroid masses usually have a well-defined outline which may be lobular. Many displace and narrow the trachea; occasionally

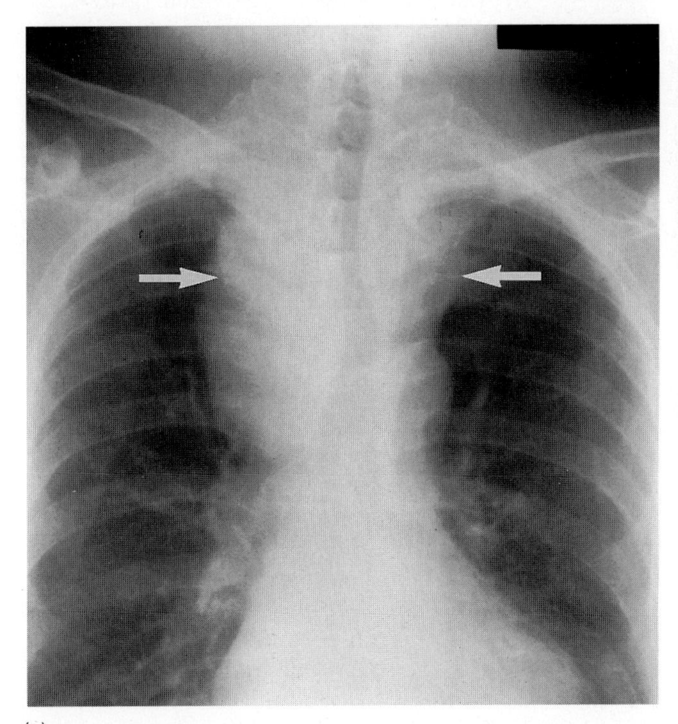

(a)

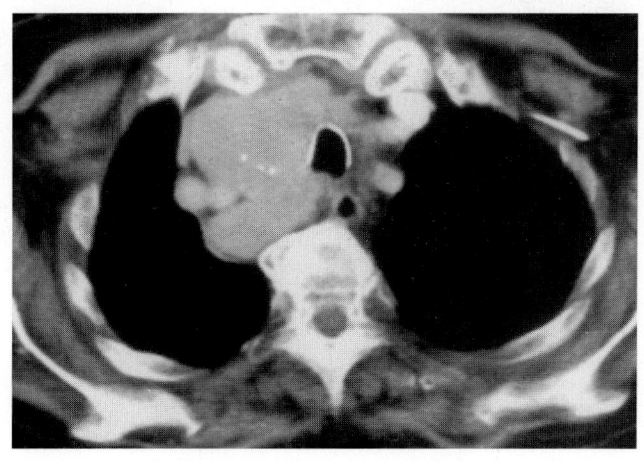

(b)

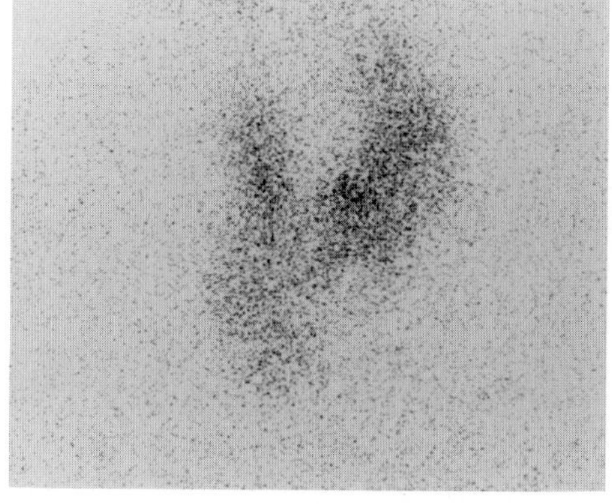

(c)

Fig. 22.46 Intrathoracic multinodular colloid goitre. (a) Note the mass (arrows) to either side of the trachea and contiguity of the mass with the neck. The trachea is deformed and narrowed by the goitre. (b) Contrast-enhanced CT scan of same patient showing a mass of almost the same density as the adjacent enhanced blood vessels. Typical small calcifications are seen within the goitre. (c) Radionuclide scan (iodine-123) showing that the intrathoracic mass concentrates the radionuclide confirming the diagnosis of a thyroid mass.

the narrowing is substantial. The pattern of displacement of the trachea depends on the location of the mass, which is usually predominantly anterior or lateral to the trachea, but is posterior to it in as many as a quarter of cases.

CT scanning demonstrates the shape, size and position of the mass which can be followed to the thyroid gland in the neck. A useful sign indicating a thyroid origin is the relatively high attenuation value of thyroid tissue compared to that of the adjacent muscles on both pre-and post contrast CT images. The attenuation of the normal thyroid tissue within a goitre is the same as thyroid tissue in the neck.

Calcification, which is better seen at CT than on plain film, is a common finding that further aids differential diagnosis from other causes of mediastinal mass. Rounded, focal, low-density areas, more easily visible on the postcontrast films, are equally common.

It is not possible to distinguish definitively between a benign and malignant mass at CT (or MRI) unless the tumour has clearly spread beyond the thyroid gland. If such spread is unequivocal, then the mass should be considered malignant. Multiple masses suggest a benign multinodular goitre.

Radionuclide imaging of the thyroid using radioiodine shows some functioning thyroid tissue in almost all intrathoracic goitres. Radionuclide imaging is very sensitive and specific for determining the thyroid nature of an intrathoracic mass. CT is, however, a useful initial test, because it provides more information should the mass turn out to be something other than thyroid and is almost as specific for diagnosing a thyroid origin.

PARATHYROID MASSES

Hyperparathyroidism may be due to parathyroid adenomas that arise in ectopic parathyroid glands in the mediastinum, usually in or near the thymus. Parathyroid adenomas are often less than 2 cm in diameter. When larger than 1.5–2.0 cm they can usually be recognized at CT, but smaller lesions may be difficult to distinguish from thymic remnants or lymph nodes. Mediastinal parathyroid glands also can be demonstrated by radionuclide imaging (page 395).

THYMIC MASSES

The size of the normal thymus varies dramatically with age, therefore size alone is an unreliable guide to pathology in younger patients. The normal thymus conforms to the shape of the adjacent great vessels on CT and MRI, whereas a thymic mass does not mould to structures such as the aorta. Also, a mass gives rise to a focal asymmetrical swelling.

The most common thymic tumour in adults is thymoma. Other tumours include thymolipoma, malignant lymphoma (notably Hodgkin's disease), thymic carcinoid (which may secrete ACTH and consequently may be responsible for Cushing's syndrome), germ cell tumours or teratomas, and thymic carcinoma.

Thymoma

Thymomas may vary in size from very small to larger than 20 cm in diameter. The tumour may be contained within a capsule or may penetrate the capsule, eventually invading the mediastinum. It is the presence or absence of spread beyond the capsule rather than the histological appearance that determines whether a tumour is labelled benign or malignant (invasive) by the pathologist.

Most patients with non-invasive thymoma have no clinical symptoms due to the tumour itself. Thymomas are, however, associated with a large variety of autoimmune diseases, most notably myasthenia gravis: approximately 35–40% of patients with thymoma have myasthenia gravis and the incidence of thymoma in patients with myasthenia gravis is approximately 10–15%. A variety of other conditions have a recognized association with thymoma, including haematologic cytopenia, notably pure red cell aplasia and hypogammaglobulinaemia.

Only the larger tumours are visible on plain film (Fig. 22.47). Most thymomas are anterior to the ascending aorta above the right ventricular outflow tract. A few are situated in the lower third of the mediastinum. Thymomas are usually spherical or have lobulated borders.

Thymic tumours are best seen with CT: thymomas are usually of homogeneous density and enhance either patchily or uniformly (Fig. 22.47). Punctate, curvilinear or ring-like calcification is frequent in both benign and invasive thymomas.

The diagnosis of thymoma depends on identifying a focal swelling rather than applying specific measurements. Before age 30, diagnosing a small thymoma can be difficult because the normal gland is variable in size and in myasthenia gravis the associated hyperplasia may lead to a bulky gland. Fortunately thymoma is so infrequent in children that the potentially difficult problem of finding a thymoma in a child with myasthenia gravis rarely arises.

Invasive thymomas invade the mediastinal fat and eventually spread to the pericardium and pleura, and may spread via the pleura and may give rise to 'drop metastases'. Blood-borne metastases are rare. Until mediastinal invasion has occurred, it is not possible to distinguish benign from invasive thymoma even with CT.

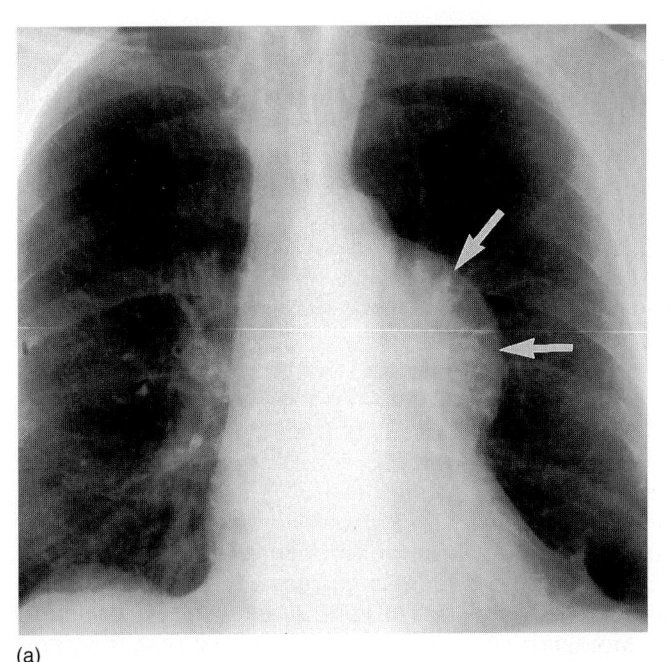

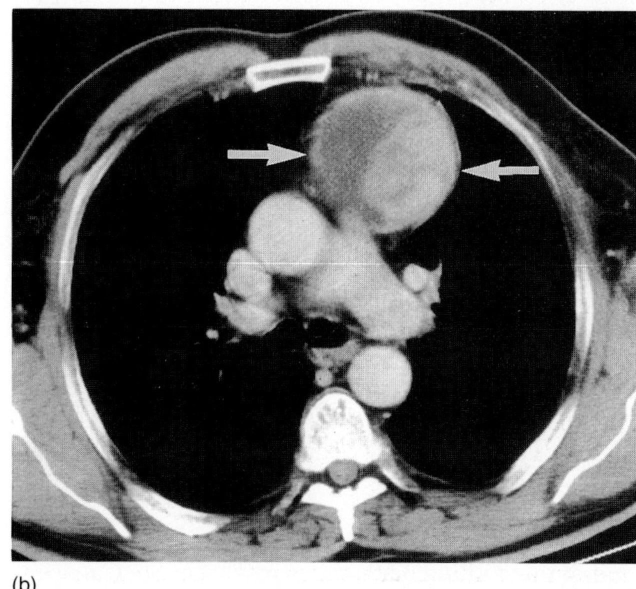

(a) (b)

Fig. 22.47 Thymoma. (a) Plain film showing the smooth, well-defined mass (arrows) projecting from the left side of the mediastinum. (b) Contrast-enhanced CT scan in the same patient showing the thymoma (arrows). In this case there is variable contrast enhancement in different parts of the tumour.

Thymic cysts

Thymic cysts are usually simple cysts, some of which may be congenital origin, within an otherwise normal or hyperplastic gland. Simple thymic cysts may be unilocular or multilocular. They are most frequently encountered in children and are usually asymptomatic. Thymic cysts may also be found within thymomas, lymphoma or thymic germ cell tumours, or may be due to radiotherapy.

On plain film, simple thymic cysts are indistinguishable from other non-lobulated thymic masses, notably thymoma. CT and MRI may demonstrate the presence of pure fluid within the cyst (Fig. 22.48), but some thymic cysts may be of higher CT density, depending on the nature of the fluid, and be misdiagnosed as solid.

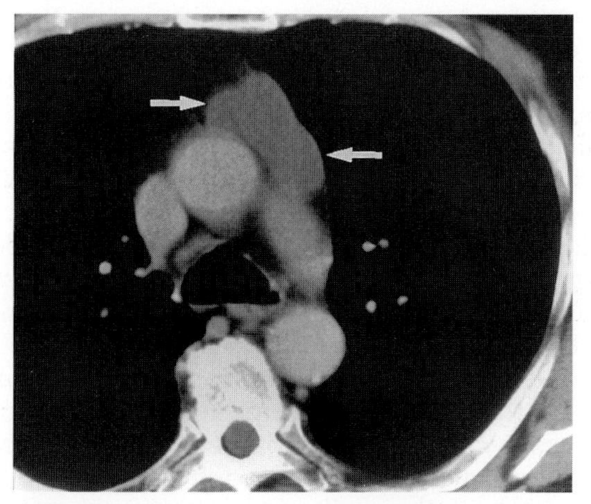

Fig. 22.48 Thymic cyst. Contrast-enhanced CT scan showing a lobular-shaped, fluid density mass (arrows) centred on the thymus.

Thymic hyperplasia

Thymic hyperplasia is rarely recognizable on any imaging modality. CT and MRI may show enlargement of both lobes of an otherwise normally shaped gland with density/signal compatible with normal thymus.

The thymus may atrophy rapidly in response to stress or to therapy with steroids and antineoplastic drugs. The gland usually grows back to its original size upon recovery or cessation of treatment. In the phenomenon known as rebound thymic hyperplasia, the gland grows back to become larger than normal.

When rebound thymic hyperplasia is seen in patients previously treated for a malignant neoplasm, there may be difficulty in distinguishing thymic involvement by neoplasm from thymic rebound. The diagnosis depends on the absence of clinical or other features indicating recurrence of tumour in a patient with a reason for thymic rebound. Helpful features on CT are that the gland, though enlarged, has normal density, retains a normal shape with a smooth outline, conforms to the shape of adjacent structures, and is symmetrical in shape.

TERATOMA AND GERM CELL TUMOURS OF THE MEDIASTINUM

Benign cystic teratomas usually produce a well-defined, rounded or lobulated mass in the anterior

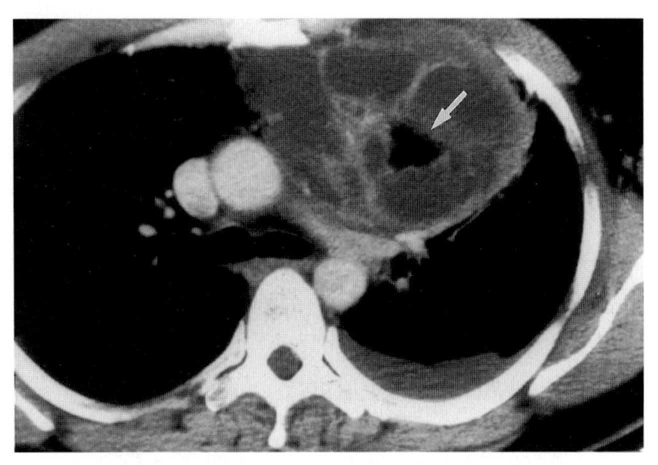

Fig. 22.49 Benign cystic teratoma of mediastinum. Contrast-enhanced CT scan showing a large oval-shaped anterior mass containing a combination of densities: fluid, fat (arrow) and enhancing septa.

mediastinum. Most teratomas project mainly to one side of the midline; sometimes markedly so. Calcification, ossification or even teeth may be visible on plain chest radiograph and, occasionally, sufficient fat is present to be detectable radiographically.

CT and MRI show the shape and contents of the mass to advantage (Fig. 22.49). Fat and fluid contents are readily identified. The combination of a large anterior mediastinal mass, which is wholly or predominantly cystic, together with a well defined wall, is highly suggestive of the diagnosis of benign cystic teratoma. The presence of teeth or unequivocal fat within the mass is pathognomonic.

The plain film findings of **malignant germ cell tumours** are similar to benign teratomas except that the mass is often lobular in outline, fat density is not noted and calcification is a rare finding. Unlike benign teratoma, the malignant forms grow rapidly, and metastases may be seen in the lungs, bones or pleura. CT and MRI show an asymmetrical mass which may have a lobular outline. The adjacent mediastinal fat planes may be obliterated and extensive local invasion may be identified. The tumours show either homogeneous soft tissue density or multiple areas of contrast enhancement interspersed with rounded areas of decreased attenuation due to necrosis and hemorrhage. Rarely, coarse tumour calcification may be seen.

MEDIASTINAL CYSTS

Most mediastinal cysts are developmental in origin. The usual entities included in this category are bronchogenic (bronchial) cysts, oesophageal duplication cysts, neurenteric cysts and pericardial cysts. The distinction between these cysts is not always clear cut. On rare occasions, a pancreatic pseudocyst extends into the posterior mediastinun.

On plain film all these cysts are usually predominantly spherical or oval in shape. Most bronchogenic cysts are in intimate contact with a major airway, whereas oesophageal cysts contact the oesophagus, pericardial cysts contact the pericardium and neurenteric cysts lie between the oesophagus and the spine. CT and MRI show a thin-or thick-walled cyst containing fluid, but the fluid content may be difficult to diagnose if previous haemorrhage has occurred.

INTRATHORACIC NEURAL TUMOURS

Intrathoracic neural tumours can be divided into nerve sheath tumours, ganglion cell tumours and paragangliomas (e.g. phaeochromocytoma)

Nerve sheath tumours comprise schwannomas (neurilemmoma), neurofibromas and their malignant counterparts. All are more common in patients with neurofibromatosis. Nerve sheath tumours arise predominantly from either the intercostal or the sympathetic nerves; some arise from the phrenic or vagus nerves. Many arise close to the spine and may extend through the neural exit foramina into the spinal canal (the so-called 'dumb-bell tumour')

The **ganglion cell tumours** form a spectrum, with neuroblastoma at the malignant end and ganglioneuroma at the benign end, ganglioneuroblastoma being an intermediate form. Neuroblastoma and ganglioneuroblastoma are essentially tumours of childhood. Ganglioneuroma shows a wider and more even age distribution, ranging from 1 to 50 years.

Nerve sheath and ganglion cell tumours appear as well-defined masses with a smooth or lobulated outline. When they are localized, it is not possible to distinguish benign from malignant tumours. The tumours may be almost any size; some are very large, occupying most of a hemithorax. Except for vagal and phrenic nerve tumours, and the occasional neuroblastoma, neural tumours are situated in the posterior mediastinum (Fig. 22.50). An important diagnostic feature is pressure deformity and displacement of the adjacent ribs and vertebrae, and the intervertebral foramina may appear widened.

On CT scanning, many neural tumours have mixed density, including low attenuation regions. Being vascular lesions, they enhance on images taken after the administration of intravascular contrast medium. Calcification is a feature of the ganglion cell tumours. One great advantage of CT is the superior demonstration of spinal and intraspinal involvement compared to plain films. MRI is even better than CT at demonstrating or excluding intraspinal involvement.

Fewer than 2% of **phaeochromocytomas** occur in the chest. Most are found in the posterior mediastinum or adjacent to the heart and pericardium, particularly in the wall of the left atrium or the interatrial septum. They form rounded soft tissue

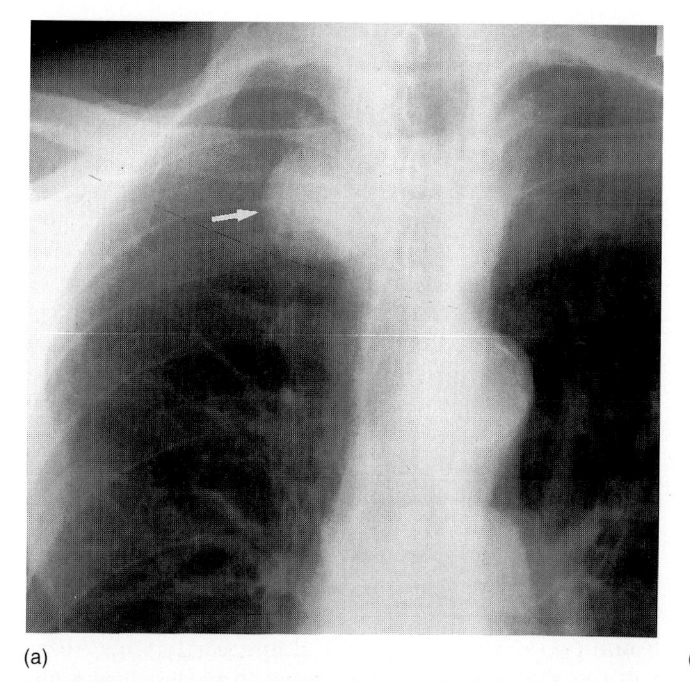
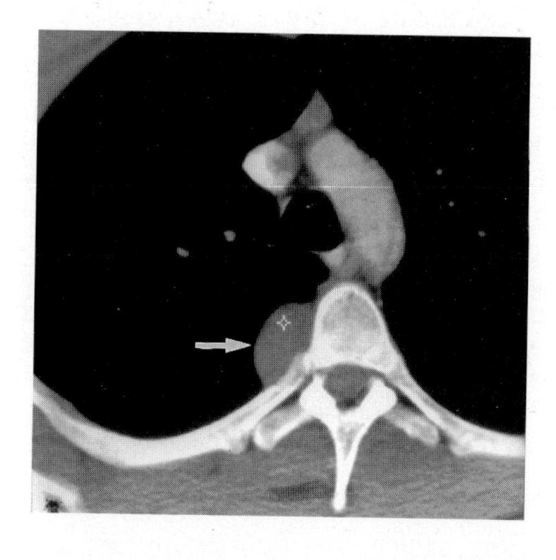

(a) (b)

Fig. 22.50 Neural tumour in the posterior mediastinum. (a) Plain film showing a smooth, round, right paravertebral mass (arrow). (b) Contrast-enhanced CT scan showing the precise location of the tumour (arrow). The small cross is a cursor used to measure density. In this case the measured density was in the low soft tissue range.

masses which are usually extremely vascular and, therefore, enhance brightly at CT after administration of intravenous contrast material. Radioiodine MIBG (meta-iodobenzylguanidine) and somatostatin receptor scintigraphy are good methods of identifying extra-adrenal phaeochromocytomas.

On MRI, phaeochromocytomas show signal intensity similar to muscle on T_1-weighted images and very high signal intensity on T_2-weighted images. MRI is particularly useful for demonstrating intracardiac phaeochromocytomas.

THORACIC AORTIC ANEURYSMS

This subject is discussed on page 548.

OESPHAGEAL RUPTURE

This subject is discussed on page 60.

PNEUMOMEDIASTINUM

Air in the mediastinum indicates a tear in the oesophagus or an air leak from the bronchi, which may be spontaneous or follow trauma from, for example, swallowed foreign bodies or endoscopy.

Spontaneous leakage of air from the bronchial tree is most commonly seen in patients with asthma or following severe vomiting when air tracks through the interstitial tissues of the lung into the mediastinum after rupture of a small airway. The air is seen as fine streaks of transradiancy within the mediastinum, often extending upward into the neck (Fig. 22.51).

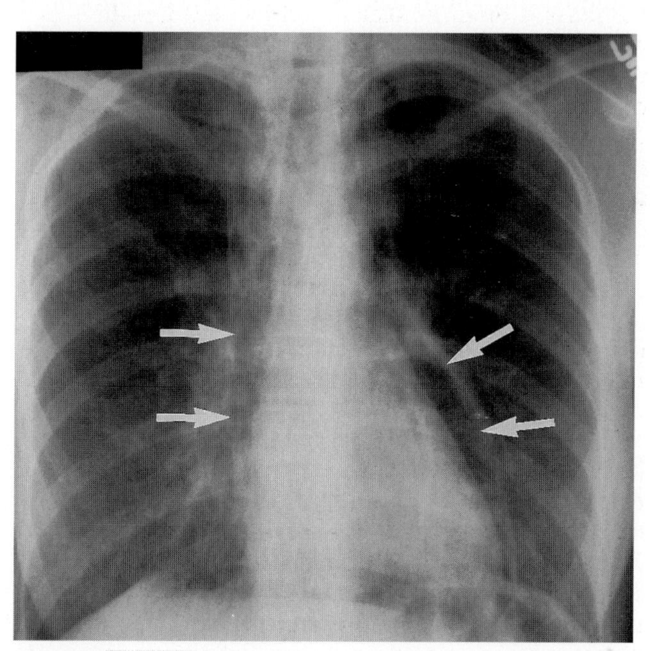

Fig. 22.51 Pneumomediastinum. The streaky air throughout the mediastinum has displaced the mediastinal pleura laterally (arrows).

THE DIAPHRAGM

The position of the diaphragm may reflect disease: both domes may be pushed up by abdominal distension, whereas unilateral elevation of a hemidiaphragm occurs with loss of volume of the ipsilateral lung or it may be due to abdominal pathology, such as an abdominal mass or a subphrenic abscess. It is important to realize that minor or moderate elevation of a hemidiaphragm is a relatively common incidental finding of no significance. The cause of a substantially elevated hemidiaphragm should be sought from the clinical features or from chest or abdominal films. It should always be borne in mind that subpulmonary effusion may mimic elevation of one or both hemidiaphragms. Marked elevation of one hemidiaphragm with no other visible abnormality suggests either paralysis or eventration.

Paralysis of the diaphragm results from disorders of the phrenic nerves, e.g. invasion by carcinoma of the bronchus. The signs are elevation of one hemidiaphragm which on fluoroscopy or ultrasound shows paradoxical movement, i.e. it moves upward on inspiration.

Eventration of the diaphragm is a congenital condition in which the diaphragm lacks muscle and becomes a thin membranous sheet. Except in the neonatal period it is almost always an incidental finding and does not cause symptoms. When the whole of one hemidiaphragm is involved, almost invariably the left, that hemidiaphragm is markedly elevated. On fluoroscopy or ultrasound, the hemidiaphragm may remain fixed during inspiration and expiration, but when more severely involved it moves paradoxically and cannot be distinguished from paralysis. The eventration may only involve part of one hemidiaphragm, resulting in a smooth 'hump'.

Rupture of the diaphragm is discussed on page 513.

THE CHEST WALL

The chest wall should be examined for evidence of soft tissue swelling or rib abnormality. Because ribs are curved structures, some portions are always foreshortened on plain chest radiographs. Therefore, if a rib abnormality is suspected, oblique views should be obtained.

Rib metastases from a tumour of the bronchus, breast, kidney, thyroid and prostate are common. All except prostatic and breast cancers produce mainly or exclusively lytic metastases. Sclerotic metastases in an elderly man suggest a prostatic primary cancer. Sclerotic or mixed lytic and sclerotic deposits in a woman suggest that the primary carcinoma is in the breast.

Destruction of the cortex, particularly the upper border of a rib, is the best sign of lytic metastases. Care should be taken when diagnosing destruction of the lower borders of the posterior portions of the ribs, since these regions are poorly seen even in normal people. When in doubt it is always wise to compare with the opposite side. Another pitfall in the diagnosis of rib metastases is that blood vessels in the lungs may cause confusing shadows. This cannot arise at the edges of the chest where the lung does not project over the ribs, so the edge of the chest is a useful place to look for bone destruction. Soft tissue swelling is frequently seen adjacent to a rib deposit. When sclerotic metastases are suspected the best place to look is in the medulla of the ribs, particularly where no lung overlies the rib.

Congenital abnormalities of the ribs are common but rarely of clinical significance. It is important not to mistake bifid ribs or fused ribs for lung shadows.

Soft tissue swelling occurs with a number of rib lesions: fractures, infections and neoplasms. The soft tissue swelling may be more obvious than the rib lesion on a chest radiograph. If an opacity suggesting soft tissue swelling is seen arising from the chest wall, it is vital to obtain a good view of the underlying ribs using oblique views or CT where necessary.

CT or MRI can be very useful in elucidating chest wall disease. The greatest advantage is in the display of soft tissue masses and bone destruction, particularly chest wall invasion from an underlying carcinoma of the lung.

TRAUMA TO THE CHEST

RIB FRACTURE

The best view to demonstrate a rib fracture varies with the location of the fracture. The standard chest film, which provides information about intrathoracic injury as well as chest wall damage, serves as the frontal view of those ribs which are not obscured by the diaphragm or heart. Oblique views of symptomatic ribs can be added. For ribs below the diaphragm and behind the heart, penetrated frontal and oblique views are necessary. It is, therefore, essential that the clinician informs the radiographer precisely which ribs are to be evaluated.

Recognizing a rib fracture depends on noting the loss of continuity of the cortex of the rib. There is usually a step across the fracture site. Haematomas that accompany rib fractures are frequently visible as extrapleural soft tissue swellings. Such swelling may be the most obvious or sometimes the only sign of fracture. Not infrequently, rib fractures are invisible because there is no displacement, or because the projection is suboptimal. Fractures through costal cartilage or costochondral junctions cannot be diagnosed with conventional radiographic techniques.

Because fractures of the upper three ribs indicate severe trauma, their presence requires careful evaluation for bronchial or aortic injury. Similarly, fracture of the lower two ribs should raise suspicion of damage to the liver, spleen and kidney. Serious intrathoracic injury can, however, occur without rib fracture, particularly in children.

LUNG CONTUSION AND LACERATION

Lung contusion appears on plain chest radiographs within six hours of injury as a non-segmental patchy or homogeneous consolidation, usually, but not invariably, on the traumatized side. Resolution begins within 48 hours and is complete within three to four days. If the consolidation does not clear within 72 hours, an alternative diagnosis for the pulmonary shadow should be considered, e.g. continued bleeding, pneumonia or atelectasis. Rib fracture and pleural fluid (haemothorax) are frequently present but many patients with clinically significant and even life-threatening pulmonary contusion do not have rib fractures.

Lung laceration may be seen with both blunt and penetrating trauma. The tear in the lung may fill with haematoma or may expand with air to become a **pneumatocele**. Pneumatocoeles often contain an air–fluid level due to blood in the air space. The lung laceration may be hidden by the contusion. As the contusion clears, haematoma may persist as a fairly well-defined rounded or oval density. Pneumatocoeles are seen as rounded air lucencies that appear soon after the injury and usually disappear quickly. Their rapid appearance after injury distinguishes them from lung cavitation.

The CT features of lung contusion and laceration are similar to the plain film findings discussed above. There is little practical information to be gained from evaluating these lesions by CT, even though CT, as in so many conditions, shows their extent more accurately.

PLEURAL AND CHEST WALL ABNORMALITIES FOLLOWING TRAUMA

Fluid in the pleural cavity following trauma is usually blood or, very rarely, chyle from thoracic duct injury. The radiology of haemothorax and chylothorax is identical to that of pleural effusion (p. 498). Haemothorax after trauma may be caused by laceration of the lung, intercostal vessels, great vessels, or diaphragm or may accompany a lung contusion. Massive or persistent bleeding suggests serious mediastinal blood vessel or intercostal artery injury.

Pneumothorax following trauma can be due to lung laceration from penetrating injury or from the sharp end of a rib fracture. When seen in cases of blunt trauma, it may be due to shearing or compression forces. Accompanying blood in the pneumothorax space is common and is recognized by noting an air–fluid level. The radiology of pneumothorax has been described on page 503.

In trauma victims, CT scans may show a pneumothorax not visible on plain chest radiographs. This is partly because of the inherent advantages of CT, but also because chest radiographs in a trauma setting are so often single views in the supine position exposed with mobile machines. With CT examinations, by comparison, the standard procedure is much the same for both the traumatized and non-traumatized patient. Chest CT is almost never required exclusively to look for pneumothorax as any sizeable pneumothorax will be recognized on a chest radiograph.

In pneumothorax, the air rises to the uppermost portion of the pleural cavity which, in the supine patient, is just above the diaphragm. Thus, if an abdominal CT has been obtained, the sections through the lower chest may show a significant pneumothorax that may have been overlooked or invisible on a plain chest radiograph.

CHEST WALL EMPHYSEMA

Subcutaneous emphysema of the chest wall is usually, in itself, of no significance, but its recognition may lead to the finding of significant abnormality such as fractured rib with associated pneumothorax or tear of a major bronchus.

TRACHEOBRONCHIAL TEAR

Tracheobronchial tears occur only with major thoracic trauma, usually an anterior chest wall deceleration injury. The major problem with bronchial tear is the late complication of significant bronchostenosis.

Pneumomediastinum, lobar collapse and pneumothorax, particularly one that does not respond to chest tube suction, are the important imaging signs. It should be remembered, however, that a significant proportion of patients who subsequently develop bronchostenosis have no radiographic evidence of a bronchial tear, probably because the integrity of the bronchial sheath is maintained.

RUPTURED DIAPHRAGM

Ruptured diaphragm is usually the result of blunt trauma to the lower chest and upper abdomen; 95% of cases involve the left hemidiaphragm. Rib fracture and ruptured spleen are commonly associated.

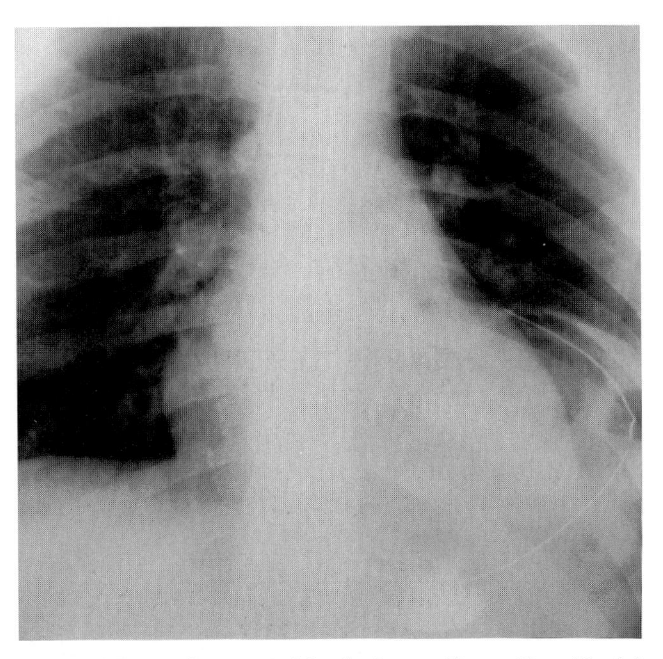

Fig. 22.52 Traumatic rupture of the diaphragm. The position of the left hemidiaphragm is ambiguous. In this case the course of the nasogastric tube shows that the stomach lies within the chest. What appears to be elevated left hemidiaphragm is in fact the stomach herniated through a rent in the left hemidiaphragm.

The radiological signs are pleural effusion and herniation of abdominal contents through the diaphragm. The tear itself is not visualized, even at CT, though it can sometimes be recognized on ultrasound. The diagnosis is frequently difficult, since it is often impossible to be sure of the position of the diaphragm on plain radiography or even on CT, especially if pleural effusion develops. Therefore, it is not easy to say if bowel or stomach are above or below the diaphragm. If a nasogastric tube has been inserted, the course of the tube may show herniated stomach (Fig. 22.52). Ultrasound can be a useful technique to search for a diaphragmatic rupture. In clinical practice, many cases of ruptured diaphragm are missed initially.

TRAUMATIC RUPTURE OF THE AORTA

Traumatic rupture of the aorta is usually due to sudden deceleration injury, which produces severe shearing stresses. In almost all patients who survive the initial accident, the rupture is at the aortic isthmus just beyond the origin of the left subclavian artery. The next most common site of injury is the origin of the brachiocephalic artery.

The plain chest film signs of aortic injury are purely those of the resulting haematoma. The haemorrhage results in mediastinal widening and lack of clarity of the aortic arch. The trachea and left main bronchus may be displaced away from the bleeding site. The mediastinal haematoma may dissect extrapleurally and can be recognized over the lung apex, almost invariably the left. Free pleural fluid will be noted if the haematoma has ruptured into the pleural space. Because the initial injury is severe, other signs of chest trauma, such as fractured ribs and pulmonary contusion, are frequently seen. Post-traumatic aneurysms only occur several weeks after the initial injury and, therefore, immediately after the accident the contours of the aorta itself may not be recognizably abnormal.

Whenever the possibility of traumatic rupture of the aorta is being seriously entertained on combined clinical and plain film grounds, aortography should be considered. It is the most sensitive and the most specific test available.

The laceration itself is rarely demonstrated on CT, but may, on occasion, be seen as a small pseudoaneurysm or a linear lucency caused by the torn intima within the lumen of the aorta, provided intravenous contrast opacification has been used. What CT shows is mediastinal haemorrhage, either diffuse mediastinal haemorrhage or a focal haematoma close to the laceration. Mediastinal haemorrhage alone is not enough to establish the diagnosis of laceration of the aorta or great vessels since the haemorrhage may be from damage to smaller branches of the aorta or rupture of mediastinal veins. Spiral CT with multiplanar reformatting appears a promising technique and may replace angiography as may MRI once the technique is widely available to very sick patients.

There is one situation in which CT may obviate aortography, namely in a patient in whom the clinical probability of a ruptured aorta is very low, but in whom the plain chest radiographs show non-specific mediastinal widening. CT scanning may then be able to demonstrate an alternative, clinically unimportant, reason for the plain film findings such as fat deposition or aortic unfolding.

INTERVENTIONAL RADIOLOGY OF THE CHEST

Virtually all image-guided interventional techniques used in other parts of the body have been adapted for interventional radiology of chest disease.

PERCUTANEOUS NEEDLE BIOPSY OF THE LUNG

The usual methods of obtaining a sample of lung tissue for histological, cytological or bacteriological examination are open lung or thoracoscopic biopsy, transbronchoscopic biopsy and percutaneous needle biopsy. The most appropriate technique depends on the site, size and likely nature of the pulmonary lesion.

Percutaneous needle biopsy is usually performed to confirm a suspected lung cancer, to obtain micro-organisms from an area of consolidation or lung abscess or to diagnose the nature of a mediastinal mass.

Percutaneous needle biopsy is clearly useful in patients with suspected pulmonary malignancy that is inoperable because of metastatic disease, tumours too extensive to resect, poor lung function or general debility. The value of percutaneous needle biopsy in patients with suspected lung cancer that is considered operable is less certain. A clear-cut benign diagnosis which would obviate the need for surgery is rare based on needle biopsy samples. Patient management is, therefore, rarely influenced by the percutaneous needle biopsy.

Although there are no absolute contraindications to percutaneous needle biopsy, a number of factors significantly increase the risk of complications. The most important are an uncooperative patient, severe chronic obstructive pulmonary disease, pulmonary arterial hypertension, a contralateral pneumonectomy and a significant coagulopathy.

Technique

Percutaneous biopsy needles can be broadly categorized into those that are used to aspirate material for cytological examination and those that have a cutting action and so provide a core of tissue for histological examination.

Fluoroscopy is the most common method for guidance of percutaneous needle biopsy, but CT can be used and ultrasound control can be useful for lesions in contact with the chest wall.

Before a fluoroscopic-guided biopsy is performed, the lesion must be accurately localized using postero-anterior and lateral radiographs. If the lesion is not visible on a lateral radiograph (and therefore unlikely to be seen on the lateral projection of biplane fluoroscopy), CT is used to gauge the precise depth of the lesion. Tests to exclude a coagulation defect are desirable but not essential. Premedication is rarely necessary if the procedure has been carefully explained to the patient. Discussing the risks of the procedure with the patient is essential, including the chance of pneumothorax, which may require a chest drain, and the possibility of haemoptysis. It is also helpful to warn the patient before starting the procedure that several needle passes may be necessary.

The needle is marked to an appropriate level before insertion so that its tip will lie within the lesion. Measurements are taken from either the lateral radiograph, which must include an allowance for magnification, or from CT. The needle is advanced smoothly along the line of the central X-ray beam with the breath held. On single-plane fluoroscopy a satisfactory position is suggested when the lesion is seen to move synchronously and with the same excursion as the tip of the needle.

An expiratory chest radiograph is usually obtained within the first 3 hours after the procedure. If no pneumothorax has developed at 4 hours and the patient is asymptomatic, many centres allow outpatients to leave the hospital, since the subsequent development of a pneumothorax becomes increasingly unlikely.

Complications of percutaneous needle biopsy

The most common complications of percutaneous needle biopsy are pneumothorax and minor haemoptysis. Rarer complications include air embolism, major haemoptysis, haemothorax, empyema formation, cardiac tamponade and implantation of tumour in the needle track.

Even though the number of patients requiring a chest drain following percutaneous needle biopsy is small (well under 10%), percutaneous needle biopsy should not be performed unless the operator is prepared to treat an iatrogenic pneumothorax instantly.

Accuracy of percutaneous needle biopsy

The cytological or histopathological statement 'no evidence of malignant disease' encompasses two different circumstances:

- a nodule from which no malignant cells are identified but for which no specific pathological diagnosis is offered;
- a nodule in which a specific benign diagnosis can be reached, e.g. pulmonary infarct or hamartoma.

It should be noted that a definitive benign biopsy by percutaneous needle biopsy is rare. Percutaneous needle biopsy specimens that are reported as containing 'inflammatory' or necrotic material should be considered non-specific and should not be considered as equivalent to excluding malignancy.

PERCUTANEOUS DRAINAGE OF INTRATHORACIC FLUID COLLECTIONS

Percutaneous drainage techniques of fluid collections within the thorax have increased with improved image guidance, particularly ultrasonography and CT. An advantage of cross-sectional imaging is the ability to identify loculations and, in the case of ultrasonography, septations within the pleural collection that may alter the management strategy. Supplementary techniques include the instillation of fibrinolytic agents for the treatment of loculated empyemas and sclerotherapy for malignant effusions.

The indications for the percutaneous drainage of an intrathoracic fluid collection include relief of symptoms caused by the mass effect of a large effusion;

drainage of an empyema; drainage of a mediastinal pus collection (most often post-sternotomy), and drainage of a sterile chronic pleural collection, e.g. a malignant effusion.

There are no absolute contraindications to the percutaneous drainage of intrathoracic fluid collections apart from a patient who is unable to cooperate. Impaired haemostasis is a relative contraindication.

Technique

The most commonly used drainage catheters are 8F to 16F catheters with a large internal luminal diameter and a number of side holes. Larger bore drainage catheters are less likely to clog when the collection contains fibrinous material, blood clots or necrotic debris. Smaller bore tubes are better tolerated by patients, especially children, and drainage catheters as small as 8F are satisfactory for non-viscous fluid collections.

Image guidance

The choice of image guidance is determined by the site and size of the collection, as well as the operator's preference.

Fluoroscopy can be used to guide the positioning of catheters in large collections. CT allows more precision in placing the catheter, whereas ultrasonography is a quick and efficient technique for identifying pleural collections and placing the catheter, provided that no subcutaneous air or calcification is in the pleural rind to prevent sonographic access and no bone blocks the path of the ultrasound beam.

Once the route of access has been chosen, the skin is cleaned and the proposed entry site is infiltrated with local anaesthetic. A 22-gauge needle may then be inserted directly into the cavity to confirm that there is no bony obstacle and to aspirate fluid for analysis. The needle can then be exchanged for a percutaneously placed drainage catheter into the most dependent portion of the cavity. Track dilatation is necessary if a guidewire is used.

Complications of drainage procedures

Serious complications of percutaneous catheter drainage are rare, the most important being severe haemorrhage. Kinking and blockage of the catheter occur frequently but can often be rectified without replacement of the catheter. Inadvertent puncture of major cardiovascular structures or the liver is less frequent with CT guidance and a guidewire technique.

TRACHEOBRONCHIAL STENTS

Stenting is indicated in patients with major airway obstruction in whom other treatments have failed to provide long-term palliation, particularly stenosis of a main airway by bronchial carcinoma which is a significant and distressing cause of severe breathlessness and recurrent infections.

The most widely, currently available, expanding metallic stents are the Gianturco and the Wallstent. Both of these stents are positioned through a sheath. Because these stents are collapsed and preloaded in a cartridge, they are relatively easy to position. Metallic stents can cross the orifice of an adjacent bronchus without obstructing that airway. Although placement can be performed under either fluoroscopic or bronchoscopic control alone, in practice the procedure is best performed by a combination of the two techniques.

Metallic mesh stents rapidly become covered by epithelium, usually within one month. They are most effective when the stenosis is caused by extrinsic neoplastic compression of the airways or for holding open a floppy malacic segment. Multiple stents can be placed for long stenoses.

SUPERIOR VENA CAVA STENTS

This topic is discussed on page 567.

CARDIAC IMAGING TECHNIQUES

Echocardiography, radionuclide examinations and plain films are the standard non-invasive imaging cardiac investigations. Angiography and angiocardiography are specialized techniques for visualizing the coronary arteries and the left ventricle in acquired heart disease and for demonstrating a large variety of congenital heart disorders. MRI provides both functional and anatomical information but is only available in specialized centres and requires specific indications.

CARDIAC ECHOCARDIOGRAPHY

Standard echocardiography demonstrates a fan-shaped slice of the heart in motion, which can be recorded on video tape with still images when necessary. By angling the transducer, the 'slice' can be moved through the heart to allow the observer to build up a mental picture of a three-dimensional image. Since tiny bubbles of air accompany the injection of almost any liquid and because ultrasound reliably detects even tiny gas bubbles within the blood stream, injections of saline can be used as a harmless intravascular 'contrast agent'.

The routine examination consists of a combination of short- and long-axis views, together with the so-called four-chamber view (Fig. 22.53). The short- and long-axis views show a cross-section of the left ventricle and mitral and aortic valves. These views

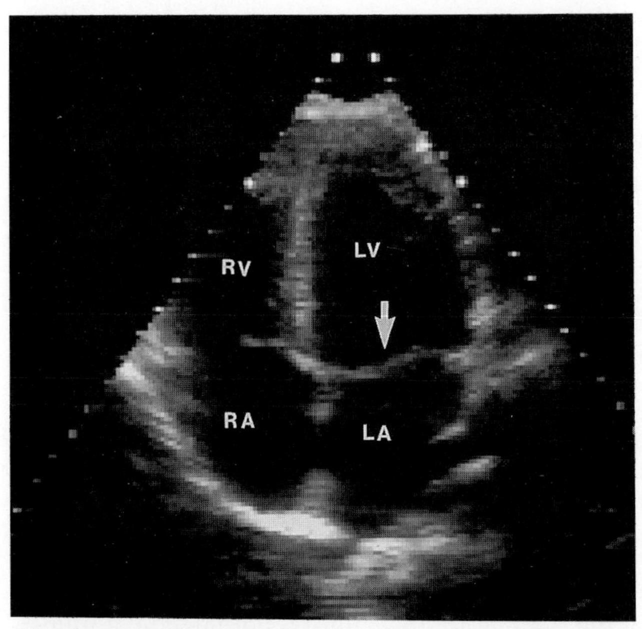

Fig. 22.53 Echocardiography. Normal four-chamber view of heart. Note the normal mitral valve (arrow) between the left atrium (LA) and left ventricle (LV). RA = right atrium; RV = right ventricle. (Courtesy of Mrs Jackie Richardson, Nottingham.)

are obtained by placing the transducer in an intercostal space just to the left of the sternum (or in some individuals, in a subcostal position). The four-chamber view, which shows both ventricles and both atria together with the mitral and tricuspid valves, is obtained by placing the transducer over the cardiac apex and aiming upward and medially. A recently introduced device is the oesophageal ultrasound probe, which looks at the cardiac structures from within the oesophagus behind the heart.

DOPPLER ECHOCARDIOGRAPHY

As discussed on page 6, when sound waves are reflected from a moving object, the frequency of the reflected waves is altered, depending on the velocity of the reflecting surface. Red blood cells can be used as reflecting surfaces and the velocity of blood flow in a given direction can be calculated. The accuracy of the technique depends on the angle of flow with respect to the ultrasound beam, flow directly in line with the beam being the most accurately measured.

Doppler flow measurements are used to:

- quantify pressure gradients across stenotic valves;
- quantify flow;
- measure cardiac output or left to right shunts;
- detect and quantify valvular regurgitation.

Pressure gradients are derived mathematically from formulae that convert velocity across a valve into a pressure gradient. Flow measurements depend on measuring the velocity by Doppler methods and then, using standard ultrasound techniques, calculating the cross-sectional areas of the structure through which the blood is flowing.

A relatively newly introduced technique is colour Doppler where the direction and velocity of a flow are colour-coded allowing the observer to appreciate the direction and magnitude of flow in specific anatomical sites. Colour Doppler is particularly useful in complex congenital heart disease, e.g. finding multiple or unusually situated ventricular septal defects.

CARDIAC CATHETERIZATION AND ANGIOGRAPHY

Catheters can be introduced under fluoroscopic control into the various chambers of the heart and into vessels that lead in and out of these chambers. Contrast injected through such catheters provide images of the heart and great vessels. An injection into the left ventricle gives information on ventricular contractility. From images in systole and diastole the ejection fraction can be calculated. Cardiac angiography is a specialized topic which will not be discussed further.

Coronary angiography, which provides detailed information about coronary artery stenoses, occlusions and collateral or anomalous vessels, is widely practised in patients being considered for cardiac surgery, particularly for coronary artery revascularization. The transfemoral route is standard; catheters being introduced by the Seldinger technique and passed selectively into the orifices of each coronary artery. Separate catheters are usually needed for the left and right sides; 4–7 ml of contrast medium are injected and observed fluoroscopically with video and cine recordings being made simultaneously.

CARDIAC DISEASE

CARDIAC CHAMBER ENLARGEMENT

Diagnosing ventricular enlargement or distinguishing ventricular hypertrophy from dilation by looking at the external contours of the heart on plain films is fraught with problems. Estimation of ventricular volumes has, therefore, become the province of echocardiography.

Assessment of atrial size on the plain chest radiographs, particularly left atrial enlargement, is easier (Fig. 22.54). The right border of an enlarged left atrium is visible as a double contour adjacent to the right heart border, usually within the main cardiac shadow. The left border is rarely visible, though the left atrial appendage, when dilated, is seen as a bulge below the

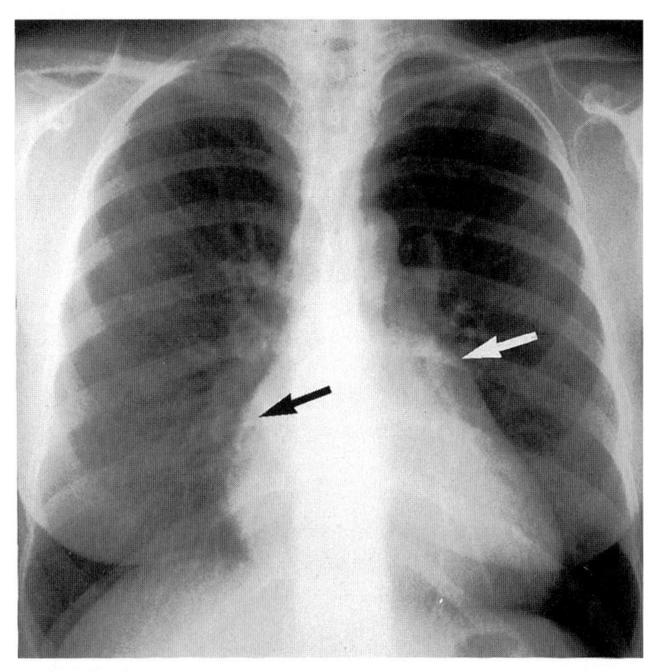

Fig. 22.54 Enlargement of the left atrium in a patient with mitral valve disease recognizable on plain chest radiograph by observing the bulge on the left heart border (white arrow) due to enlargement of the left atrial appendage, and by noting the double contour on the right side of the cardiac shadow representing the edge of the enlarged left atrium (black arrow).

main pulmonary artery on the frontal PA view. With massive left atrial enlargement the left main bronchus is pushed upwards.

Right atrial enlargement causes an increase in the curvature of the right heart border and is often accompanied by enlargement of the superior vena cava. As with ventricular volumes, accurate assessment of atrial volumes is best performed by cardiac ultrasound.

VENTRICULAR CONTRACTILITY

Real-time echocardiography, radionuclide angiocardiography and cine-MRI are all good non-invasive methods of assessing ventricular wall motion. Two major patterns of **decreased contractility** (hypokinesis) are seen:

- Generalized uniform reduction in contractility, which is usually due to valvular disorder or congestive cardiomyopathy. The ventricles in these conditions are usually dilated. Occasionally, multivessel coronary artery disease can also cause a similar pattern.
- Focal reduction in contractility, which may or may not be accompanied by dilatation, is seen with ischaemic heart disease.

Increased contractility of the left ventricle indicates hypertrophy, which can be primary (hypertrophic cardiomyopathy) or secondary to other conditions such as aortic stenosis or systemic hypertension.

PULMONARY OEDEMA AND HEART FAILURE

There are two main causes of pulmonary oedema: oedema due to circulatory problems, e.g. acute left ventricular failure and fluid overload, and non-cardiogenic pulmonary oedema, the mechanism seen in adult respiratory distress syndrome (ARDS). ARDS is discussed separately on page 493.

Pulmonary oedema due to circulatory problems occurs when the pulmonary venous pressure is above 24–25 mm Hg (the oncotic pressure of plasma). Initially, pulmonary oedema is seen in the interstitial tissues but, when more severe, the oedema is also visible in the alveoli.

Interstitial oedema causes thickening of the interstitial tissues of the lungs. Septal lines and thickening of the fissures are the hallmarks of interstitial pulmonary oedema. Septal lines are divided into Kerley A and B lines. The latter are short, horizontal, 1–2 cm lines at the extreme edge of the lungs, best appreciated at the bases. A lines are 3–6 cm long and radiate from the hila mainly in the middle and upper zones.

Alveolar oedema causes pulmonary shadowing maximal close to the hila which fades out peripherally, leaving a relatively clear zone around the edges of the lobes. This pattern is sometimes called the 'butterfly' or the 'bat's wing' pattern (Fig. 22.55).

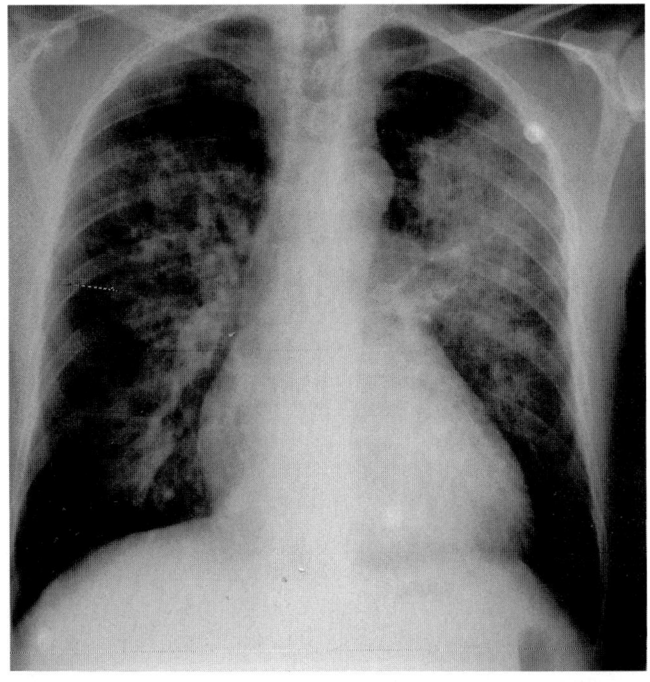

Fig. 22.55 Pulmonary oedema. Plain chest radiograph showing the 'butterfly' or 'bat's-wing' pattern of alveolar oedema, in this case due to acute left ventricular failure following a myocardial infarction.

Although the classic radiographic description of alveolar oedema is a bilaterally symmetrical appearance, symmetry is in fact unusual, and alveolar oedema often predominates on one side or the other and varies in severity from lobe to lobe. It is possible to recognize raised pulmonary venous pressure even in the absence of visible pulmonary oedema when the pulmonary vessels in the upper zones enlarge. The diagnosis needs to be made with caution, however, since it may be difficult to decide whether the vessels are truly enlarged. Also, other causes of redistribution of blood flow to the upper zones, e.g. basal pulmonary emboli and basal emphysema, need to be considered.

Heart failure is recognized radiographically by cardiac enlargement, evidence of raised pulmonary venous pressure and bilateral pleural effusions (Fig. 22.56). Sometimes the effusion on one or both sides may be too small to recognize. In severe cases these changes are accompanied by pulmonary oedema.

Non-cardiogenic oedema (see p. 493) may initially appear identical to 'cardiogenic' pulmonary oedema, but in ARDS the pulmonary shadowing becomes uniform over a period of days, until eventually all parts of the lungs are fairly equally affected. A helpful feature in distinguishing 'cardiogenic' pulmonary oedema from ARDS or widespread pulmonary exudates is the rapidity with which the oedema appears and disappears on treatment. Substantial changes in the severity of air–space filling in a 24-hour period strongly suggest 'cardiogenic' pulmonary oedema.

Widespread pneumonia and pulmonary haemorrhage may give an appearance identical to pulmonary oedema.

VALVULAR DISEASE

Information regarding valve movement and deformity is best obtained by echocardiography. Normally, the leaflets of all the valves are thin and give rise to clearly defined echoes. Valve stenosis causes thickening of the valve leaflets, restriction of movement and narrowing of the orifice (Fig. 22.57). Calcification, which is often present, is seen as a multiplicity of bright echoes arising within the leaflets. Pressure gradients across valves and the severity of any regurgitation can be calculated using Doppler techniques.

The only plain film information directly relating to the morphology of the valves is calcification which is an important feature of aortic stenosis. Calcification is better seen at fluoroscopy than on plain films.

The only imaging techniques that are capable of diagnosing the infective vegetations of **subacute bacterial endocarditis** as opposed to the accompanying valvular regurgitation, are echocardiography and MRI. The resolution of these techniques, however, is insufficient to exclude small vegetations. Vegetations

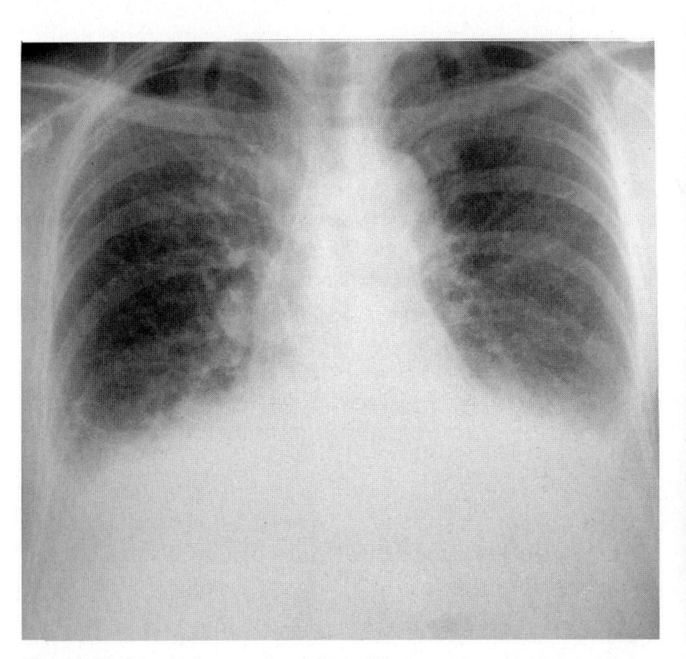

Fig. 22.56 Congestive cardiac failure. The heart is enlarged and there are bilateral effusions. The lung vessels are enlarged, particularly those in the upper zones indicating raised pulmonary venous pressure.

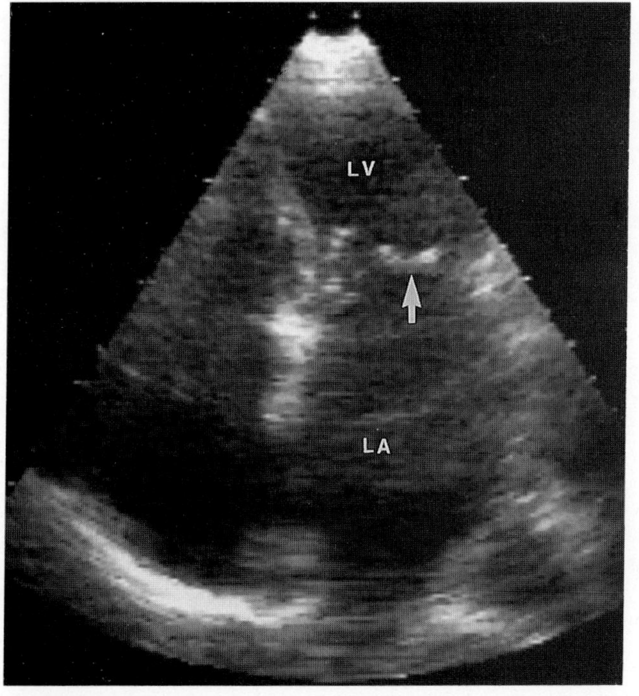

Fig. 22.57 Mitral stenosis shown by echocardiography (four-chamber view). Note the large left atrium (LA) and the greatly thickened and deformed mitral valve (arrow). LV = left ventricle. (Courtesy of Mrs Jackie Richardson, Nottingham.)

on prosthetic valves are extremely difficult to identify.

PERICARDIAL DISEASE

Echocardiography is ideally suited to detect pericardial fluid which is recognized as an echo-free space between the wall of the left ventricle and the pericardium. The nature of the fluid cannot usually be ascertained, and needle aspiration of the fluid may be necessary; such aspiration is best performed under ultrasound control.

Pericardial effusion is also readily diagnosed at CT; it is often seen in patients being examined for other reasons. The examination is rarely recommended specifically to detect pericardial effusion since echocardiography is a quicker and easier method of diagnosis, particularly in an emergency setting. When pericardial thickening or tumour is suspected, CT and magnetic resonance imaging (MRI) may provide more information than echocardiography.

It is unusual to be able to diagnose a pericardial effusion from the plain chest radiograph. Indeed, a patient may have sufficient pericardial fluid to cause life-threatening tamponade, but only have mild cardiac enlargement with an otherwise normal contour. A marked increase or decrease in the transverse cardiac diameter within a week or two, particularly if no pulmonary oedema occurs, is virtually diagnostic of the condition. Pericardial effusion should also be considered when the heart is greatly enlarged and there are no features to suggest specific chamber enlargement.

LEFT ATRIAL MYXOMA

Intracardiac tumours are rare: left atrial myxoma is the most frequently encountered. It is a benign tumour which usually arises in the interatrial septum or in the wall of the left atrium. As it enlarges, the myxoma becomes pedunculated and floats in the left atrial cavity. The myxoma may, therefore, interfere with the function of the mitral valve and mimic mitral stenosis or regurgitation both clinically and on plain chest radiograph. Echocardiography has proved to be an excellent tool for its diagnosis. A mass of echoes is seen in the cavity of the left atrium just behind the mitral valve. The mass usually prolapses into the mitral valve orifice during diastole. The only differential diagnosis is left atrial thrombus in patients with rheumatic mitral stenosis. MRI has also proved to be an excellent method of demonstrating left atrial myxoma and other intracardiac tumours.

ISCHAEMIC HEART DISEASE

Most patients with angina or myocardial infarction have a normal plain chest film and a normal echocardiogram. The signs which may be present on plain chest radiograph include signs of raised pulmonary venous pressure, pulmonary oedema, cardiac enlargement, and left ventricular aneurysm formation. Atheromatous calcification may be seen in the coronary arteries but, as elsewhere in the body, arterial calcification, though indicating the presence of atheroma, is a poor indicator of its severity.

Conventional echocardiography can demonstrate the volume of the left ventricle and the motion of the various segments of its wall. Areas of diminished movement due to infarction can be seen, as can aneurysm formation. Blood clot contained within an aneurysm can be recognized as numerous constant echoes in the cavity of the aneurysm.

Thallium-201 myocardial scintigraphy can determine areas of myocardial ischaemia and from their location it is sometimes possible to predict which of the coronary arteries is compromised. Thallium scanning not only enables a diagnosis of ischaemia to be made but it can also help distinguish ischaemic muscle from scar due to infarction. Ischaemic areas seen on the exercise scan show normal activity on the resting scan. Infarcted areas in which there is little, if any, remaining viable myocardium will show a defect on both the exercise and the resting scans. This ability to distinguish ischaemia and infarction may be useful when planning cardiac surgery.

Radionuclide-gated blood pool studies use red blood cells labelled in vivo with technetium-99m. This technique is used as an alternative to thallium-201 scintigraphy in order to diagnose myocardial ischaemia, to assess changes in ejection fraction between rest and exercise, and to diagnose aneurysm formation. Ischaemic but viable areas may move normally at rest but not on exercise, whereas infarcted areas move poorly both at rest and on exercise, and aneurysms appear as an area of paradoxical movement which bulges outward when the remainder of the ventricle contracts.

Demonstrating the state of the coronary arteries is the province of coronary arteriography; a detailed description is beyond the scope of this book.

CHAPTER 23

Arteries and lymphatics

Roger H.S. Gregson

Arteriography is an invasive radiological procedure, which involves the injection of a radiopaque liquid into an artery resulting in the production of exquisite diagnostic information. Modern diagnostic arteriography owes its widespread development to Seldinger, a Swedish radiologist, who described the technique of percutaneous catheterization of the femoral artery in 1953. The unrivalled position of arteriography has been eroded over the last 20 years by the introduction of non-invasive imaging techniques such as ultrasound, radionuclide studies, computed tomography (CT) and magnetic resonance imaging (MRI). Today arteriography is undergoing a renaissance owing to the development of therapeutic interventional vascular techniques, many of which were originally pioneered by Dotter, an American radiologist.

ARTERIAL CATHETERIZATION

EQUIPMENT

The requirements for the percutaneous catheterization of an artery are a needle, a guide wire and a catheter.

Diagnostic and Interventional Radiology in Surgical Practice. Edited by P. Armstrong and M.L. Wastie. Published in 1997 by Chapman & Hall, London. ISBN 0 412 61960 1 (HB) 0 412 61970 9 (PB)

Needles

The needle is used to produce a direct percutaneous channel into the artery. There are two types of arterial puncture needle in common usage – a one-piece disposable needle with a sharp bevelled tip and a two-piece disposable needle with an outer cannula and an inner stylette. Most needles are 18–20 gauge in size and 6–10 cm in length. A guidewire is passed through the needle or cannula into the lumen of the artery.

Guidewires

The guidewire is initially used to carry the catheter through the skin and subcutaneous soft tissues into the artery and then to carry the catheter through the arterial system itself. There are many types of guidewire, but they all have a single basic design – a short, soft, flexible tip at one end, that is relatively atraumatic to the arterial intima; a long, firm, flexible wire in the middle and a short stiffer rigid tip at the other end, onto which the catheter is threaded. Most guidewires are coated with Teflon to reduce friction, are 0.035–0.038 in in diameter and 100–150 cm in length. The flexible tip is either straight or J-shaped with a radius of curvature between 1.5 and 15 mm. A guidewire with a straight tip is suitable for a non-diseased vessel, whereas a guidewire with a 3 mm J-shaped tip is best in an atheromatous vessel.

There is also a variety of specialist guidewires:

- smaller calibre guidewires with diameters of 0.014–0.025 in for thinner catheters;
- fixed core heavy duty guidewires for added stiffness;
- moveable core guidewires for variable stiffness and shape;
- extra long guidewires with lengths of 200–260 cm for catheter exchanges to avoid losing the position of the catheter in the arterial system;
- steerable guidewires for difficult manipulations in tortuous or stenosed vessels;
- hydrophilic coated guidewires for interventional vascular techniques;
- guidewires with a central lumen for injections.

Catheters

The catheter is used to inject the contrast medium at a precise site within the arterial system. There are also many types of angiographic catheter, but again they all have a single basic design – a tapered tip with an end hole or an end hole and side holes at a specially shaped end, a length of flexible tubing in the middle and a flattened hub at the other end with a locking connection, through which contrast medium or heparinized saline is injected. Most catheters are made of polyethylene or polyurethane but some are made of Teflon or nylon. They are usually 4–7F in size and 60–100 cm in length. The shape of the tip of the catheter is designed for use in a particular artery. A straight catheter with an end hole and multiple side holes is used for abdominal aortography, but a pig-tail catheter with an end hole and multiple side holes is used for cardiac chamber angiography, thoracic and abdominal aortography, because a pig-tail catheter is more stable in position during an injection of contrast medium. Single or double curve catheters with an end hole or an end hole and two side holes are used for selective arteriography, such as the cobra and sidewinder catheters for mesenteric and renal arteriography and the mani and headhunter catheters for carotid and subclavian arteriography.

There are also specialist catheters mainly used for interventional vascular techniques:

- balloon catheters for angioplasty;
- co-axial catheters for embolization and thrombolysis;
- 2–3F microcatheters for superselective arteriography;
- 8–12F macrocatheters for embolectomy and stent insertion.

Dilators and vascular sheaths

A **dilator** is used to produce a tunnel through the subcutaneous soft tissues and arterial wall prior to the insertion of the catheter over the guidewire to prevent damage to the tip of the catheter in patients with scar tissue at the site of arterial puncture, in patients with heavily calcified vessel walls and in obese patients. Most dilators are made of Teflon with a smooth tapered tip and are usually 4–12F in size.

A dilator can also be used with an introducer **vascular sheath** which reduces trauma to the arterial wall in patients requiring multiple catheter exchanges. Most introducer sheaths have a very thin wall and a haemostatic valve.

Contrast media

The new non-ionic contrast media such as iopamidol (Niopam), iohexol (Omnipaque) and iopramide (Ultravist) have become the media of choice for angiography. These contrast media have a low osmolality (290 mOsm/kg water), which is only two to three times that of plasma, in comparison to the high osmolality of the ionic contrast media, which is five to seven times that of plasma. The non-ionic contrast media do, however, have a higher viscosity than the ionic contrast media, but this can be reduced by warming them to body temperature before injection.

A contrast medium containing 340–370 mg iodine/ml is used for conventional film aortography and a contrast medium containing 300 mg iodine/ml is used for conventional film arteriography. However, for intra-arterial angiography with a digital subtraction technique, a less concentrated contrast medium containing 150–300 mg iodine/ml is suitable, although for intravenous digital subtraction angiography, a contrast medium containing 340–370 mg iodine/ml is required, because of the dilution that occurs in the vascular system.

The contrast medium is injected through the catheter by a pressure injector for thoracic and abdominal aortography and pulmonary, mesenteric, renal and pelvic arteriography, but is injected by hand for carotid, coronary and superselective arteriography. The volume of contrast medium used during an examination should not exceed 4–5 ml/kg body weight.

TECHNIQUE

Arteriography is generally performed as an inpatient procedure, but is also being done as either a day case or an outpatient procedure in increasing numbers.

Patient care

A 24-hour hospital admission is ideal for patients undergoing arteriography and allows the radiologist the opportunity of visiting the patient before the procedure in order to explain the technique and its risks, obtain informed consent and examine the proposed puncture site, which is usually the femoral artery in the groin. Patients with a history of a previous hypersensitivity reaction to intravascular contrast media require corticosteroid cover for the procedure or an alternative imaging study, and oral anticoagulant therapy should be withdrawn at least 3 days before the procedure so that the INR is < 1.4. Preangiographic investigations include the haemoglobin level, platelet count, urea and electrolytes and clotting studies, but other investigations such as ECG, blood sugar, sickle test and hepatitis antigen are occasionally needed.

The patient requires a groin shave and must not eat any solid food for 6 hours before the procedure, but can continue with free oral fluids to within 2 hours of coming to the angiography suite.

Arteriography is usually done under local anaesthetic in adults, but a general anaesthetic is required for babies and children and some long complex vascular interventional procedures such as embolization. A premedication of 10 mg temazepam orally, 10 mg papaveretum (Omnopon) intramuscularly and 12.5 mg prochlorperazine (Stemetil) intramuscularly is useful in the majority of adults 1 hour before the procedure. Antibiotic cover is also occasionally needed.

After the procedure the patient requires 12 hours bed rest and regular observation of the puncture site, the pulse and blood pressure every 15 minutes for 1 hour, hourly for 4 hours and then 4-hourly to 12 hours. The hospital admission also allows the radiologist to visit the patient after the procedure to check for complications and discuss the results and proposed management.

Contraindications to arteriography

There are no absolute contraindications to arteriography, but relative contraindications include a previous hypersensitivity reaction to contrast media, severe hypertension with a diastolic blood pressure > 120 mmHg, anticoagulant treatment, a bleeding diathesis, severe anaemia with a haemoglobin level < 8 g/dl and pregnancy.

Arteriography also carries more risk in patients with cardiac failure, respiratory failure, renal failure, hepatic failure, thyrotoxicosis and dehydration, and requires great care in children and elderly patients.

Catheterization of the femoral artery in the groin may be contraindicated by the presence of an occlusion or an aneurysm of the common femoral artery, a synthetic graft and scar formation or infection in the soft tissues overlying the artery. Marked obesity can also make the procedure rather difficult.

Femoral arterial catheterization

The common femoral artery is the best vessel to use for percutaneous arterial catheterization, because it is a large superficial vessel, which allows access to the whole arterial tree.

The artery is catheterized in the groin under local anaesthetic with sterile conditions in the following stages:

1. The artery is palpated in the right or left groin and 5–10 ml of 1% lignocaine is injected into the skin and soft tissues around the artery at the point of maximum pulsation below the inguinal ligament, but not necessarily in the skin crease in the groin because it is variable in position.
2. A 19-gauge thin-wall one-piece needle is introduced into the artery at an angle of 30–45° with one hand whilst the artery is held in position by the index and middle fingers of the other hand. The needle is advanced through both the anterior and posterior walls of the artery in Seldinger's original description, but today the needle is often just advanced through the anterior wall of the vessel.
3. A 0.035 in guidewire with a 3 mm J-shaped tip is advanced through the tip of the needle and up into the abdominal aorta, once a good backflow of arterial blood has been obtained.
4. The needle is withdrawn over the guidewire, whilst compression is applied to the groin by the fingers of one hand.
5. A 5F catheter (or dilator and introducer vascular sheath) is advanced over the guidewire and into the artery, whilst compression is still maintained.
6. The guidewire is removed leaving the catheter within the arterial tree. The catheter is flushed with heparinized saline containing 5000 units of heparin/l and positioned for arteriography.
7. The catheter is removed at the end of the procedure and compression is again applied at the arterial puncture site for 5–10 min to prevent the formation of a haematoma.

Some bruising in the groin often becomes apparent a few days later in the majority of patients.

This technique is described as a retrograde catheterization of the common femoral artery with passage of the guidewire and catheter into the iliac arteries and abdominal aorta, but it is also possible to catheterize the common femoral artery in an antegrade direction with passage of the guidewire and catheter into the superficial femoral and popliteal arteries for the purpose of angioplasty.

Other arterial catheterization sites

In the majority of patients at least one of the femoral pulses is present. When there is only one weak femoral pulse, it is still possible to catheterize the common femoral artery using fluoroscopy to localize any arterial calcification or using ultrasound to visualize the artery directly.

When both femoral pulses are absent it is advisable to use other arteries for catheterization or direct needle puncture. The axillary or brachial artery can be catheterized in either arm using an identical technique to that already described for femoral arterial catheterization. A puncture site in the right arm gives access to the thoracic aorta and the carotid and coronary arteries, whereas the left arm gives access to the abdominal aorta and the distal part of the arterial tree.

Direct needle puncture of the upper or lower abdominal aorta, so-called translumbar aortography, is now only occasionally performed, because it inevitably results in a significant retroperitoneal haematoma and is often done under general anaesthetic.

Direct needle puncture of the carotid or subclavian arteries is no longer performed, but direct needle puncture of the femoral artery can be very useful in a scarred groin when it is difficult to catheterize the artery because of the fibrous tissue.

An arteriotomy of the brachial artery in the catheter suite is still used for coronary arteriography as an alternative to the transfemoral route. An arteriotomy of the femoral artery in theatre is useful in combined vascular surgical and interventional radiological procedures.

Venous catheterization

The femoral vein can be catheterized in the groin using an identical technique to that already described for femoral arterial catheterization. Femoral vein catheterization gives access to the pulmonary arteries.

The technique of intravenous digital subtraction angiography is used to produce images of the arteries following a central venous injection of contrast medium into the superior vena cava or right atrium, despite the dilution of the contrast medium that occurs. The procedure is usually performed after catheterization of the median basilic or cephalic veins in the cubital fossa of either arm, but can also be done following catherization of the femoral vein.

COMPLICATIONS OF ARTERIOGRAPHY

Arteriography carries a small degree of risk to the patient. Because of the high quality diagnostic information that is produced the benefits of arteriography are invariably much greater than the risks and therefore outweigh the morbidity and mortality of the procedure, which are both extremely low. Not all problems that develop after an arteriogram are necessarily caused by the procedure; many of the patients undergoing arteriography have generalized vascular disease or multiple medical problems.

Contrast medium reactions (page 4)

A fatal reaction is commoner after an intravenous than an intra-arterial injection. Patients who have had a previous major reaction to contrast media and require further angiography should be covered by corticosteroid treatment or should undergo an imaging procedure that does not require contrast media such as duplex ultrasound or magnetic resonance angiography.

Adverse reactions to other drugs

Reactions to drugs used during angiography are rare but include complications related to the premedication, the local anaesthetic and any drug given during the procedure. Intravenous diazepam can produce a respiratory arrest in an elderly patient, lignocaine can produce convulsions and cardiac dysrhythmias and glyceryl trinitrate can produce hypotension.

Arterial puncture site complications

Complications at the arterial puncture site occur in about 5% of patients undergoing arteriography and include haemorrhage, haematoma, arterial spasm, subintimal dissection (Fig. 23.1), thrombosis, perivascular extravasation of contrast medium, false aneurysm, arteriovenous fistula, nerve trauma and local sepsis. However, only 0.2% of these complications require surgical treatment.

Haemorrhage from the puncture site with external bleeding or the formation of a subcutaneous haematoma is the commonest complication of arterial catheterization. It is more likely to occur with poor angiographic technique, in hypertensive patients and in patients with clotting disorders. Some bruising in the groin a few days after the procedure is normal. The

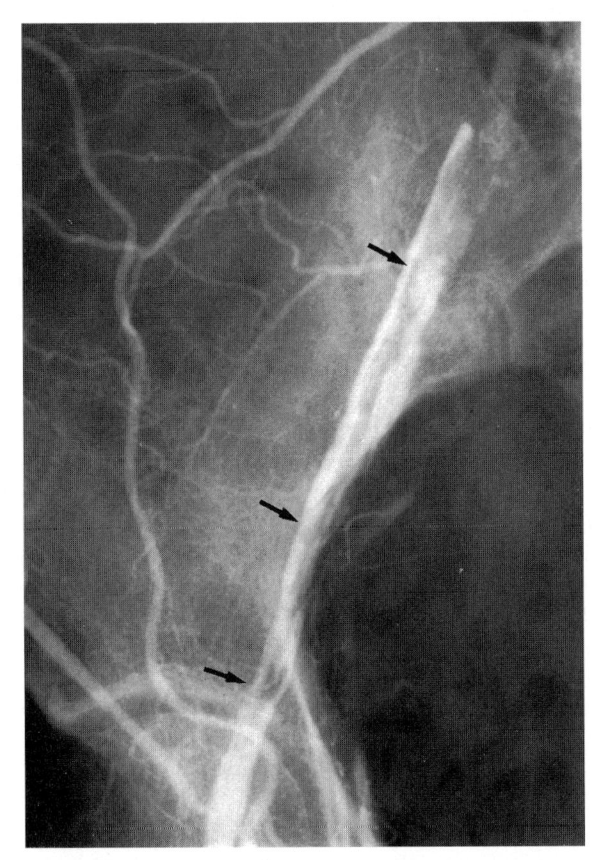

Fig. 23.1 Femoral arteriography showing a subintimal dissection in the whole of the right external iliac artery (arrows) produced by a straight guidewire.

formation of a false aneurysm is uncommon and the development of an arteriovenous fistula is rare. Subintimal dissection and local arterial spasm at the puncture site are not usually clinically significant, but can produce thrombosis which is also an uncommon complication. It is more likely to occur with poor angiographic technique, in atheromatous vessels and in patients with thrombotic tendencies.

Perivascular extravasation of contrast medium produces pain at the arterial puncture site. Nerve trauma is rare but is most likely to occur with transaxillary arteriography. Local sepsis at the puncture site is also rare.

Complications within the arterial system

Complications due to the catheter being within the arterial system occur in about 0.5% of patients and include:

- embolization (Fig. 23.2),
- subintimal dissection
- arterial spasm
- thrombosis
- perforation of the arterial wall
- vasovagal reactions
- subacute bacterial endocarditis
- septicaemia
- guidewire or catheter fracture
- organ infarction

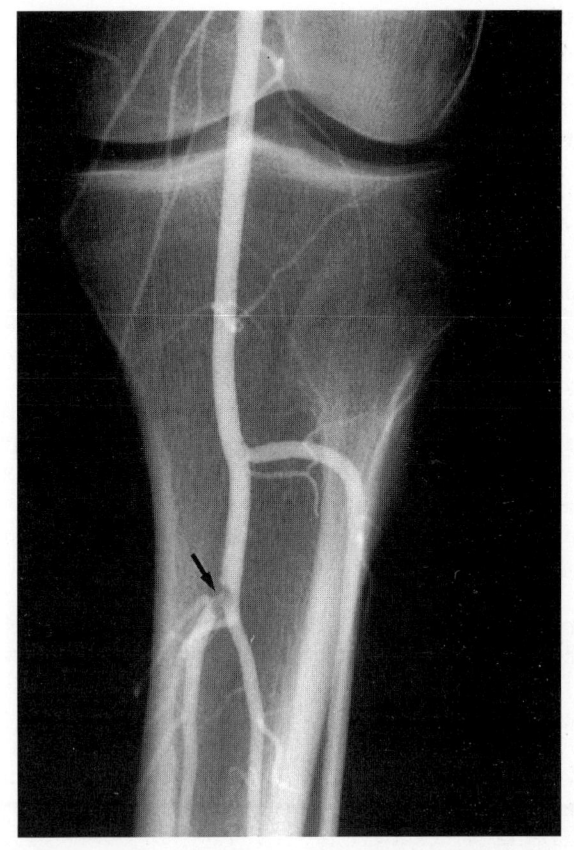

Fig. 23.2 Femoral arteriography showing a distal embolus in the left tibioperoneal trunk (arrow) produced by a large catheter.

However, only 0.1% of these complications require surgical treatment.

Distal embolization into the arterial tree is caused by dislodging an atheromatous plaque from the arterial wall or by stripping thrombus off the guidewire or catheter, but is an uncommon complication. Embolization is more likely to occur with poor angiographic technique and the absence of heparin in the flushing solution. Embolization of cholesterol crystals or air can be fatal. Guidewire or catheter fracture is rare.

Thrombosis within the arterial system is also uncommon. It is usually caused by subintimal dissection or arterial spasm and is more likely to occur with poor angiographic technique, in atheromatous vessels and in patients having angioplasty. Perforation of the arterial wall by the catheter or guidewire is rare.

Subacute bacterial endocarditis is commoner after cardiac angiography and septicaemia is more likely to occur with long procedure times, but both are rare complications. Vasovagal reactions also occur during arteriography and pyrogenic reactions can occur after the procedure.

Damage or infarction of specific organs is rare, but is usually caused by subintimal dissection during selective arteriography or embolization during aortography or arteriography. Renal function can deteriorate following renal arteriography, myocardial infarction is likely to occur after dissection of the left or right coronary artery and leg ischaemia is likely to develop after a popliteal artery embolus.

Arteriography is best performed by the transfemoral route because the overall complication rate is 1.7%, with a mortality rate of 0.03%. This is significantly lower than for transaxillary arteriography, which has an overall complication rate of 3.3% and a mortality rate of 0.09%. Translumbar aortography has an overall complication rate of 2.9% and a mortality rate of 0.05%.

RADIOLOGICAL INVESTIGATION OF ARTERIAL DISEASE

The investigation of the patient with vascular disease obviously begins with a good history and thorough clinical examination and includes a number of laboratory tests, in addition to the preangiographic investigations, such as thrombophilia screen, and blood cholesterol and serum fibrinogen estimation. The radiological imaging techniques available include:

- plain films
- ultrasound

- arteriography
- computed tomography
- magnetic resonance imaging
- radionuclide imaging
- other imaging techniques.

PLAIN FILMS

Plain films are of limited value in the investigation of arterial disease, because the arteries have a similar radiographic density to the surrounding soft tissues and therefore cannot be seen. The demonstration of calcification in the arterial wall, however, indicates the presence of arterial disease. Intimal calcification has an irregular amorphous pattern in atherosclerotic vessels and is common in elderly patients. It is diagnostic of an aneurysm when there is a curvilinear element to the calcification (Fig. 23.3). Calcification in the media has a regular tubular pattern in atherosclerotic vessels and is seen in patients with diabetes mellitus, characteristically in the tibial and foot vessels. This type of vascular calcification also occurs in hyperparathyroidism.

The presence of a soft-tissue mass can be due to a true or false aneurysm or an arteriovenous malformation, which can also produce pressure erosion of adjacent bones. Phleboliths in an unusual site are diagnostic of an arteriovenous malformation.

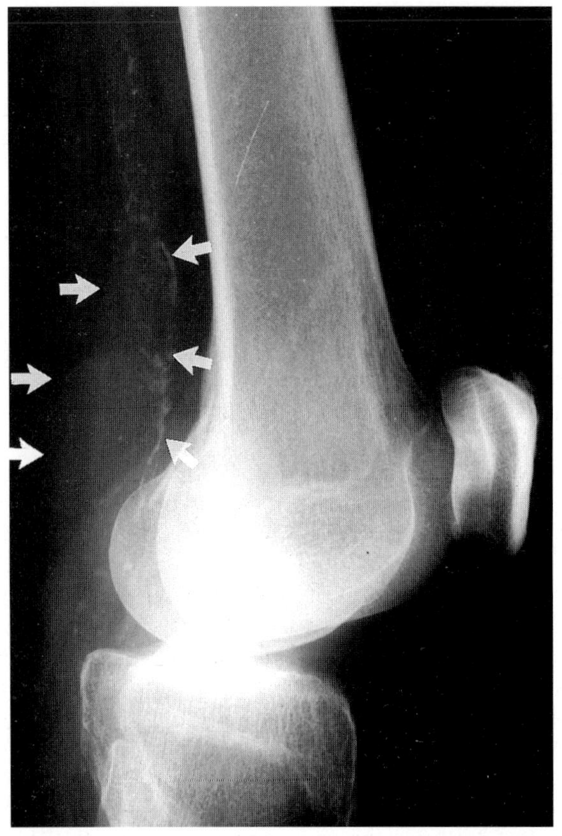

Fig. 23.3 Lateral radiograph of the knee showing calcification in an aneurysm of the popliteal artery (arrows).

ULTRASOUND

Ultrasound is an extremely useful imaging modality in the investigation of arterial disease, because it is a non-invasive technique that does not use ionizing radiation and is therefore safe. Real-time ultrasound produces an anatomical image of a blood vessel, whereas duplex ultrasound combines pulsed Doppler with an image of a blood vessel to produce a physiological image by colour coding the blood flow. This is called colour flow mapping, with the flow of blood away from the transducer conventionally coded red and the flow of blood towards the transducer coded blue.

Real-time ultrasound is mainly used to assess the size, extent and rate of growth of an abdominal aortic aneurysm (Fig. 23.4) or any other peripheral aneurysm, and has been used in screening studies. Ultrasound is also used in the follow-up of aortic grafts, to measure the size of ectatic arteries and in the investigation of a pulsating mass in the neck, groin, axilla or popliteal fossa, to see whether the mass is a true or false aneurysm or a soft-tissue mass simply transmitting the arterial pulsation. Real-time ultrasound is also occasionally used to aid the vascular radiologist in performing an arterial or venous puncture, by actually visualizing the needle tip passing through the soft tissues to enter the blood vessel.

Duplex ultrasound is mainly used to detect and assess the severity of stenoses in the peripheral arteries and femoropopliteal grafts, and stenoses in

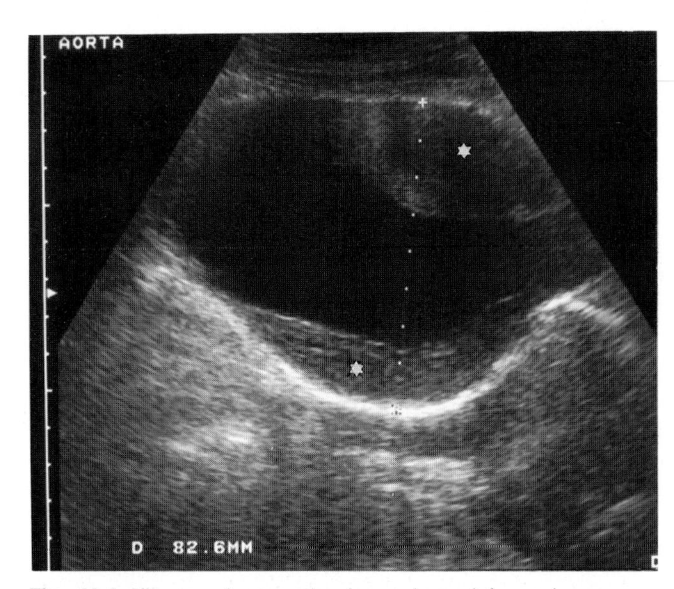

Fig. 23.4 Ultrasound scan showing a large infrarenal aneurysm measuring 8 cm in diameter of the lower abdominal aorta containing thrombus(✻).

the extracranial carotid arteries in the neck (Plates 9 and 10, opposite page 562) and the renal and mesenteric arteries in the abdomen. Duplex ultrasound is also used to see whether the tibial arteries are patent in the calf before a femorodistal graft and to assess the patency of the long saphenous vein before the by-pass is performed.

ARTERIOGRAPHY

Arteriography is still the most useful imaging modality in the investigation of arterial disease, but it requires the use of a large volume of contrast medium (100–250 ml) and is an X-ray imaging technique, which therefore results in a radiation dose to the patient.

The commonest indications for arteriography are:

- peripheral vascular disease
- ischaemic heart disease
- cerebrovascular disease.

Femoral arteriography, coronary arteriography and carotid arteriography account for well over 90% of the workload of most angiographic units, but arteriography is also indicated in:

- the investigation of the ischaemic arm;
- the investigation of renovascular hypertension and mesenteric ischaemia;
- the assessment of abdominal aortic and other aneurysms;
- the staging of both primary and secondary malignant tumours;
- the localization of the site of bleeding from any organ system;
- the investigation of pulmonary emboli;
- the investigation of trauma;
- the assessment of arteriovenous malformations.

There are three slightly different methods of producing the arterial images:

- conventional arteriography
- intra-arterial digital subtraction angiography
- intravenous digital subtraction angiography.

The advantage of intravenous digital subtraction angiography over either conventional arteriography or its intra-arterial counterpart is that it is an outpatient procedure. The disadvantages of intravenous digital subtraction angiography are that the total volume and iodine load of the contrast medium are greater than for a similar conventional arteriographic procedure and the image quality is less than for a similar arterial digital subtraction technique. The procedure is also, in essence, a right-heart catheter and for satisfactory images it is necessary to make the injection with a catheter in the superior vena cava.

Conventional arteriography is the classic form of arteriography in which the arterial images are recorded directly on radiographic film. Conventional arteriography has the best spatial resolution and is therefore used when high-definition images of the arteries are required as in coronary arteriography, intracerebral arteriography and arteriography involving analysis of the finest vessels, such as tumour vascularity and angiodysplasia. The conventional arteriogram image can be visually enhanced by the manual process of photographic subtraction, which highlights the arterial image by removing from the arteriogram film the unwanted images of bone, soft tissue and gas-filled structures, with the use of a mask film. The mask is obtained by producing a film with a reverse image to that normally seen on a radiograph (i.e. black bones instead of white bones) from the initial film of the angiographic series, which has no contrast medium in the arteries. The mask film is exactly superimposed on one of the later films from the angiographic series, which will therefore have contrast medium in the arteries. This is quite easy to do as long as there has been no movement of the patient between the two films. The effect is that the unwanted images of bone, soft tissue and gas-filled structures are cancelled out from an optical viewpoint by different densities on the two films (i.e. white bones cancelled by black bones). The subtraction film is obtained from these two exactly superimposed films and results in a reverse image of the arteries (i.e. black arteries instead of white arteries).

Intra-arterial digital subtraction angiography is the modern form of arteriography and all new angiographic units now have this facility, which uses a computer to produce an electronic subtraction of the arterial image by a similar process to manual photographic subtraction just described. The images are initially recorded by an image intensifier coupled to a television camera. This analog data is then digitized and the mask image is subtracted from the subsequent arterial images and displayed. These images can be manipulated by computer processing, before being recorded on radiographic film. Once again it is very important that no movement occurs during the angiographic series. Digital subtraction angiography therefore requires cooperative patients who do not move and are able to hold their breath. Examinations of the abdomen are done after an intravenous injection of 20 mg hyoscine butylbromide (Buscopan) to prevent peristaltic movement, examinations of the neck are done without swallowing and examinations of the chest can be done with ECG gating to eliminate the effects of cardiac pulsation. The advantages of intra-arterial digital subtraction angiography over conventional arteriography include reductions in:

- the volume and iodine concentration of the contrast medium used for each angiographic series, which is beneficial in reducing side-effects;
- the total volume and iodine load of the contrast medium used for the whole examination, which is beneficial in children and patients with impaired cardiac and renal function;
- the length of the procedure due to rapid acquisition of each angiographic series, which is likely to reduce complications;
- the diameter of the catheters used, to 3–4F, which facilitates day case and outpatient procedures;
- the amount of radiographic film used;

and also the ability to:

- use carbon dioxide gas as a contrast medium in patients with a previous hypersensitivity reaction to intravascular contrast medium, although the spatial resolution with carbon dioxide is lower than when conventional contrast agents are used;
- produce measurements such as the grade of stenosis in an artery and the cardiac output.

Intra-arterial digital subtraction angiography is being increasingly used for all types of arteriography but is particularly useful in interventional vascular procedures, such as embolization and angioplasty, and paediatric arteriography.

Intravenous digital subtraction angiography results in the production of arterial images following an intravenous injection of contrast medium. The images are produced in exactly the same way as for intra-arterial digital subtraction angiography but a delay is required before the angiographic series is obtained, as the contrast medium has to travel from the superior vena cava, inferior vena cava or right atrium, through the lungs and left side of the heart, before reaching the arteries. The contrast medium has been diluted in the blood by this stage, but because of the high contrast resolution of a digital subtraction system, an acceptable arterial image is produced, if the cardiac output is normal.

Intravenous digital subtraction angiography is used for:

- screening for carotid and renal artery disease;
- follow-up peripheral angiography after a by-pass graft or angioplasty;
- thoracic outlet syndrome and aortic disease in young patients;
- angiography in older patients with no femoral pulses;
- venography in patients with venous occlusion in the pelvic veins, inferior vena cava, subclavian and brachiocephalic veins and superior vena cava.

COMPUTED TOMOGRAPHY

CT is also a useful imaging modality in the investigation of arterial disease, but requires the use of large volumes of contrast medium (100–150 ml) and is a digital X-ray imaging technique with a significant radiation dose to the patient. The recent introduction of slip ring technology for CT (spiral or helical CT) allows a volume of tissue 10–25 cm in length to be scanned very rapidly in 10–25 s. Images of tissue slices of any thickness from 1–10 mm thick can then be produced. The advantages of spiral CT over conventional CT for demonstrating arterial disease are the improved contrast enhancement that is produced with a smaller volume of contrast medium (50–100 ml) and the very high quality reconstructed images that can be obtained.

CT is mainly used for:

- confirming the diagnosis and indicating the type of a dissecting thoracic aortic aneurysm;
- assessing the size and extent of an abdominal aortic aneurysm and its relationship to the renal and iliac arteries;
- assessing the size and extent of a thoracic aortic aneurysm;
- confirming the diagnosis of a ruptured thoracic aorta;
- the follow-up of aortic graft complications;
- the investigation of a pulsating mass in the neck or groin.

MAGNETIC RESONANCE IMAGING

MRI is a potentially very useful imaging modality in the investigation of arterial disease, but is not yet widely available. It is a non-invasive technique that does not use ionizing radiation.

MRI using a T1-weighted spin-echo sequence with cardiac gating is used for:

- diagnosing and indicating the type of a dissecting thoracic aortic aneurysm;
- showing the location and severity of a coarctation of the aorta;
- assessing the size and extent of a thoracic or abdominal aortic aneurysm.

Magnetic resonance angiography, with the use of fast-gradient echo sequences such as the time of flight and phase contrast techniques, is used for showing the location and severity of stenoses and occlusions in peripheral vascular disease and for confirming the diagnosis of carotid artery disease, renal artery stenosis and mesenteric ischaemia (Fig. 23.5).

In T1-weighted spin-echo sequences, flowing blood produces a signal void and therefore appears black,

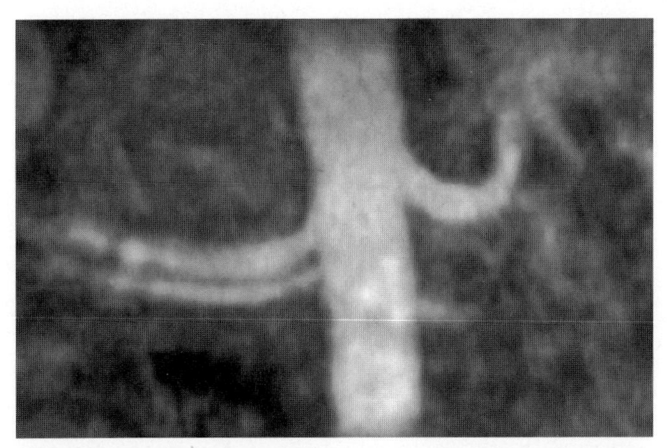

Fig. 23.5 Magnetic resonance angiography showing normal renal arteries with an accessory artery to the right kidney on this 3D time-of-flight study.

but in fast-gradient-echo sequences flowing blood produces a high signal and therefore appears white. The main advantages of MRI over CT as regards arterial disease are the multiplanar imaging capability, which includes axial, coronal, sagittal and oblique image planes, and the lack of requirement for any contrast medium. However, the paramagnetic agent gadolinium-DTPA, when injected intravenously, can be used to increase the signal intensity of flowing blood.

RADIONUCLIDE IMAGING

Radionuclide studies are a useful imaging modality in the investigation of specific problems in arterial disease but involve the use of ionizing radiation.

The diagnosis of an infected arterial graft can most easily be confirmed with a radiolabelled white cell scan (Fig. 23.6). The site of active bleeding from the gastrointestinal tract can be located with ^{99m}Tc-labelled red cells or ^{99m}Tc-labelled colloid. A radionuclide scan is an adjunct to arteriography.

OTHER TECHNIQUES

Intravascular ultrasound is performed by introducing a catheter with a crystal transducer mounted at its tip into the arterial system through a vascular sheath. It produces radial ultrasound images of the arterial wall and is at present used as a research tool to study atheromatous plaque morphology before and after angioplasty. **Angioscopy** is also performed by introducing an angioscope catheter, containing optical fibres, into the arterial system through a vascular sheath. The field of view is continually obscured by blood which has to be flushed away. Angioscopy does, however, produce spectacular visualization of the normal arterial wall, arterial graft, atheroma, thrombus and blood-flow patterns.

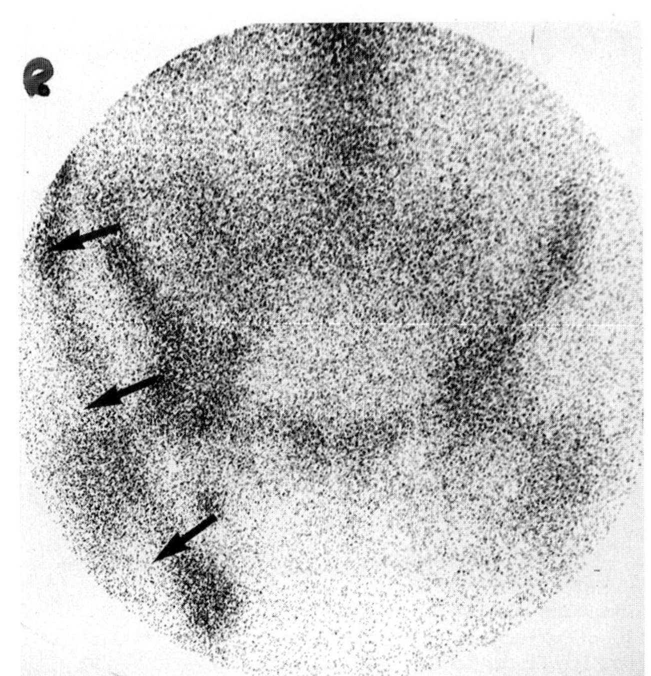

Fig. 23.6 Radionuclide study using indium-labelled white blood cells showing isotope activity in an infected right axillofemoral Dacron graft (arrows). Normal uptake is seen in the bone marrow in the lumbar spine and pelvis.

NEOPLASTIC DISEASE

Arteriography is useful in the management of tumours, but its diagnostic role has been significantly reduced by the non-invasive imaging modalities, such as ultrasound, CT, radionuclide studies and MRI, which are used for diagnosis and staging often in conjunction with needle biopsy under ultrasound or CT guidance. The indications for arteriography include both the diagnosis and localization of primary tumours, preoperative assessment of primary and secondary tumours, and therapeutic intervention.

Arteriography can be used to distinguish between an atypical benign cyst, an abscess, and a cystic or necrotic tumour, because, in a tumour, pathological circulation may be demonstrated in the wall of the tumour. Arteriography can also localize a small endocrine tumour, which has not been demonstrated by non-invasive imaging modalities, but is known to be present because of positive biochemical tests. An insulinoma or a glucagonoma in the pancreas and an ectopic parathyroid adenoma in the mediastinum all tend to be hypervascular and, therefore, demonstrable by arteriography (Fig. 23.7).

In the preoperative assessment of patients with primary or secondary hepatic tumours and ampullary tumours in the head of the pancreas, arteriography is

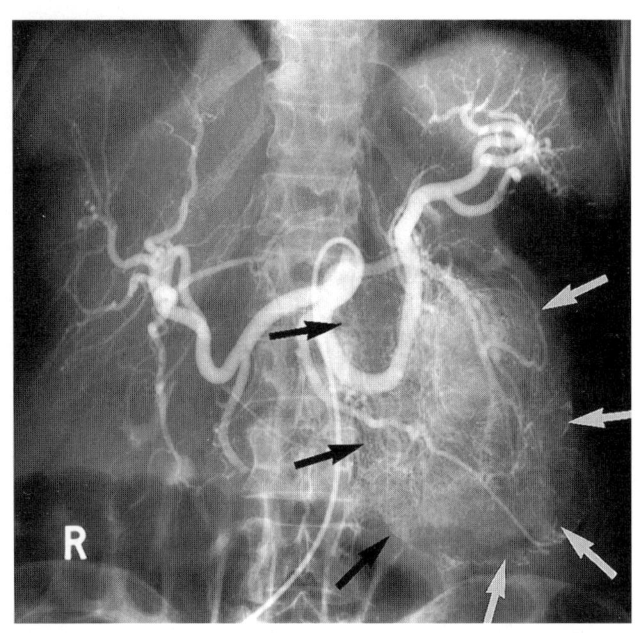

Fig. 23.7 Coeliac arteriography showing a large hypervascular tumour in the body and tail of the pancreas (arrows) due to a VIPoma.

used to map out the vascular anatomy and to identify encasement of the vessels that would make the tumour inoperable. Arteriography is also occasionally used to demonstrate the blood vessels supplying very large intra-abdominal tumours and soft-tissue tumours in the limbs.

Embolization is used to prevent bleeding from an inoperable renal or bladder tumour; to devascularize primary tumours prior to surgery such as an angiofibroma in the nasopharynx or an intracranial meningioma and to ablate the function of hepatic metastases from a carcinoid tumour. Arteriography is also useful in positioning a catheter in the main feeding artery to a tumour for intra-arterial chemotherapy.

HAEMORRHAGE

Arteriography can be extremely useful in localizing the site of bleeding from the gastrointestinal tract, the urinary tract and the respiratory tract, and occasionally in patients following severe trauma.

Acute gastrointestinal haemorrhage presents clinically with haematemesis, melaena, rectal bleeding and hypovolaemic shock. The initial investigations are endoscopy which has a diagnostic accuracy of 90% and flexible sigmoidoscopy/colonoscopy which has a diagnostic accuracy of 50–90%. Arteriography is indicated in patients who continue to bleed severely, particularly when the initial investigations have failed to demonstrate the site of the bleeding. Arteriography has a diagnostic accuracy of 50–75%, but this approaches 90% if the procedure is performed whilst the patient is actively bleeding. Arteriography demonstrates active bleeding when the rate of blood loss exceeds 0.5–1 ml/min, but radionuclide studies using either ^{99m}Tc-labelled colloid or ^{99m}Tc-labelled red cells are more sensitive and can detect active bleeding when the rate of blood loss is as low as 0.1–0.5 ml/min. Radionuclide studies have a diagnostic accuracy of 30–90% and can be used prior to arteriography.

In acute upper gastrointestinal haemorrhage, arteriography may show extravasation of contrast medium onto the gastroduodenal mucosa from a gastric or duodenal ulcer, gastro-oesophageal varices, a false aneurysm in pancreatitis or the nipple-like projection of an aortoenteric fistula. In acute lower gastrointestinal haemorrhage, arteriography may show a small intestinal leiomyoma, a small intestinal arteriovenous malformation, caecal angiodysplasia, or extravasation of contrast medium onto the colonic mucosa from a colonic diverticulum (Fig. 23.8) or ulcer.

Bleeding from erosive gastritis or a colonic diverticulum can be controlled by an intra-arterial infusion of vasopressin, which produces vasoconstriction, and bleeding from a peptic ulcer or a false aneurysm within the pancreas or liver can be treated by embolization with sponge foam fragments and steel

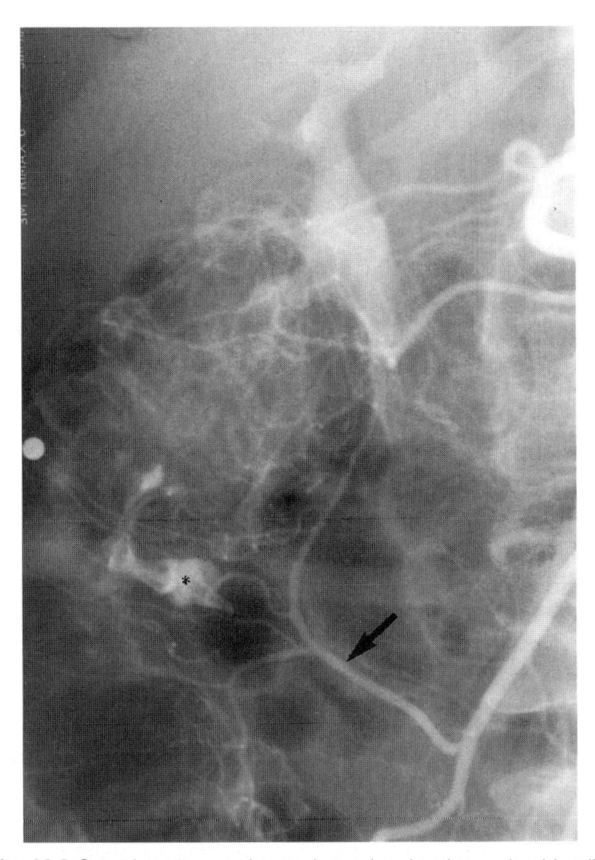

Fig. 23.8 Superior mesenteric arteriography showing active bleeding from a branch of the right colic (arrow) artery into a diverticulum in the ascending colon(✻).

coils. Tumours, arteriovenous malformations and an aortoenteric fistula are treated surgically. A small intestinal arteriovenous malformation can be very difficult to locate during a laparotomy, but if an angiographic catheter is selectively placed in its feeding artery before surgery, an injection of either methylene blue or fluorescein through the catheter will visualize the abnormal loop of small intestine during the operation. Arteriography is also useful in the investigation of both chronic and obscure gastrointestinal haemorrhage, because it may show a vascular abnormality as the cause of the anaemia or recurrent bleeding.

Renal arteriography is indicated in patients with severe haematuria following a renal biopsy. The arteriography may show a false aneurysm or an arteriocaliceal fistula which can be treated by embolization with steel coils or a detachable balloon. Renal arteriography is also indicated in patients with recurrent haematuria who have a normal intravenous urogram and cystoscopy, because an arteriovenous malformation may be present within the kidney. Embolization is used to control haematuria in patients with an inoperable renal or bladder tumour.

Bronchial arteriography is indicated in patients with chronic fibrotic lung diseases, such as tuberculosis, bronchiectasis and cystic fibrosis, who have severe haemoptysis. Arteriography shows hypertrophied bronchial arteries with extravasation of the contrast medium into the bronchial tree and the haemoptysis can be treated by embolization with sponge foam fragments.

TRAUMA

Blunt trauma, such as soft-tissue injury or bone fracture, and penetrating trauma, such as gunshot and stab wounds as well as iatrogenic needle injuries, can all produce damage to the vascular system. Arteriography may be required to characterize the acute vascular injury, but it should not delay resuscitation or treatment of the patient. Arteriography is also occasionally used to assess the blood supply to a limb in the patient who requires orthopaedic surgery, but may be compromised by peripheral vascular disease.

The types of arterial injury that can occur in acute trauma include:

- arterial spasm;
- extrinsic compression and displacement of the artery from a haematoma;
- narrowing of the artery from an intramural bleed;
- intimal damage to the artery with or without occlusion;
- partial tear or complete transection of the artery with the formation of a false aneurysm or an arteriovenous fistula.

Blunt trauma to the chest, in the form of a rapid deceleration injury during a road traffic accident or an air crash, produces a partial tear in the arch of the aorta distal to the origin of the left subclavian artery with the formation of a false aneurysm in the survivors. An aneurysm is usually apparent on a chest radiograph as widening of the mediastinum, but occasionally presents years later as a mediastinal mass. Care must be taken when interpreting portable films as magnification factors may result in a widened mediastinum. Urgent CT and aortography confirms the diagnosis of a false aneurysm. Chest injury may also damage any of the large arteries or veins in the mediastinum.

Blunt trauma to the abdomen fractures solid organs such as the spleen and tears the blood vessels in the mesentery producing haemorrhage and haematoma formation, whereas penetrating trauma to the liver and kidney from a stab wound or biopsy produces a false aneurysm or arteriovenous fistula as well. Both of these can be treated by embolization with steel coils or detachable balloons. Embolization is particularly important and may be life-saving in patients with pelvic fractures (Fig. 23.9) where partial tears in the internal iliac arteries or their branches can produce massive haemorrhage that may not be controlled by external fixation of the fractures.

Arteriography is rarely required in patients with long bone fractures in the upper or lower limbs, unless the limb is ischaemic and even this may resolve with

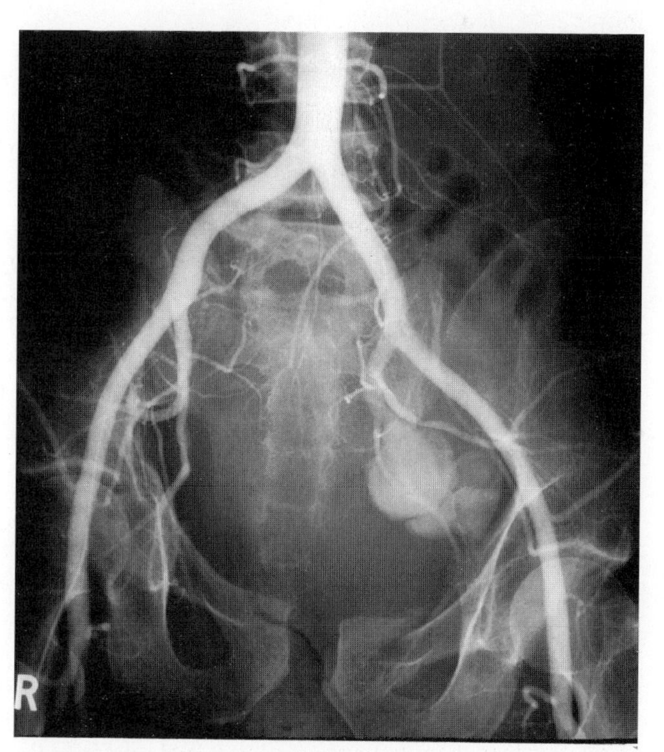

Fig. 23.9 Pelvic arteriography showing a large false aneurysm of the left internal iliac artery in a patient with fractures of the pelvis sustained in a road traffic accident.

reduction of the fracture. The ischaemia may be due to arterial spasm or occlusion. Stab wounds or other penetrating injuries to the limbs produce a false aneurysm or arteriovenous fistula, whereas gunshot wounds produce arterial occlusion and occasionally embolization of bullet fragments within the vascular system. Vascular spasm and mycotic aneurysms may occur following arterial injuries in drug abuse.

VASCULAR MALFORMATIONS

Congenital vascular malformations are a type of benign vascular tumour consisting of a collection of abnormal blood vessels, which do not have the normal anatomical pattern of development with blood passing from an artery through arterioles, capillaries and venules to a vein. Vascular malformations can be classified according to their angiographic characteristics into a high-flow arteriovenous malformation and a low-flow capillary venous malformation or venous haemangioma.

Clinically, arteriovenous malformations present in children and young adult patients as a pulsatile soft-tissue mass with a bruit in the head and neck or in one of the limbs. Arteriovenous malformations may be complicated by cutaneous ulceration and haemorrhage, limb hypertrophy or even cardiac failure. Arteriovenous malformations can also occur in any internal organ and tend to present with bleeding, but pulmonary arteriovenous malformations are usually seen as an incidental finding on a chest radiograph. Pulmonary arteriovenous malformations occur in the Osler–Rendu–Weber syndrome. Presentation may be as a cerebral abscess when infected material is shunted through the lungs and not filtered by the pulmonary capillaries.

Arteriography of arteriovenous malformations shows a single or several hypertrophied tortuous feeding arteries, a network of abnormal vessels with arteriovenous shunting and aneurysm formation, and enlarged draining veins filling in the arterial phase of the study (Fig. 23.10). Arteriovenous malformations can be treated by either surgery or embolization with polyvinyl alcohol particles, sponge foam fragments or steel coils.

Capillary venous malformations present clinically in children and young adult patients as non-pulsatile swellings in the head and neck or limbs; they are easily compressed and fill when gravity dependent. They may be complicated by pain and thrombosis. Capillary venous malformations can also occur in any internal organ and are usually seen as an incidental finding on an arteriogram. Capillary venous malformations occur in the Klippel–Trenaunay and Parkes–Weber syndromes. Arteriography of capillary venous malformations shows a normal artery and either venous pooling or enlarged veins in the venous phase of the study. Direct puncture venography is more useful in delineating the venous side of the malformation, but MRI demonstrates both the blood vessel and soft-tissue components and is therefore the most useful investigation. Capillary venous malformations

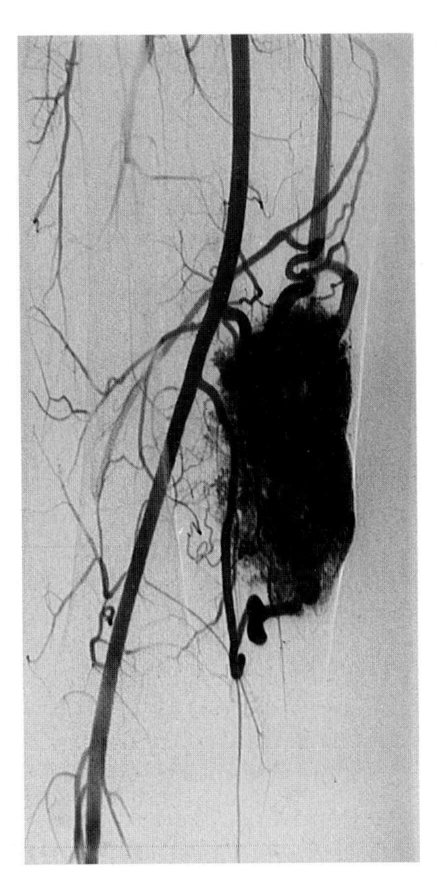

Fig. 23.10 Femoral arteriography showing an arteriovenous malformation in the lower thigh supplied by hypertrophied branches of the right superficial femoral artery and draining into the long saphenous vein.

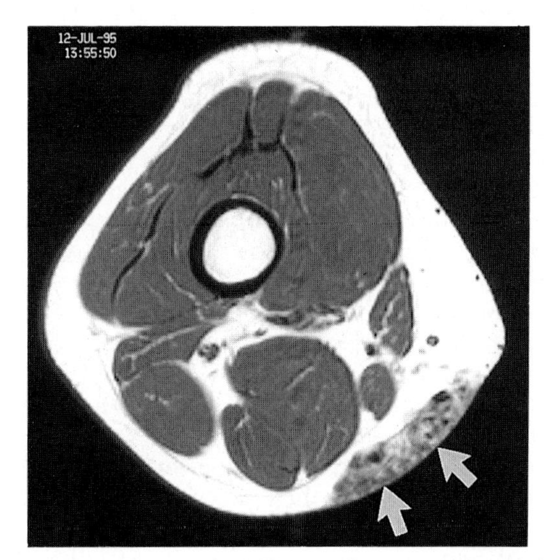

Fig. 23.11 Axial T1-weighted MRI scan (in same patient as in Fig. 23.10) showing that the arteriovenous malformation (arrows) does not involve the muscles in the thigh.

are difficult to treat surgically, because they are often more extensive than demonstrated clinically but are well shown on MRI (Fig. 23.11). They tend to recur and do not respond to embolization.

TRANSIENT ISCHAEMIC ATTACKS

Patients with carotid artery stenosis present clinically with either a transient ischaemic attack or a stroke which may produce loss of vision, loss of speech, sensory disturbances and/or loss of motor power in an arm or a leg. Recovery occurs within 24 hours in the transient ischaemic attack, but not after a stroke.

The initial investigation of patients with a bruit in the neck due to suspected carotid artery stenosis includes duplex ultrasound, magnetic resonance angiography or intravenous digital subtraction angiography. Duplex ultrasound is a non-invasive method of imaging the carotid and vertebral arteries in the neck with a high sensitivity and specificity for carotid artery stenosis, but can still misinterpret a high-grade stenosis as an occlusion. Magnetic resonance angiography is also a non-invasive method of imaging which has the advantage of being able to demonstrate both the intrathoracic and intracranial vessels, although it also tends to overestimate the degree of stenosis. Intravenous digital subtraction angiography is an invasive method of imaging with a lower sensitivity and specificity for carotid artery stenosis than duplex ultrasound and has the disadvantage of demonstrating all the intracranial arteries simultaneously which overlap on the images.

Patients with a low-grade stenosis of less than 30% are treated conservatively with antiplatelet therapy, such as aspirin, but patients with a high-grade stenosis of > 70% should be considered for surgery or possibly angioplasty (Fig. 23.12). The management of patients with a stenosis between 30–70% varies between centres.

Arteriography is performed only in patients being assessed for carotid endarterectomy, because it carries a risk of permanent neurological damage of about 1%. Selective carotid arteriography may show an atheromatous stenosis or an ulcerating plaque at the origin of the internal carotid artery or, less commonly, a stenosis at the origin of the external carotid artery, in the common carotid artery and occasionally even in the intracerebral arteries. Arch aortography may show an atheromatous stenosis at the origin of one of the great vessels arising from the arch of the aorta; an arteritis with multiple stenoses; occlusions in the carotid and subclavian arteries, or even the subclavian steal syndrome when there is occlusion of the left subclavian artery and reverse flow down the left vertebral artery.

Patients with a pulsatile lump in the neck also require investigation with either duplex ultrasound or carotid arteriography. CT may also be helpful. The lump is commonly due to a tortuous carotid artery in an elderly hypertensive patient, but may be due to a chemodectoma, carotid body tumour, or an aneurysm of the internal carotid artery.

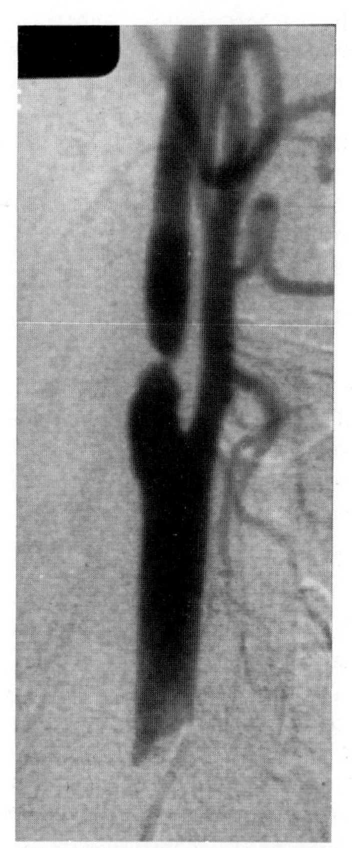

Fig. 23.12 Carotid digital subtraction arteriography showing a 75% stenosis of the right internal carotid artery.

RENOVASCULAR HYPERTENSION

A renovascular cause of hypertension occurs in about 5% of hypertensive patients. As hypertension is such a common condition, investigation has to be limited to:

- patients whose blood pressure is difficult to control with conventional medical treatment;
- patients whose renal function deteriorates on medical treatment with angiotensin-converting enzyme inhibitors such as captopril;
- patients with malignant hypertension;
- young hypertensive patients <30 years.

The use of excretion urography as a screening test for renal artery stenosis has been replaced by duplex ultrasound, magnetic resonance angiography or intravenous digital subtraction angiography. Duplex ultrasound is a non-invasive method of imaging the renal

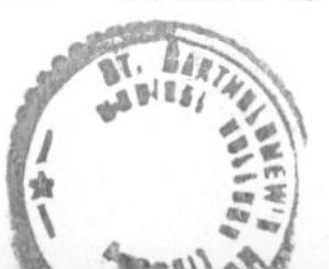

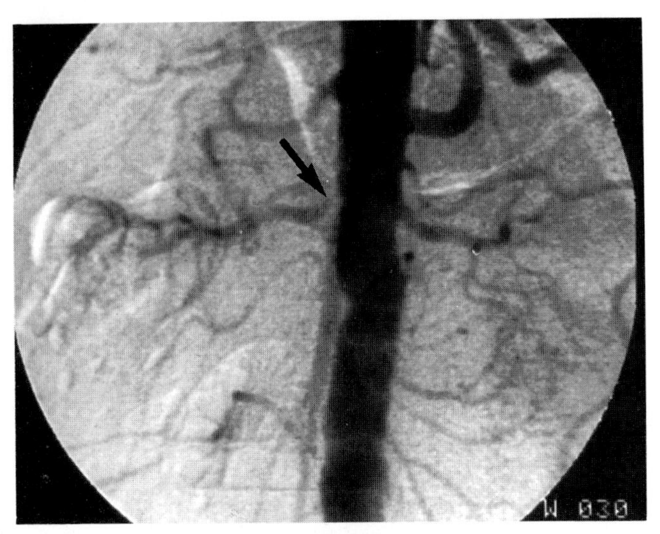

Fig. 23.13 Intravenous digital subtraction angiography showing a significant stenosis of the right renal artery (arrow).

arteries, which are often difficult to demonstrate. Magnetic resonance angiography is also a non-invasive method of imaging giving good visualization of the renal arteries; but it has the disadvantage that it cannot identify fibromuscular disease. Intravenous digital subtraction angiography is an invasive method of imaging, but can be combined with renal vein sampling, particularly in patients with a high plasma renin level. A ratio of at least 1.5 : 1 of renin in the renal veins of each kidney, suggests that there is a renal artery stenosis causing the hypertension (Fig. 24.13).

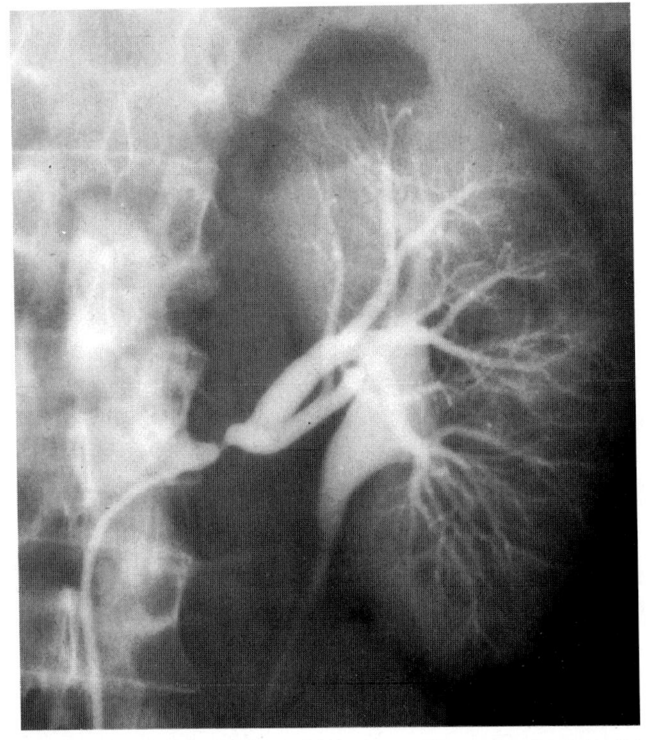

Fig. 23.14 Renal arteriography showing a 75% stenosis of the left renal artery.

Renal arteriography, however, remains the definitive diagnostic investigation for renovascular hypertension and may show an atheromatous stenosis at the origin of the vessel (Fig. 23.14) or the typically beaded appearance of fibromuscular disease more distally in the vessel. Both these types of renal artery stenosis can be treated by angioplasty, but fibromuscular disease responds better than atheromatous disease, which may require a vascular stent. Other causes of renovascular hypertension that may be demonstrated include a renal artery aneurysm, arteriovenous fistula, embolus or a renal vasculitis such as polyarteritis nodosa.

Renal artery angioplasty can be used to treat patients with deteriorating chronic renal failure, from either bilateral or unilateral renal artery stenosis (when the other renal artery is already occluded), or transplant artery stenosis.

PERIPHERAL VASCULAR DISEASE

THE ISCHAEMIC LEG

Patients with chronic ischaemia of the lower limb present with symptoms ranging from intermittent claudication and rest pain to ischaemic ulceration and gangrene; they have reduced or absent pulses below the stenosis or occlusion, whereas patients with an acutely ischaemic leg present with severe pain, altered sensation, loss of motor power and a cold leg. They also have no pulses below the occlusion.

The assessment of these patients includes clinical investigations such as relevant blood tests, urine analysis and ECG, tests in the vascular laboratory such as Doppler arterial pressure measurements, plethysmography and treadmill testing together with radiological investigations such as duplex ultrasound, MRI and arteriography.

Duplex ultrasound can be used to image the lower limb arteries, but it is very time-consuming to assess fully both legs for stenoses, occlusions and aneurysms and it can be difficult to demonstrate the iliac arteries because of overlying bowel gas. Duplex ultrasound is however most useful in the follow-up of patients who have had a surgical bypass graft or an angioplasty; in the assessment of a pulsating mass that could be due to a true or false aneurysm; and in vein mapping prior to a surgical bypass graft. Magnetic resonance angiography can also be used to image the lower limb arteries, but its availability is limited.

Arteriography, therefore, remains the best method of imaging the lower limb arteries with digital subtraction enhancing visualization of the tibial arteries and even the vessels in the foot can be well visualized. Arteriography is usually performed via catheterization of the femoral artery, as long as one of

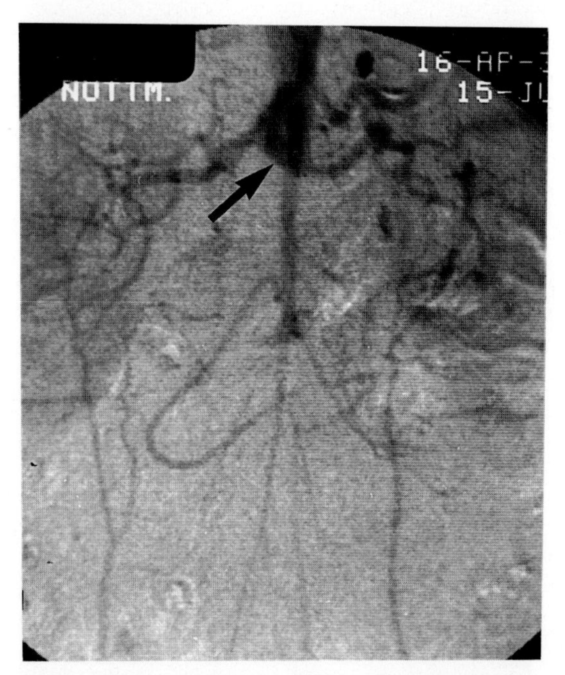

(a)

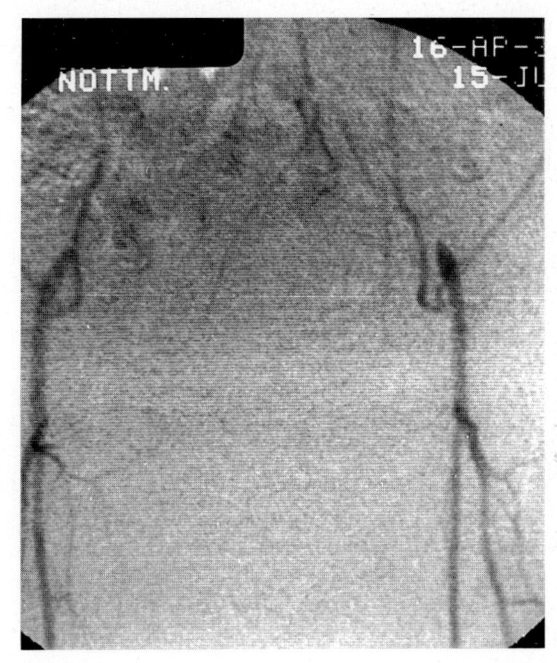

(b)

Fig. 23.15 Intravenous digital subtraction angiography showing (a) an infrarenal occlusion of the lower abdominal aorta (arrow) extending into the iliac arteries and (b) patent common, superficial and deep femoral arteries filling through collateral vessels.

the femoral pulses is present in the groin. If neither of the femoral pulses are present in the groins, as in patients with the Leriche syndrome, in which there is aortoiliac occlusive disease and impotence, the arteriography can be performed by catheterization of the brachial or axillary artery or by catheterizing an arm vein and using intravenous digital subtraction angiography (Fig. 23.15). Translumbar aortography is now rarely performed, because of the inevitable retroperitoneal bleeding that occurs on withdrawal of the needle from the aorta.

Femoral arteriography may show various patterns of atheromatous disease with stenoses or thrombotic occlusions in the aortoiliac segment, the superficial femoral artery, the popliteal artery and distal vessels or combinations of these patterns in one or both legs. Ectatic arteries with slow flow and unsuspected aneurysms in the lower abdominal aorta and iliac arteries, as well as the common femoral and popliteal arteries, may also be demonstrated. Embolic occlusions are also occasionally demonstrated. The popliteal entrapment syndrome, which is due to medial displacement and extrinsic compression of the popliteal artery by the medial head of the gastrocnemius muscle, cystic adventitial disease of the popliteal artery and an arteritis, such as Buerger's disease, are rare causes of peripheral vascular disease.

Significant stenoses of >50% in the lower limb arteries, short chronic occlusions up to 5–7 cm in length in the iliac arteries and long chronic occlusions up to 10–15 cm in length in the superficial femoral and popliteal arteries are suitable for treatment by percutaneous transluminal angioplasty. Longer occlusions in the lower limb arteries can be treated by angioplasty, but really require a surgical bypass with either a synthetic or vein graft; the choice of graft material depending upon the site. Short or long acute occlusions can be treated by either surgical embolectomy or thrombolysis.

SURGICAL GRAFTS

There are two types of surgical graft material – synthetic grafts with either Dacron or polytetrafluoroethylene and vein grafts using either *in situ* or reversed saphenous vein, or processed human umbilical vein. Radiological imaging techniques play a central role in the management of patients who have had a surgical bypass graft.

All patients who have undergone either a femoropopliteal or a femorodistal vein bypass should enter a graft surveillance programme consisting of duplex ultrasound examinations at intervals of 1 month, 3 months, 6 months, 1 year and 2 years after the surgery, in order to look for the development of stenoses which can lead to graft failure, at the proximal or distal anastomoses or within the graft itself (Plate 10, opposite page 562).

Immediate graft failure, within the first month, is usually due to a technical complication during the operation, but can be due to unsuitable patient selection. Early graft failure, within the first year, is usually due to graft stenosis, and late graft failure,

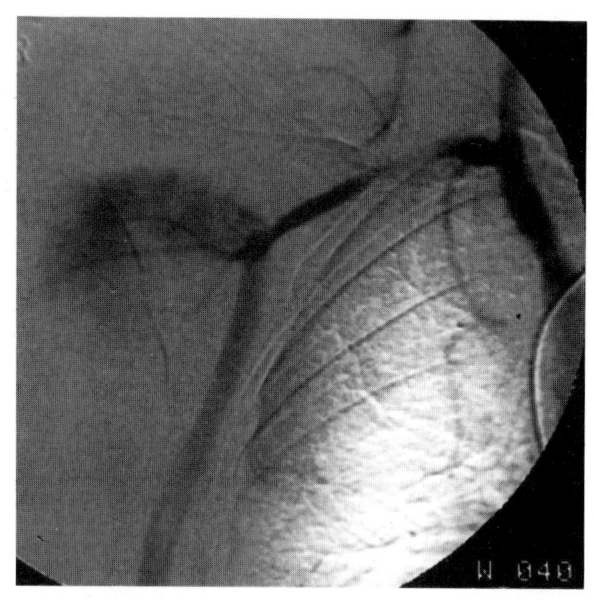

Fig. 23.16 Intravenous digital subtraction angiography showing a false aneurysm at the proximal anastomosis of an axillofemoral Dacron graft with compression of the right brachial artery.

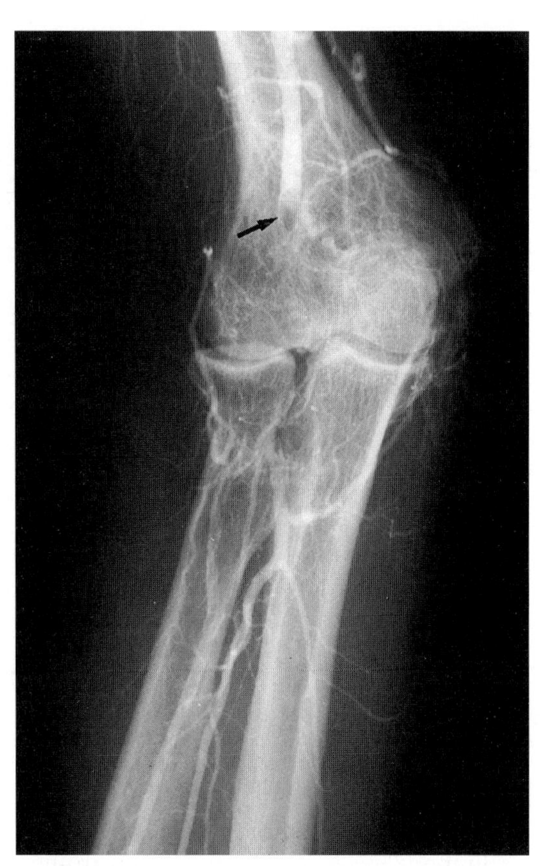

Fig. 23.17 Brachial arteriography showing an embolus in the right brachial artery (arrow).

after the first year, is commonly due to progression of distal disease and occasionally due to development of proximal disease.

Duplex ultrasound will also detect arteriovenous fistulae in the *in situ* vein graft (Plate 11, opposite page 562) and false aneurysms at the proximal or distal anastomoses of the synthetic grafts. Subsequent angiography may also be required and this can be performed either by intravenous digital subtraction angiography (Fig. 23.16) or by arteriography via the contralateral femoral artery. It is, however, possible to perform arteriography by direct puncture of the graft itself, if this provides the most suitable or only vascular access.

Graft stenoses can be treated by either vein patch or balloon angioplasty, and graft arteriovenous fistulae can be treated by either ligation or embolization. Occluded vein and synthetic grafts can be salvaged with thrombolysis but false aneurysms usually require surgery.

Radionuclide studies using radio-labelled white cells can be used to confirm the diagnosis of an infected graft and CT can be used in the assessment of false aneurysms within the abdomen and pelvis.

THE ISCHAEMIC ARM

Patients with an acutely ischaemic arm present with severe pain, altered sensation and loss of motor power and have no pulses below the occlusion as in the lower limb, but patients with chronic ischaemia of the upper limb can present with either Raynaud's phenomenon in the fingers or pain in the arm. The assessment of these patients is similar to that in the lower limbs, but once again arteriography remains the best method of imaging the upper limb arteries.

The arteriography can be performed either as an arch aortogram with selective subclavian arteriography, or as intravenous digital subtraction angiography. Selective brachial arteriography is required to demonstrate the arteries in the hand. Subclavian arteriography may show embolic occlusions (Fig. 23.17), or stenoses, thrombotic occlusions due to atheromatous disease, vasculitis or radiotherapy. Aneurysms and a thoracic outlet syndrome, which is due to extrinsic compression of the subclavian artery by a cervical rib or fibrous band as it passes over the first rib, can also be demonstrated.

Significant stenoses of >50% and short chronic occlusions in the subclavian, axillary or brachial arteries are suitable for treatment by angioplasty, but longer occlusions require a surgical bypass. Acute occlusions are usually treated by embolectomy, but can be treated by thrombolysis.

THERAPEUTIC EMBOLIZATION

Vascular embolization is a therapeutic radiological procedure, which involves the injection of embolic material through a catheter selectively positioned in a blood vessel to produce thrombus, which results in the deliberate occlusion of that blood vessel or vascular bed.

Embolization requires an experienced and skilled vascular radiologist to position the catheter and inject the embolic material safely using high-quality angiographic apparatus, preferably with a digital subtraction facility. Close monitoring of the patient's pulse rate, blood pressure and peripheral oxygen saturation is required and clotting abnormalities should be corrected. Bladder catheterization is also advised as the procedure is frequently protracted. Embolization is used as an alternative method of treatment to surgery but tends to carry less risk, because it is performed percutaneously under local anaesthetic in many cases. It can, however, be a time-consuming procedure, lasting several hours. The ideal embolic material should be:

- thrombogenic, but not toxic
- produce a permanent occlusion
- easy to inject through a catheter
- available in a wide range of sizes and shapes
- sterile
- radiopaque.

Many different solid and liquid agents have been used for embolization, but none are absolutely ideal although the ones used most commonly include:

- gelatin
- sponge fragments
- polyvinyl alcohol particles
- spiral metal coils
- detachable balloons
- hypertonic dextrose solution
- absolute ethyl alcohol
- tissue adhesives, such as bucrylate.

These embolic agents can be used either on their own or in combination cocktails, which should include antibiotics. Gelatin sponge has to be cut into small 1–2 mm fragments which are then suspended in contrast medium before injection because it is not radiopaque. Gelatin sponge fragments only produce a temporary occlusion with recanalization of the artery occurring within a few weeks. Polyvinyl alcohol particles are available in a range of sizes from 100–250, 250–500 and 500–1000 μm, and also have to be suspended in contrast medium before injection because they are not radiopaque. Polyvinyl alcohol particles do, however, produce a permanent occlusion of small arteries.

Metal coils made of steel or tungsten are available in a range of sizes with the diameter of the spiral from 1–20 mm. The steel coils are radiopaque and often have silk, wool or synthetic fibrils attached to them to increase their thrombogenicity. They are pushed through the catheter by a guidewire and produce permanent occlusion of large arteries. Detachable balloons made of latex or silicone are available in 1 and 2 mm sizes with the diameter of the inflated balloon reaching up to 4 or 8 mm. The balloon is filled with contrast medium before detachment from its microcatheter and this produces a permanent occlusion of aneurysms and arteriovenous fistulae.

Hypertonic dextrose solution, absolute alcohol and bucrylate all permeate into the smallest arterial branches because they are liquids and, although they are very effective at producing a permanent occlusion, they are also more likely to reach critical vessels close to the target organ. Hypertonic 50% dextrose solution and absolute alcohol can be mixed with contrast medium to make them radiopaque, but bucrylate is mixed with either tantalum powder or ethiodol to make it radiopaque and this also prolongs its polymerization time.

The indications for arterial embolization include the treatment of:

- acute haemorrhage management
- tumour therapy
- arteriovenous malformations
- hypersplenism
- priapism.

The indications for venous embolization include the treatment of:

- gastro-oesophageal varices
- testicular varicocoeles
- some adrenal tumours.

Embolization is used in the management of patients who are bleeding, but are unfit for surgery or in whom the surgery would be difficult. Active bleeding from the stomach, duodenum or rectum can be stopped by embolizing the left gastric, gastroduodenal or superior rectal arteries with very little risk of infarction because of the good collateral supply to these organs, unless there has been previous surgery. However, this risk of infarction is much greater in the small intestine and colon, where embolization is relatively contraindicated.

A false aneurysm within the liver or kidney following either penetrating trauma or a biopsy can be treated by selectively embolizing a branch of the hepatic or renal artery. A false aneurysm within the pancreas following recurrent pancreatitis can be treated by embolizing the gastroduodenal artery. Intractable haematuria from an inoperable renal tumour or a bladder tumour previously treated with radiotherapy can be treated by embolizing the renal arteries or both internal iliac arteries. Embolization has also been used to control haemoptysis from chronic fibrotic lung disease, epistaxis, vaginal bleeding and internal haemorrhage from a pelvic fracture (Fig. 23.18).

Embolization is used in the management of patients with neoplastic disease to control bleeding from the

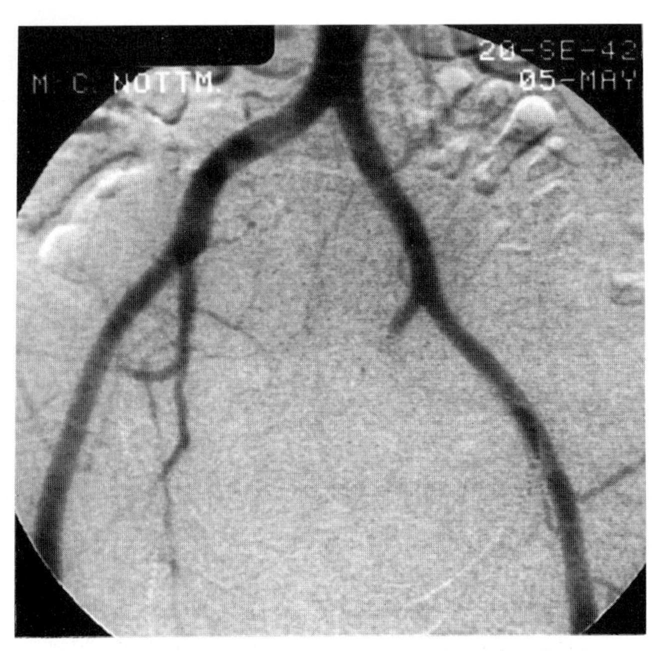

Fig. 23.18 Intravenous digital subtraction angiography showing no filling of the false aneurysm of the left internal iliac artery following embolization (in same patient as in Fig. 23.9).

tumour as already discribed, and to devascularize a tumour prior to surgery, such as an intracranial meningioma, a nasopharyngeal angiofibroma or a malignant bone tumour. Embolization of the liver is useful in ablating the function of hepatic metastases from carcinoid tumours, insulinomas and glucagonomas, reducing the size of the liver in patients with painful hepatomegaly from metastases and controlling haemobilia from metastases. Hepatic artery embolization is, however, contraindicated if the hepatic portal vein is occluded.

Congenital arteriovenous malformations, particularly those with a large arterial component, are best treated by embolization. Traumatic arteriovenous fistulae and false aneurysms are also suitable for treatment.

Embolization of the splenic artery can be used in patients with hypersplenism who are a poor surgical risk owing to their clotting abnormalities. The internal pudendal artery is embolized in patients with priapism where medical treatment has failed.

Embolization of the gonadal vein can be used to manage patients with infertility who have a testicular varicocele and embolization of the adrenal vein has been performed in patients to ablate a functioning adrenal tumour.

The complications of embolization include those of arteriography and the use of contrast media as well as accidental embolization of an adjacent critical normal organ, abscess formation in the infarcted tissue, renal failure and death. A postembolization syndrome of pain, fever and leucocytosis also develops within a few days of the procedure owing to tissue necrosis. An embolic agent, such as a steel coil or a detachable balloon misplaced within the vascular system can be retrieved with a snare.

PERCUTANEOUS TRANSLUMINAL ANGIOPLASTY

Vascular dilatation or angioplasty is a therapeutic radiological procedure, which involves the inflation of a balloon catheter positioned at the site of a stenosis or an occlusion in a blood vessel to increase blood flow through the vessel and improve perfusion to a limb or organ. Angioplasty requires an experienced and skilled vascular radiologist to cross the stenosis or recanalize the occlusion and inflate/deflate the balloon safely. High-quality angiographic apparatus should be used, preferably with a digital subtraction facility. Angioplasty is the commonest vascular interventional procedure and is an alternative method of treatment to a surgical bypass graft, but carries less risk because it is performed percutaneously under local anaesthetic. However, it can also be used to treat patients whose symptoms are not severe enough to merit reconstructive surgery and in patients to prevent amputation. It is also used in combination with a surgical bypass graft to improve the inflow or outflow in the adjacent arteries.

The indications for angioplasty include:

- peripheral vascular disease of the lower or upper limbs with stenoses or short occlusions in the peripheral arteries;
- ischaemic heart disease with stenosis in the coronary arteries;
- hypertension or chronic renal failure with renal or transplant artery stenosis;
- mesenteric and even carotid artery stenosis.

The technique, which can be performed in conjunction with a diagnostic arteriogram or as a separate procedure, which is really quite simple in theory, but can be more complex to perform in practice. The contraindications to angioplasty in patients with peripheral vascular disease are the presence of fresh thrombus, which should be treated by thrombolysis, an aortic occlusion and long occlusions in the iliac, femoral, popliteal and tibial arteries.

The ideal lesion for angioplasty is a short, smooth, central stenosis in a large artery, such as the iliac artery, with normal distal arteries, although most patients tend to have more generalized vascular disease with stenoses and occlusions in several arteries (Fig. 23.19).

After catheterization of the femoral artery, a guidewire and catheter are gently used to cross the stenosis or recanalize the occlusion; the artery is then dilated up to the size of the adjacent vessel by a suitable balloon. This is then deflated again and if the blood

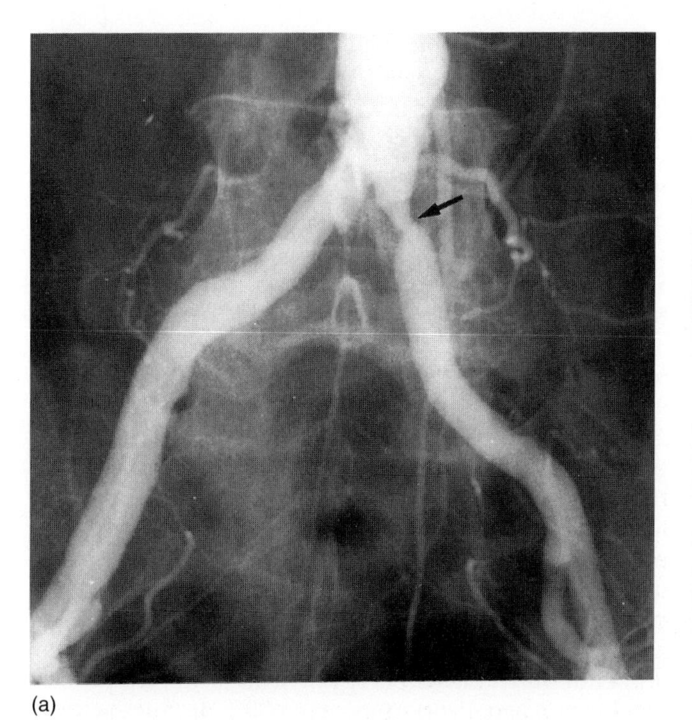
(a)

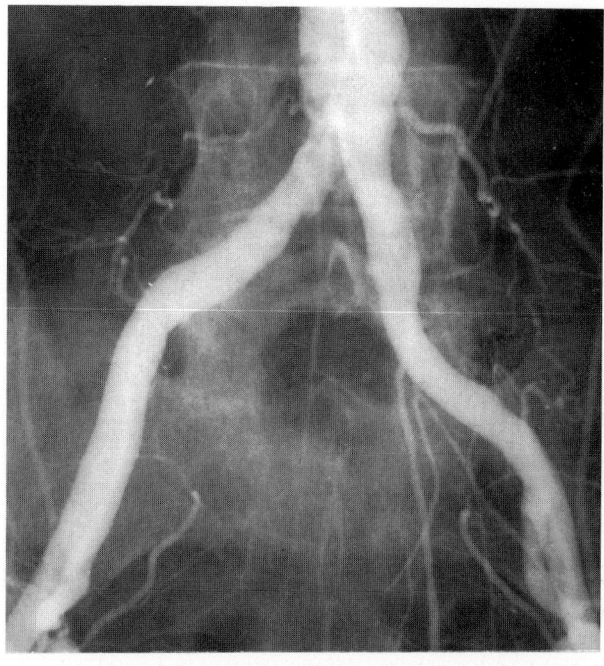
(b)

Fig. 23.19 Iliac arteriography showing (a) a 50% stenosis of the left common iliac artery (arrow) before angioplasty and (b) the result 2 years after angioplasty.

flow has been improved the balloon catheter is removed. The process can be repeated several times if there is a residual stenosis. Patients undergoing angioplasty should be started on an antiplatelet drug such as aspirin or dipyridamole about 24 hours before the procedure and this should be continued after a successful procedure for at least 3–6 months and possibly forever. During the angioplasty, patients should receive 3000–5000 units of heparin intra-arterially. The success of the procedure is based on eliminating the pressure gradient across a stenosis and producing a good angiographic result with no residual stenosis at arteriography. Endovascular ultrasound and angioscopy have been used to assess the effectiveness of angioplasty. Iliac artery stenoses and short iliac artery occlusions up to 5–7 cm in length are usually approached from below following a retrograde catheterization of the ipsilateral common femoral artery, but can be approached from above following a retrograde catheterization of the contralateral common femoral artery and crossing of the aortic bifurcation, or following catheterization of the axillary or brachial artery. Stenoses in the internal iliac, common femoral, proximal superficial and deep femoral arteries are best approached across the aortic bifurcation, but stenoses or short occlusions up to 10–15 cm in length in the distal superficial femoral and popliteal arteries are usually approached from above following an antegrade catheterization of the ipsilateral common or proximal superficial femoral arteries; they can be approached from below following catherization of the ipsilateral popliteal artery. Stenoses in the lower abdominal aorta and stenoses or short occlusions up to 5 cm in length in the tibial arteries are also suitable for angioplasty.

Coronary, renal, mesenteric, subclavian and carotid artery stenoses are usually approached from below following a retrograde catheterization of the femoral artery, but can be approached from above following catheterization of the axillary or brachial artery.

Before angioplasty a pressure gradient of >20 mmHg at rest across an iliac artery stenosis or occlusion is significant, but if it is only 10 mmHg at rest a vasodilator such as papaverine, tolazoline or glyceryl trinitrate should be injected through the catheter. An increase in the pressure gradient to >20 mmHg indicates that the stenosis is significant and requires angioplasty. Following angioplasty the ideal result is no gradient at all, but a residual gradient of <10 mmHg is often acceptable. Pressure monitoring across femoral and popliteal artery stenoses and occlusions is not accurate in an antegrade direction and angiography is, therefore, used to monitor the procedure. Following angioplasty the ideal result is no residual stenosis, but a slight narrowing of the arterial lumen up to 25% of its diameter is often acceptable.

The complications of angioplasty are the same as the complications of arteriography and can therefore occur at the arterial puncture site, at the angioplasty site, distal to the site of the angioplasty, and in the systemic circulation. The complications at the puncture site are:

- haemorrhage and haematoma formation
- thrombosis
- false aneurysm formation
- nerve trauma
- local infection.

The complications at the site of the angioplasty include arterial subintimal dissection, which is not usually significant with angioplasty performed in a retrograde direction, as the flow of blood tends to close the flap; it can be significant in the antegrade direction as the flow of blood tends to open the flap and lead to thrombus formation. Perforation of the artery within an occlusion is not usually significant, but rupture of an iliac or renal artery produces significant haemorrhage which can be life-threatening.

Complications distal to the site of angioplasty are arterial spasm and distal embolization of atheromatous or thrombotic debris. Systemic complications include:

- vasovagal reaction
- hypotension
- cardiac arrythmias
- myocardial infarction
- cerebrovascular accident
- cholesterol crystal embolization
- renal failure
- septicaemia
- death.

Restenosis occurs more frequently after coronary and renal artery angioplasty, than following iliac, femoral or popliteal artery angioplasty. Recurrent stenosis can be treated by angioplasty or with an arterial stent. Acute reocclusion at the site of the angioplasty is an indication for thrombolysis, but chronic reocclusion can be treated by repeat angioplasty. The initial technical success for iliac artery angioplasty is 90–95% for stenoses and 80–90% for occlusions with a patency rate of 50–90% at 5 years, whereas the initial technical success for femoral and popliteal angioplasty is 85–95% for stenoses, 60–90% for occlusions and 20–70% patency rate at 5 years.

OTHER TECHNIQUES FOR TREATING ARTERIAL OBSTRUCTION

There are a number of new techniques or devices that have been developed to either assist or replace balloon angioplasty, but these tend to be expensive and should therefore produce either a higher initial technical success rate or a better long-term patency rate to be of any real clinical value.

Most of these new devices are used to recanalize complete occlusions in the femoral and popliteal arteries, which then still require balloon angioplasty of the recanalized channel. The Rotational Transluminal Angioplasty Catheter System (ROTACS) is a low-speed rotating mechanical device, which rotates at about 100 rpm and produces recanalization in about 80% of cases. The Kensey catheter is a high-speed rotating mechanical device, which rotates at speeds up to 10 000 rpm and produces recanalization in up to 90% of occlusions where a guidewire and catheter system has previously been unsuccessful. Long-term patency is 50–70% at 2 years. The Rotablator is a very high-speed rotating mechanical device, rotating at over 100 000 rpm and is used over a guidewire. It produces a recanalization in over 90% of cases, but tends to produce peripheral emboli. Long-term patency is only 25–40% at 2 years. Laser-assisted angioplasty using continuous or pulsed wave lasers and either direct laser energy, hybrid or hot-tip probes produces recanalization in up to 90% of cases with a high risk of arterial perforation of about 20%. Long-term patency is 60–70% at 2 years.

The Transluminal Endarterectomy Catheter (TEC) is used over a guidewire for either stenoses or occlusions. The atheroma is aspirated through the catheter to produce a recanalization in about 80% of cases. Long-term patency is compromised by a high restenosis rate of 25–40%. The Simpson atherectomy catheter is used over a guidewire for eccentric stenoses. The atheroma is collected in a small chamber, which limits its use in occlusions.

Vascular stents are used for intraluminal mechanical arterial support to prevent an acute occlusion or improve long-term patency in the iliac arteries. The indications for their use include acute occlusion due to an initimal flap after angioplasty, residual stenosis after angioplasty, and following the successful recanalization of an occlusion in the iliac arteries (Fig. 23.20). Types include the flexible Wallstent, the Strecker stent and the rigid Palmaz stent. Long-term patency is 80–95% at 2 years. The Gianturco Z stent is used in the treatment of superior vena caval obstruction and has been used in the endovascular stenting of abdominal aortic aneurysms. Dacron-covered stents have been used successfully in the treatment of selected cases of infra-renal abdominal aortic aneurysms. Similarly, aortocaval fistulae can be treated with endoluminal stents.

THROMBOLYSIS

Thrombolysis is a new technique that can be used in the treatment of the acutely ischaemic leg or arm and

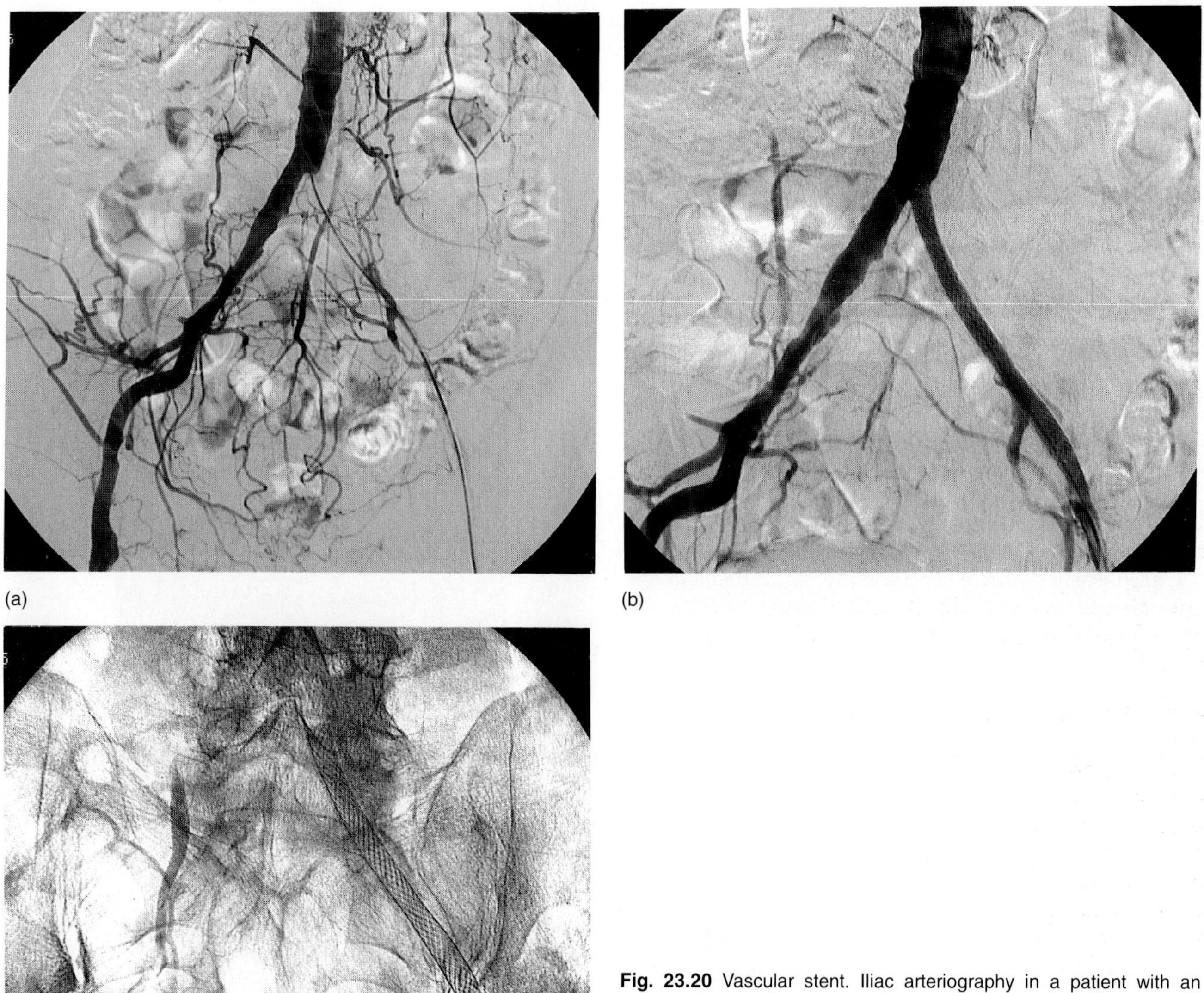

(a) (b) (c)

Fig. 23.20 Vascular stent. Iliac arteriography in a patient with an occlusion of the left common iliac artery. (a) A guidewire has been introduced across the occlusion and angioplasty subsequently performed. (b) The result after angioplasty and insertion of a vascular stent. (c) The vascular Wallstent (Schneider) in place extending from the aortic bifurcation to the external iliac artery.

may well be the most effective form of treatment for patients with a critically ischaemic limb, because the results of reconstructive vascular surgery are poor in these patients who have a mortality rate of 15–50% and an amputation rate of 20–60%. Embolectomy, however, produces a limb salvage rate of 95% with a mortality rate of about 12%, but most of the acute occlusions are caused by thrombus from underlying atherosclerotic disease.

The indications for intra-arterial thrombolytic therapy include:

- distal arterial thrombosis or embolus involving the popliteal artery with extension into the tibial arteries;
- proximal arterial thrombosis of the iliac, femoral and popliteal arteries (Fig. 23.21);
- thrombosis of a vein or a synthetic graft;
- thrombosis at the site of a recent angioplasty;
- proximal or distal arterial thrombosis in a patient at risk from vascular surgery.

The indications for vascular surgery include:

- proximal arterial embolus involving the aortic bifurcation, the iliac and the femoral arteries;
- proximal arterial thrombosis of the iliac and femoral arteries if there is insufficient time for intra-arterial thrombolysis to work in a severely ischaemic leg;
- thrombosis of a synthetic or vein graft.

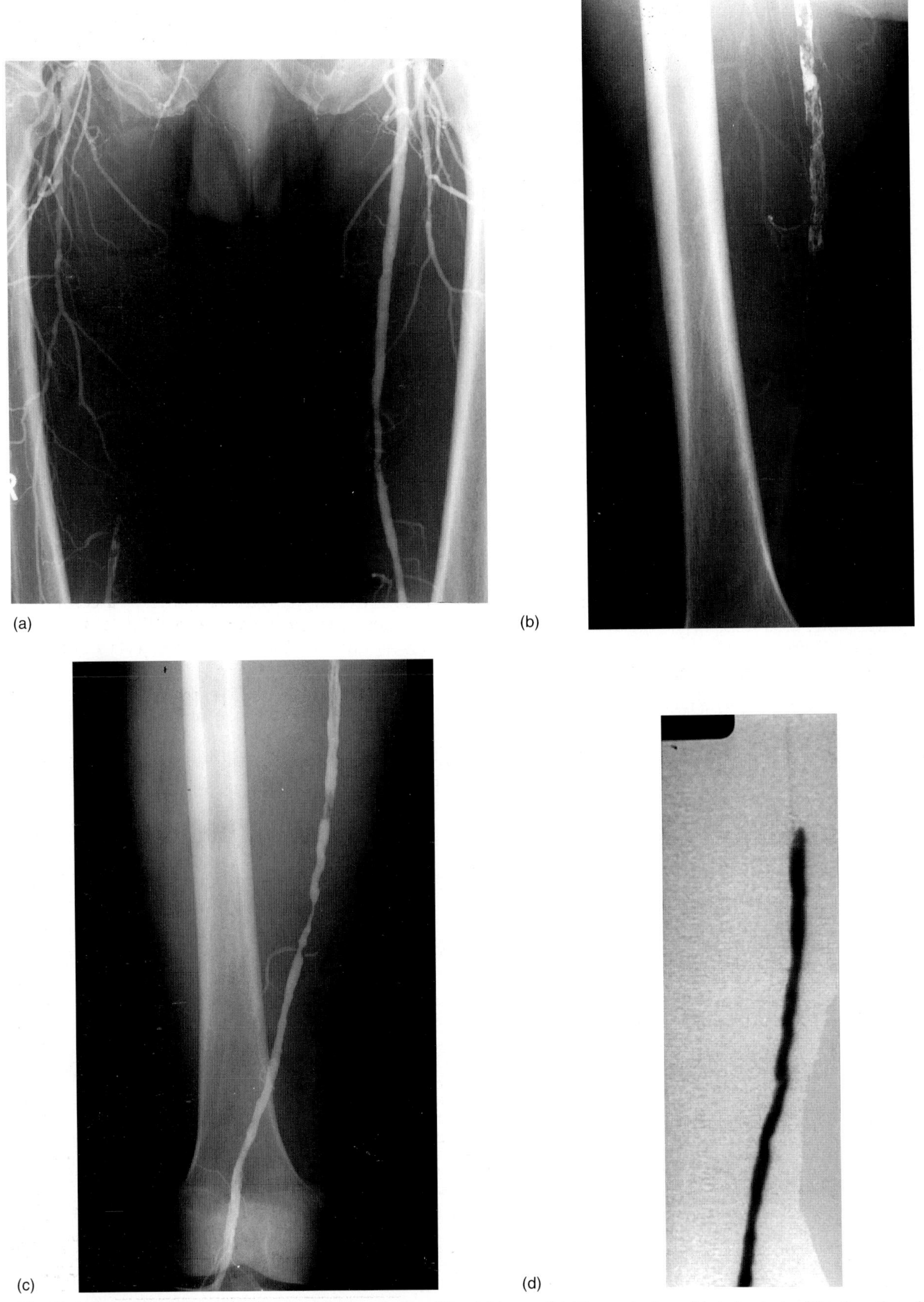

(a) (b) (c) (d)

Fig. 23.21 Femoral arteriography showing (a) an occlusion of the right superficial femoral artery; (b) during lysis of the thrombus; (c) after lysis, revealing 50–75% stenoses; (d) the result after angioplasty.

The contraindications to thrombolysis are:

- recent bleeding from any site;
- a stroke within the last three months;
- recent major surgery or trauma;
- coagulation defect;
- potential bleeding site.

Thrombolysis is performed following diagnostic arteriography with the tip of the catheter positioned in the occlusion either across the aortic bifurcation for proximal occlusions or following an ipsilateral antegrade catheterization for distal occlusions.

With the low-dose infusion technique that uses 5000 units streptokinase/h, 50 000 units urokinase/h or 0.5 mg recombinant tissue plasminogen activator/h, the catheter can be advanced as the thrombus lyses. Lysis is monitored by arteriography and any underlying stenosis revealed requires immediate angioplasty. With the high-dose infusion or bolus technique that uses 20 000 units streptokinase/h, 240 000 units urokinase/h or 10 mg recombinant tissue plasminogen activator/h, the time taken for the thrombus to lyse falls from 25–40 to 6–18 h. A new development of these accelerated thrombolytic regimens is pulse spray pharmacomechanical thrombolysis. This involves injecting 0.2 ml of fluid every 30 s into the thrombus through multiple slits in the catheter and results in a lysis time of about 90 min.

The complications of thrombolysis include:

- groin haematoma and haemorrhage from the puncture site;
- distal embolization of thrombus;
- gastrointestinal and retroperitoneal haemorrhage;
- acute renal failure owing to the release of myoglobin from necrotic muscle;
- cerebrovascular accident;
- death.

Intra-arterial thrombolysis results in limb salvage in 70–80% of patients with a critically ischaemic limb with an amputation rate of 5–10% and a mortality rate of about 10%. Thrombolysis has also been used in the treatment of renal artery occlusions, superior vena caval obstruction and deep vein thrombosis. Small amounts of fresh thrombus can be aspirated through a catheter with a large internal luminal diameter and large amounts of fresh thrombus can be removed by a rotating mechanical device or disintegrated with an ultrasonic probe.

LYMPHATICS

LYMPHOGRAPHY

Lymphography is an invasive radiological procedure, involving the injection of contrast medium into a lymphatic to give diagnostic information about not only the lymphatics but also the lymph nodes. Lymphography has been largely replaced by various non-invasive radiological imaging techniques, but is still used in the investigation of patients with lymphoedema, lymphatic leaks and the demonstration of diseased lymph nodes. An advantage of lymphography is that it can demonstrate metastatic disease or lymphoma in normal-sized glands, but its disadvantage is that many nodal groups in the abdomen and pelvis, such as the internal iliac and mesenteric lymph nodes, are not demonstrated at all by the technique.

Lymphography only demonstrates the retroperitoneal and some pelvic and inguinal lymph nodes. It may show focal deposits typically in metastatic disease or diffusely enlarged glands with abnormal internal architecture as in lymphoma (Fig. 23.22). The appearances are however not specific for malignant disease as fibrolipomatosis produces a focal deposit in the inguinal nodes in elderly patients and reactive hyperplasia produces diffusely enlarged glands.

Technique

Lymphography is performed as an in- or outpatient procedure and involves the cannulation of a lymphatic in the foot; this procedure is quite difficult, because these vessels are very small and lymph is a colourless fluid. In order to identify the lymphatics, a non-toxic dye, such as Patent Blue Violet, is injected subcutaneously into the first and second web spaces between the toes on both feet. The dye is taken up into the lymphatics within 10–20 minutes, which then become visible through the skin.

The subcutaneous tissues on the dorsum of the foot are infiltrated with local anasthetic and an incision is

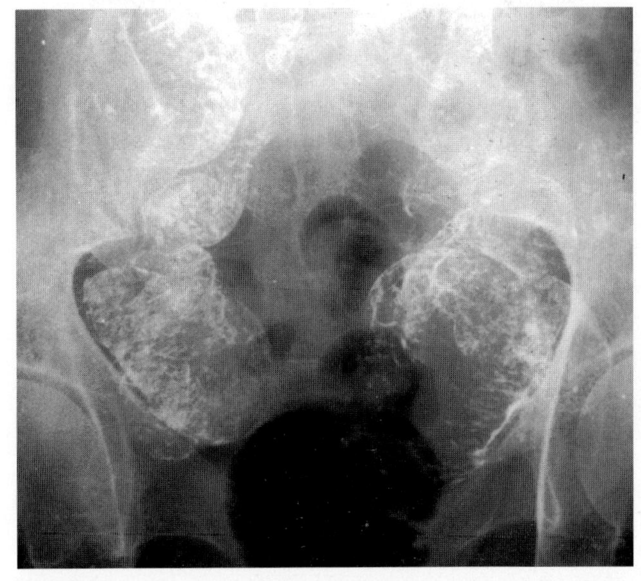

Fig. 23.22 Lymphography showing abnormal enlarged iliac lymph nodes infiltrated by non-Hodgkin's lymphoma.

made in the skin. A lymphatic vessel, which now appears blue in colour, is then very carefully dissected free from the surrounding tissues and cannulated with a 27- or 30-gauge lymphography needle attached to a soft, fine, plastic tubing with a hub at the other end. The needle is tied in position with black silk and the tubing is secured to the skin of the foot. About 1–2 ml of a non-ionic contrast medium is injected slowly by hand in order to check for leaks and then 6–8 ml of Lipiodol Ultra Fluid is injected by a pump over 1 hour.

In the investigation of nodal disease in the abdomen and pelvis, contrast medium is injected into both feet until it reaches the level of the sacroiliac joints. In the investigation of lymphoedema water-soluble contrast medium can be used instead of the oily Lipiodol and this may be sufficient to examine only the swollen leg. The patient should be warned that skin and urine will become blue in colour for 24–48 h. Lymphography can be performed in the arm by cannulating a lymphatic on the dorsum of the hand.

In patients with lymphoedema, radiographs are taken of the lower and upper leg (or arm) at the end of the procedure to show the lymphatics, but in the investigation of patients with suspected nodal disease, radiographs are taken of the abdomen and pelvis at the end of the procedure to show the lymphatic phase (Fig. 23.23) and then repeated the next day in association with an intravenous urogram to show the nodal phase (Fig. 23.24) of the investigation. Chest radiographs taken at the end of the procedure show the thoracic duct and, if repeated the next day, oil emboli in the lungs. The oily Lipiodol will remain in the opacified lymph nodes for up to a year.

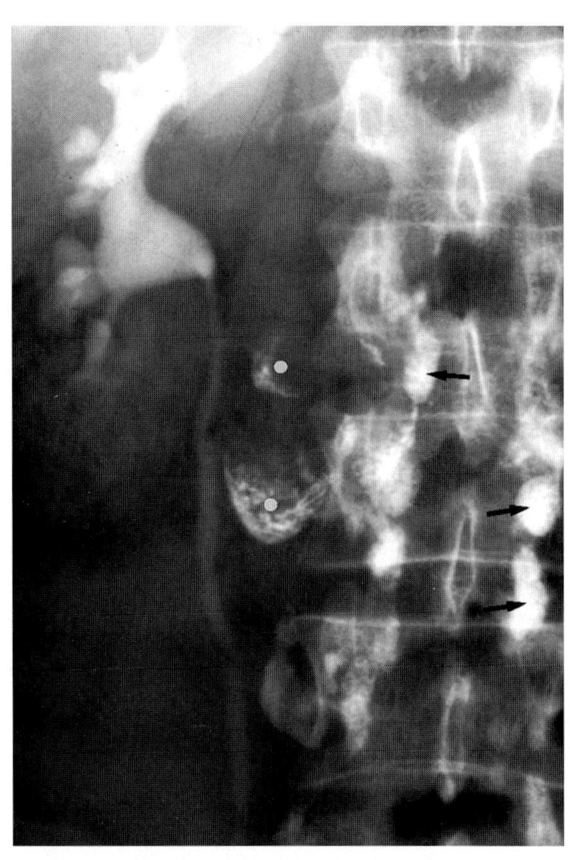

Fig. 23.24 Lymphogram showing both normal (arrows) and abnormal enlarged para-aortic lymph nodes (circles) in the nodal phase of the study, due to metastatic deposits from testicular teratoma.

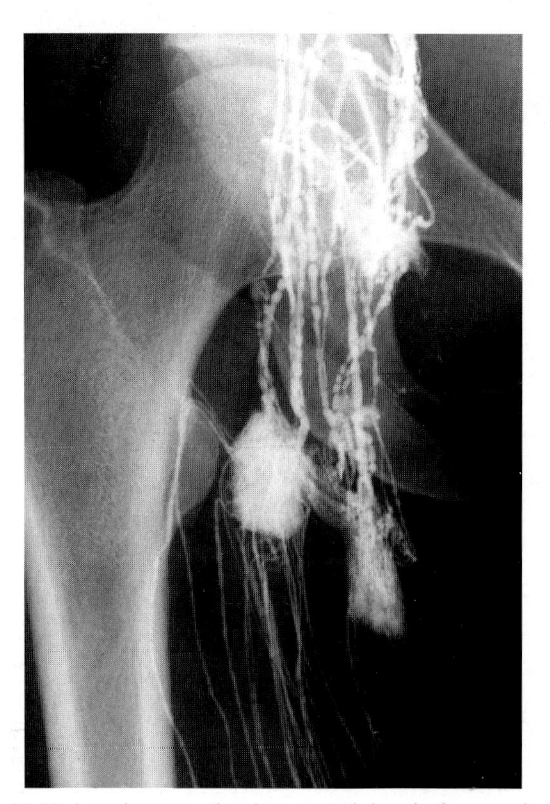

Fig. 23.23 Lymphogram showing normal lymphatic vessels and femoral lymph nodes in the lymphatic phase of the study.

The contraindications to lymphography include:

- soft-tissue infection in the foot;
- venous thrombosis in the leg;
- previous hypersensitivity reaction to contrast media;
- right-to-left cardiac shunts;
- pulmonary arteriovenous malformations;
- severe chest disease with compromised lung function;
- radiotherapy to the lungs.

Complications include:

- leg pains during the infusion of the contrast medium;
- mild symptoms such as headache, nausea and pyrexia the following day;
- pulmonary oil emboli which reduce lung function for 24–48 h;
- hypersensitivity reactions to the local anaesthetic, dye and contrast media;
- blue skin on the feet lasting several weeks.

LYMPHOEDEMA

Lymphoedema can be either congenital or acquired in origin and is one of the few remaining indications for lymphography. Congenital lymphoedema is due to aplasia, hypoplasia or hyperplasia of the lymphatics in the leg and these can be distinguished by lymphography. In aplasia there are no lymphatic vessels found in the foot which becomes rapidly stained blue due to dermal backflow of the dye. In hypoplasia there are only one or two lymphatic vessels in the leg (Fig. 28.2) instead of the usual five and in hyperplasia there are numerous dilated lymphatic vessels in the leg. Lymphatic hypoplasia is the cause of the swollen leg in 87% of patients with congenital lymphoedema. Acquired lymphoedema may be secondary to neoplastic disease or the surgery or radiotherapy associated with it, chronic infections such as filariasis and trauma.

Lymphatic flow can be assessed in patients with lymphoedema by lymphoscintigraphy using ^{99m}Tc-labelled antimony colloid and imaging with a gamma camera. The labelled colloid is injected into the web spaces between the second and third toes and is rapidly taken up into the lymphatic system so that the lymphatics in the legs and the pelvic lymph nodes are

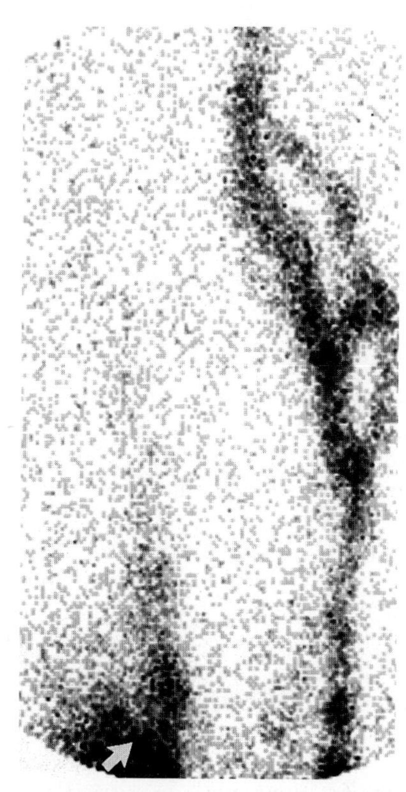

Fig. 23.26 Radionuclide study using technetium-labelled antimony colloid, showing lymphatic aplasia in the right calf with no lymphatics visualized and isotope remaining at the injection site in the right foot (arrow). Normal lymphatics are present in the left leg.

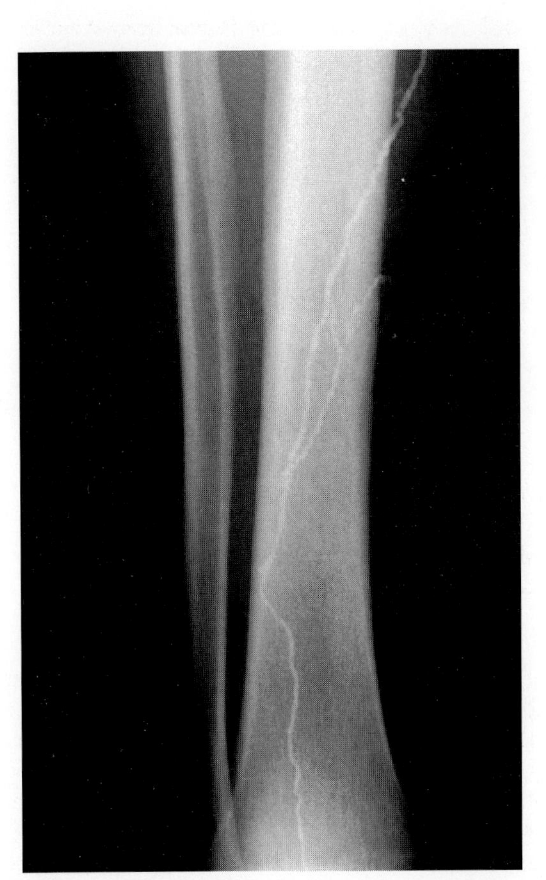

Fig. 23.25 Lymphogram showing lymphatic hypoplasia with only one lymphatic vessel visualized instead of the normal five vessels.

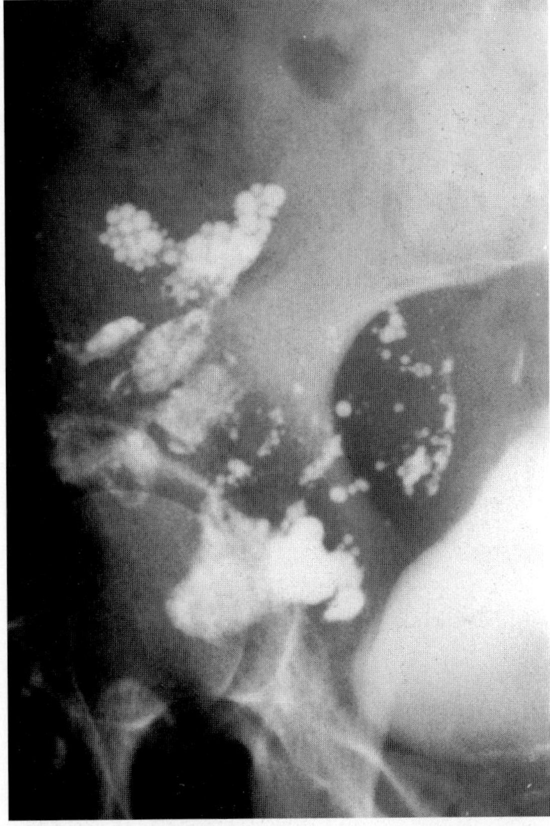

Fig. 23.27 Lymphogram showing globules of oily contrast in a large lymphocele in the pelvis following a hysterectomy for uterine carcinoma. (Contrast given for an IVU is present in the urinary bladder.)

visualized within 1 hour. In lymphoedema the usual pattern is for no lymphatics to be demonstrated (Fig. 23.26).

LYMPHATIC LEAKS AND COLLECTIONS

A **lymphocele** is a localized collection of lymph which usually occurs after pelvic lymph node dissection for neoplastic disease, but occasionally after renal transplantation, vascular reconstructive surgery and trauma. Ultrasound and CT both show a localized fluid collection in the pelvis that can be drained using image guidance. Lymphography will demonstrate a lymphocele or a cystic lymphangioma as a localized collection of oily Lipiodol in the pelvis or leg (Fig. 23.27) and lymphoscintigraphy can also demonstrate a lymphocoele or lymphangioma.

A **chylous pleural effusion**, **chylous ascites** and **chyluria** are the remaining indications for lymphography, to demonstrate the site of the leak and the cause of the obstruction. A chylothorax and chylous ascites are usually congenital in children and due to neoplastic and chronic inflammatory disease, surgery or trauma in adults. Chyluria is usually due to filariasis and is caused by a communication between the obstructed lymphatics and the pelvicalyceal system. Lymphovenous communications also occur in lymphatics obstructed by neoplastic or chronic inflammatory disease.

CHAPTER 24

Aorta

Simon C. Whitaker

THORACIC AORTA:
COARCTATION
ANEURYSM
AORTIC DISSECTION
INFLAMMATORY DISEASE

ABDOMINAL AORTA:
ANEURYSM
AORTOENTERIC FISTULA

THORACIC AORTA

COARCTATION

Coarctation refers to congenital narrowing of the thoracic aorta in the region of the isthmus. It is usually classified into pre- and post ductal types, depending upon whether the stenosis is proximal or distal to the ductus arteriosus. The condition is commonest in males and there are important associations with bicuspid aortic valve and with aneurysms of the circle of Willis. In severe cases, cardiac failure may occur in the neonatal period but most patients are asymptomatic at the time of detection. Symptoms are usually related to cardiac failure, bacterial endocarditis, aortic dissection or intracranial haemorrhage from a ruptured aneurysm.

The chest radiograph may show a dimple in the lateral aspect of the aortic arch at the site of the coarct and in severe cases there may be evidence of cardiac failure but the classic radiological sign of coarctation is notching of the ribs (Fig. 24.1). This is due to erosion of the inferior surfaces of the ribs by the pulsation of enlarged and tortuous intercostal arteries which, in tandem with the subclavian and internal mammary arteries, act as collateral supply to the aorta below the coarctation. Rib notching is not usually seen until the patient is about 10 years old and normally affects the fourth to eighth ribs bilaterally.

Diagnostic and Interventional Radiology in Surgical Practice. Edited by P. Armstrong and M. L. Wastie. Published in 1997 by Chapman & Hall, London. ISBN 0 412 61960 1 (HB), 0 412 61970 9 (PB)

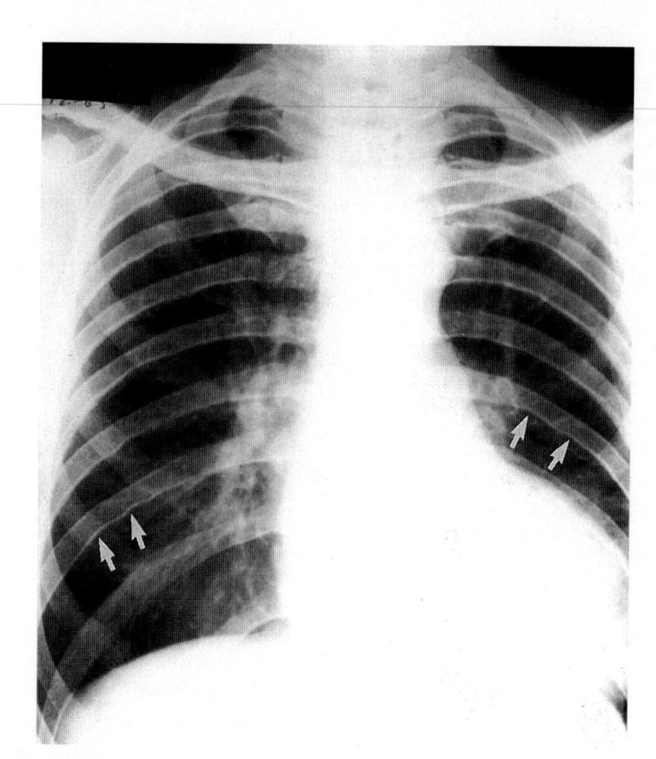

Fig. 24.1 Coarctation. This chest radiograph in a patient with coarctation shows classic erosion of the undersurfaces of the ribs due to pulsation of enlarged, tortuous intercostal arteries (arrows).

Most patients will require surgery preceded by radiological assessment of the site and severity of the coarctation. Aortography with measurement of the pressure gradient across the coarctation is the principal investigation for this purpose (Fig. 24.2) but non-invasive assessment with magnetic resonance imaging

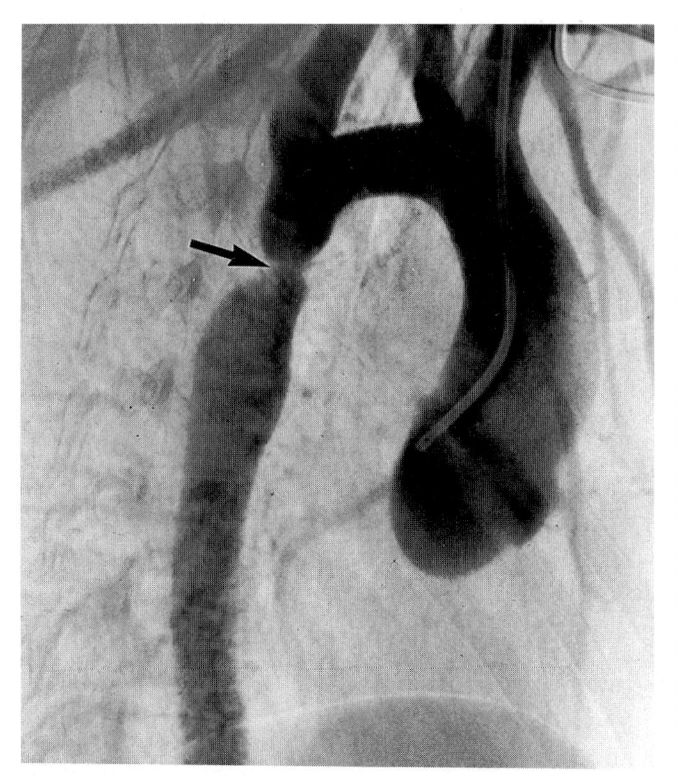

Fig. 24.2 Arch aortogram showing coarctation (arrow).

may well become the investigation of choice. Oblique sagittal T1 views along the plane of the aortic arch provide detailed anatomical information about the site of the coarctation and phase-contrast magnetic resonance angiography provides functional information in the form of measurements of velocity within the post-stenotic jet caused by the coarct. For a complete study, a magnetic resonance angiogram to look for aneurysms of the circle of Willis may also be performed. Echocardiography should be performed in all patients to look for a bicuspid aortic valve

ANEURYSM

A quarter of aortic aneurysms occur above the diaphragm. Some 70% of thoracic aneurysms are due to atherosclerosis, 15% are traumatic and the rest are due to conditions such as medial necrosis, syphilis, mycotic aneurysmse and Takayasu's arteritis.

True aneurysms result from local or diffuse weakening of the aortic wall, caused by degeneration of medial elastic fibres, and are bounded by the aortic intima. False aneurysms are usually secondary to trauma and are due to a breach in one or more layers of the aortic wall. They are bounded by adventitia, perivascular connective tissue or haematoma. Aneurysms may be saccular or fusiform in shape, saccular aneurysms having the greater risk of rupture.

DEGENERATIVE (ATHEROSCLEROTIC) ANEURYSM

Atherosclerosis is now the commonest cause of aortic aneurysm. Atherosclerotic aneurysms are more common in the abdominal aorta than in the thorax but may occur at the aortic arch or in the descending thoracic aorta. They are more common in males, with increasing age and in patients with hypertension. The presence of an aneurysm is usually evident on the

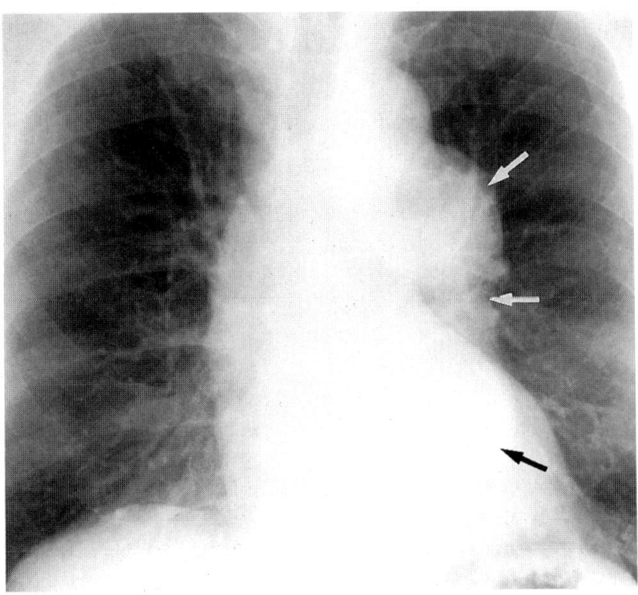

Fig. 24.3 Thoracic aortic aneurysm. Chest radiograph showing dilatation of the descending portion of the thoracic aorta (arrows).

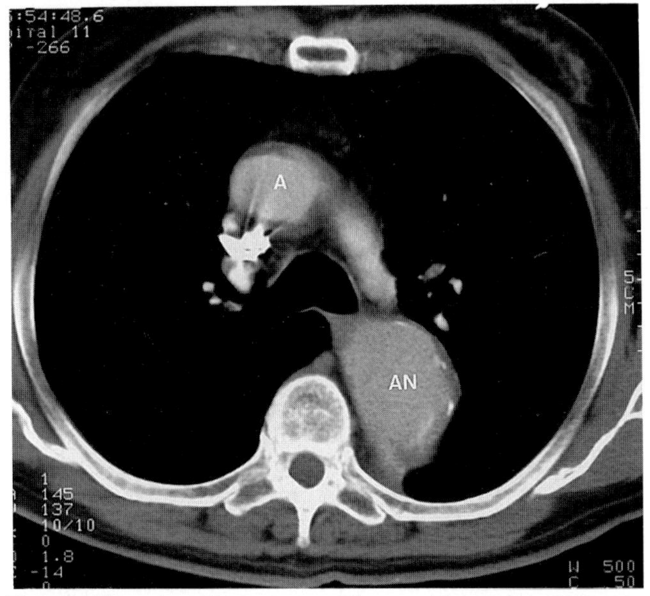

Fig. 24.4 Thoracic aortic aneurysm. CT scan of the same patient as in Fig. 24.3 confirming aneurysmal dilatation of the thoracic aorta (AN). Compare the diameter of the descending aorta at this level with that of the ascending aorta (A).

chest radiograph (Fig. 24.3). Ultrasound, CT or MRI may be used to demonstrate the size and extent of the aneurysmal sac in patients in whom surgery is considered (Fig. 23.4).

TRAUMATIC FALSE ANEURYSM

Thoracic aortic rupture occurs as a result of a blunt, decelerating injury to the chest, usually following a road traffic accident. The aortic injury is generally considered to be caused by a differential deceleration of fixed and non-fixed parts of the thoracic aorta, but momentary crushing of the aortic arch between sternum and thoracic spine may also play a part. The mechanism of injury sustained by the patient is a valuable clue to the possibility of aortic rupture. Disruption of one or more layers of the aortic wall occurs, usually at the site of the ligamentum arteriosum but occasionally at the level of the aortic valve or pericardial reflection. The result in 85% of cases is death at the scene of the accident with only 15% surviving to reach hospital. In this latter group of patients the adventitia is intact, but they will still die from delayed rupture if the injury is not detected and repaired.

The chest radiograph is rarely normal in cases of aortic rupture and may show superior mediastinal widening, left apical pleural shadowing, downward displacement of the left main bronchus or tracheal displacement (Fig. 24.5). These signs indicate mediastinal haematoma owing to associated injury of smaller vessels in the mediastinum. Fractures of the first or second ribs or of the upper thoracic spine indicate a severe thoracic injury in which aortic injury becomes more probable.

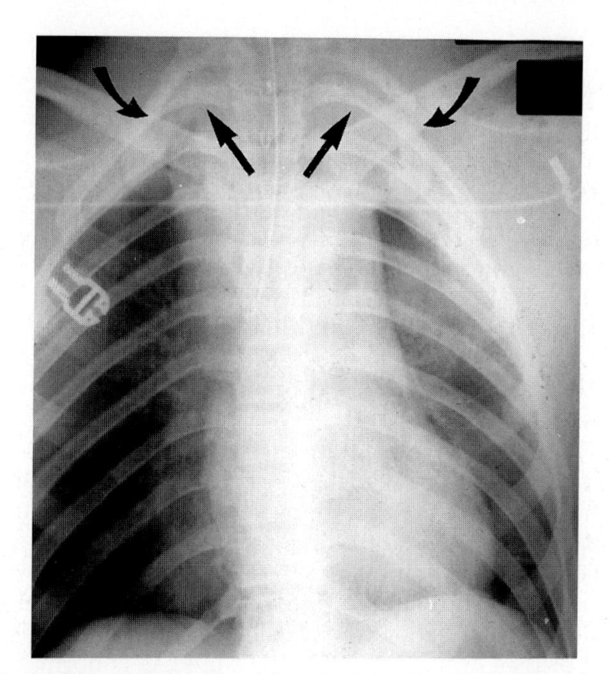

Fig. 24.5 Traumatic rupture of thoracic aorta. Chest radiograph shows bilateral first rib fractures (curved arrows), an indication of severe thoracic trauma. The mediastinum is widened and there are bilateral apical pleural caps due to haematoma (arrows).

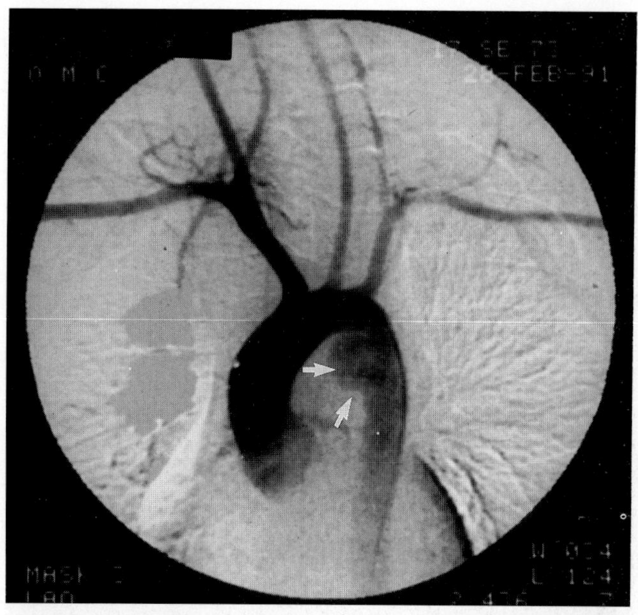

Fig. 24.6 Traumatic rupture of thoracic aorta. Arch aortography showing a classic false aneurysm (arrows) just distal to the left subclavian artery.

The diagnosis of aortic rupture is made by arch aortography and this examination should be performed without delay whenever aortic injury is suspected. Only 15 to 20% of such examinations will be positive but this low yield is justified by the consequences of missing the diagnosis. The usual angiographic finding is the presence of a false aneurysm just distal to the left subclavian artery (Fig. 24.6) but transverse lucencies representing intimal edges or extravasation may also be seen. Aortography may also reveal significant vascular injury outside the aorta (Fig. 24.7).

Conventional contrast-enhanced CT may also be used to demonstrate the sac of a false aneurysm but small intimal tears may be missed. Modern spiral CT scanners can produce high quality contrast-enhanced images of the aorta that may be reconstructed in any plane. For the assessment of aortic injury, these reconstructions are superior to those obtained with conventional (non-spiral) CT and probably rival the accuracy of angiography. The imaging method that is used will in each case depend upon the local facilities and expertise as well as the nature and extent of other injuries that may be present.

MYCOTIC ANEURYSMS

Mycotic aneurysms are due to focal destruction of the aortic wall by bacterial infection. The normal aorta is relatively resistant to infection and pre-existing aortic

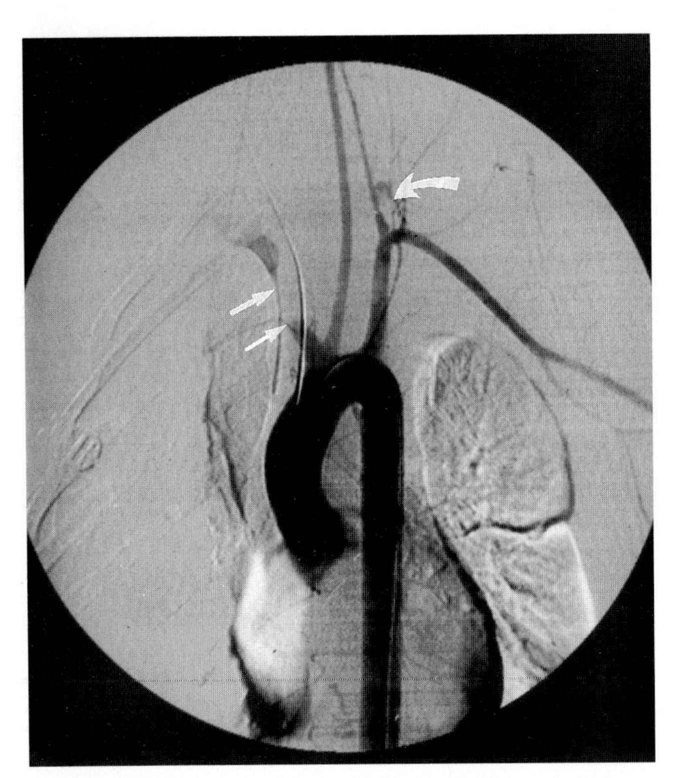

Fig. 24.7 Arch aortogram performed following chest trauma because aortic rupture was suspected. There is occlusion of the right brachiocephalic artery (straight arrows) and active haemorrhage from the left thyrocervical trunk (curved arrow) but the aorta itself is normal.

disease such as atherosclerosis is usually present. Pre-existing conditions include bacterial endocarditis, intravenous drug abuse, coarctation and local trauma to the vessel (e.g. catheter-related). Infection may also arise from direct spread of an adjacent focus. The commonest sites for mycotic aneurysms in the thoracic aorta are the sinuses of Valsalva and the ascending aorta. Because the mural destruction is focal, such aneurysms are usually saccular in shape. They may enlarge rapidly and their presence may be suggested by the rapid appearance of aneurysmal dilation of the aorta between successive chest radiographs. The diagnosis is readily confirmed by CT (Fig. 24.8). Prompt surgical repair is essential because of the very high risk of rupture.

SYPHILITIC ANEURYSMS

Cardiovascular syphilis is part of the spectrum of tertiary syphilis and is caused by an obliterative endarteritis of the vasa vasorum leading to necrotic changes in the aortic media. Typically, this results in fusiform dilation of the ascending aorta which also shows a fine line of calcification within its wall. Dilation of the aortic valve ring may give rise to aortic regurgitation. With modern methods of treatment, syphilis is now a rare cause of thoracic aneurysm.

MARFAN'S SYNDROME

Marfan's syndrome is an inherited autosomal dominant condition in which production of collagen is defective. Cystic medial necrosis in the wall of the aorta leads to widening of the aortic root and valve ring with accompanying aortic regurgitation. This condition also predisposes to aortic dissection (see below).

AORTIC DISSECTION

Aortic dissection occurs when a breech in the intima allows blood under arterial pressure to form an intramural channel or haematoma. In most cases there is pre-existing degenerative disease of the media caused by atherosclerosis or cystic medial necrosis. Dissection is more commonly seen in male patients over the age of 50 years. Hypertension, trauma, Marfan's and Ehlers–Danlos syndromes, coarctation, pregnancy, bicuspid aortic valve and aortic valve surgery all predispose to aortic dissection. The intramural track may burst through the adventitia into the pericardial sac, pleural space or the mediastinum or back through the intima to re-enter the aortic lumen at another site. The dissection may also extend into the branches of the aorta, such as the major branches in the chest or the mesenteric and renal arteries in the abdomen.

Aortic dissection may be classified according to two schemes. The best known is that of DeBakey who proposed three categories:

- **Type I**. Involvement of both ascending and descending aorta;
- **Type II**. Involvement of the aorta proximal to the ligamentum arteriosum;
- **Type III**. Involvement of the aorta distal to the ligamentum arteriosum.

In 1970, Daley and colleagues proposed a simpler classification into **type A** (involving the ascending aorta – DeBakey types I and II) and **type B** (confined to the descending aorta – DeBakey type III) to reflect the usual management strategy which is urgent surgical repair for type A dissections and conservative management for type B.

The clinical presentation is sudden onset of chest and interscapular back pain with collapse. Other clinical features are determined by adventitial rupture (which may be fatal) or aortic branch occlusion. Involvement of branches from the aortic arch may lead to a blood pressure difference between the arms. Unless the dissection track has involved and occluded one of the coronary artery ostia the ECG is normal.

The initial radiological examination is the chest radiograph which may show evidence of mediastinal haematoma in the form of mediastinal widening

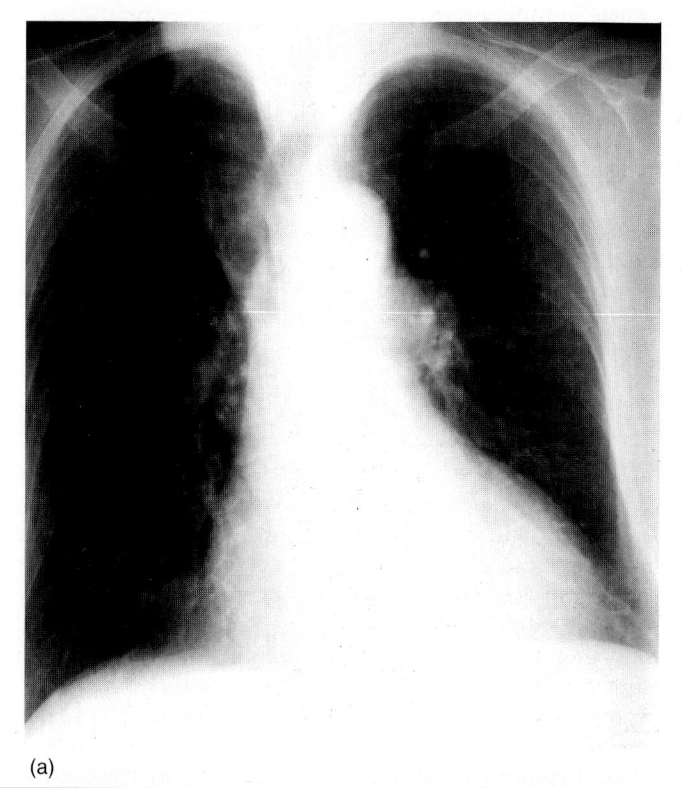
(a)

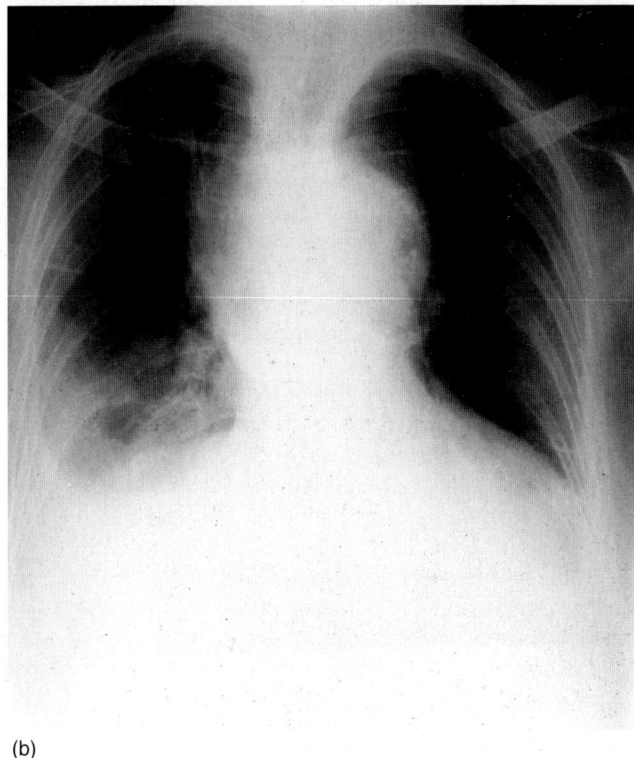
(b)

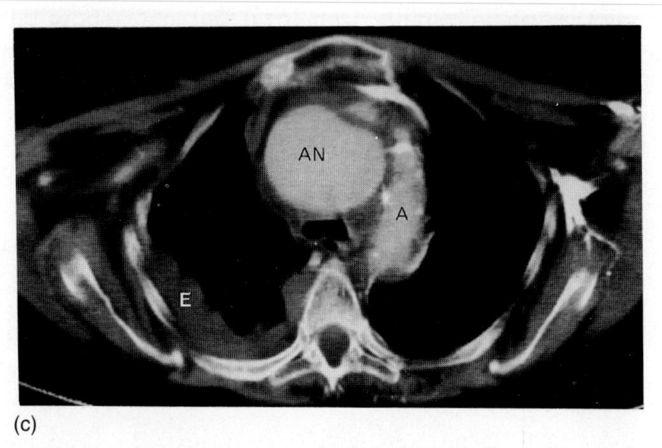

(c)

Fig. 24.8 Mycotic aortic aneurysm. (a) and (b) Two chest radiographs performed 2 weeks apart in this patient with salmonella septicaemia show rapid development of mediastinal widening. (c) Contrast-enhanced CT shows the mycotic aneurysm of the aortic arch. The aortic arch (A) is displaced to the left by a large aneurysm sac (AN) arising from the right lateral aspect of the ascending aorta. There is also a right pleural effusion (E) which could represent some leakage from the aneurysm.

(50–70%), left pleural effusion, left apical pleural cap, displacement of the trachea to the right and loss of definition of the aortic arch. Intimal calcification, if present, may rarely be seen to be displaced into the aortic lumen. Confirmation of the diagnosis is made by echocardiography, angiography, contrast enhanced CT or MRI.

2D-echocardiography is quick, non-invasive and sensitive for dissections that involve the aortic root. The dissection flap is shown within the aortic lumen together with other important features such as dilatation of the valve ring, aortic regurgitation or pericardial effusion. More distal dissections will not be visible unless bi-plane transoesophageal echocardiography is used. For transoesophageal echocardiography, the ultrasound probe is introduced into the oesophagus and is therefore in close proximity to the heart and great vessels. The accuracy of ultrasound diagnosis is comparable to CT with the advantages that additional information such as the presence of aortic regurgitation is gained and the examination can take place at the bedside. Unfortunately, the transoesophageal technique is not widely available but it is considered by many to be the initial investigation of choice, reserving CT or angiography for preoperative planning in those patients where additional information is needed.

In most centres, conventional contrast-enhanced CT is the method of diagnosis. This must be performed with care to avoid false negative studies. Adequate opacification of the aorta is essential and various methods have been described to achieve this. The usual technique is to inject a large volume of contrast of between 100 and 150 ml via a cannula in the antecubital vein while axial scans are performed from just above the arch to the level of the diaphragm. Modern spiral CT is particularly useful in aortic dissection. With this technique, in which data are acquired in a three-dimensional block rather than individual slices, the entire thorax may be scanned in one breath-hold. The speed of the examination allows for greater and more uniform contrast enhancement of the aortic lumen.

The dissection may be shown as a thin band representing the intimal flap traversing the aortic lumen, separating the true and false channels (Fig. 24.9), or as a non-opacified crescent around the edge of the true lumen. The presence of mediastinal haematoma, pleural or pericardial effusions may also be visible. The dissection flap may be quite thin and easily confused with linear artifacts that are commonly present. Where any doubt exists, a repeat scan concentrating at the level in question should be performed for clarification. If a dissection of the descending aorta is found, the scan can be continued into the abdomen to look for renal and mesenteric arterial involvement.

For many years, arch aortography has been the mainstay of diagnosis, but is now superseded by CT for initial assessment. At aortography the intimal flap may be visible as a thin radiolucent line within the aortic lumen or there may be distortion of the true lumen by a thrombosed false channel. It is also possible to identify aortic regurgitation and involvement of aortic branches at aortography. There are a number of diagnostic pitfalls and the examination must be performed by an experienced operator.

Where facilities are available, MRI may also be used and is an excellent method of imaging for the thoracic aorta. Cardiac-gated axial as well as oblique sagittal scans are made to show the aortic arch in cross-section and in profile.

INFLAMMATORY DISEASE

Takayasu's disease is a form of autoimmune vasculitis which may affect the thoracic aorta, abdominal aorta, aortic branches or the pulmonary arteries in various combinations. Females are affected eight times more commonly than men. It has a world-wide distribution but is commonest in young oriental females. Fibrosis and degeneration of elastic fibres in the media occur together with thickening of the adventitia and intima. Symptoms commence in adolescence with fever, malaise, pain and fatigue. Bruits may be audible and hypertension or cardiac failure may occur. The chest radiograph is usually unhelpful but may show rib notching or aortic calcification. Angiography shows various combinations of stenoses of the aorta or its branches and saccular or fusiform dilatation of the aorta, usually of its ascending portion.

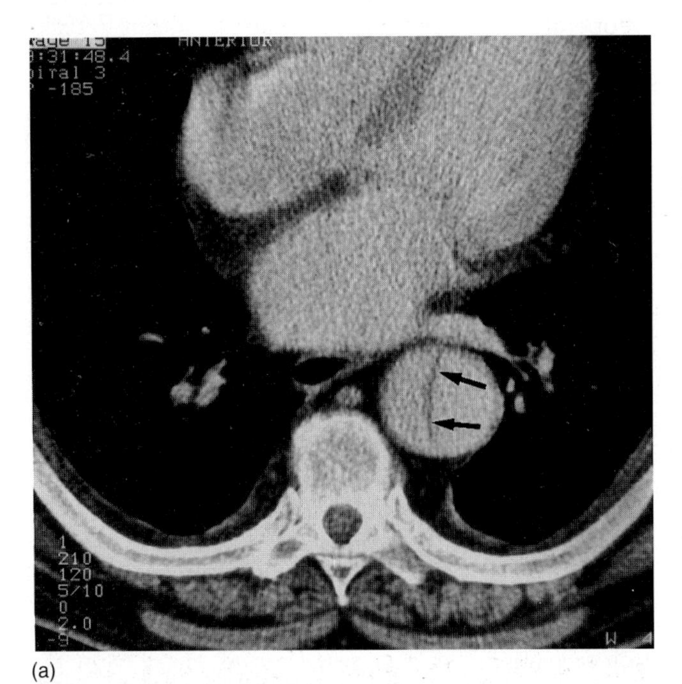

(a)

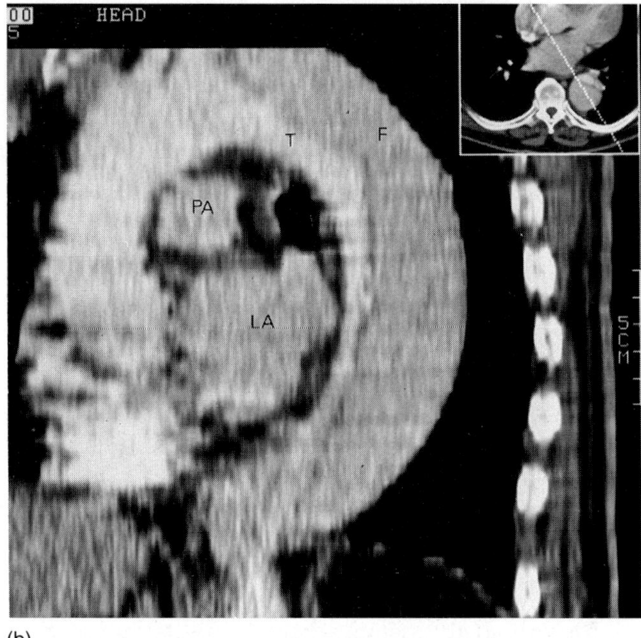

(b)

Fig. 24.9 Aortic dissection in two different patients. (a) CT showing a thin line traversing the descending thoracic aorta (arrows) which is the dissection flap, separating the true and false lumens. (b) Spiral CT allows reconstruction of an image along the plane of the aorta which clearly shows the true (T) and false (F) lumen of a type B dissection (DeBakey type III). PA=pulmonary artery; LA=left atrium.

ABDOMINAL AORTA

ANEURYSM

Abdominal aortic aneurysm may be asymptomatic or present as an acute abdomen following rupture. The incidence of asymptomatic abdominal aortic aneurysms >4 cm in diameter in the 55–75-year-old age group is 2–3%. Ruptured aneurysm has a mortality of 75–95% and accounts for some 10 000 deaths per annum in England and Wales. Conventional surgical aneurysm repair is a major undertaking which in specialist units has a mortality of between 1 and 7%, a figure that can be significantly higher in non-specialist units. Techniques for the endovascular repair of aortic aneurysms are now emerging. Over 50% of patients with abdominal aortic aneurysm have coronary artery disease and serious, potentially fatal complications of surgery are usually cardiovascular in nature, precipitated by the tremendous change in haemodynamics that occurs with aortic clamping and unclamping.

Some 5–15% of abdominal aneurysms are **inflammatory aneurysms**. These are characterized by excessive fibrotic thickening of the aneurysm wall which becomes glistening and pearly white in external appearance and shows lymphocytic infiltration microscopically. Surrounding fibrosis and adhesions may lead to problems such as renal hydronephrosis. The aetiology of inflammatory aneurysms is uncertain but it appears to be an immune response, possibly to atheromatous material in the aortic wall. Inflammatory aneurysms are associated with an increase in morbidity and mortality from surgical repair.

An asymptomatic aneurysm may be detected on a plain abdominal radiograph as a soft tissue density with a thin peripheral rim of calcium (Fig. 24.10). Aneurysms may also be detected or assessed at ultrasound, CT or angiography.

Ultrasound is well suited to the examination of aortic aneurysms and allows accurate measurement of the aneurysm in sagittal and coronal planes. Associated complications such as hydronephrosis can also be identified as well as potential risk factors for surgery such as an inflammatory aneurysm or the presence of a horseshoe kidney. The likelihood of aneurysm rupture increases as the aneurysm increases in size and surgery is usually planned once the aneurysm diameter exceeds 5.5 cm. When surgery is not contemplated, the size of the aneurysm can be monitored by serial ultrasound scans.

Abdominal aortic aneurysms are readily demonstrated by CT. Inflammatory aneurysms are characterized by a rind of soft-tissue density around them and may be associated with hydronephrosis (Fig. 24.11). CT is not usually necessary prior to elective open surgical repair if there has been adequate preoperative ultrasound assessment. Various techniques for minimally invasive endovascular aneurysm repair are emerging in which a tubular delivery system is used to place a graft within the aorta using

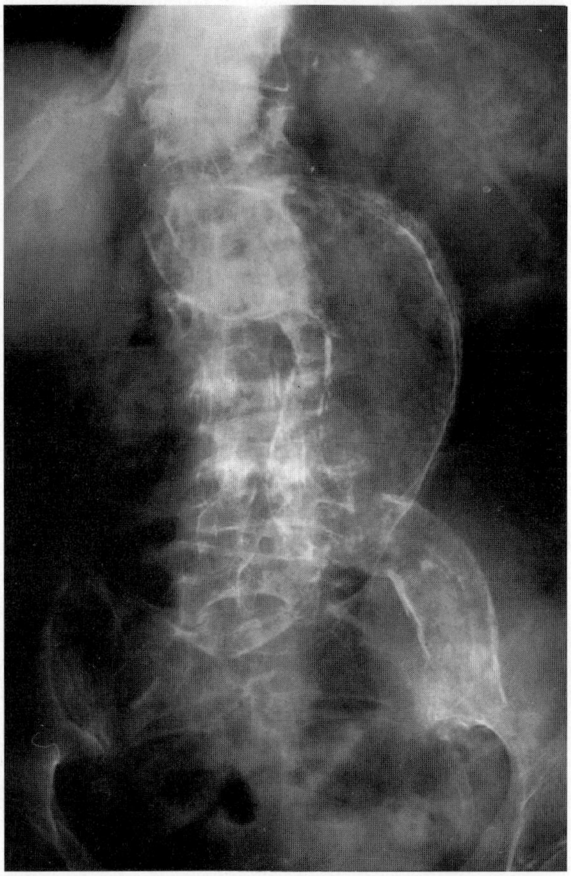

Fig. 24.10 Aortic aneurysm. Plain abdominal radiograph showing calcification in the walls of aortic and left iliac artery aneurysms.

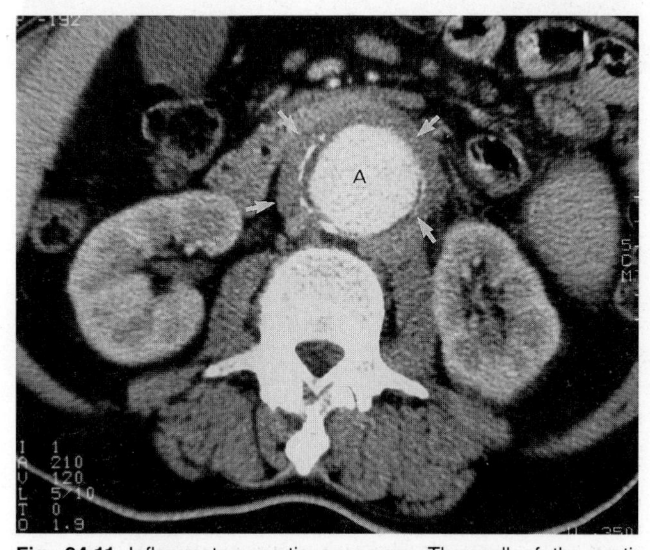

Fig. 24.11 Inflammatory aortic aneurysm. The wall of the aortic aneurysm (A) shows marked thickening (arrows).

femoral arteriotomies for access. The graft is held in place by expandable metallic stents that are sutured to the graft openings before its insertion. The graft can be straight (aortoaortic or aortoiliac) or bifurcated. Correct sizing of the graft for each patient is critical to the success of these procedures and requires detailed preoperative assessment of the size and shape of the abdominal aorta and iliac arteries with CT (preferably spiral CT).

Aortic aneurysms may be identified on the initial frames of a femoral angiogram performed for lower limb ischaemia. The lumen may be obviously widened (Fig. 24.12) but the angiogram does not give a true impression of the external diameter of the aneurysm because of the variable amount of mural thrombus that may be present. Indeed, the aorta may look almost normal in calibre, the clue to the presence of an aneurysm being the thin rim of calcification that marks the true site of the aortic wall. Angiography should be performed with care when an aneurysm is present in case a thrombus is dislodged from the aneurysm sac. Angiography is not usually required prior to conventional surgical repair but is valuable prior to endovascular repair.

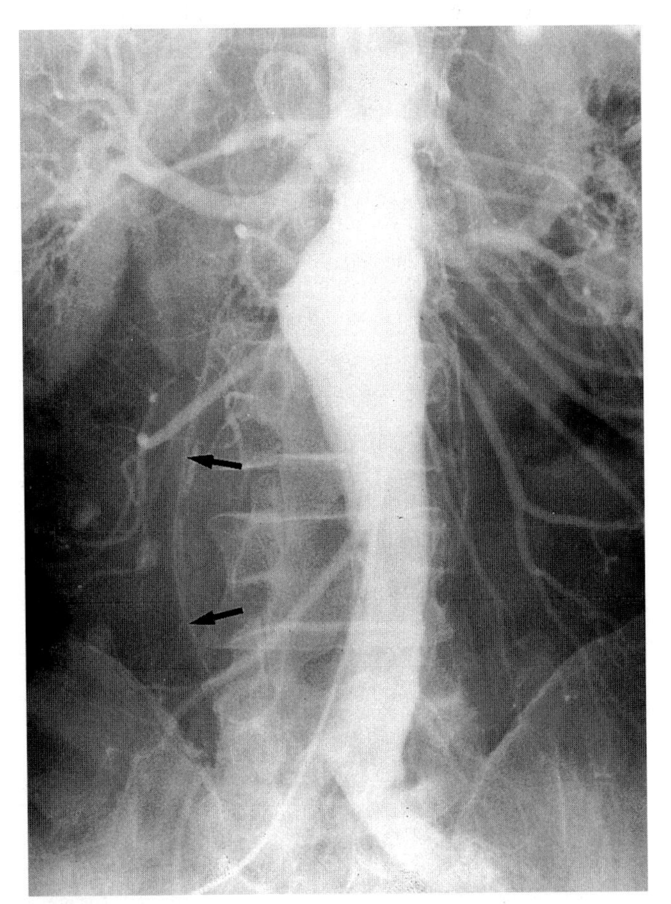

Fig. 24.12 Angiogram of aortic aneurysm. The contrast shows the lumen only. There is a large amount of thrombus lining the wall of the and the true diameter of the aneurysm can only be inferred from the thin line of calcification in the aneurysm wall (arrows).

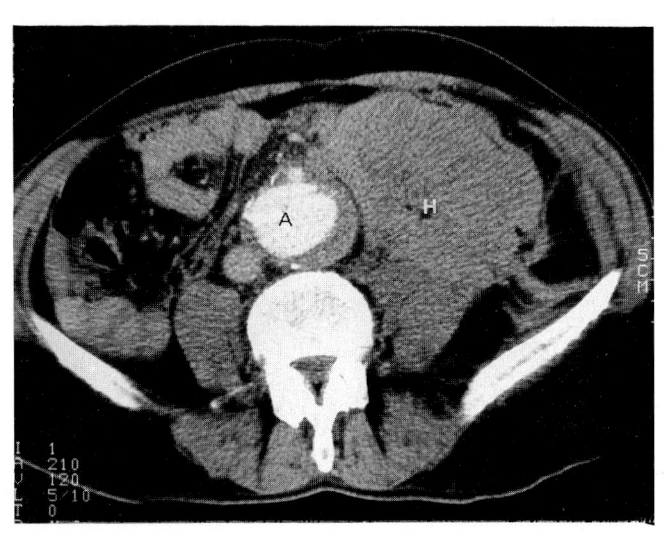

Fig. 24.13 Ruptured aortic aneurysm. In this example, the CT scan shows a large haematoma (H) adjacent to the aortic aneurysm (A).

Ruptured aneurysm presents with acute onset of abdominal and back pain with cardiovascular collapse. The plain abdominal radiograph often shows the characteristic curvilinear calcification in the aneurysm wall and the psoas muscle outlines may be obscured by retroperitoneal haematoma. The mortality is high and the best chance of survival lies with urgent surgical repair. When an abdominal aneurysm is palpable and the clinical picture is consistent with rupture, further investigation is usually unnecessary and serves only to delay surgery. Ultrasound or CT may, however, be helpful when there is doubt about the diagnosis of aortic aneurysm, for instance if the patient is obese. Ultrasound can detect large retroperitoneal haematomas but is an unreliable means of excluding the possibility of rupture for which the best investigation is abdominal CT. The indications and contraindications for preoperative investigation of ruptured aortic aneurysms may change in the future if endovascular techniques of repair become more widely used in the emergency setting (Fig. 24.13).

AORTOENTERIC FISTULA

A fistulous communication between the aortic lumen and the gastrointestinal tract is a rare but potentially fatal cause of gastrointestinal bleeding. The condition most commonly occurs in patients who have previously had a abdominal aortic aneurysm repair, particularly if the graft has become infected. The fistula usually communicates between the proximal anastomotic suture line of the graft and the third part of the duodenum. Primary aortoenteric fistulae may also occur and again these are usually in association with an aortic aneurysm. Despite the potential for severe, life-threatening haematemesis and melaena, there is often a history of smaller herald episodes of gastrointestinal bleeding which should always raise the possibility of the diagnosis when there has been previous aortic surgery or if an aneurysm is palpable. Preoperative diagnosis can be difficult. Endoscopy should be the preliminary investigation but may fail to identify the fistula if the third part of the duodenum cannot be reached. Other potentially useful investigations are barium meal, CT or aortography with a lateral series to demonstrate the anterior aortic wall. False negative imaging is not uncommon in aortoenteric fistulae and the diagnosis may not be confirmed until laparotomy.

CHAPTER 25

Veins

Simon C. Whitaker

The venous system may be assessed by venography, ultrasound or, in selected cases, by computed tomography or magnetic resonance imaging. The presence of thrombus may also be imaged with radionuclide techniques.

IMAGING TECHNIQUES

VENOGRAPHY

A venogram is a series of radiographs of one or more veins, taken while radiopaque contrast medium is injected into a tributary. The technique of the examination varies according to the part of the venous system that is being studied.

LOWER LIMB VENOGRAPHY

Lower limb venography is performed in a fluoroscopy room with a tilting table. A tourniquet is applied at the ankle and a cannula inserted into a suitable vein on the dorsum of the foot. Leaving the ankle tourniquet in place to occlude the superficial veins and encourage preferential filling of the deep system, 50 ml of non-ionic contrast agent is injected by hand with a head-up table tilt of about 45° to slow the dissipation of the contrast agent. The process is observed with fluoroscopy and, when the venous opacification is sufficient, frontal and oblique radiographs are taken of the calf together with frontal views of the knee and thigh (Fig. 25.1). Finally, a film of the pelvis is taken as the patient is returned to the horizontal position and the leg elevated to show the iliac veins and the lower inferior vena cava (IVC).

Normal appearances

In the normal subject (Fig. 25.1) there are three columns of veins in the calf. From medial to lateral these are: the posterior tibial, peroneal and anterior tibial veins. These veins are usually paired and run alongside their respective arteries. The popliteal and superficial femoral veins are usually single but may also be duplicated as variations in venous anatomy are common. The common femoral vein is formed a few centimetres below the inguinal ligament by the confluence of the deep and superficial femoral veins. In the pelvis, the external and internal iliac veins join to form the common iliac veins which pass over their corresponding arteries to unite at the level of L5 to form the IVC. The long and short saphenous veins constitute the superficial venous system of the leg. The long saphenous passes medially in the calf and thigh

Diagnostic and Interventional Radiology in Surgical Practice. Edited by P. Armstrong and M. L. Wastie. Published in 1997 by Chapman & Hall, London. ISBN 0 412 61960 1 (HB), 0 412 61970 9 (PB)

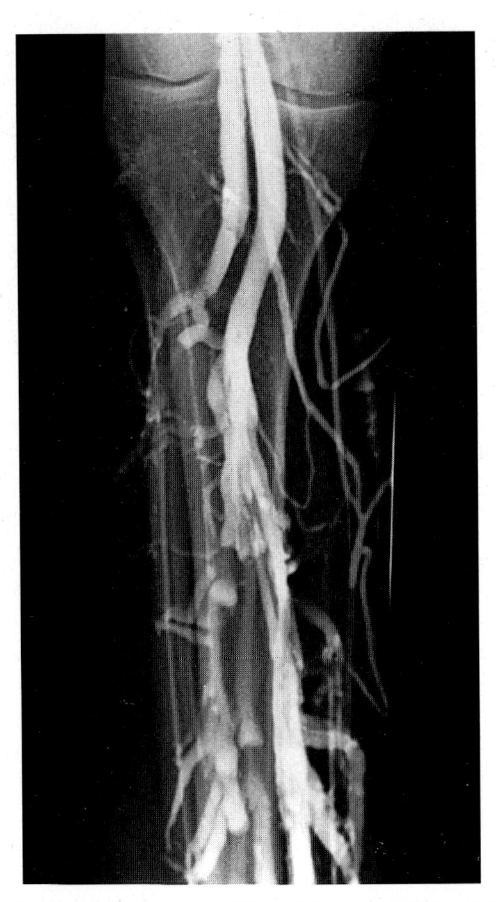

Fig. 25.1 Lower limb venogram. Normal study showing contrast within the calf veins.

to join with the common femoral vein via the saphenous opening in the deep fascia. The short saphenous vein passes posteriorly in the calf and usually joins the popliteal vein just above the level of the knee joint. The saphenous veins and their superficial tributaries communicate with the deep veins via a number of small perforating veins.

The superficial and deep venous systems of the leg contain a number of valves which allow flow in a cranial direction only. Perforating veins also contain valves which allow flow from superficial to deep veins.

Contraindications and complications

The risk of serious complication following venography with modern contrast agents is remote and consequently there are few contraindications to the procedure. However, the use of intravenous contrast does carry a small risk of adverse reaction. The development of deep vein thrombosis, as a consequence of lower limb venography, is a rare but recognized complication when ionic contrast agents are used. It has also been reported following non-ionic contrast but, even if a causal relationship exists, the risk is very much smaller with non-ionic agents.

INFERIOR VENA CAVOGRAPHY

The pelvic veins and the lower IVC are normally shown in a good quality conventional lower limb venogram. To show these structures specifically, a short cannula is placed in the femoral vein using the Seldinger technique. Sequential radiographs of the pelvis are taken as contrast medium is injected by hand or with the use of a pump. Simultaneous injection into both common femoral veins may be made if both sides of the pelvis are to be examined. If the IVC is the principal interest, contrast injection may be made using a pig-tail catheter placed at the confluence of the common iliac veins (Fig. 25.2). Intravenous catheters should be used with caution in the pelvic veins and IVC when proximal deep vein thrombosis is suspected, to avoid dislodgement of thrombus and subsequent pulmonary embolism.

The IVC receives lumbar veins, the right gonadal vein, two renal veins (the left renal vein receiving the left adrenal and gonadal veins), right adrenal vein, hepatic veins and phrenic veins before passing through the caval opening in the diaphragm at the

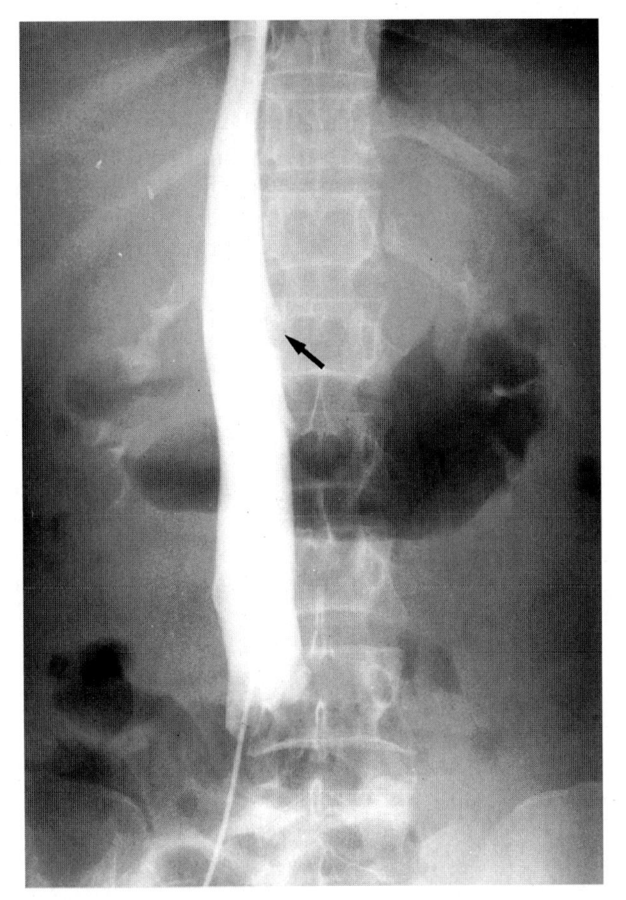

Fig. 25.2 Inferior vena cavogram. An angiographic catheter has been placed via the right common femoral vein with its tip at the confluence of the iliac veins. The arrow indicates the position of the left renal vein, shown by the stream of unopacified blood entering the IVC.

level of T8. The position of these tributaries is shown on contrast studies of the IVC by the stream of non-opacified blood from them entering the main lumen.

SUPERIOR VENA CAVOGRAPHY

In a similar manner to inferior vena cavography, the superior vena cava (SVC) can be demonstrated by contrast injection into one or both median antecubital veins or by injection at its origin using an angiographic catheter.

The SVC is quite short and is the final common pathway for venous drainage from the head, neck and upper limbs, being formed by the junction of the right and left brachiocephalic veins. Its single tributary is the azygos vein which ascends alongside the lower thoracic vertebral bodies before passing forwards in the right lateral aspect of the mediastinum, passing over the origin of the right main bronchus and entering the SVC posteriorly.

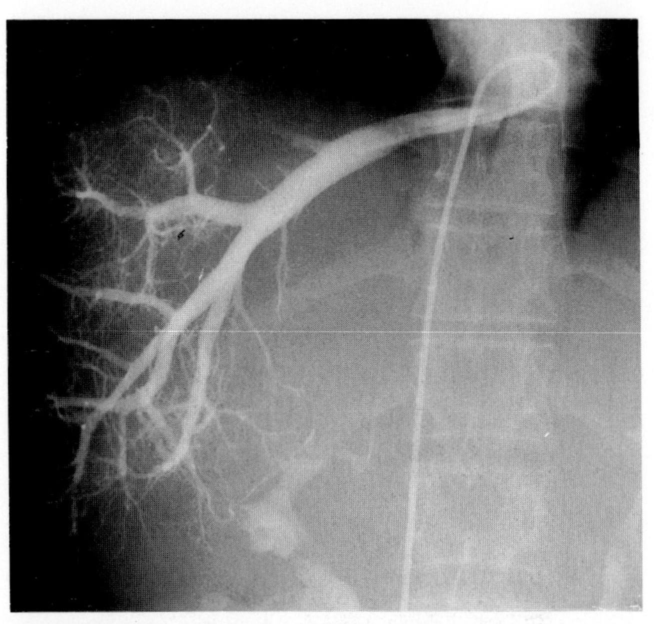

Fig. 25.3 Hepatic venogram. A catheter has been passed from the femoral vein in the groin, up the IVC and into the hepatic vein.

UPPER LIMB VENOGRAPHY

To demonstrate the axillary and subclavian veins, a cannula is inserted into the ipsilateral median antecubital vein and sequential images of the shoulder/upper chest are taken as contrast is injected with the patient supine. To show the forearm veins, the injection may be made into a vein on the dorsum of the hand with a tourniquet around the upper arm.

VISCERAL VENOGRAPHY

The **hepatic veins** are demonstrated by retrograde injection of contrast into one or more of the veins, using a curved catheter introduced from a femoral vein or from the right internal jugular vein (Fig. 25.3). With a catheter in the hepatic vein it is also possible to perform pressure measurements with the catheter tip wedged in a distal tributary to give an indirect measurement of the pressure in the portal vein.

The **renal veins** are also shown by selective retrograde contrast injection using a curved angiographic catheter. It is usual to perform an inferior vena cavogram first, to make sure that there is no clot protruding into the IVC lumen that might be dislodged.

The **portal vein** may be demonstrated by indirect portography, direct transhepatic portography or, in the past, by splenoportography. **Indirect portography** is the most straightforward and is performed by selective contrast injection into the splenic artery. Images are taken during the late, venous phase as contrast passes from the spleen into the portal vein. **Direct portography** is performed by introducing a catheter into the portal vein itself either by a percutaneous transhepatic route or via a transjugular, intrahepatic route. In both cases the portal vein must be patent, so direct portography cannot be used to demonstrate portal vein occlusion. Direct methods are technically more difficult than indirect and carry a greater risk of bleeding. For these reasons, direct portography is generally reserved for specific purposes such as portal vein sampling (see below) or as part of the transjugular intrahepatic portosystemic shunt procedure (p. 264). **Splenoportography**, a method that is no longer used, involved direct contrast injection into the body of the spleen. Excellent views of the portal vein were obtained but splenic puncture carried the risk of haemorrhage or splenic rupture.

CROSS SECTIONAL IMAGING

ULTRASOUND

Most veins are visible at ultrasound, the one notable exception being the SVC. Doppler and, in particular, colour Doppler ultrasound (Plate 12, opposite page 562), are important facilities for venous imaging which allow non-invasive confirmation of occlusion or venous incompetence. The IVC is normally visible at ultrasound but its orientation at right angles to the ultrasound probe makes Doppler assessment of blood flow difficult except in thin patients. There are no contraindications to the use of ultrasound but difficulty may be encountered in obese patients or if there is marked oedema. The use of ultrasound is discussed in more detail below.

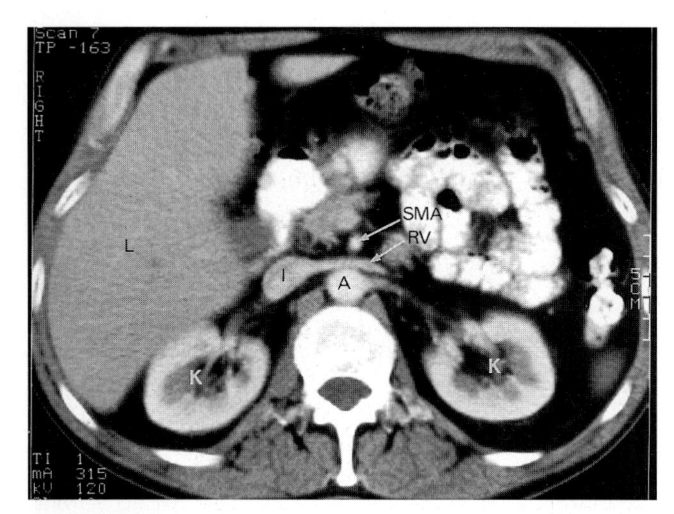

Fig. 25.4 IVC shown on a CT of the abdomen. I=inferior vena cava; RV=renal vein; A=aorta; SMA=superior mesenteric artery; L=liver; K=kidney.

COMPUTED TOMOGRAPHY

Contrast-enhanced CT may be used to show veins and their neighbouring structures and is particularly useful for the central veins such as the SVC, IVC (Fig. 25.4) and portal vein. Thrombus is identified as a filling defect within the vessel lumen and compression by an adjacent masses is readily demonstrated.

MAGNETIC RESONANCE ANGIOGRAPHY

Modern magnetic resonance scanners have the ability to detect and display movement of blood. The techniques in common use for angiography, 2D or 3D time-of-flight (TOF) and phase contrast (PC) angiography, provide angiographic images without the use of intravenous contrast agents. Magnetic resonance angiography is commonly used to display arterial blood flow (for instance in the carotid or intracranial arteries) but can also be used to display the slow flow in the venous system (Fig. 25.5). Magnetic resonance scanners are still expensive and there is heavy demand for their use from various specialties. Their use for investigation of venous disease is likely to remain limited to selected cases.

RADIONUCLIDE SCANNING

Isotope techniques have been advocated to demonstrate the venous system and venous occlusion due to thrombus in cases of suspected pulmonary embolus. The ^{99m}Tc-labelled macroaggregates used for the lung perfusion scan are injected into a vein on the dorsum of the foot and the venous system imaged with a gamma camera during the passage of the radionuclide to the lungs.

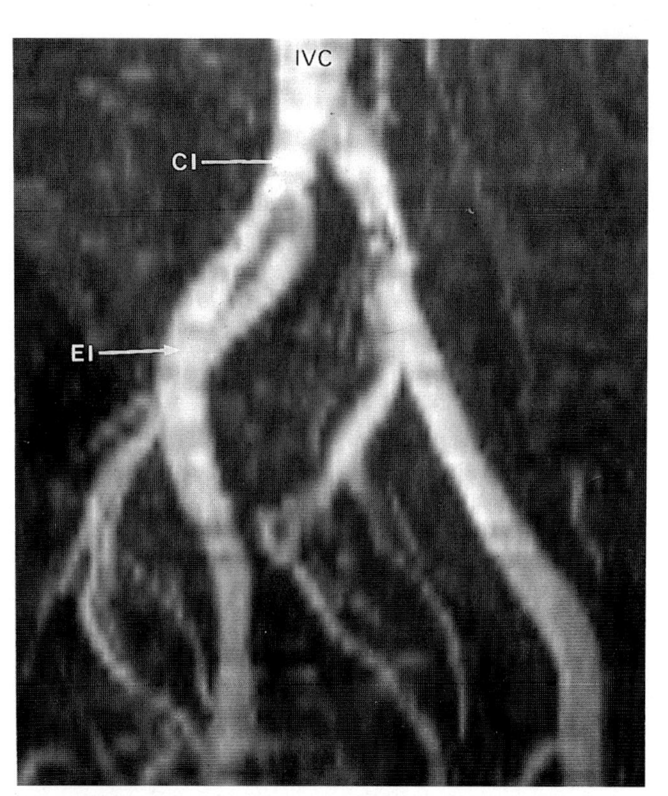

Fig. 25.5 Magnetic resonance angiography of pelvic veins. 2D time-of-flight study showing the pelvic veins and the IVC. EI=external iliac vein; CI=common iliac vein; IVC=inferior vena cava.

VENOUS DISEASE

LOWER LIMB

DEEP VEIN THROMBOSIS

Conditions that predispose to the development of deep vein thrombosis include recent surgery or trauma (particularly orthopaedic procedures involving the lower limb), pregnancy, oral contraceptives, immobility, obesity and malignant disease. Confirmation of the diagnosis is necessary before commencing treatment with anticoagulants because the accuracy of clinical diagnosis on its own is poor. The main imaging methods are venography and ultrasound.

Lower limb venography

Thrombus shows as a serpiginous filling defect within the vessel lumen on the venogram. As clot retraction occurs, the thrombus does not occupy the entire cross-section of the vein and is outlined by 'tram-lines' of contrast between it and the vein wall (Fig. 25.6). When

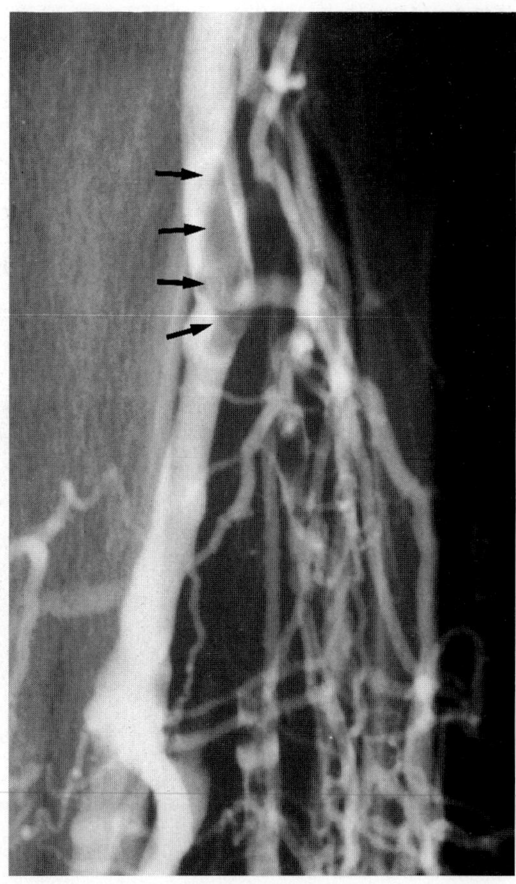

Fig. 25.6 Lower limb venogram showing thrombus (arrows).

the thrombosis is very extensive, obstruction of the deep veins may be complete with the result that the venogram shows only a mesh of fine collateral veins with no filling of the deep veins.

Ultrasound

Deep vein thrombosis may be detected with conventional ultrasound alone. Fresh thrombus is difficult to distinguish from normal blood but with time, thrombus becomes more echogenic and therefore visible (Fig. 25.7). Thrombus of any age within a vein prevents its collapse when the vein is subjected to compression by the ultrasound probe. This compression test can, with reasonable reliability, detect thrombus in the femoral and popliteal veins with the exception of the segment within the adductor canal.

Colour Doppler ultrasound

Colour Doppler ultrasound increases both the speed and reliability of detection of deep vein thrombosis. Thrombus is shown by an absence of flow, at rest or in response to gentle calf compression, or by flow that is only present in part of the lumen (Plate 13, opposite page 562). The femoral and popliteal veins are readily demonstrated in most subjects, as are the calf veins (Plate 14, opposite page 562).

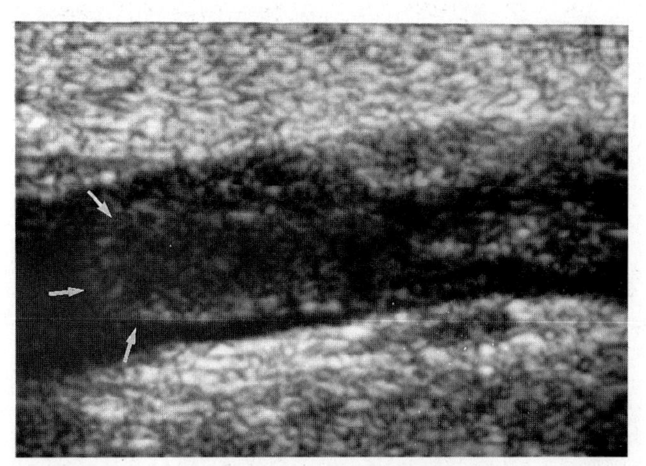

Fig. 25.7 Deep vein thrombosis. Ultrasound of the common femoral vein showing the echogenic column of thrombus in the vein lumen (arrows).

The pelvic veins are more difficult to examine with ultrasound because of overlying bowel. If, however, the common femoral vein is patent and shows normal variation in flow with the cardiac and respiratory cycles, it is likely that the iliac veins are patent as well. When there is doubt about the integrity of the pelvic veins, a conventional venogram should be performed to resolve the issue.

Doppler ultrasound versus venography

Venography provides excellent visualization of the deep veins and for many years has been the 'gold standard' for the detection of deep vein thrombosis. There are, however, some important disadvantages to venography. Ionizing radiation is used, venepuncture is uncomfortable and there is a small risk of complications of the procedure itself. Children tolerate venography poorly and some causes of lower limb swelling, such as ruptured Baker's cyst (Fig. 25.8) or muscle haematoma show indirectly or not at all. For these reasons venography is now being superseded by Doppler ultrasound.

In comparison, Doppler ultrasound is painless and does not carry any risk for the patient or operator. Ionizing radiation is not involved and the procedure is well tolerated, making it ideal for use during pregnancy and in children. Doppler ultrasound is capable of detecting deep vein thrombosis with an accuracy close to 100% for clot in the femoral or popliteal veins. Diagnosis of Baker's cyst, muscle haematoma and other soft-tissue abnormalities that are commonly mistaken for deep vein thrombosis may be made and the distinction between cellulitis and deep vein thrombosis is usually readily apparent. The disadvantage of vascular ultrasound is that, perhaps more so than for ultrasound of other sites, its success is dependent upon the skill and experience of the operator and the quality of equipment

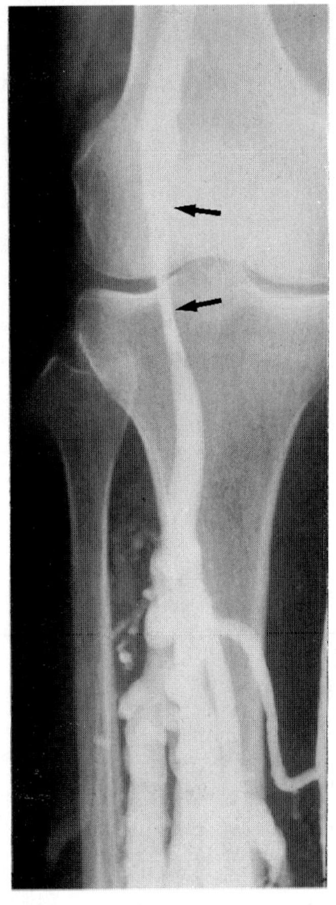

(a)

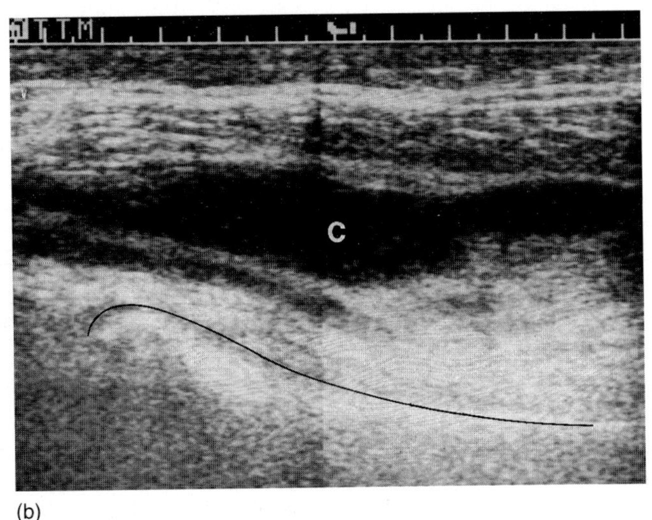

(b)

Fig. 25.8 Baker's cyst. (a) Venography shows lateral deviation of the popliteal vein (arrows). (b) Ultrasound in the same patient confirms rupture of a Baker's cyst (C) with fluid tracking down into the calf. The posterior surface of the tibia has been drawn in.

used. Ultrasound of the pelvic veins and the inferior vena cava may be difficult because of overlying bowel gas and the SVC cannot be seen at all.

Investigation of aetiology

In some cases, if extensive deep vein thrombosis involving the iliac veins has occurred without an obvious predisposing cause, a search for an underlying abnormality, such as an abdominal or pelvic mass compressing the proximal veins should be made, starting with an abdominal ultrasound. Abdominal and/or pelvic CT may be helpful for further evaluation if an abnormality is detected.

VARICOSE VEINS

Varicose veins of the lower limb may be either primary or secondary. The commonest cause of secondary venous disease is deep vein thrombosis. Whether primary or secondary, superficial varicosities are associated with one or more incompetent communications with the deep venous system, the identification of which is essential for successful treatment. Typical sites of incompetence are the saphenofemoral junction, the saphenopopliteal junction and perforating veins in the thigh or calf. Clinical examination can detect simple saphenofemoral and saphenopopliteal incompetence and the larger perforating veins but, in complex cases (e.g. recurrence of varicose veins after surgery), further information will be needed from Doppler ultrasound or venography.

Doppler ultrasound

The patient is first examined in the supine position to show the femoral veins and the saphenofemoral junction. Deep venous or saphenofemoral incompetence is shown by asking the patient to perform a Valsalva manoeuvre whilst the vein is observed with colour Doppler. In normal veins antegrade flow reduces or ceases when the intra-abdominal pressure rises, whereas incompetent veins show reversal of flow (Plate 15, opposite page 562). Long saphenous incompetence may stem from the saphenofemoral junction or from a mid-thigh perforator. Patients who have had previous saphenofemoral ligation may develop recurrent long saphenous incompetence as a result of the development of new collateral vessels

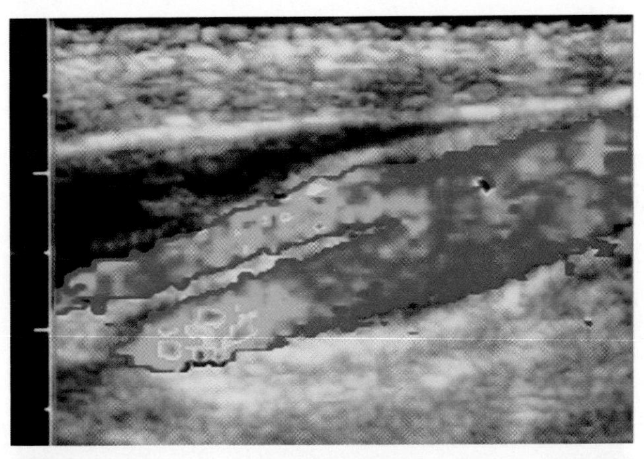

Plate 9 Duplex ultrasound scan showing the bifurcation of a normal common carotid artery into the internal and external carotid arteries.

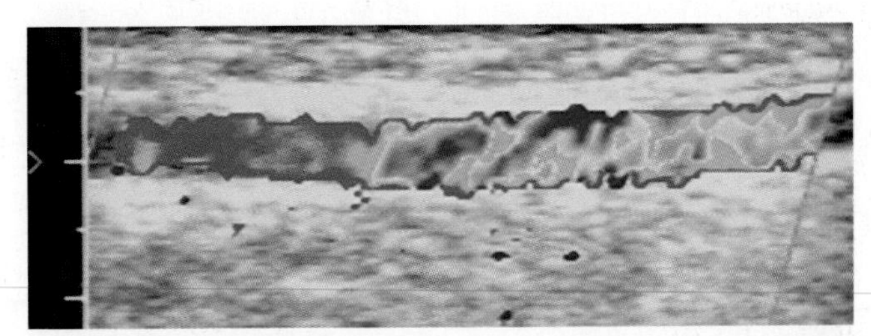

Plate 10 Duplex ultrasound scan showing a colour change from red to blue in a femoropopliteal vein graft due to turbulent flow at the site of a significant stenosis.

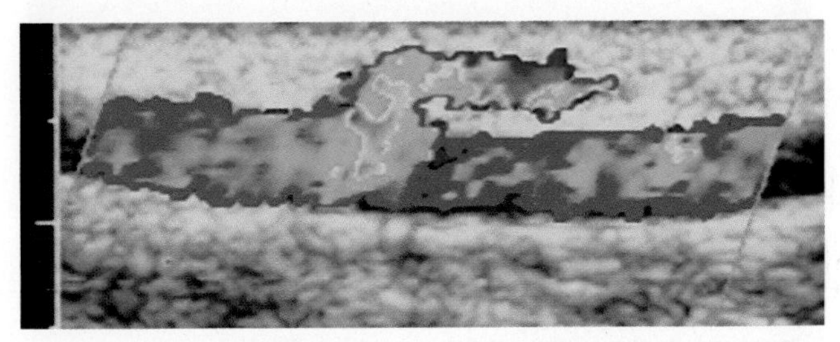

Plate 11 Duplex ultrasound scan showing a fistula in a femoropopliteal vein graft.

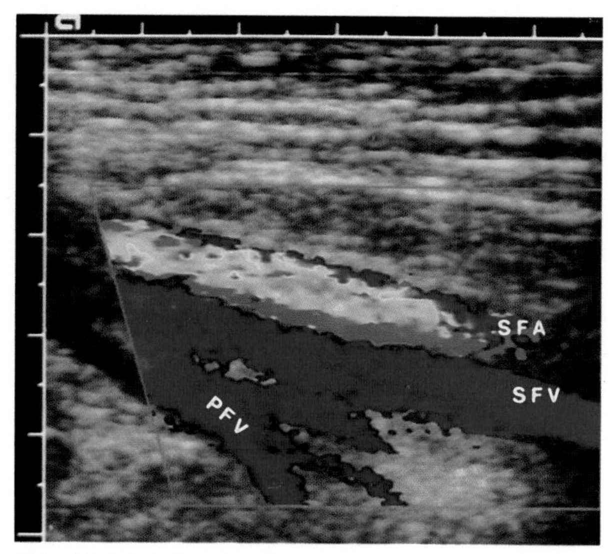

Plate 12 Colour Doppler ultrasound showing the normal confluence of the profunda femoris (PFV) and superficial femoral (SFV) veins. The superficial femoral artery is also shown (SFA).

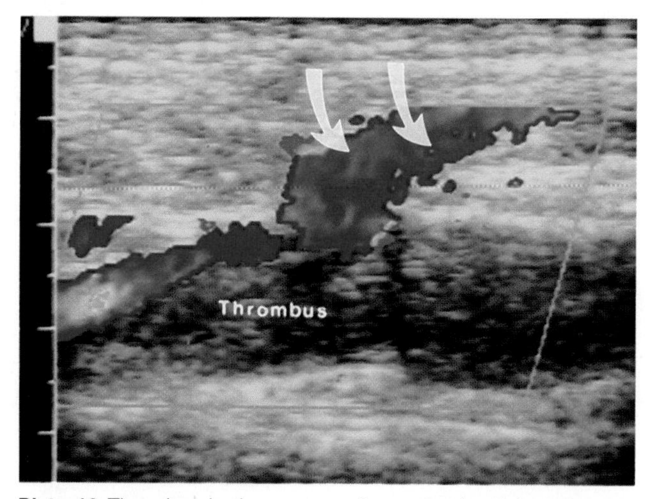

Plate 13 Thrombus in the common femoral vein. Colour Doppler ultrasound in the same patient as in Fig. 25.7. The thrombus is outlined by blood flow into the common femoral vein from the long saphenous vein (curved arrow).

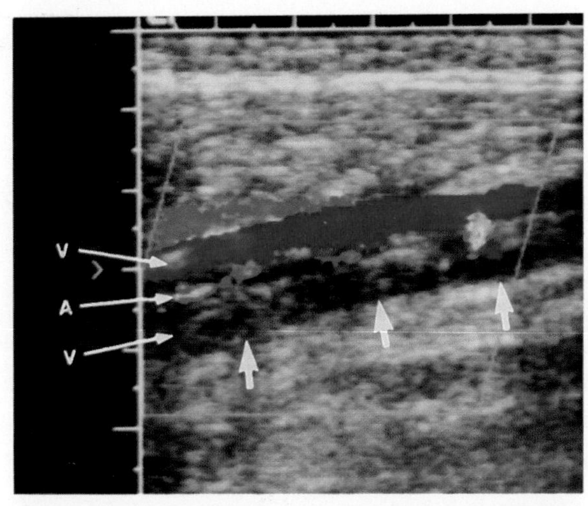

Plate 14 Colour Doppler ultrasound in calf vein thrombosis. Paired posterior tibial veins (V) are seen on either side of the posterior tibial artery (A). Flow is absent from one vein (arrows) due to thrombosis.

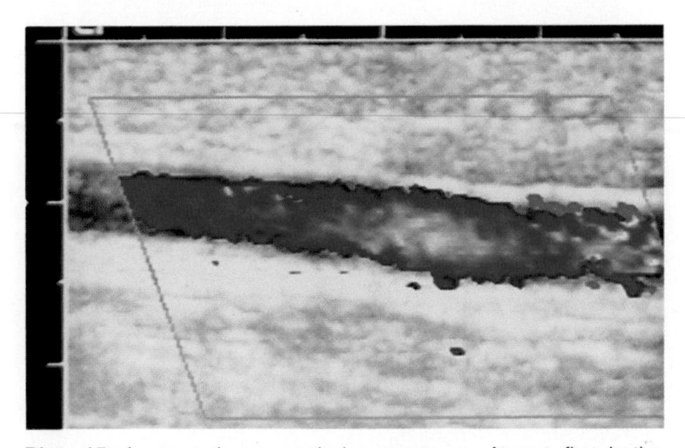

Plate 15a Long saphenous vein incompetence. At rest, flow in the long saphenous vein is towards the heart represented as blue.

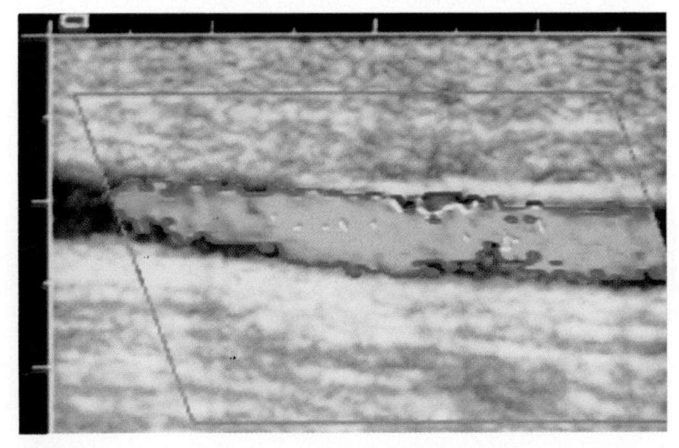

Plate 15b When the patient performs a Valsalva manoeuvre the flow reverses in direction, the representation then changing to orange, confirming venous incompetence.

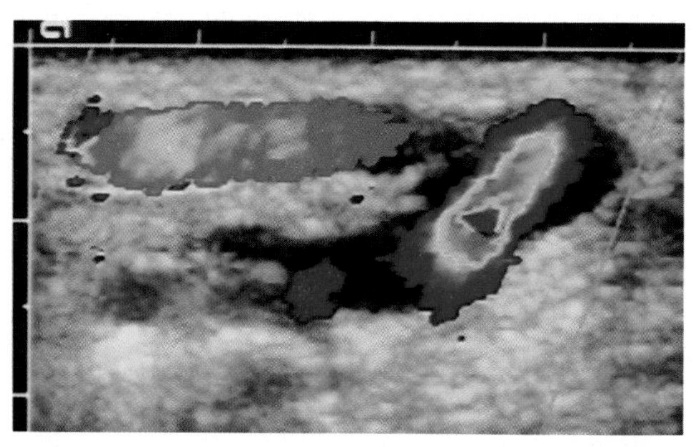

Plate 16 Incompetent perforating vein. Flow in a deep to superficial direction (coded here in blue) confirming incompetence.

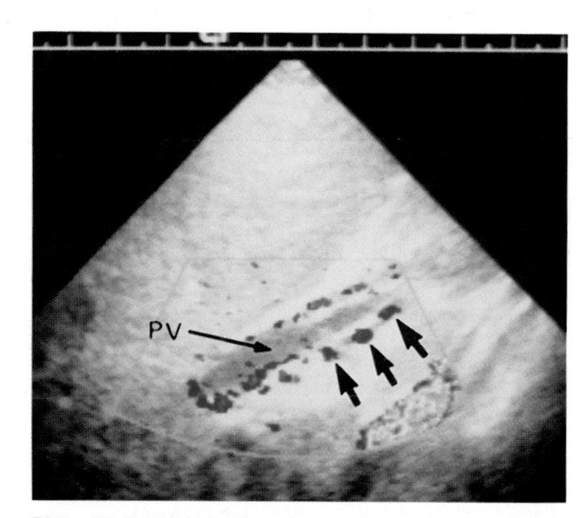

Plate 17 Portal vein thrombosis. Colour Doppler image showing small venous collaterals (arrows) that surround the occluded main portal vein (PV). (By kind permission of Dr S Amar, Nottingham.)

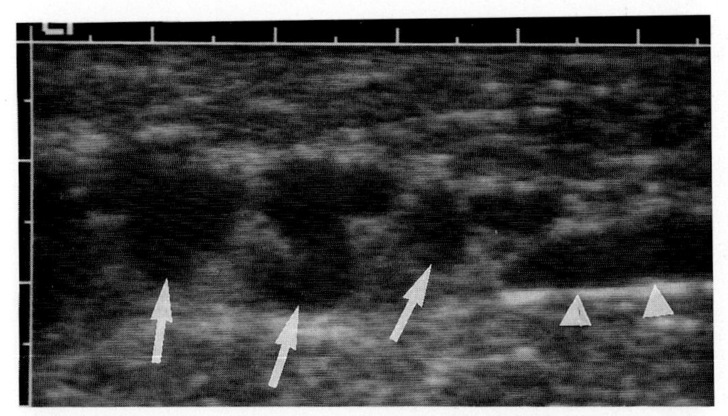

Fig. 25.9 Recurrent long saphenous incompetence following surgery. A tortuous collateral has developed (arrows) which connects the long saphenous vein (arrowheads) to the common femoral vein.

between the common femoral vein and remnant of the long saphenous vein (Fig. 25.9).

The patient is then asked to sit or stand and the calf is examined for short saphenous incompetence and the presence of perforating veins. Perforators are visible as vessels crossing the plane of the deep fascia (Fig. 25.10; Plate 16, opposite page 562). Those that are clinically significant communicate with subcutaneous varicose vessels and are usually dilated. Most will also show deep to superficial blood flow in response to calf compression but flow patterns in varicose veins can be complex and some significant perforators will be missed if this criterion is used alone.

Venography

Modifications to the technique of lower limb venography may be employed in the investigation of chronic venous disease. These include:

- the application of tourniquets at different levels in the calf during venography to determine the level of incompetent perforators;
- descending venography to detect venous reflux when contrast is injected into the common femoral vein as the patient performs a Valsalva manoeuvre;
- varicography to identify individual perforators when contrast is injected directly into a superficial varicose vein.

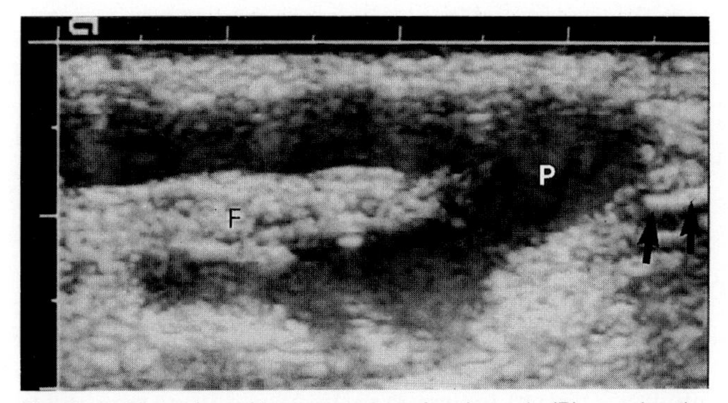

Fig. 25.10 Plain view of incompetent perforating vein (P) crossing the deep fascia (F). The arrows also point to the deep fascia.

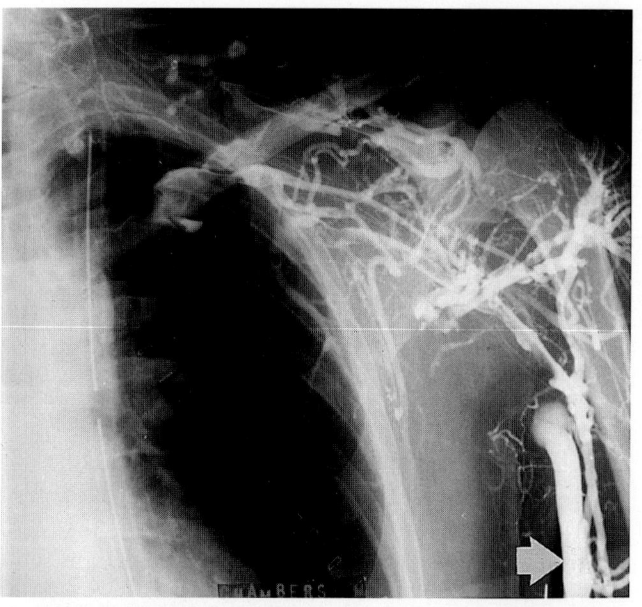

Fig. 25.11 Axillary vein thrombosis. The brachial vein is patent (arrow) but the axillary vein is occluded by thrombus. A mass of fine collateral veins around the axilla is shown instead.

When used in the assessment of chronic venous disease, both ultrasound and venography require experienced operators but, in experienced hands, they give results that are comparable to each other. Venography and varicography are, however, less pleasant for the patient.

UPPER LIMB

Axillary or subclavian vein thrombosis can occur because of indwelling catheters, extension of central venous thrombosis secondary to mediastinal disease, thrombotic syndromes or vasculitis but may also occur in otherwise fit patients. Either Doppler ultrasound or venography (Fig. 25.11) may be used to confirm the diagnosis. Thrombus within the axillary or subclavian veins has the same radiographic or ultrasonic appearance as in the lower limb with the exception that compression ultrasound cannot be used since the axillary and subclavian veins are protected from compression by the clavicle

CENTRAL VEINS

IVC OBSTRUCTION

IVC obstruction occurs as a result of thrombosis or involvement by adjacent lesions. It is usually the result of extension of thrombus from pelvic or lower limb veins (Fig. 25.12) but may also arise from extension of clot from other thrombosed tributaries, particularly the renal veins. Renal tumours are noted

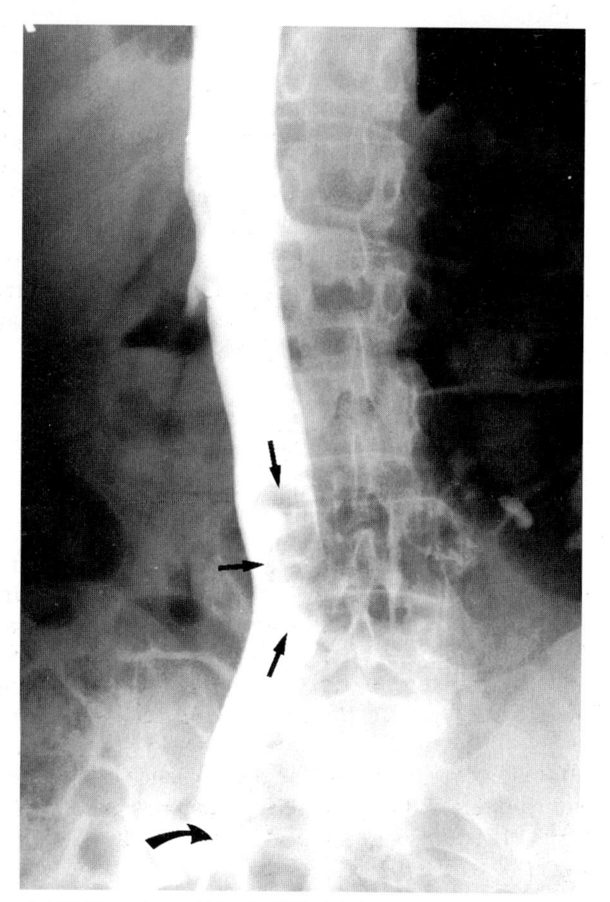

Fig. 25.12 Thrombus within the IVC. Inferior vena cavogram showing thrombus arising out of the left common iliac vein orifice (arrows). The angiographic catheter (curved arrow) has been passed into the IVC from the right common femoral vein.

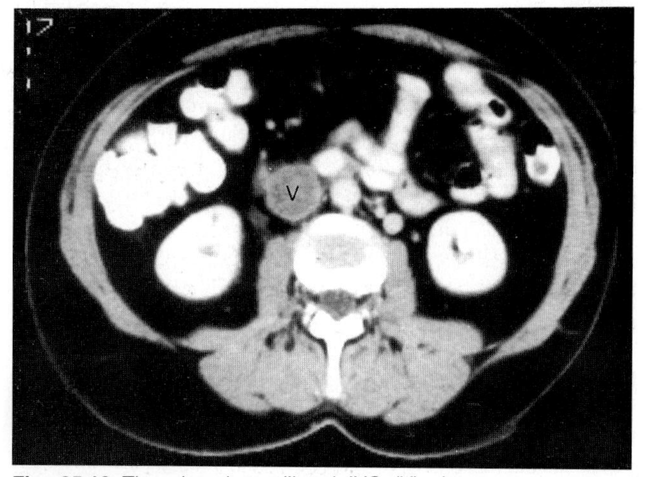

Fig. 25.13 Thrombus in a dilated IVC (V) shown on a contrast-enhanced CT. There is a thin rim of contrast visible between the thrombus and vein wall.

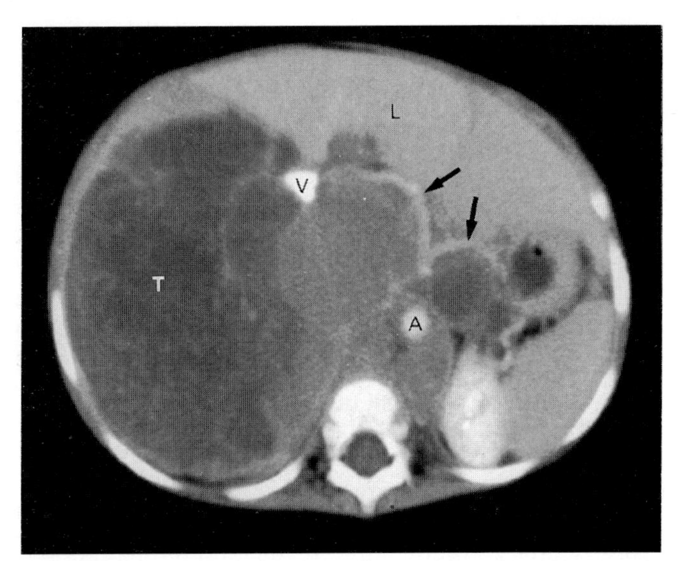

Fig. 25.14 Contrast-enhanced CT scan of the abdomen of a child showing an enormous retroperitoneal and para-aortic tumour (T) (neuroblastoma) with anterior displacement of the IVC (V) and aorta (A). The liver (L) is pushed across to the left. The branches of the coeliac axis (arrows) are also displaced.

for their ability to spread along the lumen of the renal vein and into the IVC, an event that may also lead to secondary thrombosis. Adjacent pathologies that may cause narrowing, displacement or obstruction of the IVC include retroperitoneal disease such as lymphadenopathy or retroperitoneal fibrosis, neoplasia such as hepatic, adrenal, renal, duodenal or pancreatic tumours and other masses such as aortic aneurysms.

Ultrasound and CT are usually the first investigations in the assessment of IVC occlusion. Thrombus can be seen on ultrasound as echogenic material and on contrast-enhanced CT as a non-enhancing defect within the lumen (Fig. 25.13). CT is particularly useful when there is extrinsic involvement of the IVC (Fig. 25.14). In comparison, inferior cavography is invasive and does not give information about the nature and extent of pathology outside the IVC lumen and it is generally reserved as a preliminary examination prior to the insertion of a vena cava filter (see below).

SVC SYNDROME

In contrast to the IVC, the SVC cannot be assessed with ultrasound and superior vena cavography or contrast-enhanced CT of the chest are the first investigations in suspected occlusion. Collateral pathways open up in the anterior and posterior chest wall which become opacified when contrast is injected into an arm vein. Associated mediastinal lesions can also be demonstrated with CT. The condition and its treatment with stent insertion is discussed in greater detail on page 567.

VISCERAL VEINS

BUDD-CHIARI SYNDROME

The Budd–Chiari syndrome refers to thrombosis or occlusion of the main hepatic veins and the clinical sequelae which are usually abdominal pain, ascites and hepatomegaly. The condition can occur as a result of hypercoagulable states such as polycythaemia rubra vera, tumours or trauma, but in many cases the cause is unknown. A similar clinical presentation to Budd–Chiari syndrome may result from membranous obstruction of the terminal portion of the IVC. The caudate lobe of the liver is usually spared as it drains directly into the IVC by a number of small veins that remain patent. As a consequence of impaired function of the rest of the liver, caudate lobe hypertrophy often results. The diagnosis of Budd–Chiari syndrome may be made by colour Doppler ultrasound, hepatic venography, contrast-enhanced CT or MRI. Characteristic changes are also present on liver biopsy.

Colour Doppler ultrasound

The normal hepatic veins are clearly visible and flow within them is readily demonstrated using colour Doppler ultrasound. When the hepatic veins are occluded, they are difficult to visualize and no flow can be shown. Instead, many small collateral vessels are seen. In established cases of Budd–Chiari syndrome the caudate lobe may become markedly hypertrophied.

Hepatic venography

Until the advent of CT and MRI, the diagnosis of Budd–Chiari syndrome was made with hepatic venography or liver biopsy. When the main hepatic veins are occluded, they may be difficult or impossible to catheterize but if cannulation is successful, contrast injection shows a mass of fine collaterals instead of the usual branching pattern of the normal veins (Fig. 25.15a).

CT and MRI

The appearances on contrast-enhanced CT may be diagnostic. There is a characteristic mottling to the pattern of contrast enhancement of the hepatic parenchyma and occluding material may also be visible in the IVC (Fig. 25.15b). Features that may be detected on MRI include inhomogeneity of signal intensity and intrahepatic anastomoses. Both CT and MRI detect general hepatic enlargement, disproportionate caudate lobe enlargement and ascites.

PORTAL VEIN DISORDERS

Portal vein thrombosis

Patency of the portal vein may be demonstrated in a number of ways. The easiest non-invasive method is to use colour Doppler ultrasound, patency being confirmed by the demonstration of blood flow (Plate 17, opposite page 562). However, colour Doppler ultrasound is not completely reliable as very slow flow may not be detected. If the vein appears normal but blood flow is not shown, confirmatory evidence of portal vein occlusion such as the presence of collateral veins should be sought. In these instances it is best to confirm the diagnosis by some other method, such as contrast-enhanced CT (Fig. 25.16).

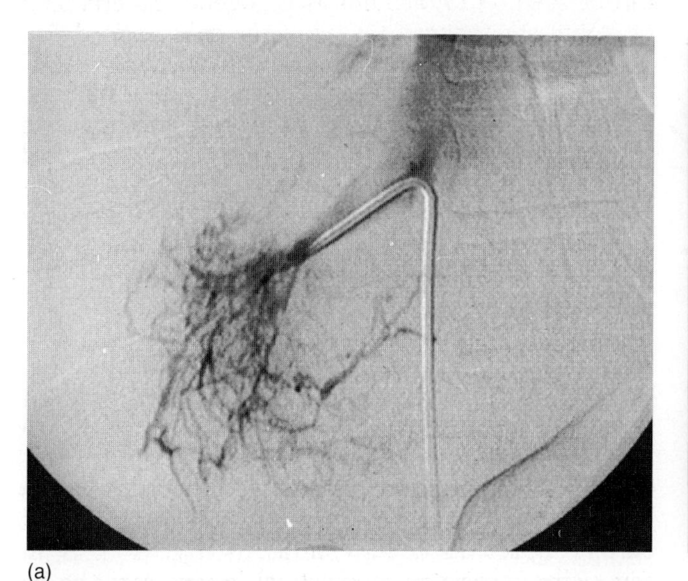

(a)

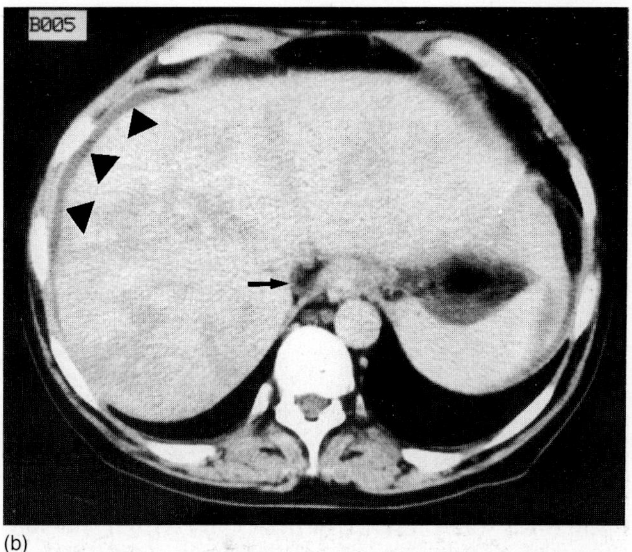

(b)

Fig. 25.15 Budd–Chiari syndrome. (a) Hepatic venogam showing angiographic catheter in right hepatic vein. Although the main vein is patent, the normal branching pattern is lost and a mesh of fine collaterals shown instead. Compare with a normal hepatic venogram (Fig. 25.3). (By kind permission of Dr G. Steele, Derbyshire Royal Infirmary.) (b) CT in another patient showing patchy contrast enhancement of the liver. The IVC also contains thrombus (arrow) and there is some ascites (arrowheads)

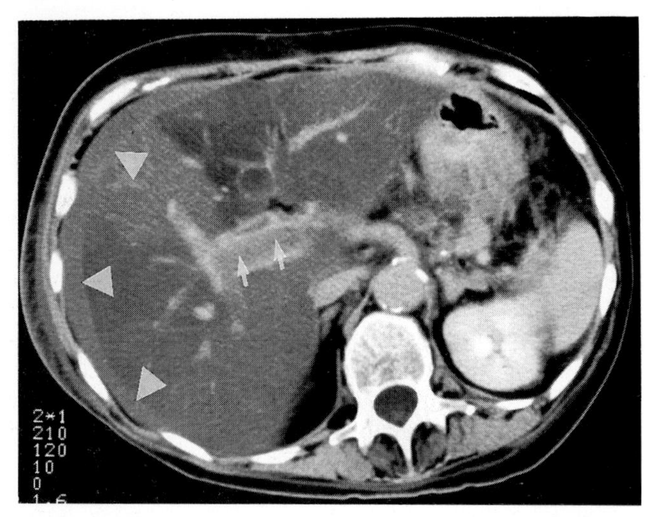

Fig. 25.16 CT scan showing recent portal vein thrombosis. Clot is visible as a filling defect within the vein (arrows). The scan also shows fatty change within most of the liver and a small amount of ascites (arrowheads). (By kind permission of Dr S. Amar, Nottingham.)

Portal Hypertension

Portal hypertension may be due to extrahepatic causes such as portal vein occlusion but is usually due to hepatic disease. Hepatic abnormalities leading to elevated portal pressure may be presinusoidal (such as schistosomiasis), sinusoidal (cirrhosis) or post-sinusoidal (Budd–Chiari syndrome or hepatic veno-occlusive disease). The commonest cause is alcoholic cirrhosis.

The main adverse effect of portal hypertension is the development of varices which are enlarged tortuous venous collaterals between the portal and systemic circulations.

RENAL VEINS

Renal vein thrombosis may occur in a number of conditions such as:

- dehydration
- hypercoagulable states
- renal tumours
- renal parenchymal disease
- renal trauma
- caval thrombosis.

It may be sudden and complete (leading to venous infarction of the kidney) or subacute, in which case, perfusion of the kidney is maintained but nephrotic syndrome occurs as a sequel. In complete renal vein thrombosis, the presence of thrombus within the vein may be visualized with ultrasound, CT, MRI or venography and the intravenous urogram will show an enlarged, poorly or non-functioning kidney with a reduced or absent nephrogram. In subacute renal vein thrombosis, thrombus may be confined to tributaries of the main renal vein, requiring selective renal venography for its demonstration.

INTERVENTIONAL PROCEDURES

VENOUS SAMPLING

Venous sampling is a technique for localizing small endocrine tumours whose presence has been confirmed by the biochemical demonstration of inappropriately high hormone levels but conventional imaging methods have failed to demonstrate. An angiographic catheter is introduced into the relevant vein (systemic or portal) and multiple samples taken in a careful, systematic manner from along the vein. The level of hormone is measured in each sample and the results are plotted on an image of the venous anatomy (Fig. 25.17).

Abnormally high hormone levels are found in the veins draining the tumour. In some cases, the sensitivity of the test may be increased by performing venous sampling after injection of the appropriate secretagogue. Venous sampling is applicable to many different hormone-secreting lesions such as pituitary, parathyroid, thyroid, adrenal, pancreatic and carcinoid

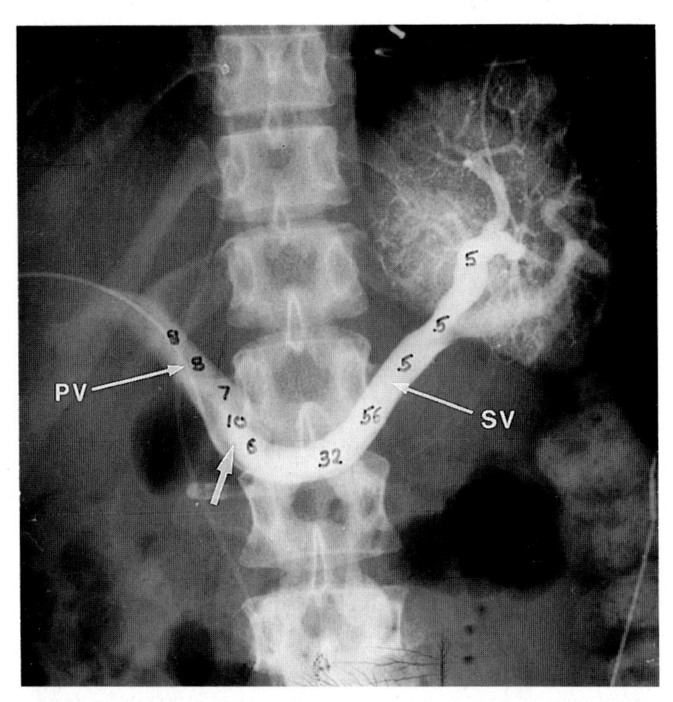

Fig. 25.17 Direct percutaneous transhepatic portography and venous sampling in a patient with suspected insulinoma. After the catheter has been introduced, contrast injection is made into the splenic vein (SV) which also shows the main portal vein (PV). The superior mesenteric vein is not shown but non-opacified blood can be seen entering the portal vein from it (arrow). The numbers indicate the levels of insulin from samples taken at each site and show a step-up in concentration in the distal splenic vein. An insulinoma was subsequently removed from the tail of the pancreas.

umours. It is, however, a difficult and expensive test to perform. There is scope for error, largely because of the considerable variability in venous anatomy and patterns of drainage. Venous sampling is therefore a facility that is generally available only in specialist centres.

SUPERIOR VENA CAVA SYNDROME

Stenosis or occlusion of the SVC lead to the distressing condition of superior vena cava syndrome which is characterized by cyanosis and oedema of the head, neck and arms, with orbital oedema and proptosis. Some patients complain of headache. SVC obstruction may be due to benign strictures of the SVC (such as may occur in mediastinal fibrosis or in vasculitic syndromes) but in most cases obstruction is due to neoplastic lesions in the mediastinum. SVC stenosis may also occur as a result of long-term central venous catheters. Radiotherapy is used to treat malignant strictures but relief is not achieved immediately. Benign strictures may be treated by surgical bypass but these have a poor record of long-term patency. Treatment of both benign and malignant strictures is now much easier with the advent of expandable metallic stents which are placed within the lesion and, once in place, provide internal support that maintains the SVC lumen.

Expandable metallic stents are cylindrical in shape and constructed from stainless steel or nitinol in such a way that they can be collapsed into or onto a narrow diameter delivery device. Examples are the Wallstent (Fig. 25.18) and the Gianturco stent. When deployed in strictures smaller than their maximum diameter, stents generate a constant radial dilating force within the lesion. As a result, significant expansion of the stent often occurs in the days following insertion, even in lesions that have proved resistant to balloon dilatation. Pathological examination of stents that have been in place for weeks or months has shown that they become incorporated into the vessel wall during this period.

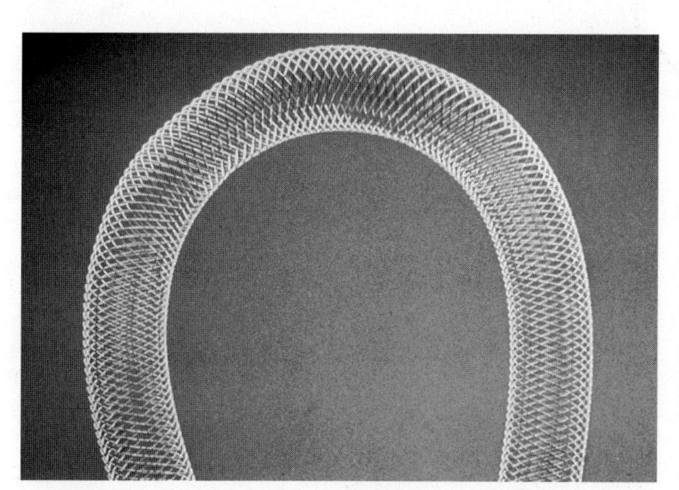

Fig. 25.18 Wallstent (Schneider). The stent comes mounted in a 7F or 9F delivery system (2.3 mm or 3 mm diameter) for insertion. Once deployed the stent expands to its natural diameter (as in the illustration) which can be anything from 5 to 16 mm in diameter. (By kind permission of Schneider).

The position and extent of the stricture is first delineated using superior vena cavography. Thrombus may be present above the stricture and this must be cleared before stent insertion by thrombolysis using local infusion of streptokinase or recombinant tissue plasminogen activator. With the lumen free of clot, the stricture is traversed using a guidewire and catheter advanced from either the right internal jugular vein or the groin. Once a guidewire is across the stricture, the stent delivery system may then be introduced and the stent deployed under fluoroscopic guidance (Fig. 25.19).

The results are usually very gratifying with immediate relief of headache and resolution of oedema over 24 hours. The long-term patency of the SVC after stent insertion is good. Most patients with malignant strictures will die from the underlying condition without recurrence of the symptoms of SVC obstruction but in a small number of cases signs of obstruction will return caused by overgrowth of tumour at the stent margins. Encouraging long-term patency has also been reported in benign disease.

INFERIOR VENA CAVA FILTERS

The majority of patients with deep vein thrombosis or pulmonary embolism can be managed satisfactorily with anticoagulation alone. Difficulties arise when pulmonary embolism occurs despite effective anticoagulation or when anticoagulant treatment is complicated or contraindicated. In these circumstances, or when the patient has a greater than usual risk of pulmonary embolism, such as the presence of a large mass of thrombus protruding into the IVC, an IVC filter is inserted to act as a trap for emboli originating in the pelvis and lower limbs.

There are a number of varieties of filter (Fig. 25.20). Most are permanent implants such as the Greenfield filter, the Antheor filter and the Bird's Nest filter. The Greenfield and Antheor filters both present funnel-shaped cages to the venous flow from the pelvis. The funnel shape causes trapped emboli to be held in the central portion of the filter, away from the vein wall; this seems to reduce the likelihood of IVC occlusion. The Bird's Nest filter consists of two V-shaped wire barbs which fix to the IVC wall, connected by a fine wire mesh. The mesh fills the IVC lumen and traps embolic particles.

The right femoral vein is usually used for access unless the lower IVC or right iliac veins are occluded

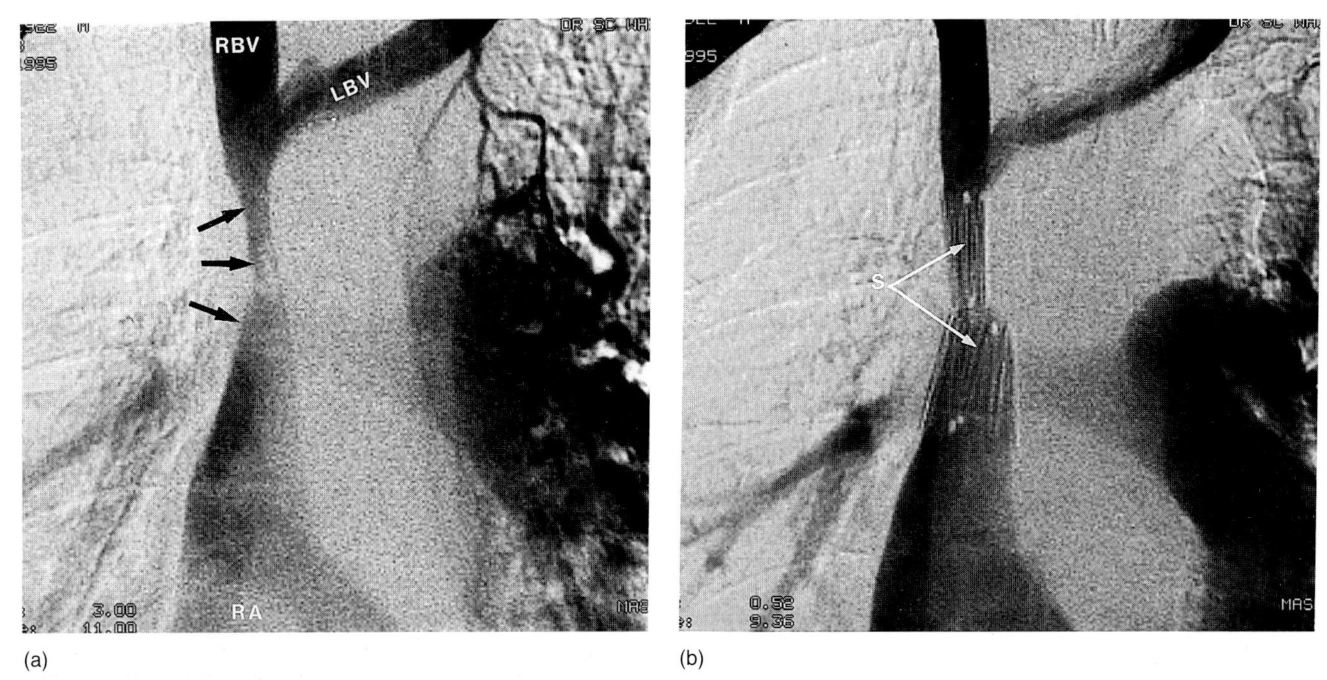

(a) (b)

Fig. 25.19 Superior vena canal stenosis due to a mediastinal tumour. (a) Simultaneous contrast injection into both antecubital veins shows the stenosis (arrows). (b) Superior vena cavogram performed 4 days after insertion a self-expanding metallic stent (S) within the stricture. Dilatation of the stricture by the Gianturco Z-stent (Cook Inc.) has occurred over several days. RBV=right brachiocephalic vein; LBV = left brachiocephalic vein; RA = right atrium.

in which case the right internal jugular vein is used. Preliminary inferior vena cavography is essential to show the level of the renal veins, to demonstrate the presence and extent of any thrombus within the IVC itself and to measure the size of the IVC. With the exception of the Bird's Nest filter which has no predefined shape and can be used in any size cava, vena cava filters should not be used if the diameter of the IVC is too large since this would result in inadequate stability and possible migration. The fil-

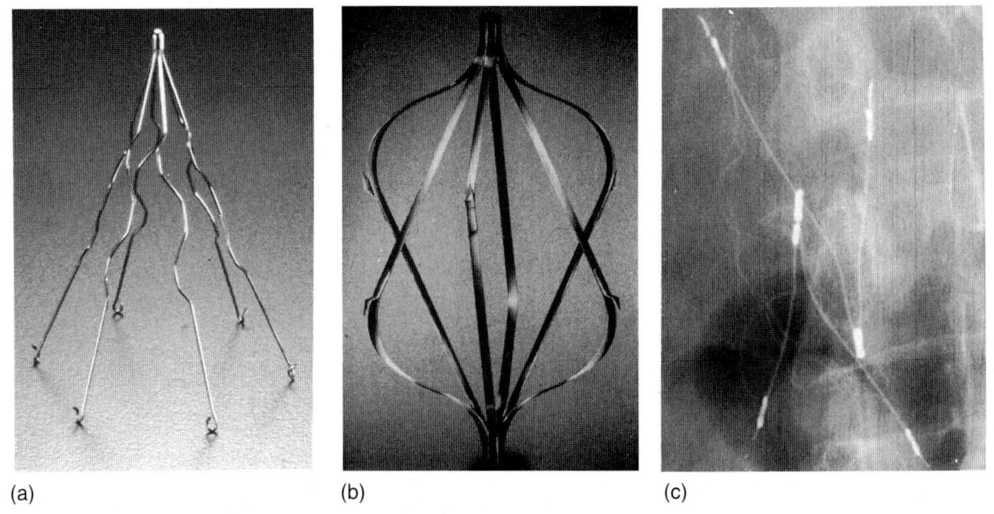

(a) (b) (c)

Fig. 25.20 Types of vena cava filters. (a) Greenfield filter (Boston Scientific); (b) Antheor filter (Boston Scientific); (c) Bird's Nest filter (Cook Inc.).

ter itself is normally deployed below the level of the renal veins so that, should IVC thrombosis occur, the renal veins will not be affected. In some circumstances where the lower IVC contains thrombus, it may not be possible to place a filter below the renal veins, necessitating placement in the suprarenal cava. This is less satisfactory because of the additional risk of renal vein occlusion should the filter occlude. As in all interventional procedures, the potential risks and benefits should be considered carefully.

The main risks of IVC filters are IVC occlusion and migration of the filter but with modern filters, the risk of complication is low. Typically, the rate of recurrent pulmonary embolism is reduced to less than 5%. Some manufacturers have introduced temporary vena cava filters which remain attached to an intravenous catheter for later removal. These filters are used to provide temporary protection when a procedure that has a high risk of pulmonary embolism is being undertaken.

HICKMAN LINE INSERTION

A Hickman line is a central venous catheter, inserted via a subclavian vein, which is used for long-term venous access. Typical uses for Hickman lines are the administration of chemotherapy or parenteral nutrition. In order to reduce the chance of infection, the entry points at the skin and the subclavian vein wall are kept as far apart as practical by passing the catheter through a 10–15 cm long subcutaneous tunnel before it enters the vein. The tip of the catheter lies in the SVC where the flow rate and the lumen calibre are greatest.

In many centres, Hickman line insertion is performed in the radiology department where digital angiographic facilities allow quicker and more accurate placement. A venogram is performed first via an antecubital vein. Using the venogram for guidance, the point where the subclavian vein crosses the undersurface of the clavicle is identified and the vein is punctured at this point. A guidewire is passed into the subclavian vein and then into the SVC. Next, a 10–15 cm subcutaneous track is created from the venepuncture site to a point above and lateral to the nipple. The Hickman catheter is passed through this track and then advanced into the vein through a removable sheath until its tip is in the SVC. The catheter hub is fixed to the skin and the skin wounds are sutured.

The most important complication is catheter infection and septicaemia. If infection cannot be controlled the catheter should be removed. For this reason, insertion is always performed under antibiotic prophylaxis. Other complications include catheter malposition, catheter thrombosis and cutaneous inflammation at the entry point.

REMOVAL OF INTRAVASCULAR FOREIGN BODIES

The vascular system may play host to a variety of foreign bodies. Most are iatrogenic, such as catheter fragments or misplaced embolization coils. The site at which the foreign body lodges depends on its size, shape and pliability. Venous foreign bodies will commonly pass to the central veins and from there to the right ventricle and pulmonary arteries. Percutaneous removal using an intravascular retrieval device is the best method of managing intravascular foreign material.

A variety of retrieval devices exist. The simplest is a snare which is constructed of a wide-bore catheter and a thin, looped guidewire. The loop is manipulated around the foreign body and then tightened by traction on the external ends. Once grasped, the foreign body can be pulled back to the catheter entry site. If small enough it can be simply pulled out but large objects may require a cut down. The Goose Neck snare (Fig. 25.21) is a purpose-designed commercially available version of the snare principle. The Dormier basket has been used for many years for stone retrieval from the biliary and urinary tracts and is also available for intravascular use. Biopsy forceps of the type used in endoscopy may also be used to grasp an offending object. Fortunately, percutaneous catheter removal has a high rate of success. Complications are few but there is the potential for vascular injury. Catheter manipulation across the right heart may lead to arrhythmias and care must be employed in retrieving objects from the right ventricle to avoid injury to the chordae tendinae.

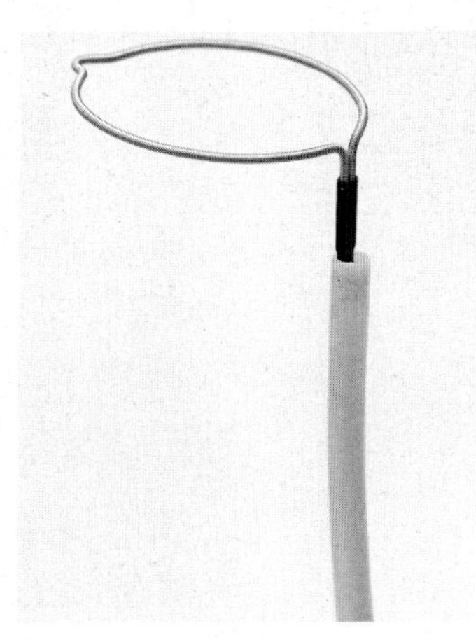

Fig. 25.21 Goose Neck snare (Microvena) used for retrieval of intravascular foreign bodies. The loop is manipulated around the object and tightened by withdrawing it into the catheter.

Index

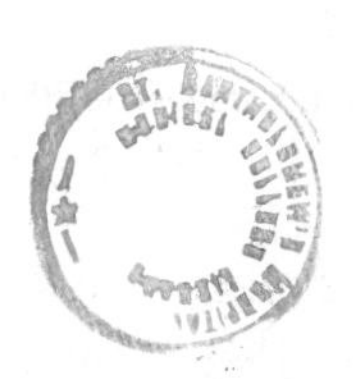